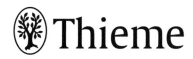

Tumors of the Nose, Sinuses, and Nasopharynx

Valerie J. Lund, CBE, MS, FRCS, FRCSEd
Professor of Rhinology
University College London
and
Honorary Consultant ENT Surgeon
Royal National Throat, Nose and Ear Hospital
University College, Royal Free, and
Moorfields Eye Hospitals
London, UK

David J. Howard, BSc, MB BS, FRCS, FRCSEd
Professor of Head and Neck Oncology
Imperial College NHS Trust Hospitals, London
and
Honorary Consultant Head and Neck Surgeon
Royal National Throat, Nose and Ear Hospital
London, UK

William I. Wei, MS, FRCS, FRCSEd, FRACS (Hon), FACS (Hon)
Emeritus Professor of Surgery
The University of Hong Kong
and
Honorary Consultant
Li Shu Pui ENT Head and Neck Surgery Centre
Hong Kong Sanatorium and Hospital
Hong Kong SAR, China

686 illustrations

Thieme
Stuttgart · New York

Library of Congress Cataloging-in-Publication Data
Lund, Valerie J., author.
 Tumors of the nose, sinuses, and nasopharynx / Valerie J.
Lund, David J. Howard, William I. Wei.
    p. ; cm.
 Includes bibliographical references and index.
 ISBN 978-3-13-147191-8 (hardback : alk. paper)—ISBN
978-3-13-164561-6 (eISBN)
 I. Howard, David J., author. II. Wei, William I., author. III.
Title.
 [DNLM: 1. Otorhinolaryngologic Neoplasms. WV 190]
 RC280.N6
 616.99′421—dc23
                                                            2013042503

Illustrators: Katja Dalkowski, MD, Buckenhof, Germany, and Adrian Cornford, Reinheim-Zeilhard, Germany

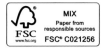

© 2014 Georg Thieme Verlag KG,
Rüdigerstrasse 14, 70469 Stuttgart, Germany
http://www.thieme.de
Thieme Medical Publishers, Inc., 333 Seventh Avenue,
New York, NY 10001, USA
http://www.thieme.com

Cover design: Thieme Publishing Group
Typesetting by Prepress Projects, Perth, UK
Printed in China by Everbest Printing Co. Ltd.

ISBN 978-3-13-147191-8

Also available as an e-book:
eISBN 978-3-13-164561-6

Important note: Medicine is an ever-changing science undergoing continual development. Research and clinical experience are continually expanding our knowledge, in particular our knowledge of proper treatment and drug therapy. Insofar as this book mentions any dosage or application, readers may rest assured that the authors, editors, and publishers have made every effort to ensure that such references are in accordance with **the state of knowledge at the time of production of the book.**
Nevertheless, this does not involve, imply, or express any guarantee or responsibility on the part of the publishers in respect to any dosage instructions and forms of applications stated in the book. **Every user is requested to examine carefully** the manufacturers' leaflets accompanying each drug and to check, if necessary in consultation with a physician or specialist, whether the dosage schedules mentioned therein or the contraindications stated by the manufacturers differ from the statements made in the present book. Such examination is particularly important with drugs that are either rarely used or have been newly released on the market. Every dosage schedule or every form of application used is entirely at the user's own risk and responsibility. The authors and publishers request every user to report to the publishers any discrepancies or inaccuracies noticed. If errors in this work are found after publication, errata will be posted at www.thieme.com on the product description page.

Contributors

K. Kian Ang, MD, PhD[1]
Senior Head and Neck Medical Oncologist/Radiotherapist
Professor of Radiation Oncology
The University of Texas M. D. Anderson Cancer Center
Houston, Texas, USA

Nafi Aygun, MD
Associate Professor of Radiology
Director, Neuroradiology Fellowship Program
Division of Neuroradiology
Johns Hopkins University
Baltimore, Maryland, USA

Daniel T. T. Chua, MD, FRCR, FHKCR, FHKAM
Associate Director
Comprehensive Oncology Centre
Hong Kong Sanatorium and Hospital
Hong Kong SAR, China

Steven J. Frank, MD
Associate Professor
Director of Advanced Technology
Department of Radiation Oncology
The University of Texas M. D. Anderson Cancer Center
Houston, Texas, USA

Adam S. Garden, MD
Professor
Department of Radiation Oncology
The University of Texas M. D. Anderson Cancer Center
Houston, Texas, USA

Anna E. Nidecker, MD
Department of Radiology
The University of California Davis Medical Center
Sacramento, California, USA

S. James Zinreich, MD
Professor of Radiology: Otolaryngology/Head & Neck
Surgery
Johns Hopkins Hospital
Baltimore, Maryland, USA

[1]Since writing his chapter, Professor Kian Ang has very sadly died. We would like to pay tribute to his tremendous contribution to radiation oncology throughout the world.

Foreword

This volume is an exhaustive, masterly crafted storehouse of invaluable information on the tumors of the nose, paranasal sinuses, and nasopharynx. In the spirit of completeness and thoroughness that characterized the original book, *Tumors of the Upper Jaw*, authored by Professor Valerie Lund and the late Sir Donald Harrison, this up-to-date text goes into extensive detail on all the common and virtually all the unusual pathological entities that may involve this complex and difficult area.

The introductory chapter by Professor David Howard, based on an earlier chapter by Professor Philip Stell, is a fascinating, often humorous, and extremely informative chapter describing the history behind the development of surgery of the maxilla and paranasal sinuses. Many of the myths attributing the original diagnoses of certain pathological entities and the origins of certain operative procedures to specific individuals, beliefs held by many of us throughout our professional careers, are "blown out of the water" by Professor Howard's historical revelations.

Each individual chapter in this book is a treasure trove of valuable up-to-date information on each pathological entity. The format of each chapter—naming the disease process, listing the other common synonyms for the tumor or inflammatory processes, discussing the etiology and pathophysiology, and reviewing diagnostic procedures, particularly radiography, all followed by treatment, complications, and results, and finally by citations of survivals from the world literature—is excellent. Regarding complications and survival results, the authors have had the good fortune of being able to draw from an extensive personal experience of their own, augmented by that of their mentors.

The section on the treatment of malignancies of the paranasal sinuses is extremely instructive. The techniques of endoscopic resection, both subcranially and intracranially, is well detailed. It is quite easy to then contrast these techniques with the subcranial and combined transfacial–intracranial open approaches to sinus malignancies with and without skull base involvement.

The section on the management of nasopharyngeal lesions, especially nasopharyngeal carcinoma by Professor William Wei is especially valuable. His extensive experience with this tumor, coupled with having practiced in the same institution for most of his career, has enabled him to follow his patients for long periods of time and formulate a best treatment strategy.

This volume will be an important addition to the libraries of residents, (registrars), and fellows in both endoscopic sinus surgery and head and neck oncological surgery and consultants in otolaryngology, plastic surgery, and oromaxillofacial surgery, as well as the ancillary services of therapeutic radiology, medical oncology, diagnostic radiology, and pathology.

Paul J. Donald, MD, FRCSC

Table of Contents

7 Epithelial Nonepidermoid Neoplasms

8 Mesenchymal Neoplasms and Other Lesions

9 Vasoform Neoplasms and Other Lesions

10 Neoplasms of Muscle

11 Cartilaginous Tumors

12 Odontogenic Tumors and Other Lesions

1 Introduction and Acknowledgments

When we three, Valerie, David, and William, decided to undertake this project 3 years ago, we knew that it was going to be a major undertaking. *Tumours of the Upper Jaw* had been published by Valerie with Professor Sir Donald Harrison (**Fig. 1.1**) in 1993 and in the intervening period there had been a significant number of changes in the evaluation and management of tumors in the sinonasal and nasopharyngeal areas. Unfortunately, tumors in these areas still present late and their cure provides huge challenges. In addition to our own substantial experience, we have conducted an extensive review of the literature to identify all significant contributions since the last book and have tried to use the best evidence available.

We recognize that level I or II randomized placebo-controlled trials are absent in the literature for virtually any treatment used for these tumors due to a combination of ethical considerations and the rarity of the conditions. Even the acquisition of large prospective cohorts of tumor patients has proved difficult, although there are now several centers, including our own, that have published data that are adequate for statistical analysis. Nonetheless, there are a large number of pathologies that are represented only by case reports or small retrospective series. It is also worth noting that journals willing to publish these types of report are now few because of the pursuit of scientific credibility and improved impact factors. Thus it may become increasingly difficult to gather information on the rarest pathologies but this situation also supports the view that there should be a degree of centralization of many sinonasal, skull base, and nasopharyngeal neoplasms. This is particularly underlined by the proliferation of endoscopic techniques and has led to the development of collaborative multicenter networks and prospective data collection.[1] Along with accurate records of long-term follow-up, this will greatly facilitate future evaluation of results. Similarly, the majority of the tumors covered in this book are now managed by multidisciplinary teams which include input from neurosurgeons, ophthamologists, plastic and maxillofacial surgeons, radiation oncologists, and a range of other experts.

We have included a few additional clinical conditions that strictly speaking do not come under the definition of neoplasms but are difficult to manage, may mimic tumors, and at times are life-threatening in their own right.

While odontogenic tumors are normally the province of oral pathologists, oral surgeons, and maxillofacial surgeons, they are also seen and treated by ENT and plastic surgeons in many parts of the world and accordingly have been included.

In undertaking this project we have been helped by a large number of individuals, not only through the excellent contributions from Professors Zinreich, Ang, Chua and their colleagues but also from friends and coworkers. This list is by no means complete but we would like to thank our long-suffering secretaries, Angela Constantinou, Trisha Holness, and Anne Oliphant; colleagues including Tim Beale, Lloyd Savy, Gita Madani, Anne Sandison, Peter Clarke, Dawn Carnell, Simon Stewart, Richard Welfare, Geoff Rose, and other colleagues at Moorfields; and Fellows and trainees Humera Babar-Craig, Ed Chisholm, Jo Rimmer, Adin Selcuk, and Matteo Trimarchi.

Finally we would like to pay tribute to several individuals whose unique clinical expertise and support have enormously enhanced the treatment of our patients: Tony Cheesman, Sir Donald Harrison, Glyn Lloyd, Leslie Michaels, and Margaret Spittle (**Figs. 1.2, 1.3, 1.4, 1.5**).

Reference

1. Lund VJ, Stammberger H, Nicolai P, et al. European position paper on endoscopic management of tumours of the nose, paranasal sinuses and skull base. Rhinol Suppl 2010;(22):1–143

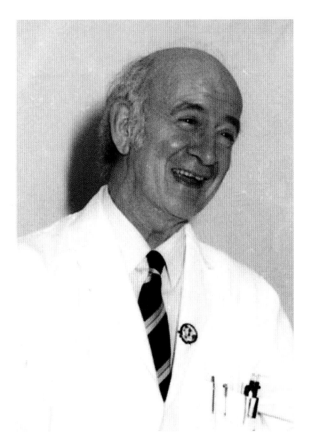

Fig. 1.1 Professor Sir Donald Harrison.

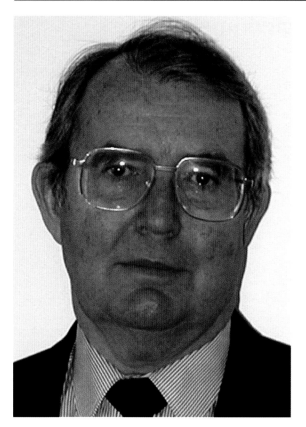

Fig. 1.2 Tony Cheesman.

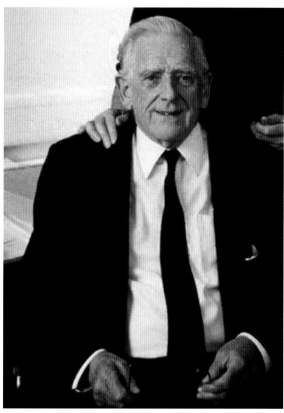

Fig. 1.3 Glyn Lloyd.

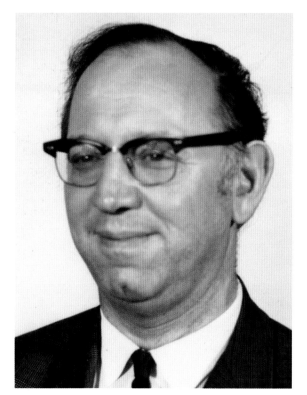

Fig. 1.4 Leslie Michaels.

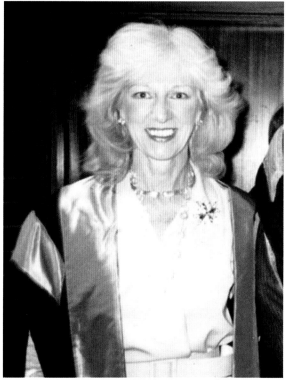

Fig. 1.5 Margaret Spittle OBE.

2 Historical Aspects of Surgery in the Sinonasal Area

D. J. Howard and P. Stell

In an earlier book entitled *Tumours of the Upper Jaw* written by Valerie Lund and Sir Donald Harrison and published in 1993,[1] Professor Philip Stell, then Professor of Otolaryngology at the University of Liverpool, was asked to contribute a chapter on the history of the surgery of the upper jaw. I have chosen to reproduce and add further to that chapter here for several extremely good reasons. Following his appointment to the Chair in Liverpool in 1979, Philip Stell confined his practice largely to laryngology and all aspects of head and neck malignancies. He developed his own extensive computerized database and was a strong advocate of statistical analysis of all surgical results. He established the journal *Clinical Otolaryngology and Allied Sciences* in 1978 and founded the UK Otorhinolaryngological Research Society. He published more than 300 peer review papers and was a superb linguist, being fluent in Spanish, French, German, and Dutch. He lectured extensively in Europe and was honored by many European countries.

Following his early retirement at the age of 57 on health grounds in 1992, he subsequently moved to York where he enrolled for an MA in history at York University and his thesis was entitled "Medical care in late Medieval York." He achieved his degree with distinction and in 1996 commenced further research in the Centre for Medieval Studies in the University of York, establishing a unique database for medieval Yorkshire wills, names, and other early documents. He was subsequently honored with invitations to become a Fellow of the Society of Antiquaries and also of the Royal Historical Society. He received an MBE for his contributions to medical history shortly before his death in 2004.

For all of the above reasons, it would be extremely difficult to improve on his superbly researched historical chapter which follows, but as there have been substantial and wide ranging developments since the 1980s, I have taken the liberty of adding an overview of the more recent developments. For consistency of style, the spelling and other conventions of the present volume have been adopted in the reproduced text.

History of Surgery of the Upper Jaw

(PM Stell. History of surgery of the upper jaw. In: Harrison DFN, Lund VJ. *Tumours of the Upper Jaw*. Edinburgh, London, Madrid, Melbourne, New York, Tokyo: Churchill Livingstone; 1993:1–15)

An historical introduction to major articles or textbooks has become commonplace. Sadly, most of these historical vignettes are, for various reasons, inaccurate, the commonest reason being that the author failed to read the original articles. For example, it is often stated that Patrick Heron Watson did the first laryngectomy for syphilis, in 1865. But, the original paper shows that Watson described the larynx, trachea, and bronchi of a patient who had syphilis; the only operation performed during life was a tracheotomy.[2] A second source of error is an inability to read languages other than English. It is often said that adenoid cystic carcinoma was first described by Billroth in 1859 by the term "Zylindrome."[3] This is untrue: the tumor was first described by two Frenchmen, Robin and Laboulbene, as "tumeur heteradenique" in 1853.[4]

A third source of error is to ignore the context of the historical events. It is stated repeatedly[5] that cancer of the ear was first discussed ca. 1775 by Wilde and Schwartz. Apart from the fact that Wilde was born in 1815 and Schwartz in 1837, this statement ignores the fact that in 1775, histopathological diagnosis still lay almost a century ahead, so that no such discussion was possible.

A specific example of historical inaccuracy is the large monograph on malignant tumors of the maxilloethmoidal region written by Oehngren in 1933.[6] His extensive historical introduction is marred by two facts: first it is obvious that he did not personally read all the original reports for he misquotes names, e.g., Lizzard for Lizars; second, he gives no references to the authors he quotes.

In compiling this account of the development of upper jaw surgery, I have read and searched widely through the available literature, attempting to resolve these writings to the technology and politics of the relevant times. The development of the single-lens microscope by Antonie van Leeuwenhoek around 1665 and the discovery of aniline dyes ca. 1856 by Perkin, an Englishman working in Germany, eventually made histopathology possible.[7] Normal histology developed mainly in Germany, throwing up such well-known names as Schwann and Henle. They were followed by Virchow, who laid the foundations of histopathology with his book *Cellular Pathology*. Virchow was the first to emphasize that classification based on external appearances was arbitrary and rather it should be based on normal cellular structures. He was one of the first to use terms such as epithelioma for squamous carcinoma.[8]

By around 1860 economic and technological advances initiated a German surgical school led by famous men such as Conrad Langenbeck, his nephew Bernard Langenbeck, Billroth, Thiersch, Kocher, Trendelenburg, Czerny, Mululicz, and others (**Figs. 2.1 and 2.2**). This was the

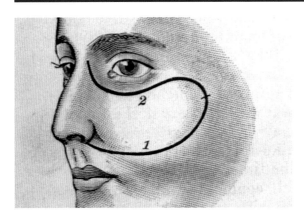

Fig. 2.1 B. Langenbeck's osteoplastic flap procedure described in 1861 to treat a 15-year-old boy with an angiofibroma. The object of this approach was to hinge the maxilla on the lateral aspect of the nose without interfering with the alveolar and palatine tissues or the floor of the orbit.

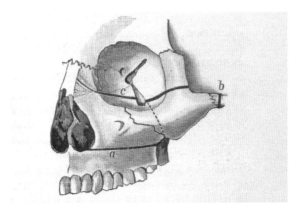

Fig. 2.2 This drawing shows the lines in Langenbeck's operation for the saw cuts through the upper jaw and zygoma followed by elevation of the bone by means of an instrument introduced under the malar bone.
"The growth was completely exposed and removed. The operation took one hour, was attended with much hemorrhage, most of which stopped spontaneously. The wounds healed well."

golden age of excisional surgery, and all the first major excisions of the internal organs such as gastrectomy, total laryngectomy, glossectomy, and so on were described at that time in Germany.

Between 1825 and 1875 when maxillectomy was developed, the main contributors came from the French and three British schools: Edinburgh, London, and Dublin. The outstanding names were those of Gensoul and Dupuytren in France; Syme, Liston, and Lizars of Edinburgh; the English school led by Fergusson; and the Dublin school under Stokes and Butcher. The German schools only contributed toward the end of this period. The school that flourished in Dublin from ca. 1800–1830 produced such well-known names as Wilde, the father of modern otology (and of Oscar Wilde), Stokes, Adams,

Colles, Corrigan, Cheyne, Graves, and the now forgotten Butcher, who in his time was preeminent in the field of maxillectomy. Why this school sprang up where and when it did is an historical mystery. Dublin society had been greatly depleted by the departure for London of diplomats and politicians after the Act of Union in 1800. Furthermore, Ireland had an entirely agricultural economy, whereas Europe was rapidly becoming industrialized and therefore more prosperous.

Surgical Practice in the 19th Century

It is virtually impossible to imagine how primitive were the conditions under which the pioneers of upper jaw surgery worked. Despite the incredible differences in pathology, anesthesia, instrumentation and, not least, operating facilities, between the early part of the 19th century and today, almost all the fundamental concepts of surgery in this region were during a period of 50 years.

Operating Conditions

If we could step back in time to 1830, perhaps the first difference that would be apparent would be the surgeon's dress. At that time it was usual to wear an old frock coat that hung on the back of the theater door: the more encrusted with blood and pus the more honorable it was. Surgical gowns and gloves belong to this century: even after the introduction of asepsis by Lister in 1867 it was usual for surgeons to operate with bare hands until at least 1895.[9]

Resection of the upper jaw was classified as a "capital operation," so called because the patient could, and often did, die during or immediately after the operation. It was usual to give notice, not only to the medical profession but also to society in general, of forthcoming operations of this type. Thus the audience included not only medical students but curious bystanders: the famous violinist Paganini performed a tour of England and Scotland in 1831–32, and attended a maxillectomy performed by Earle in 1831. At the end of the operation, Earle came forward and was greeted by "deserved applause." This operation had to be postponed because the rumor of it had brought together such a multitude that even after an adjournment to the anatomy theater, it was impracticable to continue with the operation.[10] The operation performed by Liston in 1835 attracted several hundred spectators. The operating theater was so called because the seats were arranged in ascending rows, as in an ordinary theater, for easier viewing. For similar reasons, it was called an amphitheater in France (**Fig. 2.3**).

Pathology

The second enormous difference between the present day and the 50-year period from 1820 to 1870 during

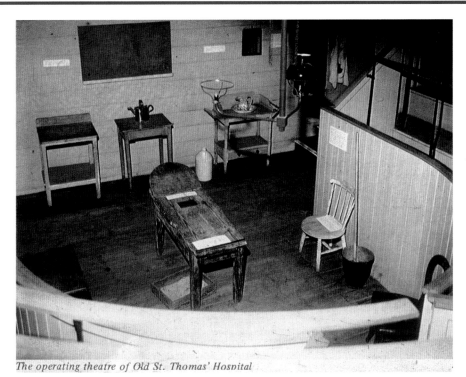

The operating theatre of Old St. Thomas' Hospital

Fig. 2.3 A photograph showing the operating theater of the old St Thomas' Hospital, London, which was used between 1822 and 1861 (and which can still be visited). From PM Stell. History of surgery of the upper jaw. In: Harrison DFN, Lund VJ. *Tumours of the Upper Jaw*. Edinburgh: Churchill Livingstone; 1993:1–15. With permission from Elsevier.

which maxillectomy was developed, was in pathological diagnosis. Surgeons had no histopathological description of the tumor on which to base their classification until ca. 1855, and the terms used were merely descriptions of the macroscopic appearance of the tumor. Histopathology was not placed on a firm basis until the publication of Virchow's book in 1856. He was the first to describe tumors on the basis of their cellular appearance.[8] Gross descriptive terms were still being used as late as 1863 when Barton stated that maxillary tumors may be divided into medullary, scirrhous, melanoid, or epithelial.[11] Furthermore, even after histopathology became generally available around 1860, histological examination was restricted to postoperative examination.[12] The examination of a biopsy belongs to this century: indeed, as late as 1923 Ochsner was vigorously maintaining that preoperative biopsy with a knife led to the setting up of metastases.[13]

A patient described by Dickson in 1840, though not subjected to operation, gives useful insight into the appreciation of gross pathology at that time. The patient was described as having a "fungus of the antrum with lymphatic contamination, but not visceral taint." The lymphatic contamination was a lymph node enlarged to the size of an almond in the digastric space. It was clearly appreciated that this was a malignant tumor which had spread to the lymph nodes so that the tumor was therefore incurable. A necropsy was performed 12 hours after death showing no "visceral taint," that is, no distant metastases.[14]

In 1833 there were three indications for resection of the upper jaw:[15]

- "Malignant disease"
- "Augmented growth of the bony parts"
- "A sort of dropsy"

The terms used for "malignant disease" were often so vague that it is now impossible to know what they described. They included tumor, intumescence, malignant disease, medullary disease, sarcoma, and so on. The term carcinoma was not used in relation to the maxilla until 1878 by a German, Koerte.[15] However, it is clear that the lesions were often carcinoma, and that the terms medullary tumor and sarcoma were squamous carcinomas. The word sarcoma was often used in its literal Greek meaning, that is a "fleshy tumor." It did not take on the connotation of a tumor of mesodermal origin until the latter part of the 19th century. Virchow in his classic *Cellular Pathology* tells us that the term medullary disease arose from the idea that it originated in the nerves and resembled nervous matter. This tumor was originally thought to arise from the body of the sphenoid bone or other bones of the base of the cranium, but Heath showed that it did indeed originate in the maxillary antrum itself.[16] A review of 160 maxillectomies published between 1830 and 1880[11,14,15,17–145] shows that ~50 of the 160 were done for carcinoma, although it was said that "cancer is certainly a very unusual form of growth to occur in the upper jaw."[71]

"Augmented growth of the bony parts" may refer either to bony tumors or to fibrous dysplasia. Of the first

160 cases, 19 were described as being bony tumors of some sort, such as exostosis, and many are described as osteosarcoma. Of 14 patients described by Dieffenbach, 6 were classed as osteosarcoma.[47] This description was not based on histology, and it is unlikely that almost half his patients suffered from so rare a disease. However, some of the bony tumors described were clearly osteomas; for example, the antral tumor described by Bickersteth in 1857, which could only be examined by sawing it in half.[25] It is interesting to speculate why osteomas (or exostoses) appear to have been so common in the early part of the 19th century.

"A sort of dropsy" was almost certainly expansion of the antrum and erosion of its bony walls by an expanding retention cyst. A patient who had undergone resection of the entire upper jaw for a cyst via a Fergusson type of incision on the face was shown at a meeting of the Medical Society of London in 1874.[70] The surgeon was strongly criticized for carrying out an operation that was more serious than the disease required. Another member pointed out that many of these cysts were of dentigerous origin, and were cured by the removal of the offending teeth, an opinion which would hold good to this day. Another dentigerous cyst of the antrum was described by Bryant, who said that doubtless upper jaws had been removed in former times for this affection, its true pathology not having been understood.[146]

Another common diagnosis not included in Guthrie's classification[15] was fibroid tumor or fibroplastic disease. Thirty of the first 160 maxillectomies were for such tumors. From detailed descriptions this tumor had a firm consistency with thin adherent bone, that had been eroded by pressure. Many of these tumors presented with a nonulcerated swelling of the palate; some later histological studies described fibrous tissue. Many of these tumors are clearly what would now be called angiofibromas, and a series of them is described by the Irish surgeon Butcher.[31–34] However, not all these tumors were angiofibromas as they appear to have arisen in both sexes and at all ages. Microscopy of one of these fibrous tumors showed elongated cells forming fibers, calcareous matter deposited along the course of the fibers, and a central hard portion infiltrated by earthy salts converting it into a stony mass.[90] This tumor was almost certainly an ossifying fibroma. A fibrous tumor, described as a fibrosarcoma, was removed from the upper jaw of a man of 58 by the well-known Irish surgeon Stokes in 1873.[147] The histological appearances showed tough fibrous tissue with a few small blood vessels.

At least a dozen maxillectomies were performed for what was described as necrosis or caries of the upper jaw, due to syphilis,[27,117] typhus,[148] or occupational exposure to phosphorus.[149]

Microscopical examination of tissue removed surgically began in the 1850s: Brainard in 1852 in the United States was one of the earliest practitioners describing

the tumor as presenting no trace of cancerous tissue and said that no cancer cells were detected under the microscope.[150] This examination was not necessarily based on examination of a section, because Craven in 1863 comments "under the microscope the juice scraped from the cut surfaces exhibited no fibrous element but simply a confused mass of broken up cells and granular matter."[39] Thus, in the early stages it appears that some form of cytology was practiced on cells scraped from the tumor. Furthermore, examination of sections as we know it did not develop until the end of the 19th century. Until then specimens for histology were preserved in alcohol[20] and cut by hand, but in ca. 1866 His made his sliding microtome, which was improved in the following decade. Automatic machines began with Threlfall's, made in 1883. These demanded rigid embedding of the specimen in substances such as paraffin wax.[7]

Early histological reports include that by Clark in 1856, who described a tumor "under the microscope as presenting cells and nuclei of every size and shape. A few commencing characteristics of epithelial cancer were present sufficiently distinctly to show positively that the tumor belonged to that class."[36] Another tumor[94] was encased in true bone, and histologically showed "oily globules compressed together but rather more irregular and oval in form, ~1/300th inch in the long diameter. The walls were made of closely packed cellules 1/2000th inch in diameter. No true bony cells could be found. When examined under polarized light at a power of 400 it showed a structure similar to that of horn or ivory."

Histological descriptions then followed rapidly: of a fibronucleated tumor,[151] "a section of the mass hardened in spirit showed bundles of fibrous tissue but not arranged so as to form a cancerous stroma; several simple round cells and masses of spindle shaped cells";[51] a "globular epithelioma";[152] a small round cell carcinoma;[153] and a myxosarcoma including a woodcut of the histological appearances.[116] Heiberg in 1861 described an adenoid cystic carcinoma under the then current term of cylindroma; this view was based on histological examination.[154] Other probable adenoid cystic carcinomas were soon described.[49,138] In the latter case histology showed "an epitheliomatous epulis resembling an adenoma of the breast."[12] In another case recorded as a cubular epithelioma,[22] histology showed "the ground work to consist of well-developed fibrous tissue with large groups of cells arranged in some parts like a racemose gland and in other parts like tubular glands. In the center of most of these groups there was a lumen." This was probably an adenoid cystic carcinoma, although it might have been an adamantinoma as it was said to resemble identically a "multilocular epithelioma" previously described in the upper jaw.

Sir William Fergusson must have had an interesting career, spanning as it did the development of both pathology and anesthesia. The circumstances when he performed his first operation in 1842[53] must have been very different from those when he removed a maxilla in 1872.[67,155] On the latter occasion histology was available to show that the tumor was composed of fibrous tissue with islandlike and spindle-shaped nuclear bodies with a calcareous nodule in its center, which was probably an ossifying fibroma. He was certainly using chloroform by 1863.[61]

Anesthesia

In the early days the patient was held or tied down. Nobody records "dulling the patient with alcohol" but this must surely have been common; laudanum (i.e., morphine) appears to have been given only after the operation. Chloroform was introduced in 1847 and ether in 1842, but chloroform was usually the sole agent used for maxillectomy (**Fig. 2.4**).

Chloroform was in frequent use by the 1860s, even in the provinces. Unfortunately, the patient was often conscious during the greater part of the operation: "chloroform was administered to its full extent to begin with, but its inhalation was not continued afterwards."[52] Another report from Australia in 1868 tells us that it "was tried but abandoned."[156]

It was often necessary to allow the patient to wake up during the operation if he or she was bleeding profusely. As late as 1870 it was customary to fix patients in the armchair as a precaution in case they did wake up.[111] Patients often recovered from the chloroform and "spat the blood as is often the case on all bystanders."[157]

Some thought that chloroform was dangerous because "the irritability of the glottis is weakened if not wholly lost, so that there must be the danger of the trickling of blood from the mouth into the glottis without the excitement of a cough for expelling it from the windpipe."[76] It was often necessary to suspend the administration of chloroform and allow the patient to recover consciousness because of the "danger of strangulation from the great amount of blood poured out." For this reason Rose recommended carrying out the operation with the head hanging.[158] Some surgeons remained unwilling to use chloroform until late in the century.[159]

In the early days chloroform was administered by sprinkling it on a piece of lint,[79] but by 1860 it was being administered by a tube passed through one nostril.[58] Later a special tubular inhaler was developed to be passed through one nostril[45] but this method was rapidly displaced by Trendelenberg's cannula. Trendelenberg had introduced a tracheostomy tube with a cuff in 1870.[160] This cannula had been used for the administration of an anesthetic through a tracheostomy to the first patient to undergo total laryngectomy by Billroth in 1873,[161] and it was used for a maxillectomy for a cylindroma by Heiberg in Germany in 1872.[154] This method is the obvious way to avoid the dangers of hemorrhage during the

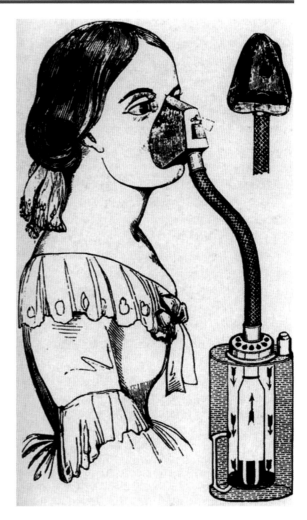

Fig. 2.4 An illustration from John Snow's book "On chloroform and other anaesthetics" (1858) on anesthesia showing an apparatus for inhaling the vapor from liquid chloroform. By 1831 ether, nitrous oxide gas, and chloroform had all been discovered and in 1842 ether was first used medically. In 1853 Queen Victoria was given chloroform by John Snow for childbirth and its use spread worldwide within months!

administration of chloroform, and had become established by the 1880s: Bellamy in 1883 said "I was first inclined to do a prophylactic tracheotomy and to use Trendelenberg's tamponade apparatus."[162]

A further means of preventing pain was to freeze the line of incision with ether.[156]

Instruments

Although surgical instruments of many kinds had been available and used for centuries (**Fig. 2.5**) there were nonetheless some instances of great differences between the early 19th century and the present day. Two examples might suffice to emphasize this: first, the only form of illumination was natural daylight. Only one paper in the

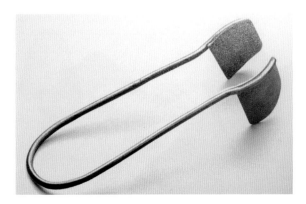

Fig. 2.5 Ludwig Johann Thudicum (1829–1901 from London) designed his speculum in 1868 and it remains in use in many ENT departments worldwide for initial anterior rhinoscopy.

first 50 years comments on illumination. In Irving's case in 1824 the patient was placed in an armchair opposite a window.[163] The question of illumination is not otherwise discussed. Lighting must have been very difficult as efficient illumination, either by gas or electric light, did not come into general use until the 1880s. Second, artery forceps for the control of hemorrhage were not invented until the latter part of the century, although ligatures were available for the arteries, and indeed were used by Nivison in 1824.[163] Fergusson's textbook of 1870 shows that the vessel was held by a forceps and the ligature was applied.[66]

A common instrument was the cautery, of which there were two types: the actual cautery and the potential cautery. The actual cautery was a hot branding iron, whereas the potential cautery consisted of caustics of different sorts. Division of cautery into these two types was of ancient origin, and their use was described by Parey in the 17th century.[164] The actual cautery was used to deal with carious bone. Parey felt that it was more effective than potential cauteries such as sulfuric acid, scalding oil, and molten sulfur, because it could be used more precisely, but that the potential cautery often had to be used because of the pain produced by the actual cautery! In the 19th century discussions as to the relative merits of the two continued: Liston (1821) felt that the actual cautery was preferable in maxillectomy because it was effective and the pain it produced was greater but momentary, whereas the pain of potential cautery persisted for several days.[105]

The term "actual cautery" continued to be used into this century: Ochsner wrote a paper entitled "Treatment of cancer of the jaw with the actual cautery" in 1923.[10] The cautery he used was a simple soldering iron heated to red heat in a gas flame. He felt that it was important to hold the iron in place for at least a minute to destroy tissue up to 2 cm away. Also, he thought that the necrotic tissue thus formed stimulated the production of antibodies that attacked the cancer, a concept which reemerged

some 50 years later with the cryosurgical probe. However, by 1926 the diathermy had almost completely replaced the use of soldering irons, as it requires no protection for the surrounding tissues, and may be employed with greater facility.[165] The electrocoagulation was produced by a bipolar high-frequency current of the d'Arsonval type.[166] A further extension of the principle of the actual cautery is cryosurgery, which was first used for maxillary carcinoma around 1970.[167]

An interesting illustration of the use of potential cautery is provided by a patient from Wales with a tumor of the palate who was eventually subjected to excision of the jaw in 1843, but who for some time had been under the care first of a "wild wart" doctor and then a wild wart doctress. These two practitioners had treated the tumor with external applications consisting of a mixture of clay, French brandy, and a caustic fluid, probably sulfuric acid.[168] The Welsh wild wart doctors survive to this day and still have a successful practice for the treatment of basal cell carcinomas of the skin using mixtures of this kind.

There was much discussion about the best way of removing the bone; one of the common methods was the use of the lion-jawed forceps designed by Sir William Fergusson (**Fig. 2.6**).[20] The use of the "chain saw" (i.e., Gigli's saw) was popularized by Davies in 1858[46] and Heyfelder in 1857.[169] The latter devised a blunt needle passed into the sphenomaxillary fissure to emerge in the zygomatic fossa, allowing a chain saw to be pulled through for division of the malar bone. He pointed out the advantages of the chain saw over the ordinary saw: the greater ease and rapidity with which the bones can be divided; the avoidance of splintering; and the facts that the parts are cut from behind forward, avoiding unintentional division by the saw, that corners can be rounded, and that the division of the bony parts can be effected in a very small space. He strongly criticized Desault's procedure of boring a hole into the antrum with a punch and enlarging it with a short curved knife ("instrument tranchant en forme serpette") because the walls of the antrum in many cases are not thinned. He clearly understood the principle of total excision for cancer when he stated that

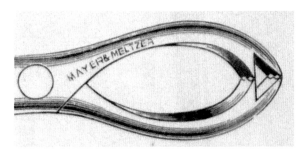

Fig. 2.6 A drawing from Meyer & Phelps's catalogue in 1931 of the distal end of Sir William Fergusson's lion-jawed forceps.

"all pathologists and operators on the upper jaw seem with one consent to deprecate the removal of tumors and especially cancerous with a sparing or niggardly hand, their usual counsel in practice being the extirpation of the whole jaw." Another commonly used means of dividing bone was the Hayes saw.[156]

The speed with which these operations were performed can but leave us breathless. The length of the operation is only rarely recorded, but Hancock resected the entire upper jaw in 8 minutes in 1847,[78] and Key in 20 minutes in 1833.[96]

Development of Surgery for Maxillary Cancer

This surgery developed in three phases: first, piecemeal removal of tumors, a phase lasting until 1825; second, the establishment of formal excision of the upper jaw beginning about 1825; third there followed the development of more refined procedures such as lateral rhinotomy in the latter part of the 19th and early 20th centuries.

The controversy as to who performed the first maxillectomy was most aptly summed up by Butcher: "the operations on the upper jaw may, in reality, be classed under two heads, that of exsection and that of disarticulation of the bone."[31]

Localized Removal

The first recorded partial removal of a maxillary tumor was that performed by Wiseman, surgeon to Charles II, reported in 1676:[170]

A man about twenty-eight years of age came out of the Country recommended to me with a Cancer of his left Cheek, stretching itself from the side of his nose close under the lower Eye-lid to the external Canthus, so making a compass downwards. It was broad in its basis, and rose copped like a Sugarloaf. It gleeted, and was accompanied with Inflammation and much pain. He had also some scirrhous glands under that Jaw. The extirpation of this Cancer had been attempted in the Country; but it growing afterwards bigger and threatening his Eye lately with inflammation, he hastned up, and importuned me to undertake it. I complied with his desire, and four or five days after having prepared all things ready, viz actual Cauteries, Digestives, Defensatives, Bandage, etc. Doctor Walter Needham and my Kinsman Jaques Wiseman being assisting. I pulled the Tumour toward me with one hand, during which I made my Incision close by the Eye-lid, and cut it smooth off as close to the Os jugulare as I could doe it, avoiding the Periosteum. The blood at first spurt out forcibly from many capillaries besides two considerable Arteries: we permitted them to bleed awhile. The lesser Vessels stopped

of themselves, and we cauterized the greater afterwards. Then viewing our work, and observing some relique of the Cancer remaining above the external Canthus, we consumed it by actual cautery, and dressed up the Wound with our Digestive, with Embrocations, Desensatives, and moderate bandage to retain them. The third day we took off Dressings, saw it well disposed to digest, and dressed it as before. The second day after, dressing it again, the Cancer appeared rising from the side of the nose and Eye-lid; it also overspread the Cheekbone. I dressed it as I had done the time before, and the next time came prepared with actual cauteries, and consumed it all, then dressed it up with Lenients. From that time the Ulcer healed daily, and contracted in ten days space to the half; yet since then it begins to bud again here and there, which will put me upon a necessity of using the actual Cautery: and what account to give of it I yet know not.

According to Butcher a part of the upper jaw was removed by Acoluthus, a physician at Breslau in 1693. A woman had a turnout on the jaw after the extraction of a tooth. He enlarged the mouth with a cut, removed part of the swelling, together with four teeth, but was unable at once to get completely round it; "he attacked it several times at intervals of a few days, sometimes with cutting instruments, and sometimes with the actual cautery, and at last succeeded in curing his patient."[31] In 1770, White described a turnout of the antrum of two years' standing. He removed it by a semicircular incision in the face, scooping away "matter like rotten cheese and many fragments of rotten bones"; the bony walls of the orbit were already destroyed. He preserved the eye, the optic nerve and part of the alveolus, but stopped at the dura which he could see and feel![171]

Operations for tumors of the upper jaw were thus rarely attempted before 1800, and they are not mentioned at all in the standard 18th-century texts such as those by Bell, Heister, Hunter, and Pott.[172-175] However, between 1800 and 1820 sporadic attempts were made with increasing frequency at localized excision of diseased tissue.

Localized removal of a turnout after elevating skin flaps, was performed by Dupuytren in 1818,[176] by Liston in Edinburgh in 1821,[105] by Irving a surgeon in Annan, Scotland on November 1, 1822,[88,163] by Rogers in 1824 in New York,[177] by Ballingal in 1827 in Edinburgh,[21] and by Velpeau of Paris in 1829 and 1830.[178] In all of these cases an incision was made in the face, the soft tissues of the cheek were elevated, and a tumor of the antrum was removed by traction on the tumor itself. No deliberate attempt was made to divide the bony attachments of the maxilla and such cases could not really qualify as maxillectomies.

Butcher also tells us that the scooping operation was practiced by Desault, Garengeot, Jourdain, Plaque and others, and has been "in modern times more especially brought under notice by Dupuytren, in 1820, and since by many surgeons."[31] Although Dupuytren argued that the greater part of the jaw might be excised, he did not do the operation himself.

A similar operation was being performed as late as 1837 in Germany: Dieffenbach described 17 cases, but only one of these could be classed as a subtotal maxillectomy, the remainder being localized resections of tumors affecting the hard palate or alveolus. The exception was an osteoma probably arising in the ethmoid sinuses which he removed preserving the alveolus and hard palate.[47]

Formal Maxillectomy

Guthrie in 1835 said that maxillectomy was one of the great improvements in modern surgery over the previous 16 years for which we were mainly indebted to the French.[15] This statement suggests that the operation began to develop around 1820.

Lizars of Edinburgh, in 1826, proposed the entire removal of the superior maxillary bone, and described the procedure.[108] Speaking of "polypi, or sarcomatous tumors, which grow in the antrum," he says:

> All the cases which have come within my knowledge (with the exception of one) wherein these sarcomatous tumors have been removed by laying open the antrum, have either returned or terminated fatally. I am, therefore, decidedly of opinion, that unless we remove the whole diseased surface, which can only be done by taking away the entire superior maxillary bone, we merely tamper with the disease, put our patient to excruciating suffering, and ultimately to death. An incision should be made through the cheek, from the angle of the mouth backward or inwards, to the masseter muscle, carefully avoiding the parotid duct, then to divide the lining membrane of the mouth, and to separate the soft parts from the bone, upwards to the floor of the orbit; second, to detach the half of the velum palati from palate bone. Having thus divested the bone to be removed of its soft coverings, the mesial incisive tooth of the affected side is to be removed; then the one superior maxillary bone to be separated from the other, at the mystachial and longitudinal palatine sutures, and also the one palate bone from the other at the same palatine suture, as the latter bone will also require to be removed either by the cutting pliers or a saw; third, the nasal process of the superior maxillary bone should be cut across with the pliers; fourthly, its malar process, where it joins the cheek bone; fifthly the eye, with its muscles and cellular cushion, being carefully held up by a spatula, the floor of the orbit is to be cleared of its soft connections, and the superior maxillary bone separated from the lacrymal and ethmoid bones with a strong scalpel. The only objects now holding the diseased mass are, the pterygoid processes of the sphenoid bone, with the pterygoid muscles. These bony processes will readily yield by depressing or shaking the anterior part of the bone, or they may be divided by the pliers, and the muscles cut with a knife. After the bone with its diseased tumor has been removed, the flap is to be carefully replaced, and the wound in the cheek held together by one or two stitches, adhesive plaster, and bandage. In no other way do I see that this formidable disease can be eradicated.

Lizars attempted the operation in December 1827 "for a medullary sarcomatous tumor of the antrum, from a miner or collier", but had to abandon the operation because of bleeding. He tried again on August 1, 1829 and this time succeeded. He first tied the trunk of the temporal and internal maxillary arteries, and also the external jugular vein which had been divided in the first incision. He cut through the alveolar process and bony plate on the left side of the palatine suture, and completely separated the upper jaw with the saw, Liston's forceps, and strong scissors, but the orbital plate was separated from the eyeball by the handle of the knife. The tumor was medullary sarcomatous, and a portion of it, attached to the pterygoid process of the sphenoid bone, could not be detached, but part of the malar bone involved in the disease was removed. On the 16th day the wound had healed and she left the house on that day. Three days after "she expired suddenly, but no examination was permitted." He performed a further successful operation on 10 January 1830.[179]

A very similar procedure was performed by Syme, also at the Edinburgh Royal Infirmary on May 15, 1829.[131] He made a cruciate incision and, after exposing the tumor, divided the malar bone with a saw and pliers, divided the nasal process of the maxillary bone, and cut through the hard palate using cutting pliers after having extracted one of the incisor teeth. He therefore probably did the operation a few weeks before Lizars, although Lizars gave the first description.

The early French literature is reviewed very thoroughly by Gensoul in his monograph of 1833.[180] He describes operations performed by Garengeot, Desault, and Dupuytren up to 1824. He records the great pains he took to find out what operations were actually performed, both by reading the contemporary accounts and by talking to those present at these operations. His research can be summarized as showing that all the procedures performed to 1827 consisted of an incision on the face followed by piecemeal removal of diseased tissue; no formal excision had been attempted. Gensoul then described his own patient, a 17-year-old boy with a 2-year history of a swelling in the superior part of the canine fossa, which he described as a hyperostosis (**Fig. 2.7**). The tumor measured 7¾ × 7½ inches (197 mm × 190 mm) with a circumference of 16¼ inches (413 mm). After much thought and consultation with colleagues he embarked on an operation on May 26, 1827, at the Hotel Dieu in Lyon. After making three incisions in the skin of the face he elevated skin flaps. Then he used a mallet and chisel to divide the lateral wall of the orbit close to the frontozygomatic suture, passed the chisel as far as the pterygomaxillary fissure, and divided the frontal process of the zygoma. Next he applied a very large chisel to the inner canthus and passed it through the lacrimal bone. He divided the ascending process of the nasal bone in a similar manner. He used the knife to divide the soft tissues of the nasal ala from the maxilla, removed the first upper incisor on the left side, and divided the hard palate. Finally, to detach the maxilla from the pterygoid process,

he plunged the chisel through the orbit and through the tumor, dividing the superior maxillary nerve, and used the chisel to bevel the specimen into the mouth. Shortly afterwards the patient fainted, but ultimately recovered! This is clearly the first account of a deliberate excision of the upper jaw.

Gensoul also did at least six other similar procedures, some for cancer, one with a 5-year cure. Unusually for that time, he followed his patients for upwards of 5 years and also recorded the size of the tumors, and at one point frankly admits a diagnostic mistake! Even more unusually, he deliberately delayed publication for 6 years to assess the long-term effects. His monograph runs to 77 pages, and in addition describes excision of the lower jaw. Gensoul also acknowledged Lizars' claim to have done the first operation, an apparent reference to Lizars' *System of Anatomical Plates*, published in 1826.

In the early 1850s there was a fairly vicious correspondence under pseudonyms such as "studens chirugiae" or "chirurgus"[130,181] in the medical press about the question of who did the first maxillectomy: Lizars, Syme, or Gensoul. Who it was is of little consequence, except perhaps to Lizars, Syme, and Gensoul at the time! Such claims for scientific precedence are common: they tell us that the procedure was not a "maverick" out of its time, but rather that surgery had progressed to the point where the operation was feasible and several surgeons in different countries had decided to try it, indicating that the topic was one of general interest. The main countries contributing to this development were France and Great Britain and, to a lesser extent, Germany. The US Surgeon General's Catalogue tells us that the procedure did not spread to other European countries until the second half of the 19th century.[182] It was first performed in Belgium in 1845 by Heylen,[183] in Poland in 1852 by Klose,[184] in Italy in 1857 by Gianflone[185] (a previous resection for necrosis had been reported in 1850 by Moretti),[186] in the Netherlands in 1857 by Leonides van Praag,[102] in Austria in 1857 by Dehler,[187] in Portugal in 1862 by Barbosa,[188] in Russia in 1862 by Kade,[95] in Spain in 1864 by Rosa[189] (one case for necrosis had been performed by Toca in 1858[190]), and in Finland in 1873 by Estlander.[191]

Resection of both upper jaws was first performed by Heyfelder in Erlangen, Germany in 1844.[84] A report was given in English by his son Oscar in 1857 in the *Dublin Journal of Medical Science*; Dublin being one of the main centers for this procedure, notably under Butcher, a name now forgotten. The operation was performed for a large "pseudo-plasma" arising from the palate, pushing the nose forward. He raised a large bilateral flap up to the inferior orbital margin and then formally excised both maxillae, preserving the nose. No attempt was made to provide a prosthesis. The patient returned to work but died 15 months later of a recurrence in the frontal

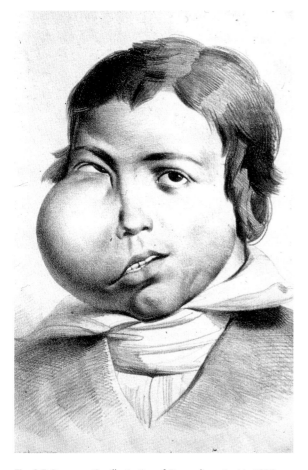

Fig. 2.7 Pre-operative illustration of Gensoul's patient in 1827. The operation was performed without anesthesia. This was almost certainly the first total maxillectomy and was undertaken for an osteosarcoma.

bone.[169] Oscar Heyfelder stated that the indications for the removal of both upper jaws included the following:

- Necrosis and caries
- Benign tumors including enchondroma and osteo-sarcoma
- Malignant tumors including epithelial cancer (cancroid of Virchow), cancer gelatiniforme, carcinoma medullare, and cystocarcinoma.

Incision

Many incisions have been described for maxillectomy, but they can be divided into two main types. The first is an incision passing from the outer canthus to the angle of the mouth. This was used in the early years—by Ballingal in 1827,[21] Lizars in 1829,[179] Velpeau in 1832,[178] Key in 1834,[96] and Liston in 1835[106]—but appears to have been abandoned by about 1840. The second is an incision passing down the lateral side of the nose. This was first used in 1827 by Gensoul[180] and has become the standard incision. Gensoul brought the incision through the upper lip at the level of the first incisor tooth, and Fergusson, in 1842, brought it through the upper lip in the midline.[53] The French school also developed a similar incision without division of the upper lip for partial operations on the upper part of the maxilloethmoidal complex, first described in 1865 by Legouest.[192] A further lateral limb through the lower eyelid was soon added. Farabeuf ascribes to Blandin of Paris an incision running from the inner to the outer canthus at the level of the infraorbital margin,[193] to join the incision running down the side of the nose, but this incision is *not* included in Blandin's original paper of 1834.[26] An incision passing from the inner to the outer canthus within the lower eyelid and through the conjunctiva at the oculopalpebral fold was described by Michaux in 1854, the purpose being to prevent retraction of the lower eyelid.[194] The incision through the external surface of the lower eyelid just below the lashes is usually ascribed to Weber. However, the source of this attribution is a mystery: a careful search has failed to reveal any record of a description of this incision by Weber, and the reference to his work[195] relates to fractures of the jaws. The so-called Weber–Fergusson incision would be more accurately termed the Blandin-Gensoul incision (**Fig. 2.8**). The incision described by Dieffenbach, splitting the patient down the midline, did not catch on![47]

Ligation of the Carotid Arteries

In the earlier operations it was customary to ligate the common or external carotid artery before the operation. For example, Earle, in 1831, ligated the common carotid artery on the affected side, apparently with no ill effects,[10] whereas Scon in 1830 tied the external carotid artery.[196] Heath, in his textbook *Injuries and Diseases of the Jaws*, tells us that this practice had been quite abandoned by the time of writing.[16]

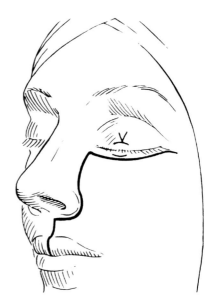

Fig. 2.8 A drawing showing the so-called Weber–Fergusson incision, which should probably be more accurately termed the Blandin–Gensoul incision.

Partial Resections

Surgery of the upper jaw continued to be developed for a further century, almost exclusively by the French, who introduced the concept of surgery "a la demande des lesions."[39]

In 1925 Comet reviewed this development dividing the upper jaw into three stages: superstructure (the ethmoido-maxillo-orbito-malar complex), a naso-sinus mesostructure, and a palatal infrastructure. He discussed the embryological basis of this division and the main histological tumor types, pointing out that about half are squamous carcinomas. He then discussed the anatomical origin of these tumors—from the ethmoids, the nasal cavity, from the antrum itself, and from the hard palate and alveolus—and the route of spread.[197] He performed experiments with Sebileau on the cadaver, demonstrating that it was impossible to clear the ethmoids via a buccal or transantral approach, and therefore recommended the paralateronasal rhinotomy described by Moure as the operation of choice for tumors of the suprastructure. Sebileau in 1906 described the clinical forms of maxillary cancer (neoplastic, suppurative and putrid) and gave a description of the routes of spread of maxillary cancer into the cheek, nose, and mouth; into the nose through the inferior meatus; into the canine fossa through the anterior walls; through the socket of an extracted tooth to appear on the upper alveolus; into the orbit through the superior wall; and into the pterygomaxillary or pterygoid fossa through the posterior wall.[197]

Superstructure

In the early years it was thought necessary to resect all of the upper jaw, because the methods of investigation had not allowed the exact point of origin and extent of the malignant tumor to be determined. However, as early as 1848 Michaux was questioning whether it was necessary to excise the hard palate when it was healthy.[198] He described partial operations for ethmoidal tumors and also preserved the floor of the orbit to maintain the function of the eye.[194] He also stressed the need to exclude extension of the tumor into the cranial cavity. In his monograph of 1854 Michaux described seven different procedures:[194]

- Ablation of the maxilla and malar bones
- Ablation of the maxilla alone
- Removal of the upper portion of the maxilla preserving the hard palate
- Removal of the inferior portion of the maxilla conserving the floor of the orbit and the ascending process of the maxilla
- Removal of the palatine arch
- Resection of the upper alveolus
- Removal of both maxillae.

In 1865 Legouest made an incision from the inner canthus descending along the nasal ala as far as the center of the upper lip. He then opened the left nostril widely and retracted the nose toward the healthy side after having divided the articulation of the nasal bone with the ascending ramus. Finally, he turned the internal wall of the maxillary sinus outward using scissors, after dividing the ascending ramus and the external and inferior part of the anterior opening of the nostril.[192] He did this operation for a boy with a nasopharyngeal polyp, presumably an angiofibroma. Until then these tumors had been treated by total maxillectomy with sacrifice of the orbit, but Legouest made a plea for a more conservative approach.

Cornet tells us that Michel of Nancy in 1869 modified the operations of Michaux and Legouest by omitting the resection of the maxilla itself and by adding an incision perpendicular to the vertical incision to allow partial excision of the orbital rim.[197]

The next development was a lateral rhinotomy described by Moure (**Fig. 2.9**) in 1902 as a radical intervention for malignant tumors arising from the upper part of the nasal fossa or from the ethmoid. He tells us that the orbital route had been previously recommended for approaching tumors of the upper jaw but advocated a different approach as follows. The nose was turned aside after making an incision from the lower part of the frontal bone to the nostril, the nasal bone being exposed using a periosteal elevator. He divided the ascending process of the maxilla and a part of the lacrimal bone after first elevating and retracting the "membranous nasal canal" so as not to damage it. He then divided the nasal bone

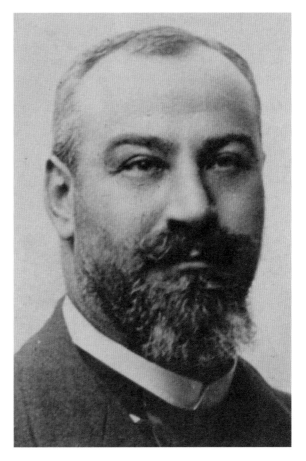

Fig. 2.9 Emile-Jean Gabriel Moure (1855–1914), inaugurator of the lateral rhinotomy.

within the nose, and finally the nasal spine of the frontal bone. To avoid opening the cranial cavity he passed a gouge parallel to the cribriform plate as far as the anterior wall of the sphenoid sinus, removing the ethmoids with a large curette working from below upwards. This step was performed using illumination from a forehead mirror. The operation finished with curettage of diseased areas of the septum, the orbit and sphenoid sinus. He counseled conserving the ridge of the nasal bone to preserve the shape of the nose, and advised packing the postnasal fossa at the start of the operation to prevent inhalation of blood. However, he said that bleeding usually stopped after removal of the tumor, and packing was then no longer necessary. He pointed out that it is possible to reach the sphenoid sinus by this route.[199]

His first patient, a cooper of 55, underwent the operation described above on July 9, 1901. One year later the patient was alive and well with no recurrence. Histology showed an "epithelioma cylindrique." Moure did not describe what he meant by this term, but the tumor is described fully in a later French paper by Hautant in 1933. From this description, including the fact that it arises from the olfactory mucosa, and from the accompanying woodcut, it is clear that "epithelioma cylindrique" would now be called an olfactory neuroblastoma. Indeed this tumor was fully described by the French.[5]

Sebileau further refined this procedure under the name of paralateronasal rhinotomy, emphasizing certain technical details and dividing rhinotomy into high, low, or total.[200] Moure's lateral rhinotomy was extended further by Hautant[201] in 1933 using an incision beginning above at the same point as Moure's incision, but then extending laterally beneath the eye. He used chisels to excise all the anterior part of the wall of the maxilla plus the floor of the orbit. This monograph was the first to include a description of the radiological appearances of these tumors.

The French were also the first to point out that sacrifice of the floor of the orbit is excessive if it is not invaded, because the physiological suspension of the eye is lost; "an eye not lying in its correct place is an eye lost."

It is interesting that St. Clair Thomson said in 1937 that lateral rhinotomy had quite replaced excision of the upper jaw,[202] and yet by 1977 it was described as a neglected operation.[203]

Mesostructure

Cornet in 1925 described unusual tumors that destroy the nasoantral wall and early invade the maxillary antrum.[197] These cases, he says, are suitable for a procedure that preserves both the floor of the orbit and hard palate. He describes a procedure that he terms an extended Caldwell–Luc antrostomy: the initial incision in the gingivobuccal sulcus between the canine and second molar tooth is extended and the entire anterior wall of the sinus is resected. Thereafter, the tumor is removed by careful and meticulous curettage of the antral cavity, whose other walls are assessed for erosion.

This was only a minor modification of the operation described by Denker in 1909.[204] After retracting the upper lip, Denker made an incision in the upper buccal sulcus of the affected side and for 2–3 cm on the opposite side. The soft tissues were then elevated from the face up to the orbital rim. He opened the maxillary antrum through the canine fossa and removed the lateral nasal wall with Luer's forceps and chisel. The lower part of the nasal bone and the nasal process of the maxilla were also resected. If necessary, he cleared the ethmoidal labyrinth and removed the anterior wall of the sphenoid.

Cornet also described a similar procedure[197] for the excision of malignant tumors arising from the inferior part of the nasal fossa (the septum and the inferior turbinate), which he ascribes to Rouge but sadly gives no reference. A careful search has failed to reveal where this procedure is recorded. The steps are as follows:

- A horizontal sublabial incision extending from one first molar to the other in the gingivolabial groove.
- Exposure of the nose: the curved periosteal elevator is used to denude the bone toward the bony orifice of the

nostrils, which it exposes on the lateral part of their circumference, exposing the anterior and inferior nasal spine.

- Division of the quadrangular cartilage from below upward using the scissors, and of the nasal spine allowing the superstructure of the nose to be elevated.
- Pterygomaxillary disarticulation, using a special shears curved on the flat.
- Extraction of the block held by a Farabeuf's forceps.

Infrastructure

Partial procedures for palatal tumors were described in 1854 by Michaux.[194] He describes resection of the upper alveolus, which he divided above the roots of the teeth with small scissors. He also describes in some detail an operation described by Nelaton of Paris, but unfortunately does not give a reference. Nelaton first elevated the palatal mucosa, providing of course that it was not diseased, and next made several holes at the anterior end of the hard palate. He introduced one blade of the scissors through this hole, dividing the hard palate and inferior edge of the septum.

Farabeuf generally made a transverse incision on the face to expose the upper alveolus. He perforated the anterior wall of the antrum to allow scissors to be introduced to cut the attachments of the alveolus.[52] He too ascribes to Nelaton the midline incision in the hard palate, but gives no reference to where Nelaton's work may be found.[193]

Barwell in 1873 removed the hard palate and alveolus from within the mouth, without opening into the nasal cavity.[23] He said that he could find no account of such an operation in any surgical work or journal, completely ignoring the fact that Michaux had given a very full description of this procedure in an extensive monograph 20 years earlier. Barwell's procedure of transoral palatectomy appears to have been empirical, rather than a systematic development based on the study of anatomy and pathology as was the case with the developments described by the French. The final development was that described by Cornet for tumors of the infrastructure. This operation was redescribed in the English literature a quarter of a century later by Wilson, who gave no credit to the French either for describing the operation or for describing the anatomical and pathological principles upon which it is based.[139]

Osteoplastic Procedures

The only other contribution from the German school, apart from resection of both maxillae and Denker's sublabial approach, was the development of an osteoplastic approach, originally described by Langenheck in 1859.[205] His patient was 18 years old, with two fibrous polyps, probably an angiofibroma of the nasopharynx. He first made a skin incision, much like that used for lateral rhinotomy, and divided the nasal cartilages from their attachments. Using a cutting bone forceps he divided the nasal bone close to the septum up to the nasal process of the frontal bone. A second incision divided the bone of the nasal process and continued into the maxillary sinus, ending at the attachment of the nasal process of the maxilla where it forms the lower border of the orbit. He used an elevator to turn the bone back on to the forehead.

In 1863 Voelckers described an osteoplastic flap, pedicled superiorly, of the anterior wall of the antrum for removal of a tumor—again probably an angiofibroma—invading the antrum from the region of the sphenoid sinus.[206]

Combined Irradiation

In the early years of the 20th century maxillectomy was also combined with the introduction of radium into the cavity. This method was popular both in England and the United States.[165,166,207,208] Jacketed tubes, steel points, or emanation seeds were used. The radium was applied directly to the tumor using a 50- or 100-mg tube within a silver tube for 15 to 20 hours.[209] An alternative was radium needles contained in a dental plate molded to fit the cavity.[207]

Prostheses

It has been customary since the earliest days to fill the defect left by maxillectomy with some form of dental prosthesis. A prosthesis was made after one of the very first maxillectomies, performed by Syme in 1835: Nasmyth made an artificial plate and a set of teeth that rendered the patient's appearance, mastication, and articulation "hardly at all defective."[132] Hart in 1862 tells us of a patient undergoing maxillectomy for scrofula for whom an artificial set of teeth was made by Hart's brother, a dentist.[81] Baker, a surgeon/dentist to Dr. Stevens Hospital in Dublin, "arranged the palate and dental apparatus in a most satisfactory manner so that the patient was enabled to eat with comfort and to articulate with perfect distinctness."[109]

By the early years of the 20th century the technique of dental restoration was well developed. Woodman describes how a plaster cast must be taken a few days before operation, to allow a temporary denture to be made with a bulbous extension to fit the cavity and prevent prolapse of the cheek. A permanent vulcanite splint, bearing teeth, is made a few months later (**Fig. 2.10**).[210,211]

Summary

Despite the dramatic technical innovations developed during the last half of the 20th century within the fields of chemotherapy, anesthesia, illumination, and instrumentation, possibly the only new major surgical procedure relevant to upper jaw neoplasia has been the craniofacial resection.

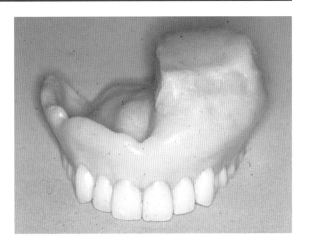

Fig. 2.10 A photograph of a permanent dental obturator (after Woodman 1923[209]).

A search through the original European literature has shown that during a period of some 50 years (1825–1875) most of the operations viewed today as standard were developed without the assistance of adequate illumination, blood replacement, anesthesia, and so on by a small number of exceptionally gifted and determined surgeons within a small number of European countries. The fact that any patients survived these traumatic experiences is a tribute to these surgeons' skills as well as the patients' own forbearance.

Despite the best efforts of the early pioneering surgeons and radiotherapists, the majority of patients with malignant disease of the nose, paranasal sinuses, and nasopharynx subsequently succumbed to their disease with high rates of locally recurrent disease within the structures of the adjacent anterior and antrolateral skull base, infratemporal fossa, clivus, orbit, and anterior and middle cranial fossae. The anatomy of the sinuses and skull base had been extensively studied and described by the end of the 19th century, notably by Onodi (**Fig. 2.11a, b**). However, it was not until the second half of the 20th century, with its dramatic technical innovations within the field of anesthesia, illumination, instrumentation, Hopkin's rod telescopes (**Fig. 2.12**), and the operating microscope, that it became possible to develop new major skull base surgical procedures, most notably the wide variety of craniofacial approaches and resections.

These new operative procedures were considerably aided by improved understanding and preoperative evaluation of the extent of both benign and malignant tumors by means of computed tomography (CT), introduced in the 1960s, and magnetic resonance imaging (MRI) introduced in the 1980s. Improved understanding of the pathological process and natural history of each disease improved our understanding of preoperative considerations in regard to treatment of the individual pathologies.

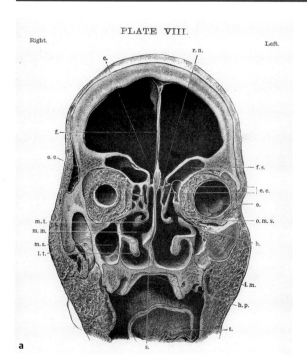

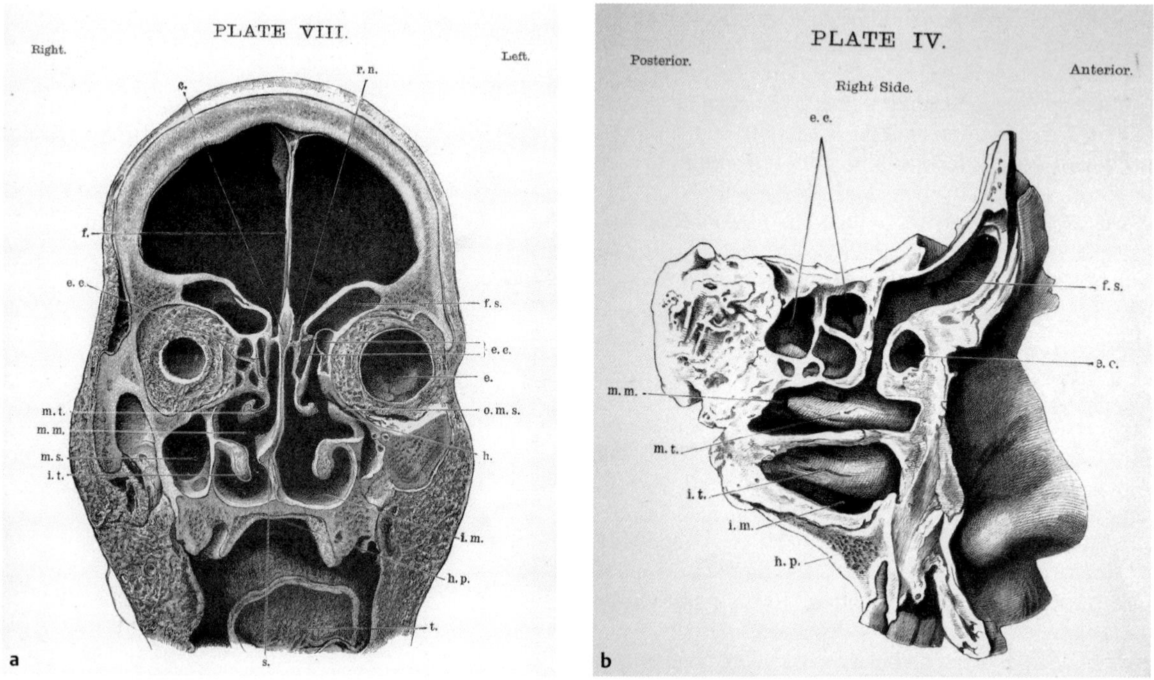

Fig. 2.11a, b

a Plate VIII Coronal section made vertically through the nose in its posterior third. (From "Dr. Onodi's Atlas of the Nasal Cavity and Sinuses" 1894, translated by St. Clair Thomson.)

b Plate IV Sagittal section through the right side of the nose external to the plane of the middle and inferior turbinals. (From Dr. A. Onodi's Atlas 1894, translated by St. Clair Thomson.)

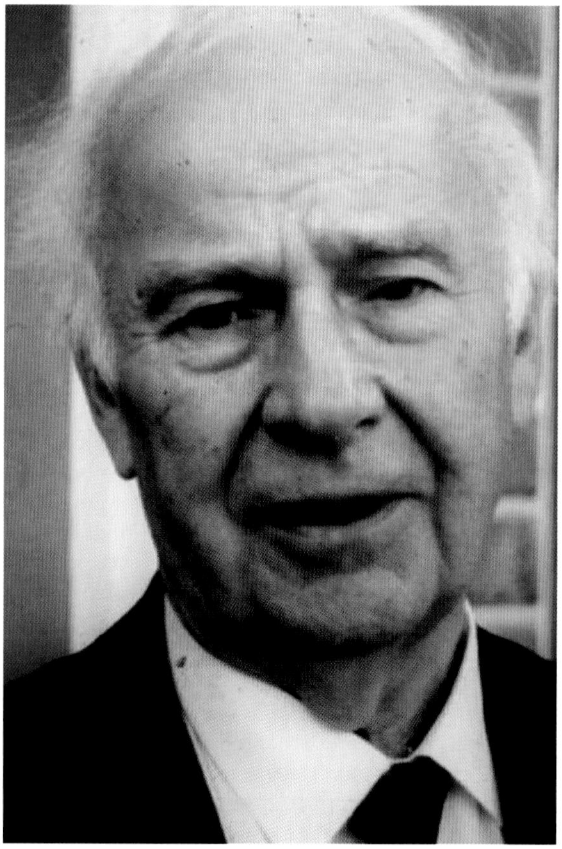

◁ **Fig. 2.12** Harold Hopkins, Professor of Optical Physics at Reading University, who developed his solid rod lens system in 1954, which allowed the development of modern endoscopic sinus surgery by Professor Walter Messerklinger of Graz.

Skull Base Surgery

Pituitary Surgery

Sir Victor Horsley is believed to be the first person to undertake in 1899 a transfrontal approach to a substantial hypophyseal tumor.[212] The technique of this operation remains the basis of the approach still used today. Just prior to Horsley's work, an Italian surgeon, Giordano,[213] approached the pituitary by turning aside the nose and frontal sinus as an osteoplastic flap and then removing the nasal septum, turbinates, and sphenoid to gain access. Schloffer in 1906[214] described the first purely transnasal approach, also removing the septum and turbinates to gain access through the sphenoid, but it was really Cushing in 1909[215] who developed this procedure over the following two decades. He described a sublabial approach coupled with a submucous resection of the nasal septum and preserved the nasal structure and function, developing the transseptal/transsphenoidal operation that is used by many to this day.

Dandy[216] is credited with the first reported anterior craniofacial resection which commenced as an orbitocraniotomy through an anterior approach, but he entered the ethmoid block to achieve resection of the tumor. Smith, Klopp, and Williams described the anterior craniofacial excision of a frontal sinus carcinoma in 1954.[217] It became increasingly well-recognized that the poor prognosis associated with malignant tumors of the nose and paranasal sinuses was a consequence of local recurrence, often related to inadequate resection. The realization that every tumor affecting the inferior surface of the cribriform plate and the roof of the ethmoid could spread intracranially became even more apparent with the advent of CT scanning. Thus, the principle of a combined craniofacial procedure became of increasing interest and was subsequently developed, most notably by the report of Ketcham and colleagues in 1963.[218] This initial report was subsequently added to by Ketcham et al in 1966 and 1973,[219,220] in Australia by Millar in 1973,[221] in the UK by Peter Clifford in 1977[222] and in the USA by Schramm, Myers & Maroon in 1979[223] and Terz et al in 1980.[224]

Our own experience at the Royal National Throat, Nose and Ear Hospital commenced with Sir Donald Harrison, who had a life-long interest in tumors of the nose and paranasal sinuses, reporting their management notably in 1973 and developing his rationale with his great friend George Sisson from the United States, who reported his 15-year experience in 1976.[225] Harrison's personal series of 85 patients with sinonasal tumors, which he reported in 1973,[226] led him to believe that ~80% of all patients with antroethmoidal tumors would have extension of their neoplasm up to and beyond the limits of conventional total maxillectomy with or without orbital exenteration. He encouraged Tony Cheesman, who already had an extensive training in ENT, skull base, and neurosurgery, to commence craniofacial resection in 1978 (**Fig. 2.13**). Our 7-year experience of 60 patients was subsequently reported in 1986.[227]

While the craniofacial procedure that we developed involved the use of a small anterior window craniotomy (**Fig. 2.14**), minimal dural retraction, and resection under operative microscope control, other colleagues wished to improve the exposure of the posterior extent of the anterior cranial fossa without retraction of the frontal lobes and the fronto-orbital band was removed in a procedure developed from craniofacial surgery for congenital craniomaxillary anomalies introduced by Tessier et al.[228] The extended anterior subcranial approach was developed by Raveh initially to manage intracranial trauma but subsequently to allow tumor resection, reported in 1993.[229]

There was an explosion of interest in the anterior approaches to tumors of the nose, paranasal sinuses, and skull base in the 1980s and many of the approaches to the skull base began to blend in with intraoral approaches and more lateral based approaches such as the infratemporal fossa approach pioneered by Fisch,[230] and Sekhar and Schramm.[231] Many institutions formed multidisciplinary

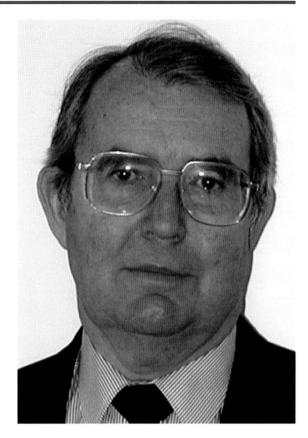

Fig. 2.13 Tony Cheesman, who has been the main promoter of craniofacial resection in the United Kingdom.

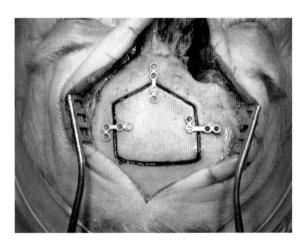

Fig. 2.14 Anterior craniofacial operation. Intraoperative photograph showing initial placement of 1.7 mm microplating prior to removal of the shield-shaped craniotomy window. This allows precise replacement of the window at the end of the craniofacial procedure.

teams around the world that continue with this work to the present day, and it becomes invidious to single out individuals and institutions as a wide variety of people continue to contribute significantly to this advancing area of surgery. However, it would be remiss not to mention the contributions of Cocke, Derome, Donald, Jackson, Janecka, and Maniglia,[232-237] who have all made substantial contributions to the wide variety of approaches now available for tumors in this region.

Endonasal and Endoscopic Surgery

Endonasal surgery has its main origins in Germany, notably with four generations of doctors in the Heerman family in the 20th century. Hans Heermann[238] demonstrated the use of the binocular Zeiss operating microscope in 1957 for endonasal ethmoid surgery. By 1974 this endonasal microscopic technique was reported to have been used in 14,000 ethmoid, maxillary, sphenoid, and frontal sinus procedures.[239]

Hirshman was reported to be the first surgeon to attempt nasal and sinus endoscopy using a modified cystoscope based on the design of Nitze in 1897.[238] This endoscope was made by Reiniger, Gebbert, and Schall in Berlin, Germany. The endoscope was initially used for diagnosis and minor procedures such as cautery and removal of foreign bodies, but essentially these rigid telescopes and other derivatives had proximal illumination with a small bulb and were used for diagnosis.

Harold Hopkins's invention of the rod endoscope, manufactured by Storz, facilitated the major developments that began in the 1960s and 1970s and this coincided with the development of endonasal surgery using the binocular operating microscope, first reported by Heerman in 1958.[239] Draf also used the microscope but additionally combined this with an angled endoscope.[240,241]

Endoscopic sinus surgery was first reported in the European literature in 1967 by Messerklinger,[242] Wigand,[243] and Stammberger.[244] The latter in particular further expanded and popularized the technique that Kennedy introduced into the United States in 1985.[245] With an abundance of new instruments to complement the improved endoscopes, it was only a matter of time before benign and malignant tumors were approached using this method.

During the last three decades, the considerable improvements in detailed scanning by CT and MRI of the skull base and recently image guidance systems, have allowed skull base surgeons to approach deeply seated tumors using minimal-access endoscopic techniques. Extended endonasal endoscopic surgical procedures are increasingly described and employed and the feasibility and low morbidity of these extended approaches have now been well established and reported in numerous studies. These expanded endonasal approaches are continuously being used throughout major centers around the world as a new method for sinonasal and skull base surgeons tackling these tumors. It is now possible to gain access to anterior, middle, and posterior cranial fossa

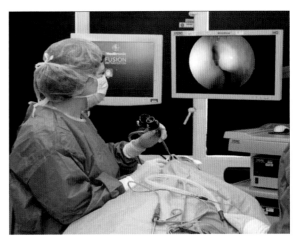

Fig. 2.15 Operating theater set-up for endoscopic sinus surgery (for a meningoencephalocele).

structures. The use of extended endoscopic approaches instead of traditional open surgery is limited by the experience of the surgical team involved and the relationship of many tumors to critical neurovascular structures (**Fig. 2.15**).

As with the open approaches, it is invidious to try to single out all colleagues who have made contributions to the development of this surgery, but the recent European position paper on the endoscopic management of tumors of the nose, paranasal sinuses, and skull base gives an excellent overview of the subject and its development by colleagues Carrau, Castelnuovo, Kassam, Lund, Nicolei, Stammberger, Stamm, and Wormald, who have made and continue to make contributions to this important area.[246] Interestingly, the two-person, four-handed technique was first promoted by May in 1990[247] but has been extensively popularized more recently.[248-250]

Multiple centers have now concentrated on all aspects of skull base surgery with an increasing emphasis on endoscopic approaches but with the retention of the wide variety of open procedures that remain necessary in combination with new developments in radiotherapy, chemotherapy, and the recently introduced novel targeted pharmacotherapies that antagonize cellular proliferation by interfering with specific cellular processes. While much is hoped for these latter therapeutic agents, guided by our increasing understanding of molecular factors, history teaches us that the early demise of surgery as the main treatment of cancer is a considerable way off as a consequence of the complexity of malignant disease. Our hope is that this publication will continue to guide surgeons and promote an increasing understanding of these diseases in a multidisciplinary team, but our expectation is that the necessary skills will be required for the present generation of young surgeons.

References

1. Harrison DFN, Lund VJ. Tumours of the Upper Jaw. New York: Churchill Livingstone; 1993:1–351
2. Watson. Ulceration of larynx, tracheotomy, haemoptysis. Edinburgh Med J 1865;xi:78
3. Billroth T. Beobachtungen ueber Geschwuelste der Speicheldrusen. Arch Pathol Anat Physiol Klin Med 1859;17:357–375
4. Robin C, Laboulbene JJA. Trois productions morbides. Compte Rendu Soc Biol 1853;5:185–196
5. Herger L, Luc G, Richard D. L"esthesioneuroepitheliome olfactif. Bull Assoc Fr Etud Cancer 1924;13:410–421
6. Oehngren LG. Malignant tumours of the maxillo ethmoidal region. Acta Oto-laryngol 1933;(Suppl):xix
7. Pledge HT. Science Since 1500. A Short History of Mathematics, Physics, Chemistry and Biology. London: Her Majesty's Stationery Office; 1966:166
8. Virchow R. Cellular Pathology as Based Upon Physiological and Pathological Histology. London: Churchill; 1858:464–465
9. Erichsen JE. Diseases of the antrum and upper jaw. In: Heck M, Johnson R, eds. The Science and Art of Surgery. 10th ed. Vol II. London: Longmans, Green; 1895:627–643
10. Earle. Osteo-sarcoma of the antrum, extirpation of the superior maxillary bone. Lancet 1831–2;i:378–379
11. Barton IK. Removal of superior maxillary bone, for malignant disease. Dublin Q J Med Sci 1863;xxxiv:32–38
12. Porter G. Excision of a large portion of the upper-jaw for epuloid disease—recovery. Dublin J Med Sci 1867;xliii:106:257–261
13. Ochsner AJ. The treatment of cancer of the jaw with the actual cautery. J Am Med Soc 1923;81:1487–1491
14. Dickson D. Fungus of the antrum: lymphatic contamination: no visceral taint. London Med Gazette 1840;ii:256–258
15. Guthrie CG. Clinical lecture on the removal of the superior maxillary, and other bones of the face. London Med Gazette 1835–1836;xvi:315–318
16. Heath C. In: Injuries and Diseases of the Jaws. 2nd ed. London: Churchill; 1872
17. Koerte W. Rescerionen des Oberkiefers. Archiv fur Klinische Chirurgie (Berlin) 1880;xxv:514–516
18. Adams. Large fibro-cellular growth in the antrum, removal of the superior maxilla (operation by single incision); recovery. Med Times Gaz 1853;vii:89
19. Aikin CA. Excision of the superior maxillary bone. Lancet 1839;ii:217–218
20. Ashurst. Case of fibroid tumour of the upper jaw. Am J Med Sci (Philadelphia) 1870;lix:121–123
21. Ballingal. Removal of a sarcomatous tumour from the superior maxillary antrum. Lancet 1827;xii:620
22. Barker AE. Notes of a specimen of tubular epithelioma. Lancet 1884;ii:827
23. Barwell R. Myeloid sarcoma of the upper jaw removed, with nearly all the alveolus of the left side, without opening the cavity of the nose into that of the mouth. Lancet 1873;ii:81
24. Beatson WB. Osseous tumour ofthe left superior maxilla; removal of the bone. Lancet 1873;i:271
25. Bickersteth E. Excision of the upper jaw. Med Times Gaz 1857;xiv:338
26. Blandin E. Case of osteosarcoma of the left upper maxillary bone. Lancet 1834;ii:353–354
27. Braun H. Ueber totale doppelte Oberkieferresectionen. Archiv fur Klinische Chirurgie 1875–1876;xix:728–748
28. Buchanan G. Excision of superior maxillary bone. Edinburgh Med J 1864;x:406
29. Buchanan G. Tumour of antrum: excision ofsuperior maxillary bone: recovery. Glasg Med J 1879;xi:143–144
30. Burow. Fibroid der fossa sphenomaxillaris; osteoplastische oberkieker resection: heilung. Berliner Klinische Wochenschrift 1877;xiv:60–63
31. Butcher RGH. On extirpation of the upper jaw. Dublin Q J Med Sci 1853;xvi:18–36
32. Butcher RGH. Excision of nearly the entire left superior maxillary bone. Dublin Q J Med Sci 1860;xxix:259–271
33. Butcher RGH. Successful excision of the entire upper jaw and malar bone, for an enormous tumour involving both, and filling the parotid region. Dublin Q J Med Sci 1861;xxxi:1–15
34. Butcher RGH. Successful excision of the entire upper jaw and palate bone for an enormous fibro-vascular tumour. Dublin Q J Med Sci 1863;xxxv:279–293
35. Canton. Disease of the left upper jaw-bone, originating primarily in a blow from the fist; successful removal of the entire bone. Lancet 1865;i:477–478
36. Clark F, Le G. Case of malignant disease of the right upper jaw;excision; recovery. Med Times Gaz 1856;xiii:171
37. Collis P. Excision ofthe upper jaw for malignant tumour of the antrum. BMJ 1869;i:377
38. Coote H. Extirpation of the upper jaw for malignant disease. Lancet 1866;ii:411
39. Craven R. Excision of the superior maxilla and malar bone. Med Times Gaz 1863;ii:669–670
40. Craven R. Excision of the superior maxilla for tumour recovery. Med Times Gaz;ii:356–357
41. Craven R. Excision ofupper jaw. Med Times Gaz 1876;ii:677
42. Crile GW. Excision of cancer of the head and neck. JAMA 1906;47:1780–1786
43. Croly HG. Excision of the entire left superior maxilla, by a single incision, for myeloid tumour. Dublin Q J Med Sci 1868;xlv:278–285
44. Crompton DW. Tumor in the left antrum. London Med Gazette 1846;i:679–680
45. Cumming AJ. Excision of superior maxilla. Lancet 1871; i:231–232
46. Davies R. Encephaloid tumour of antrum. Lancet 1858; i:85–88
47. Dieffenbach JF. On the resection of facial bones. Lancet 1837–8; i:692–699
48. Dobie W. Fibrous polypus of antrum, etc. evulsion, recovery. Monthly J Med Sci 1853;17:307–309
49. Dobson NC. Removal of greater part of both superior maxillae simultaneously for malignant disease. BMJ 1873;ii:430–432
50. Dunsmure J. Osteo-sarcoma of upper jaw; excision of superior maxilla; recovery. Edinburgh Med Surg J 1854; lxxxi:100–101
51. Brichsen JE. Fibro-plastic tumor of the right upper jaw; excision; recovery. Lancet 1872;i:611–612
52. Fearn SW. Case of fibrous tumour of the antrum, in which the jaw was excised. BMJ 1863;ii:523–524
53. Fergusson W. Tumour of the upper jaw—excision of the superior maxillary and malar bone. Lancet 1841–2; i:710–712
54. Fergusson W. Excisions of the superior maxilla. Med Times Gaz 1856;xiii:569
55. Fergusson W. Removal of the upper jaw. Lancet 1857; ii:33–34
56. Fergusson W. Excision of the upper jaw. BMJ 1857; ii:728–729
57. Fergusson W. Vascular fibrous polypus of the antrum extending into the nose—removal. Med Times Gaz 1860;i:235
58. Fergusson W. Excision of the superior maxilla—clinical remarks. Med Times Gaz 1861;i:550
59. Fergusson W. Fibrous tumour of the antrum extending through the hard palate into the mouth—successful removal. Lancet 1861;i:206–207

60. Fergusson W. Clinical remarks upon a case of removal of the upper jaw, for a tumour extending to the base of the cranium. Lancet 1862;ii:205–206
61. Fergusson W. Extensive tumour of the antrum, involving the floor of the orbit and the soft palate; excision of superior maxilla; recovery. Med Times Gaz 1863;i:159–160
62. Fergusson W. Malignant tumour of left antrum, involving left side of hard and the whole of soft palate. Lancet 1864;i:8–9
63. Fergusson W. Removal of a portion of the superior maxilla for a fibrous tumour of the antrum. Med Times Gaz 1865;i:600
64. Fergusson W. Case of removal of fibrous polypus attached to base of skull. Med Times Gaz 1868;i:211
65. Fergusson W. Two cases of disease of the superior maxillary bone; excision; clinical remarks. Lancet 1870;i:584
66. Fergusson W. Practical Surgery. 5th ed. London: Churchill; 1870:30–31
67. Fergusson W. Tumour of antrum; removal of greater portion of the superior maxilla. Med Times Gaz 1872;i:598
68. Field AG. Resection of the upper jaw. Med Times Gaz 1858;xvii:217
69. Fyffe. Encephaloid tumour ofthe antrum. Dublin Q J Med Sci 1853;xv:470–471
70. Gant FJ. Excision of the antrum of the upper jaw. Lancet 1874;i:164
71. Godlee RJ. Resection of upper jaw for carcinoma, with remarks. Med Times Gaz 1885;xl:746
72. Gott WH. Exsection of the right superior maxilla, and a portion of the left for disease of long standing. Am J Med Sci (Philadelphia) 1860;xxxix:344–348
73. Gott WA . Encephaloid disease of the right superior maxilla; resection of the bone; recovery. Am J Med Sci (Philadelphia) 1871;lxii:289–290
74. Grant J. Tumour of the antrum; removal of the upper jawbone. Lancet 1843;i:148–151
75. Greenhow TM. Excision of the upper jaw for fungoid disease. Med Times Gaz 1835–36;ix:122
76. Guthrie CG. Removal of the upper jaw. Lancet 1850;i:247–248
77. Hadden. A case of removal of left superior maxilla. Dublin Q J Med Sci 1870;1:251–254
78. Hancock H. Amputation of the upper jaw. Lancet 1847;i:359–360
79. Hancock H. Removal of the superior maxilla on the left side, with a large tumour involving that bone. Lancet 1852;i:360
80. Harrison R. Excision of the upper jaw. Liverpool Med Surg Rep 1870;iv:106–107
81. Hart E. Resection of the maxillae, without skin incision. Lancet 1862;ii:59–60
82. Hawkins C. Excision of the upper jaw. BMJ 1859;ii:716–717
83. Hewett P. Removal of the upper jaw for fibro-plastic disease. Lancet 1859;i:537
84. Heyfelder JFM. Totale resektion beider oberkiefer. J d Chir u Augenh 1844;xxxii:633–638
85. Higgens C. Sarcoma of the superior maxilla and orbit; removal; speedy recurrence, and rapid growth. BMJ 1878;ii:722
86. Howse. Removal of the superior maxillary bone. Lancet 1850;i:90–91
87. Hulke JW. Excision of superior maxilla. BMJ 1873;i:671
88. Irving J. Observations on the case of malignant tumour, successfully removed by operation, from the left antrum maxillare. Edinburgh Med Surg J 1825;xxiv:93–95
89. Jackson A. Myeloid disease of the left superior maxilla; removal of the whole bone without any external incision; recovery. BMJ 1877;ii:478–479
90. Jackson TC. Fibrous tumour of the upper jaw, removed by excision. Transact Pathol Soc 1862;xiv:236–238
91. Jalland. Tumour of the antrum; excision of the superior maxilla; cure. Lancet 1885;ii:526
92. Johnson HC. Extirpation of the upper jaw for tumour of the antrum. Lancet 1857;ii:602–603
93. Johnson HC. Malignant tumour of the upper jaw, partial excision of that bone. BMJ 1858;101
94. Johnson Z. Removal of the superior maxilla for disease of that bone. Dublin Q J Med Sci 1858;xxvi:68–86
95. Kade. Totale resection des rechten oberkiefers vollstandige heilung. St Petersburg Med Z 1862;iii:157
96. Key CA. Operations—Removal of a great portion of the upper jawbone. Lancet 1834;ii:575–576
97. Key CA. Extirpation of a tumour from the antrum maxillare with removal of the superior maxillary bone, including the palate bone. Dublin Q J Med Sci 1846;ii:552–553
98. Keyworth. Excision of the right superior maxilla on account of fibroid tumour in the antrum. Med Times Gaz 1862;i:321–322
99. Lane. Excision of both superior maxillary bones, both palatal bones, both inferior turbinated bones, vomer and part of the ethmoid bones, involved in a tumour; recovery. Lancet 1862;i:96–98
100. Lansdowne. Excision of the superior maxilla for epithelioma of the cheek and hard palate. Lancet 1871;ii:677
101. Leake WI. Exsection of the superior maxillary, together with the malar and palate bones of the right side; recovery. Am J Med Sci (Philadelphia) 1860;xxxix:348–351
102. Leonides van Praag I. Partielle resektion des oberkiefers wegen epulis. Arch Hallsender Beitrage Nationale Heilkunde Utrecht 1857–1858;i:370–398
103. Lewis JS. Tumours of the middle ear cleft and temporal bone. In: Ballantyne, Groves, eds. Scott Brown's Diseases of the Ear, Nose and Throat. Vol 3. 4th ed. London: Butterworths; 1979:385
104. Lister J. Two cases of tumour of the upper jaw; excision of the superior maxillary bone. London Edinburgh Monthly J Med Sci 1854;xix:428–433
105. Liston R. Case of polypus successfully removed by operation from the antrum maxillare. Edinburgh Med Surg J 1821;vii:397–400
106. Liston R. Osteosarcoma of the jaw; removal of the superior maxillary and malar bones. Lancet 1835;i:917–918
107. Liston R. Tumour of the upper jaw-bone; excision and recovery. Lancet 1841–2;i:67–68
108. Lizars J. The organs of sense. A System of Anatomical Plates. London: WH Lizars; 1826:164
109. McDonnell R. Case of excision of a portion of the superior maxilla. BMJ 1868;i:53
110. McFarlane J. Fungus of the antrum. Edinburgh Med Surg J 1837;xlvii:25–28
111. Mapother ED. Rhinoplasty and removal of upper jaw. BMJ 1870;1(494):622
112. Marsden F. Case of excision of the right superior maxilla, and of the palatine process of the left; recovery. Med Times Gaz 1862;i:165
113. Marshall H. Case of excision of the upper jaw. BMJ 1865;i:641–642
114. Mash B. Fibroplastic tumour of the antrum; excision of the superior maxilla; recovery. Med Times Gaz 1865;i:35–36
115. Mueller M. Fall von osteoplastischer oherkiefer-resection. Arch Klin Chir 1870;xi:323–326
116. Neilson JL. Central myxosarcoma of the right superior maxilla; removal of entire maxilla and portion of malar bone. Am J Med Sci (Philadelphia) 1880;lxxix:437–442
117. Norton AF. Removal of the frontal portion of the frontal bone, the roots of both orbits, the ethmoid bone, parts of both superior maxillae, the vomer, and palate, the left greater wing of the sphenoid bone, and the left eyeball: followed by complete restoration to health. Transact Clin Med Soc London 1880;xiii:48–51

118. Nunneley T. Excision of the superior maxillary bone for a large fibroid tumour attached to its palatal portions, and filling the mouth and fauces. Transact Pathol Soc London 1860;xi:266

119. Paget J. Fibrous tumour of the antrum, successfully removed. Lancet 1861;i:813

120. Paget J. Fibrous tumour of the antrum with pulsation excision—recovery. Med Times Gaz 1861;ii:250–251

121. Parkman P. Excision of superior maxillary bone; result unfavourable. Am J Med Sci (Philadelphia) 1851;xxi:52–53

122. Peters GA. Excision of the superior maxilla with remarks. NY Med J 1885;41:57–60

123. Quinten WM. Removal of a tumour from the antrum. Lancet 1839;i:359–360

124. Ransford R. Exostosis of the antrum; removal of superior maxilla; death. Lancet 1881;i:414–415

125. Savory WS. Removal of the superior maxilla. Lancet 1871; ii:577–578

126. Simon J. Excision of the upper jaw an account of fibrous polypus. Med Times Gaz 1858;xvii:35

127. Smith H. Tumour of the upper jaw; new operation. Med Times Gaz 1852;iv:391–392

128. Smith T. Tumour of the superior maxilla, removal; rapid recovery. Lancet 1873;i:731–732

129. Solly S. Myeloid tumour of the upper jaw; excision; recovery. Med Times Gaz 1869;i:464–465

130. Chirurgiae S. Excision of the maxillary bone. Med Times Gaz 1854;viii:69–70

131. Syme J. Excision of the superior maxillary bone. Edinburgh Med Surg J 1829;xxxii:238–239

132. Syme I. Excision of the superior maxillary bone. Edinburgh Med Surg J 1835;xliv:1–5

133. Syme J. Peculiar disease of the maxillary antrum, and removal of the bone by a single incision of the cheek. London Edinburgh Monthly J Med Sci 1843;xxx:495–497

134. Syme J. Excision of the superior maxillary bone. London Edinburgh Monthly J Med Sci 1852;xiv:530–531

135. Syme J. Excision of the greater portion of the upper jaw. Edinburgh Med J 1862–3; viii:138–139

136. Thorold H. Necrosis of an osseous growth projecting into the antrum of the upper jaw. Med Times 1849;xx:394–395

137. Trenerry C. Report of a case of extirpation of the superior maxillary bone. Lancet 1850;ii:574–575

138. Wagstaffe WW. Tumour occupying both upper jaws, removed by operation. Transact Pathol Soc London 1873;xxiv:189–191

139. Wilson CP. Growths arising primarily in the antra and anterior ethmoidal regions. Proc R Soc Med 1955;48:72–75

140. Windsor T. Cancer of the upper jaw—removal—death. Med Times Gaz 1857;xiv:564–565

141. Stokes W. Excision of the upper jaw. Med Press Circ 1868;vi:54–55

142. Stokes W. Excision of the upper jaw, along with an enormous fibro-sarcomatous tumour, which, springing from the base of the skull, passed forwards, causing extensive absorption of the osseous structures surrounding it. Med Press Circ 1872;iv:522–523

143. Tatum T. Fibrous tumour to the base of the skull: resection of the upper jaw bone: removal of the tumour. BMJ 1858;lvi:857–858

144. Thompson H. Removal of the left upper maxilla: recovery. BMJ 1870;i:601

145. Thomson St CS. Malignant disesse of the nose and sinuses. Lancet 1916;i:987–991

146. Bryant T. Tumours of the upper and lower jaws: on some cases of cystic disease of the antrum. Guy's Hosp Reports 1870;xv(3rd series):252–255

147. Stokes W. Excision of the upper jaw for the removal of a fibro-sarcomatous tumour growing from the base of the skull. Dublin J Med Sci 1873;lvi:273–287

148. Lawrie IA. Necrosis; removal of the whole of the superior maxilla; division of the masseter; repair of the gap in the cheek; cure. London Edinburgh Monthly J Med Sci 1843;ii:678–681

149. Riedinger F. Resection des oberkiefers mit erhaltung des mukores-periostealen heherzuges des harten gaumens. Berliner Klin Wochenschr 1873;10:521–524

150. Brainard D. Case of resection of the superior maxillary and malar bones. Am J Med Sci (Philadelphia) 1852;xxiv:131–132

151. Lawson G. Extirpation of tumour from the antrum of highmore. Med Times Gaz 1872;i:513

152. Lawson G. Epithelioma of mucous membrane invading the hard palate; partial excision of superior maxillary bone. Med Exam 1876;i:513

153. Walsham WJ. Tumour of the antrum; removal of the left superior maxillary bone:from a man aged sixty-seven; recovery. Lancet 1879;i:807

154. Heiberg J. Resection des oberkiefers wegen cylindoms, mit vorangeschickter tracheotomie und tamponade des larynx. Heilung. Berliner Klin Wochenschr 1872;9:432–434

155. Fergusson W. Tumour of the antrum. Med Times Gaz 1876;ii:439

156. Reid DB. Case of excision of the upper jaw. Lancet 1868; ii:7–8

157. MacLeod GHB. Excision of the upper jaw. Glasgow Med J 1871–1872;iv:329

158. Rose E. Vorschlag zur erleichterung der operationen am oberkiefer. Arch Klin Chir (Berlin) 1874;xvii:454–464

159. Carothers AE. Extirpation of both superior maxillary, left malar, and pterygoid process of left sphenoid bones. Am J Med Sci (Philadelphia) 1875;lxx:430–433

160. Trendelenburg FA. Die tamponnade der trachea. Berliner Klin Wochensch 1870;7:278–281

161. Gussenbauer C. Ueber die erste durch R. Th. Billroth am Menschen ausgefuehne kehlkopf exstirpation und die anwendung eines kuenstlichen kehlkopfes. Arch Klin Chir 1874;17:343

162. Bellamy E. Removal of the greater portion of both upper jaw bones, without external incision. Med Times Gaz 1883;ii:452–453

163. Nivison JF. Case of a malignant tumour successfully removed, by operation, from the left antrum maxillare vel Highmorianum. Edinburgh Med Surg J 1825;xxiii:290–293

164. Parey A. The Workes of that Famous Chirurgion Ambrose Parey. London: Chappell; 1695:480–481

165. New GB. Malignant tumours of the antrum of Highmore: end results of treatments. Arch Otolaryngol 1926; 4:201–214

166. Clark WL. Cancer of the oral cavity, jaws and throat. JAMA 1918;71:1365–1369

167. Holden HB, McKelvie P. Cryosurgery in the treatment of head and neck neoplasia. Br J Surg 1972;59(9):709–712

168. Williams W. Cases of extirpation of the superior maxillary bone. Guys Hosp Rep 1843;i:462–465

169. Heyfelder O. On the resection of both upper jaw bones. Dublin Q J Med Sci 1857;xxiii:107–119

170. Wiseman R. Observations of a cancer on the left cheek. Severall Chirurgicall Treatises. London: Fiesher and Macock; 1676:112

171. White C. An extraordinary tumour on the lower part of the orbit of the eye, thrusting the eye out of its socket, successfully extirpated. Cases in Surgery with Remarks. Part the First. London: W Johnston; 1770:135–139

172. Bell B. A System of Surgery. 5th ed. Edinburgh: Bell & Bradfute; 1791

173. Heister L. A General System of Surgery. 7th ed. London: Clarke, Whiston & White; 1759

174. Hunter J. The Works of John Hunter. London: Longman, Rees, Orme, Brown, Green and Longman; 1837

175. Pott P. The Chirurgical Works of Percival Pott. London: Lowndes; 1779
176. Dupuytren M. Leçons Orales de Clinique Chirurgicale. Paris: Baillière; 1839:452–453
177. Rogers DL. Case of osteosarcoma of the superior maxillary bone with the operation for its removal. NY Med Phys J 1824;iii:301–303
178. Velpeau ALM. Nouveaux Elements de Medecine Operatoire. Paris: Bailliere; 1832: 547–552
179. Lizars J. Removal of the superior maxillary bone. London Med Gaz 1829–30;v:92–93
180. Gensoul PJ. Lettre Chirurgicale sur quelques maladies graves du sinus maxillaire et de l"os maxillaire inferieur. Paris: Baillière; 1833
181. Chirurgus. Letter. Remarks on Mr. Syme being the first to perform the operation of removal of the superior maxillary bone in Europe. Med Times Gaz 1853;viii:20–21
182. Surgeon-General's Office. Index Catalogue, Vol. VII. Washington: Government Printing Office; 1886
183. Heylen JB. Tumeur cancereuse de l'os maxillaire superieur droit; extirpation; guerison, reflexions; modifications au procede operatoire de Dieffenbach. Ann Soc Med Anvers 1845;vi:409–420
184. Klose CW, Paul J. Krebs des oberkiefers; resectio maxillae superioris. Z Klin Med Bresle 1852;iii:53
185. Gianflone F. Cenno di un fatto di ablazione totale dell"osso mascellare superiore. Morgagni 1857;i:259–261
186. Moretti F. Asportazione quasi totale di ambedue i massilari superiori. Gazz Med Ital Feder Tos Firenze 1850;2 (series i):89–91
187. Dehler J. Partielle resection des oberkiefers wegen necrose. Oesterrische Z Prakt Heilkd 1857;iii:401–404
188. Barbosa AM. Reseccao de todo o osso maxillar superior do lado direito praticada pela primeira vez em Portugal. J Soc Sci Med Lisbon (2nd series) 1862;xxvi:441–443
189. Rosa E. Reseccion del maxilar superior, hecha por DF Rubio. Siglo Med Madrid 1864;xi:406
190. Toca MS. Fungas y caries de la mandibula superior del maxilar: curacion. Cron Hosp Madrid 1858;vi:469–472
191. Estlander. Resektion af ofverkaken jemte exstirpation af tumor. Finska Laksallsk Handl Helsingfors 1873;XV:271
192. Legouest. Apropos des fibromes nasopharyngiens. Bulletin Soc Imp Chirurg (2nd series) 1865;vi:523–524
193. Farabeuf L-H. Resections de la machoire superieure. In: Precis de Manuel Operatoire. 3rd ed. Paris: Masson; 1889:870–889
194. Michaux. Resections de la Machoire superieure. Bull Acad R Med Belg 1854;iii:1–118
195. Weber O. In: von Pitha F, Billroth T, eds. Handbuch der Allgemeinen und Speciellen Chirurgie. Vol III. Stuttgart: Enke; 1866:232, 247, 283, 285
196. Scott. Extirpation of the right superior maxillary bone affected with osteosarcoma. Lancet 1830–31;i:319–320
197. Cornet P. La chirurgie des tumeurs malignes du massif facial superieur "a la demande des lesions." Ann Mal Oreille Larynx 1925;xliv:574–605
198. Michaux L. Cancer de l'os maxillaire supericur droit penetrant dans la fosse nasale, l'orbite, le sinus frontal, les cellules ethmoidales et le sinus sphenoidal. Extirpation de taute la tumeur par une seule incision pratique sur le ligne mediane de la face, hemorragies consecutives, guerison. Bull Acad R Med Belg 1848–9;viii:1287–1294
199. Moure EJ. Traitment des tumeurs malignes primitives de l'ethmoide. Rev Hebdomadaire Laryngol Otol Rhinol 1902;47:402–412
200. Sebileau I. Les formes cliniques du cancer du sinus maxillaire. Ann Maladies Oreille Larynx 1906;xxxii:430–450
201. Hautant A, Monod O, Klotz A. Les epitheliomas ethmoidoorbitaires: leur traitment par l'association chirurgie-radium: resultats eloignes. Ann Oto-Laryngol 1933:385–421
202. Thomson St CS, Negus VE. Diseases of the Nose and Throat. 4th ed. London: Cassell; 1937
203. Harrison DFN. Lateral rhinotomy: a neglected operation. Ann Otol Rhinol Laryngol 1977;86(6 Pt 1):756–759
204. Denker A. Die operative behandlung der malignen tumoren der nase. Arch Laryngol Rhinol 1909;21:1–14
205. Langenbeck B. Beitrage zur osteoplastik. Deutsche Klinik 1859;ii:471–476
206. Voelckers C. Ein fall von osteoplastischer resection des oberkiefers. Arch Klin Chir 1863;iv:603–607
207. Hanner WD. Treatment of malignant disease in the upper jaw. Lancet 1935;i:129–133
208. Woodman EM. Malignant disease of the nasal accessory sinuses. J Laryngol Otol 1922;37:287–295
209. New GB. The use of heat and radium in the treatment of cancer of the jaw and cheeks. JAMA 1918;71:1369–1371
210. Woodman EM. Malignant disease ofthe upper jaw. Br J Surg 1923;II:153–171
211. Woodman EM. Plastic repair after operations on the upper jaw. Proc R Soc Med 1931;24(4):435–438
212. Horsley V. On the technique of operations on the nervous system. BMJ 1906;2:411
213. Giordano D. Compendio di chirurgia operatorio italiana. Turin: Unione Tipografico-Editrice Torinese; 1897:100
214. Schloffer H. Zur frage der operation en an der hypophyse. Beitr Klin Chir 1906;50:767
215. Cushing H. The hypophysis cerebri clinical aspects of hyperpituitarism and of hyopituitarism. JAMA 1909;LII(4):249–255
216. Dandy WE. Orbital Tumour: Results Following The Transcranial Operative Attack. New York: Oskar Piest; 1941: 168
217. Smith RR, Klopp CT, Williams JM. Surgical treatment of cancer of the frontal sinus and adjacent areas. Cancer 1954;7(5):991–994
218. Ketcham AS, Wilkins RH, Vanburen JM, Smith RR. A combined intracranial facial approach to the paranasal sinuses. Am J Surg 1963;106:698–703
219. Ketcham AS, Hoye RC, Van Buren JM, Johnson RH, Smith RR. Complications of intracranial facial resection for tumors of the paranasal sinuses. Am J Surg 1966;112(4):591–596
220. Ketcham AS, Chretien PB, Van Buren JM, Hoye RC, Beazley RM, Herdt JR. The ethmoid sinuses: a re-evaluation of surgical resection. Am J Surg 1973;126(4):469–476
221. Millar HS, Petty PG, Wilson WF, Hueston JT. A combined intracranial and facial approach for excision and repair of cancer of the ethmoid sinuses. Aust N Z J Surg 1973;43(2):179–183
222. Clifford P. Transcranial approach for cancer of the antroethmoidal area. Clin Otolaryngol Allied Sci 1977; 2(2):115–130
223. Schramm VL Jr, Myers EN, Maroon JC. Anterior skull base surgery for benign and malignant disease. Laryngoscope 1979;89(7 Pt 1):1077–1091
224. Terz JJ, Young HF, Lawrence W Jr. Combined craniofacial resection for locally advanced carcinoma of the head and neck I. Tumors of the skin and soft tissues. Am J Surg 1980;140(5):613–617
225. Sisson GA, Bytell DE, Becker SP, Ruge D. Carcinoma of the paranasal sinuses and craniofacial resection. J Laryngol Otol 1976;1:59–68
226. Harrison DFN. The management of malignant tumours affecting the maxillary and ethmoidal sinuses. J Laryngol Otol 1973;87(8):749–772
227. Cheesman AD, Lund VJ, Howard DJ. Craniofacial resection for tumors of the nasal cavity and paranasal sinuses. Head Neck Surg 1986;8(6):429–435
228. Tessier P, Guiot G, Rougerie J, Delbet JP, Pastoriza J. Cranio-naso-orbito-facial osteotomies. Hypertelorism. [Article in French] Ann Chir Plast 1967;12(2):103–118

229. Raveh J, Laedrach K, Speiser M, et al. The subcranial approach for fronto-orbital and anteroposterior skull-base tumors. Arch Otolaryngol Head Neck Surg 1993;119(4):385–393

230. Fisch U, Pillsbury HC. Infratemporal fossa approach to lesions in the temporal bone and base of the skull. Arch Otolaryngol 1979;105(2):99–107

231. Sekhar LN, Schramm VL Jr, Jones NF. Subtemporal-preauricular infratemporal fossa approach to large lateral and posterior cranial base neoplasms. J Neurosurg 1987;67(4):488–499

232. Cocke EW Jr, Robertson JH, Robertson JT, Crook JP Jr. The extended maxillotomy and subtotal maxillectomy for excision of skull base tumors. Arch Otolaryngol Head Neck Surg 1990;116(1):92–104

233. Derome PJ. Surgical management of tumours invading the skull base. Can J Neurol Sci 1985;12(4):345–347

234. Donald P. Craniofacial surgical resection: new frontiers in advanced head & neck cancer. ANZ J Surg 1989;59:523–528

235. Jackson IT, Laws ER Jr, Martin RD. A craniofacial approach to advanced recurrent cancer of the central face. Head Neck Surg 1983;5(6):474–488

236. Janecka IP. Classification of facial translocation approach to the skull base. Otolaryngol Head Neck Surg 1995;112(4):579–585

237. Maniglia AJ, Phillips DA. Midfacial degloving for the management of nasal, sinus, and skull-base neoplasms. Otolaryngol Clin North Am 1995;28(6):1127–1143

238. Heermann H. Endonasal surgery with the use of the binocular Zeiss operating microscope. Arch Klin Exp Ohren Nasen Kehlkopfheilkd 1958;171:295–297

239. Heerman J. Endonasal microsurgery of the maxillary sinus. Laryngol-Rhino-Otol 1974;53:938–942

240. Draf W. Surgical treatment of the inflammatory diseases of the paranasal sinuses. Indication, surgical technique, risks, mismanagement and complications, revision surgery. [Article in German] Arch Otorhinolaryngol 1982;235(1):133–305

241. Draf W. Practical references for surgery of inflammatory paranasal sinus diseases and postoperative complications. [Article in German] Arch Otorhinolaryngol 1982;235(2–3):367–377

242. Messerklinger W. Endoscopy of the Nose. Lippincott Williams and Wilkins; 1977:187

243. Wigand M. Endoscopic Surgery of the Paranasal Sinuses and Anterior Skull Base. Stuttgart: Thieme; 1990:152

244. Stammberger H. Functional Endoscopic Sinus Surgery: The Messerklinger Technique. Mosby; 1991: 552

245. Kennedy DW, Zinreich SJ, Rosenbaum AE, Johns ME. Functional endoscopic sinus surgery. Theory and diagnostic evaluation. Arch Otolaryngol 1985;111(9):576–582

246. Lund VJ, Stammberger H, Nicolai P, et al; European Rhinologic Society Advisory Board on Endoscopic Techniques in the Management of Nose, Paranasal Sinus and Skull Base Tumours. European position paper on endoscopic management of tumours of the nose, paranasal sinuses and skull base. Rhinol Suppl 2010;22(22):1–143

247. May M, Hoffmann DF, Sobol SM. Video endoscopic sinus surgery: a two-handed technique. Laryngoscope 1990;100(4):430–432

248. Briner HR, Simmen D, Jones N. Endoscopic sinus surgery: advantages of the bimanual technique. Am J Rhinol 2005;19(3):269–273

249. Kassam AB, Gardner P, Snyderman C, Mintz A, Carrau R. Expanded endonasal approach: fully endoscopic, completely transnasal approach to the middle third of the clivus, petrous bone, middle cranial fossa and infratemporal fossa. Neurosurg Focus 2005;19(1):E6

250. Castelnuovo P, Locatelli D, Mauri S, De Bernadis F. Extended endoscopic approacjhes to the skull base, anterior cranial base CSF leaks. In: de Divitiis E, Cappabianca P, eds. Endoscopic Endonasal Trans-Sphenoidal Surgery. New York: Springer Vienna; 2003:137–138

Section IA Nose and Paranasal Sinuses

3 Surgical Anatomy

The complex anatomy of the nose, the paranasal sinuses, and the adjacent nasopharynx and intracranial and intraorbital structures has been explored in considerable detail from the seminal works of Johannes Lang and Heinz Stammberger in several recent publications[1-8] and it seems inappropriate to reinvent the wheel. However, an intimate knowledge of the anatomy (and physiology) of the area is a prerequisite to understanding the natural history of tumor pathology and its treatment.

Intrinsic areas of weakness exist throughout the area (**Fig. 3.1**). The lamina papyracea is well named and may be dehiscent in the young and old, though the orbital periosteum is fortunately resistant (**Figs. 3.2 and 3.3**). Unfortunately, even when the orbital periosteum resists tumor spread, disease can run extraperiosteally to the apex and thence into the middle cranial fossa. The superior and inferior orbital fissures also offer routes of tumor exit and entry. The inferior fissure communicates with the pterygopalatine fossa medially and the infratemporal fossa laterally while the superior fissure leads to the cavernous sinus.

Similarly, the dura is relatively robust even when tumor infiltrates the bone of the skull base. Areas of vulnerability are found, however, in the cribriform plate with the many fenestrations for the olfactory fibrils connecting to the bulbs and tracts, together with dural prolongations and emissary veins to the sagittal sinus. The length and depth of the cribriform niche varies considerably (length

15.5 to 25.8 mm; depth 0 to 15.5 mm). The roof of the ethmoids is largely composed of hard frontal bone (**Fig. 3.4**) but the lateral lamina of the cribriform plate is effectively an extension of the vertical attachment of the middle turbinate, the depth of which has been divided into three using the Keros-Kainz classification. As this bone is very thin, it represents an easy route into the anterior cranial fossa. This situation is further compounded by the route and foramina of the anterior and posterior ethmoidal neurovascular bundles offering access to the orbit. The anterior ethmoidal artery is most vulnerable, usually running across the anterior skull base posterior to a suprabullar cell, often in a mesentery of mucosa or in a dehiscent bony canal. The posterior ethmoidal artery is generally more protected, running within the bone of the roof.

The sphenoid has important relationships with the optic nerve, carotid artery, and pituitary (**Fig. 3.5**). These structures vary in their prominence in the sinus walls and in the thickness of bony covering, which is dependent on the shape of the sinus cavity and its degree of pneumatization. The cavernous sinus also lies laterally and the foramen rotundum (V2) and pterygoid canal may impinge on the sinus cavity, especially if well pneumatized. The intersinus septum is often asymmetric and can attach to the lateral wall in the region of the carotid. Posterior to the jugum of the sphenoid, lies the optic chiasm (mean distance 21 mm).[2] In 5 to 12% of the population,

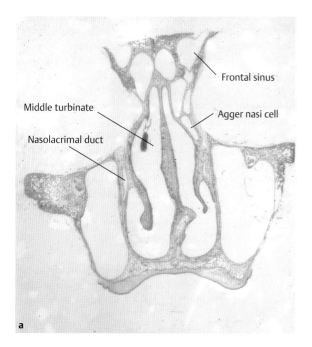

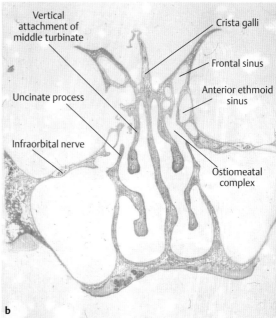

Fig. 3.1a–e Coronal sections through a midfacial block; hematoxylin and eosin. Anterior to posterior.

Fig. 3.1c–e ▷

◁ continued

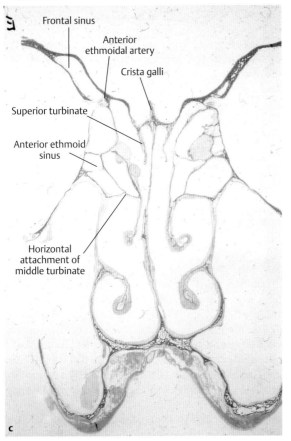

Frontal sinus

Anterior ethmoidal artery

Crista galli

Superior turbinate

Anterior ethmoid sinus

Horizontal attachment of middle turbinate

c

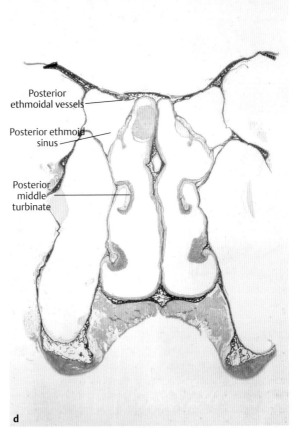

Posterior ethmoidal vessels

Posterior ethmoid sinus

Posterior middle turbinate

d

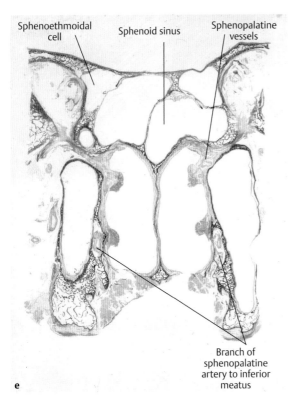

Sphenoethmoidal cell

Sphenoid sinus

Sphenopalatine vessels

Branch of sphenopalatine artery to inferior meatus

e

the posterior ethmoids may extend superiorly and laterally to the sphenoid, forming a sphenoethmoidal cell. The optic nerve and carotid artery are usually found in the lateral wall of these cells when present, rendering these structures at risk from disease and surgery.

The maxillary sinus also has areas of potential weakness, notably the medial wall through the maxillary hiatus, which in life is closed by the inferior turbinate, uncinate process, and bulla of the ethmoid, lacrimal, and perpendicular plate of the palatine (**Figs. 3.6, 3.7, 3.8, 3.9, 3.10, 3.11**). However, areas without bone such as the natural ostium, anterior and posterior fontanelles, and accessory ostia are easily breached by disease. In the sinus roof, in the infraorbital canal and foramen, and in the floor the dental roots provide access to the orbit, cheek, and oral cavity.

Attached to the posterior wall of the maxilla are the pterygoid plates, which are part of the sphenoid. The space between the plates and the sinus is the pterygomaxillary fissure, through which the maxillary artery runs. This in turn connects with the pterygopalatine fossa and the infratemporal fossa. This is an area in which angiofibromas typically arise. The pterygopalatine fossa is divided into a neural component composed of pterygopalatine ganglion and maxillary nerve and a vascular

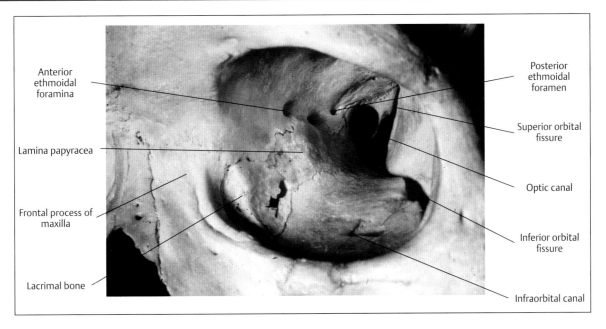

Anterior ethmoidal foramina

Lamina papyracea

Frontal process of maxilla

Lacrimal bone

Posterior ethmoidal foramen

Superior orbital fissure

Optic canal

Inferior orbital fissure

Infraorbital canal

Fig. 3.2 Photograph of a left orbit.

component containing the terminal part of the maxillary artery and its branches. The infratemporal fossa lies beneath the skull base between the side wall of the pharynx and ascending ramus of the mandible. It contains the pterygoid muscles, branches of the mandibular nerve, the maxillary artery, and the pterygoid venous plexus in the lateral pterygoid muscle. While the bone of the posterior wall of the maxillary sinus is strong, once it invaded by a malignant tumor such as a squamous cell carcinoma, the excellent blood supply of these areas rapidly facilitates tumor spread and therefore has a significant detrimental effect on prognosis.

The frontal sinus is unique in size and shape to each individual once developed and may be absent in ~1% of a white population. As it arises embryologically from the anterior ethmoids, (**Fig. 3.12**) it has a complex anatomy with asymmetric septations and a range of cellular pneumatization that has been the subject of many classifications (Kuhn). The drainage into the middle meatus is also variable, more like an hourglass than a "duct" and is referred to as the frontonasal recess. However, this is influenced by the configuration of the agger nasi and suprabullar cells. Given the complexity of these clefts and the capacity for retrograde mucociliary flow back into the sinus, it is perhaps surprising that the frontal sinus is so rarely a primary site of neoplasia.

Nasal Septum

The nasal septum is composed of a small membranous area, the quadrilateral and vomeronasal cartilages with a contributions from the upper and lower lateral cartilages and bone, including the perpendicular plate of the ethmoid, vomer, and crests of the maxilla and palatine (**Figs. 3.3, 3.6, 3.9, 3.13**). Primary tumors of the septum are rare, but it is one of the commoner sites of origin for chondrosarcoma, which can spread covertly into the skull base and/or palate. Anteroinferiorly the upper lip and gingivobuccal sulcus can also be affected.

External Nose

Tumors arising within the nasal cavity and vestibule or on the columella may readily spread into the bone and cartilaginous superstructure and can involve the subcutaneous tissues and skin. The nasal bones are united as a pair in the midline (**Fig. 3.14**) and are supported by the nasal spine of the frontal and perpendicular plate of the ethmoid. They have attachments to the frontal bone superiorly at the nasofrontal suture and with the frontal process of the maxillary bone on either side at the nasolacrimal suture. The bones themselves may be eroded, with a mass appearing at the glabella as can occur with adenocarcinoma. Inferiorly they form the pyriform aperture together with the maxillary bones, intersected by the quadrilateral septal cartilage.

In addition, upper and lower nasal cartilages form the malleable part of the lower external nose. The upper lateral cartilages lie inferior to and are overlapped by the nasal bones, the frontal processes of the maxillae, and the lower lateral cartilages in 72% of cases.[1] They are continuous medially with the septal cartilage. The lower lateral cartilages are composed of a medial and lateral crus. The medial crura contribute to the columella which lies in front of the septal cartilage. These cartilages and the

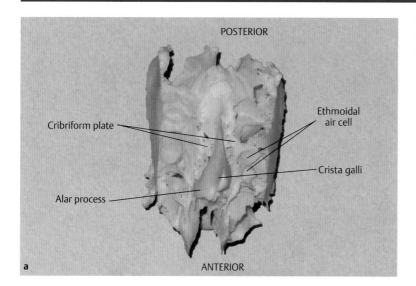

Fig. 3.3a–e Photographs of a disarticulated ethmoid bone.

a Superior view.

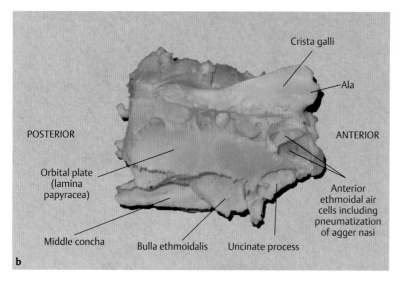

b Lateral view.

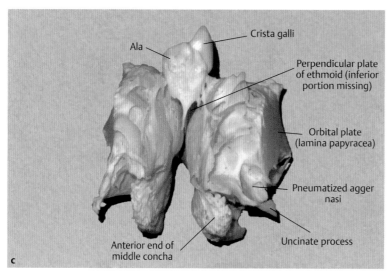

c Anterior view.

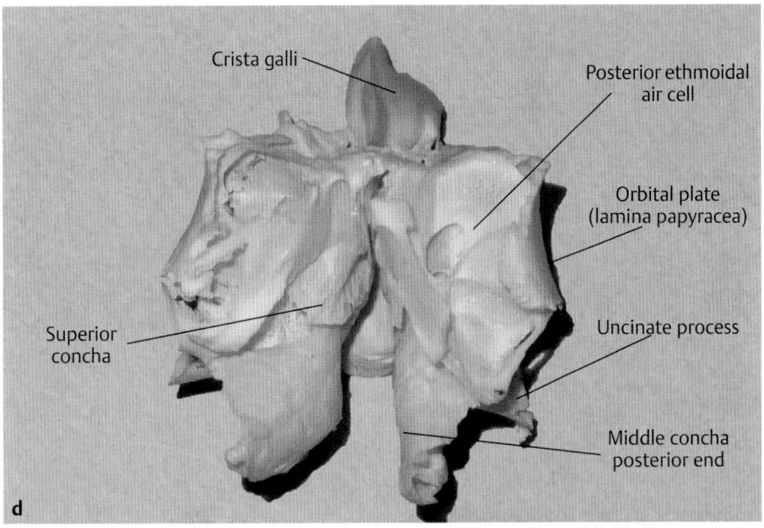
Crista galli
Posterior ethmoidal air cell
Orbital plate (lamina papyracea)
Superior concha
Uncinate process
Middle concha posterior end
d

◁ continued

d Posterior view.

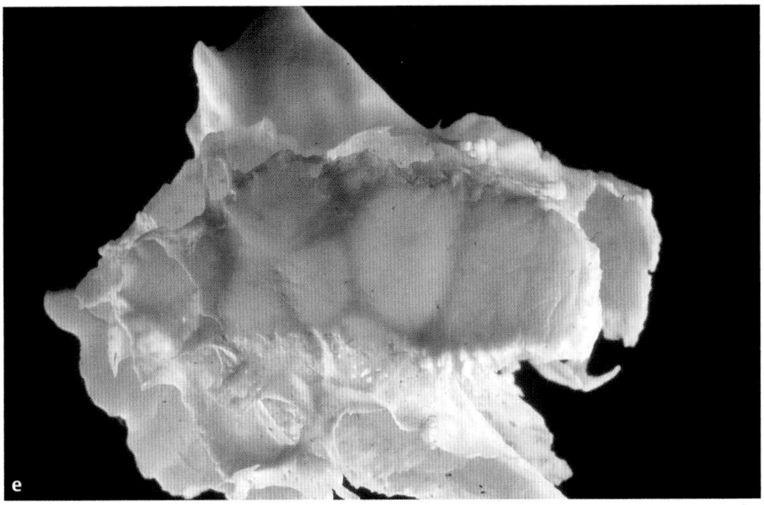
e

e Lateral view backlit to show lamina papyracea.

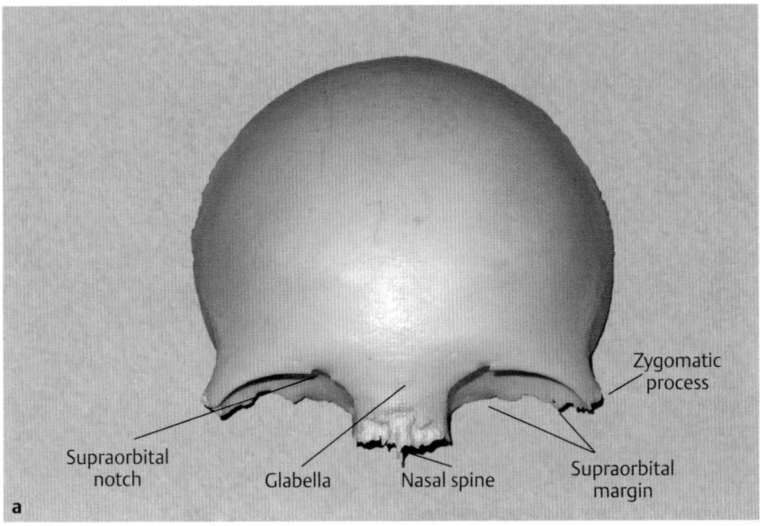
Zygomatic process
Supraorbital notch
Glabella
Nasal spine
Supraorbital margin
a

Fig. 3.4a, b Photographs of a disarticulated frontal bone.

a Anterior view.

Fig. 3.4b ▷

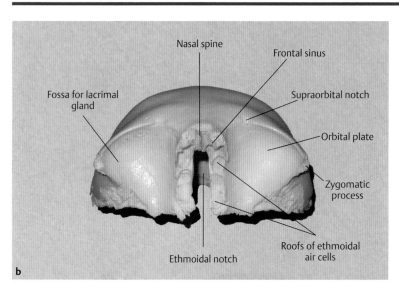

◁ continued

b Inferior view.

Nasal spine

Frontal sinus

Fossa for lacrimal gland

Supraorbital notch

Orbital plate

Zygomatic process

Roofs of ethmoidal air cells

Ethmoidal notch

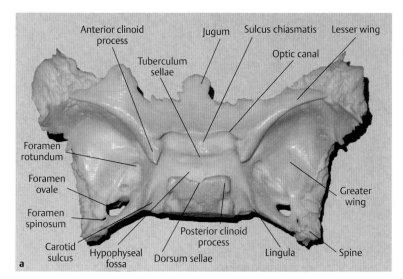

Fig. 3.5a–c Photographs of a disarticulated sphenoid bone.

a Superior view.

Anterior clinoid process

Jugum

Sulcus chiasmatis

Lesser wing

Tuberculum sellae

Optic canal

Foramen rotundum

Foramen ovale

Foramen spinosum

Greater wing

Posterior clinoid process

Carotid sulcus

Hypophyseal fossa

Dorsum sellae

Lingula

Spine

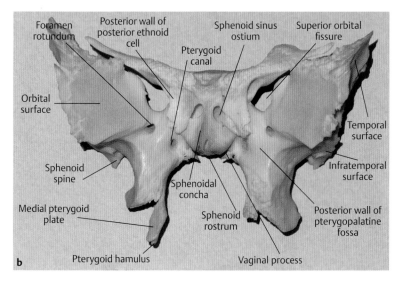

b Anterior view.

Foramen rotundum

Posterior wall of posterior ethnoid cell

Sphenoid sinus ostium

Superior orbital fissure

Pterygoid canal

Orbital surface

Temporal surface

Sphenoid spine

Infratemporal surface

Medial pterygoid plate

Sphenoidal concha

Sphenoid rostrum

Posterior wall of pterygopalatine fossa

Pterygoid hamulus

Vaginal process

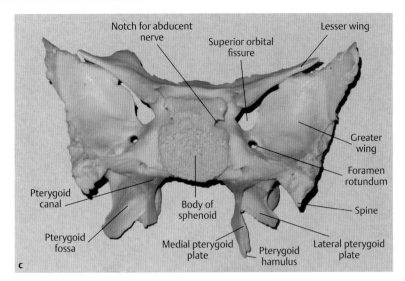

◁ continued

c Posterior view.

Notch for abducent nerve
Superior orbital fissure
Lesser wing
Greater wing
Foramen rotundum
Spine
Pterygoid canal
Body of sphenoid
Pterygoid fossa
Medial pterygoid plate
Pterygoid hamulus
Lateral pterygoid plate

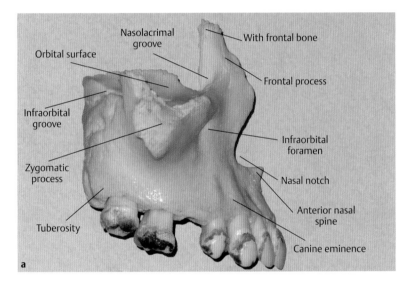

Fig. 3.6a–c Photographs of a disarticulated right maxillary bone.

a Lateral view.

Nasolacrimal groove
With frontal bone
Orbital surface
Frontal process
Infraorbital groove
Infraorbital foramen
Zygomatic process
Nasal notch
Anterior nasal spine
Tuberosity
Canine eminence

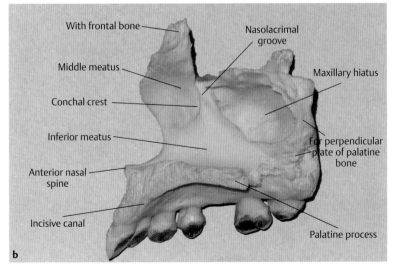

b Medial view.

With frontal bone
Nasolacrimal groove
Middle meatus
Maxillary hiatus
Conchal crest
Inferior meatus
For perpendicular plate of palatine bone
Anterior nasal spine
Incisive canal
Palatine process

Fig. 3.6c ▷

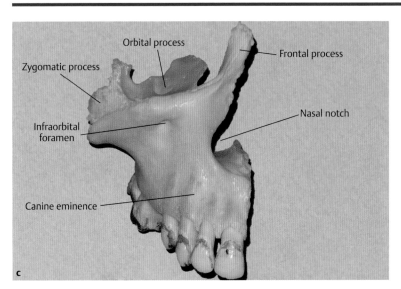

◁ continued

c Anterior view.

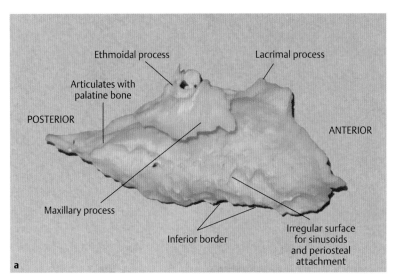

Fig. 3.7a, b Photographs of a disarticulated right turbinate bone.

a Lateral view.

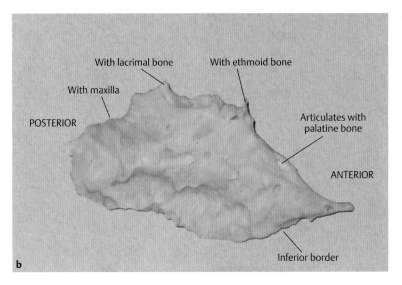

b Medial view.

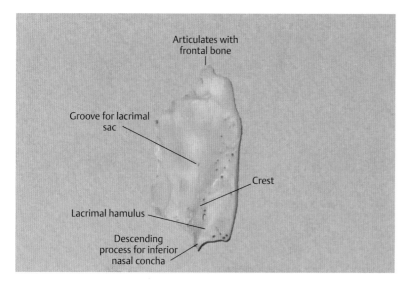

Fig. 3.8 Photograph of a disarticulated left lacrimal bone.

Articulates with frontal bone

Groove for lacrimal sac

Crest

Lacrimal hamulus

Descending process for inferior nasal concha

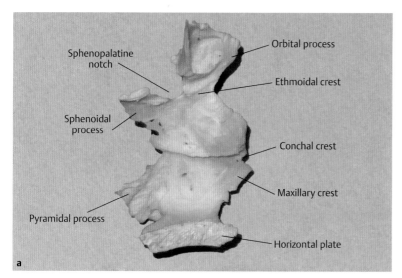

Fig. 3.9a, b Photographs of a disarticulated left palatine bone.

a Medial view.

Sphenopalatine notch

Orbital process

Ethmoidal crest

Sphenoidal process

Conchal crest

Maxillary crest

Pyramidal process

Horizontal plate

a

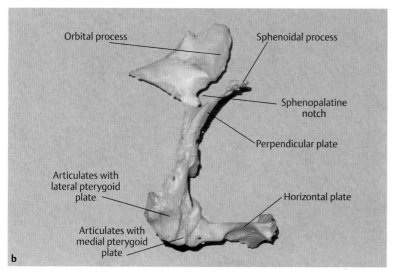

b Posterior view.

Orbital process

Sphenoidal process

Sphenopalatine notch

Perpendicular plate

Articulates with lateral pterygoid plate

Horizontal plate

Articulates with medial pterygoid plate

b

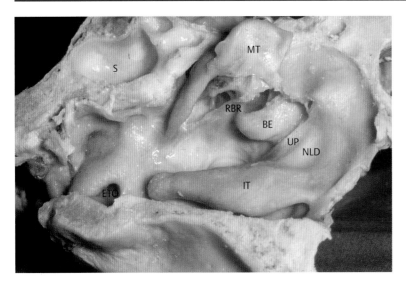

Fig. 3.10 Lateral wall of nose: cadaver specimen with middle turbinate lifted to show middle meatus. BE, bulla ethmoidalis; ETO, eustachian tube orifice; IT, inferior turbinate; MT, middle turbinate; NLD, nasolacrimal duct; RBR, retrobullar recess; S, sphenoid; UP, uncinate process.

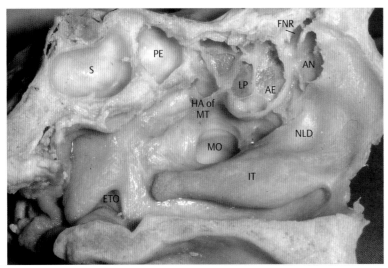

Fig. 3.11 Lateral wall of nose: cadaver specimen with dissection to show structures of lateral wall: AE, anterior ethmoid; AN, agger nasi; ETO, eustachian tube orifice; FNR, frontonasal recess; HA of MT, horizontal attachment of middle turbinate duct; IT, inferior turbinate; LP, lamina papyracea; MO, maxillary ostium; NLD, nasolacrimal; PE, posterior ethmoids; S, sphenoid.

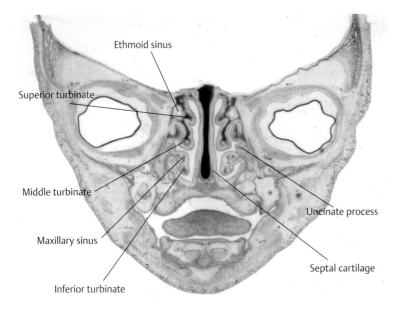

Fig. 3.12 Coronal section through a 24-week fetus (hematoxylin and eosin).

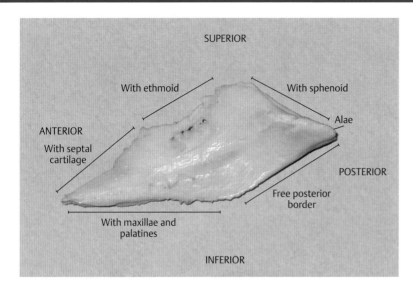

Fig. 3.13 Photograph of a disarticulated vomer.

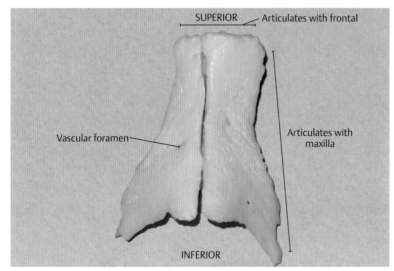

Fig. 3.14 Photograph of disarticulated nasal bones.

fibrous tissue that connects them present little resistance to tumor spread, though this is fortunately rare in the anterior nasal cavity. However, tumors that arise on the anterior septum and columella are able to spread bilaterally to the cervical lymphatics and therefore have a particularly poor prognosis.

Paranasal Sinuses

Histology

The lining of the nose and paranasal sinuses may be grossly divided into skin anteriorly, olfactory epithelium superiorly, and ciliated columnar respiratory epithelium elsewhere. In addition there may be areas of squamous metaplasia on the anterior ends of the inferior and middle turbinate, reflecting areas of aerodynamic "trauma."

Blood Supply

The blood supply of the nose and sinuses is grossly derived from the external and internal carotid with considerable overlap and crossover between the right and left sides. The sphenopalatine, greater palatine, facial, and superior labial branches supply the majority of the nasal cavity with a contribution superiorly from internal carotid via the anterior and posterior ethmoidal arteries. Sinusoids on the inferior turbinate and adjacent anterior septum (anterior septal tubercle [**Fig. 3.15**]), under autonomic control, regulate airflow. The blood supply of the septum has become more appreciated of late due to the frequent use of the Haddad nasoseptal flap based on the branches of the sphenopalatine artery in reconstruction of the larger posterior skull base defects.[9]

The cavernous venous system drains into the facial veins anteriorly, into the pterygoid plexus posteriorly,

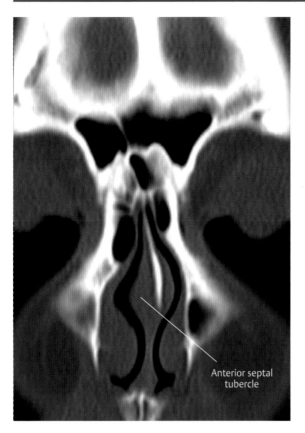

Anterior septal
tubercle

Fig. 3.15 Coronal CT scan through the anterior nasal septum, showing the anterior septal tubercle.

and superiorly has connections with the superior ophthalmic veins and superior sagittal sinus. These pathways may in part be responsible for the pattern of local spread for tumors such as olfactory neuroblastoma, which may appear in the contralateral eye or anywhere on the dura.

The maxillary sinus receives its blood supply via branches of the facial, maxillary, infraorbital, and greater palatine arteries with venous drainage to the anterior facial vein and pterygoid plexus. Once this area is infiltrated by malignancy, such as a squamous cell carcinoma, complete surgical excision is difficult. The frontal sinuses are supplied by the supraorbital and anterior ethmoidal arteries with venous connections through the diploic veins into the sagittal and sphenoparietal sinuses and also with the superior ophthalmic veins. The sphenoid sinuses are supplied by the posterior ethmoidal vessels and nerves.

Nerve Supply

The nerves may also provide routes of tumor spread, as graphically demonstrated by adenoid cystic carcinoma, whose capacity for perineural spread either directly or embolically, severely compromises attempts at curative resection. The maxillary division of the trigeminal nerve supplies the majority of the septum via the nasopalatine nerves with a contribution from the anterior superior alveolar and anterior ethmoidal branch of the nasociliary nerve anteriorly. The posteroinferior septum also receives a small supply from the nerve of the pterygoid canal and the posterior inferior nasal branch of the anterior palatine nerve. On the lateral wall again the majority is supplied by branches of the maxillary and pterygopalatine ganglion, with anterior contributions from the anterior superior alveolar, anterior ethmoidal, and infraorbital nerves. Superiorly, olfactory epithelium extends down from the olfactory niche onto the superior turbinate and septum. The extent varies between individuals and diminishes with age. Some evidence of olfactory epithelium has been reported on the medial middle turbinate, but this does not appear to be functional.

The sinuses receive their nerve supply via the supraorbital nerve (frontal), posterior ethmoidal and pterygopalatine ganglion (sphenoid), and maxillary division of the trigeminal, which supplies sensation to the maxillary sinus via the infraorbital, superior alveolar, and greater palatine nerves, all of which may act as conduits for tumor spread.

Lymphatic Drainage

Fortunately the lymphatic drainage from the sinuses is relatively poor to the retropharyngeal and jugulodigastric nodes and to the pterygopalatine fossa, but this is not true of the nasal vestibule, anterior septum, and columella, from where bilateral cervical spread can occur to the submandibular region.

References

1. Lang J. Clinical Anatomy of the Nose, Nasal Cavity and Paranasal Sinuses. Stuttgart, New York: Thieme; 1989
2. Stammberger H. Functional Endoscopic Sinus Surgery. Philadelphia: BC Decker; 1991:49–88
3. Wormald P-J. Endoscopic Sinus Surgery. Anatomy, Three-Dimensional Reconstruction and Surgical Technique. 2nd ed. New York, Stuttgart: Thieme; 2007
4. Stammberger H, Lund V. Anatomy of the nose and paranasal sinuses. In: Gleeson M et al, eds. Scott-Brown's Otorhinolaryngology, Head and Neck Surgery. 7th ed. Chicago: Hodder Arnold; 2008:1315–1343
5. Wigand M. In: Endoscopic Surgery of the Paranasal Sinuses and Anterior Skull Base. 2nd ed. Stuttgart, New York: Thieme; 2008:22–67
6. Castelnuovo P, Palma P. Anatomy of the Nose, Paranasal Sinuses and Anterior Skull Base: A Colour Atlas for Surgeons. Berlin, Heidelberg: Springer Verlag; 2012
7. Casiano R. Endoscopic Sinonasal Dissection Guide. New York, Stuttgart: Thieme; 2011
8. Stamm AC. Transnasal Endoscopic Skull Base and Brain Surgery. New York, Stuttgart: Thieme; 2011:3–47
9. Hadad G, Bassagasteguy L, Carrau RL, et al. A novel reconstructive technique after endoscopic expanded endonasal approaches: vascular pedicle nasoseptal flap. Laryngoscope 2006;116(10):1882–1886

4 Diagnostic Strategy

Presentation

While the clinical features of each specific pathology are covered in their respective chapters, a few general observations may be made. The principal problem in the diagnosis of sinonasal tumors, both benign and malignant, has been related to late presentation. Patients develop relatively innocuous symptoms, often unilateral, that are ignored by both patient and primary care physician. Unlike hoarseness or dysphagia, which are recognized as of potential significance, nasal obstruction, discharge, even serosanguinous discharge, and reduced sense of smell are common complaints more often associated with allergy, inflammation, or infection than with a tumor. With hindsight the unilateral nature and usually spontaneous onset should elicit concern, but in the case of malignancy it is more often the spread beyond the sinonasal confines to the cheek, eye, or upper alveolus that leads to diagnosis. Fortunately, with malignancy neck disease remains relatively rare, as does systemic disease with a few notable exceptions (**Table 4.1**).

Local Disease

A mass in the nasal cavity will produce unilateral nasal obstruction, discharge that is often bloodstained, a reduction in the sense of smell, and occasionally facial discomfort.[1] Frank epistaxis is less common than might be supposed, although it typically occurs with vascular lesions such as juvenile angiofibroma, olfactory neuroblastoma, and malignant melanoma.

Tumors that arise in or involve the ethmoidal labyrinths obviously affect the nasal cavity at an early stage and may spread across the midline, for example, adenocarcinomas, but more often present with orbital symptoms due to early erosion of the lamina papyracea. These include proptosis, a sign that is almost always due to a mass either within or outside the orbit. The direction and degree of displacement will depend on the position of the mass and its speed of growth. This in turn may be associated with diplopia if displacement occurs quickly but may be absent if the change in position takes place slowly. Similarly, the optic nerve and its blood supply can tolerate impressive stretching if it occurs slowly, but vision may be lost rapidly when additional inflammation or infiltration is present. Diplopia may also occur as a consequence of direct muscle infiltration or involvement of the neural supply, especially in the cavernous sinus. Once at the orbital apex, whether extra- or intraperiosteal, the disease can spread into the middle cranial fossa. Tumors that invade or arise within the skull base may directly affect the optic nerve(s) and chiasm. This can occur with meningioma and chondrosarcoma and may tragically be

bilateral. Visual loss can also result from chemosis due to corneal exposure, keratosis, and ulceration.

The incidence of orbital invasion by sinonasal malignancies will vary with the histology, but overall visual symptoms occurred in 50% of a cohort of 220 cases.[1] This rose to 62% if the tumor arose in the ethmoid, compared with 46% with malignant tumors of the nasal cavity. However, it should be noted that the orbital periosteum, unlike the lamina papyracea, is relatively resistant to penetration by malignant tumors, so the presence of orbital symptoms does not indicate intraperiosteal spread per se, nor does the lack of orbital symptoms and signs necessarily mean that the eye has not been infiltrated. A recognition of this led to a change in strategy for the management of the orbit in the 1980s.[2] It has been estimated that between 66% and 82% of patients with ethmoidal malignancy have erosion of the lamina, whereas the periosteum is involved in 30 to 50%.[3-6]

Epiphora due to nasolacrimal involvement is quite often encountered with anterior ethmoidal and maxillary lesions as a result of secondary compression or distortion of the system.

Superior extension of the tumor into the anterior cranial cavity can occur through the lateral lamella of the cribriform plate, along the anterior and posterior neurovascular bundles, or directly through the fovea, but this is generally asymptomatic. Classically this occurs with olfactory neuroblastoma. CSF leakage and meningitis are exceptionally rare and even when the dura has been breached and extensive frontal lobe infiltration occurs, any personality changes are usually too subtle to be noticed. Occasionally patients with direct involvement of the olfactory bulbs and tracts may develop reduction or distortion of the sense of smell, for example, in frontal meningioma, although this rarely attracts much attention.

Tumors arising within the anterior ethmoids/middle meatus can spread into the maxillary sinus and/or into the frontal sinus via the frontal recess, occasionally producing a mucocele, although this is a rare phenomenon in the presence of a malignant tumor. We have had three patients with sinonasal malignancies who have presented in this way (0.3%). It is not known why the frontal and sphenoid sinuses are rarely the site of primary malignant tumors and are more often involved by local spread or involvement from the surrounding bone. A frontal sinus tumor is most likely to present with swelling of the forehead, whereas sphenoid tumors produce orbital symptoms, in particular visual loss.

Malignancy of the maxillary sinus will spread medially into the nasal cavity, producing obstruction and serosanguinous discharge, as before, but may also spread superiorly, particularly into the infraorbital canal,[7]

Table 4.1 Clinical features arising from sinonasal tumors

Primary symptoms	
Nasal cavity	• Nasal blockage • Serosanguinous discharge • Hyposmia
• Inferiorly into palate	• Mass
• Anterosuperiorly into the nasal bone	• Glabellar mass
• Externally into skin	• Mass/ulceration
• Superiorly into anterior cranial fossa	• Minimal—subtle personality change • Headache
• Posteriorly into nasopharynx and eustachian orifice	• Middle ear effusion
Ethmoid sinuses	
• Medially into nasal cavity	• As above, can cross to contralateral side to produce bilateral symptoms
• Inferolaterally into maxilla	• Facial pressure due to mucus retention
• Medially into orbit	• Proptosis • Diplopia • Visual loss • Chemosis • Epiphora
• Superiorly into the anterior cranial fossa	• Minimal—subtle personality change
Maxillary sinus	
• Medially into nasal cavity	• As above
• Anteriorly into cheek directly or via infraorbital canal	• Mass or ulceration of skin • Paresthesia
• Posteriorly into pterygoid region and infratemporal fossae	• Trismus and pain
• Inferiorly into the palate or alveolar ridge	• Mass • Loosening of the teeth • Malignant oroantral fistula
• Superiorly into orbit	• As above
Secondary symptoms	
Lymphatic	• Cervical lymphadenopathy in levels I & II and facial
Systemic	• Bone pain • Dyspnea • Liver pain • Skin nodules • Localizing neurologic symptoms & signs • General malaise • Confusion

producing paresthesia of the cheek as well as orbital symptoms. Direct anterior spread through bone or via the infraorbital foramen may produce a mass in the cheek, which in turn may ulcerate. Inferior spread from the maxilla produces a mass in the oral cavity, loosening of teeth, and/or a malignant oroantral fistula. Posterior spread into the pterygoid region and infratemporal fossa is associated with trismus and pain.

Metastatic Disease

Although it is mandatory to examine the neck, fewer than 10% of epithelial malignancies present with cervical disease, reflecting the paucity of lymphatic drainage from the sinuses. This is more often a concern with tumors of the nose and some of the lymphomas and sarcomas. The submandibular, jugulodigastric, prefacial and postfacial nodes are most commonly involved by tumors from the septum and in particular the columellar region; these sometimes spread bilaterally, which is invariably associated with a poor prognosis. However, careful examination may reveal more cervical disease than had hitherto been suspected, as with olfactory neuroblastoma, and the possibility of locoregional spread should always be considered during follow-up even in unusual locations such as the cheek.[8]

Systemic metastases are generally uncommon but may occur with longer follow-up and in the presence of uncontrolled local disease. Again this is particularly true of olfactory neuroblastoma and also of malignant melanoma. Adenoid cystic carcinoma is also known to spread along perineural lymphatics, either directly or by embolization, often presenting at some distance from the original tumor, although patients can survive for some time with disseminated disease. Patients may be unaware of systemic metastases for some time and it is a matter of debate how aggressively one should seek them out in the case of tumors where the therapeutic options may be limited. Notwithstanding this, particularly at presentation, complaints of an unresolving nonproductive cough, bone pain, or significant fatigue should prompt further investigation as this can have a direct bearing on the management of the primary lesion.

Examination

In addition to a general ENT examination, including careful inspection and palpation of the oral cavity, midface, and neck, the mainstay of diagnosis remains endoscopy of the nasal cavity and nasopharynx. An initial inspection with a 4 mm 0° or 30° scope using the traditional "three passes" technique to adequately consider the inferior, middle, and superior segments of the nose may immediately determine the problem, but specific attention should be paid to the olfactory niche and middle and superior meatuses. Ideally the nasopharynx should also be examined using either a rigid or a flexible endoscope. However, in many cases the associated edema and nasal secretions obscure a good view of the tumor itself. The nose should then be anesthetized/decongested using whatever combination of topical solution is available. In our own service, a preparation containing phenylephrine hydrochloride and lidocaine hydrochloride is applied topically on a short length of ribbon gauze into either side of the nose for 5 minutes, which shrinks the lining and reduces sensation, but even this may not give adequate exposure.

Where there is any element of suspicion, imaging is undertaken (see later) followed by a formal examination and biopsy. In our own practice this is conducted as a day case under general anesthetic combined with local anesthesia/decongestion (usually using Moffatt's solution [1 mL 2% sodium bicarbonate, 2 mL 10% cocaine, 2mL 1:1000 epinephrine[9]]), which ensures that adequate

representative tissue is taken. Of course, this may be done under local anesthesia alone, but one should not succumb to the temptation of a quick "smash and grab" in a busy outpatient clinic. Under endoscopic control it is rarely necessary to use any external open approach that risks transgression of normal tissue planes. Exceptions to this would be a rare lesion in the frontal sinus lateral to the midpoint of the orbit.

Tissue must be subjected to expert histopathology. Diagnosis can usually be reached using formal saline fixation but occasionally fresh tissue may still be required in some lymphoreticular disease.

Histopathology

The sinonasal region is the region with the greatest histological diversity in the body and this is reflected in the WHO classification,[10] which has been largely used in this document (Table 4.2) and our own series (Table 4.3). However, there have been several changes to this classification over the years and sometimes the histopathological classification is at odds with clinical findings. The best example of this is the erroneous inclusion of angiofibroma in the nasopharynx, where it merely presents in common with several other areas but does not actually arise. Our own clinical and imaging studies show that angiofibroma actually originates in the pterygopalatine fossa at the anterior aspect of the pterygoid (vidian) canal and initially erodes the sphenopalatine foramen.

Immunohistochemistry is frequently required, particularly for any small cell or undifferentiated carcinoma. Due to the histological diversity, frozen section can pose some difficulties on initial biopsy, although it has an important role during subsequent resection once the diagnosis has been established.

Other Investigations

Imaging

(See also Chapter 5.)

Fine-detail three-plane computed tomography (coronal, axial and sagittal plane) combined with magnetic resonance imaging provides an accurate demonstration of tumor extent and can sometimes indicate the type of histology.[11] Although together these modalities produced an accuracy of 98% in predicting extent of tumor, the assessment of spread through the orbital periosteum and dura still requires microscopic confirmation. MRI alone is not sufficient as early erosion of the cribriform plate is still best shown on coronal CT.[12,13]

The extent to which imaging beyond the midface and brain is undertaken will be determined by the histology and patient symptoms. It is not routinely undertaken

Table 4.2 Histopathology and ICD-O codes[a] according to WHO classifications of tumors

A Nasal cavity and paranasal sinuses

(1) Malignant epithelial tumors

Squamous cell carcinoma
- Keratinizing squamous cell carcinoma ICD-O 8070/3
- Nonkeratinizing (cylindrical cell, transitional) carcinoma; currently no separate ICD-O code
- Verrucous carcinoma ICD-O 8051/3
- Papillary squamous cell carcinoma ICD-O 8052/3
- Basaloid squamous cell carcinoma ICD-O 8083/3
- Spindle cell carcinoma ICD-O 8074/3
- Adenosquamous carcinoma ICD-O 8560/3
- Acantholytic squamous cell carcinoma ICD-O 8075/3

Lymphoepithelial carcinoma ICD-O 8082/3

Sinonasal undifferentiated carcinoma ICD-O 8020/3

Adenocarcinoma
- Intestinal-type adenocarcinomas ICD-O 8144/3
- Sinonasal nonintestinal-type adenocarcinomas ICD-O 8140/3

Salivary gland-type carcinoma
- Adenoid cystic carcinoma ICD-O 8200/3
- Acinic cell carcinoma ICD-O 8550/3
- Mucoepidermoid carcinoma ICD-O 8430/3
- Epithelial-myoepithelial carcinoma ICD-O 8562/3
- Clear cell carcinoma ICD-O 8310/3
- Myoepithelial carcinoma ICD-O 8982/3
- Carcinoma ex pleomorphic adenoma ICD-O 8941/3

Neuroendocrine tumors
- Typical carcinoid ICD-O 8240/3
- Atypical carcinoid ICD-O 8249/3
- Small cell carcinoma, neuroendocrine type ICD-O 8041/3

(2) Benign epithelial tumors

Sinonasal papillomas
- Inverted papilloma (Schneiderian papilloma, inverted type) ICD-O 8121/1
- Oncocytic papilloma (Schneiderian papilloma, oncocytic type) ICD-O 8121/1
- Exophytic papilloma (Schneiderian papilloma, exophytic type, everted type) ICD-O 8121/1

Respiratory epithelial adenomatoid hamartoma; no ICD-O code

Salivary gland-type adenomas
- Pleomorphic adenoma ICD-O 8940/0
- Myoepithelioma ICD-O 8982/0
- Oncocytoma ICD-O 8290/0

(3) Malignant soft tissue tumors

Fibrosarcoma ICD-O 8810/3

Undifferentiated high grade pleomorphic sarcoma ("MFH") ICD-O 8830/3

Leiomyosarcoma ICD-O 8890/3

Rhabdomyosarcoma ICD-O 8900/3
- Embryonal ICD-O 8910/3
- Alveolar ICD-O 8920/3

Angiosarcoma ICD-O 9120/3

Kaposi's sarcoma ICD-O 9140/3

Malignant peripheral nerve sheath tumor ICD-O 9540/3

Liposarcoma ICD-O 8850/3

Synovial cell sarcoma ICD-O 9040/3

Alveolar soft part sarcoma ICD-O 9581/3

Malignant fibrous histiocytoma ICD-O 8830/3

(4) Borderline and low malignant potential tumors of soft tissue

Desmoid-type fibromatosis ICD-O 8821/1

Inflammatory myofibroblastic tumor ICD-O 8825/1

Glomangiopericytoma (sinonasal-type hemangiopericytoma) ICD-O 9150/1

Extrapleural solitary fibrous tumor IDC-O 8815/1

(5) Benign soft tissue tumors

Myxoma ICD-O 8840/0

Leiomyoma ICD-O 8890/0

Rhabdomyoma ICD-O 8900/0

Hemangioma ICD-O 9120/0

Schwannoma ICD-O 9560/0

Neurofibroma ICD-O 9540/0

Meningioma ICD-O 9530/0

(6) Malignant tumors of bone and cartilage

Chondrosarcoma ICD-O 9220/3

Mesenchymal chondrosarcoma ICD-O 9240/3

Osteosarcoma ICD-O 9180/3

Chordoma ICD-O 9370/3

(7) Benign tumors of bone and cartilage

Fibrous dysplasia; no ICD-O code

Osteoma ICD-O 9180

Osteoid osteoma ICD-O 9191/0

Osteoblastoma ICD-O 9200/0

Osteochondroma (exostosis) ICD-O 9210/0

Chondroma ICD-O 9220/0

Chondroblastoma ICD-O 9230/0

Chondromyxoid fibroma ICD-O 9241/0

Giant cell lesion; no ICD-O code

Giant cell tumor of bone ICD-O 9250/1

Ameloblastoma ICD-O 9310/0

Nasal chondromesenchymal hamartoma; no ICD-O code

(8) Hematolymphoid tumors

Extranodal NK/T cell lymphoma ICD-O 9719/3

Diffuse large B cell lymphoma ICD-O 9680/3

Extramedullary plasmacytoma ICD-O 9734/3

Extramedullary myeloid sarcoma ICD-O 9930/3

Histiocytic sarcoma ICD-O 9755/3

Langerhans cell histiocytosis ICD-O 9751/1

Juvenile xanthogranuloma; no ICD-O code

Rosai–Dorfman disease (sinus histiocytosis with massive lymphadenopathy); no ICD-O code

continued ▷

Table 4.2 Histopathology and ICD-O codes[a] according to WHO classifications of tumors (continued)

(9) Neuroectodermal tumors
Ewing's sarcoma ICD-O 9260/3
Primitive neuroectodermal tumor (PNET) ICD-O 9364/3
Olfactory neuroblastoma (esthesioneuroblastoma) ICD-O 9522/3
Melanotic neuroectodermal tumor of infancy ICD-O 9363/0
Mucosal malignant melanoma ICD-O 8720/3
Heterotopic central nervous system tissue (nasal glioma); no ICD-O code
(10) Germ cell tumors
Immature teratoma ICD-O 9080/3
Teratoma with malignant transformation ICD-O 9084/3
Sinonasal yolk sac tumor (endodermal sinus tumor) ICD-O 9071/3
Sinonasal teratocarcinosarcoma; no ICD-O code
Mature teratoma ICD-O 9080/0
Dermoid cyst ICD-O 9084/0
(11) Secondary tumors
B Nasopharynx
(1) Malignant epithelial tumors
(2) Benign epithelial tumors
(3) Soft tissue neoplasms
Nasopharyngeal angiofibroma[b] ICD-O 9160/0
(4) Hematolymphoid tumors
(5) Tumors of bone and cartilage
(6) Secondary tumors

[a] Whenever available.

[b] Although juvenile angiofibroma is known to arise from the posterior nasal cavity and not the nasopharynx, the WHO classification includes this lesion here.

for all sinonasal malignancy, but poorly differentiated tumors such as sinonasal undifferentiated carcinoma (SNUC), neuroendocrine carcinoma and lymphoreticular lesions require more extensive staging. Similarly adenoid cystic carcinoma, which has a tendency to spread to the lung, requires chest CT.

Ultrasound and Fine Needle Aspiration

Ultrasound of the neck should be offered at presentation and during follow-up to selected patients, if available, in combination with fine needle aspiration, for example, for olfactory neuroblastoma.[14,15] This is widely available but requires specialist expertise in head and neck/sinonasal pathology.[16,17]

Additional Tests

The accuracy and utility of positron emission tomography (PET) remains to be established in the nose and sinuses but may prove of value in staging and revealing recurrence, particularly as it becomes more readily available.[18,19]

A radionuclide bone scan should be considered in individuals where bone metastases are suspected and hematological investigations including bone marrow aspirate may be appropriate in cases of chloroma (leukemic deposits), lymphoma and individuals where bone and liver secondaries are suspected.

Table 4.3 Types of histopathology in our personal cohort of sinonasal neoplasia (*n* = 1506)

Classification	Type of histopathology	n
Epidermoid	• Squamous	320
	• Inverted papilloma	114
	• Other	46
Nonepidermoid	• Adenocarcinoma	117
	• Adenoid cystic	54
	• Other glandular	15
Mesenchymal	• Fibrosarcoma	23
	• Malignant fibrous histiocytoma	6
	• Alveolar soft part sarcoma	5
	• Other	6
Vasoform	• Angiofibroma	155
	• Hemangiopericytoma/glomangiopericytoma	13
	• Vascular malformations/hemangioma	21
	• Angiosarcoma	1
Muscular	• Rhabdomyosarcoma	26
	• Leiomyoma	3
	• Leiomyosarcoma	5
Cartilage	• Chondrosarcoma	42
Bone	• Osteosarcoma	12
	• Osteoma	55
	• Ossifying fibroma	31
	• Fibrous dysplasia	18
	• Other	8
Lymphoreticular	• B cell lymphoma	60
	• NK/T cell lymphoma	33
	• Extramedullary plasmacytoma	13
	• Other	6
Neuroectodermal	• Olfactory neuroblastoma	80
	• Malignant melanoma	115
	• SNUC	24
	• Schwannomas	17
	• Meningioma	11
	• Carcinoid	7
	• PNET/Ewing's sarcoma	6
	• Other	6
Germ cell tumors	• Mature teratoma	1
	• (Dermoids)	7
Odontogenic	• Ameloblastoma	6
	• Ameloblastic fibroma	5
	• Odontogenic keratocyst	3
Metastases		10

Abbreviations: PNET, primitive neuroectodermal tumor; SNUC, sinonasal undifferentiated carcinoma.

References

1. Lund VJ. Malignant tumours of the nasal cavity and paranasal sinuses. ORL J Otorhinolaryngol Relat Spec 1983;45(1):1–12

2. Suárez C, Ferlito A, Lund VJ, et al. Management of the orbit in malignant sinonasal tumors. Head Neck 2008;30(2):242–250

3. Nuñez F, Suarez C, Alvarez I, Losa JL, Barthe P, Fresno M. Sino-nasal adenocarcinoma: epidemiological and clinico-pathological study of 34 cases. J Otolaryngol 1993; 22(2):86–90

4. Suarez C, Llorente JL, Fernandez De Leon R, Maseda E, Lopez A. Prognostic factors in sinonasal tumors involving the anterior skull base. Head Neck 2004;26(2):136–144

5. Ganly I, Patel SG, Singh B, et al. Craniofacial resection for malignant paranasal sinus tumors: Report of an International Collaborative Study. Head Neck 2005;27(7):575–584

6. Iannetti G, Valentini V, Rinna C, Ventucci E, Marianetti TM. Ethmoido-orbital tumors: our experience. J Craniofac Surg 2005;16(6):1085–1091

7. Tiwari R, van der Wal J, van der Waal I, Snow G. Studies of the anatomy and pathology of the orbit in carcinoma of the maxillary sinus and their impact on preservation of the eye in maxillectomy. Head Neck 1998;20(3):193–196

8. Rinaldo A, Ferlito A, Shaha AR, Wei WI, Lund VJ. Esthe-sioneuroblastoma and cervical lymph node metastases: clinical and therapeutic implications. Acta Otolaryngol 2002;122(2):215–221

9. Moffatt A. Postural instillation. A method of inducing local anaesthesia in the nose. J Laryngol Otol 1941;56:429–436

10. Barnes L, Eveson J, Reichart P, Sidransky D. World Health Organization Classification of Tumours. Pathology and Genetics of Head and Neck Tumours. Lyon: IARC Press; 2005

11. Lund VJ, Howard DJ, Lloyd GA, Cheesman AD. Magnetic resonance imaging of paranasal sinus tumours for cranio-facial resection. Head Neck 1989;11(3):279–283

12. Lloyd GAS, Lund VJ, Howard DJ, Savy L. Optimum imaging for sinonasal malignancy. J Laryngol Otol 2000;114(7):557–562

13. Madani G, Beale TJ, Lund VJ. Imaging of sinonasal tumours. Semin Ultrasound CT MR 2009;30(1):25–38

14. Collins BT, Cramer HM, Hearn SA. Fine needle aspiration cytology of metastatic olfactory neuroblastoma. Acta Cytol 1997;41(3):802–810

15. Zanation AM, Ferlito A, Rinaldo A, et al. When, how and why to treat the neck in patients with esthesio-neuroblastoma: a review. Eur Arch Otorhinolaryngol 2010;267(11):1667–1671

16. Robinson IA, Cozens NJ. Does a joint ultrasound guided cytology clinic optimize the cytological evaluation of head and neck masses? Clin Radiol 1999;54(5):312–316

17. Kocjan G, Feichter G, Hagmar B, et al. Fine needle aspiration cytology: a survey of current European practice. Cytopathology 2006;17(5):219–226

18. Koshy M, Paulino AC, Howell R, Schuster D, Halkar R, Davis LW. F-18 FDG PET-CT fusion in radiotherapy treatment planning for head and neck cancer. Head Neck 2005;27(6):494–502

19. Agarwal V, Branstetter BF IV, Johnson JT. Indications for PET/CT in the head and neck. Otolaryngol Clin North Am 2008;41(1):23–49, v

5 Imaging of the Paranasal Sinuses and Nasopharynx

A. E. Nidecker, N. Aygun, and S. J. Zinreich

Introduction

Imaging of the paranasal sinuses and nasopharynx is essential in the diagnosis of patients with pathology in these regions. In the last three decades we have witnessed a tremendous advance in the therapy of patients with inflammatory, infectious, and neoplastic diseases of the head and neck. During the same period we have also seen revolutionary changes in imaging technology that have greatly influenced the evolving surgical and medical therapies.

The use of computed tomography (CT) imaging technology is well known for the evaluation of inflammatory disease affecting the paranasal sinuses. A combination of CT and magnetic resonance imaging (MRI), and at times positron emission tomography (PET) imaging, is obtained in the work-up of patients with suspected sinonasal and nasopharyngeal malignancy. There are many confounders in imaging, which occasionally make it difficult to distinguish inflammatory and infectious diseases from neoplasms. However, these three main imaging modalities can be used in a complementary fashion to help reduce this uncertainty and to assist with staging, biopsy, and treatment planning for tumors.

The objective of this chapter is to highlight the application of imaging information with regard to the identification of the typical findings in inflammatory, infectious, and neoplastic disorders of the paranasal sinuses and nasopharynx. Additionally, we will describe some of the pitfalls of diagnosis encountered with imaging. We will also review radiological staging of sinonasal (SN) and nasopharyngeal (NP) malignancies as well as the imaging of postsurgical and post–radiation therapy patients. The efficacy and quality of information provided by radiological assessment primarily depends on the way in which the images are acquired. For example, depending on the plane of acquisition, the slice thickness, and the presence or absence of contrast, a CT image can vary greatly in its utility in assessing a potential sinonasal or nasopharyngeal tumor patient.[1] Described in each section are the current standards for imaging of these regions. Occasionally these vary depending on the clinical requisite (i.e., contrast medium is rarely administered in patients with neutropenic fever being assessed for acute sinusitis), but for the most part they are fairly consistent and reliable.[2]

Paranasal Sinuses

Imaging Protocols

Computed Tomography

Given its superior bony resolution, CT is typically the best imaging modality for the display of the delicate regional bony anatomy as well as of the mucosal changes in the presence of inflammatory disease. It is also superior in the detection of bony involvement by pathology, in particular periosteal reaction and bony erosion. Particularly when intravenous (IV) contrast is used, CT can also provide excellent soft tissue information, although it is inferior to the soft tissue contrast resolution provided by MRI.

Images are acquired in the axial plane, preferably with 0.5 mm slice thickness. The imaging plane should start above the skull base structures and include the entirety of the paranasal sinuses and nasal cavity, the orbits, and the middle and anterior cranial fossae. Coronal and sagittal reformatted images are reconstructed from the axial imaging acquisition. If derived from the thin-section source images, these reformatted images should demonstrate excellent spatial resolution, essentially indistinguishable from the axial source images.

Coronal images represent the optimal plane for endoscopic correlation. Sagittal planes are very helpful in improving the 3D conceptualization of the regional morphology.[3] However, when employing these images for ensuring the accuracy of the spatial orientation in one's mind, the sagittal images should always be correlated with an additional orthogonal plane, that is, a coronal or axial plane image. The application of multiplanar reconstruction and the use of cross-hairs for localization purposes is especially helpful (**Fig. 5.1**).

If contrast administration is contemplated, one should first consider doing an MRI examination. Intravenous contrast is typically administered for improved soft tissue resolution. Information provided by MRI is superior for this purpose and avoids the radiation dose received with CT.

Magnetic Resonance Imaging

MRI provides excellent soft tissue contrast resolution. It offers multiplanar capabilities, and does not involve ionizing radiation, which is of particular advantage when imaging children and women of childbearing age.

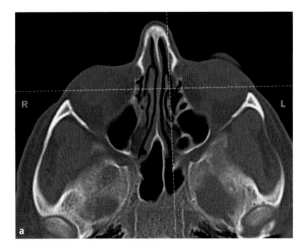

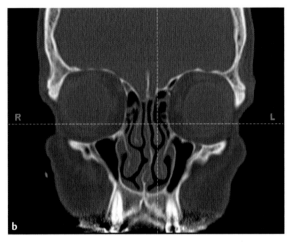

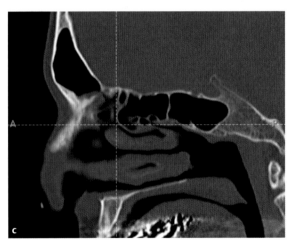

Fig. 5.1a–c Axially acquired CT imaging of the paranasal sinuses (**a**) with coronal (**b**) and sagittal (**c**) reformatted images demonstrating triangulation of planes for precise localization of anatomical structures, in this case the frontal recess.

Typically, a surface coil is used. Axial and coronal planes are acquired, pre- and postcontrast T1-weighted (T1W) (typically with fat saturation), noncontrast T2-weighted (T2W), and noncontrast STIR (a fat-saturated fluid-sensitive sequence) images being the standard protocol for evaluation.

Magnetic resonance angiography (MRA) should be considered when dealing with a vascular pathology or a pathological process affecting or in relationship with the regional vascular structures. This is an excellent noninvasive means to obtain information regarding vascular supply to pathological tissue, as well as to display vascular relationships that may be critical for performing surgery safely.

PET-CT

PET is generally reserved for staging and follow-up of sinonasal carcinomas. However, it can also be useful in the work-up of an unknown primary tumor.[4] Although PET has poor spatial resolution, this issue is compensated by the simultaneous acquisition and fusion with CT imaging. Therefore, a PET-CT study is the preferred evaluation.[5]

Imaging for Initial Diagnosis and Staging

CT is the most readily available sectional imaging modality. It provides the best resolution for bone morphology, and the first "glimpse" into the differential diagnosis of the pathology being dealt with.[6] The evaluation should focus on the integrity of the bony architecture, and the presence of bone erosion within the sinus morphology as well as the bony perimeter defining the borders of the nasal cavity and paranasal sinuses. The initial questions to be answered with CT are: "Is there a soft tissue pathology?" "Where, exactly, is it?" and "What is its influence on the bony morphology?" "Is there extension beyond the boundaries of the nasal cavity and paranasal sinuses?"[7]

Important areas assessed by CT in defining the extent of pathological invasion include the cribriform plate and planum sphenoidale; the fovea ethmoidalis; the lamina papyracea; the frontal, maxillary, and sphenoid sinus borders; and the internal bony framework of the sinuses vulnerable to direct invasion and/or destruction. Should the soft tissue and/or bony pathology penetrate the paranasal sinus boundaries, the final step is to assess the extent of "invasion": into the orbits, or into the intracranial compartment through skull base foramina, and other possible pathways of spread including the pterygomaxillary fissure and pterygopalatine fossa.

CT is also the modality of choice to initially assess bony lesions, such as benign fibro-osseous lesions as well as primary malignant bone tumors. Often the specific diagnosis can be determined by CT.

Having identified the pathology by the CT examination, its etiology as well as the precise extent may still be in question. This is where MRI can provide significant additional help. The soft tissue resolution provided by MRI may be able to further delineate the etiology of the pathological process. It may also help distinguish between the various inflammatory pathologies, and may be able to help narrow the diagnosis to a specific neoplastic entity. The use of contrast and fat suppression can significantly improve the accuracy of assessing subtler perineural spread of tumor, intraorbital invasion, and invasion of intracranial structures.[2]

In initial diagnosis, PET-CT has little utility except in the case of an unknown primary neoplasm: patients with cervical lymph node metastases in whom a primary tumor cannot be detected on physical examination or other conventional imaging. It is uncommon for sinonasal malignancy to be detected in such a way. Most of these neoplasms have a pharyngeal, hypopharyngeal, laryngeal, or tonsillar origin. However, in a small percentage of cases these tumors are sinonasal, and PET-CT has a high sensitivity for detecting such lesions. The detection of residual or recurrent neoplasm in the postoperative patient can be significantly aided by this modality.

Pathology

Nonneoplastic

Inflammation and Infection

Sinus inflammatory disease typically begins with obstruction of a sinus. This is followed by a mucosal inflammation and fluid exudation. Eventually the fluid is resorbed. However, if the obstruction persists, this mucosal inflammation can continue, at times completely opacifying the sinus.[8]

On CT, this process is demonstrated by uniform peripheral mucosal thickening and an air–fluid level. The obstruction of a sinus may also be apparent on CT. Following contrast administration, there should be uniform enhancement of the mucosa, which is in general uninterrupted.[9] With repeated infections, the inflammatory process may invade the bony framework, producing a uniform bony thickening that usually affects the perimeter of the sinuses and is referred to as "osteitis"[10] (Fig. 5.2).

On MRI, the combination of edema and retained secretions associated with inflammatory disease is typically hyperintense on T2W and iso/hypointense on T1W imaging due to the high water content.[11] T2W and T1W postcontrast images will demonstrate the uniform appearance of the mucosa, an important "hallmark" of inflammatory disease (Fig. 5.3).

Fungal inflammatory disease, due to its unique qualities including eosinophilic mucus and high concentration of metabolized ferromagnetic elements and calcium, has a totally different appearance, demonstrating low signal on T2W imaging.[12] Nevertheless, with this modality, the uniformly "thickened" sinus mucosa also remains intact. Inspissated secretions can also vary in their appearance, demonstrating intermediate signal on T1W and T2W imaging.[13] However, on contrast-enhanced MRI, sinuses containing inspissated secretions will still demonstrate intact mucosa with uniform enhancement.[14]

Neoplasms, on the other hand, tend to be low to intermediate in signal on these sequences. Furthermore,

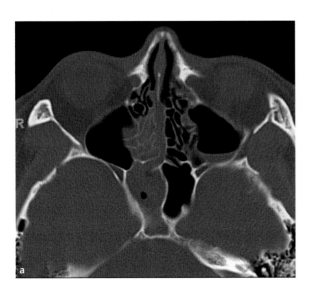
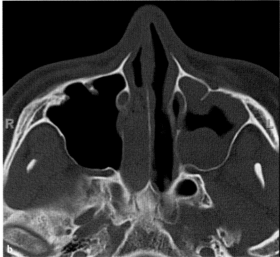

Fig. 5.2a–d CT of paranasal sinuses demonstrating acute rhinosinusitis, with mucosal thickening and air–fluid levels present (**a, b**), and chronic rhinosinusitis, with mucosal thickening and periosteal reaction or "osteitis" (**c, d**).

Fig. 5.2c–d ▷

◁ continued

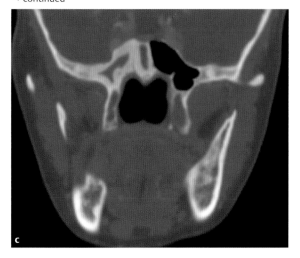

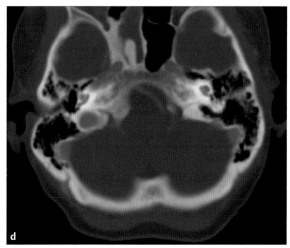

neoplasms penetrate the typically smooth and uniform mucosal thickening seen with inflammatory disease, as they extend beyond the sinus outline (**Table 5.1**).

Aggressive Infections

Aggressive infections, specifically invasive fungal (*Mucor* or *Aspergillus* being the more commonly encountered) diseases, can have a tumorlike appearance (**Fig. 5.4**). When an aggressive-appearing soft tissue process is identified, it is first important to determine the patient's history and their immune status as immunocompetent patients are less likely to develop these infections.[15] These can be associated with bone destruction, but as the fungi tend to extend along the vasculature, there may be little associated bony destruction or even mucosal inflammation.[16] Fungal infection also can have a hyperdense appearance on CT,[17] and very low signal on T2W imaging, possibly due to the ferromagnetic elements and calcium within the fungal hyphae.[18]

Granulomatous Diseases

Granulomatous diseases, such as Wegener's granulomatosis and sarcoidosis, may also have a tumorlike appearance.[19,20] The invasive soft tissue pathology and bony erosive changes can mimic the appearance of a neoplastic process, or the appearance of a patient having had extensive surgical procedures, with persistent inflammatory disease (**Fig. 5.5**). The presence of associated inflammatory disease within the orbits is not uncommon.

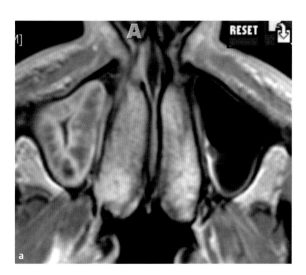

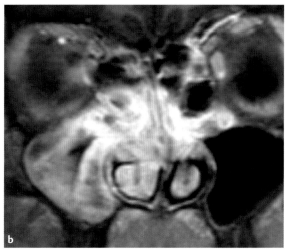

Fig. 5.3a, b Axial (**a**) and coronal (**b**) T2W MRI of the maxillary sinuses demonstrating intact and uniform sinus mucosa despite significant inflammatory disease, nearly obliterating the sinus air space. The hyperintense signal of the mucosal thickening and secretions is appreciated.

Table 5.1 The distinguishing imaging features of sinonasal neoplasms contrasted to infection and inflammation on CT, as well as MRI

Pathology	CT	T1W MRI	T2W MRI	Postcontrast T1W MRI
Neoplasm	• Bony erosion • Less intense enhancement • Obstructive opacification	Low signal Obliteration of perineural fat	Low signal Interruption or inhomogeneity of mucosal lining	Less intense enhancement
Infection and Inflammation	• Mucosal thickening • Uniform peripheral mucosal enhancement • Osteitis/bony thickening	Low signal	High signal Homogeneous and intact mucosal thickening	Intense enhancement of intact mucosa

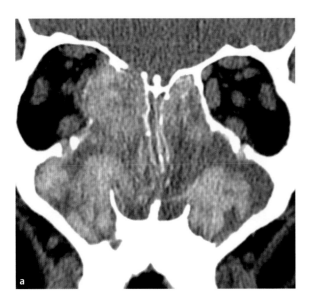
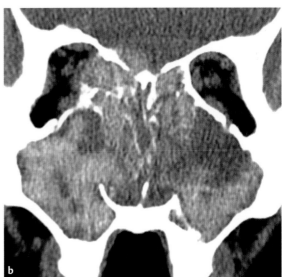

Fig. 5.4a, b Coronal CT of an immunocompromised patient with invasive fungal rhinosinusitis. Note the aggressive-appearing morphology, with invasion of adjacent structures. Also note intrinsic CT hyperdensity, a hallmark of fungal infection.

Sinonasal Organized Hematoma

Similarly, sinonasal organized hematoma represents an accumulation of blood products in the sinonasal area, primarily in the maxillary sinus.[21] The etiology is unclear but it is believed to be associated with trauma, surgery, bleeding diathesis, and/or a hemorrhagic lesion in the nasal cavity/sinuses. The CT evaluation reveals an expansile lesion eroding bone and penetrating through the sinonasal borders, with the appearance of an aggressive neoplasm. On MRI the lesion is well defined and the mucosa at the periphery is intact and enhances uniformly. Central low-intensity signal changes are characteristic of blood products, and therefore indicative of a peripheral inflammatory process (**Fig. 5.6**).

Neoplastic

Benign Bony Tumors

Benign bony lesions are the most common neoplasm of the sinonasal region, of which the most common are osteomas. These are well defined and in general homogeneous bone density lesions. They are most commonly found within or associated with the frontal and ethmoid sinuses and less commonly within the sphenoid and maxillary sinuses. These lesions are best displayed on coronal bone-windowed CT images. However, for additional help in establishing their bony adherence, axial images may also be helpful. MRI is rarely helpful in the assessment of these lesions.

Benign fibro-osseous masses are also not uncommonly encountered.[22] Ossifying fibromas are well-demarcated lesions with a central fibrous component that is peripherally surrounded by an osseous rim. They are more commonly found in the mandible and maxilla but can also be present in the sinuses.[23] Fibrous dysplasia appears as a poorly defined asymmetric expansion of the maxillofacial bony morphology with a classic "ground glass" appearance on CT, which may be homogeneous or have cystic areas (**Fig. 5.7**). In these cases, special attention is needed with respect to the ostia of the sinuses, as there is a tendency for ostial closure and the creation of mucoceles.[24] Other fibro-osseous lesions are much less common. These

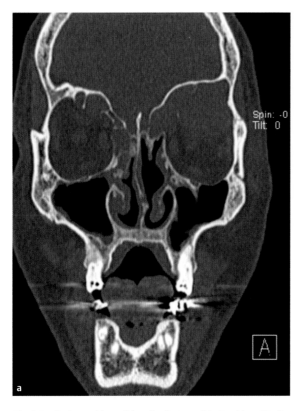

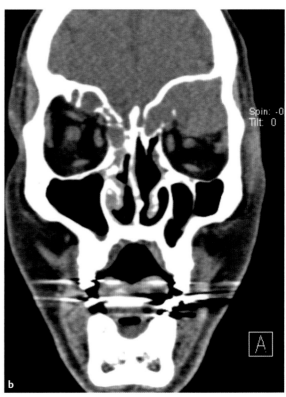

Fig. 5.5a, b Coronal bone (**a**) and soft tissue (**b**) algorithm CT of a patient with Wegener's granulomatosis, demonstrating destruction of sinonasal anatomy, erosion of bony margins, and invasion of the orbits.

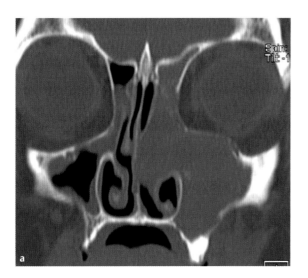

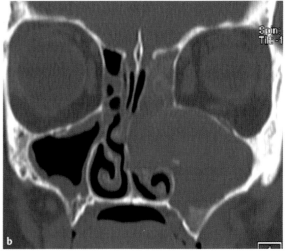

Fig. 5.6a–h

a–c Coronal CT of a sinonasal organized hematoma, demonstrating opacification of the left maxillary, ethmoid,

and frontal sinuses with thinning and dehiscence of the bony margins of the left maxillary sinus.

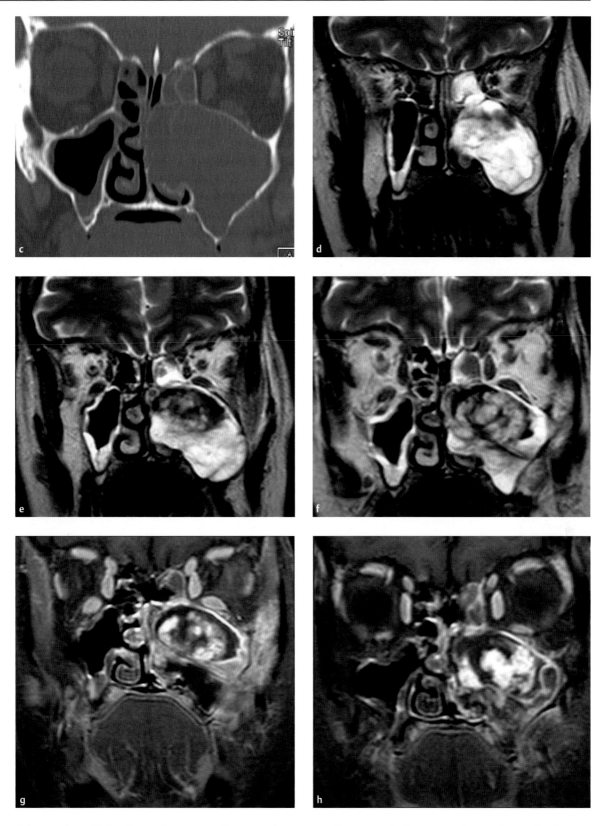

d–h Coronal T2W (**d–f**) and coronal postcontrast fat-saturated T1W (**g, h**) MRI of the same patient, demonstrating the heterogeneous signal intensity of the hematoma as well as the associated enhancement. Also note the peripheral, intact-appearing mucosal lining, high in signal on both sequences.

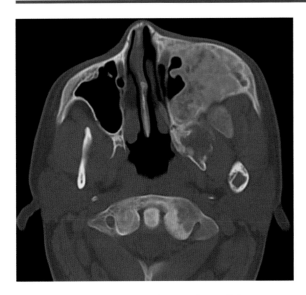

Fig. 5.7 Axial CT image showing the typical ground glass appearance of fibrous dysplasia involving the left maxilla.

lesions are best assessed with CT, and often a specific diagnosis can be rendered by CT alone. Imaging evaluation is also essential in determining their site of origin, and their connection/adherence to the bony framework of the paranasal sinuses. This specific determination will have an important effect on the surgery and the postsurgical outcome. Again, MRI is rarely helpful in these cases, and can confound the diagnosis as they can have a variable and sometimes confusing appearance on MRI.

Benign Soft Tissue Tumors

Benign soft tissue tumors of the nose and paranasal sinuses are somewhat less common entities but include papillomas and adenomas, as well as vascular lesions including hemangiomas and angiofibroma.[25]

Inverted Papillomas

Benign tumors can have a relatively distinctive appearance on imaging and are best assessed with MRI.[26] For example, inverted papillomas on postcontrast T1W MRI may demonstrate a unique "serpiginous" enhancing pattern similar to the appearance of the superficial brain gyral pattern (**Fig. 5.8**). These lesions originate most commonly from the "transitional" epithelium of the lateral nasal wall, but may also arise along the epithelium of the middle turbinate.[27] If they originate from the lateral nasal wall, they may erode through the lamina papyracea into the orbit. However, if they arise from the middle turbinate, they extend to the skull base and may be indistinguishable from an esthesioneuroblastoma (olfactory neuroblastoma).[28,29]

Angiofibroma

The angiofibroma is another lesion that, while histologically benign, can behave in an aggressive fashion. It is an intensely enhancing lesion that originates at the sphenopalatine foramen and can extend into the nasal cavity, the nasopharynx, and the pterygopalatine fossa, and into the intracranial compartment via the foramen

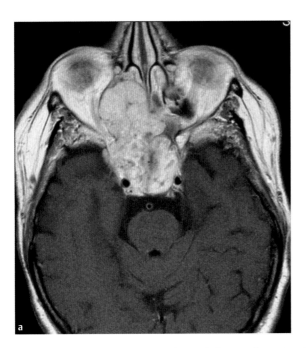
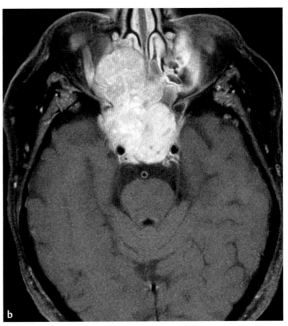

Fig. 5.8a, b Axial MRI demonstrating the cerebriform configuration of an inverting papilloma on postcontrast T1W (**a**) and fat-saturation postcontrast T1W (**b**) images.

rotundum or the vidian canal. It may also extend into the sphenoid, maxillary, and ethmoid sinuses, and may invade the masticator space and the inferior orbital fissure. CT will demonstrate bone destruction, in particular erosion of the upper part of the medial pterygoid plate. MRI with contrast best displays the extent of the lesion (**Fig. 5.9**). Angiography may be performed to establish the blood supply to the mass and plan for presurgical embolization.[30] The blood supply may arise from the external as well as the internal carotid arteries and, even though the mass may appear unilateral, it may also receive blood supply from the contralateral carotid arteries.

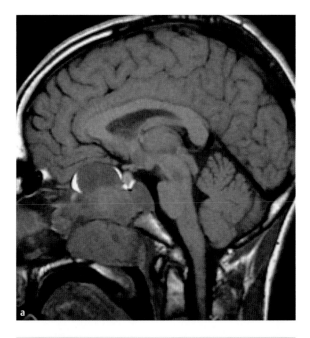

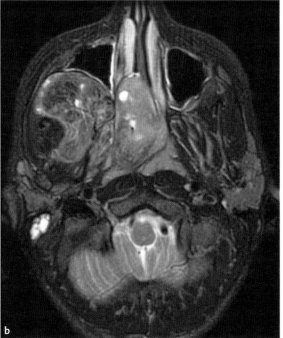

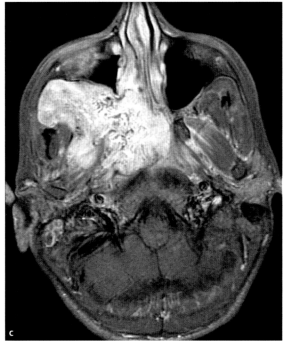

Fig. 5.9a–c Sagittal T1 (**a**), axial fat-sat T2 (**b**), and postcontrast axial fat-sat T1 (**c**) weighted MRI of a patient who presented with epistaxis, with a large mass growing into the nasal cavity, sphenoid, and maxillary sinuses found to be an angiofibroma. Note the intermediate signal on T1W and intense postcontrast enhancement due to the vascularity of the tumor.

Malignant Soft Tissue Tumors

Squamous Cell Carcinoma

Slightly more than half squamous cell carcinomas (SCCs) originate in the maxillary antrum, 30% in the nasal cavity, and 10% in the ethmoid sinuses.[31] On CT, these are iso-attenuating with a wide variety of appearances based on the site of origin and extent of spread. In general, malignancies are associated with bone erosion/destruction, which is easiest to recognize on the CT evaluation.

On MRI, these are typically intermediate in signal intensity on T1W and usually have a lower signal intensity on T2W images.[32] After contrast administration, they enhance homogeneously, but the enhancing area has a lower signal intensity than inflammatory tissue. In general, malignancies will destroy the uniform peripheral sinus mucosa and will invade neighboring structures.

Regional metastatic lymphadenopathy of SCC of paranasal sinuses is uncommon, but once the tumor has spread beyond the sinus there is greater likelihood of nodal disease or distant metastases (see later).

Minor Salivary Gland Tumors: Adenoid Cystic Carcinoma

Adenoid cystic tumors are the most common in this category, accounting for one-third to one-half of minor salivary gland malignancies. The soft palate is the most common site of origin. This tumor is known for a high incidence of perineural spread. While this tumor often tends to be slow-growing, it is relentlessly progressive. It is distinct on imaging because of its relatively high signal on T2W imaging, as opposed to the majority of other primary sinonasal malignancies, which are intermediate or low in signal.

Malignancy-Associated Inflammation

Inflammation often accompanies neoplasm, as the tumor can invade or obstruct normal sinus drainage pathways. In such cases, it is essential to distinguish inflammatory disease from tumor. MRI is the best imaging modality for this purpose, and inflammation can often be distinguished from neoplasm by its precontrast T2W hyperintense appearance. Both can enhance on postcontrast T1W imaging. However, as stated above, the inflammatory mucosa T2W signal and postcontrast enhancement reveal a brighter signal on these image sequences (**Fig. 5.10**).

Staging

Sinonasal malignancy staging is based on the TNM staging system, and the stage of the tumor depends on its size at diagnosis, the presence and characteristics of associated lymphadenopathy, invasion of adjacent structures, and the presence of distant metastases (**Table 5.2**).[33]

Nodal Metastases

Nodal disease is a poor prognostic sign. Clinical examination is notoriously inaccurate in staging, lacking both sensitivity and specificity, with only ~70% accuracy in detection of abnormal nodes in head and neck cancer.[34] Lymph node drainage for the sinonasal malignancies follows venous drainage: the anterior half of the nasal cavity drains into level Ib nodes, the posterior half drains with the nasopharynx into the retropharyngeal nodes and into levels II through V. Frontal and ethmoid sinuses drain to level I nodes, sphenoid sinuses drain to retropharyngeal nodes, and maxillary antra drain into the level Ib, II, III, and IV, as well as the parapharyngeal nodes.

Currently, size and central necrosis are the general criteria employed to determine nodal involvement, with extracapsular spread being a grave prognostic sign (**Fig. 5.11**). Either CT or MRI can be used with relatively equal accuracy to detect lymphadenopathy. However, while they have improved accuracy of nodal staging, they again have a false-negative rate anywhere between 10% and 30%. This is likely due to the dependence of detection on nodal size, central necrosis, and enhancement, characteristics that may or may not be present in metastatic nodes.

PET has a higher sensitivity and specificity than CT or MRI, alone. However, it does not improve detection of clinically occult nodes, showing similar sensitivity for detection of occult nodes on dissection when compared with CT and MRI.[35] The spatial resolution of PET is the limiting factor; at this time most available machines are only able to detect abnormal FDG uptake in nodes greater than 3 to 5 mm in size. Thus, distinguishing N0 from N1 disease with very small nodes remains difficult.[36] There are some emerging imaging modalities that may be utilized in the future, including diffusion weighted and dynamic postcontrast MRI, which may help make this distinction.[37,38] The use of superparamagnetic iron oxide nanoparticles is still in the experimental phases but also shows some promise in better detecting metastatic nodes.[39]

Perineural Spread

This is a serious prognostic feature of some malignant soft tissue tumors. Perineural spread is best assessed on thin-section fat-suppressed postcontrast T1W imaging. Subtle soft tissue obliteration of the fat in the pterygopalatine fossa, for example, and enhancement within skull base foramina along cranial nerves (i.e., CN V_3 in the foramen ovale) and insinuating into adjacent intracranial fossae and extracranial spaces can be difficult or impossible to evaluate on CT. Relatively early extension into the cranium can occur due to these "highways" of spread, and intracranial disease is again best assessed with MRI (**Fig. 5.12**).[40] Tracing in one's mind the paths taken by the various cranial nerves connecting the intracranial compartment with the infratemporal fossa, as well as comparing the symmetry and presence of fat signal in these

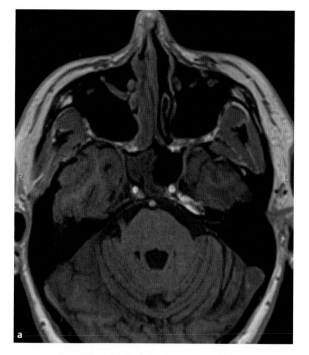

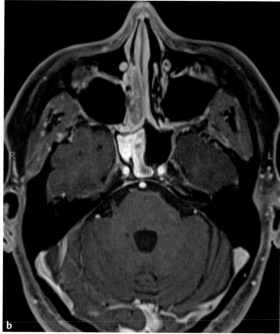

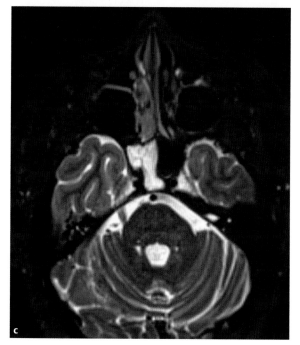

Fig. 5.10a–c High-resolution T2W (**a, b**) and postcontrast T1W (**c**) MRI demonstrating tumor (in this case, an esthesioneuroblastoma) which is less bright and enhances less than surrounding (obstructive) mucosal inflammation.

Table 5.2 TNM staging of sinonasal soft tissue malignancy

T1	Restricted to mucosa
T2	Associated with adjacent osseous erosion or destruction
T3–T4	Extend beyond the sinus into the masticator space, buccal space, adjacent sinuses, orbit, skull base, or intracranially
T4a	Anterior orbit, skin of cheek, pterygoid plates, infratemporal fossa, cribriform plate, sphenoid or frontal sinuses
T4b	Orbital apex, dura, brain, middle cranial fossa, CN other than V2, nasopharynx, or clivus
NX	Cannot be assessed
N0	None
N1	Single ipsilateral node not more than 3 cm
N2a	Single ipsilateral node 3–6 cm
N2b	Multiple ipsilateral nodes, none more than 6 cm
N2c	Bilateral or contralateral nodes, none more than 6 cm
N3	Any node greater than 6 cm

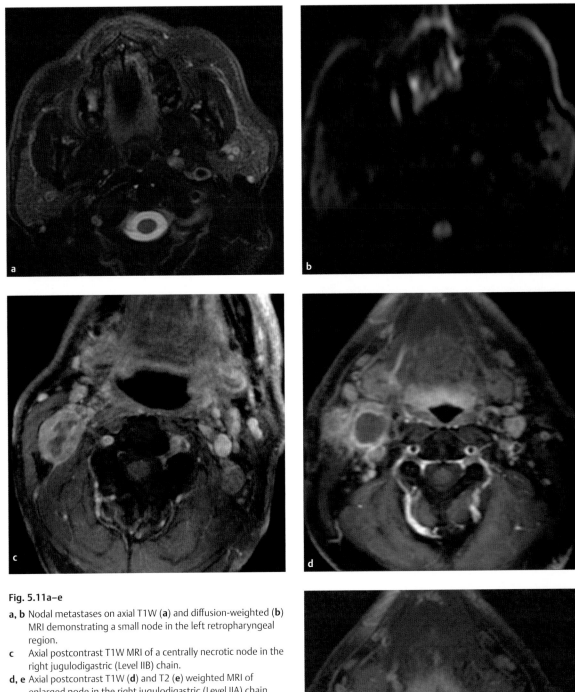

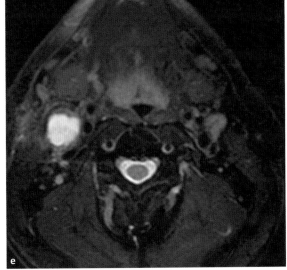

Fig. 5.11a–e

a, b Nodal metastases on axial T1W (**a**) and diffusion-weighted (**b**) MRI demonstrating a small node in the left retropharyngeal region.

c Axial postcontrast T1W MRI of a centrally necrotic node in the right jugulodigastric (Level IIB) chain.

d, e Axial postcontrast T1W (**d**) and T2 (**e**) weighted MRI of enlarged node in the right jugulodigastric (Level IIA) chain with extracapsular spread.

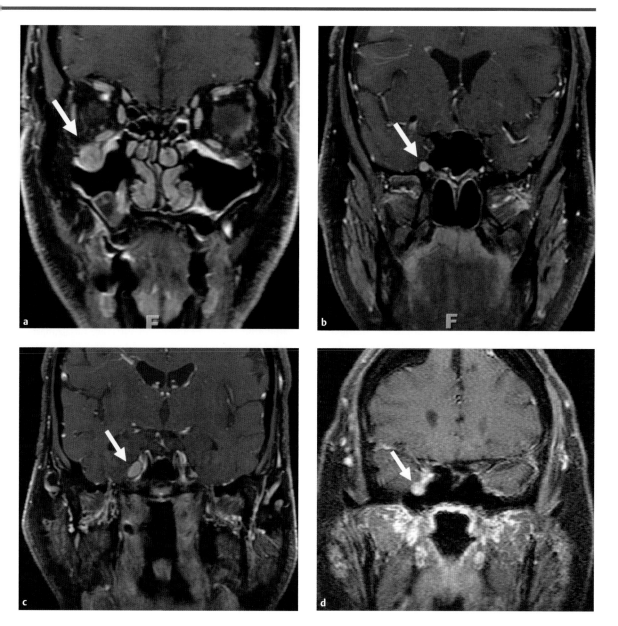

Fig. 5.12a–f Coronal postcontrast fat-saturated T1W MRI of the skull base demonstrating perineural spread along the second (V2) and third (V3) divisions of the trigeminal nerve. **a–c** Abnormal enlargement and enhancement along the infraorbital (V2) nerve (**a**), which extends posteriorly into the foramen rotundum (**b**), and into Meckel's cave (**c**). **d–f** A different patient with extension into the foramen rotundum (**d**), Meckel's cave (**e**), and the foramen ovale (**f**).

Fig. 5.12e–f ▷

◁ continued

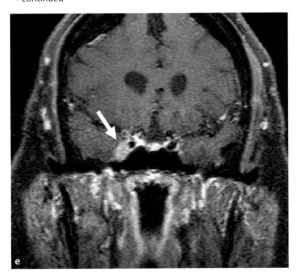

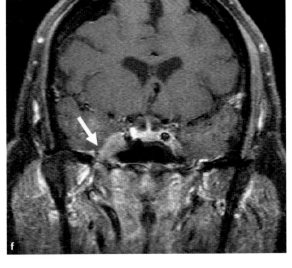

"paths" provide an excellent means to detect perineural neoplastic extension. The object is to detect areas of fat obliteration/absence, and in this quest "the presence of fat is a friendly sign" (**Fig. 5.13**). That said, the easiest way to assess perineural spread currently is with fat-saturated postcontrast T1W imaging.

Direct Skull Base Invasion

CT aptly demonstrates the bony destruction due to direct invasion through the cranial floor, including the planum sphenoidale, cribriform plate, and fovea ethmoidalis (**Fig. 5.14a–f**). MRI is still superior, however, in defining the extent of soft tissue invasion, as well as the intracranial extent of tumor. Neoplasms that tend to erode and invade the skull base include undifferentiated squamous cell carcinoma, esthesioneuroblastoma,[41] lymphomas, and sarcomas. It is important to keep in mind that benign lesions can also invade the skull base, including inverted papilloma, mucocele, and angiofibroma (**Fig. 5.14g–j**).

Imaging Following Treatment, Including Surgery and Radiation

Imaging Approach

Following surgical, radiotherapy, and chemotherapy treatment of patients with malignant sinonasal tumors, a combined close interval clinical and radiological follow-up is often employed. This is both to assess for tumor recurrence and to detect treatment-related pathology, which will be discussed below.

Distinguishing postsurgical scarring or granulation tissue from residual or recurrent neoplasm is the most challenging aspect of follow-up imaging. Inflammatory disease can often be distinguished by its T2W hyperintense appearance on MRI. Early granulation tissue can also have a hyperintense appearance on T2W imaging. However, granulation tissue can have similar CT and MRI appearance to neoplasm, demonstrating hypointensity on T2W imaging and enhancing after contrast administration. A posttreatment MRI (usually at 3 months) provides a baseline appearance for subsequent studies, which may help distinguish these by demonstrating stability or even retraction of scar tissue.

In cases where scar tissue and neoplasm cannot be distinguished on MR, PET-CT can be employed to evaluate for FDG uptake, which will be avid in cases of recurrence.[42,43]

Pathology

Postradiation Osteonecrosis

Osteonecrosis of bone in the radiation field is a not infrequent complication of radiotherapy. For this, CT is recommended as a first-line imaging modality.

Gliosis

Gliosis in the radiation field can be encountered months or even years after treatment. The temporal lobes are most often affected, given their proximity to the sinuses.[44] This can occur early on, during treatment, or can occur months or years after treatment. There is typically T2W hyperintensity within the affected areas, representing edema, which can be reversible. Later on, demyelination and inflammation can be encountered, demonstrated by T2W hyperintensity as well as patchy or peripheral

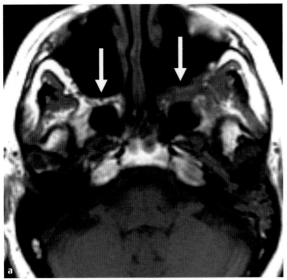
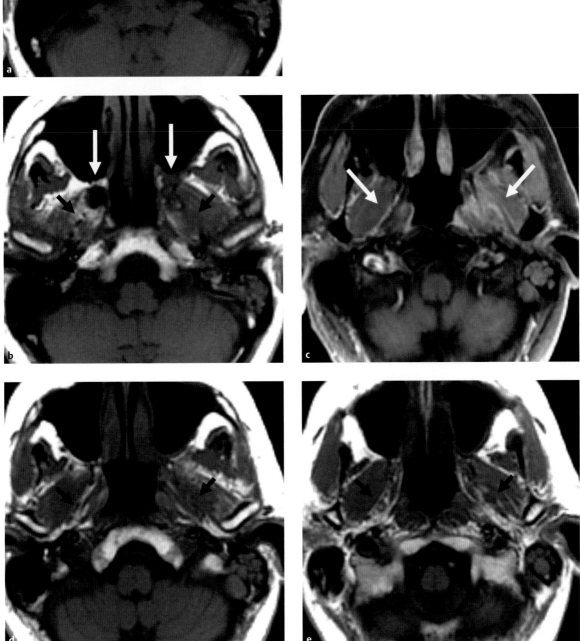

Fig. 5.13a–e Axial T1W MRI of the skull base in a patient with squamous cell carcinoma of the left maxillary antrum, demonstrating obliteration of normal fat pads in cases of subtle perineural tumoral extension. Obliteration of normal bright signal of fat in the right pterygopalatine fossa (**a** and **b**, white arrows), along the course of the third division of the fifth cranial nerve (**b**, **d** and **e**, black arrows). Axial fat-saturated postcontrast T1W image demonstrates this even more (**c**).

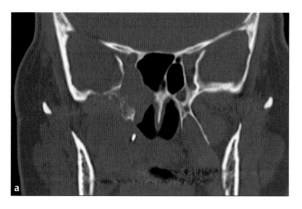
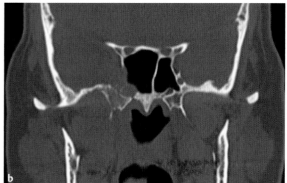
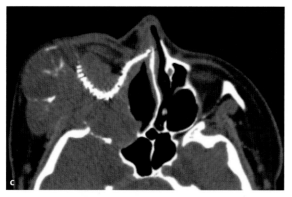
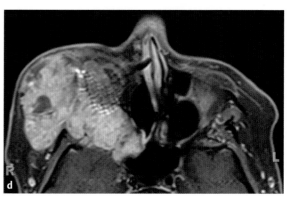
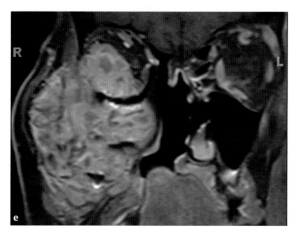

Fig. 5.14a–j

a–f CT (**a–c**) and MRI (**d–f**) demonstrating direct skull base and orbital invasion of an adenoid cystic carcinoma. Note the intrinsic T2 hyperintensity of the lesion, unusual among sinonasal soft tissue malignancies.

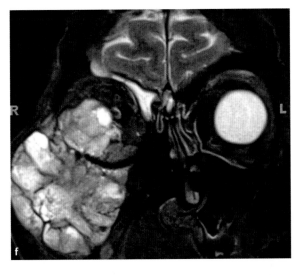

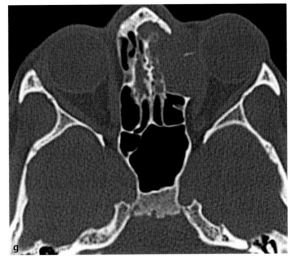

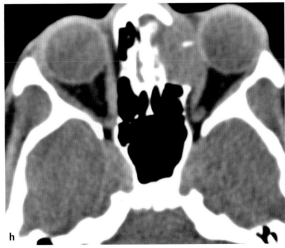

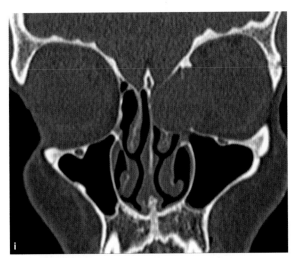

g–j Axial (**g, h**) and coronal (**i, j**) bone and soft tissue algorithm CT of a left anterior ethmoidal mucocele, demonstrating thinning/dehiscence of the fovea ethmoidalis, cribriform plate, and lamina papyracea, and invasion of the medial left orbit.

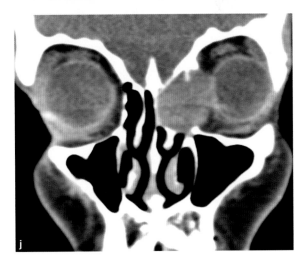

enhancement around a necrotic cavity. This is best assessed with MRI (**Fig. 5.15**).

Ischemia

Radiation can cause necrosis of the deep perforating arteries, leading to ischemia in the basal ganglia, thalami, brainstem, and deep white matter. This is also best assessed with MRI, including diffusion-weighted imaging.

Cranial Neuropathy

Patients can present following treatment with cranial neuropathies that are not related to tumor spread.[45] When this affects nerves supplying efferent motor fibers (i.e., trigeminal, facial), the muscles can show denervation edema and then atrophy, a finding best seen on MRI. High-resolution MRI of the skull base can be employed to demonstrate enlargement and enhancement of the involved nerves, as well.

The Nasopharynx

Imaging Approach and Protocols

The patient undergoing imaging for a suspected nasopharyngeal pathology will in most cases come to the imaging department after having been evaluated by an ENT specialist, and the request for imaging usually specifies the suspected nasopharyngeal area of involvement.[46] The

location of a nasopharyngeal mass can be determined by how it is positioned in relation to the adjacent spaces of the neck (**Table 5.3**).

Imaging for Initial Diagnosis and Staging

Computed Tomography

In general, the imaging evaluation of the nasopharynx is part of a neck evaluation. A noncontrast examination is sufficient when determining the presence of a foreign body or the status of the airway. However, when evaluating a possible nasopharyngeal malignancy, the CT of the neck should only be performed after administration of intravenous contrast, and should extend from just above the skull base to the aortic arch.[47] CT will afford optimal evaluation of the skull base bony morphology, and given the density differences of most of the neck soft tissues, this evaluation will provide adequate information regarding the presence of a pathological process. The presence of contrast within the vasculature affords initial identification of potential vascular involvement, and commonly aids in the diagnosis of pathological involvement of lymph nodes.

Magnetic Resonance Imaging

MRI with axial and coronal T1W and fat-saturated T2W images as well as axial and coronal postcontrast T1W

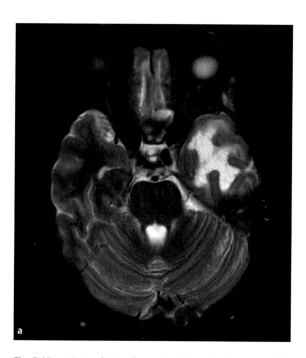
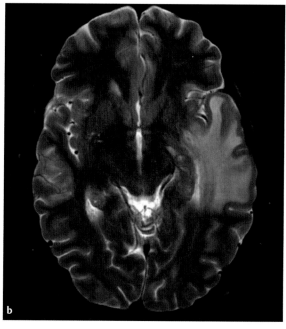

Fig. 5.15a–c Postradiation changes involving the left temporal lobe on axial T2W (**a, b**) and postcontrast T1W (**c**) MRI in this patient who was treated with radiation 1.5 years earlier for invasive squamous cell carcinoma of the right maxillary sinus.

Table 5.3 Imaging characteristics which define that a mass originates from the pharyngeal mucosal space

The mass is medial to the parapharyngeal space
The mass causes mass effect on the parapharyngeal space from medial to lateral
The mass breaks through the normal pharyngomucosal space and submucosal architecture (pharyngobasilar fascia)
Caution, do not mistake a fluid-filled lateral pharyngeal recess with neoplasm If there is no mass effect, it is probably a fluid-filled recess, and can be proven by a Valsalva maneuver

images are best for the evaluation of the neck soft tissues including the pharyngeal mucosal space. MRI is superior to CT in demonstrating direct invasion of neoplasm as well as perineural tumor spread, bone marrow infiltration, and retropharyngeal cervical node metastases. Extracapsular spread of pathological lymph node involvement is also best detected with MRI.

Positron Emission Tomography–Computed Tomography

PET-CT examinations can be particularly helpful when dealing with an unknown primary neoplasm in the neck, as well as when evaluating patients after surgery with suspicion of local recurrence that is not clearly detected with MRI, or with distant metastasis (**Fig. 5.16**). This imaging modality may also be very useful in assessing the

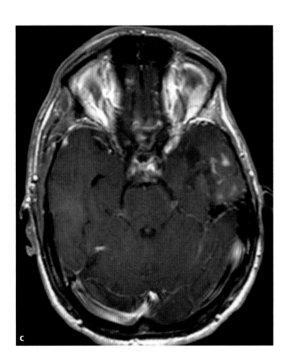

c

response to therapy. PET-MRI is the most recent application of nuclear medicine technology to improve detection of neoplasm in this area. MRI has demonstrated a higher accuracy than FDG PET-CT in detecting residual and/or recurrent NPC at the primary tumor site.

Pathology

Nonneoplastic

Thornwaldt's Cyst

This is a developmental nasopharyngeal midline cyst covered by mucosa anteriorly and bordered posteriorly by the longus colli muscles. It is the most common lesion in the nasopharynx, found in 4% of autopsies and 5% of routine brain MRIs. It is therefore often an incidental finding on diagnostic evaluations performed for other than nasopharyngeal-related concerns. It becomes a clinical concern when it becomes infected or grows in size.

On CT, this is demonstrated as a midline, typically fluid-density, round structure. The rim of the cyst may enhance. On MRI, the cyst will be high intensity on T2W images, and is homogeneous but can be variable in T1W intensity (**Fig. 5.17**), depending on cyst contents.[48] A thin rim of peripheral enhancement may be detected after contrast administration.

Adenoidal Hyperplasia

Enlargement of the nasopharyngeal lymphoid tissue is common in preadolescent and adolescent children and is thought to be a response to repeated infections. On MRI, an obstruction of the nasopharyngeal airway is noted with a sharp demarcation of the pharyngobasilar fascia. This needs to be distinguished from pathology in this region, including epithelial malignancies as well as lymphoma, which may be suspected when the patient is older, or when there is asymmetry or invasion of adjacent structures (**Fig. 5.18**).

Retention Cyst

A retention cyst of the pharyngeal mucosal space represents a benign, usually asymptomatic, epithelium-lined mucosal cyst, most commonly found in the lateral pharyngeal recess when it occurs in the nasopharynx. On CT, these cysts have a low density and do not enhance after contrast administration. Axial and coronal T2W MRI images reveal a hyperintense cyst within the lateral pharyngeal recess, which provides the diagnosis. In common with adenoidal hypertrophy, these cysts may also obstruct the eustachian tube, causing middle ear and mastoid fluid accumulation/infection.

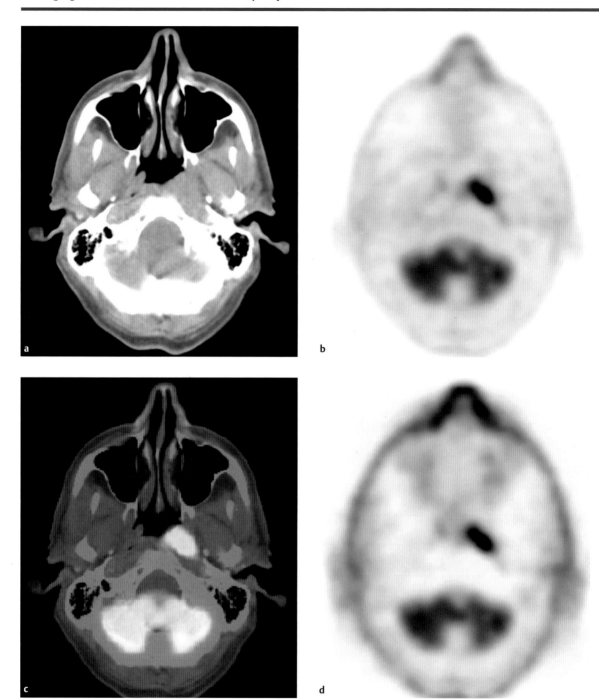

Fig. 5.16a–d PET-CT demonstrating a hypermetabolic lesion in the left fossa of Rosenmüller. While the axial CT images (**a**) do demonstrate some asymmetry of the nasopharynx, this lesion was occult clinically and on initial radiographic examination. The hypermetabolic activity of the lesion makes it relatively easy to detect on PET (**b, d**) and the fused PET-CT (**c**) localizes the area of activity to the correct anatomical structure.

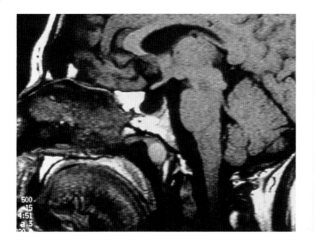
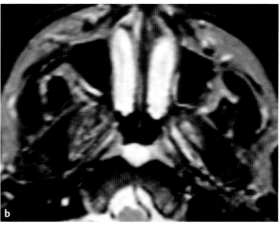

Fig. 5.17a, b Sagittal T1W (**a**) and axial T2W (**b**) weighted MRI demonstrating a Thornwaldt's cyst in the midline nasopharynx. Note the bright signal on T1W, likely reflective of proteinaceous contents, and T2W, reflective of cystic nature.

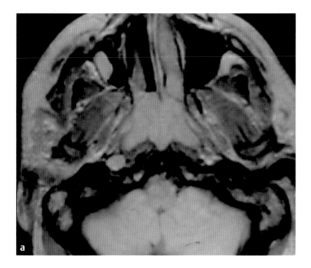
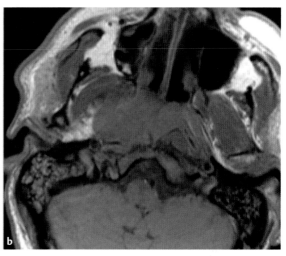

Fig. 5.18a, b Adenoidal hyperplasia in a young patient, demonstrating relatively homogeneous symmetric hyperplasia (**a**); note intact nasopharyngeal landmarks including posterior nasopharyngeal margins and parapharyngeal space. Nasopharyngeal carcinoma in the right posterior nasopharynx, demonstrating asymmetry and prevertebral extension (**b**).

Neoplastic

Benign

Benign Mixed Tumor—Pleomorphic Adenoma

On CT this tumor of minor salivary gland origin has a sharply demarcated solitary appearance, and is isodense to muscle with minimal enhancement after contrast administration.[49] Given its slow growth, it can remodel the bony architecture. On MRI it is isointense on T1W and hyperintense on T2W images. Central low-intensity areas on T2W images may represent focal calcifications. On T1W C+ images in general the enhancement is homogeneous. They are found, in decreasing order, in the soft palate, lingual and faucial tonsils, and nasopharynx. It is the most common salivary gland tumor and 85% are in the parotid gland; 6.5% arise from the minor salivary glands along the pharyngeal and oral mucosal spaces.

Malignant

Squamous Cell Carcinoma

This entity arises from the mucosa of the nasopharynx and has three histological subtypes: keratinizing squamous cell carcinoma (SCCa) (WHO type 1), nonkeratinizing SCCa (WHO type 2), and undifferentiated SCCa (WHO type 3).

This lesion may be asymptomatic and may come to the clinician's attention as a result of metastatic lymphadenopathy, unilateral conductive hearing loss due to otitis media, or possibly nasal bloody discharge. However, it is often clinically occult early in the course of the disease and may be detected incidentally on imaging for other reasons (Fig. 5.19).

On CT with contrast, nasopharyngeal carcinoma typically appears as a mildly enhancing mass arising in the lateral pharyngeal recess and/or posterolateral nasal wall. The lesion may be focal and mucosal in location; however, lateral extension into the parapharyngeal space and masticator space is common. In more advanced cases the lesion will extend into the carotid space, with subsequent extension to the intracranial compartment. The presence of metastatic nodes is common. With increased size and extension, the lesion may erode the clival cortex, pterygoid plates, and posterior skull base (Fig. 5.20a–c).

On MRI, the mass is typically isointense to muscle on T1W imaging. Bone invasion is shown as abnormally low signal intensity (Fig. 5.20d–f). Asymmetric fat obliteration is the "sign" of perineural neoplastic spread (see Fig. 5.13). These lesions are also typically mildly hyperintense on T2W imaging, but remain lower in signal intensity compared with inflammatory disease. Lesions typically demonstrate mild enhancement on postcontrast T1W imaging. Axial and coronal images are optimal for distinguishing the neoplasm from adjacent normal structures. Coronal imaging is optimal for detecting cavernous sinus and intracranial extension.

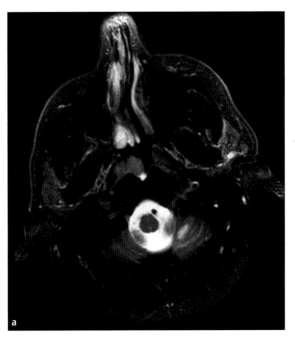
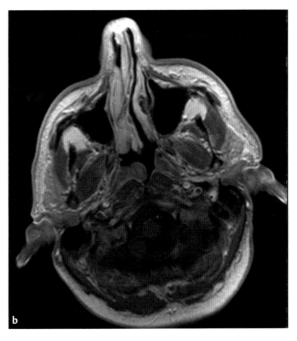

Fig. 5.19a, b Axial T2W (**a**) and postcontrast axial T1W (**b**) MRI demonstrating a small lobular mass in the right fossa of Rosenmüller, in an MRI of the brain performed for follow-up evaluation of a primary brain tumor.

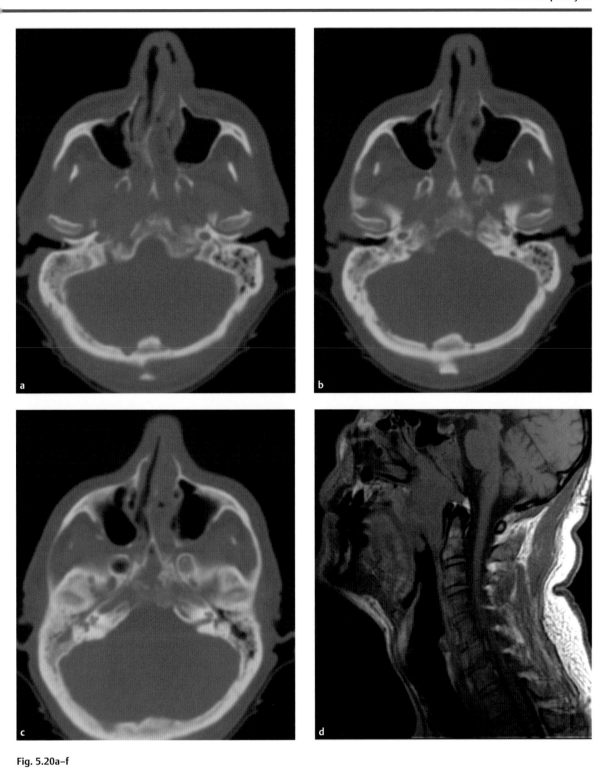

Fig. 5.20a–f

a–c Axial CT of the skull base demonstrating an infiltrating soft tissue mass, in this case a squamous cell carcinoma, eroding and invading the occiput and clivus.

d Sagittal T1W MRI demonstrating an isointense mass in the posterior nasopharynx; note the low signal within the mildly expanded clivus, a sign of bony extension.

Fig. 5.20e–f ▷

◁ continued

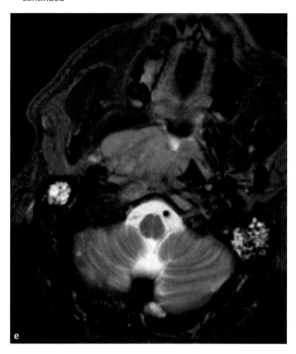

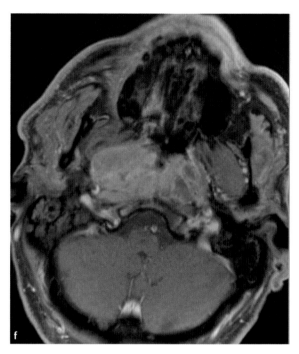

e Axial T2W MRI demonstrating relatively isointense signal of a large posterior nasopharyngeal mass; also note the bilateral mastoid effusions.

f Axial postcontrast T1W MRI of the same mass, demonstrating mild heterogeneous enhancement.

Minor Salivary Gland Malignancies

These are aggressive neoplasms arising from the minor salivary glands in the pharyngomucosal space and typically infiltrate deeply into the adjacent spaces. The most common location is the soft palate area, but these can also occur in the mucosa of the sinonasal tract, the tongue, the lingual tonsil, and the pharyngeal mucosa. On CT and MRI these lesions are characterized by an invasive lesion with infiltrating margins. Moderate enhancement is present on postcontrast images.[50]

Non-Hodgkin's lymphoma

This is an extranodal lymphatic neoplasm, and in the nasopharynx arises in the Waldeyer ring. Non-Hodgkin's lymphoma is five times more common in the head and neck area than is Hodgkin's lymphoma.[51] The pharyngomucosal space is its most common extranodal site, with 35% in the nasopharyngeal adenoid.[52]

On imaging studies it presents as a large mass in the pharyngomucosal space with associated cervical lymphadenopathy in >50% of cases.

On CT, a bulky mass will be present in the nasopharynx, with minimal enhancement without deep extension into the adjacent spaces. The mass is likely to be bilateral and associated with enlarged nonnecrotic nodes. If the associated nodes are necrotic, an association with AIDS needs to be considered.

On MRI, T1W imaging reveals a large mass that is typically isointense to muscle. On T2W imaging, the lesion is usually homogeneously hyperintense. Lesions will demonstrate homogeneous enhancement on postcontrast imaging.

Staging

MRI is optimal for the evaluation and staging of known nasopharyngeal SCCa. Bone-windowed CT images are optimal for evaluation of bone erosion due to direct invasion, although noncontrast T1W MRI is superior for showing the extent of bone involvement.[53] MRI is optimal for the evaluation of intraorbital and intracranial direct perivascular and/or perineural extension.[54]

Direct Patterns of Spread

Anteriorly, lesions typically extend into the pterygopalatine fossa and the nasal cavity, with associated obstruction of the eustachian tube. Superiorly, lesions can spread into the sphenoid sinus, the anterior clivus, the foramen lacerum tracking along the carotid canal, and perineurally along V_3 through the foramen ovale. Posteriorly, tumors can extend through the retropharyngeal space into the prevertebral musculature. This is an ominous extension best diagnosed with MRI, which shows the neoplasm "piercing" into the musculature. Laterally, lesions can extend into the parapharyngeal space, which affords a direct extension to the skull base and intracranial compartment. Inferiorly, the mass may extend into the oropharynx.[55]

Nodal Metastatic Disease

Lymph node metastases are present in 90% of squamous cell carcinoma patients upon presentation, affecting the retropharyngeal, deep cervical, and spinal accessory nodes.[56] This high percentage is due to the fact that these tumors remain clinically occult until they become quite large and begin impinging upon other structures.

The lymphatic drainage of the nasopharynx is largely through the retropharyngeal and jugulodigastric nodes. Occasionally lymphatic vessels will pass to the spinal accessory and midjugular nodes. Postcontrast T1W and T2W imaging is optimal for retropharyngeal nodes. However, in all other neck areas contrast-enhanced CT is equivalent to MRI for pathological node detection.

Imaging Following Treatment, Including Surgery and Radiation

As with sinonasal malignancy, following surgical, radiation, and chemotherapy treatment of patients with malignant nasopharyngeal tumors, a combined close interval clinical and radiological follow-up is typically employed.[57] This is both to assess for tumor recurrence and to detect treatment-related pathology, which was discussed in the previous section.

As with sinonasal malignancies, distinguishing postsurgical scarring or granulation tissue from residual or recurrent neoplasm in the nasopharynx is the most challenging aspect of follow-up imaging. Inflammatory disease can often be distinguished by its hyperintense appearance on T2W MRI. Early granulation tissue can also have a hyperintense appearance on T2W imaging. However, granulation tissue can have similar CT and MRI appearance to neoplasm, demonstrating hypointensity on T2W imaging and enhancing after contrast administration. Posttreatment MRI at 3 months can provide a baseline for subsequent studies, which may help distinguish these by demonstrating stability or even regression of scar tissue.

PET-CT examinations can be particularly helpful when local recurrence or distant metastasis are suspected post treatment which may not be easily detected with MRI. This imaging modality may also be useful in assessing the response to therapy. MRI also demonstrates a high degree of accuracy in detecting residual and/or recurrent NPC at the primary tumor site. Combined use of MRI and FDG PET/CT may be more accurate for tumor restaging than when either modality is used independently.[58]

Conclusion

Imaging techniques and technology are essential in the diagnosis of patients with sinonasal disease as well as nasopharyngeal pathology. In the last three decades, imaging has revolutionized the care of patients with inflammatory, infectious, and neoplastic diseases of the paranasal sinuses, maxillofacial area, and neck. The introduction of routine CT and MRI assessment has had a significant impact on the management of patients with various pathologies, and has had a great influence on the treatment of neoplasms within the head and neck area.

Typically, a combination of CT and MRI is performed in the work-up of patients with suspected malignancy. There are many confounders in imaging, which occasionally make it difficult to distinguish inflammatory and infectious diseases from neoplasm. However, these two main imaging modalities can be used in a complementary fashion to help reduce this uncertainty, and to help stage, biopsy, and plan treatment of the wide variety of tumors.

In this chapter, we have described the current practice with regard to methods of imaging of the nose and paranasal sinuses and the nasopharynx; typical findings of the more common neoplasms of the nose and paranasal sinuses; and some of the pitfalls of diagnosis with imaging.

References

1. Branstetter BF IV, Weissman JL. Role of MR and CT in the paranasal sinuses. Otolaryngol Clin North Am 2005;38(6):1279–1299, x
2. Lloyd G, Lund VJ, Howard D, Savy L. Optimum imaging for sinonasal malignancy. J Laryngol Otol 2000; 114(7):557–562
3. Zinreich SJ, Kennedy DW, Rosenbaum AE, Gayler BW, Kumar AJ, Stammberger H. Paranasal sinuses: CT imaging requirements for endoscopic surgery. Radiology 1987;163(3):769–775
4. Mukherji SK, Drane WE, Mancuso AA, Parsons JT, Mendenhall WM, Stringer S. Occult primary tumors of the head and neck: detection with 2-[F-18] fluoro-2-deoxy-D-glucose SPECT. Radiology 1996;199(3):761–766
5. Rusthoven KE, Koshy M, Paulino AC. The role of fluoro-deoxyglucose positron emission tomography in cervical lymph node metastases from an unknown primary tumor. Cancer 2004;101(11):2641–2649
6. Rao VM, el-Noueam KI. Sinonasal imaging. Anatomy and pathology. Radiol Clin North Am 1998;36(5):921–939, vi
7. Zinreich SJ. Paranasal sinus imaging. Otolaryngol Head Neck Surg 1990;103(5 Pt 2):863–868, discussion 868–869
8. Laine FJ, Smoker WR. The ostiomeatal unit and endoscopic surgery: anatomy, variations, and imaging findings in inflammatory diseases. AJR Am J Roentgenol 1992;159(4):849–857
9. Rao VM, Sharma D, Madan A. Imaging of frontal sinus disease: concepts, interpretation, and technology. Otolaryngol Clin North Am 2001;34(1):23–39
10. Zinreich SJ. Imaging for staging of rhinosinusitis. Ann Otol Rhinol Laryngol Suppl 2004;193:19–23
11. Hähnel S, Ertl-Wagner B, Tasman AJ, Forsting M, Jansen O. Relative value of MR imaging as compared with CT in the diagnosis of inflammatory paranasal sinus disease. Radiology 1999;210(1):171–176

12. Aribandi M, McCoy VA, Bazan C III. Imaging features of invasive and noninvasive fungal sinusitis: a review. Radiographics 2007;27(5):1283–1296

13. Mafee MF, Tran BH, Chapa AR. Imaging of rhinosinusitis and its complications: plain film, CT, and MRI. Clin Rev Allergy Immunol 2006;30(3):165–186

14. Som PM, Shapiro MD, Biller HF, Sasaki C, Lawson W. Sinonasal tumors and inflammatory tissues: differentiation with MR imaging. Radiology 1988;167(3):803–808

15. Rassi SJ, Melkane AE, Rizk HG, Dahoui HA. Sinonasal mucormycosis in immunocompromised pediatric patients. J Pediatr Hematol Oncol 2009;31(12):907–910

16. Silverman CS, Mancuso AA. Periantral soft-tissue infiltration and its relevance to the early detection of invasive fungal sinusitis: CT and MR findings. AJNR Am J Neuroradiol 1998;19(2):321–325

17. DelGaudio JM, Swain RE Jr, Kingdom TT, Muller S, Hudgins PA. Computed tomographic findings in patients with invasive fungal sinusitis. Arch Otolaryngol Head Neck Surg 2003;129(2):236–240

18. Fellows DW, King VD, Conturo T, Bryan RN, Merz WG, Zinreich SJ. In vitro evaluation of MR hypointensity in Aspergillus colonies. AJNR Am J Neuroradiol 1994; 15(6):1139–1144

19. Grindler D, Cannady S, Batra PS. Computed tomography findings in sinonasal Wegener's granulomatosis. Am J Rhinol Allergy 2009;23(5):497–501

20. Lohrmann C, Uhl M, Warnatz K, Kotter E, Ghanem N, Langer M. Sinonasal computed tomography in patients with Wegener's granulomatosis. J Comput Assist Tomogr 2006;30(1):122–125

21. Kim EY, Kim HJ, Chung SK, et al. Sinonasal organized hematoma: CT and MR imaging findings. AJNR Am J Neuroradiol 2008;29(6):1204–1208

22. Eller R, Sillers M. Common fibro-osseous lesions of the paranasal sinuses. Otolaryngol Clin North Am 2006; 39(3):585–600, x

23. MacDonald-Jankowski DS. Fibro-osseous lesions of the face and jaws. Clin Radiol 2004;59(1):11–25

24. Ricalde P, Horswell BB. Craniofacial fibrous dysplasia of the fronto-orbital region: a case series and literature review. J Oral Maxillofac Surg 2001;59(2):157–167, discussion 167–168

25. Goyal N, Jones M, Sandison A, Clarke PM. Maxillary haemangioma. J Laryngol Otol 2006;120(2):e14

26. Yousem DM, Fellows DW, Kennedy DW, Bolger WE, Kashima H, Zinreich SJ. Inverted papilloma: evaluation with MR imaging. Radiology 1992;185(2):501–505

27. Melroy CT, Senior BA. Benign sinonasal neoplasms: a focus on inverting papilloma. Otolaryngol Clin North Am 2006;39(3):601–617, x

28. Ojiri H, Ujita M, Tada S, Fukuda K. Potentially distinctive features of sinonasal inverted papilloma on MR imaging. AJR Am J Roentgenol 2000;175(2):465–468

29. Schuster JJ, Phillips CD, Levine PA. MR of esthesioneuroblastoma (olfactory neuroblastoma) and appearance after craniofacial resection. AJNR Am J Neuroradiol 1994;15(6):1169–1177

30. Schick B, Kahle G. Radiological findings in angiofibroma. Acta Radiol 2000;41(6):585–593

31. Resto VA, Deschler DG. Sinonasal malignancies. Otolaryngol Clin North Am 2004;37(2):473–487

32. Raghavan P, Phillips CD. Magnetic resonance imaging of sinonasal malignancies. Top Magn Reson Imaging 2007;18(4):259–267

33. Greene FL. The American Joint Committee on Cancer: updating the strategies in cancer staging. Bull Am Coll Surg 2002;87(7):13–15

34. Loevner LA, Sonners AI. Imaging of neoplasms of the paranasal sinuses. Neuroimaging Clin N Am 2004; 14(4):625–646

35. Kau RJ, Alexiou C, Laubenbacher C, Werner M, Schwaiger M, Arnold W. Lymph node detection of head and neck squamous cell carcinomas by positron emission tomography with fluorodeoxyglucose F 18 in a routine clinical setting. Arch Otolaryngol Head Neck Surg 1999;125(12):1322–1328

36. Kutler DI, Wong RJ, Schoder H, Kraus DH. The current status of positron-emission tomography scanning in the evaluation and follow-up of patients with head and neck cancer. Curr Opin Otolaryngol Head Neck Surg 2006;14(2):73–81

37. Sumi M, Sakihama N, Sumi T, et al. Discrimination of metastatic cervical lymph nodes with diffusion-weighted MR imaging in patients with head and neck cancer. AJNR Am J Neuroradiol 2003;24(8):1627–1634

38. Fischbein NJ, Noworolski SM, Henry RG, Kaplan MJ, Dillon WP, Nelson SJ. Assessment of metastatic cervical adenopathy using dynamic contrast-enhanced MR imaging. AJNR Am J Neuroradiol 2003;24(3):301–311

39. Anzai Y. Superparamagnetic iron oxide nanoparticles: nodal metastases and beyond. Top Magn Reson Imaging 2004;15(2):103–111

40. Eisen MD, Yousem DM, Montone KT, et al. Use of preoperative MR to predict dural, perineural, and venous sinus invasion of skull base tumors. AJNR Am J Neuroradiol 1996;17(10):1937–1945

41. Yu T, Xu YK, Li L, et al. Esthesioneuroblastoma methods of intracranial extension: CT and MR imaging findings. Neuroradiology 2009;51(12):841–850

42. Lapela M, Eigtved A, Jyrkkiö S, et al. Experience in qualitative and quantitative FDG PET in follow-up of patients with suspected recurrence from head and neck cancer. Eur J Cancer 2000;36(7):858–867

43. Greven KM, Williams DW III, Keyes JW Jr, et al. Positron emission tomography of patients with head and neck carcinoma before and after high dose irradiation. Cancer 1994;74(4):1355–1359

44. Chong VE, Fan YF. Radiation-induced temporal lobe necrosis. AJNR Am J Neuroradiol 1997;18(4):784–785

45. Martí-Fàbregas J, Montero J, López-Villegas D, Quer M. Post-irradiation neuromyotonia in bilateral facial and trigeminal nerve distribution. Neurology 1997;48(4):1107–1109

46. Weber AL, al-Arayedh S, Rashid A. Nasopharynx: clinical, pathologic, and radiologic assessment. Neuroimaging Clin N Am 2003;13(3):465–483

47. Chong VF, Khoo JB, Fan YF. Imaging of the nasopharynx and skull base. Neuroimaging Clin N Am 2004;14(4):695–719

48. Ikushima I, Korogi Y, Makita O, et al. MR imaging of Tornwaldt's cysts. AJR Am J Roentgenol 1999;172(6):1663–1665

49. Becelli R, Frati R, Cerulli G, Perugini M, Frati A, Lannetti G. Pleomorphic adenoma of the minor salivary glands of the palate. J Exp Clin Cancer Res 2001;20(1):25–28

50. Sigal R, Monnet O, de Baere T, et al. Adenoid cystic carcinoma of the head and neck: evaluation with MR imaging and clinical-pathologic correlation in 27 patients. Radiology 1992;184(1):95–101

51. Weber AL, Rahemtullah A, Ferry JA. Hodgkin and non-Hodgkin lymphoma of the head and neck: clinical, pathologic, and imaging evaluation. Neuroimaging Clin N Am 2003;13(3):371–392

52. King AD, Lei KI, Richards PS, Ahuja AT. Non-Hodgkin's lymphoma of the nasopharynx: CT and MR imaging. Clin Radiol 2003;58(8):621–625

53. Daffner RH, Lupetin AR, Dash N, Deeb ZL, Sefczek RJ, Schapiro RL. MRI in the detection of malignant infiltration of bone marrow. AJR Am J Roentgenol 1986;146(2):353–358

54. Nishioka T, Shirato H, Kagei K, et al. Skull-base invasion of nasopharyngeal carcinoma: magnetic resonance imaging

findings and therapeutic implications. Int J Radiat Oncol Biol Phys 2000;47(2):395–400

55. Dubrulle F, Souillard R, Hermans R. Extension patterns of nasopharyngeal carcinoma. Eur Radiol 2007;17(10): 2622–2630

56. Gross ND, Ellingson TW, Wax MK, Cohen JI, Andersen PE. Impact of retropharyngeal lymph node metastasis in head and neck squamous cell carcinoma. Arch Otolaryngol Head Neck Surg 2004;130(2):169–173

57. Ng SH, Liu HM, Ko SF, Hao SP, Chong VF. Posttreatment imaging of the nasopharynx. Eur J Radiol 2002;44(2):82–95

58. Comoretto M, Balestreri L, Borsatti E, Cimitan M, Franchin G, Lise M. Detection and restaging of residual and/or recurrent nasopharyngeal carcinoma after chemotherapy and radiation therapy: comparison of MR imaging and FDG PET/CT. Radiology 2008;249(1):203–211

Section IB Histological Types of Tumor

6 Epithelial Epidermoid Tumors

Benign Epidermoid Tumors

- Squamous papillomas of the nasal vestibule
- Everted squamous papilloma ICD-O 8121/1
- Cylindrical cell papilloma
- Inverted papilloma ICD-O 8121/1

Squamous Papillomas of the Nasal Vestibule

These lesions are very common and can occur at any age. They occur equally in men and women. Small, solitary cauliflower-like pedunculated lesions, they are similar to verrucous warts elsewhere in the body. They may be viral in origin and have been reported as undergoing spontaneous regression. They are composed of exophytic squamous proliferation associated with marked proliferation. They do not undergo malignant change and are locally resected. However, if they recur, the area may need to be "cauterized" with a laser.

Papillomas of the Nasal Cavity and Paranasal Sinuses

These are usually divided into three types:
1. Everted
2. Cylindrical cell
3. Inverted

Originally it was thought that all papillomas had a similar derivation and they were often lumped together as "schneiderian" papilloma, but subsequent investigation suggests that they are three distinct entities.[1] The term "schneiderian" refers to an anatomist, Victor Conrad Schneider, from the early 17th century. The sinonasal epithelium is derived from ectoderm, unlike the rest of the respiratory tract, which is endodermal and is sometimes referred to as "transitional" but should not be confused with urogenital epithelium. In fact, both terms (schneiderian and transitional) are best avoided. In 1847 Kramer used the term "papillae" to describe a cauliflower-like tumor of the mucous membrane.[2] Billroth probably first described a true papilloma in the nasal cavity, but Ringetz described the inverting nature of a papilloma in 1938.[3,4]

Everted Squamous Papilloma

Definition

Wartlike exophytic or fungiform squamous papilloma.

Etiology

There has been some confusion in the literature due to the consideration of different types of papilloma, but on balance there is evidence that everted papillomas are associated with human papilloma virus (HPV) 6/11[5] and are regarded by some as a simple wart.

Synonyms

Exophytic, squamous, transitional, and fungiform are all sometimes applied to these papillomas.

Incidence and Site

Everted papillomas usually grow on the septum though are occasionally found on the lateral wall of the nose and rarely in the maxillary sinus. Overall they are rare in ENT, comprising only 6 cases compared with 114 inverted papillomas in our own series.

Diagnostic Features

Clinical

A unilateral warty lesion growing in the anterior nose is often visible and results in nasal obstruction (**Fig. 6.1**). The lesion is more common in men and at a slightly younger age than with other papillomas. There were 5 men and 1 woman in our group, average age 47.3 years (age range 40 to 59 years).

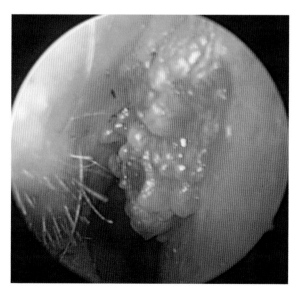

Fig. 6.1 Endoscopic view of everted papilloma in the right nasal vestibule.

Imaging

Imaging is rarely undertaken due to the superficial and accessible nature of the lesions, but they have the non-specific appearances of a benign soft tissue mass.

Histological Features and Differential Diagnosis

The exophytic pink lesions may have a firm, convoluted surface arising from a broad base and are characterized by numerous branching fronds of mucosa over a fibro-vascular connective tissue core, covered by stratified squamous epithelium. Large cystic mucus-filled spaces can be seen throughout the epithelium and occasionally microabscesses.

They must be distinguished from papillary squamous cell carcinoma, from inverted and cylindrical papillomas, and also from the squamous papillomas that grow on vestibular skin, which are identical to those which occur elsewhere on the skin.

Natural History

The everted papillomas may recur but virtually never become malignant.

Treatment and Outcome

Surgical removal with a small cuff of normal mucosa is usually adequate to obtain cure. However, in one case report concerning an HIV-positive patient, a combination of surgery and topical cidofovir was employed.[6]

Cylindrical Cell Papilloma

Definition

A papilloma composed of papillae lined with columnar epithelium.

Etiology

These lesions are not associated with human papillomavirus.

Synonyms

Oncocytic schneiderian papilloma, columnar cell papilloma, transitional cell papilloma, microcystic papillary adenoma.

Incidence

This lesion constitutes only 5% of sinonasal papillomas, being less frequent than its inverted counterparts. In our cohort of papillomas, there were 10 cylindrical cell papillomas compared with 114 inverted lesions.

Site

The lesion is found on the lateral nasal wall or within a sinus cavity.

Diagnostic Features

Clinical

These papillomas are usually unilateral and are reportedly equally commonly in men and women; our cases included 7 men and 3 women. They are rarely found in children; most patients are in their fifth and sixth decades. It is often broad-based with a finely granular surface. Our 10 cases have a mean age of 60 years (range 39 to 82 years).

Imaging

There are no specific features.

Histological Features and Differential Diagnosis

There is a mixture of endophytic and exophytic features and the tumor is characterized by a columnar oncocytic epithelium due to finely granular eosinophilic cytoplasm together with numerous intraepithelial mucinous cysts. These are larger than those found in inverted papilloma. Goblet cells are not present but microabscesses are seen.

Natural History

The tumor can be associated with squamous cell carcinoma or mucoepidermoid carcinoma.[7]

Treatment and Outcome

Complete excision is not associated with recurrence but has been reported in up to one-third of cases. All of our cases underwent local endoscopic excision without recurrence over a 2- to 12-year follow-up.

Inverted Papilloma

Definition

Inverted papilloma (IP) is a relatively uncommon benign epithelial tumor of the nasal cavity that is notorious for recurrence and malignant transformation.

Etiology

The role of human papilloma virus (HPV) has been investigated in inverted papilloma and its DNA has been found in both the inverted papilloma and the cells of neighboring normal-appearing mucosa.[8] This has led to the suggestion that all neighboring normal-appearing predisposed mucosa should be removed to reduce the rate of recurrence.[9] HPV 6 and 11 have been linked to the aggression of the papilloma in terms of presence of dysplasia, carcinoma in situ, and recurrence.[10] HPV57b has also been implicated in the etiology of the tumor.[11] It has also been suggested that Epstein-Barr virus may play a role.[12]

A case–control study of risk factors associated with sinonasal inverted papilloma in 50 patients suggested that outdoor and industrial occupations were associated with IP development.[13]

Malignant Transformation

The exact cause of malignant transformation has yet to be identified. Tumors with HPV positivity have been shown to be associated with significantly increased epidermoid growth factor receptor (EGFR) and Ki-67 index and, in turn, elevated levels of EGFR and transforming growth factor-α (TGF-α) are associated with early carcinogenesis.[14] Chao et al have also shown that EGFR is raised in IP both with and without malignant change compared with control tissue and proposed that this plays a role in malignant transformation.[15] In a review of the literature in 2008, Lawson and colleagues found that higher rates of HPV detection were found in dysplastic IP and those associated with malignant change.[16] Koo et al have recently shown that decreased expression of E-cadherin and β-catenin in the cell membrane may be associated with carcinogenesis of IP.[17]

Mutation of the *p53* tumor suppressor gene has been implicated as a risk factor for malignant transformation[18,19] and significantly increased staining of p21 and p53 has been observed in IP with severe dysplasia, carcinoma in situ, and frank carcinoma compared with normal controls,[20,21] and it has been suggested that screening for p21 might identify those at risk.[22] Serial measurement of fascin, an actin-binding protein that is raised in IP and strongly raised with associated malignant change, has also been proposed.[23]

A study by Huang et al has shown mRNA expression level for desmoglein 3 is significantly higher in IP than normal control tissue and strongly present in areas of malignant transformation, which might be helpful in prediction of change.[24]

Synonyms

Inverting papilloma, schneiderian papilloma.

Incidence

The frequency with which inverted papilloma (IP) is found in surgically removed nasal tumors varies from 0.5 to 4%,[25,26] with an incidence ranging from 0.6 to 1.5 cases per 100,000 inhabitants per year.[27,28] Another series considered the local population of Nottingham and, excluding tertiary referral cases, found the incidence was 4.3 cases per million per year.[29]

The frequency of IP in ostensibly normal bilateral polyps varies between 0% and 0.92%. Van Den Boer and colleagues examined material from 1,944 endoscopic procedures and found 37 unsuspected diagnoses, of which 18 were IP.[30] From this they concluded that routine examination of all tissue was not justified, a conclusion that we find surprising and which we do *not* endorse. Age, sex, and number of recurrences did not influence the frequency of this diagnosis.[31]

Site

It can be difficult to determine the precise site of origin with large lesions, but the ethmoid region, the lateral wall of the nasal fossa, and the maxillary sinus are the most frequent sites of origin of inverted papilloma. There is some radiological evidence that many IPs arise within the middle meatus and spread into the adjacent sinuses. The frontal sinus is exceedingly rare as a primary site of origin. IP is thought to originate in the ethmoid region in 48%, the maxillary sinus in 28%, the sphenoid sinus in 7.5%, the frontal sinus in 2.5%, the inferior turbinate in 2.5%, and the septum in 2.5%.[32,33] Distinction should be made between extension into the sinuses, with and without mucosal involvement, which can have a bearing on ease of removal and the surgical approach and may only be determined at operation.

In most cases IP is unilateral, although separate lesions can occasionally be seen seeded within the nasal cavity. However, bilateral involvement of the sinonasal tract is very rare, being reported in less than 1%[34-36] to 9%[37] of patients and in these instances malignancy should be suspected. In a personal series of 114 cases, there were 2 bilateral cases, both of which were associated with malignant change at presentation. In one case both frontal sinuses were separately affected and in the second the lateral wall and the floor of the nasal cavities.

Although IP most commonly arises from the lateral wall of the nasal cavity and extends into the paranasal sinuses, occasionally it may extend to the nasopharynx, and more rarely traverse the cribriform plate or orbit. While this may indicate malignant change, the authors have seen both significant intracranial and intraorbital extension in histologically proven benign IP, albeit extradural and extraperiosteal. Even intradural and intraperiosteal invasion has been described.[38] IPs rarely arise from the nasal septum[39] and this diagnosis would warrant close inspection as to whether the lesion is really inverted or not.

Diagnostic Features

Clinical

In the literature the age at onset ranges from 15 to 96 years, with the highest incidence occurring in the 5th and 6th decades of life.[40] The male-to-female ratio is reported as between 2:1 and 5:1[35,41] and no significant racial differences have been noted.[33] This has also been our experience (Table 6.1).

Inverted papilloma presents primarily with nasal obstruction and sometimes epistaxis. When the sphenoid is involved, patients may in addition experience neurological symptoms such as headache, visual disturbance, and even hearing loss due to eustachian obstruction.[32] The tumor can extend from any origin into the nasopharynx, mimicking an antrochoanal polyp. There may be epiphora if the papilloma affects the drainage of the nasolacrimal system. As it obstructs the adjacent sinuses it can occasionally cause a mucocele or expand sufficiently into the orbit to produce proptosis, but, as this occurs slowly, there is rarely diplopia. The duration of symptoms can vary from 5 months to 20 years with a mean duration of 3.9 years.[40] Conversely, some patients are asymptomatic and the papilloma is a chance finding.

Table 6.1 Inverted papilloma: personal series 1986–2010

n	Age		M:F	MFD	LR	ESS	ESS + AA or EFE	Recurrence	
	Range (y)	Mean (y)						Open	ESS
114	24–89	52.6	78:36	15	20	66	13	19%	8%

Abbreviations: EFE, external frontoethmoidectomy; ESS, endoscopic sinus surgery; ESS + AA or EFE, endoscopic sinus surgery + anterior antrostomy or external frontoethmoidectomy; F, female; LR, lateral rhinotomy; M, male; MFD, midfacial degloving; y, year(s).

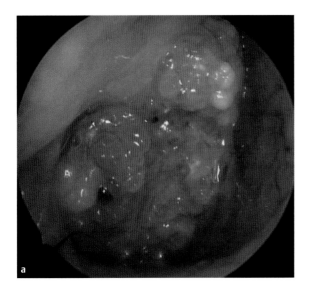

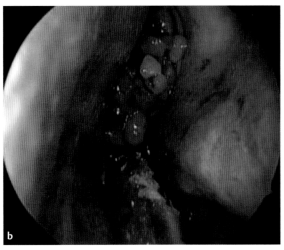

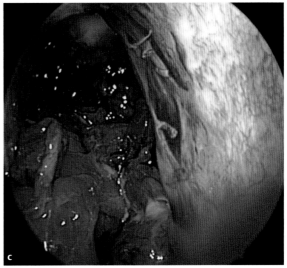

Fig. 6.2a–c Endoscopic views of inverted papilloma (IP).

a IP in the right middle meatus.

b IP in the left nasal cavity with a microdebrider.

c Recurrent IP coming out of the left maxillary sinus through a previous antrostomy.

In one patient in our series, a sphenoidal IP came to light as part of a routine work-up prior to liver transplantation.

The diagnosis of IP should be suspected in anyone with a unilateral nasal polyp.[42] On close inspection with endoscopy, they differ from "normal" polyps in that they have a cerebriform appearance often with small vessels running on the surface and are generally firm as opposed to the translucent or edematous softer polyps (**Fig. 6.2**).

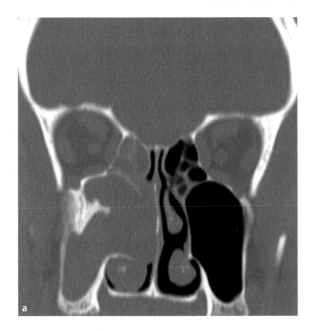

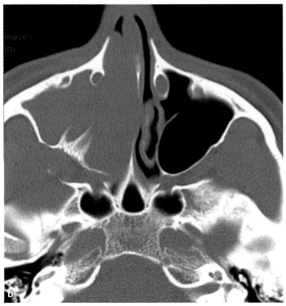

Fig. 6.3a, b

a Coronal CT scan showing inverted papilloma arising in the right maxilla and presenting in the nasal cavity with an area of hyperdensity on the lateral maxillary sinus wall.

b Axial CT scan in the same patient showing conelike areas of hyperdensity at the site of origin.

However, this is not always the case, especially with recurrent polyps, and papilloma may also be mixed with polypoid change. Therefore, when dealing with polypoid disease, it is important to send off for histology as much tissue as possible so as not to miss the diagnosis of IP and also to confirm or exclude malignancy.[42] Many patients give a history of repeated unilateral polypectomies before the diagnosis is finally made.

Imaging

CT is the principal mode of imaging as it will demonstrate a soft tissue mass and any bone erosion. Although this can occur without malignant transformation, it is more likely and more extensive when present. The characteristic features on CT are a lobulated mass continuous from the middle meatus into the adjacent maxillary antrum through a widened maxillary ostium. This gives a recognizable shape somewhat similar to that of the continent of Africa (**Fig. 6.3a**). The other even more classic signs of IP are the presence of hyperostosis or irregular sclerosis at the periosteal bone–tumor interface and flecks of hyperdensity within the papilloma, presumed to be calcification.[43–45] Two types of localized thickening have been described, a focal plaquelike hyperostosis and more prominent "cone-shaped" areas (**Fig. 6.3b, Fig. 6.4**).[46] There is a high correlation between the areas of hyperostosis and the tumor origin.[45–47]

MRI is helpful in determining the extent of the tumor from retained mucus and inflamed mucosa when there is opacification within the sinuses on CT[43,48] as this will assist in deciding the best surgical approach. This particularly applies to the lateral maxillary sinus, the frontal

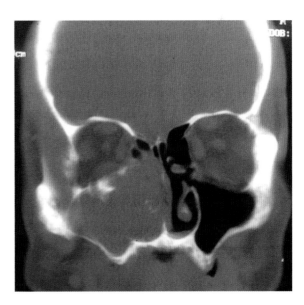

Fig. 6.4 Coronal CT scan showing opacification of the right maxillary sinus due to inverted papilloma with en-plaque area of hyperdensity on the roof of the sinus, which must be encompassed in subperiosteal dissection.

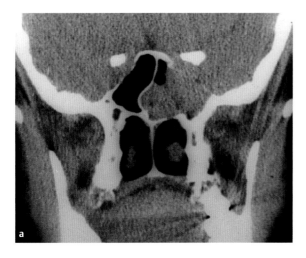
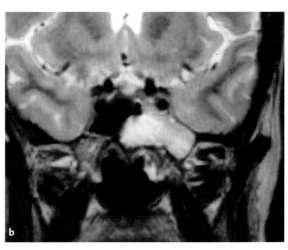

Fig. 6.5a, b

a Coronal CT scan showing opacification of the left sphenoid with bone erosion adjacent to the optic nerve and carotid artery.

b Coronal MRI scan (T2W) in the same patient showing the extent of papilloma and its relationship to lateral structures and excluding possible carotid aneurysm.

sinus, and, to a lesser extent, the orbit and skull base (**Fig. 6.5**). Enhanced T1W and T2W MRI is very accurate in this respect,[43,49] often showing a convoluted cerebriform pattern, whereas the areas of hyperostosis appear hypodense on T1W images. In addition the tumor often shows a striated or columnar pattern that is strongly associated with

IP (**Fig. 6.6**).[50,51] Thus the surgical approach can be more accurately determined by a combination of CT and MRI.[52]

Although IP usually shows homogeneous enhancement with intravenous gadolinium, there are no distinctive features that differentiate this tumor from others or show foci of malignancy[53] unless there are areas of

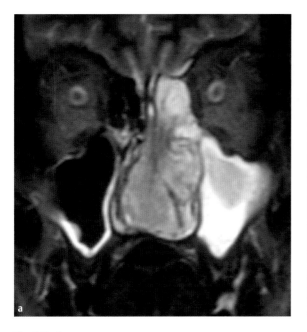
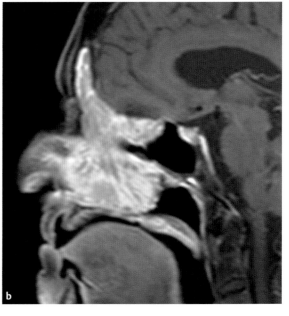

Fig. 6.6a, b

a Coronal MRI scan (STIR sequence) delineating inverted papilloma in the nasal cavity and adjacent sinuses from inflammatory mucosa and secretions.

b Sagittal MRI (T1W post gadolinium contrast) in the same patient showing classical striations in IP.

marked hypodensity.[51] Focal loss of the cerebriform pattern may also suggest malignant change.[49,50] Bone thinning and dehiscence can be seen in benign IP, but irregular erosion and infiltration into the adjacent soft tissues suggest malignant change (**Fig. 6.7**). It was thought that PET scanning might be useful in this respect but it has not fulfilled its early promise.[54,55]

The differential diagnosis on imaging includes acute on chronic rhinosinusitis as sclerosis of adjacent sinus bone can be seen in chronic inflammation/infection. The heterogeneous hyperdensity must be distinguished from allergic/eosinophilic fungal rhinosinusitis and chondrosarcoma. Other malignancies should be considered in the presence of bone erosion and soft tissue infiltration.

Histological Features and Differential Diagnosis

The term "inverted papilloma" describes the histological appearance of the epithelium inverting into the stroma with a distinct and intact basement membrane that separates and defines the epithelial component from the underlying connective tissue stroma. There are numerous twisting ducts within the stroma lined with maturing stratified squamous epithelium. Keratinization is usually absent as are submucous glands. Residual respiratory epithelium can be seen in the duct lining, which may be ciliated and have goblet cells.

Michaels and Hellquist (see ref. 1: pp. 179–181) regard the lesion as a severe form of squamous metaplasia, initially characterized by microcyst formation with marked apoptotic activity in the inflammatory cells that accumulate there.

Microscopically the tumor can be associated with atypia, dysplasia, carcinoma in situ, as well as overt squamous cell carcinoma, but in the past the frequency with which these changes occur has been overestimated, most likely due to the underdiagnosis of well-differentiated squamous cell carcinoma. Certain factors raise suspicion of malignant change,[56,57] including:

- Significant bone erosion
- Absence of inflammatory polyps
- Increased ratio of neoplastic epithelium to stroma
- Increased hyperkeratosis
- Presence of squamous hyperplasia
- High mitotic index
- Low numbers of eosinophils
- The presence of plasma cells

Malignancy can occur under two main circumstances:
1. Synchronous carcinoma—the carcinoma may arise from the papilloma itself or it may be found as a separate lesion.[58]
2. Metachronous carcinoma—the carcinoma arises at the site of a previously benign inverted papilloma.

In the literature the incidence of carcinoma associated with IP ranges from 0%[59] to 53%.[60] In an updated review of 65 published case series (3,181 patients)[61] (**Table 6.2**), 11 series found atypia in a total of 88 cases out of 958 patients (1.1%), 9 series noted dysplasia in 9 cases out of 454 patients (1.9%), and 10 series found carcinoma in situ in 15 cases out of 494 patients (3%). Overall 6.8% had synchronous carcinoma and 3.6% developed metachronous carcinoma. The majority were squamous cell carcinomas but there were also cases of transitional cell carcinoma, adenocarcinoma, mucoepidermoid carcinoma, and verrucous carcinoma. The mean time interval to developing

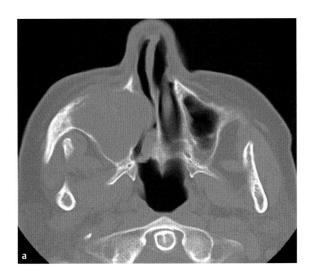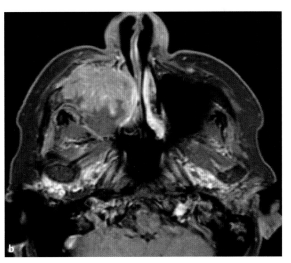

Fig. 6.7a, b

a Axial CT showing inverted papilloma with malignant change eroding the anterior wall of the maxilla and extending into the soft tissues of the cheek.

b Axial MRI (T1W post gadolinium fat saturation sequence) in the same patient showing tumor mass adjacent to the anterior wall with classical striations.

Table 6.2 Incidence of pathological changes in inverted papilloma

Pathology	Incidence/case series	Percentage
Atypia/number in case series	88/958	1.1
Dysplasia/number in case series	9/454	1.9
Carcinoma in situ/number in case series	15/494	3.0
Synchronous carcinoma/number in case series	165/2444	6.8
Metachronous carcinoma/number in case series (mean follow-up 52 months)	76/2114	3.6
Source: Modified from reference 61 with permission from *Rhinology*.[8,9,13,27,29,35,37,39,41,59–112]		

a metachronous carcinoma was 52 months (range 6–180 months). In our series we had 3 patients with carcinoma in situ change (2.6%), 8 with synchronous change (7%), and 5 (4%) with metachronous change.

No significant association between atypia or dysplasia and recurrence or malignant transformation was found, but the estimated malignant potential for recurrent disease is up to 11%.[29] However, these series are mainly from tertiary referral centers and are potentially biased to the more aggressive cases.

Some reports suggest that the development of squamous cell carcinoma in IP is heralded by a reduced cellular apoptosis, which is triggered by HPV infection.[113]

IP must be distinguished from well-differentiated squamous cell carcinoma, with which it may easily be confused (and vice versa) on small biopsies. While frozen section may be helpful in the diagnosis of IP,[114] determination of malignancy is a more difficult proposition. Nasal contact endoscopy may be applied as a noninvasive technique to diagnosis for IP and squamous cell carcinoma.[115]

Natural History

Generally IP is a slow-growing lesion that invaginates into the clefts of the lateral wall and ostia of adjacent sinuses, often forming a dumbbell mass between the maxillary sinus and nasal cavity. This leads to obstruction and mucus stasis within the sinuses. Initially the papilloma conforms to the anatomy but with time remodeling occurs, leading to expansion and bone erosion of the lateral wall and eventually the skull base. In addition, wherever the periosteal reaction of hyperostosis is seen on CT, IP should be assumed to be involving the adjacent mucosa. Failure to remove the affected periosteum and bone potentially leaves behind microscopic disease, hence most recurrences are in fact residual tumor although field change may also be a factor in some cases.[8] Thus the frequency of "recurrence" and malignant transformation has been exaggerated in the literature, but there is no question that it does occur and may do so after many years, so long-term follow-up is recommended except in the most straightforward of cases.

Staging

An inverted papilloma sometimes has a narrow pedicle, so it has been suggested by some that the site of tumor attachment, not volume,[116,117] should determine staging. However, of the various systems, the Krouse[118] and Cannady[119] systems seemed to correlate best with outcome according to Gras-Cabrerizo et al (**Table 6.3**).[120]

Treatment

Inverted papilloma requires surgical removal but, whatever the approach, all macroscopic tumor must be removed together with adjacent periosteum and any abnormal bone as well as a margin of "normal" mucosa, all of which should be submitted for detailed histopathology. This means that there must be access to facilitate a subperiosteal dissection and drilling of the underlying bone.

The choice of approach will depend on the extent of the disease. In the literature, surgery has ranged from a headlight intranasal polypectomy, to open approaches such as Caldwell-Luc procedures, lateral rhinotomy, midfacial degloving, and various external procedures on the frontal sinus (**Table 6.4**). The endoscopic resections may also be combined with external approaches such as anterior antrostomy.

In recent years, the majority of cases have been amenable to a completely endonasal endoscopic approach that encompasses an endoscopic medial maxillectomy,[105,124,125] median frontal sinus procedures (Draf III),[111] and resection of the skull base. This provides similar access to the major external procedures but with lower postoperative morbidity; as a consequence, IP was among the first and commonest tumors for which endoscopic surgery was undertaken. Endoscopic techniques avoid a facial or sublabial incisions, paresthesia or facial pain, epiphora, and diplopia and are associated with a shorter inpatient stay. In addition, the endoscope offers improved visualization with enhanced discrimination of tumor from normal tissue. With modern camera systems the magnification gives better visibility and the lens systems allow visualization around corners.

Table 6.3 Staging systems for inverted papilloma

Author	Staging system
Krouse[118]	**Type 1**: Tumor totally confined to the nasal cavity. The tumor can be localized to one wall or region of the nasal cavity, or can be bulky and extensive within the nasal cavity, but must not extend into the sinuses or into any extranasal compartment. There must be no concurrent malignancy
	Type 2: Tumor involving the ostiomeatal complex, and ethmoid sinuses, and/or the medial portion of the maxillary sinus, with or without involvement of the nasal cavity. There must be no concurrent malignancy
	Type 3: Tumor involving the lateral, inferior, superior, anterior, or posterior walls of the maxillary sinus, the sphenoid sinus, and/or the frontal sinus, with or without involvement of the medial portion of the maxillary sinus, the ethmoid sinuses, or the nasal cavity. There must be no concurrent malignancy
	Type 4: All tumors with any extranasal/extrasinus extension to involve adjacent, contiguous structures such as the orbit, the intracranial compartment, or the pterygomaxillary space. All tumors associated with malignancy
Han et al[121]	**Group 1**: Tumor involvement limited to the nasal cavity, lateral nasal wall, medial maxillary sinus, ethmoid sinus, and sphenoid sinus
	Group 2: Same as group 1 except that tumor extends lateral to the medial maxillary wall
	Group 3: Tumor extends to involve the frontal sinus
	Group 4: Tumor extends outside the sinonasal cavities (i.e., orbital or intracranial extension)
Kamel et al[122]	**Type 1**: Tumor originating from the nasal septum or lateral nasal wall
	Type 2: Tumor originating from the maxillary sinus
	(This classification focuses on origin and not size/extent of tumor—does not analyze frontal sinus separately)
Oikawa et al[123]	**T1**: Tumor limited to nasal cavity
	T2: Tumor limited to ethmoid sinus and/ or medial and superior portions of maxillary sinus
	T3: Tumor involves lateral, inferior, anterior, or posterior walls of maxillary sinus, sphenoid sinus, or frontal sinus
	T3-A: Without extension to frontal sinus or supraorbital recess
	T3-B: Involving frontal sinus or supraorbital recess
	T4: Tumor extends outside sinonasal cavities (orbital or intracranial extension) or associated with malignancy
Cannady et al[119]	**Group A**: Inverted papilloma confined to the nasal cavity, ethmoid sinuses, or medial maxillary wall
	Group B: Inverted papilloma with involvement of any maxillary wall (other than the medial wall), or frontal sinus, or sphenoid sinus
	Group C: Inverted papilloma with extension beyond the paranasal sinuses

Source: Modified from reference 61 with permission from *Rhinology*.

Table 6.4 Treatment strategies for excision of inverted papilloma

Tumor extent	Approach
Limited to middle meatus, ethmoids, sphenoid, frontonasal recess	Endoscopic
Extension to lateral, inferior, anterior wall of maxillary sinus	Endoscopic medial maxillectomy ± anterior antrostomy
Extension to skull base, nasolacrimal region and orbit	Extended radical endoscopic resection ± preservation of nasolacrimal duct ± repair skull base
Extension into frontal sinus with mucosal involvement up to midpoint of orbit	Endoscopic frontal sinus procedure, e.g., Draf III
Extension into frontal sinus with mucosal involvement beyond midpoint of orbit	Endoscopic and external frontal sinus procedures

However, there are circumstances when the endoscopic approach may need to be combined with additional surgery. If mucosal involvement by tumor extends laterally beyond the midpoint of the orbit, an additional small external incision is required. If the anterior, inferior, or lateral walls of the maxillary sinus are extensively involved, an anterior antrostomy (modified Caldwell-Luc) may also be done to facilitate complete periosteal resection and drilling of adjacent bone. However, as mentioned above, the endoscopic medial maxillectomy has reduced the need for additional open approaches.[124,125]

More extensive surgery may also be necessitated by scarring of the frontal recess, distortion from previous surgery, very advanced disease, and associated malignancy.[33] In a series of 87 cases of IP, 78% of whom had primary disease, 70% could be removed by an endonasal endoscopic approach but 23% required combined procedures. These were mainly those who were undergoing revision surgery.[107]

Outcome

It is hardly surprising that recurrence rates of up to 78% have been reported for conservative surgery comprising polypectomy or local excision.[41] However, historically, external procedures such as lateral rhinotomy and midfacial degloving represented the "gold-standard."[39,69,126] Vrabec[8] reported a recurrence rate of only 2% using a lateral rhinotomy with a modified Weber–Fergusson incision with a mean follow-up of 8.9 years, although a meta-analysis of the literature suggests an overall figure of 17% with a mean follow-up of over 5 years (**Table 6.5**). This is somewhat less than the 20% suggested by Busquets and Hwang.[127]

Comparable data are now available for endoscopic resection since it has now been undertaken for at least 25 years.[128] Mirza et al found that recurrence rates in 63 case series was 12.8% for endoscopic procedures (n = 484), 17.0% for lateral rhinotomy with medial maxillectomy (n = 1025) and 34.2% for limited resections such as nasal polypectomy (n = 600).[29] Giotakis and colleagues found very similar results in a cohort of 67 patients.[112] **Table 6.5** demonstrates that notwithstanding a shorter reported period of follow-up, similar results can be achieved

endoscopically with 14.7% recurring with a mean follow-up of 3 years and 3 months in a similar-sized cohort.

As recurrent disease usually occurs in the first 9 months[105] and generally with a mean of 30 months (range 14–48 months),[129] the recurrence rates for the endoscopic group can legitimately and favorably be compared with the external group.

There is less data for combined endoscopic and external techniques. However, Woodworth et al describe 24 patients who had undergone a combined endoscopic and Caldwell-Luc approach with one recurrence (mean follow-up of 40 months for the entire series of 114 patients).[130] In the Minovi et al series of 87 cases, during a follow-up period of 12 to 75 months (mean 74 months), overall recurrence was 10.3%—10% in the endonasal cases and 15% in those undergoing combined procedures.[107]

Many factors influence recurrence of IP: tumor location, extent, histology, multicentricity, method of removal, and length of follow-up; but the most important is the thoroughness of removal[39] irrespective of the approach.[41] In other words, the "recurrence" is most often at the original site (**Table 6.6; Figs. 6.8 and 6.9**).[128] In addition, Batsakis and others have cited a mitotic index of >2/high-power microscopic field, abundant plasma cells, cellular atypia, and keratosis.[131,132] Smoking has also been implicated, with a trend to multiple recurrence found by Jardine et al and Moon et al.[94,133]

Recurrence rates are higher in revision cases,[47,130] and once IP has recurred, the risk of subsequent recurrence increases to up to 58%.[76]

Based on the literature, follow-up should be for a minimum of 3 years. In primary cases where excision is considered complete and there are no other confounding factors, 3 years is adequate as most "recurrences" occur within the first 9 months and mean recurrence time in general with endoscopic surgery is 28 months.[107] However, if the case has already recurred, if a combined approach was needed, if there are concerns about the adequacy of the excision, or if the tumor shows signs of aggressiveness in its behavior or histology, long-term observation is required. Histologically, this would include hyperkeratosis, squamous epithelial hyperplasia, and a high mitotic index.[56,57,131,132] Postoperative follow-up

Table 6.5 Recurrence rates of inverted papilloma

Surgical approach	Recurrence/case series	Percentage	Mean follow-up
Endoscopic resection	226/1532	14.7	3 y 3 mo (documented in 952)
Open procedures, e.g., lateral rhinotomy, mid facial degloving	234/1371	17	5 y 2 mo (documented in 899)
Limited resection such as nasal polypectomy	208/606	34.4	Inadequate data
Abbreviations: mo, month(s); y, year(s). Source: Modified from reference 61 with permission of *Rhinology*.[8,9,27,29,33,35,37,39,41,47,59–111,113,126–153]			

Table 6.6 When "recurrence" is residual disease

Not suspected (e.g., multiple "polypectomies")
Length of follow-up <3 years
Inadequate removal • Site of origin • Involved bone
Extent of origin/multifocal
Wrong diagnosis—bilateral (e.g., well-differentiated squamous cell carcinoma)

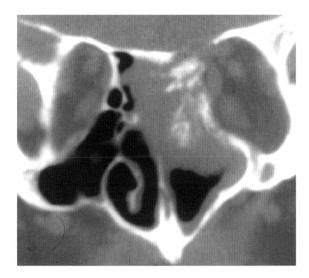

Fig. 6.8 Coronal CT showing recurrent inverted papilloma after multiple operations with areas of hyperdensity and bone erosion of the adjacent skull base and orbit.

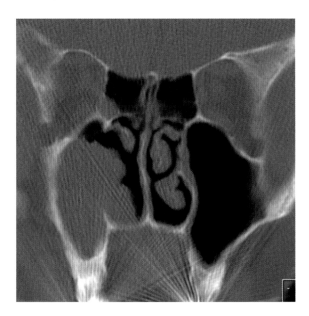

Fig. 6.9 Coronal CT showing "recurrent" or residual inverted papilloma in the right maxillary sinus with hyperostosis of the lateral wall.

imaging is not usually needed unless there are areas of concern that cannot be directly inspected endoscopically, such as the lateral frontal sinus. MRI would then be preferred to CT for sequential scans (**Fig. 6.10**).

If histology shows dysplasia or carcinoma in situ, a complete surgical resection may be sufficient provided the patient is available for long-term follow-up and the area is accessible to observation. However, if squamous cell carcinoma (or other malignancy) is demonstrated, a full oncological work-up and follow-up is indicated and postoperative radiotherapy at the least is recommended.[22] This is offered even in some cases of carcinoma in situ; for example, when the frontal sinus or skull base are affected. Experience and the literature suggest that malignancy ex inverted papilloma can be an aggressive tumor and requires radical treatment, so a more radical surgical excision may also be indicated depending on the initial resection.[113] About 40% of patients will die of their disease within the first 3 years in these circumstances.

Key Points

- Malignant transformation occurs but has been overestimated and occurs in <5%.
- All tissue should be submitted for histopathological examination.
- Recurrence can occur but usually represents residual disease.
- When complete removal is attempted, recurrence is found in 15 to 17% irrespective of the approach but is rare if subperiosteal resection ± adjacent bone is removed.
- A review of the literature shows that endoscopic removal of inverted papilloma gives results as good as, if not better than, those from external approaches.
- Three year follow-up is adequate if primary resection is complete, but should be continued longer if there are any concerns.
- Long-term follow-up is required for "recurrent" and extensive cases and those with hyperkeratosis, squamous epithelial hyperplasia, and a high mitotic index.

References

1. Michaels L, Hellquist H. Ear, Nose and Throat Histopathology. 2nd ed. Springer: London; 2001:177–179, 179–181
2. Kramer J [1847] Quoted in Kramer R, Som M. True papillomas of the nasal cavity. Arch Otolaryngol 1935;22:22–43
3. Billroth T. Ueber dem Bau des Schleimpolyp. Reimer: Berlin; 1870:11
4. Ringetz N. Pathology of malignant tumours arising in the nasal and paranasal cavities and maxilla. Acta Otolaryngol 1938;(Suppl 27):31–42
5. Gaffey MJ, Frierson HF, Weiss LM, Barber CM, Baber GB, Stoler MH. Human papillomavirus and Epstein-Barr virus in sinonasal Schneiderian papillomas. An in situ hybridization and polymerase chain reaction study. Am J Clin Pathol 1996;106(4):475–482

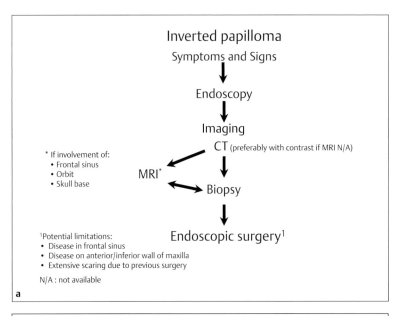

Inverted papilloma
Symptoms and Signs

Endoscopy

Imaging

CT (preferably with contrast if MRI N/A)

MRI*

Biopsy

Endoscopic surgery[1]

* If involvement of:
• Frontal sinus
• Orbit
• Skull base

[1]Potential limitations:
• Disease in frontal sinus
• Disease on anterior/inferior wall of maxilla
• Extensive scaring due to previous surgery

N/A : not available

a

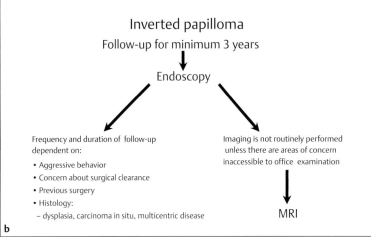

Inverted papilloma
Follow-up for minimum 3 years

Endoscopy

Frequency and duration of follow-up dependent on:
• Aggressive behavior
• Concern about surgical clearance
• Previous surgery
• Histology:
  – dysplasia, carcinoma in situ, multicentric disease

Imaging is not routinely performed unless there are areas of concern inaccessible to office examination

MRI

b

Fig. 6.10a, b Algorithms for management of inverted papilloma. (From Lund, Stammberger, Nicolai et al[61] with permission of *Rhinology*.)

6. Capaccio P, Ottaviani F, Cuccarini V, et al. Surgery and topic cidofovir for nasal squamous papillomatosis in HIV+ patient. Eur Arch Otorhinolaryngol 2009;266(6):937–939
7. Ward BE, Fechner RE, Mills SE. Carcinoma arising in oncocytic Schneiderian papilloma. Am J Surg Pathol 1990;14(4):364–369
8. Vrabec DP. The inverted Schneiderian papilloma: a 25-year study. Laryngoscope 1994;104(5 Pt 1):582–605
9. Yoon JH, Kim CH, Choi EC. Treatment outcomes of primary and recurrent inverted papilloma: an analysis of 96 cases. J Laryngol Otol 2002;116(9):699–702
10. Beck JC, McClatchey KD, Lesperance MM, Esclamado RM, Carey TE, Bradford CR. Presence of human papillomavirus predicts recurrence of inverted papilloma. Otolaryngol Head Neck Surg 1995;113(1):49–55
11. Wu TC, Trujillo JM, Kashima HK, Mounts P. Association of human papillomavirus with nasal neoplasia. Lancet 1993;341(8844):522–524
12. Macdonald MR, Le KT, Freeman J, Hui MF, Cheung RK, Dosch H-M. A majority of inverted sinonasal papillomas carries Epstein-Barr virus genomes. Cancer 1995;75(9):2307–2312

13. Sham CL, Lee DL, van Hasselt CA, Tong MC. A case-control study of the risk factors associated with sinonasal inverted papilloma. Am J Rhinol Allergy 2010;24(1):e37–e40
14. Katori H, Nozawa A, Tsukuda M. Markers of malignant transformation of sinonasal inverted papilloma. Eur J Surg Oncol 2005;31(8):905–911
15. Chao JC, Fang SY. Expression of epidermal growth factor receptor in the inverted papilloma and squamous cell carcinoma of nasal cavity. Eur Arch Otorhinolaryngol 2008;265(8):917–922
16. Lawson W, Schlecht NF, Brandwein-Gensler M. The role of the human papillomavirus in the pathogenesis of Schneiderian inverted papillomas: an analytic overview of the evidence. Head Neck Pathol 2008;2(2):49–59
17. Koo BS, Jung BJ, Kim SG, Liang ZL, Yeong MK, Rha KS. Altered expression of E-cadherin and beta-catenin in malignant transformation of sinonasal inverted papillomas. Rhinology 2011;49(4):479–485
18. Califano J, Koch W, Sidransky D, Westra WH. Inverted sinonasal papilloma : a molecular genetic appraisal of its putative status as a precursor to squamous cell carcinoma. Am J Pathol 2000;156(1):333–337

19. Eggers G, Mühling J, Hassfeld S. Inverted papilloma of paranasal sinuses. J Craniomaxillofac Surg 2007;35(1):21–29

20. Katori H, Nozawat A, Tsukuda M. Relationship between p21 and p53 expression, human papilloma virus infection and malignant transformation in sinonasal-inverted papilloma. Clin Oncol (R Coll Radiol) 2006;18(4):300–305

21. Altavilla G, Staffieri A, Busatto G, Canesso A, Giacomelli L, Marioni G. Expression of p53, p16INK4A, pRb, p21WAF1/CIP1, p27KIP1, cyclin D1, Ki-67 and HPV DNA in sinonasal endophytic Schneiderian (inverted) papilloma. Acta Otolaryngol 2009;129(11):1242–1249

22. Mendenhall WM, Hinerman RW, Malyapa RS, et al. Inverted papilloma of the nasal cavity and paranasal sinuses. Am J Clin Oncol 2007;30(5):560–563

23. Wang AL, Liu HG, Zhang Y. Increased expression of fascin associated with malignant transformation of sinonasal inverted papilloma. Chin Med J (Engl) 2007; 120(5):375–379

24. Huang CC, Lee TJ, Chang PH, et al. Desmoglein 3 is overexpressed in inverted papilloma and squamous cell carcinoma of sinonasal cavity. Laryngoscope 2010;120(1):26–29

25. Lampertico P, Russell WO, MacComb WS. Squamous papilloma of upper respiratory epithelium. Arch Pathol 1963;75:293–302

26. Skolnik EM, Loewy A, Friedman JE. Inverted papilloma of the nasal cavity. Arch Otolaryngol 1966;84(1):61–67

27. Buchwald C, Franzmann MB, Tos M. Sinonasal papillomas: a report of 82 cases in Copenhagen County, including a longitudinal epidemiological and clinical study. Laryngoscope 1995;105(1):72–79

28. Outzen KE, Grøntveld A, Jørgensen K, Clausen PP, Ladefoged C. Inverted papilloma: incidence and late results of surgical treatment. Rhinology 1996;34(2):114–118

29. Mirza S, Bradley PJ, Acharya A, Stacey M, Jones NS. Sinonasal inverted papillomas: recurrence, and synchronous and metachronous malignancy. J Laryngol Otol 2007;121(9):857–864

30. van den Boer C, Brutel G, de Vries N. Is routine histopathological examination of FESS material useful? Eur Arch Otorhinolaryngol 2010;267(3):381–384

31. Garavello W, Gaini RM. Incidence of inverted papilloma in recurrent nasal polyposis. Laryngoscope 2006;116(2):221–223

32. Guillemaud JP, Witterick IJ. Inverted papilloma of the sphenoid sinus: clinical presentation, management, and systematic review of the literature. Laryngoscope 2009;119(12):2466–2471

33. Lawson W, Patel ZM. The evolution of management for inverted papilloma: an analysis of 200 cases. Otolaryngol Head Neck Surg 2009;140(3):330–335

34. Chatterji P, Friedmann I, Soni NK, Solanki RL, Ramdeo IN. Bilateral transitional-type inverted papilloma of the nose and paranasal sinuses. J Laryngol Otol 1982;96(3):281–287

35. Phillips PP, Gustafson RO, Facer GW. The clinical behavior of inverting papilloma of the nose and paranasal sinuses: report of 112 cases and review of the literature. Laryngoscope 1990;100(5):463–469

36. Hosal SA, Freeman JL. Bilateral lateral rhinotomy for resection of bilateral inverted papilloma. Otolaryngol Head Neck Surg 1996;114(1):103–105

37. Weissler MC, Montgomery WW, Turner PA, Montgomery SK, Joseph MP. Inverted papilloma. Ann Otol Rhinol Laryngol 1986;95(3 Pt 1):215–221

38. Bignami M, Pistochini A, Meloni F, Delehaye E, Castelnuovo P. A rare case of oncocytic Schneiderian papilloma with intradural and intraorbital extension with notes of operative techniques. Rhinology 2009;47(3):316–319

39. Lawson W, Kaufman MR, Biller HF. Treatment outcomes in the management of inverted papilloma: an analysis of 160 cases. Laryngoscope 2003;113(9):1548–1556

40. Bhandary S, Singh RK, Sinha AK, Badhu BP, Karki P. Sinonasal inverted papilloma in eastern part of Nepal. Kathmandu Univ Med J (KUMJ) 2006;4(4):431–435 (KUMJ)

41. Bielamowicz S, Calcaterra TC, Watson D. Inverting papilloma of the head and neck: the UCLA update. Otolaryngol Head Neck Surg 1993;109(1):71–76

42. Diamantopoulos II, Jones NS, Lowe J. All nasal polyps need histological examination: an audit-based appraisal of clinical practice. J Laryngol Otol 2000;114(10):755–759

43. Savy L, Lloyd G, Lund VJ, Howard D. Optimum imaging for inverted papilloma. J Laryngol Otol 2000;114(11):891–893

44. Chiu AG, Jackman AH, Antunes MB, Feldman MD, Palmer JN. Radiographic and histologic analysis of the bone underlying inverted papillomas. Laryngoscope 2006;116(9):1617–1620

45. Bhalla RK, Wright ED. Predicting the site of attachment of sinonasal inverted papilloma. Rhinology 2009;47(4):345–348

46. Lee DK, Chung SK, Dhong HJ, Kim HY, Kim HJ, Bok KH. Focal hyperostosis on CT of sinonasal inverted papilloma as a predictor of tumor origin. AJNR Am J Neuroradiol 2007;28(4):618–621

47. Sham CL, King AD, van Hasselt A, Tong MC. The roles and limitations of computed tomography in the preoperative assessment of sinonasal inverted papillomas. Am J Rhinol 2008;22(2):144–150

48. Yousem DM, Fellows DW, Kennedy DW, Bolger WE, Kashima H, Zinreich SJ. Inverted papilloma: evaluation with MR imaging. Radiology 1992;185(2):501–505

49. Jeon TY, Kim HJ, Chung SK, et al. Sinonasal inverted papilloma: value of convoluted cerebriform pattern on MR imaging. AJNR Am J Neuroradiol 2008;29(8):1556–1560

50. Ojiri H, Ujita M, Tada S, Fukuda K. Potentially distinctive features of sinonasal inverted papilloma on MR imaging. AJR Am J Roentgenol 2000;175(2):465–468

51. Maroldi R, Farina D, Palvarini L, Lombardi D, Tomenzoli D, Nicolai P. Magnetic resonance imaging findings of inverted papilloma: differential diagnosis with malignant sinonasal tumors. Am J Rhinol 2004;18(5):305–310

52. Oikawa K, Furuta Y, Oridate N, et al. Preoperative staging of sinonasal inverted papilloma by magnetic resonance imaging. Laryngoscope 2003;113(11):1983–1987

53. Roobottom CA, Jewell FM, Kabala J. Primary and recurrent inverting papilloma: appearances with magnetic resonance imaging. Clin Radiol 1995;50(7):472–475

54. Shojaku H, Fujisaka M, Yasumura S, et al. Positron emission tomography for predicting malignancy of sinonasal inverted papilloma. Clin Nucl Med 2007;32(4):275–278

55. Jeon TY, Kim HJ, Choi JY, et al. 18F-FDG PET/CT findings of sinonasal inverted papilloma with or without coexistent malignancy: comparison with MR imaging findings in eight patients. Neuroradiology 2009;51(4):265–271

56. Katori H, Nozawa A, Tsukuda M. Histopathological parameters of recurrence and malignant transformation in sinonasal inverted papilloma. Acta Otolaryngol 2006;126(2):214–218

57. Sauter A, Matharu R, Hörmann K, Naim R. Current advances in the basic research and clinical management of sinonasal inverted papilloma (review). Oncol Rep 2007;17(3):495–504

58. Kerschner JE, Futran ND, Chaney V. Inverted papilloma associated with squamous cell carcinoma and adenocarcinoma: case report and review of the literature. Am J Otolaryngol 1996;17(4):257–259

59. Mansell NJ, Bates GJ. The inverted Schneiderian papilloma: a review and literature report of 43 new cases. Rhinology 2000;38(3):97–101

60. Yamaguchi KT, Shapshay SM, Incze JS, Vaughan CW, Strong MS. Inverted papilloma and squamous cell carcinoma. J Otolaryngol 1979;8(2):171–178

61. Lund VJ, Stammberger H, Nicolai P, et al. European position paper on endoscopic management of tumours of the nose, paranasal sinuses and skull base. Rhinol Suppl 2010;(22):1–143

62. Norris HJ. Papillary lesions of the nasal cavity and paranasal sinuses. I. Exophytic (squamous) papillomas. A study of 28 cases. Laryngoscope 1962;72:1784–1797

63. Oberman HA. Papillomas of the nose and paranasal sinuses. Am J Clin Pathol 1964;42:245–258

64. Cummings CW, Goodman ML. Inverted papillomas of the nose and paranasal sinuses. Arch Otolaryngol 1970;92(5):445–449

65. Snyder RN, Perzin KH. Papillomatosis of nasal cavity and paranasal sinuses (inverted papilloma, squamous papilloma). A clinicopathologic study. Cancer 1972; 30(3):668–690

66. Lasser A, Rothfeld PR, Shapiro RS. Epithelial papilloma and squamous cell carcinoma of the nasal cavity and paranasal sinuses: a clinicopathological study. Cancer 1976;38(6):2503–2510

67. Ridolfi RL, Lieberman PH, Erlandson RA, Moore OS. Schneiderian papillomas: a clinicopathologic study of 30 cases. Am J Surg Pathol 1977;1(1):43–53

68. Suh KW, Facer GW, Devine KD, Weiland LH, Zujko RD. Inverting papilloma of the nose and paranasal sinuses. Laryngoscope 1977;87(1):35–46

69. Calcaterra TC, Thompson JW, Paglia DE. Inverting papillomas of the nose and paranasal sinuses. Laryngoscope 1980;90(1):53–60

70. Kelly JH, Joseph M, Carroll E, et al. Inverted papilloma of the nasal septum. Arch Otolaryngol 1980;106(12):767–771

71. Barnes L, Bedetti C. Oncocytic Schneiderian papilloma: a reappraisal of cylindrical cell papilloma of the sinonasal tract. Hum Pathol 1984;15(4):344–351

72. Majumdar B, Beck S. Inverted papilloma of the nose. Some aspects of aetiology. J Laryngol Otol 1984;98(5):467–470

73. Abildgaard-Jensen J, Greisen O. Inverted papillomas of the nose and the paranasal sinuses. Clin Otolaryngol Allied Sci 1985;10(3):135–143

74. Eavey RD. Inverted papilloma of the nose and paranasal sinuses in childhood and adolescence. Laryngoscope 1985;95(1):17–23

75. Kristensen S, Vorre P, Elbrønd O, Søgaard H. Nasal Schneiderian papillomas: a study of 83 cases. Clin Otolaryngol Allied Sci 1985;10(3):125–134

76. Christensen WN, Smith RR. Schneiderian papillomas: a clinicopathologic study of 67 cases. Hum Pathol 1986; 17(4):393–400

77. Mickelson SA, Nichols RD. Denker rhinotomy for inverted papilloma of the nose and paranasal sinuses. Henry Ford Hosp Med J 1990;38(1):21–24

78. Myers EN, Fernau JL, Johnson JT, Tabet JC, Barnes EL. Management of inverted papilloma. Laryngoscope 1990; 100(5):481–490

79. Benninger MS, Lavertu P, Levine H, Tucker HM. Conservation surgery for inverted papillomas. Head Neck 1991; 13(5):442–445

80. Furuta Y, Shinohara T, Sano K, et al. Molecular pathologic study of human papillomavirus infection in inverted papilloma and squamous cell carcinoma of the nasal cavities and paranasal sinuses. Laryngoscope 1991;101(1 Pt 1):79–85

81. Outzen KE, Grøntved A, Jørgensen K, Clausen PP. Inverted papilloma of the nose and paranasal sinuses: a study of 67 patients. Clin Otolaryngol Allied Sci 1991;16(3):309–312

82. Dolgin SR, Zaveri VD, Casiano RR, Maniglia AJ. Different options for treatment of inverting papilloma of the nose and paranasal sinuses: a report of 41 cases. Laryngoscope 1992;102(3):231–236

83. Pelausa EO, Fortier MA. Schneiderian papilloma of the nose and paranasal sinuses: the University of Ottawa experience. J Otolaryngol 1992;21(1):9–15

84. Waitz G, Wigand ME. Results of endoscopic sinus surgery for the treatment of inverted papillomas. Laryngoscope 1992;102(8):917–922

85. McCary WS, Gross CW, Reibel JF, Cantrell RW. Preliminary report: endoscopic versus external surgery in the management of inverting papilloma. Laryngoscope 1994; 104(4):415–419

86. Kamel RH. Transnasal endoscopic medial maxillectomy in inverted papilloma. Laryngoscope 1995;105(8 Pt 1):847–853

87. Lawson W, Ho BT, Shaari CM, Biller HF. Inverted papilloma: a report of 112 cases. Laryngoscope 1995;105(3 Pt 1): 282–288

88. Raveh E, Feinmesser R, Shpitzer T, Yaniv E, Segal K. Inverted papilloma of the nose and paranasal sinuses: a study of 56 cases and review of the literature. Isr J Med Sci 1996;32(12):1163–1167

89. Hwang CS, Yang HS, Hong MK. Detection of human papillomavirus (HPV) in sinonasal inverted papillomas using polymerase chain reaction (PCR). Am J Rhinol 1998;12(5):363–366

90. Ingle R, Jennings TA, Goodman ML, Pilch BZ, Bergman S, Ross JS. CD44 expression in sinonasal inverted papillomas and associated squamous cell carcinoma. Am J Clin Pathol 1998;109(3):309–314

91. Chee LW, Sethi DS. The endoscopic management of sinonasal inverted papillomas. Clin Otolaryngol Allied Sci 1999;24(1):61–66

92. Kaza S, Capasso R, Casiano RR. Endoscopic resection of inverted papilloma: University of Miami experience. Am J Rhinol 2003;17(4):185–190

93. Mirza N, Nofsinger YC, Kroger H, Sato Y, Furth EE, Montone KT. Apoptosis and p53 in inverting papilloma of the sinonasal tract. Am J Rhinol 1999;13(6):427–434

94. Orvidas LJ, Lewis JE, Olsen KD, Weiner JS. Intranasal verrucous carcinoma: relationship to inverting papilloma and human papillomavirus. Laryngoscope 1999; 109(3):371–375

95. Jardine AH, Davies GR, Birchall MA. Recurrence and malignant degeneration of 89 cases of inverted papilloma diagnosed in a non-tertiary referral population between 1975 and 1995: clinical predictors and p53 studies. Clin Otolaryngol Allied Sci 2000;25(5):363–369

96. Klimek T, Atai E, Schubert M, Glanz H. Inverted papilloma of the nasal cavity and paranasal sinuses: clinical data, surgical strategy and recurrence rates. Acta Otolaryngol 2000;120(2):267–272

97. Lund VJ. Optimum management of inverted papilloma. J Laryngol Otol 2000;114(3):194–197

98. Kaufman MR, Brandwein MS, Lawson W. Sinonasal papillomas: clinicopathologic review of 40 patients with inverted and oncocytic schneiderian papillomas. Laryngoscope 2002;112(8 Pt 1):1372–1377

99. Baruah P, Deka RC. Endoscopic management of inverted papillomas of the nose and paranasal sinuses. Ear Nose Throat J 2003;82(4):317–320

100. Kraft M, Simmen D, Kaufmann T, Holzmann D. Long-term results of endonasal sinus surgery in sinonasal papillomas. Laryngoscope 2003;113(9):1541–1547

101. Llorente JL, Deleyiannis F, Rodrigo JP, et al. Minimally invasive treatment of the nasal inverted papilloma. Am J Rhinol 2003;17(6):335–341

102. Lee TJ, Huang SF, Huang CC. Tailored endoscopic surgery for the treatment of sinonasal inverted papilloma. Head Neck 2004;26(2):145–153

103. Pasquini E, Sciarretta V, Farneti G, Modugno GC, Ceroni AR. Inverted papilloma: report of 89 cases. Am J Otolaryngol 2004;25(3):178–185

104. Tomenzoli D, Castelnuovo P, Pagella F, et al. Different endoscopic surgical strategies in the management of inverted papilloma of the sinonasal tract: experience with 47 patients. Laryngoscope 2004;114(2):193–200

105. Von Buchwald C, Larsen AS. Endoscopic surgery of inverted papillomas under image guidance—a prospective study of 42 consecutive cases at a Danish university clinic. Otolaryngol Head Neck Surg 2005;132(4):602–607

106. Eggers G, Eggers H, Sander N, Kössling F, Chilla R. Histological features and malignant transformation of inverted papilloma. Eur Arch Otorhinolaryngol 2005;262(4):263–268

107. Minovi A, Kollert M, Draf W, Bockmühl U. Inverted papilloma: feasibility of endonasal surgery and long-term results of 87 cases. Rhinology 2006;44(3):205–210

108. Holzmann D, Hegyi I, Rajan GP, Harder-Ruckstuhl M. Management of benign inverted sinonasal papilloma avoiding external approaches. J Laryngol Otol 2007;121(6):548–554

109. Mortuaire G, Arzul E, Darras JA, Chevalier D. Surgical management of sinonasal inverted papillomas through endoscopic approach. Eur Arch Otorhinolaryngol 2007; 264(12):1419–1424

110. Tanna N, Edwards JD, Aghdam H, Sadeghi N. Transnasal endoscopic medial maxillectomy as the initial oncologic approach to sinonasal neoplasms: the anatomic basis. Arch Otolaryngol Head Neck Surg 2007;133(11):1139–1142

111. Yoon BN, Batra PS, Citardi MJ, Roh HJ. Frontal sinus inverted papilloma: surgical strategy based on the site of attachment. Am J Rhinol Allergy 2009;23(3):337–341

112. Giotakis E, Eleftheriadou A, Ferekidou E, Kandiloros D, Manolopoulos L, Yiotakis I. Clinical outcomes of sinonasal inverted papilloma surgery. A retrospective study of 67 cases. B-ENT 2010;6(2):111–116

113. Tanvetyanon T, Qin D, Padhya T, Kapoor R, McCaffrey J, Trotti A. Survival outcomes of squamous cell carcinoma arising from sinonasal inverted papilloma: report of 6 cases with systematic review and pooled analysis. Am J Otolaryngol 2009;30(1):38–43

114. Chen C-M, Tsai Y-L, Chang C-C, Chen H-C, Chen M-K. Is planned surgery important in sinonasal inverted papilloma? B-ENT 2009;5(4):225–231

115. Prado FA, Weber R, Romano FR, Voegels RL. Evaluation of inverted papilloma and squamous cell carcinoma by nasal contact endoscopy. Am J Rhinol Allergy 2010;24(3):210–214

116. Lee TJ, Huang SF, Lee LA, Huang CC. Endoscopic surgery for recurrent inverted papilloma. Laryngoscope 2004;114(1):106–112

117. Landsberg R. Attachment-oriented endoscopic surgical approach for sinonasal inverted papilloma. Oper Tech Otolaryngol Head Neck Surg 2006;17:87–96

118. Krouse JH. Development of a staging system for inverted papilloma. Laryngoscope 2000;110(6):965–968

119. Cannady SB, Batra PS, Sautter NB, Roh HJ, Citardi MJ. New staging system for sinonasal inverted papilloma in the endoscopic era. Laryngoscope 2007;117(7):1283–1287

120. Gras-Cabrerizo JR, Montserrat-Gili JR, Massegur-Solench H, León-Vintró X, De Juan J, Fabra-Llopis JM. Management of sinonasal inverted papillomas and comparison of classification staging systems. Am J Rhinol Allergy 2010;24(1):66–69

121. Han JK, Smith TL, Loehrl T, Toohill RJ, Smith MM. An evolution in the management of sinonasal inverting papilloma. Laryngoscope 2001;111(8):1395–1400

122. Kamel R, Khaled A, Kandil T. Inverted papilloma: new classification and guidelines for endoscopic surgery. Am J Rhinol 2005;19(4):358–364

123. Oikawa K, Furuta Y, Nakamaru Y, Oridate N, Fukuda S. Preoperative staging and surgical approaches for sinonasal inverted papilloma. Ann Otol Rhinol Laryngol 2007;116(9):674–680

124. Jurado-Ramos A, Jodas JG, Romero FR, et al. Endoscopic medial maxillectomy as a procedure of choice to treat inverted papillomas. Acta Otolaryngol 2009; 129(9):1018–1025

125. Liu Q, Yu H, Minovi A, et al. Management of maxillary sinus inverted papilloma via transnasal endoscopic anterior and medial maxillectomy. ORL J Otorhinolaryngol Relat Spec 2010;72(5):247–251

126. Syrjänen KJ. HPV infections in benign and malignant sinonasal lesions. J Clin Pathol 2003;56(3):174–181

127. Busquets JM, Hwang PH. Endoscopic resection of sinonasal inverted papilloma: a meta-analysis. Otolaryngol Head Neck Surg 2006;134(3):476–482

128. Karkos PD, Fyrmpas G, Carrie SC, Swift AC. Endoscopic versus open surgical interventions for inverted nasal papilloma: a systematic review. Clin Otolaryngol 2006;31(6):499–503

129. Anari S, Carrie S. Sinonasal inverted papilloma: narrative review. J Laryngol Otol 2010;124(7):705–715

130. Woodworth BA, Bhargave GA, Palmer JN, et al. Clinical outcomes of endoscopic and endoscopic-assisted resection of inverted papillomas: a 15-year experience. Am J Rhinol 2007;21(5):591–600

131. Woodson GE, Robbins KT, Michaels L. Inverted papilloma. Considerations in treatment. Arch Otolaryngol 1985;111(12):806–811

132. Batsakis JG, Suarez P. Schneiderian papillomas and carcinomas: a review. Adv Anat Pathol 2001;8(2):53–64

133. Moon IJ, Lee DY, Suh M-W, et al. Cigarette smoking increases risk of recurrence for sinonasal inverted papilloma. Am J Rhinol Allergy 2010;24(5):325–329

134. Segal K, Atar E, Mor C, Har-El G, Sidi J. Inverting papilloma of the nose and paranasal sinuses. Laryngoscope 1986;96(4):394–398

135. Smith O, Gullane PJ. Inverting papilloma of the nose: analysis of 48 patients. J Otolaryngol 1987;16(3):154–156

136. Stankiewicz JA, Girgis SJ. Endoscopic surgical treatment of nasal and paranasal sinus inverted papilloma. Otolaryngol Head Neck Surg 1993;109(6):988–995

137. Tufano RP, Thaler ER, Lanza DC, Goldberg AN, Kennedy DW. Endoscopic management of sinonasal inverted papilloma. Am J Rhinol 1999;13(6):423–426

138. Schlosser RJ, Mason JC, Gross CW. Aggressive endoscopic resection of inverted papilloma: an update. Otolaryngol Head Neck Surg 2001;125(1):49–53

139. Thorp MA, Oyarzabal-Amigo MF, du Plessis JH, Sellars SL. Inverted papilloma: a review of 53 cases. Laryngoscope 2001;111(8):1401–1405

140. Terzakis G, Vlachou S, Kyrmizakis D, Helidonis E. The management of sinonasal inverted papilloma: our experience. Rhinology 2002;40(1):28–33

141. Wormald PJ, Ooi E, van Hasselt CA, Nair S. Endoscopic removal of sinonasal inverted papilloma including endoscopic medial maxillectomy. Laryngoscope 2003;113(5):867–873

142. Poetker DM, Toohill RJ, Loehrl TA, Smith TL. Endoscopic management of sinonasal tumors: a preliminary report. Am J Rhinol 2005;19(3):307–315

143. Peng P, Har-El G. Management of inverted papillomas of the nose and paranasal sinuses. Am J Otolaryngol 2006;27(4):233–237

144. Sautter NB, Cannady SB, Citardi MJ, Roh HJ, Batra PS. Comparison of open versus endoscopic resection of inverted papilloma. Am J Rhinol 2007;21(3):320–323

145. Zhang G, Rodriguez X, Hussain A, Desrosiers M. Outcomes of the extended endoscopic approach for management of inverted papilloma. J Otolaryngol 2007;36(2):83–87
146. Cansz H, Tahamiler R, Yener M, et al. Modified midfacial degloving approach for sinonasal tumors. J Craniofac Surg 2008;19(6):1518–1522
147. Kim YM, Kim HS, Park JY, Koo BS, Park YH, Rha KS. External vs endoscopic approach for inverted papilloma of the sino-nasal cavities: a retrospective study of 136 cases. Acta Otolaryngol 2008;128(8):909–914
148. Stange T, Schultz-Coulon HJ. [Surgical management of inverted papillomas of the nose and paranasal sinuses]. HNO 2008;56(6):614–622
149. Durucu C, Baglam T, Karatas E, Mumbuc S, Kanlikama M. Surgical treatment of inverted papilloma. J Craniofac Surg 2009;20(6):1985–1988
150. Reh DD, Lane AP. The role of endoscopic sinus surgery in the management of sinonasal inverted papilloma. Curr Opin Otolaryngol Head Neck Surg 2009;17(1):6–10
151. Kim WS, Hyun DW, Kim C-H, Yoon J-H. Treatment outcomes of sinonasal inverted papillomas according to surgical approaches. Acta Otolaryngol 2010;130(4):493–497
152. Philpott CM, Dharamsi A, Witheford M, Javer AR. Endoscopic management of inverted papillomas: long-term results—the St. Paul's Sinus Centre experience. Rhinology 2010;48(3):358–363
153. Nakamaru Y, Furuta Y, Takagi D, Oridate N, Fukuda S. Preservation of the nasolacrimal duct during endoscopic medial maxillectomy for sinonasal inverted papilloma. Rhinology 2010;48(4):452–456

Squamous Cell Carcinoma

Definition

The respiratory mucosa of the nasal cavity and paranasal sinuses gives rise to two basic types of epithelial neoplasm—squamous and glandular. Squamous cell carcinoma (SCC) is by far the commonest type, arising from metaplastic epithelium, while the rarer group of primary tumors in this region arise from the mucous glands. Squamous carcinoma within the nose and sinuses displays the same range of histological appearances as elsewhere in the body, being graded according to the degree of differentiation and mitotic activity. This is often of little clinical significance since this type of grading is essentially subjective and influenced by variations in the biopsy material, often obtained from only a small proportion of the tumor mass.

Approximately 80% of squamous carcinomas of the nose and paranasal sinuses present as well-differentiated or moderately well-differentiated tumors.[1] The WHO classification of tumors of 2005 classifies squamous cell carcinoma under the following variants.

ICD-O codes

- Squamous cell carcinoma 8070/3
- Verrucous carcinoma 8051/3
- Papillary squamous carcinoma 8052/3
- Basaloid squamous carcinoma 8083/3
- Spindle cell carcinoma 9074/3
- Adenosquamous carcinoma 8560/3
- Acantholytic squamous cell carcinoma 8075/3

Etiology

Etiological factors have naturally attracted considerable interest, but the relative rarity of these diseases, particularly the nonkeratinizing forms of squamous carcinoma, make definitive conclusions difficult to reach. Furthermore, changes in working practices in industry, working conditions, and the increasing mobility of populations in the modern world make the effects of occupational risks more difficult to ascertain, particularly as the onset of the disease may be associated with lengthy induction times, as is notably the case with the well-known association between adenocarcinoma of the ethmoid and the woodworking industry.[2,3]

Essentially, environmental agents may affect the nose and paranasal sinuses by three routes:
1. Direct inhalation of particles whose effects depend upon their size and density, and the host's breathing pattern.[4]
2. Direct absorption. Radium has been reported to be absorbed from the oral mucosa into the facial bones.[5]
3. Parenteral, as a consequence of administration of toxins such as dioxane, nitrosamines or nickel compounds.[6]

Occupational

Historically, three occupations have a proven linkage with squamous carcinoma of the nose and paranasal sinuses. The first two, radium dial painting and mustard gas production, are now no longer undertaken, but nickel refining remains a potential risk.[7,8] In contrast to the usual requirement of longstanding exposure, a high risk has been demonstrated with even short exposures in the nickel industry, particularly for those workers involved in the sintering and roasting processes. The risk increases with age and duration of exposure.[9]

Exposure to chlorophenols, textile dust, and asbestos,[10] and exposure in the baking industry[11] have also been implicated but the numbers of substantiated cases are small.

Non-Occupational Risks

Again, in the historical context, the adverse effect of direct irradiation from thorium dioxide (Thorotrast), which was used as a radiological contrast agent that was injected directly into the maxillary antrum until 1954, has been recognized. Peak radioactivity from this material is not obtained until ~15 years after exposure and the direct association with subsequent squamous cell carcinoma was reported by Rankow et al in 1974.[12]

Snuff

Reports associating snuff-taking as a causation of squamous sinonasal cancer continue up to the present day. The most definitive report on the subject comes from South Africa, where the indigenous Bantu race use a home-made snuff containing quantities of hard wood ash that is associated with one of the highest reported incidences of advanced antroethmoidal squamous carcinoma in the world literature.[13] Acherson et al also associated snuff-taking in their classic epidemiological studies of sinonasal cancer in the boot and shoe industry.[14]

Smoking

The role of smoking in the etiology of sinonasal squamous carcinoma is not as definitive as in other areas of the respiratory tract, such as larynx and lung. Hayes et al in their study within the Netherlands suggested a relative risk of 3:1 in the development of sinonasal cancer related to smoking.[15] The effects of smoking can be a potential confounding factor in studies looking at occupational risks. In a similar vein, the relationship between chronic infection and malignancy within the nose and sinuses remains uncertain as chronic rhinosinusitis is extremely common throughout the world, whereas malignant disease of the nose and sinuses is rare.

Human Papilloma Virus

Over the last decade, there have been increasing reports of human papilloma virus (HPV) in squamous cell carcinomas, particularly those associated with inverted papilloma. Most recently, this subgroup of HPV-positive patients has not unexpectedly been found to have a better prognosis than those who are HPV-negative. Epstein-Barr virus has also been isolated from some cases of squamous carcinoma. The definite etiological role for these viruses has not been clearly established.[16]

Molecular and Clinicopathological Studies

Molecular studies of head and neck squamous carcinoma have likewise increased considerably over the last decade and many of these studies have noted genetic differences between conventional squamous carcinoma and the entire spectrum of the other morphological subtypes. Overall, the less aggressive types of carcinoma such as verrucous, papillary, and the conventional well-differentiated squamous carcinoma, have a significantly lower loss of heterozygosity (LOH) than the more aggressive high-grade conventional squamous carcinoma and basaloid and sarcomatous types.

While there is general agreement that the commonest genetic alterations are on the short arm of chromosome 9, attempts to identify a small set of specific markers on specific chromosomes that show a highly significant association between clinicopathological factors and the prognosis of the patient have not yet been reliably agreed between a wide number of research workers. Obviously, it is to be hoped that these markers will prove useful in the future and perhaps allow early detection of high-risk individuals or, more appropriately, guide specific treatment in individual patients.[17]

Synonyms

Squamous cell carcinoma of the nose and paranasal sinuses includes both keratinizing and nonkeratinizing types. Among the latter, the terms schneiderian carcinoma, cylindrical cell carcinoma, and transitional cell carcinoma have been used; the last is particularly confusing and should be confined to the epithelium of the urogenital tract. Ringertz carcinoma and respiratory epithelial carcinoma are terms that are best abandoned altogether.

Incidence

Sinonasal squamous cell carcinoma is a rare disease accounting for <1% of all cancer deaths within the United States and the United Kingdom from national studies.[18–20] The incidence figures in the literature of many countries quote a figure of 1:100,000 population, but detailed data from the International Agency for Research show considerable ethnic variations. The disease is more common in Japan, with a figure of 2.6:100,000 for men, and similar high rates are found for the indigenous populations of Nigeria and the West Indies.[21]

The disease is extremely rare in children; in adults the age range is generally between 40 and 90 years with a peak incidence between 55 and 65 years. The overall male-to-female ratio for squamous carcinoma is generally quoted as 1.5:1, but there are some variations depending on the site of origin of the tumor. Nasal vestibular carcinoma is almost exclusively a male disease, while within the nasal cavity itself, squamous carcinoma is more common in females.

Site and Classification

Sinonasal squamous cell carcinomas are often advanced at presentation and the exact site of origin is not always accurately discernible. As a consequence, figures vary considerably in the literature; the most frequently reported site is the maxillary sinus (60 to 70%) followed by the nasal cavity and ethmoid sinuses, with figures varying between 10% and 25% for these areas. In contrast, the disease is extremely rare in both the sphenoid and frontal sinuses with <1% of cases reported as originating from these areas (**Fig. 6.11**).[22] Nasal cavity and ethmoid sinus cancers are approximately equal in frequency, although the nasoethmoidal complex was only defined as a second separate site within the sinuses in the AJCC classification of 2002.

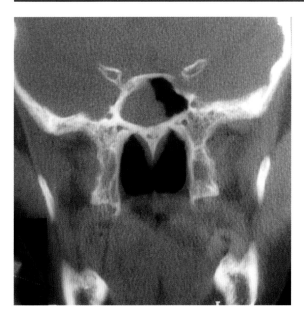 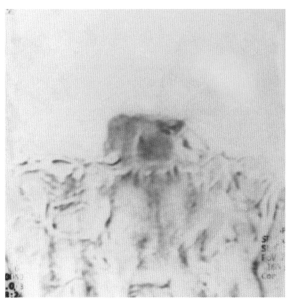

Fig. 6.11 Coronal CT and subtraction MRI showing squamous cell carcinoma presenting in the lateral wall of the right sphenoid sinus with infiltration of the cavernous sinus.

The nasal cavity is divided into four subsites: vestibule, septum, floor, and lateral nasal wall. The ethmoids are further subdivided into two subsites, left and right, separated by the nasal septum.

Our cohort comprises 320 cases, 271 squamous cell carcinoma and 49 variants. The 271 are divided into 21 cases of vestibular lesions (8%), 28 arising on the nasal septum (10%), 96 on the lateral wall and ethmoids (35%), and 126 in the maxillary sinus (47%) (Table 6.7).

The WHO classification of head and neck tumors 2005 considers that squamous cell carcinoma of the nasal vestibule should be considered as carcinoma of the skin rather than of the sinonasal mucosal epithelium. While this may be true from a theoretical point of view for those tumors confined to skin, clinically the situation may be far more complex as the nasal vestibule is bounded laterally by the alar cartilages and medially by the lower part of the nasal septum. Squamous carcinoma may arise from either the mucosa or skin of the area and a clear distinction is not always possible. The same may be said clinically for carcinomas arising from the anterior part of the nasal septum and involving the nasal vestibule. As a consequence of this unique location, vestibular carcinomas can present specific problems in diagnosis and treatment and larger lesions may have a poor prognosis.

Nasal Vestibular Carcinoma

The nasal vestibule is the recess immediately within the nostrils bounded by the medial and lateral crura of the

Table 6.7 Squamous cell carcinoma: personal series 1970–2010

Site	n	Age		M:F	Surgery + DXT	Surgery	Surgery + DXT + CT	DXT	DXT+ CT	No RXª
		Range (y)	Mean (y)							
All	271	14–93	59. 7		129	54	44	25	6	12
Vestibule	21	36–81	53. 8	3:2	10	4	1	5	1	
Nasal septum	28	32–86	61. 3	1:1	16	3	4	4		1
Lateral wall and ethmoid	96	14–79	50. 3	1. 8:1	44	14	27	8		3
Maxilla	126	20–93	56. 5	1. 7:1	59	33	12	8	5	8

Abbreviations: CT, chemotherapy; DXT, radiotherapy; F, female; M, male; RX, treatment; y, year(s).
ª Palliative treatment only in advanced disease at presentation.

alar cartilages and extending to the apex of the nose. Within the recess there is both hair-bearing skin and mucous membrane, and in some reported series this area represents ~7% of sinonasal neoplasms (**Fig. 6.12**).[23] Various series report a further ~15% of SCC tumors on the nasal septum, some of which extend to involve the nasal vestibule.

Diagnostic Features

Clinical Features

These rare malignancies are not uncommonly misdiagnosed and may be reported either in the skin literature or the sinonasal literature. There is a definite male predominance, with over 90% of tumors occurring in patients over 50 years of age with a predominance of white patients and smokers. The male to female ratio was 3:2 in our cases, with an age range of 36 to 81 years, mean of 53.8 years, and 87% were over 50 years old at diagnosis. Prolonged exposure to sunlight has also been cited as an etiological factor.[24,25] These cancers may present initially as a small raised lesion in the vestibule, which may be misdiagnosed as a viral wart when it is in fact a well-differentiated squamous carcinoma. Alternatively, there may be initial crusting and mild ulceration with minimal bleeding that rarely attracts attention until there is significant involvement of the adjoining nasal septum, nasal floor, alar skin, or cartilage. Local invasion in this area, particularly spread to the upper lip, allows access to rich lymphatic channels and spread to facial, submandibular, submental, and even parotid nodes. Such metastases can be contralateral or bilateral and may occur relatively early in the disease and are a major factor in the potential poor prognosis. Seven of our 21 cases (30%) presented with cervical lymphadenopathies, of which one was bilateral.

Once the lesion has filled the nasal vestibule, it is frequently impossible to determine its site of origin with any accuracy.

Staging

There is no wholly accepted classification for tumors in this area, although Wang in 1975[25] proposed a system in which patients were simply grouped according to the overall extent of their disease.

- T1: lesion limited to the nasal vestibule, superficial, involving one or more sites within the nasal cavity
- T2: lesion extending to involve the upper lip, dorsal nasal skin, and nasolabial fold, but without extension to underlying bone
- T3: large tumor with extension to the hard palate, alveolar and buccal sulcus, turbinates, maxillary sinus, or bone involvement.

Lymph node metastases were classified according to the TNM system.

The most recent UICC and AJCC classifications are identical (**Table 6.8**[26,27]), but multiple publications confirm the difficulties of assessing the prognostic significance of the differing classifications. The favorable early T1 lesions occupy a wide range between 50% and 90% of the cases reported.[28–30] Barzan et al found a delay in diagnosis averaging 17 months (range 1–24 months) in their 12 patients and this is a recurrent comment throughout the literature.[31]

Imaging

CT scanning using 2 mm axial and coronal cuts with contrast is essential for high-quality definition of this difficult area. Additional MRI, again with contrast using gadolinium-DPTA, adds to the CT study to give the maximum information on the extent of invasion by these tumors. The imaging, of course, complements careful clinical examination.

Histological Features and Differential Diagnosis

Most lesions are well-differentiated squamous cell carcinomas, but when the gross initial appearance is of a papillary or warty lesion, there may be confusion with dysplastic changes in a benign squamous papilloma. True verrucous carcinoma may also occur, characterized by an exophytic growth of extremely well-differentiated squamous epithelium with little cellular atypia. Invasion may be difficult to ascertain and inadequate biopsy material may lead to a diagnosis of a benign lesion rather than a well-differentiated squamous carcinoma. Poorly differentiated squamous cell carcinoma and spindle cell carcinoma may also present in this area, and in the past the latter has been confused with fibrosarcoma.[32]

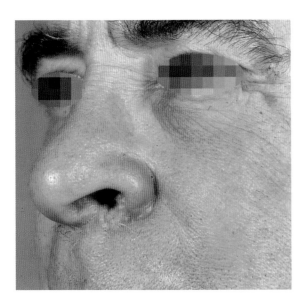

Fig. 6.12 Clinical photograph of patient with vestibular carcinoma.

Table 6.8 TMN classification[26,27]

Primary tumor (T)	
Maxillary sinus	
TX	Primary tumor cannot be assessed
T0	No evidence of primary tumor
Tis	Carcinoma in situ
T1	Tumor limited to the maxillary sinus mucosa with no erosion or destruction of bone
T2	Tumor causing bone erosion or destruction including extension into the hard palate and/or middle nasal meatus, except extension to the posterior wall of the maxillary sinus and pterygoid plates
T3	Tumor invades any of the following: bone of the posterior wall of the maxillary sinus, subcutaneous tissues, floor or medial wall of the orbit, pterygoid fossa, ethmoid sinuses
T4a	Tumor invades the anterior orbital contents, skin of the cheek, pterygoid plates, infratemporal fossa, cribriform plate, sphenoid or frontal sinuses
T4b	Tumor invades any of the following: orbital apex, dura, brain, middle cranial fossa, cranial nerves other than maxillary division of trigeminal nerve V_2, nasopharynx or clivus
Nasal cavity and ethmoid sinus	
TX	Primary tumor cannot be assessed
T0	No evidence of primary tumor
Tis	Carcinoma in situ
T1	Tumor restricted to any one subsite, with or without bony invasion
T2	Tumor invading two subsites in a single region within the nasoethmoidal complex, with or without bony invasion
T3	Tumor extends to invade the medial wall or floor of the orbit, maxillary sinus, palate, or cribriform plate
T4a	Tumor invades any of the following: anterior orbital contents, skin of the nose or cheek, minimal extension to anterior cranial fossa, pterygoid plates, sphenoid or frontal sinuses
T4b	Tumor invades any of the following: orbital apex, dura, brain, middle cranial fossa, cranial nerves other than V_2, nasopharynx, or clivus
Regional lymph nodes (N)	
NX	Regional lymph nodes cannot be assessed
N0	No regional lymph node metastasis
N1	Metastasis in a single ipsilateral lymph node, 3 cm or less in greatest dimension
N2	Metastasis as described below:
N2a	Metastasis in a single ipsilateral lymph node, more than 3 cm but not more than 6 cm in greatest dimension
N2b	Metastasis in multiple ipsilateral lymph nodes, none more than 6 cm in greatest dimension
N2c	Metastasis in bilateral or contralateral lymph nodes, none more than 6 cm in greatest dimension
N3	Metastasis in a lymph node, more than 6 cm in greatest dimension
Distant metastasis (M)	
MX	Distant metastasis cannot be assessed
M0	No distant metastasis
M1	Distant metastasis

Natural History

A lack of understanding of the natural history of these lesions leads not only to delayed diagnosis but to the distinct possibility of undertreatment. Although small lesions respond well to initial treatment, deep extension into surrounding tissues rapidly occurs without necessarily producing significant symptoms. Metastases to the regional lymph nodes remains a major cause of failure to cure in all reported series, although the incidence rates vary considerably, depending obviously on the percentage of early patients in any reported series.

Treatment

Nasal vestibular carcinomas may be treated with either radiation therapy or surgery and, indeed, in early nasal vestibular lesions reported from the 1980s, more or less equal treatment results were obtained.[29,33,34] As a consequence of surgical removal of even early carcinomas of the vestibule having a significant impact on cosmesis, radiotherapy has generally been reported as the treatment of choice. Because these lesions are rare, reports are often gathered over a long period of time and may contain a mix of primary tumors and recurrences, which makes definitive conclusions difficult.[35–37] Radiation treatment has consisted of external beam radiotherapy (EBRT) or brachytherapy of several types. In some series, patients have received elective radiation therapy to regional lymph nodes while other series have included these nodes for T4 or recurrent lesions.[38,39]

Landgendijk et al in 2004[40] reported a relatively recent series of 56 patients with T1 and T2 tumors (Wang classification) treated with external beam radiotherapy with or without a boost using endocavitary brachytherapy. Even in this group of early patients, 32 were treated with EBRT with an additional boost with intermediate dose-rate brachytherapy, 15 with EBRT and a boost with high-dose brachytherapy, and 9 with EBRT alone. The local control rate at 2 years was 80% and further cases were successfully salvaged with surgery, but 12% even of these early patients developed lymph node metastases. As with other centers reporting results, they had used EBRT with an intermediate dose of endocavitary boost up until 1997, when this type of boost was replaced with a fractionated high-dose-rate endocavitary brachytherapy. With the advent of intensely modulated radiation therapy (IMRT), further changes are to be expected in lesions reported since 2000 and additional details can be seen in Chapter 20 on radiotherapy.

Surgery

Early lesions may be excised and the ala, septum, and any minor involvement of the upper lip can be reconstructed using local mucosal and pedicled skin flaps such as the nasolabial flap. Additional conchal cartilage may be required as a free graft.

Larger lesions and those recurring after radiotherapy may need substantial resections to achieve oncologically sound margins. This may involve extensive loss of the nasal tip, dorsum, and columella up to and including total rhinectomy.[41] Additional extensive septal resection, partial maxillectomy (which may be bilateral), and full-thickness excision of the upper lip may be required. Reconstruction of this extensive midfacial loss is difficult with at best moderate functional and cosmetic results. A wide variety of local, pedicled, and free flaps have been used but each patient has to be assessed individually and achieving a long-term acceptable aesthetic result with good skin color-matching and minimal scarring can be a challenge. Donor site morbidity is an important consideration, notably if any type of forehead flap is required.

High-quality prosthetic replacement may be the best choice for many patients. However, satisfactory bone, needed to place osseointegrated implants to retain prostheses, may be lacking in radiotherapy failure patients and those requiring large midfacial resections.

In our 21 cases, 10 received surgery and radiotherapy, 5 radiotherapy alone, 4 surgery alone, 1 chemoradiation, and 1 combined surgery and chemoradiation. Surgery ranged from local excision to rhinectomy and the cohort has been treated over 40 years, during which medical oncology has improved significantly. This, combined with the wide range of tumor extent, makes it difficult to draw conclusions. Suffice to say that there are no long-term survivors among patients who presented with lymphatic spread. There are 6 "long-term" survivors (2–7 years)—3 treated with combined therapy (2 with surgery plus radiotherapy, 1 with chemoradiotherapy) and 3 with radiotherapy alone.

The Nasal Septum

Most published series of nasal septal carcinoma from tertiary referral centers have been gathered over many years and Echeverria-Zumarraga et al[42] found that no more than 300 cases of primary septal carcinoma had been reported in the literature at that time (1988), giving an incidence of ~9% of all malignant tumors arising within the nasal cavity. The majority of cases reported have been between 40 and 60 years of age with a slight male predominance.[43,44] In our cohort of 28 cases (**Table 6.7**), men and women were equally affected. The age range was 32 to 86 years with a mean of 61.3 years, somewhat older than that reported.

Etiology and Site

There are no particularly strong etiological factors associated with septal cancer other than snuff-taking and repeated trauma by nose picking. Both smokers and non-smokers are represented in most series.

Early lesions are most commonly reported to arise from the anterior septum close to the mucocutaneous junction. This is logically the area where particulate matter from the atmosphere is most likely deposited (Fig. 6.13).

Septal tumors spread to involve the nasal vestibule, making separation from this site of origin difficult at times, and additionally spread in all directions on the septum to involve the nasal floor and nasal framework. Two of our cases arose on the columella. The tumors notably spread submucosally beyond the obvious margins without marked accompanying symptoms to suggest the extent of spread. Hence, in a manner similar to vestibular carcinoma, there is a potential for undertreatment of these tumors and, indeed, cervical metastases have been reported occurring in up to 44% of the patients,[44] which was double that reported by Beatty et al[43] and 4 times the generally quoted rate for nose and paranasal sinus tumors. Although in some series few patients present with lymph node disease, local recurrence is common and the development of lymph node metastases reflects an extremely poor prognosis, often in association with recurrent local disease. Three of our cohort of 28 patients presented with cervical lymphadenopathy, bilateral in one individual.

LeLeive et al reported a high correlation between tumors larger than 2 cm in overall diameter and eventual prognosis.[44]

Diagnostic Features

Clinical Features

In a similar manner to vestibular carcinoma, the lesions may present in a variety of ways on the septum, ranging from fungating friable masses which bleed easily and may infiltrate the soft tissues of the external nose (Figs. 6.14 and 6.15), to small ulcerated fissured lesions, or in association with a septal perforation.[42,43] Anterior lesions extending into the vestibule may be associated with crusting covering superficial ulceration. Again, as with

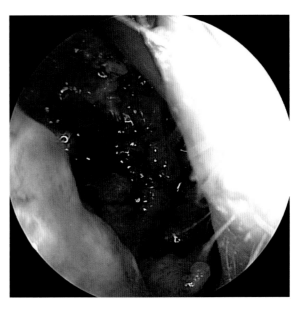

Fig. 6.14 Endoscopic photograph showing squamous cell carcinoma on the anterior nasal septum. (Courtesy of R. Almeyda.)

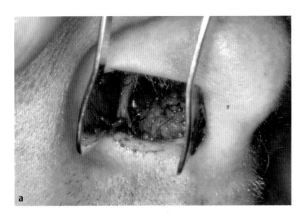

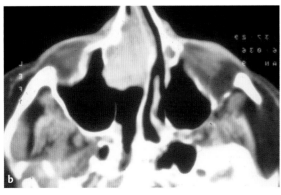

Fig. 6.13a, b
a Clinical photograph of anterior nasal septal squamous cell carcinoma extending to the columella.
b Axial CT scan of the same patient.

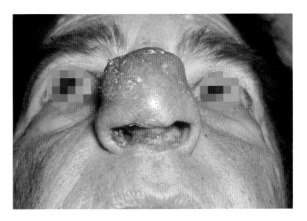

Fig. 6.15 Clinical photograph of a patient with very extensive squamous cell carcinoma of the nasal septum infiltrating the overlying soft tissues of the nose.

vestibular carcinoma, the literature reports considerable delay in diagnosis with a range varying from 1 month to 6 years.[45]

Imaging

Imaging considerations are the same as for vestibular lesions (p. 95).

Differential Diagnosis

A wide variety of pathological conditions are found on the nasal septum, and these commonly provide confusion and further delay in diagnosis. Benign lesions such as mycosis, tuberculosis, syphilis, leishmaniasis, leprosy, and sarcoid may all mimic septal carcinoma. In addition, all variants of squamous carcinoma, amelanotic malignant melanoma, chondrosarcoma, adenoid cystic carcinoma, adenocarcinoma, mucoepidermoid carcinoma, plasmacytoma, and T cell lymphoma have all been reported. Adequate biopsy material and expert specialist histopathology assessment are therefore essential.

Treatment

The literature reports from the 1970s and 1980s show considerable variation in treatment strategies, follow-up times, details of tumor extent, and histopathology. These reports were mainly made before the advent of high-quality CT and MRI and the routine use of nasal endoscopes. What they do clearly show is that primary septal carcinoma is a serious disease and that primary treatment by surgery or radiotherapy often failed to control the disease with the best survival figures from this period obtained by combined treatment. LeLiever et al[44] gave an absolute 5-year survival rate for their 18 patients of 66% with a median survival time of 45 months.

While in all areas of cancer treatment there are examples of both over- and undertreatment, a modern multidisciplinary team with specialist radiology, pathology, and multiple treatment skills has the opportunity to notably improve on past results with this disease. The fact that is beyond any doubt from the previous 40 years of literature is that this disease is often undertreated. There has been a failure to appreciate the true extent of the lesion, and the desire on the part of the patient and the treating physician to avoid severe cosmetic disability means that with both the smaller and larger tumors, total local eradication of disease is frequently not obtained. As is so often the case with tumors of the nose and paranasal sinuses, it is important to understand the natural history of the disease, particularly its pattern of spread into adjacent surrounding tissues, and in the case of nasal septal carcinoma there may be significant submucosal spread that makes excision incomplete. There is potential for spread to the nasal vestibule and upper lip, with the lymphatics of the lip, soft tissues of the angle of the mouth, and the mental and submental region being involved, and an increased possibility of cervical node disease. With these important points in mind, any proposed endoscopic excision of early nasal septal lesions must adequately encompass the entire lesion to obtain definitive free margins. Even if this is the case, it is probably best followed by radiotherapy; depending on the size of the resected lesion and its detailed pathology, the radiotherapy fields may need to include the vestibule, upper lip, bilateral soft

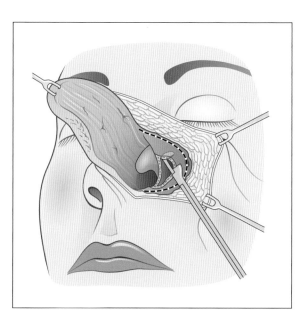

Fig. 6.16 Drawing showing the incision for lateral rhinotomy.

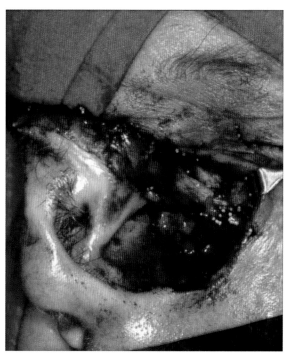

Fig. 6.17 Clinical photograph showing the view into the nose during lateral rhinotomy.

tissues of the lower face, and level I nodes. Accurate ultrasound evaluation combined with fine needle aspiration should now be able to assess nodes as small as 4 mm in major centers where these techniques are available.

The most evident point from the older literature is that tumors larger than 2 cm in diameter have a poorer potential prognosis.[44] Although lateral rhinotomy was widely used in the past to approach septal tumors (Figs. 6.16 and 6.17), better access may be obtained by a midfacial degloving procedure, particularly for tumors extending onto the floor of the nose, into the superior framework, and more posteriorly to the vomer.

For those lesions extending into the vestibule or to a greater degree into the nasal framework, total rhinectomy was an operation rarely used in the past because of its perceived cosmetic sequelae.[41] While total rhinectomy remains a considerable decision for patients (Fig. 6.18), modern osseointegrated prosthetics and soft tissue

plastic surgery procedures have lessened the concerns with regard to the procedure. Certainly it is preferable to consider it as an effective primary procedure rather than for recurrent disease following failure of both surgery and radiotherapy. In even more extensive tumors, particularly with superior and posterior extension, craniofacial resection may be required in addition to total rhinectomy.

In our cohort, the majority had combined therapy, either surgery + radiotherapy (57%) or surgery + chemoradiotherapy (14%), 3 (11%) had surgery alone, 4 (14%) had radiotherapy, and one very advanced case had none. Surgery included lateral rhinotomy,[9] rhinectomy (3 cases), craniofacial resection (2 cases), midfacial resection (1 case), and endoscopic surgery (1 case) with additional neck dissections where required. As with vestibular carcinoma, it is difficult to draw definitive conclusions from the outcomes. However, there were more long-term survivors (10 for 3–16 years; 5 for >5 years), all but one treated with combined therapy. All patients with cervical nodes died of disease.

Lateral Nasal Wall and Ethmoid Sinus Carcinoma

It was not until 2002 that the AJCC committee included the nasoethmoid complex as a second site for nose and paranasal sinus tumors in their staging system. Within this nasoethmoid site, there was further division into nasal cavity and ethmoid sinuses. As previously mentioned, the nasal cavity was divided into four subsites: septum, floor, lateral wall, and vestibule. The ethmoid sinus was divided into two subsites: right and left. The ease with which squamous carcinoma of the maxillary sinus invades the ethmoid or enters the nasal cavity often renders imprecise an assessment of the relative frequency of primary lateral nasal wall or ethmoidal carcinoma, and in the past we and others have frequently reported the lesions overall as "antroethmoidal." A recurring theme throughout the literature is the high proportion of patients presenting with advanced stage disease at the time of diagnosis. In a substantial study published in 2007, Mackay et al[46] noted that 67% of their patients with sinonasal squamous cell carcinoma presented with advanced disease (T4a or T4b). Obviously with improved modern imaging techniques, along with endoscopic assessment, there is a tendency for recently published studies to up-stage the disease, purely because of our improving ability to detect the precise limits and hopefully thereby to improve the treatment of these patients.

Incidence

While the literature contains multiple accounts of patients seen at tertiary referral centers over a long period, a more accurate study of the natural history of

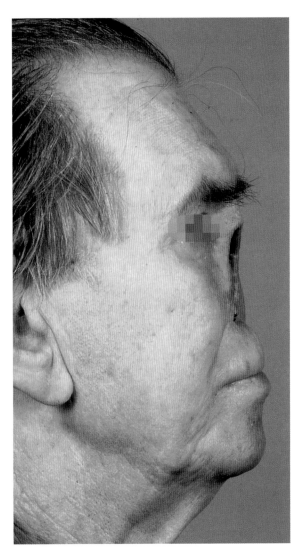

Fig. 6.18 Clinical photograph of a patient after a total rhinectomy.

individual neoplasms is obtained from cancer registries evaluating large numbers of a local population. Robin et al in their classical study published in the United Kingdom in 1979 evaluated all cases of nasal and paranasal sinus tumors from the Birmingham Regional Cancer Registry from 1957 to 1972.[47] These figures were based on a local population within the United Kingdom of more than 5 million with a registration rate of at least 95%. In all, 602 patients were studied and, although larger numbers have been recorded from tertiary referral centers, the data from cancer registries based on a specific population present a more accurate picture of incidence rates. Robin et al tabled the number of patients and incidence rates per 100,000 population for age groups from 0 to 90 years and then calculated the incidence rates using the population at risk. They gave a figure of 10% for lateral nasal wall and ethmoid tumors with a male-to-female ratio of 1:0.6. In contrast, Hopkin et al, reporting from the Royal Marsden Hospital, a UK tertiary referral center, in 1984 analyzed 561 patients seen at this institution over a 15-year period from the 1960s and 1970s and quoted an incidence of 19% for tumors in this region and a male predominance of 3:2.[48] These variations from two studies in the United Kingdom emphasize the problems of site assessment and statistical presentation when unusual tumors are evaluated.

In our cohort of 96 cases (**Table 6.7**) there was a moderate male preponderance (1.8:1) and an age range of 14 to 79 years with a mean of 50.6 years, and with 76% older than 50 years at presentation.

All ethnic groups are represented in the literature overall, but there are considerable variations in age-adjusted incidence rates around the world, and particular areas of high incidence, such as the snuff-induced squamous cell carcinoma of the lateral nasal wall reported in the South African Bantu community.[49]

Etiology

Although wood dust is well recognized as a carcinogen in humans, being responsible for the production of ethmoidal adenocarcinoma, there are no particular etiological factors for squamous cell carcinoma in this area beyond those already mentioned for nose and paranasal sinus carcinoma in general.

Considerable research has been undertaken with regard to formaldehyde; research in rats exposed to formaldehyde vapor for 24 months showed that they developed nasal squamous metaplasia and, in a single animal, a squamous cell carcinoma.[50] However, human mortality studies from a variety of institutions, notably the U.S. National Cancer Institute, which studied 26,561 industrial workers exposed to formaldehyde vapor, have not shown any increased incidence of sinonasal cancer.[51]

Diagnostic Features

Clinical Features and Natural History

As in other sites of the nose and paranasal sinuses, the early course of disease in the nasoethmoidal area is often accompanied by trivial symptoms such as nasal obstruction and discharge. Slight bleeding is common and again it is the unilateral nature of these symptoms that should give rise to concern. However, diagnosis is not usually made until there is a substantial intranasal mass or extension to produce facial swelling, numbness or paresthesia in relation to the infraorbital nerve, or effects on the orbit such as proptosis, diplopia, or epiphora (**Fig. 6.19**). Twelve percent of our patients presented with cervical lymphadenopathy.

On examination, the intranasal mass may vary enormously, being exophytic, fungating, papillary, or indurated. The lesion may be relatively well demarcated or infiltrative and often friable, necrotic, and hemorrhagic, notably with biopsy.

Additional clinical features will depend on the overall natural history of a given tumor. Tumor expansion generally occurs circumferentially along the path of least resistance. The ethmoid is intimately related to the orbit laterally and the thin lamina papyracea offers little resistance to orbital invasion. Although penetration of the orbital periosteum is a rare entity, it is an extremely important clinical point, as what appears on imaging as an intraorbital tumor may be extraperiosteal. This important point relates closely to prognosis, as disease that has breached the orbital periosteum and is truly intraorbital is associated with a marked reduction in prognosis.[52]

Imaging

Even with the most modern CT and MRI, one aspect of skull base imaging remains difficult—has microscopic disease invaded through the orbital periosteum? (**Figs. 6.20 and 6.21**) In a similar manner, the roof of the ethmoid is intimately related to the anterior cranial fossa dura and the cribriform plate (**Figs. 6.21, 6.22, 6.23**). Extension to the dura and subsequently through the dura is also of important prognostic significance. The same point therefore applies even to the best modern imaging where difficulties can still arise with regard to the certainty of knowing whether disease has breached the cribriform plate or the dura and is truly intradural or invading the frontal lobes.[53,54] Extension to the middle cranial fossa may then occur through the orbital apex, ethmosphenoid region or from the anterior cranial fossa (**Fig. 6.24**).

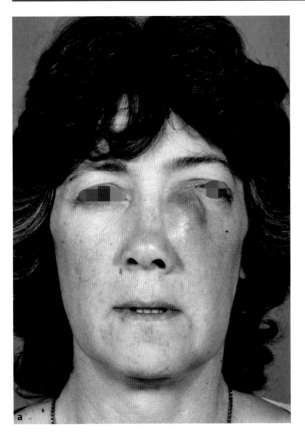

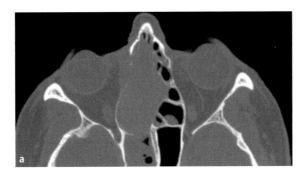

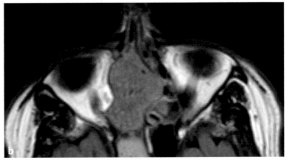

Fig. 6.19a, b

a Clinical photograph of a patient with large tumor probably arising on the lateral wall of the nose and ethmoids, extending laterally into the maxillary sinus and anteriorly into the soft tissues of the cheek, displacing the eye laterally and superiorly.

b Coronal CT scan of the same patient showing a large "antroethmoidal" tumor.

Fig. 6.20a, b

a Axial CT scan of ethmoidal squamous cell carcinoma with expansion into the medial orbit but probably extraperiosteal.

b Axial MRI (T1W post gadolinium fat saturation sequence) in the same patient showing the line of delineation between tumor and orbital contents with fluid in the sphenoid, highly suggestive that the lesion remains extraperiosteal.

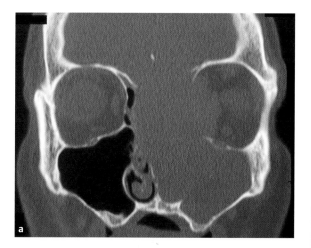

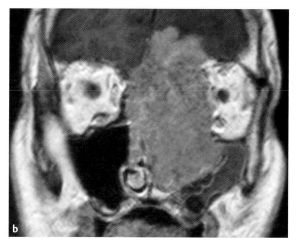

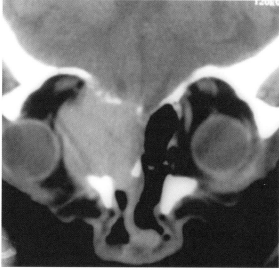

Fig. 6.22 Coronal CT scan showing squamous cell carcinoma of the right anterior ethmoid probably infiltrating through the orbital periosteum and showing early bone erosion of the skull base.

Fig. 6.21a, b

a Coronal CT scan showing extensive squamous cell carcinoma involving the medial antrum and ethmoids, probably infiltrating through the dura and orbital periosteum.

b Coronal MRI (T1W post gadolinium fat saturation sequence) in the same patient strongly suggestive that the tumor has penetrated into the contents of the anterior cranial fossa and orbit.

Treatment and Prognosis

General considerations

Early lesions of the lateral nasal wall and ethmoid sinuses may be amenable to wide local excision, with surgery being the only treatment required or with additional postoperative radiotherapy should the histopathology evaluation merit this. However, **with the all too common advanced lesions, the complexity of these cases is most effectively discussed in a multidisciplinary tumor board.** While treatment decisions will essentially be based on the location, stage, and histology of the squamous carcinoma, the presence of significant patient comorbidities may alter the treatment plan as radical surgery, orbital exenteration, or craniotomy, and possibly flap reconstruction, all raise morbidity and occasionally produce mortality. The overall aim of any surgery must be complete tumor removal. The proximity of orbital, neurological, and vascular structures within the skull base and cranium means that the indications for surgery remain somewhat controversial.

Even with experience of craniofacial surgery now extending into the fourth decade in many centers, areas of debate with regard to contraindications are extensive involvement of the nasopharynx, clivus, optic nerve, optic chiasma, cavernous sinus, and carotid artery. They all require considerable discussion in a given patient. A point in favor of squamous carcinomas originating from a sinonasal origin is that they tend to spread in a continuous manner, albeit at times with additional perineural spread, but this is in contrast to primary brain malignancies and does make the possibility of local resection a reality. Additionally, even with advanced lesions, cervical metastases are rare and generalized metastases even more so, so that discussion mainly relates to the control of local disease. For example, penetration of the anterior cranial fossa dura by squamous carcinoma, even into

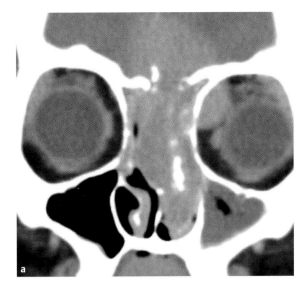

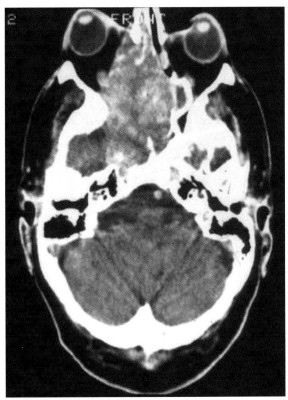

Fig. 6.24 Axial CT showing extensive ethmoidal tumor infiltrating the orbit, sphenoid, cavernous sinus, and middle cranial fossa.

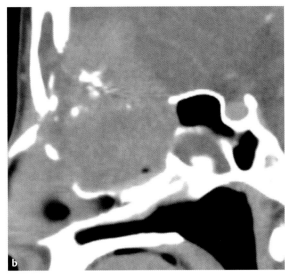

Fig. 6.23a, b

a Coronal CT scan showing squamous cell carcinoma infiltrating into the anterior cranial fossa from the nasal cavity and involving the left orbit.

b Sagittal CT scan in the same patient showing massive destruction of the posterior frontal sinus and adjacent skull base.

the frontal lobe, may allow adequate resection including the involved frontal lobe portion with only minimal functional deficit for the patient. In contrast, surgical resection of the internal carotid artery, cranial nerves, and cavernous sinus, while possible at times, carries an extremely high morbidity and mortality. The final choice of any surgery will also depend on the abilities and experience of the surgical team. This is also true with regard to both the availability of modern radiotherapeutic techniques and the experience of the radiation oncologist. Chemotherapy for squamous carcinoma of the nose and paranasal sinuses has not yet reached an established and proven place in the same way that it has for lesions of the oral cavity and pharyngolarynx.

Surgical Therapy

If total resection of the tumor seems possible, surgical procedures for sinonasal squamous carcinomas are based on the approach to the lesion. Transfacial approaches may be undertaken by variations of several different facial incisions, for example, lateral rhinotomy and the variations of the Weber–Fergusson incision. In midfacial degloving, the approach via a bilateral sublabial incision allows for subperiosteal elevation of the soft tissues of the midface when combined with complete transfixion and intercartilaginous and pyriform aperture incisions. This avoids facial incisions and with adequate bony removal the exposure can be extended to allow visualization of the whole nasal cavity, maxilla and ethmoidal sinuses, nasopharynx, pterygomaxillary space, and infratemporal fossa.

Intracranial approaches via a variety of craniotomies may be undertaken through bilateral coronal incisions or a variety of butterfly incisions across the nasal bridge and beneath the eyebrows, which also allows a subcranial approach. The details of these approaches and more extensive craniofacial resection are described in Chapter 19 on surgical treatment.

Endoscopic Surgery

As yet, there are few studies reported of treatment of squamous cell carcinoma of the lateral wall and ethmoids exclusively by endoscopic excision. Generally, endoscopically assisted surgery has been combined with conventional open surgery or done in combination with radiotherapy or chemotherapy. In studies reporting endoscopic resection of malignant tumors of the sinonasal complex, overall there are frequently only a small number of squamous cell carcinoma cases, giving insufficient numbers to provide detailed analyses.[55–59]

Management of the Orbit, Reconstruction and Prosthesis

These issues will be discussed in Chapter 19 (p. 505).

Radiotherapy and Chemotherapy

The published clinical outcomes for radiotherapy and chemotherapy for tumors of the lateral nasal wall suffer from the same inherent difficulties as for those patients receiving surgery. The studies are mainly confined to retrospective reviews of single-institution experience and precise evaluation of this particular primary site has only recently been better defined. While most studies have combined surgery and radiotherapy, a small proportion of patients treated with a nonsurgical approach have shown great variation in the published studies. Chemotherapy has been added to postoperative radiotherapy as an adjuvant treatment, but again using different agents within differing protocols.

As with primary surgery, in the older series primary radiotherapy has been associated with apparently higher treatment-related complications and with notable recurrence despite the ability to adequately encompass gross disease without potentially damaging important surrounding structures such as the eye, optic nerve, and brainstem. Notable complications even from experienced major tertiary referral units include brain necrosis, conjunctivitis, keratitis, late (persistent) mucositis, retinopathy, optic neuropathy, trismus, and oromaxillary fistula. Chemotherapy-induced sepsis and brain necrosis may cause death.[60] However, for patients who are medically unfit or deemed to have inoperable tumors, definitive radiotherapy with or without additional chemotherapy does provide an alternative approach, although overall there is general agreement that the reported outcomes are less favorable than those from combined treatment with surgery and radiotherapy.[61]

Recently, intensity modulated radiation therapy (IMRT) has offered the ability to administer a higher tumoricidal dose of radiation to the tumor volume with minimal involvement of the surrounding important normal tissues. To date, published articles, mainly of single-institutional series, suggest that despite short follow-up, both the clinical outcomes and decreased toxicity offer a definitive improvement for patients. Clearly, larger, long-term prospective studies will further evaluate the potential for treatment with IMRT and other new techniques such as proton therapy.[61–64]

Further details of radiotherapy and chemotherapy treatment can be found in Chapter 20 (p. 515).

In our cohort of 96 individuals, surgery was the principal treatment (88.5%), usually in combination with radiotherapy or chemoradiotherapy (Table 6.7). Eight patients received radiotherapy alone, largely for palliation, and 3 received no treatment due to the extent of disease at presentation. Surgery included craniofacial resection, lateral rhinotomy in the earlier cases, midfacial degloving, maxillectomy, and more recently endoscopic resection (Table 6.9). In addition, there were 9 orbital clearances and 8 neck dissections. The craniofacial resection results are the most robust, showing a 5-year actuarial survival of 53%, which drops to 35% at 10 years and remains at 35% thereafter. Intracranial involvement, particularly frontal lobe infiltration, is the most important determinant of outcome. Death from disease usually occurred between 6 and 24 months, which must be regarded as residual disease; however, as seen from the craniofacial series, genuine recurrence can occur up to 10 years later and we have one case which recurred at 25 years.

Table 6.9 Surgical management of squamous cell carcinoma:[a] personal series 1970–2010

	N	CFR	Maxil	LR	MFD	ESS	Orbit	ND
Lateral nasal wall and ethmoid	85/96	31	4	51	4	8	9	8
Maxillary sinus	103/126	4	75	20	4	—	44	8

Abbreviations: CFR, craniofacial resection; ESS, endoscopic sinus surgery; LR, lateral rhinotomy; Maxil, maxillectomy; MFD, midfacial degloving; Orbit, orbital clearance; ND, neck dissection.
[a] Multiple operations in some patients.

Maxillary Sinus

There have been many attempts in the past at classification schemes for squamous carcinoma of the maxillary sinus, with a critical look at all those proposed.[65,66] The best known was that of Ohngren[67] who highlighted the significantly decreased survival of patients with posterior and superior extension of maxillary carcinoma. This was defined in a simple way via a line termed the Ohngren line running from the medial canthus to the angle of the mandible. Locally advancing disease from the posterosuperior region extends into the orbit and pterygomaxillary fossa and is associated with a worse outcome. His classification scheme, described in 1933, also incorporated histological grading and the presence of metastases.

Diagnostic Features

Clinical Features

The signs and symptoms of maxillary sinus carcinoma depend on the stage of the disease and the direction and extent of invasion of the important surrounding structures. Initially the symptoms may be vague, with minimal nasal obstruction, unilateral rhinorrhea which may be blood-stained, and, occasionally, minor epistaxis. Symptoms may often be diagnosed as "sinusitis." Further

symptoms depend on whether the tumor extends intranasally, orally, into the soft tissues of the face, into the orbit, or through the skull base intracranially. Unfortunately, the pattern of spread from the maxillary sinus is extremely variable. Anterior spread through the relatively thin anterior maxillary wall may cause swelling and pain associated with the soft tissues of the face. Inferior spread may take longer to result in oral and dental symptoms, which may occur either through direct bony destruction or through involvement of the dental roots. Superior spread into the orbit may occur through the infraorbital canal, with associated paresthesia or numbness of the cheek, or through destruction of the orbital floor itself, with associated proptosis, visual disturbance, swelling of the eyelids, or excessive tearing (**Fig. 6.25**). Further extension into the pterygopalatine fossa and infratemporal area may be associated with trismus, pain, and malocclusion (**Fig. 6.26**).

With additional spread, other clinical findings may include a neck mass, indicative of nodal spread. Approximately 10 to 15% of patients will present initially with positive regional lymph nodes, although the literature

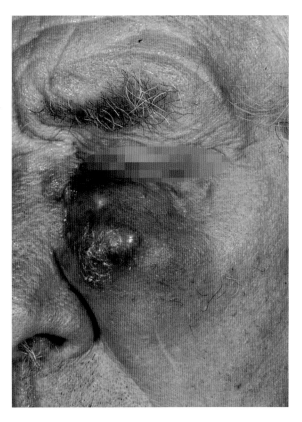

Fig. 6.25 Clinical photograph showing maxillary squamous cell carcinoma extending into the soft tissues of the face.

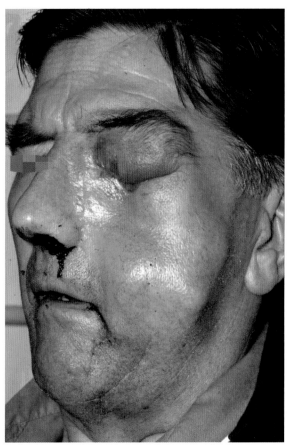

Fig. 6.26 Clinical photograph showing recurrent maxillary squamous cell carcinoma extending into the soft tissues of the face, bloody discharge from nose, trismus, and submandibular lymphadenopathy. Previous maxillectomy and orbital clearance.

reports a range of 5 to 20%.[22,68–77] Distant metastases at the time of diagnosis are uncommon, being usually reported as less than 5%[22,68,71,72,74,75,77] although this figure may change with the increasing use of PET-CT. If the tumor extends to the nasopharynx and involves the eustachian tube, then serous otitis media may be apparent at presentation. All notable series describing maxillary carcinoma comment on an average delay in the past of up to 9 months before diagnosis is established and somewhere between 60 to 95% of patients present with advanced T3 and T4 tumors.[22]

The incidence and etiological factors are described earlier in this chapter but between 60 and 70% of sinonasal squamous cell carcinomas occur in the maxilla, predominantly in men with a median age of around 65 years. Our cohort of 126 cases constitutes 46.5% of our sinonasal squamous carcinomas due to larger number of lateral wall lesions, reflecting our interest in craniofacial resection. In this cohort, there was a moderate male preponderance (1.7:1) similar to that for the lateral wall lesions with an age range of 20 to 93 years, mean 56.5 years. Again >80% were over 50 years old at diagnosis. The majority of our patients presented with T3/T4 disease (90%) and 7% had cervical lymphadenopathy.

It cannot be overemphasized that a detailed history and examination of the nose, face, orbit, oral cavity, cranial nerves, and neck are necessary for thorough evaluation of these patients. If an intranasal mass is visible, it may be exophytic, fungating, papillary, or indurated and vary from being well demarcated to obviously friable, infiltrative, necrotic, or hemorrhagic. Unilateral symptoms and the presence of polypoid change in the nasal cavity should always raise the suspicion of malignancy. While endoscopically guided biopsies of the nasal mass may be undertaken under local anesthetic, these can result in severe hemorrhage and nowadays are best delayed until after appropriate imaging, particularly if PET-CT is to be included among the initial studies. If no intranasal lesion is visible but other features in the history and examination give rise to concern, then CT and MRI imaging are essential.

While reports of bilateral primary squamous cell carcinomas of the maxilla are extremely rare, colleagues in Japan, where the incidence of squamous cell carcinoma is high generally, do see occasional cases and Miyaguchi et al[78] noted 10 patients (1.2%) with bilateral tumors in their study of 802 patients.

Imaging

Because of the low incidence of distant metastases at the time of diagnosis, the recent use of PET scanning remains debatable, but CT and MRI are indispensable and complementary in determining the extent of disease and the type of treatment appropriate to individual patients. As the majority of cases are advanced at the time of diagnosis,

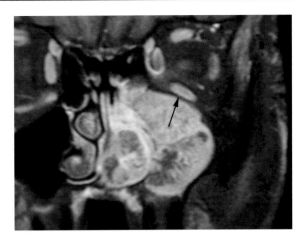

Fig. 6.27 Coronal MRI (T1W post gadolinium contrast) showing squamous cell carcinoma of the left maxillary sinus abutting the orbit but not penetrating through the orbital periosteum (the arrow indicates the area of concern) and subsequently confirmed at surgery and histologically.

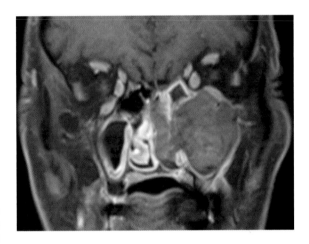

Fig. 6.28 Coronal MRI (T1W post gadolinium contrast) showing squamous cell carcinoma of the left maxillary sinus penetrating through the orbital periosteum adjacent to the inferior rectus muscle and confirmed at surgery and histologically after orbital clearance.

destruction of the bony walls of the maxillary sinus and extension of the disease into multiple surrounding areas are all too common. The important differentials were outlined earlier in the section on imaging (Chapter 5, p. 47), but extension into the orbit, through the skull base and into the intracranial cavity both have a profound effect on prognosis (**Figs. 6.27 and 6.28**). The other area of involvement that carries serious prognostic consequences is the pterygopalatine fossa, which can be well visualized by a combination of CT and MRI (**Fig. 6.29**). These combined imaging modalities are required before considering any form of primary surgical treatment and MRI remains extremely useful in the long term during follow-up.

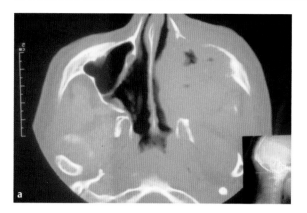

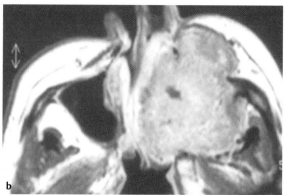

Fig. 6.29a, b

a Axial CT scan showing extensive squamous cell carcinoma extending through the anterior wall and posterior wall into the pterygopalatine and infratemporal fossae.

b Axial MRI (T1 post gadolinium contrast) in the same patient confirming the extent of disease.

Histological Features and Differential Diagnosis

The majority of squamous carcinomas of the maxilla, in all areas of the world, are reported as either well or moderately differentiated. Poorly differentiated tumors are uncommon and there is no histological evidence that these squamous cell carcinomas differ from other mucosal sites in the head and neck. Squamous differentiation may be apparent, with both extracellular or intracellular keratin. The tumor morphology varies between arrangement in groups of cells, in nests, or in masses with, at times, the classical "mosaic tile" arrangement. There may be an associated desmoplastic stromal reaction and variable degrees of obvious invasion that is usually irregular. This is in contrast to nonkeratinizing carcinoma, which, among its differing features, tends to invade into adjacent tissue with a smooth and somewhat delineated edge.

Treatment

Squamous cell carcinoma of the maxillary sinus is generally advanced at the time of diagnosis and, indeed, it can be difficult to differentiate from those squamous carcinomas arising in the lateral wall of the nose and ethmoids as most cases are generally advanced (stage III or IV) at the time of diagnosis. The standard approach over the past 40 years, in the majority of patients, has been a combination of surgery and radiotherapy; more recently with or without chemotherapy. Given the advanced stage and often complex nature of the spread of these lesions in a group of patients of widely varying age, planning is most effectively developed in a multidisciplinary team-based approach. Essentially, treatment is based on the extent of spread and the specific histology of the lesion. However, advanced age of a patient and the presence of other comorbidities may significantly alter treatment considerations as there is considerable variation in a patient's ability to withstand radical surgical procedures, possible flap or prosthetic reconstruction and the combined use of chemotherapy and radiotherapy. Surgery for lesions extending outside the maxilla and involving the skull base with all its critical neurovascular structures requires careful consideration of postoperative function and cosmetic restoration, even more so if the disease is recurrent and extensive (**Fig. 6.26**).

Contraindications for surgery of extensive lesions of the maxillary sinus invading the orbit, skull base, pterygomaxillary, infratemporal fossa, and oral cavity remain controversial and the details are often ill-defined in the long-term retrospective reported series in the literature. Contraindications to surgery also remain different in different institutions, depending on the experience and availability of various members of the surgical team and the possibility or otherwise of adopting advanced radiotherapy techniques, with or without chemotherapy. In many centers, spread of a maxillary squamous carcinoma to extensively involve the nasopharynx, clivus, bilateral orbital cavities (particularly the orbital apex), optic canal, optic nerve, the skull base passage of the internal carotid artery, the cavernous sinus, or the brain is generally considered inappropriate for surgery, although in younger patients lacking any notable comorbidity surgical treatment has been described that may include these areas.[79]

Involvement of the intracranial cavity, and subsequently, the brain, from squamous carcinoma of the maxilla or lateral wall of the nose and ethmoid is almost exclusively by local spread in a continuous fashion. While surgical resection of structures such as the cavernous sinus, internal carotid artery, and cranial nerves carries a high morbidity and an overall poor outcome, resection of a portion of the frontal lobe adjacent to the floor of the anterior cranial fossa may result in either minimal or no noticeable deficit in a patient.

Notwithstanding these limitations and irrespective of the surgical approach, it is well recognized that the overall poor prognosis for squamous carcinoma of the maxillary sinus does require an aggressive surgical approach to remove the entire microscopic disease if at all possible. In addition to the obvious obstacle of having to perform wide local excision in the proximity of multiple, critical neurovascular structures, the propensity for squamous carcinoma to undergo perineural spread is not always appreciated. While this problem is often mentioned with regard to the much rarer adenoid cystic carcinoma, it is almost certainly underreported in squamous carcinoma and may be responsible for a portion of the poor results seen following what appeared to be successful surgery. The surgeon's goal of obtaining negative margins frequently requires multiple frozen section specimens intraoperatively and revision of the extent of resection. This is obviously particularly difficult when bone of the skull base is involved as it may not be possible to evaluate these specimens intraoperatively.

The most common spread of squamous carcinoma of the maxilla into the intracranial cavity is by direct tumor extension through skull base bone. For those maxillary tumors extending upward through the ethmoid complex and the nasal cavity, the easiest access is through the thin osseous floor of the anterior cranial cavity via the cribriform plate or the roof of the ethmoid. The cribriform plate has multiple perforations through which the dural sleeves of the olfactory filaments pass. These structures allow direct spread of carcinoma to the olfactory bulbs, which are, of course, actual extensions of the brain. Fortunately, they are distinct and separated from the gyri of the frontal lobes above and while squamous carcinoma may spread to them, it may remain separate from the actual frontal lobes themselves. Additional extension may be from the ethmoid via the lamina papyracea along the route provided by the ethmoid foramina, which allow passage of the ethmoid neurovascular bundles from the orbits into the nasal cavity. The anterior and posterior ethmoidal arteries pierce the lamina papyracea at the suture line between the ethmoid and frontal bone then enter the intracranial cavity on the floor of the anterior cranial fossa before entering the nasal vault.

While orbit invasion is initially held in check by the orbital periosteum, the orbital apex provides three routes of access into the intracranial cavity via the optic canal, the superior orbital fissure, and the inferior orbital fissure. Spread along the optic canal may reach the optic chiasm, which lies in close proximity to the distal internal carotid artery and the anterior midbrain. Additionally, invasion

out of the optic canal may allow penetration into the middle cranial fossa. The superior orbital fissure spread may gain access to the cavernous sinus and the medial aspect of the middle fossa; and via the inferior orbit, the infraorbital canal leads to the foramen rotundum and from there to the trigeminal ganglion in Meckel's cave. Indeed, the fifth cranial nerve branch foramina probably provide the most common route of intracranial spread and malignancy from a squamous carcinoma of the maxilla. This is hardly surprising when one considers that the sensory supply to the face is principally through the branches of the trigeminal nerve and perineural spread can occur along these nerve sheaths. It is now almost 30 years since the excellent paper of Carter et al[80] on perineural spread by squamous carcinomas of the head and neck, which showed that these carcinomas have the ability to run along an affected nerve in a discontinuous manner with intervening skip areas that may have one centimeter or more of intervening normal nerve between one focus of perineural tumor and the next focus. Subsequent studies have shown that tumor may remain in this perineural space for a considerable period of time and occasionally notable aggregations of perineural spread may be seen on modern MRI imaging. There is still a great deal to learn about this potential method of spread from squamous carcinoma in addition to the more publicized adenoid cystic tumors.

While extensive maxillary carcinomas may spread to involve the jugular and carotid foramina in the floor of the middle fossa, the carotid canal has substantial periosteum, which is thought to resist tumor penetration, particularly in the region of the so-called "fibrous ring."[81] However, should tumor penetrate this area, it gains entry into the cavernous sinus where the internal carotid artery media is easily penetrated as the outer adventitial layer becomes much thinner. An additional vascular pathway exists via the ophthalmic veins, which join at the orbital apex and drain into the anterior inferior aspect of the cavernous sinus such that tumor in the orbital apex can pass through the superior orbital fissure via these veins into the cavernous sinus.

Endoscopic Surgery

Consideration of all the above modes of spread and the overall condition of the patient allows a wide variety of surgical therapy to be considered for squamous carcinoma of the maxilla. While endoscopic surgery may be undertaken for some squamous carcinomas of the nasal cavity, lateral nasal wall, ethmoid, and skull base, it is rare to be able to utilize these techniques in carcinoma of the maxillary sinus due to the extent and directions of spread at presentation.[82]

Midfacial Degloving

Midfacial degloving allows exposure of the entire mid-face and maxilla without external facial incisions.[83] This essentially sublabial approach requires periosteal elevation of the soft tissues over the anterior maxilla and therefore cannot be used when the maxillary sinus squamous carcinoma has perforated the anterior wall and is involving the soft tissues of the cheek. This technique gives an excellent exposure of the nasal cavity as the soft tissues of the nasal dorsum are elevated by a combination of transfixion, intercartilaginous, and piriform aperture incisions. The approach may be used in combination with a transcranial approach with either a frontal craniotomy or anterior subcranial approach. Following removal of the maxilla, excellent access can then be obtained to the pterygomaxillary space, infratemporal fossa, and adjacent skull base.

Anterior Transfacial Approaches

A variety of incisions have been recommended for the procedure of lateral rhinotomy and the medial component of the maxilla, lateral nasal wall, and nasal cavity can be accessed satisfactorily through this incision. The access is further improved if the incision is extended to encompass the orbit when orbital clearance or exenteration is undertaken at the same time as partial maxillectomy. Indeed, once the orbit is removed, total maxillectomy can be achieved via this combined lateral rhinotomy and palpebral incisions. More commonly, a Weber–Fergusson incision is used to undertake total maxillectomy with or without orbital extension. Occasional lesions presenting below Ohngren's line and encompassing the maxillary floor, anterior alveolus, hard palate, and lower lateral nasal wall can be removed through a midfacial degloving or unilateral sublabial approach. More commonly, these tumors actually arise from the oral cavity with secondary involvement of the inferior aspect of the maxillary sinus.

In all of these anterior facial approaches, multiple reconstruction options are possible with the well-established use of obturators, or the more recent use of free tissue transfer with or without subsequent osseointegrated support for dentition. Further details of these procedures are to be found in Chapter 19, p. 451.

Craniofacial Resection

This operative procedure has allowed a major advance in the surgical treatment of tumors of the nasal cavity and paranasal sinuses that have spread to involve the skull base in the manner outlined above.[52] In addition to tumors originating in the maxilla, it is frequently necessary for advanced tumors of the anteroethmoidal complex, lateral aspect of the nose, and nasal cavity and those rare tumors arising in the frontal and sphenoid sinuses. The procedure usually requires a multidisciplinary team

approach with head and neck surgeons and neurosurgeons. A head and neck surgeon may be from otorhinolaryngology, maxillofacial surgery, or plastic surgery or indeed combinations of any of these three disciplines. The facial approaches outlined above are used in combination with a craniotomy to achieve a complete resection of the anterior skull base in addition to orbit, affected dura, and, if necessary, adjacent brain. The sinonasal portion of the operation is usually performed first to delineate the tumor margins from inferiorly. Prior to opening the intracranial cavity following the appropriate extracranial osteotomies, the bulk of the tumor may be removed, which frequently assists in the delineation required for intracranial and skull base osteotomies prior to removal of this component of the tumor. Considerable variations in the techniques for this still-developing area of surgery are described in detail in Chapter 19.

In our cohort of 126 cases, the majority were treated with surgery (82.5%), either alone (26%), in combination with radiotherapy (47%) or with chemoradiation (9.5%) (Table 6.7). Six percent received radiotherapy alone, largely for palliation, and in 8 patients (6%) the disease was too advanced for them to receive anything other than symptomatic relief.

Surgery consisted mainly of radical maxillectomy with or without orbital clearance, as well as lateral rhinotomy, craniofacial resection, and midfacial degloving (Table 6.9). Given the advanced state of disease at presentation and the fact that 47% had had failed previous treatment, it is not surprising that the results overall are poor, with only 28% long-term survivors despite radical treatment. The majority died of residual disease within the first 2 years, most within the first 12 months, although three developed true recurrence at 7 and 10 years.[2]

References

1. Hellquist HB. Pathology of the Nose and Paranasal Sinuses. London: Butterworths;1990:88
2. Acheson ED, Cowdell RH, Hadfield E, Macbeth RG. Nasal cancer in woodworkers in the furniture industry. BMJ 1968;2(5605):587–596
3. MacBeth RG. Malignant disease of the paranasal sinuses. J Laryngol Otol 1965;79:592–612
4. Andersen HC, Andersen I, Solgaard J. Nasal cancers, symptoms and upper airway function in woodworkers. Br J Ind Med 1977;34(3):201–207
5. Roland RE. The risk of malignancy from internally deposited radio-isotopes. Radiation Research—Biomedical, Chemical & Physical Perspectives. New York: Academic Press; 1975:146–155
6. Boysen M, Solberg LA, Torjussen W, Poppe S, Høgetveit AC. Histological changes, rhinoscopical findings and nickel concentration in plasma and urine in retired nickel workers. Arch Otolaryngol 1984;97(1–2):105–115
7. Wada S, Miyanishi M, Nishimoto Y, Kambe S, Miller RW. Mustard gas as a cause of respiratory neoplasia in man. Lancet 1968;1(7553):1161–1163
8. Doll R, Morgan LG, Speizer FE. Cancers of the lung and nasal sinuses in nickel workers. Br J Cancer 1970;24(4):623–632

9. Pedersen E, Hogetveit AC, Andersen A. Cancer of respiratory organs among workers at a nickel refinery in Norway. Int J Cancer 1973;12(1):32–41

10. Stell PM, Magill T. Asbestos and cancer of the head and neck. Lancet 1973;1(7804):678

11. Roush GC. Epidemiology of cancer of the nose and paranasal sinuses: current concepts. Head Neck Surg 1979;2(1):3–11

12. Rankow RM, Conley J, Fodor P. Carcinoma of the maxillary sinus following thorotrast instillation. J Maxillofac Surg 1974;2(2-3):119–126

13. Harrison DFN. Snuff—its use and abuse. BMJ 1964;2(5425):1649–1651

14. Acheson ED, Cowdell RH, Jolles B. Nasal cancer in the Northamptonshire boot and shoe industry. BMJ 1970;1(5693):385–393

15. Hayes RB, Kardaun JW, de Bruyn A. Tobacco use and sinonasal cancer: a case-control study. Br J Cancer 1987;56(6):843–846

16. Alos L, Moyano S, Nadal A, et al. Human papillomaviruses are identified in a subgroup of sinonasal squamous cell carcinomas with favorable outcome. Cancer 2009;115(12):2701–2709

17. Choi HR, Roberts DB, Johnigan RH, et al. Molecular and clinicopathologic comparisons of head and neck squamous carcinoma variants: common and distinctive features of biological significance. Am J Surg Pathol 2004;28(10):1299–1310

18. Wenig B. Tumors of the upper respiratory tract. Part A: Nasal cavity, paranasal sinuses and nasopharynx. In: Fletcher CDM, ed. Diagnostic Histopathology of Tumors. London: Churchill Livingstone; 2000:50–66

19. Mason TJ, Mackay FW. In: US Cancer Mortality by County 1950–1969. Washington DC: DHEW Publications; 1974: 74–615

20. Osmond C, Gardener MJ, Acherson ED. Trends in Cancer Mortality, Analysis by Period of Birth and Death 1951–1980. London: HMSO; 1983

21. Curado M, Edwards B, Shin HR. Cancer Incidence in Five Continents. Vol IX. Lyon: IARC (IARC Scientific Publications No.160) 2007

22. Robin PE, Powell DJ. Regional node involvement and distant metastases in carcinoma of the nasal cavity and paranasal sinuses. J Laryngol Otol 1980;94(3):301–309

23. Shiffman NJ. Anterior intranasal carcinoma. Can J Surg 1979;22(2):159–160

24. Hopkin N, McNicoll W, Dalley VM, Shaw HJ. Cancer of the paranasal sinuses and nasal cavities. Part I. Clinical features. J Laryngol Otol 1984;98(6):585–595

25. Wang CC. Treatment of carcinoma of the nasal vestibule by irradiation. Cancer 1975;38(1):100–106

26. Sobin L, Gospodarowicz M, Wittekind C, eds.UICC TNM Classification of Malignant Tumours. 7th ed. Chichester: Wiley Blackwell; 2009:46–50

27. Edge S, Byrd D, Compton C, Fritz A. AJCC Cancer Staging Manual. New York, Dodrecth, Heidelberg, London: Springer; 2011

28. Johansen LV, Hjelm-Hansen M, Andersen AP. Squamous cell carcinoma of the nasal vestibule. Treatment results. Acta Radiol Oncol 1984;23(2-3):189–192

29. Kagan AR, Nussbaum H, Rao A, et al. The management of carcinoma of the nasal vestibule. Head Neck Surg 1981;4(2):125–128

30. Goepfert H, Guillamondegui OM, Jesse RH, Lindberg RD. Squamous cell carcinoma of nasal vestibule. Arch Otolaryngol 1974;100(1):8–10

31. Barzan L, Franchin G, Frustaci S, De Paoli A, Comoretto R. Carcinoma of the nasal vestibule: report of 12 cases. J Laryngol Otol 1990;104(1):9–11

32. Michaels L. Malignant neoplasms of surface epithelium. Ear, Nose and Throat Histopathology. Berlin: Springer Verlag; 1987:171–176

33. Schalekamp W, Hordijk GJ. Carcinoma of the nasal vestibule: prognostic factors in relation to lymph node metastasis. Clin Otolaryngol Allied Sci 1985;10(4):201–203

34. Wong CS, Cummings BJ. The place of radiation therapy in the treatment of squamous cell carcinoma of the nasal vestibule. A review. Acta Oncol 1988;27(3):203–208

35. Mendenhall NP, Parsons JT, Cassisi NJ, Million RR. Carcinoma of the nasal vestibule treated with radiation therapy. Laryngoscope 1987;97(5):626–632

36. Weinberger JM, Briant TD, Cummings BJ, Wong CS. The role of surgery in the treatment of squamous cell carcinoma of the nasal vestibule. J Otolaryngol 1988;17(7):372–375

37. McCollough WM, Mendenhall NP, Parsons JT, et al. Radiotherapy alone for squamous cell carcinoma of the nasal vestibule: management of the primary site and regional lymphatics. Int J Radiat Oncol Biol Phys 1993;26(1):73–79

38. Kummer E, Rasch CR, Keus RB, Tan IB, Balm AJ. T stage as prognostic factor in irradiated localized squamous cell carcinoma of the nasal vestibule. Head Neck 2002; 24(3):268–273

39. Mendenhall WM, Stringer SP, Cassisi NJ, Mendenhall NP. Squamous cell carcinoma of the nasal vestibule. Head Neck 1999;21(5):385–393

40. Langendijk JA, Poorter R, Leemans CR, de Bree R, Doornaert P, Slotman BJ. Radiotherapy of squamous cell carcinoma of the nasal vestibule. Int J Radiat Oncol Biol Phys 2004;59(5):1319–1325

41. Harrison DF. Total rhinectomy—a worthwhile operation? J Laryngol Otol 1982;96(12):1113–1123

42. Echeverria-Zumarraga M, Kaiser C, Gavilan C. Nasal septal carcinoma: initial symptom of nasal septal perforation. J Laryngol Otol 1988;102(9):834–835

43. Beatty CW, Pearson BW, Kern EB. Carcinoma of the nasal septum: experience with 85 cases. Otolaryngol Head Neck Surg 1982;90(1):90–94

44. LeLiever WC, Bailey BJ, Griffiths C. Carcinoma of the nasal septum. Arch Otolaryngol 1984;110(11):748–751

45. Ringertz W. Pathology of malignant tumours arising in the nasal cavity, paranasal sinuses and maxilla. Acta Otolaryngol 1938;27(Suppl):1–495

46. McKay SP, Shibuya TY, Armstrong WB, et al. Cell carcinoma of the paranasal sinuses and skull base. Am J Otolaryngol 2007;28(5):294–301

47. Robin PE, Powell DJ, Stansbie JM. Carcinoma of the nasal cavity and paranasal sinuses: incidence and presentation of different histological types. Clin Otolaryngol Allied Sci 1979;4(6):431–456

48. Hopkin N, McNicoll W, Dalley VM, Shaw HJ. Cancer of the paranasal sinuses and nasal cavities. Part I. Clinical features. J Laryngol Otol 1984;98(6):585–595

49. Higginson J, Oettle AG. Cancer incidence in the Bantu and "Cape Colored" races of South Africa: report of a cancer survey in the Transvaal (1953–55). J Natl Cancer Inst 1960;24:589–671

50. Holmström M, Wihelmsson B. Respiratory symptoms and pathophysiological effects of occupational exposure to formaldehyde and wood dust. Scand J Work Environ Health 1988;14(5):306–311

51. Blair A, Stewart P, O'Berg M, et al. Mortality among industrial workers exposed to formaldehyde. J Natl Cancer Inst 1986;76(6):1071–1084

52. Howard DJ, Lund VJ, Wei WI. Craniofacial resection for tumors of the nasal cavity and paranasal sinuses: a 25-year experience. Head Neck 2006;28(10):867–873

53. Lloyd G, Lund VJ, Howard D, Savy L. Optimum imaging for sinonasal malignancy. J Laryngol Otol 2000; 114(7):557–562

54. Lund VJ, Howard DJ, Lloyd GA, Cheesman AD. Magnetic resonance imaging of paranasal sinus tumors for craniofacial resection. Head Neck 1989;11(3):279–283
55. Castelnuovo PG, Belli E, Bignami M, Battaglia P, Sberze F, Tomei G. Endoscopic nasal and anterior craniotomy resection for malignant nasoethmoid tumors involving the anterior skull base. Skull Base 2006;16(1):15–18
56. Lund V, Howard DJ, Wei WI. Endoscopic resection of malignant tumors of the nose and sinuses. Am J Rhinol 2007;21(1):89–94
57. Podboj J, Smid L. Endoscopic surgery with curative intent for malignant tumors of the nose and paranasal sinuses. Eur J Surg Oncol 2007;33(9):1081–1086
58. Shipchandler TZ, Batra PS, Citardi MJ, Bolger WE, Lanza DC. Outcomes for endoscopic resection of sinonasal squamous cell carcinoma. Laryngoscope 2005;115(11):1983–1987
59. Nicolai P, Battaglia P, Bignami M, et al. Endoscopic surgery for malignant tumors of the sinonasal tract and adjacent skull base: a 10-year experience. Am J Rhinol 2008;22(3):308–316
60. Blanco AI, Chao KS, Ozyigit G, et al. Carcinoma of paranasal sinuses: long-term outcomes with radiotherapy. Int J Radiat Oncol Biol Phys 2004;59(1):51–58
61. Harrison LB, Pfister DG, Kraus D, et al. Management of unresectable malignant tumors at the skull base using concomitant chemotherapy and radiotherapy with accelerated fractionation. Skull Base Surg 1994;4(3):127–131
62. Daly ME, Chen AM, Bucci MK, et al. Intensity-modulated radiation therapy for malignancies of the nasal cavity and paranasal sinuses. Int J Radiat Oncol Biol Phys 2007;67(1):151–157
63. Hoppe BS, Stegman LD, Zelefsky MJ, et al. Treatment of nasal cavity and paranasal sinus cancer with modern radiotherapy techniques in the postoperative setting—the MSKCC experience. Int J Radiat Oncol Biol Phys 2007;67(3):691–702
64. Chen AM, Daly ME, Bucci MK, et al. Carcinomas of the paranasal sinuses and nasal cavity treated with radiotherapy at a single institution over five decades: are we making improvement? Int J Radiat Oncol Biol Phys 2007;69(1):141–147
65. Sisson GA, Johnson NE, Amiri CS. Cancer of the maxillary sinus. Clinical classification and management. Ann Otol Rhinol Laryngol 1963;72:1050–1059
66. Harrison DF. Critical look at the classification of maxillary sinus carcinomata. Ann Otol Rhinol Laryngol 1978;87(1 Pt 1):3–9
67. Ohngren L. Malignant tumours of the maxilloethmoid region. Acta Otolaryngol 1933;(Supp 19):1
68. St-Pierre S, Baker SR. Squamous cell carcinoma of the maxillary sinus: analysis of 66 cases. Head Neck Surg 1983;5(6):508–513
69. Kondo M, Inuyama Y, Ando Y, et al. Patterns of relapse of squamous cell carcinoma of the maxillary sinus. Cancer 1984;53(10):2206–2210
70. Knegt PP, de Jong PC, van Andel JG, de Boer MF, Eykenboom W, van der Schans E. Carcinoma of the paranasal sinuses. Results of a prospective pilot study. Cancer 1985;56(1):57–62
71. Lavertu P, Roberts JK, Kraus DH, et al. Squamous cell carcinoma of the paranasal sinuses: the Cleveland Clinic experience 1977–1986. Laryngoscope 1989;99(11):1130–1136
72. Giri SP, Reddy EK, Gemer LS, Krishnan L, Smalley SR, Evans RG. Management of advanced squamous cell carcinomas of the maxillary sinus. Cancer 1992;69(3):657–661
73. Stern SJ, Goepfert H, Clayman G, et al. Squamous cell carcinoma of the maxillary sinus. Arch Otolaryngol Head Neck Surg 1993;119(9):964–969
74. Alvarez I, Suárez C, Rodrigo JP, Nuñez F, Caminero MJ. Prognostic factors in paranasal sinus cancer. Am J Otolaryngol 1995;16(2):109–114
75. Miyaguchi M, Sakai S, Takashima H, Hosokawa H. Lymph node and distant metastases in patients with sinonasal carcinoma. J Laryngol Otol 1995;109(4):304–307
76. Myers LL, Nussenbaum B, Bradford CR, Teknos TN, Esclamado RM, Wolf GT. Paranasal sinus malignancies: an 18-year single institution experience. Laryngoscope 2002;112(11):1964–1969
77. Bhattacharyya N. Cancer of the nasal cavity: survival and factors influencing prognosis. Arch Otolaryngol Head Neck Surg 2002;128(9):1079–1083
78. Miyaguchi M, Sakai S-I, Mori N, Kitaoku S. Multiple primary malignancies in patients with malignant tumours of the nasal cavities and paranasal sinuses. J Laryngol Otol 1990;104(9):696–698
79. Jackson K, Donald P, Gandour-Edwards R. Pathophysiology of skullbase malignancies. In: Donald P, ed. Surgery of the Skull Base. Philadelphia: Lippincot, Williams and Wilkins; 1998:51–72
80. Carter RL, Foster CS, Dinsdale EA, Pittam MR. Perineural spread by squamous carcinomas of the head and neck: a morphological study using antiaxonal and antimyelin monoclonal antibodies. J Clin Pathol 1983;36(3):269–275
81. Prasad S, Barnes L, Janecka I. Anatomy of the internal carotid artery. Presented at the 3rd meeting of the North Americal Skullbase Society: Acapulco, Mexico; February 16–20 1992
82. Lund VJ, Stammberger H, Nicolai P, et al. European position paper on endoscopic management of tumours of the nose, paranasal sinuses and skull base. Rhinol Suppl 2010;(22):1–143
83. Howard DJ, Lund VJ. The role of midfacial degloving in modern rhinological practice. J Laryngol Otol 1999;113(10):885–887

Squamous Cell Carcinoma Variants

The Association of Human Papilloma Virus with Benign and Malignant Sinonasal Neoplasms

Human papilloma viruses (HPVs) are prevalent pathogens, and their epidemiology has been mostly studied in the uterine cervix and the vagina, beginning as long ago as the 1950s. The carcinogenicity of HPV infection in this area is well established and recent details of this large area of research are covered in detail in the IARC monograph (volume 90) published in 2007.[1] Even this excellent monograph on human papilloma viruses shows that there are considerable areas where we do not have a full understanding of the major steps necessary for carcinogenesis subsequent to HPV infection, persistence of that infection, progression to precancerous lesions, and eventually invasion. We now understand that provided invasion has not taken place, this process is reversible by clearance of HPV infection and regression of the precancerous change. HPV infection can be separated into low viral load infections that do not produce any microscopically evident abnormalities, and higher viral load infections that do. Most of our knowledge refers to HPV16, which is the type most frequently found in tumors in the general population.

The role of human papilloma viruses in head and neck lesions has been far less extensively studied, but even within the research that has been done there are widely varying reports with regard to the incidence of HPV involvement in both benign and malignant lesions. The literature can be contradictory and confusing. It is widely accepted that persistence of HPV infection is essential for the development of cervical precancerous lesions and cancer, but from the extensive studies in this area we know that most HPV infections are transient and become undetectable within 1 to 2 years, even by sensitive PCR assays. Consequently, these anogenital HPV infections tend to resolve spontaneously, as indeed do warts anywhere else on the body. We can assume, therefore, that they are cleared completely by the cell-mediated immune system or are self-limited or are suppressed into long-term latency. These issues remain a significant unresolved question when considering the natural history of HPV and which infections are cleared. It may be that small foci of cells can maintain infection with low DNA copy numbers, even when no HPV DNA is detectable by the variety of molecular tests. There are still many answers required to these questions. Persistence of HPV infection appears to be uncommon compared with clearance and there is certainly no consensus on the length of time of perceived persistence that goes on to produce precancerous or cancerous lesions. The supposition is that the longer duration of infection with high-risk types of HPV may have obvious implications for the production of cancer, but as yet there is no agreement on a uniform definition of HPV persistence.

There are now over 100 types of human papilloma viruses described and infection is so common worldwide that it is far from straightforward to assess whether the presence of HPV contributes to tumor formation. Advances in the understanding of the natural history of HPV are still required and, while intensive efforts have been made to standardize accurate and reliable measurements of HPV DNA, most of the variable results from the late 1980s and 1990s in the study of cervical cancer were caused by unsuspected misclassification of HPV status in the original large-scale molecular epidemiological studies. In the area of the head and neck, which has been studied to a far lesser degree, it is therefore not surprising that results using different methods on smaller numbers of specimens have produced varying conclusions. In the future, with further additional improvements in cytology and serology, it will be important to optimize methods to improve our interpretation of the patterns of viral involvement, viral clearance, persistence, and progression of disease.

HPV Prevalence in Squamous Cell Carcinoma of the Head and Neck

At the time of writing, the previous decade of research related to HPV prevalence in association with squamous carcinoma has shown between 20% and 30% correlation for oropharyngeal, hypopharyngeal, and laryngeal squamous carcinomas, with a correlation up to 50% with squamous cell carcinoma of Waldeyer's tissue within the tonsil ring. The evidence is particularly compelling for oropharyngeal carcinomas, particularly those of the tonsil.[2-5]

Clear identification of this subset of tumors has been of considerable clinical interest because although it initially appeared that these lesions presented more aggressive behavior, with the HPV-positive patients usually presenting with a higher lymph node status (which normally is a strong predictor for decreased survival times), the converse was found to be true and HPV positivity was related to increased times to recurrence and improved overall survival times following treatment.

In contrast to the oropharynx, the evidence with regard to the larynx or sinonasal cavities is far less conclusive and the IARC 2007 monograph stated that the evidence for the larynx was limited and that there is inadequate evidence in the sinonasal area.[1] Of the previous reports suggesting possible implication of HPV in the development of carcinomas in the sinonasal region, those of Hoffman et al, Syrojanen et al, El-Mofty and Lu, and Alos et al are of note.[6-9] In the most recent of these studies from Barcelona,[9] 60 squamous cell carcinomas of the sinonasal tract seen between 1981 and 2006 were reviewed retrospectively. HPV infection was determined and typed by amplification of HPV DNA by PCR. P16 expression was determined by immunohistochemistry. HPV DNA was detected in tumor tissue of 12 of 60 patients (20%). HPV16 was identified in 11 tumors.

Immunohistochemistry for P16 stained all HPV-positive and no HPV-negative tumors. In 12 cases, the carcinoma was said to develop on a sinonasal inverted papilloma that coexisted in 11 cases and had previously been excised in one case. This is certainly a very high incidence of this association with squamous carcinoma and leads to some concern about the validity of the data. Only one of the carcinomas arising on a sinonasal inverted papilloma tested positive for HPV16.

On the basis of Kaplan-Meier estimates, HPV-positive tumors statistically had a significantly better survival than HPV-negative tumors, being 62% at 5 years in contrast to 20%. On multivariant analysis, HPV status retained statistical significance. This publication appears to be the first evidence of better survival of HPV-positive tumors in sinonasal squamous cell carcinomas, but the conclusions drawn from this relatively small series of patients remain to be confirmed by further studies.

Verrucous Carcinoma

Definition

(ICD-O code 8051/3)

Verrucous carcinoma is a rare, low-grade variant of squamous cell carcinoma and characteristically has a warty or papillary appearance, producing an exophytic mass that is composed of keratinizing, well-differentiated epithelium.

Etiology

Friedell and Rosenthal[10] were the first to describe 8 cases in the oral cavity with a papillary verrucoid appearance. However, it was Ackerman[11] who coined the term "verrucous carcinoma" and recognized its clinical significance and good prognosis when treated by surgery.

Hanna and Ali[12] implicated use of snuff, use of chewing tobacco, and poor oral hygiene as etiological factors in verrucous carcinoma. A more recent report by Karthikeya et al[13] from India also associated intranasal snuff and smoking with an extensive intranasal verrucous carcinoma.

Human papilloma virus has been identified in many benign and malignant lesions of the upper aerodigestive tract, and colleagues at the Mayo Clinic[14] in 1999 reported a retrospective group of 13 patients with intranasal verrucous carcinomas seen between 1960 and 1996. Ten presented with nasal obstruction and the maxillary sinus was the extranasal site most often involved. Five patients had verrucous carcinoma developing in inverted papilloma and one a squamous carcinoma with a verrucous component. In 7 patients (10 specimens), DNA was successfully amplified for PCR testing and *no* HPV DNA was detected. No role for HPV in the etiology of these tumors was found.

Synonyms

Ackerman tumor.

Incidence

Verrucous carcinoma of the nose and sinus is a very rare tumor and overall the maxillary sinus appears to be the most common site, followed by the nasal fossa. We have only treated two cases, both in elderly women (75 and 90 years old, respectively). Nasopharyngeal lesions encroaching into the nasal cavities have been reported.[15]

Diagnostic Features

Clinical

By far the majority of patients in the literature are men and most are smokers or users of snuff as noted above. The most common presenting symptom is nasal obstruction in ~75% of the cases, in addition to the majority being aware of an intranasal lesion. Approximately one-third present with pain that is more common in those with disease developing in the maxilla. Unilateral mucopurulent rhinorrhea may be long-standing and swelling of the cheek, loosening of the teeth, the inability to fit dentures, trismus, and a visible lesion presenting in the oral cavity are all found in those patients with maxillary involvement.

Verrucous carcinoma generally presents in the 50- to 80-year-old age group and the symptoms may be long-standing, with reports of symptoms for up to 2 years prior to presentation.

Intranasal examination usually reveals an extensive, expansile exophytic lesion, often visible in the nostrils, with the lateral wall of the nose being the commonest site in those lesions where the site of origin can be discerned.[14] Approximately half the patients with intranasal lesions will have evidence of further spread into the maxilla and ethmoid sinuses. A careful intraoral examination is necessary to evaluate teeth, the possibility of a sinus tract, simple edema, or a definitive mass. It may be difficult to know whether some of the more extensive lesions arose in the oral cavity or intranasally.

The literature contains examples of these lesions appearing in association with both inverted papilloma and benign nasal polyps and, although the lesions are extremely rare, this once again demonstrates the need for accurate histology on all nasal polypoid masses and adequate examination of the nasal cavity at the time of removal of any benign nasal polyposis.

Imaging

Depending on the extent of the lesion, CT, MRI scans, and orthopantomograms are all useful. Indeed, simple sinus plain radiographs may show diffuse radiopacity and bone destruction, particularly for those lesions within the maxillary sinus. Coronal CT sections are particularly useful for showing destruction within areas such as the floor of the maxillary antrum or nasal cavity as well as spread into the ethmoid sinuses. MRI may be indicated in addition if the lesions are large enough to encroach on the orbit or skull base.

Histological Features and Differential Diagnosis

Verrucous carcinoma is a lesion that continues to be difficult to diagnose on occasions. Diagnosis from a small or superficial biopsy may be impossible, with only hyperkeratosis, acanthosis, and apparently benign papillomatosis in the material. Cooper et al[16] showed that mean cell and nuclear areas were significantly higher in verrucous carcinoma than in squamous papillomas, giving a mean cell area above 300 μm^2 as a useful dividing point to establish malignancy. Foci of typical squamous carcinoma may occur within a tumor, which otherwise looks exclusively verrucous. This subgroup has a higher recurrence rate. The surgeon must provide the pathologist with not only the details of the history, which is often prolonged, but an ample representative sample or excisional biopsy to aid in an accurate diagnosis.

The differential diagnosis of verrucous carcinoma includes exophytic squamous cell carcinoma, papillary squamous cell carcinoma, and keratinizing inverted papilloma.

Natural History

Verrucous carcinoma is a slow but locally invasive neoplasm that can cause extensive local destruction if left untreated. True verrucous carcinoma does not metastasize, but, when it is associated with squamous carcinoma, the potential for lymph node metastasis is present and clearly these patients should be managed as if they had squamous cell carcinoma. These rare cases of verrucous carcinoma within the nose and sinuses have an excellent prognosis but they must be fully excised as recurrence with inadequate treatment remains a problem.

Treatment and Outcome

Patients with verrucous carcinoma may be treated by a wide variety of excisional surgery and, not surprisingly, depending on the size and site of the presenting lesion, surgical options have included endoscopic excision, lateral rhinotomy, total rhinectomy, maxillectomy, with and without orbital exenteration, and craniofacial resection. Those with extensive disease in particular, may require further surgery for recurrence but in the Mayo Clinic series[14] with follow-up ranging from 2 months to 32 years (mean 6.5 years), none of the 13 patients with nose and paranasal sinus verrucous carcinoma had metastases and none died because of the tumor. While the literature still has a tendency to quote the fear of anaplastic transformation of verrucous carcinoma after radiotherapy, critical review of these reports has shown that many are unrecognized, hybrid verrucous carcinoma associated with squamous carcinoma. They have been inappropriately labeled as verrucous carcinoma.[14,17,18] Radiotherapy can be an effective treatment for this disease and indeed was the treatment given to our two patients with good results, both surviving longer than 5 years.

Papillary Squamous Cell Carcinoma

Definition

(ICD-O code 8052/3)

Papillary squamous cell carcinoma (PSCC) is a distinct variant of squamous cell carcinoma that has an exophytic, papillary configuration with thin fingers of malignant epithelium overlying a central fibrovascular core. The surface epithelium may resemble that seen in intraepithelial neoplasia or high-grade dysplasia with minimal keratosis.

Etiology

The majority of papillary squamous cell carcinomas of the head and neck have been reported in the larynx and hypopharynx, and both smoking and alcohol have been implicated as factors.[19,20] However, the rarity of lesions presenting in the nose and sinuses does not allow extrapolation of this data as an etiological factor in the sinonasal tumors.

As with other variants of squamous carcinoma, human papilloma virus, notably HPV16, has been suggested as an etiological factor, but the prevalence of HPV in a wide variety of studies of head and neck tumors commencing in the 1980s has reported a prevalence of HPV varying from 0 to 48% in papillary squamous carcinoma.[21] Comparison of HPV DNA detection rates between the published studies is confounded by the different molecular biological techniques used, different sites and patient details, and the often small sample sizes. In general a reciprocal relationship has been found between p53 and HPV prevalence. The role of HPV in the etiology of papillary squamous carcinoma therefore still requires further investigation. Indeed, papillary squamous cell carcinoma of the sinonasal region is a poorly understood variety of squamous carcinoma in this region and, because of its very low incidence, it may be confused with verrucous carcinoma, exophytic conventional squamous cell carcinoma, or inverted papilloma.

Incidence and Site

Papillary squamous cell carcinoma may be derived from preexisting papillary mucosal hyperplasia or squamous cell papilloma, although in the report of Suarez et al[21] of 38 cases from all sites in the head and neck, only 2 papillary squamous cell carcinomas exhibited histological evidence of a preexisting papilloma. However, 34% of the patients had a history of previous papillomas at the site of the subsequent papillary carcinoma. Unfortunately, the paper does not contain precise clinical details of the 11 sinonasal cases and 5 nasopharyngeal cases (out of 38), nor of the length of time over which these cases were collected.

Diagnostic Features

Clinical

Unilateral nasal obstruction and epistaxis are the commonest presenting symptoms and, on examination, the lesions within the nasal cavity are usually soft, friable, pedunculated, exophytic papillary masses. The base of the pedicle is often small, but broad-based lesions have been reported. Less than 10% of patients with papillary squamous cell carcinoma of the entire head and neck area present with cervical metastases and pulmonary metastases are extremely rare.

Histological Features and Differential Diagnosis

The multiple papillary projections of these lesions have a central fibrovascular core covered by the malignant epithelium, which is usually composed of nonkeratinized, immature basaloid cells or more pleomorphic cells. Multiple papillary squamous carcinoma has been reported along with evidence of papillary precursor lesions. Of considerable importance is the finding of stromal invasion, which may consist of single or multiple nests of tumor cells with a chronic lymphoplasma cellular infiltrate in the lamina propria adjacent to the carcinoma, but minimal elsewhere within the papillary cores. These findings are in contrast to squamous papilloma and verrucous carcinoma, which, although having similar architecture, do not have the same findings of atypia of the epithelium. The most notable difficulty reported by colleagues in pathology seems to be differentiating between exophytic SCC and papillary SCC, but in general the papillary stalks of PSCC are much better defined than in exophytic SCC.[22]

Treatment and Prognosis

While the available literature describes the prognosis of these lesions in the larynx as favorable, the sinonasal papillary carcinomas were found by Suarez et al[21] to be the most lethal. Detail is missing from their publication, but 11 of 25 patients (44%) with a median long-term follow-up of 3 years died of disease. Recurrence and sinonasal tumor site were the only factors related to outcome. All patients had been treated with surgery and radiotherapy, but no details were available and it is not possible to draw definite conclusions on treatment from a paper whose aim was to define the clinicopathological characteristics of papillary squamous cell carcinoma.

Basaloid Squamous Cell Carcinoma

Definition

(ICD-O code 8083/3)

Basaloid squamous cell carcinoma is a generally aggressive high-grade variant of squamous cell carcinoma, having both basaloid and squamous cells, usually closely packed and in a solid pattern.

Etiology

While tobacco use and alcohol use have been strongly implicated in basaloid squamous cell carcinoma (BSCC) in pharyngeal and laryngeal sites, it is difficult to be certain

of their relevance for the rare cases reported in the sinonasal complex.[23–25] It remains controversial whether Epstein-Barr virus (EBV) or human papilloma virus (HPV) are contributory factors in BSCC. Wan et al reported three cases of nasopharyngeal BSCC in which they detected EBV.[26]

Synonym

The terms basaloid carcinoma and adenoid cysticlike carcinoma have both been used in the past.

Incidence and Site

BSCC was initially described by Wain et al[27] in 1986 in cases involving the tongue, hypopharynx, and larynx. Subsequent reports have confirmed that the head and neck is the most frequently involved area but with larynx, pharynx, and oral cavity sites predominating. Nasopharynx and sinonasal tract cases are extremely rare and we have only one case in a series of 320 squamous carcinomas and variants, a 75-year-old man. In 20 head and neck cases reported in the year 2000 from the combined departments of the University of Michigan, Ann Arbor, and the Memorial Sloane Kettering Cancer Center, New York, from between 1975 and 1997,[25] only 2 cases occurred in the nose and one in the nasopharynx (the latter in a nonsmoker).

Diagnostic Features

Clinical

Basal cell carcinoma presents predominantly in men between 60 and 80 years of age.

In contrast to verrucous and papillary carcinoma, BSCCs within the nasal cavity usually appear as a solid mass, often with considerable induration and ulceration with easily induced bleeding on examination. The clinical history of nasal obstruction and epistaxis is more often accompanied by pain and of significantly shorter duration than other forms of squamous carcinoma. Again, in contrast to the other variants, they appear to present with advanced T stage in all reports; metastases to the regional lymph nodes are more common and distant metastases involving the lungs, bones, skin, and brain have been reported to occur in as many as 50% of the patients. As a consequence of the aggressive nature of these lesions, nasal and cheek deformities, paresthesia, proptosis and diplopia are more likely to be clinical features of this rare form of squamous carcinoma.

Imaging

CT and MRI are often required to delineate the full extent of the lesion as there is frequently significant bone invasion and extension to neighboring structures such as the

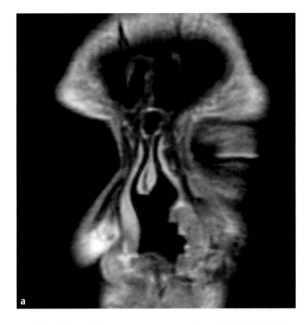

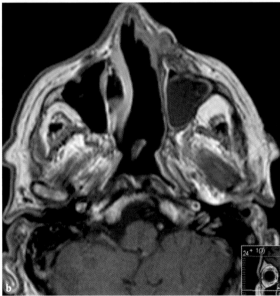

Fig. 6.30a, b

a Coronal MRI (T1W post gadolinium contrast) showing recurrent basaloid squamous cell carcinoma in the anterior nasal cavity, vestibule, and lateral wall after previous resection elsewhere.

b Axial MRI (T1W post gadolinium contrast) in the same patient showing tumor in the anterior nasal cavity extending into the soft tissues of the cheek. Benign retention cyst in the adjacent maxillary sinus.

orbit, pterygopalatine fissure, infratemporal space, and anterior cranial fossa (**Fig. 6.30**). The lesions may extend bilaterally prior to diagnosis with involvement of the opposite ethmoid complex and substantial erosion of the nasal septum.

Histological Features and Differential Diagnosis

As a consequence of its extreme rarity in the sinonasal tract,[27] BSCC is rarely suspected clinically and has to be differentiated from other aggressive sinonasal malignancies. Weineke et al[28] identified only 14 cases from the sinonasal tract in the files of the Otolaryngologic Head and Neck Pathology Tumor Registry at the Armed Forces Institute of Pathology over a 21-year period between 1975 and 1996.

Difficulties arise as a consequence of the fact that basaloid squamous cell carcinoma is frequently associated with a more standard well- or moderately differentiated squamous cell carcinoma component, which may in itself be associated with in situ carcinoma or frank invasive keratinizing squamous cell carcinoma. There may also be areas of squamous differentiation within the basaloid tumor islands, with an abrupt change from basaloid to squamous cells. The basaloid cells are frequently in rounded nests and are highly atypical with hypochromatic nuclei and considerable mitotic activity. There are often areas of comedo-type necrosis and a pseudoglandular arrangement that can cause confusion with adenoid cystic carcinoma.

Metastases may be composed of basaloid carcinoma, keratinizing squamous cell carcinoma, or both.[28,29]

The differential diagnosis includes adenoid cystic carcinoma, adenosquamous carcinoma, and neuroendocrine carcinoma. While modern immunohistochemistry and electron microscopy can help considerably here, it is important to remember that adenoid cystic carcinoma only very rarely spreads to cervical lymph nodes and only in the solid variant with advanced disease. Palpable metastatic nodes in association with BSCC are quite common, even from sinonasal lesions. Immunohistochemistry may require a variety of cytokeratin antibodies, but the antibody 34 β E12 directed against the high molecular weight cytokeratins is said to be the most sensitive for the detection of basaloid cells. The presence of dotlike vimentin expression in BSCC can also be helpful, and the absence of any myoepithelial cells helps to distinguish between BSCC and adenoid cystic carcinoma.[23]

In a substantial report published in 2004, the multidisciplinary team from the MD Anderson Cancer Center reported a study that performed molecular analysis on 92 squamous cell carcinoma variants from the head and neck.[30] These comprised 44 primary, untreated, conventional squamous cell carcinomas between 1985 and 2001, and 48 variant carcinomas (18 verrucous, 6 papillary,

7 basaloid, and 17 sarcomatoid). These were assessed using microsatellite markers and loss of heterozygosity (LOH). Overall, a higher than average incidence of LOH was found at most (15/21) of the markers tested in the basaloid squamous cell carcinomas. These differences were significant and distinguished between the other variant carcinomas, particularly at markers D9 S157 and D11 S4167. This study showed significant association between certain clinicopathological factors and LOH with significant statistical associations being found between the incidence of LOH, age, size, site, stage, and patient survival. This study is an example of markers that might prove to be useful in the future and might assist with the early detection and diagnosis in individuals in the future.

Treatment and Natural History

Of the 14 sinonasal cases of Wieneke et al,[28] 13 received primary surgery (no details) and 5 adjuvant radiotherapy. Chemotherapy was given to 2 patients; 7 had recurrence within 2 years of diagnosis, with 4 having distant metastases to bone and lung that are regional lymph node metastases. In 2 patients dura and brain were directly invaded and 10 (71%) either died of disease[7] or were alive with disease[3] at last follow-up. The average and median times to death were 33 months and 12 months.

As a consequence of the features outlined above, basaloid squamous cell carcinoma in sinonasal sites follows the pattern seen elsewhere in the head and neck and has a poor prognosis. While precise statistics from this rare variant are difficult to gain because of the small numbers involved, some authors feel that it appears to be more aggressive than conventional squamous cell carcinoma when matched stage for stage,[27,28,31] but others feel that stage for stage BSCC is similar to conventional squamous carcinoma.[23,32] It certainly appears to be the case that modern multimodality therapy must be tried and assessed in these cases. Our patient received radiotherapy following surgical excision and has survived 3 years so far.

Spindle Cell Carcinoma

Definition

(ICD-O code 9074/3)

Spindle cell carcinoma (SPCC) is a tumor that is composed of elements of squamous cell carcinoma, either invasive or in situ, and an additional, usually larger, component of malignant spindle cells that are of epithelial origin but often have a mesenchymal appearance, which has given rise to considerable confusion and misdiagnosis in the past.

Synonyms

These have been multiple and include pseudosarcoma, sarcomatoid carcinoma, metaplastic carcinoma, carcinosarcoma, biphasic tumor, and collision tumor.

Etiology

This rare variant of squamous cell carcinoma has been most commonly described in the glottic area of the larynx and less frequently in the hypopharynx. It is very rare in the sinonasal complex. The laryngopharyngeal tumors have been linked to cigarette smoking and alcohol consumption and radiation, but there is insufficient evidence to link these factors with the production of SCC in the sinonasal area.[33,34]

Incidence

Of the rare variant tumors of squamous cell carcinoma in the sinonasal tract, spindle cell carcinoma is the commonest variant reported from the largest centers. Of the 48 variant tumors studied in the MD Anderson series reported in 2004, 18 were verrucous, 6 were papillary, 7 were basaloid, and 17 were spindle cell carcinomas (sarcomatoid). These variants were seen over a period of 16 years from 1985 to 2001.[35] In our series, there were 9 patients out of a total of 320 squamous cell carcinomas and variants. They were predominantly male (8:1), with ages ranging from 39 to 64 years (mean 54.3 years).

Site

These lesions are rare within the sinonasal tract and most commonly present within the nasal cavity. However, in 6 patients the ethmoids and skull base were affected and in the other 3 the maxilla was the primary site of origin.

Diagnostic Features

Clinical Features and Imaging

These tumors most commonly present with unilateral nasal obstruction associated with rhinorrhea and minor epistaxis; on examination they are frequently polypoidal but may have significant ulceration of the surface and pronounced infiltration at the base. There are no specific features on imaging, but with the larger lesions there will be extensive bone erosion and invasion into the adjacent sinuses.

Histological Features and Differential Diagnosis

The most commonly used synonym for these tumors in the past has been "sarcomatoid," and when the spindle cell pattern dominates the histopathological picture SPCC can be mistaken for a true sarcoma. Foci of osteosarcomatous, chondrosarcomatous, or rhabdosarcomatous differentiation may be present, but the most common resemblance of these tumors is to fibrosarcoma or malignant fibrous histiocytoma. While the spindle cell pattern usually forms the bulk of the tumor, the squamous component is often seen either as in situ carcinoma or as invasive SCC. Ulceration makes the evaluation of carcinoma in situ difficult and multiple sections may be required to demonstrate the infiltration of the squamous cell component. Further difficulties may be encountered with biopsies of metastases, which may only contain squamous cell carcinoma, a mixture of spindle cell and squamous cell, or rarely only the spindle cell component.[34]

When the squamous cell component is not apparent in a spindle cell lesion, it is important to investigate for evidence of epithelial differentiation and the tumor cells can express both epithelial and mesenchymal markers. The most useful epithelial markers are currently AE1, AE3, CK1, and CK18, and epithelial membrane antigen. Cytokeratin expression can be demonstrated in spindle cells in up to 90% of cases. Occasionally, spindle cell carcinomas can be confused with other spindle cell proliferations such as inflammatory myofibroblastic sarcoma and myoepithelial carcinoma.[35] The recent molecular evidence has shown a significantly higher frequency of LOH at marker D4 S2632 for spindle cell carcinoma compared with the other variant forms and the overall molecular evidence would suggest that SPCC is a monoclonal epithelial neoplasm with divergent mesenchymal differentiation.[36,37] However, continuing debate on this subject is fierce and it is at the very center of our traditional histological classification of tumors.

Treatment

The limited literature on spindle cell carcinoma in the head and neck region, mainly the larynx, places it in the more aggressive forms of variant along with basaloid carcinoma and poorly differentiated squamous carcinoma with lymph node metastases in up to 25% of cases, but distant metastases are less common, between 5 and 15%.[36] There are insufficient numbers of sinonasal lesions reported to provide any firm figures or statements with regard to prognosis. Irradiation is generally unrewarding as a primary treatment for laryngeal spindle cell carcinomas and complete surgical excision of the rare sinonasal lesions would seem to be the most appropriate form of treatment with radiotherapy as an adjunct guided by the postoperative histopathology findings.

All 9 of our patients underwent radical surgery (6 craniofacial resection, 3 maxillectomies plus one orbital clearance). In addition 5 received radiotherapy and 3 chemotherapy. Despite this, outcome was universally poor, with only one patient surviving beyond 5 years and eventually dying of their disease at 70 months, while survival of the others ranged from only a few months to 3 years.

Adenosquamous Carcinoma

Definition

(ICD-O code 8560/3)

This rare variant of squamous carcinoma contains both true adenocarcinoma and squamous cell carcinoma, but characteristically the two components are generally separate; this differentiates this rare lesion from mucoepidermoid carcinoma, which has a notably different natural history.

Incidence

Gerughty et al[38] described 2 patients with nasal disease (out of 10 head and neck cases) in the defining publication of 1968. The excellent 2002 review by Keelawat et al[39] of their own 12 cases from the head and neck and a further 46 cases from the anglophone literature, showed only 4 cases originating from the nose and sinuses.

Diagnostic Features

Histological Features

The surface mucosal element may be either squamous cell carcinoma or in situ change. The adenocarcinomatous component tends to be deeper and usually consists of tubular areas where mucin is present, either within the lumen of the tubular structures or within the cells. The latter may form signet ring cells. Mucin is not a strict requirement if there is obvious glanduloductal formation.

The diagnosis of this very rare variant is best made after resection of the entire lesion and subsequent thorough overall histological examination.

Treatment and Prognosis

Local surgery and irradiation in the two nasal cases of Gerughty et al was followed by rapid recurrence requiring radical surgery (total maxillectomy, ethmoidectomy, and orbital exenteration) and radical neck dissection. Precise details of the nasal cases in the review by Keelawat et al are not available but overall the head and neck cases were treated with primary surgery (total 58) with 10 receiving additional postoperative irradiation and only a single case receiving chemotherapy.

The laryngeal, pharyngeal, and floor of mouth tumors in these reports generally appeared to be very aggressive and are currently thought to have a poorer prognosis than squamous cell carcinoma, with up to 75% of patients having regional lymph node metastases and 25% of patients having distant metastases, most commonly to the lungs.[38] However, stage-for-stage comparison with conventional squamous cell carcinoma has not been studied carefully and this is another example of a rare tumor from the older literature that may benefit from modern multimodality therapy.

Acantholytic Squamous Cell Carcinoma

This rare variant of squamous cell carcinoma occurs most commonly in the sun-exposed skin of the head and neck and has been reported in the larynx, nasopharynx, hypopharynx, and oral cavity, but is unknown in the sino-nasal tract. The tumor is characterized by acantholysis of the tumor cells, which produces pseudolumina and areas of apparent glandular differentiation.

Nonkeratinizing Squamous Cell Carcinoma (Cylindrical Cell, Transitional Cell)

The term "nonkeratinizing carcinoma" (NKC) has become considerably more widely used over the last decade and is now the official description sanctioned by the World Health Organization, although it has no assigned ICD code. The developing knowledge and discussions around this particular variant of squamous cell carcinoma illustrate both the progress of our understanding and the considerable confusion that is apparent at times in the literature of the last three decades, where a wide variety of different terms have been used to describe this lesion. Its incidence also varies considerably in older reported series as a consequence of our incomplete understanding; recently, in keeping with the other rarer variants, there have been widely conflicting results with regard to possible etiological factors such as HPV and EBV. However, the situation is becoming clearer, and this is important from a clinical point of view as true cases of this tumor have a better prognosis than conventional squamous carcinoma and other rare variants such as SNUC (sinonasal undifferentiated carcinoma) with which it has been confused in the past.

Definition

Nonkeratinizing carcinoma is currently thought to be a distinctive variant of squamous cell carcinoma derived from the respiratory epithelium and usually composed of substantial ribbons of nonkeratinized mitotically active epithelial cells. These produce invaginations of surface epithelium and the elongated cells perpendicular to the basement membrane are multilayered (hence the incorrect term "transitional," which should be confined to the urogenital tract) and at times the cells create a cylindrical appearance (hence the synonym "cylindrical cell carcinoma").

Synonyms

Anaplastic carcinoma, cylindrical cell carcinoma, transitional cell carcinoma, schneiderian carcinoma, respiratory epithelial carcinoma, and Ringertz carcinoma.

Etiology

As indicated in the introduction, considerable research and debate still surrounds this area. There is no definitive evidence for risk factors such as smoking and alcohol, and attention in recent times has concentrated on the possible roles of human papilloma and Epstein-Barr viruses.

Epstein-Barr Virus

While Epstein-Barr virus has a well-established association with nasopharyngeal carcinoma, its association with sinonasal carcinomas is still controversial. Hwang and colleagues[40] from Taiwan evaluated the potential value of EBER in situ hybridization techniques in specimens of sinonasal carcinoma and the nasopharynx. The EBER in situ hybridization was performed on paraffin-embedded tissues using PCR-derived digoxigenin-labeled EBR-1 DNA probes. EBV was detected in all 31 carcinomas of the nasopharynx including (according to their classification) 1 keratinizing squamous cell carcinoma, 15 nonkeratinizing carcinomas, 14 undifferentiated carcinomas, and 1 adenocarcinoma. In contrast, EBV was detected in only 2 of 31 surgical specimens of sinonasal carcinoma including 1 normal keratinizing squamous cell carcinoma and 1 adenocarcinoma. This study did **not** support the role of EBV in the development of sinonasal carcinoma.

In direct contrast to the above study, Leung et al[41] from the Department of Pathology, Queen Mary Hospital, University of Hong Kong, studied 29 sinonasal carcinomas from Hong Kong Chinese patients. Their study also used in situ hybridization using an EBER probe. Seven of their 29 tumors were shown to be strongly positive for EBV RNA. The tumors displayed a wide morphological spectrum, being classified as 1 cylindrical cell carcinoma, 1 intestinal type adenocarcinoma, 4 nonkeratinizing squamous cell carcinomas (these four would probably now include the one cylindrical cell carcinoma), and 1 undifferentiated carcinoma. Interestingly, 3 of these 7 patients had complete remission of disease after radiotherapy. They concluded **the exact opposite** of the Taiwanese study, suggesting that EBV **may** play a role in the pathogenesis of a diverse spectrum of sinonasal carcinomas.

In contrast to these results, some further clarification has been obtained in the last decade and it is now more clearly recognized that a small proportion of patients, particularly from Asia, have primary sinonasal nasopharyngeal type undifferentiated carcinoma, which is now officially termed lymphoepithelial carcinoma. Further confusion in the past has been due to the similarities to sinonasal undifferentiated carcinoma (SNUC) and both tumors were reported to be associated with EBV. Jeng and colleagues[42] in Taiwan undertook further studies evaluating the clinicopathological features and EBV status of 36 SNUC and 13 lymphoepithelial carcinomas from the sinonasal region. All 36 SNUC tumors proved to be negative for EBER-1 by in situ hybridization and their median survival was 10 months. All 13 lymphoepithelial tumors were positive for EBER-1 by in situ hybridization. Eight of these patients achieved disease-free survival. Clearly these two tumor groups in this study were very different in relation to EBV and their prognosis and response to radiotherapy. This study confirmed the usefulness of EBV studies in these two rare tumors and the work has subsequently been confirmed by others.[43,44]

Human Papilloma Virus

El-Mofty and Lu[8] from the University of Washington commented on the varying reports of HPV viruses, particularly types 16 and 18, occurring in anything between 0 to 40% of carcinomas of the sinonasal tract in previous studies. They evaluated a further 21 cases of keratinizing squamous cell carcinoma, 8 cases of nonkeratinizing carcinoma, and 10 cases of SNUC. PCR techniques were used to detect the presence of HPV DNA in addition to a panel of immunohistochemical stains including P16, P53 and Ki-67 antibodies. They found that 50% (i.e., 4 out of 8) nonkeratinizing carcinomas contained HPV16, HPV18, or HPV45 in direct contrast to only 10% of the SNUCs being positive for the virus and 19% of the keratinizing squamous carcinomas. As with other studies, this indicates a possible link to HPV, particularly in the nonkeratinizing carcinomas, but is far from conclusive. The keratinizing squamous cell carcinoma cases were more likely to be positive and more strongly reactive to P53; in contrast, the SNUC tumors had high Ki-67 labeling scores. These observations add to the suggestion of others that nonkeratinizing carcinoma of the sinonasal tract may be a distinct histopathological and molecular disease entity with an etiological relationship to high-risk HPV.[8] This report has been further added to by Alos et al,[9] showing a subset of HPV-positive patients in 12 out of their 60 sinonasal cancers (see section on HPV, p. 113).

Incidence

Precise figures for the incidence of nonkeratinizing carcinoma are complicated by past difficulties with the exact histological assessment and the use of many synonyms such as cylindrical cell carcinoma and transitional cell carcinoma. However, taking these factors into account, three large series published in the 1970s and 1980s[45–47] reported incidences between 8% and 16% of their large collections of sinonasal cancers in the United Kingdom. In our cohort of 320 squamous-type tumors, there were 37 cases of nonkeratinizing carcinoma.

Site

The tumors most commonly present unilaterally in the nasal cavity and more rarely in the maxillary sinus, in contrast to keratinizing squamous cell carcinoma (Table 6.10).

Diagnostic Features

Clinical Features and Imaging

Nonkeratinizing carcinomas have been described in a wide age range of patients from 20 to 90 years of age with an average around 60 years. Our patients ranged from 23 to 81 years (mean 57.9 years). In the literature, in contrast to squamous carcinoma they are described as approximately equal in male and female, although our own group continued to show a male preponderance (2.1:1). Most commonly they present as a unilateral polypoidal mass associated with nasal block. The unilateral solitary polypoid appearance may lead the clinician to believe that they are a simple sinonasal polyp or inverted papilloma. Auerbach et al found evidence of multifocal intranasal lesions in 23% of their patients.[48]

There are no specific features on imaging, and neither the lack of substantial maxillary involvement, nor the extensive disease so commonly seen with presentation of SNUCs, are pointers toward the possibility of this lesion (Figs. 6.31 and 6.32).

Histological Features and Differential Diagnosis

The most common area of confusion in the past has been with inverted papilloma, particularly with low-magnification hematoxylin and eosin studies. However, at higher

Table 6.10 Nonkeratinizing squamous cell carcinoma (NKC): personal series 1970–2010

Site	n	Age		M:F	Surgery + DXT	Surgery	Surgery + DXT & CT	DXT	CT	No RX[a]
		Range (y)	Mean (y)							
All	37	23–81	59.7	2.1:1	20	7	6	2	1	1
Nasal cavity	13				7					
Ethmoid	15				8					
Maxilla	9				4					

Abbreviations: CT, chemotherapy; DXT, radiotherapy; F, female; M, male; RX, treatment; y, year(s).
[a] Palliative treatment only in advanced disease at presentation.

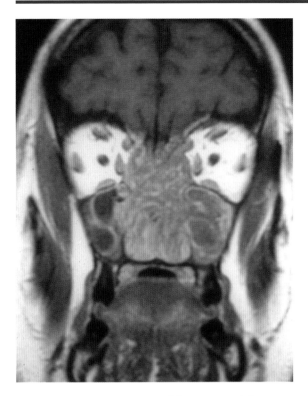

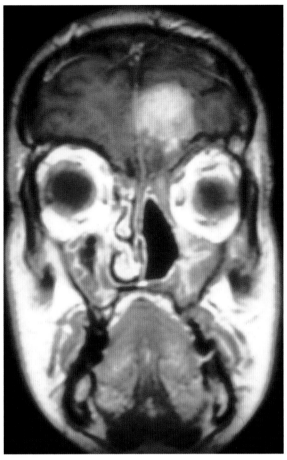

Fig. 6.31 Coronal MRI (T1W post gadolinium contrast) showing a large nonkeratinizing squamous cell carcinoma filling both sides of the nose and ethmoids, and bulging into the maxillary sinuses bilaterally. The maxillary sinuses are filled with inflamed mucosa and secretions. Originally reported as "transitional cell carcinoma" with a striated pattern reminiscent of inverted papilloma.

Fig. 6.32 Coronal MRI (T1W post gadolinium contrast) showing recurrent nonkeratinizing squamous cell carcinoma in the left frontal sinus; inflammatory change in the left maxillary sinus after lateral rhinotomy.

magnifications, the pleomorphic nature and markedly increased mitotic activity in NKC contrasts with inverted papilloma. Nonkeratinizing carcinomas often have a corrugated papillary surface, and the multiple layers of nonkeratinized cells and the cylindrical appearance aid further in the histopathological diagnosis. The cells may appear to be surrounded by an intact basement membrane and it is necessary to evaluate sufficient biopsy material to elicit focal and diffuse invasion.

Cytokeratin Expression

Franchi et al[49] have aided understanding of the potentially difficult differential diagnosis of these tumors by evaluating the differing cytokeratin (CK) expression, which can be used for diagnostic purposes. They compared the expression of a large panel of CKs in a series of 6 SNUCs, 10 poorly differentiated keratinizing squamous cell carcinomas, 10 nonkeratinizing squamous cell carcinomas, and 5 nasopharyngeal undifferentiated carcinomas (lymphoepithelial carcinoma). The nonkeratinizing carcinomas are typically positive for CK5/6, 8, 14, and 19, and negative for CK4, 7, and 10. The squamous cell carcinomas in their series expressed CK7 (60% of cases) and CK4 (30% of cases), which were absent in nonkeratinizing

squamous cell carcinoma and lymphoepithelial carcinoma. Nonkeratinizing squamous cell carcinomas have rarely been described arising with concurrent inverted papilloma and in their series there were three nonkeratinizing squamous cell carcinomas associated with papillomas. The results of immunostaining were similar in the two lesions, with the exception of CK4 and CK7, which were expressed by the papilloma and not by the carcinoma. The SNUCs were characterized by the exclusive expression by CKs of simple epithelia such as CK8 (100% of cases). This work has added to our knowledge demonstrating some significant differences in the pattern of CK expression between these tumor groups, which further supports the hypothesis that SNUCs are a separate entity from squamous cell carcinoma and lymphoepithelial carcinoma.

Natural History and Treatment

Osbourne,[50] reviewing a series of tumors described under the heading of transitional cell carcinoma, noted that metastases to regional lymph nodes were <10% and rare to more distant sites, and this is true of the more modern series reported under the heading of nonkeratinizing carcinoma. These lesions are more likely to be confined to the nasal cavity, making their complete surgical removal more achievable. Generally, these lesions have been thought to have a better prognosis than conventional squamous cell carcinoma, and Alos et al[9] reported a notably improved survival in 12 cases of sinonasal carcinoma that were HPV positive out of a group of 60 evaluated over a 25-year period. Definite conclusions cannot be drawn from this relatively small group of 12 patients, which included 2 keratinizing squamous cell carcinomas (out of 42), 6 nonkeratinizing (out of 11), 2 basaloid (out of 5), and 2 papillary (out of 2). However, this group of 12 cases had a significantly improved survival, the HPV status remaining statistically significant on multivariant analysis. Further work in this area may assist in amending the treatment regime for this rare group of tumors in the future.

In our cohort the majority were treated with a combination of radiotherapy and surgery (68%). In all cases the surgery was radical and ranged from lateral rhinotomy (35%) through endoscopic resection, rhinectomy, and midfacial degloving, to maxillectomy and craniofacial resection (22%). Seven patients also received chemotherapy; 7 received surgery alone; and a few patients were so advanced at presentation that they received either only radiotherapy or no treatment. Two underwent orbital clearance and one needed a neck dissection.

Sixteen patients died of disease between 2 months and 4 years after treatment (mean survival 14 months); 8 are alive and well with follow-up of 2 to 20 years (mean 8.3 years); 4 died of intercurrent disease; and 9 of the earliest patients have been lost to follow-up. This does not suggest an improved prognosis as compared with keratinizing SCC, but it should be noted that the HPV status of these cases is not known.

Key Points

- The term "nonkeratinizing carcinoma" (NKC) is now the official World Health Organization term covering transitional and cylindrical cell carcinomas, although it has no assigned ICD code.
- There has been considerable confusion in the literature of the last three decades, where a wide variety of different terms have been used to describe this lesion, making an accurate assessment of its true incidence difficult.
- There have been widely conflicting results with regard to possible etiological factors such as HPV and EBV. While Epstein-Barr virus has a well-established association with nasopharyngeal carcinoma, its association with sinonasal carcinomas is still controversial and the possible link to HPV is far from conclusive.

- The unilateral solitary polypoid appearance may lead the clinician to believe that the lesion is a simple sinonasal polyp or inverted papilloma. However, at higher magnifications, the pleomorphic nature and markedly increased mitotic activity in NKC contrasts with inverted papilloma.
- There are some significant differences in the pattern of CK expression that further support the hypothesis that SNUCs are a separate entity from squamous cell carcinoma and lymphoepithelial carcinoma.
- When these lesions are confined to the nasal cavity, their complete surgical removal is more achievable, leading to a better prognosis than for conventional squamous cell carcinoma. When the antrum or skull base is affected, however, as in our own cohort, the results are of the same order.

References

1. International Agency for Research on Cancer (IARC). Natural history and epidemiology of HPV infection. IARC Monographs on the Evaluation of Carcinogenic Risk to Humans. Vol. 90: Human Papilloma Viruses. Lyon: IARC; 2007:68–92
2. Gillison ML, Koch WM, Capone RB, et al. Evidence for a causal association between human papillomavirus and a subset of head and neck cancers. J Natl Cancer Inst 2000;92(9):709–720
3. Herrero R, Castellsagué X, Pawlita M, et al; IARC Multicenter Oral Cancer Study Group. Human papillomavirus and oral cancer: the International Agency for Research on Cancer multicenter study. J Natl Cancer Inst 2003;95(23):1772–1783
4. Hoffmann M, Görögh T, Gottschlich S, et al. Human papillomaviruses in head and neck cancer: 8 year-survival-analysis of 73 patients. Cancer Lett 2005;218(2):199–206
5. Chaturvedi AK, Engels EA, Anderson WF, Gillison ML. Incidence trends for human papillomavirus-related and -unrelated oral squamous cell carcinomas in the United States. J Clin Oncol 2008;26(4):612–619
6. Hoffmann M, Klose N, Gottschlich S, et al. Detection of human papillomavirus DNA in benign and malignant sinonasal neoplasms. Cancer Lett 2006;239(1):64–70
7. Syrjänen KJ. HPV infections in benign and malignant sinonasal lesions. J Clin Pathol 2003;56(3):174–181
8. El-Mofty SK, Lu DW. Prevalence of high-risk human papillomavirus DNA in nonkeratinizing (cylindrical cell) carcinoma of the sinonasal tract: a distinct clinicopathologic and molecular disease entity. Am J Surg Pathol 2005;29(10):1367–1372
9. Alos L, Moyano S, Nadal A, et al. Human papillomaviruses are identified in a subgroup of sinonasal squamous cell carcinomas with favorable outcome. Cancer 2009;115(12):2701–2709
10. Friedell H, Rosenthal L. The aetiologic role of chewing tobacco in cancer of the mouth. JAMA 1941;116:2130–2133
11. Ackerman LV. Verrucous carcinoma of the oral cavity. Surgery 1948;23(4):670–678
12. Hanna GS, Ali MH. Verrucous carcinoma of the nasal septum. J Laryngol Otol 1987;101(2):184–187
13. Karthikeya P, Mahima VG, Bhavna G. Sinonasal verrucous carcinoma with oral invasion. Indian J Dent Res 2006;17(2):82–86
14. Orvidas LJ, Lewis JE, Olsen KD, Weiner JS. Intranasal verrucous carcinoma: relationship to inverting

papilloma and human papillomavirus. Laryngoscope 1999;109(3):371–375

15. Newman AN, Colman M, Jayich SA. Verrucous carcinoma of the frontal sinus: a case report and review of the literature. J Surg Oncol 1983;24(4):298–303

16. Cooper JR, Hellquist HB, Michaels L. Image analysis in the discrimination of verrucous carcinoma and squamous papilloma. J Pathol 1992;166(4):383–387

17. McCaffrey TV, Witte M, Ferguson MT. Verrucous carcinoma of the larynx. Ann Otol Rhinol Laryngol 1998;107(5 Pt 1):391–395

18. Koch BB, Trask DK, Hoffman HT, et al; Commission on Cancer, American College of Surgeons; American Cancer Society. National survey of head and neck verrucous carcinoma: patterns of presentation, care, and outcome. Cancer 2001;92(1):110–120

19. Crissman JD, Kessis T, Shah KV, et al. Squamous papillary neoplasia of the adult upper aerodigestive tract. Hum Pathol 1988;19(12):1387–1396

20. Thompson LD, Wenig BM, Heffner DK, Gnepp DR. Exophytic and papillary squamous cell carcinomas of the larynx: A clinicopathologic series of 104 cases. Otolaryngol Head Neck Surg 1999;120(5):718–724

21. Suarez PA, Adler-Storthz K, Luna MA, El-Naggar AK, Abdul-Karim FW, Batsakis JG. Papillary squamous cell carcinomas of the upper aerodigestive tract: a clinicopathologic and molecular study. Head Neck 2000;22(4):360–368

22. Barnes L, Eveson J, Reichart P, Sidransky D, eds. World Health Organization Classification of Tumours. Pathology and Genetics of Head Neck Tumours. Lyons: IARC Press; 2005:126

23. Banks ER, Frierson HF Jr, Mills SE, George E, Zarbo RJ, Swanson PE. Basaloid squamous cell carcinoma of the head and neck. A clinicopathologic and immunohistochemical study of 40 cases. Am J Surg Pathol 1992;16(10):939–946

24. Barnes L, Ferlito A, Altavilla G, MacMillan C, Rinaldo A, Doglioni C. Basaloid squamous cell carcinoma of the head and neck: clinicopathological features and differential diagnosis. Ann Otol Rhinol Laryngol 1996;105(1):75–82

25. Paulino AF, Singh B, Shah JP, Huvos AG. Basaloid squamous cell carcinoma of the head and neck. Laryngoscope 2000;110(9):1479–1482

26. Wan S-K, Chan JK, Lau W-H, Yip TT. Basaloid-squamous carcinoma of the nasopharynx. An Epstein-Barr virus-associated neoplasm compared with morphologically identical tumors occurring in other sites. Cancer 1995; 76(10):1689–1693

27. Wain SL, Kier R, Vollmer RT, Bossen EH. Basaloid-squamous carcinoma of the tongue, hypopharynx, and larynx: report of 10 cases. Hum Pathol 1986;17(11):1158–1166

28. Wieneke JA, Thompson LD, Wenig BM. Basaloid squamous cell carcinoma of the sinonasal tract. Cancer 1999;85(4):841–854

29. Raslan WF, Barnes L, Krause JR, Contis L, Killeen R, Kapadia SB. Basaloid squamous cell carcinoma of the head and neck: a clinicopathologic and flow cytometric study of 10 new cases with review of the English literature. Am J Otolaryngol 1994;15(3):204–211

30. Choi HR, Roberts DB, Johnigan RH, et al. Molecular and clinicopathologic comparisons of head and neck squamous carcinoma variants: common and distinctive features of biological significance. Am J Surg Pathol 2004;28(10):1299–1310

31. Winzenburg SM, Niehans GA, George E, Daly K, Adams GL. Basaloid squamous carcinoma: a clinical comparison of two histologic types with poorly differentiated squamous cell carcinoma. Otolaryngol Head Neck Surg 1998;119(5):471–475

32. Luna MA, el Naggar A, Parichatikanond P, Weber RS, Batsakis JG. Basaloid squamous carcinoma of the upper

aerodigestive tract. Clinicopathologic and DNA flow cytometric analysis. Cancer 1990;66(3):537–542

33. Lewis JE, Olsen KD, Sebo TJ. Spindle cell carcinoma of the larynx: review of 26 cases including DNA content and immunohistochemistry. Hum Pathol 1997;28(6):664–673

34. Thompson LD, Wieneke JA, Miettinen M, Heffner DK. Spindle cell (sarcomatoid) carcinomas of the larynx: a clinicopathologic study of 187 cases. Am J Surg Pathol 2002;26(2):153–170

35. Choi HR, Roberts DB, Johnigan RH, et al. Molecular and clinicopathologic comparisons of head and neck squamous carcinoma variants: common and distinctive features of biological significance. Am J Surg Pathol 2004;28(10):1299–1310

36. Thompson L, Chang B, Barsky SH. Monoclonal origins of malignant mixed tumors (carcinosarcomas). Evidence for a divergent histogenesis. Am J Surg Pathol 1996;20(3):277–285

37. Torenbeek R, Hermsen MA, Meijer GA, Baak JP, Meijer CJ. Analysis by comparative genomic hybridization of epithelial and spindle cell components in sarcomatoid carcinoma and carcinosarcoma: histogenetic aspects. J Pathol 1999;189(3):338–343

38. Gerughty RM, Hennigar GR, Brown FM. Adenosquamous carcinoma of the nasal, oral and laryngeal cavities. A clinicopathologic survey of ten cases. Cancer 1968;22(6):1140–1155

39. Keelawat S, Liu CZ, Roehm PC, Barnes L. Adenosquamous carcinoma of the upper aerodigestive tract: a clinicopathologic study of 12 cases and review of the literature. Am J Otolaryngol 2002;23(3):160–168

40. Hwang TZ, Jin YT, Tsai ST. EBER in situ hybridization differentiates carcinomas originating from the sinonasal region and the nasopharynx. Anticancer Res 1998;18(6B):4581–4584

41. Leung SY, Yuen ST, Chung LP, Kwong WK, Wong MP, Chan SY. Epstein-Barr virus is present in a wide histological spectrum of sinonasal carcinomas. Am J Surg Pathol 1995;19(9):994–1001

42. Jeng YM, Sung MT, Fang CL, et al. Sinonasal undifferentiated carcinoma and nasopharyngeal-type undifferentiated carcinoma: two clinically, biologically, and histopathologically distinct entities. Am J Surg Pathol 2002;26(3):371–376

43. Thompson LDR. Sinonasal carcinomas. Curr Diagn Pathol 2006;12:40–53

44. Trabelsi A, Tebra S, Abdelkrim S, et al. Lymphoepithelial carcinoma of the nasal cavity with EBV infection in a North African man. World J Oncol 2010;1:91–93

45. Lewis JS, Castro EB. Cancer of the nasal cavity and paranasal sinuses. J Laryngol Otol 1972;86(3):255–262

46. Robin PE, Powell DJ, Stansbie JM. Carcinoma of the nasal cavity and paranasal sinuses: incidence and presentation of different histological types. Clin Otolaryngol Allied Sci 1979;4(6):431–456

47. Hopkin N, McNicoll W, Dalley VM, Shaw HJ. Cancer of the paranasal sinuses and nasal cavities. Part I. Clinical features. J Laryngol Otol 1984;98(6):585–595

48. Auerbach MJ, Adair CF, Kardon D, et al. Respiratory epithelial carcinoma: a clinicopathologic study. Mod Pathol 2002;15:215A [abstract 902]

49. Franchi A, Moroni M, Massi D, Paglierani M, Santucci M. Sinonasal undifferentiated carcinoma, nasopharyngeal-type undifferentiated carcinoma, and keratinizing and nonkeratinizing squamous cell carcinoma express different cytokeratin patterns. Am J Surg Pathol 2002;26(12):1597–1604

50. Osborn DA. Nature and behavior of transitional tumors in the upper respiratory tract. Cancer 1970;25(1):50–60

Lymphoepithelial Carcinoma

Definition

Lymphoepithelial carcinoma (LEC) of the sinonasal area is morphologically similar to the undifferentiated variant of the well-known nasopharyngeal carcinoma. It is essentially a poorly differentiated or undifferentiated carcinoma accompanied by a prominent reactive lymphoplasmacytic infiltrate.

Synonyms

Additional names that have been applied to this tumor include nasopharyngeal undifferentiated carcinoma, lymphoepithelial carcinoma-like carcinoma, undifferentiated carcinoma with lymphocytic stroma, or simply undifferentiated carcinoma.

Etiology

Lymphoepithelial carcinoma is a rare and relatively unrecognized tumor within the nasal cavity and paranasal sinuses that, other than its location in the sinonasal tract, in contrast to the nasopharynx, is otherwise histologically identical to the undifferentiated form of nasopharyngeal carcinoma. Almost all the cases have originated from South-East Asia, although isolated individual cases have been reported in Europeans and recently from North Africa.[1,2] The literature since 2000 has improved our understanding of this rare sinonasal tumor, allowing us to separate it from SNUC and nonkeratinizing carcinoma (see individual sections).[3-8] Almost all cases of sinonasal lymphoepithelial carcinomas, including those outside of Asia, have been associated with EBV using in situ hybridization to EBV-encoded RNA. Immunohistochemical expression of EBV latent membrane protein 1 (LMP1) is also increasingly being used. While the precise role that EBV plays in the formation of lymphoepithelial carcinoma remains unknown, the considerable amount of indirect evidence already gained from the long-term study of nasopharyngeal tumors makes it likely that EBV and host hereditary and environmental factors play a role in the genesis of this tumor.

Incidence

At the time of writing, ~30 cases of this tumor have been recorded in the sinonasal cavity, but this number can be expected to rise significantly with our increasing ability to differentiate these tumors from nonkeratinizing SCC and SNUC.

Site

While the tumor most often originates in the nasal cavity, in the reports to date it clearly invades the nasal septum and ethmoids and the adjacent orbit and cranial cavity.

Diagnostic Features

Clinical Features and Imaging

The tumor occurs in an age group above 30 years of age, the most common being between 45 and 55 years of age. There are no reports of the bimodal distribution seen with nasopharyngeal undifferentiated carcinoma. Patients typically present with nasal obstruction, blood-stained rhinorrhea, and epistaxis, but in the 13 patients reported by Jeng et al[8] from Taiwan additional orbital invasion was seen in 4 cases and intracranial invasion in 2 cases. In contrast to the far more common nasopharyngeal lymphoepithelial carcinoma, only 23% of cases presented with cervical node metastases and only a single case from the 13 had evidence of distant metastases. This important series of cases was compared in the same publication with 36 SNUCs from the same department and there was no substantial difference in these main clinical features or in the age group of the patients. Interestingly, 5 of the SNUC patients had a history of previous nasopharyngeal carcinoma treated with irradiation from 6 to 26 years earlier.

While CT and MRI are essential for accurate evaluation of the sinonasal structures involved and any extension into the orbit, skull base, and intracranial structures, there were no particularly defining features between the two groups of tumors. Cervical node metastases were detected in 17% of the SNUCs, but in contrast to the LEC cases, distant metastases to liver, lung, bone, and other sites were found in 31% of the SNUC patients.

Histological Features and Differential Diagnosis

There is some notable variation in the reporting of the microscopic findings in LEC and, as outlined in the sections on nonkeratinizing carcinomas and SNUC, this has led to considerable difficulties in the past. In general, the tumors are composed of individual cells having eosinophilic cytoplasm with oval or large round nuclei and medium-sized nucleoli. The tumor cells may be spindle-shaped and arranged in a streaming pattern, and these spindle cells are hypochromatic with indistinct nucleoli. Intraepithelial carcinoma was detected in 3 of the 13 cases of Jeng et al.[8] Although most reports describe prominent inflammatory infiltrates composed of lymphocytes and plasma cells permeating the tumor, this was not the case in 5 out of 13 of the cases of Jeng et al. However, there were no cases with necrosis of tumor nests, in contradistinction to the often extensive necrosis seen in SNUC tumors, which additionally have high levels of mitosis and angiolymphatic invasion.

Immunohistochemistry

The papers of Zong et al[6] (Gwangzhous, China), Franchi et al[7] (Florence, Italy) and Jeng et al[8] (Taiwan) have considerably improved our ability to differentiate between SNUC,

LEC and NKSCC. In summary, LEC is almost always positive for EBV, CK5/6, and CK13, and in addition, Franchi et al found positivity for CK8 and CK19. LECs are positive for pankeratin and epithelial membrane antigen. In contrast, SNUC is usually negative for EBV, CK5/6, and CK13. Additionally, LEC is usually negative for CK4, CK7, CK10, and CK14.[7]

Natural History, Prognosis, and Treatment

These rare tumors are the perfect example of how accurate pathology diagnosis is an essential cornerstone of treatment in head and neck tumor patients. In the series of Jeng et al,[8] at the time of treatment their clarification between the SNUC tumors and primary sinonasal lymphoepithelial carcinomas was not fully understood and the EBV findings were not available to the treating physicians in all cases. Hence the treatment program was varied, with 7 of the 13 LEC patients undergoing surgery. Radiotherapy was used in only 10 of 13 cases. Chemotherapy was given to 3 additional cases, but the details were not available. Despite this varied treatment, 8 of the LEC patients who had received radiotherapy were disease-free with a median follow-up time of 48 months. This was in complete contrast to the group of patients who were subsequently placed in the SNUC group by their detailed pathology investigations. Of the 36 SNUC patients, there was no standardized treatment approach, but surgery was the primary modality in 17 patients (47%), radiation therapy was given to 23 patients, with an additional 9 receiving high-dose chemotherapy (respectively 64% and 25% of the patients). The prognosis of this group was extremely poor, with a median survival of only 10 months. Only 14% of the patients were disease-free with a median follow-up time of 31 months. Interestingly, all of these 5 patients had received surgical resection. It is interesting to consider what the results for the sinonasal LECs would have been had they all received combined chemoradiation appropriate to this rare tumor.

Key Points

- Lymphoepithelial carcinoma of the sinonasal area (LEC) is a rare and relatively unrecognized tumor that is morphologically similar to the undifferentiated variant of the well-known nasopharyngeal carcinoma.
- It is likely that EBV and host hereditary and environmental factors play a role in the genesis of this tumor.
- These rare tumors are the perfect example of how accurate pathology diagnosis is an essential cornerstone of treatment in head and neck tumor patients.

References

1. Hajiioannou JK, Kyrmizakis DE, Datseris G, Lachanas V, Karatzanis AK, George Velegrakis AA. Nasopharyngeal-type undifferentiated carcinoma (lymphoepithelioma) of paranasal sinuses: Rare case and literature review. J Otolaryngol 2006;35(2):147–151
2. Trabelsi A, Tebra S, Abdelkrim S, et al. Lymphoepithelial carcinoma of the nasal cavity with EBV infection in a North African man. World J Oncol 2010;1:91–93
3. Lopategui JR, Gaffey MJ, Frierson HF Jr, et al. Detection of Epstein-Barr viral RNA in sinonasal undifferentiated carcinoma from Western and Asian patients. Am J Surg Pathol 1994;18(4):391–398
4. Leung SY, Yuen ST, Chung LP, Kwong WK, Wong MP, Chan SY. Epstein-Barr virus is present in a wide histological spectrum of sinonasal carcinomas. Am J Surg Pathol 1995;19(9):994–1001
5. Dubey P, Ha CS, Ang KK, et al. Nonnasopharyngeal lymphoepithelioma of the head and neck. Cancer 1998;82(8):1556–1562
6. Zong Y, Liu K, Zhong B, Chen G, Wu W. Epstein-Barr virus infection of sinonasal lymphoepithelial carcinoma in Guangzhou. Chin Med J (Engl) 2001;114(2):132–136
7. Franchi A, Moroni M, Massi D, Paglierani M, Santucci M. Sinonasal undifferentiated carcinoma, nasopharyngeal-type undifferentiated carcinoma, and keratinizing and nonkeratinizing squamous cell carcinoma express different cytokeratin patterns. Am J Surg Pathol 2002;26(12):1597–1604
8. Jeng YM, Sung MT, Fang CL, et al. Sinonasal undifferentiated carcinoma and nasopharyngeal-type undifferentiated carcinoma: two clinically, biologically, and histopathologically distinct entities. Am J Surg Pathol 2002;26(3):371–376

Transitional Cell Papilloma and Carcinoma of the Lacrimal Sac

Definition

Although not strictly arising in the nose or paranasal sinuses, tumors of the lacrimal sac may come within the remit of the rhino-oncological surgeon. Tumors of the lacrimal sac are rare and cover a wide variety of pathology. Transitional cell papillomas (TCPs) are considered benign but may evolve into transitional cell carcinoma (TCC), which has been associated with high mortality.

Etiology

As with other papillomas, human papilloma virus (HPV) has been implicated in their pathogenesis. HPV DNA was found in all of 11 transitional cell tumors (5 TCPs and 6 TCCs) by Sjo et al.[1] This included HPV 6, 11, and 16.

Incidence

TCPs and TCCs are exceptionally rare tumors. In a series of 377 biopsy specimens taken during dacryocytorhinostomy in 316 patients, there were only 4 (1.1%) TCPs and 2 cases of TCC (0.5%).[2] In another study, routine biopsy of 164 patients revealed one TCP.[3] In a series of 15 patients with lacrimal neoplasms,[4] there were one TCP and 2 TCCs, and in a meta-analysis of 420 primary lacrimal sac tumors, epithelial tumors accounted for 70% of which 50% were malignant.[5] In our personal series of 30 lacrimal sac tumors, we have managed 11 TCPs and 9 TCCs.

Site

The lacrimal canaliculi are lined by stratified squamous epithelium that merges with a double-layered columnar epithelium in the lacrimal sac, which then continues inferiorly into the nasolacrimal duct. The lacrimal sac and duct are derived from an invagination of embryonic ectoderm and may be grouped with the mucosa of the nose and paranasal sinuses as "Schneiderian" mucosa.[6] This common embryological origin has been used to justify classifying pathology in this area together with that of the nose,[7] but this has not been accepted generally and tumors of the lacrimal sac are sufficiently rare and varied to be considered as separate entities.

Diagnostic Features

Clinical

Patients classically present with unilateral epiphora and dacryocystitis. They may develop a mass in the medial canthal region.[8] As they are often mistaken for dacryoceles, they may already have undergone one or more unsuccessful dacryocystorhinostomies before a biopsy of the sac lining is performed revealing the tumor. Rarely a papilloma will present in the upper or lower canaliculus, appearing in the medial corner of the eye. The disease is painless unless there is an associated dacryocystitis. The lesions may be seen on endoscopic examination of the nasal cavity (Fig. 6.33).

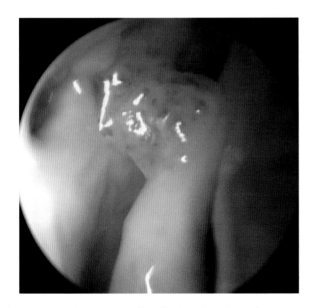

Fig. 6.33 Endoscopic view of papilloma in the right nasal cavity, related to dacryocystorhinostomy.

In our series of 20 patients (11 TCPs, 9 TCCs), there were 8 male and 12 female patients, median ages 50 years and 53.3 years, respectively (range 29–82 years) (Table 6.11). This is the same demographic as that in the Mayo Clinic series.[9] All of our cases had epiphora for 1 to 3 years, and were initially biopsied at the time of dacryocystorhinostomy. Half went on to develop a palpable mass and two developed a papillary lesion at the site of the rhinostomy.

Imaging

Many patients will have undergone a dacryocystogram as part of the investigation of epiphora, which will demonstrate obstruction.

CT reveals a soft tissue mass in the region of the lacrimal sac, which may be interpreted as a dacryocele. This is best seen on axial cuts (Fig. 6.34). MRI may suggest a mass rather than fluid; it is not sufficiently discriminatory to be mandatory but can discriminate between lesions confined within the sac and infiltration beyond this.

Histological Features and Differential Diagnosis

Various classifications have been described for tumors of the lacrimal sac, the most widely accepted being that of Ryan and Font,[10] who classified tumors by growth pattern (exophytic, inverted, or mixed) and histological type (Table 6.12). The transitional cell papillomas typically display a mixed growth pattern and are composed of elongated epithelial cells without clear-cut epidermoid (squamous) cells with abundant eosinophilic cytoplasm and intercellular bridges.[11] They have been termed "transitional" because their morphology is intermediate between squamous cells and columnar respiratory cells and resembles that of transitional cell tumors of the vesicoureteric mucosa.[10] Nonetheless, the use of the term "transitional" is felt by some to be misleading as they do not arise from a histologically specific transitional epithelium.[6]

Malignancy in the nasolacrimal system may arise from the epithelium, as either squamous cell carcinoma or transitional cell carcinoma, or as an adenocarcinoma arising from underlying glandular tissue. However, controversy remains as to whether carcinoma can arise de novo and, if so, whether these malignant tumors might not represent a distinct group from those developing within preexisting papillomas.

Transitional cell carcinoma may be difficult to distinguish histologically from poorly differentiated squamous cell carcinoma.[11] It is important that an adequate biopsy is taken as in five of our cases the transitional cell papilloma had foci of malignant change; this can lead to underdiagnosis because of sampling problems.

Table 6.11 Lacrimal sac tumors: personal series

	n	Age		M:F	LR	Orbit	ESS	DXT	FU (y)	Outcome
		Range (y)	Mean (y)							
TCP	11	29–82	50	4:7	10	–	1	–	1–14 (mean 6.5)	10 NSR, 1 multiple recurrences
TCC	9	47–71	53.3	4:5	9	1	–	4	1.5–10 (mean 6.4)	8 NSR, 1 recurrence Rx ESS
CCC	3	54,66,71	63.6	2:1	2	1	–	1	3,6,10	2 A&W 1 DOD
SCC	7	40–68	55.4	4:3	6	3	–	5	3–11 (mean 4.5)	5 A&W 1 DOD 1 lost

Abbreviations: A&W, alive and well; CCC, cylindrical cell carcinoma; DOD, dead of disease; DXT, radiotherapy; ESS, endoscopic sinus surgery; F, female; FU, follow-up; LR, lateral rhinotomy; M, male; NSR, no sign of recurrence; Orbit, orbital exenteration; SCC, squamous cell carcinoma; TCC, transitional cell carcinoma; TCP, transitional cell papilloma; y, year(s).

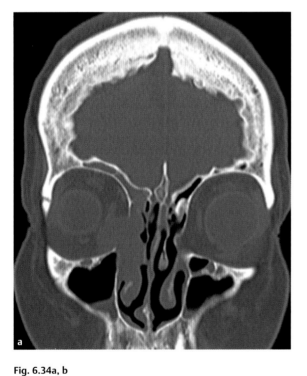
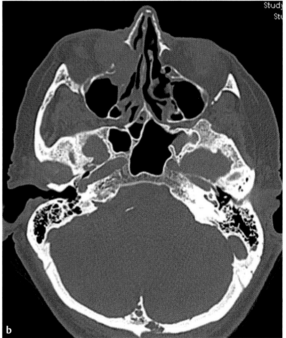

Fig. 6.34a, b

a Coronal CT scan showing smooth expansion of the right nasolacrimal sac.

b Axial scan in the same patient.

Table 6.12 The classification of lacrimal sac tumors described by Ryan and Font[10]

Papillomas		
Growth pattern	Exophytic	
	Inverted	
	Mixed	
Histology	Squamous cell	
	Transitional	
	Mixed	
Papilloma with carcinoma		
Growth pattern	Exophytic	
	Inverted	
	Mixed	
Histology	Squamous cell	
	Transitional	
	Mixed	
Carcinoma		
Growth pattern	Papillary	
	Nonpapillary	
Histology	Squamous cell	
	Transitional	
	Adenocarcinoma	

Natural History

In our series of 11 patients with transitional cell papilloma of the lacrimal sac, 3 showed carcinoma in situ and 9 presented with overt malignant change. This malignancy has in previous series been associated with high mortality and aggressive behavior,[12] although this has not been our experience. As in the nose, exophytic papillomas are less likely to undergo malignant change than inverted or mixed pattern papillomas.[10]

Treatment

Anything less than removal of the entire sac, canaliculi, and duct will result in "recurrence," so debulking, fulguration, and other strategies within the sac are doomed to failure. As the tumors can spread down the nasolacrimal duct, it is also important to resect this structure completely down to its entry into the nasal cavity in the inferior meatus.[8]

Complete excision of the sac will disrupt the orbital periosteum and expose orbital fat. The extent of resection of the orbital periosteum will depend on the histology. A papilloma completely contained within the sac requires clearance of the nasolacrimal system, whereas those that have undergone malignant change should have a wider resection of adjacent orbital periosteum and fat. However,

unless there is macroscopic invasion of the orbital fat, it has not proved necessary in our experience to remove the eye. Nonetheless, significant enophthalmos will result from extrusion of the orbital contents into the ethmoid region and repair of the area may be appropriate. This can be achieved using a free graft of nasal mucosa (from the contralateral inferior or middle turbinate) or using a small split skin graft applied directly to the fat and held in place with some biological glue, Gelfoam soaked in antibiotic solution, and a small ribbon gauze pack soaked in Whitehead's varnish that is left in place for 7 to 10 days. (Whitehead's varnish is compound iodoform paint: iodoform, benzoin, prepared storax, tolu balsam, and solvent ether.)

Although the area may be approached endoscopically, better overall visualization is offered by a small external incision (i.e., the upper half of a lateral rhinotomy, which heals well) combined with an endoscopic endonasal approach.[13] Any preexisting dacryocytorhinostomy scar can be incorporated into this. A routine anterior ethmoidectomy exposes the lamina papyracea, which is then removed to expose the sac and duct. This can then be sharply dissected free from the underlying orbital fat with a peripheral cuff of orbital periosteum. The duct is followed down into the lateral wall of the nose, which can also be removed to expose the duct's opening at the genu of the inferior turbinate into the meatus. Frozen section can sometimes be helpful in determining the limits of the resection.

All 20 patients underwent a wide-field resection mainly via a modified lateral rhinotomy. If malignant change is present and not encompassed by the surgery, additional radiotherapy is offered, as occurred in four of our cases.

If patients develop "recurrence" it may occur at the site of the resection, within the nasal cavity at the site of the rhinostomy, or on adjacent septum, or it may seed anywhere on the nasal mucosa. It may also present in the caruncle. Further local/endoscopic resection combined with coagulating laser ablation (e.g., KTP or argon laser) of the adjacent mucosa is recommended.

There are also reports of the use of topical and intralesional interferon for recurrent papillomas,[14] and cidofovir might have a role. Mitomycin C has been reported as adjuvant therapy in maintaining lacrimal flow used as a peroperative irrigation.[15]

Outcome

All 20 patients remain well at a median follow-up of 6.5 years (range 18 to 168 months). In one patient, a small local recurrence of transitional cell carcinoma was resected endoscopically 4 months after the lateral rhinotomy. One patient with TCP has had multiple local recurrences of papilloma on the lateral wall and adjacent septum treated with KTP laser under endoscopic control.

There was no disturbance of orbital function and complications were limited to epiphora and persistent crusting of the surgical cavity. The epiphora, which was often the presenting symptom, may be managed by a permanent Lester Jones tube (a small glass funnel) or the creation of a permanent rhinostomy, although some patients find this cosmetically suboptimal. In those who receive subsequent radiotherapy, epiphora may be less of a problem due to the reduction in tear production from the lacrimal gland.

Aggressive treatment at this early stage appears to be associated with a significantly better prognosis than has traditionally been described with these tumors, and therefore seems justified even in the presence of histopathological uncertainty. The two largest published series of lacrimal sac TCC each comprise 6 cases[9,12] and in both, there was 100% tumor-related mortality. In the Mayo Clinic series (collected over 39 years)[9] only one patient survived 9 years, the rest less than 3 years. Ni and coauthors included 6 cases in a series of 82 primary lacrimal sac carcinomas treated over a 25-year period,[12] and found TCC to have the worst outcome. They noted metastatic spread to both lung (9 years) and esophagus (2 years) following resection of the primary, but individual details of patient presentation, treatment, and survival were not given. It is probable that the patients presented with more advanced disease than in our series, and that they were treated with both surgery and radiotherapy. The apparently reduced morbidity and mortality in our series probably emphasizes the importance of early diagnosis and appropriate radical treatment, particularly when transitional cell papilloma is associated with carcinoma.

References

1. Sjö NC, von Buchwald C, Cassonnet P, et al. Human papillomavirus: cause of epithelial lacrimal sac neoplasia? Acta Ophthalmol Scand 2007;85(5):551–556
2. Anderson NG, Wojno TH, Grossniklaus HE. Clinicopathologic findings from lacrimal sac biopsy specimens obtained during dacryocystorhinostomy. Ophthal Plast Reconstr Surg 2003;19(3):173–176
3. Merkonidis C, Brewis C, Yung M, Nussbaumer M. Is routine biopsy of the lacrimal sac wall indicated at dacryocystorhinostomy? A prospective study and literature review. Br J Ophthalmol 2005;89(12):1589–1591
4. Parmar DN, Rose GE. Management of lacrimal sac tumours. Eye (Lond) 2003;17(5):599–606
5. Heindl LM, Jünemann AG, Kruse FE, Holbach LM. Tumors of the lacrimal drainage system. Orbit 2010;29(5):298–306
6. Batsakas JG, Suarez P. Schneiderian papillomas and carcinomas: a review. Adv Anat Pathol 2001;8(2):53–64
7. Karcioglu ZA, Caldwell DR, Reed HT. Papillomas of lacrimal drainage system: a clinicopathologic study. Ophthalmic Surg 1984;15(8):670–676
8. Valenzuela AA, Selva D, McNab AA, Simon GB, Sullivan TJ. En bloc excision in malignant tumors of the lacrimal drainage apparatus. Ophthal Plast Reconstr Surg 2006;22(5):356–360
9. Henderson JW. Secondary epithelial neoplasms. In: Orbital Tumours, 3rd ed. New York: Raven Press; 1994:343–360
10. Ryan SJ, Font RL. Primary epithelial neoplasms of the lacrimal sac. Am J Ophthalmol 1973;76(1):73–88
11. Hornblass A, Jakobiec FA, Bosniak S, Flanagan J. The diagnosis and management of epithelial tumors of the lacrimal sac. Ophthalmology 1980;87(6):476–490
12. Ni C, D'Amico DJ, Fan CQ, Kuo PK. Tumors of the lacrimal sac: a clinicopathological analysis of 82 cases. Int Ophthalmol Clin 1982;22(1):121–140
13. Sullivan TJ, Valenzuela AA, Selva D, McNab AA. Combined external-endonasal approach for complete excision of the lacrimal drainage apparatus. Ophthal Plast Reconstr Surg 2006;22(3):169–172
14. Parulekar MV, Khooshabeh R, Graham C. Topical and intralesional interferon therapy for recurrent lacrimal papilloma. Eye (Lond) 2002;16(5):649–651
15. Woodcock M, Mollan SP, Harrison D, Taylor D, Lecuona K. Mitomycin C in the treatment of a Schneiderian (inverted) papilloma of the lacrimal sac. Int Ophthalmol 2010;30(3):303–305

7 Epithelial Nonepidermoid Neoplasms

The WHO classification of the epithelial nonepidermoid tumors includes the following conditions:
- **Benign epithelial (nonepidermoid) tumors**
  - Salivary gland type adenomas
    - Pleomorphic adenoma ICD-O 8940/0
    - Myoepithelioma ICD-O 8982/0
    - Oncocytoma ICD-O 8290/0
  - Respiratory epithelial adenomatoid hamartoma; no ICD-O
- **Malignant epithelial (nonepidermoid) tumors**
  - Adenocarcinoma
    - Intestinal-type adenocarcinomas ICD-O 8144/3
    - Sinonasal nonintestinal type adenocarcinomas ICD-0 8140/3
  - Salivary gland type carcinoma
    - Adenoid cystic carcinoma ICD-O 8200/3
    - Acinic cell carcinoma ICD-O 8550/3
    - Mucoepidermoid carcinoma ICD-O 8430/3
    - Epithelial-myoepithelial carcinoma ICD-O 8562/3
    - Clear cell carcinoma ICD-O 8310/3
    - Myoepithelial carcinoma ICD-O 8982/3
    - Carcinoma ex pleomorphic adenoma ICD-O 8941/3

Benign Epithelial (Nonepidermoid) Tumors

Adenomas

Definition

(ICD-O code 8940/0)

Benign salivary gland type epithelial tumors of one or mixed cell type (monomorphic or pleomorphic).

Etiology

The etiology is unknown. There is no evidence to support an early suggestion that they arise from the vomeronasal organ,[1] especially as glandular elements are found throughout the sinonasal tract.[2] There is one report in the literature suggesting a relationship of a pleomorphic adenoma on the nasal septum with Epstein-Barr virus.[3]

Synonyms

First described by Billroth in 1859, pleomorphic adenomas have been referred to as complex or mixed adenomas.[4] The first one described in the nose was probably by Eichler in 1898.[5]

Incidence

The lesion is rare in the sinonasal region, constituting around 5% of all glandular tumors. Pleomorphic adenomas are somewhat more common than monomorphic. However, between 1949 and 1974 only 40 cases were referred to the Armed Forces Institute of Pathology.[6] Since 1971, ~ 60 sinonasal cases have been reported in the literature.[7–40]

Site

These lesions most often arise on the septum but they have been reported on the lateral wall on the inferior turbinate[21,31] and within the sinuses (occasionally maxillary or ethmoids). They have also been reported on the columella,[33] in the pterygopalatine fossa,[16] and in the nasopharynx[27,28] but are much more commonly encountered in minor salivary tissue on the palate.

Diagnostic Features

Clinical Features

Slow growth eventually produces unilateral nasal obstruction, occasionally epistaxis, or serosanguinous discharge, or produces a mass on the palate affecting denture fitting, but the lesions can achieve spectacular proportions if neglected (**Fig. 7.1**). In the series of Compagno and Wong[6] the patient age range for sinonasal pleomorphic adenomas was 3 to 82 years, mean 42 years, with only a slight female preponderance in contrast to the situation in the major salivary glands where it is most frequent in women. In the 56 reported cases, the ages ranged from 5 to 67 years (mean 42.3 years) and the male-to-female ratio was 1.2:1. Fifty-two percent arose on the septum and 31% on the lateral wall (usually the inferior turbinate); one case affected the rostrum of the sphenoid, one the columella, and two the nasopharynx.

Imaging

The features are those of any benign unilateral solid mass and are not specific (**Fig. 7.2**).[14] There can be some local excavation of adjacent bone on CT, but there is little if any active destruction.[35,37] Calcified foci and irregular enhancement has been described on CT with contrast.[17] The tumor may be multilobulated and better defined on MRI. Fat-suppressed contrast-enhanced T1-weighted (T1W) spin-echo images showed marked curvilinear enhancement with small unenhanced foci.[17] In the 9 patients reported by Wu et al[40] there was low intensity on T1W images but intermediate to high on T2W sequences.

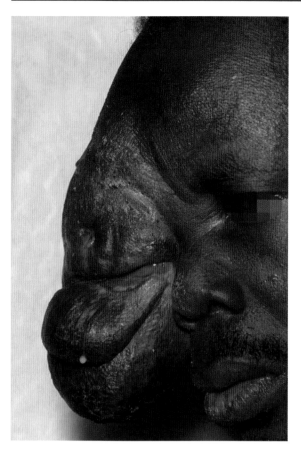

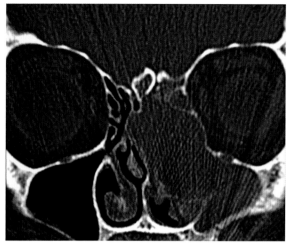

Fig. 7.2 Coronal CT scan showing a pleomorphic adenoma mass occupying the left nasal cavity with opacification of adjacent sinuses, displacement of the septum and lateral wall. The tumor arose from the middle turbinate and was completely removed endoscopically.

Fig. 7.1 Photograph of patient with an extremely advanced pleomorphic adenoma.

Histological Features and Differential Diagnosis

Monomorphic adenomas can be divided into myoepithelial, basaloid, trabecular/tubular, or oncocytic.

The diagnosis of pleomorphic adenoma requires the demonstration of epithelial (glandular) and mesenchymal (or myoepithelial) components. It is usually a lobulated and circumscribed lesion composed of epithelial tissue mixed with mucoid, myxoid or chondroid material, but a true capsule is rarely present.[15] Intranasal pleomorphic adenomas have a similar immunohistochemical profile to their counterparts in the major salivary glands that depends on the dominant phenotype of the tumor. Most of the epithelial components will express various cytokeratins, whereas the myoepithelial component will express smooth muscle actin, S100, GFAP, CD10, and p63.[19,41–43] Very occasionally the myoepithelial component is such that the tumor is designated as a *myoepithelioma*, which carries a separate ICD code in the WHO classification (ICD-O 8982/0). This is an exceptionally rare tumor in the sinonasal region and is more often encountered in the parotid and palate. It may be regarded as part of the spectrum of pleomorphic adenomas, being benign but more likely to recur.

The most important differentiation for pleomorphic adenoma is from malignant glandular tumors such as adenoid cystic type, adenocarcinoma, and the occasional carcinoma ex pleomorphic or true malignant mixed tumor.

Natural History

The normal course is slow insidious growth with conformity of the adjacent anatomy. Occasionally malignant transformation has been reported, although it is possible in some cases that the tumor was undercalled ab initio. A 5% rate of change has been estimated in general.

Carcinoma Ex Pleomorphic Adenoma and Malignant Mixed Tumors

These extremely rare malignant variants can arise either within an existing pleomorphic adenoma or de novo. Only a handful of cases (<20) have been reported, mainly arising on the palate or septum.[44–57] Although factors relating to the prognosis of these tumors elsewhere have been discussed[46,54] it is not known whether they can be extrapolated to this site.

Treatment and Outcome

Complete surgical excision by whatever approach is appropriate and will cure benign sinonasal adenomas. In the Compagno and Wong series, 3 out of 31 that were followed up for 1 to 41 years recurred and all were controlled with further surgery.[6] Therefore, in many instances, cure can now be accomplished by endonasal endoscopic surgery,[19,20,22,24,27,29,30,36,38–40] although lateral rhinotomy, midfacial degloving, and even craniofacial approaches

Table 7.1 Pleomorphic adenomas of the nasal cavity: personal cases

Age (y)	Sex	Symptoms	Site	Treatment	Follow-up (y)
41	F	Nasal obstruction	Septum	Septectomy	A&W 4
44	M	Massive swelling of cheek, eye, nose	Maxillary, ethmoid and orbit	Craniofacial resection and orbital clearance	A&W 6
57	M	Nasal obstruction and swelling	Maxillary and ethmoid	Lateral rhinotomy	A&W 17
65	F	Nasal obstruction and epistaxis	Lateral wall: middle turbinate	Endoscopic sinus surgery	A&W 5

Abbreviation: A&W, alive and well; y, year(s).

have been required in some instances. In our five cases, all underwent surgical excision (3 by lateral rhinotomy, 1 by craniofacial resection and 1 by endoscopic resection) and none has recurred with 48 to 204 months' follow-up (**Table 7.1**).

In the reported malignant cases, wide local excision has been the primary treatment combined with radiotherapy in ~50% of cases, but despite this outcomes have been poor with <50% alive and well and the rest either dead of disease or alive with recurrence at the time of reporting. As there are fewer than 20 cases, it is difficult to make any objective comment about optimum treatment.

References

1. Stevenson H. Mixed tumour of the nasal septum. Ann Otol Rhinol Laryngol 1932;41:563–570
2. Tos M. Goblet cells and glands in the nose and paranasal sinuses. In: Proctor D, Andersen I, eds. The Nose: Upper Airway Physiology and the Atmospheric Environment. Amsterdam: Elsevier; 1982:99–144
3. Malinvaud D, Couloigner V, Badoual C, Halimi P, Bonfils P. Pleomorphic adenoma of the nasal septum and its relationship with Epstein-Barr virus. Auris Nasus Larynx 2006;33(4):417–421
4. Billroth T. Beobachtungen uber Gerschwulste der Speicheldrusen. Virchows Arch 1859;17:357–375
5. Eichler W. Adenom einen von der Nasenschleimhaut ausgehenden Polypen vortäuschend. Arch Laryngol 1898;7:134
6. Compagno J, Wong RT. Intranasal mixed tumors (pleomorphic adenomas): a clinicopathologic study of 40 cases. Am J Clin Pathol 1977;68(2):213–218
7. Majed MA. Pleomorphic adenoma of nasal septum. J Laryngol Otol 1971;85(9):975–976
8. Worthington P. Pleomorphic adenoma of the nasal septum. Br J Oral Surg 1977;14(3):245–252
9. Bergström B, Biörklund A. Pleomorphic adenoma of the nasal septum. Report of two cases. J Laryngol Otol 1981;95(2):179–181
10. Baraka ME, Sadek SA, Salem MH. Pleomorphic adenoma of the inferior turbinate. J Laryngol Otol 1984;98(9):925–928
11. Kamal SA. Pleomorphic adenoma of the nose: a clinical case and historical review. J Laryngol Otol 1984;98(9):917–923
12. Haberman RS II, Stanley DE. Pleomorphic adenoma of the nasal septum. Otolaryngol Head Neck Surg 1989;100(6):610–612
13. Freeman SB, Kennedy KS, Parker GS, Tatum SA. Metastasizing pleomorphic adenoma of the nasal septum. Arch Otolaryngol Head Neck Surg 1990;116(11):1331–1333
14. Clark M, Fatterpekar GM, Mukherji SK, Buenting J. CT of intranasal pleomorphic adenoma. Neuroradiology 1999;41(8):591–593
15. Jassar P, Stafford ND, MacDonald AW. Pleomorphic adenoma of the nasal septum. J Laryngol Otol 1999;113(5):483–485
16. Kanazawa T, Nishino H, Ichimura K. Pleomorphic adenoma of the pterygopalatine fossa: a case report. Eur Arch Otorhinolaryngol 2000;257(8):433–435
17. Motoori K, Takano H, Nakano K, Yamamoto S, Ueda T, Ikeda M. Pleomorphic adenoma of the nasal septum: MR features. AJNR Am J Neuroradiol 2000;21(10):1948–1950
18. Yiotakis I, Dinopoulou D, Ferekidis E, Manolopoulos L, Adamopoulos G. Pleomorphic adenoma of the nose. Rhinology 2001;39(1):55–57
19. Hirai S, Matsumoto T, Suda K. Pleomorphic adenoma in nasal cavity: immunohistochemical study of three cases. Auris Nasus Larynx 2002;29(3):291–295
20. London SD, Schlosser RJ, Gross CW. Endoscopic management of benign sinonasal tumors: a decade of experience. Am J Rhinol 2002;16(4):221–227
21. Unlu HH, Celik O, Demir MA, Eskiizmir G. Pleomorphic adenoma originated from the inferior nasal turbinate. Auris Nasus Larynx 2003;30(4):417–420
22. Kumagai M, Endo S, Koizumi F, Kida A, Yamamoto M. A case of pleomorphic adenoma of the nasal septum. Auris Nasus Larynx 2004;31(4):439–442
23. Mackle T, Zahirovic A, Walsh M. Pleomorphic adenoma of the nasal septum. Ann Otol Rhinol Laryngol 2004;113(3 Pt 1):210–211
24. Pasquini E, Sciarretta V, Frank G, et al. Endoscopic treatment of benign tumors of the nose and paranasal sinuses. Otolaryngol Head Neck Surg 2004;131(3):180–186
25. Tahlan A, Nanda A, Nagarkar N, Bansal S. Pleomorphic adenoma of the nasal septum: a case report. Am J Otolaryngol 2004;25(2):118–120
26. Narozny W, Kuczkowski J, Mikaszewski B. Pleomorphic adenoma of the nasal cavity: clinical analysis of 8 cases. Am J Otolaryngol 2005;26(3):218
27. Roh JL, Jung BJ, Rha KS, Park CI. Endoscopic resection of pleomorphic adenoma arising in the nasopharynx. Acta Otolaryngol 2005;125(8):910–912
28. Lee SL, Lee CY, Silver SM, Kuhar S. Nasopharyngeal pleomorphic adenoma in the adult. Laryngoscope 2006;116(7):1281–1283
29. Sciarretta V, Pasquini E, Frank G, et al. Endoscopic treatment of benign tumors of the nose and paranasal sinuses: a report of 33 cases. Am J Rhinol 2006;20(1):64–71
30. Karakus MF, Ozcan KM, Dere H. Endoscopic resection of pleomorphic adenoma of the nasal septum. Tumori 2007;93(3):300–301
31. Mercante G, Di Lella F, Corradi D, Rindi G, Oretti G, Ferri T. Endoscopic surgical treatment of pleomorphic

adenoma of the inferior nasal turbinate. J Otolaryngol 2007;36(3):E12–E14

32. Uğuz MZ, Onal K, Demiray U, Ekinci N. Tumoral mass presenting in the nasomalar region arising from the lateral nasal wall: pleomorphic adenoma. Eur Arch Otorhinolaryngol 2007;264(11):1377–1379

33. Ceylan A, Celenk F, Poyraz A, Uslu S. Pleomorphic adenoma of the nasal columella. Pathol Res Pract 2008;204(4):273–276

34. Gana P, Masterson L. Pleomorphic adenoma of the nasal septum: a case report. J Med Case Reports 2008;2:349

35. Oztürk E, Sağlam O, Sönmez G, Cüce F, Haholu ACT. CT and MRI of an unusual intranasal mass: pleomorphic adenoma. Diagn Interv Radiol 2008;14(4):186–188

36. Sciandra D, Dispenza F, Porcasi R, Kulamarva G, Saraniti C. Pleomorphic adenoma of the lateral nasal wall: case report. Acta Otorhinolaryngol Ital 2008;28(3):150–153

37. Olajide TG, Alabi BS, Badmos BK, Bello OT. Pleomorphic adenoma of the lateral nasal wall—a case report. Niger Postgrad Med J 2009;16(3):227–229

38. Acevedo JL, Nolan J, Markwell JK, Thompson D. Pleomorphic adenoma of the nasal cavity: a case report. Ear Nose Throat J 2010;89(5):224–226

39. Ng T-Y, Tsai M-H, Tai C-J. Pleomorphic adenoma of nasal septum: a case report. B-ENT 2010;6(1):53–54

40. Wu F, Huang CC, Fu CH, Chen YL, Lee TJ. Transnasal endoscopic surgery for intranasal pleomorphic adenomas. B-ENT 2010;6(1):43–47

41. Erlandson RA, Cardon-Cardo C, Higgins PJ. Histogenesis of benign pleomorphic adenoma (mixed tumor) of the major salivary glands. An ultrastructural and immunohistochemical study. Am J Surg Pathol 1984;8(11):803–820

42. Bilal H, Handra-Luca A, Bertrand JC, Fouret PJ. P63 is expressed in basal and myoepithelial cells of human normal and tumor salivary gland tissues. J Histochem Cytochem 2003;51(2):133–139

43. Eveson J, Kusafuka K, Stenman G, et al. Pleomorphic adenoma. In: Barnes L, Eveson J, Reichert P, Sidransky D, eds. World Health Organization Classification of Tumours. Pathology and Genetics of Head and Neck Tumours. Lyon: IARC Press; 2005:254–258

44. Hjertman L, Eneroth CM. Tumours of the palate. Acta Otolaryngol Suppl 1969;263:179–182

45. Goepfert H, Luna MA, Lindberg RD, White AK. Malignant salivary gland tumors of the paranasal sinuses and nasal cavity. Arch Otolaryngol 1983;109(10):662–668

46. Tortoledo ME, Luna MA, Batsakis JG. Carcinomas ex pleomorphic adenoma and malignant mixed tumors. Histomorphologic indexes. Arch Otolaryngol 1984;110(3):172–176

47. Hellquist H, Michaels L. Malignant mixed tumour. A salivary gland tumour showing both carcinomatous and sarcomatous features. Virchows Arch A Pathol Anat Histopathol 1986;409(1):93–103

48. Cho KJ, el-Naggar AK, Mahanupab P, Luna MA, Batsakis JG. Carcinoma ex-pleomorphic adenoma of the nasal cavity: a report of two cases. J Laryngol Otol 1995;109(7):677–679

49. Freeman SR, Sloan P, de Carpentier J. Carcinoma ex-pleomorphic adenoma of the nasal septum with adenoid cystic and squamous carcinomatous differentiation. Rhinology 2003;41(2):118–121

50. Chaudhry AP, Vickers RA, Gorlin RJ. Intraoral minor salivary gland tumors. An analysis of 1,414 cases. Oral Surg Oral Med Oral Pathol 1961;14:1194–1226

51. Bergman F. Tumors of the minor salivary glands. A report of 46 cases. Cancer 1969;23(3):538–543

52. Rafla S. Mucous gland tumors of paranasal sinuses. Cancer 1969;24(4):683–691

53. Frable WJ, Elzay RP. Tumors of minor salivary glands. A report of 73 cases. Cancer 1970;25(4):932–941

54. Spiro RH, Koss LG, Hajdu SI, Strong EW. Tumors of minor salivary origin. A clinicopathologic study of 492 cases. Cancer 1973;31(1):117–129

55. Gnepp DR. Malignant mixed tumors of the salivary glands: a review. Pathol Annu 1993;28(Pt 1):279–328

56. Chimona TS, Koutsopoulos AV, Malliotakis P, Nikolidakis A, Skoulakis C, Bizakis JG. Malignant mixed tumor of the nasal cavity. Auris Nasus Larynx 2006;33(1):63–66

57. Yazibene Y, Ait-Mesbah N, Kalafate S, et al. Degenerative pleomorphic adenoma of the nasal cavity. Eur Ann Otorhinolaryngol Head Neck Dis 2011;128(1):37–40

Oncocytomas

Definition

(ICD-O code 8290/0)

An oncocytoma is an epithelial tumor composed of large cells containing a granular eosinophilic cytoplasm.

Etiology

Oncocytes are found in major and minor salivary glands and throughout the body in glandular tissue including adrenal, pituitary, thyroid, liver, pancreas, ovary, and stomach.[1] In the head and neck, they have been found in the larynx, tonsillar fossa, and lacrimal gland.

Synonyms

Oxyphil adenoma, oncocytic cell adenoma, eosinophilic granular cell tumor have all been used for this rare lesion. Hamperl first used the term "oncocyte" in 1931 to describe large cells in major salivary glands filled with acidophilic granular cytoplasm.[2] The first reference to an oncocytoma was by Gruenfeld and Jorsted in 1936.[3]

Incidence

These are rare lesions in the nose and sinuses with only around 30 reported as single case reports in the literature and account for <1% of all salivary gland tumors. We have only seen three cases in our cohort of 1,700 sinonasal tumors.

Site

Oncocytomas can occur on the septum or lateral nasal wall or within the maxillary and ethmoid sinuses (Table 7.2).[4–24]

Diagnostic Features

Clinical Features

Sinonasal oncocytomas occur equally in men and women, the reported age range being 12 to 84 years (mean 64 years), whereas elsewhere in the body they are more common in the elderly and in women.[25] Two of our three patients were female. Patients present with nasal

Table 7.2 Oncocytomas of the upper jaw: world literature and personal cases

Author	Age (y)	Sex	Symptoms	Duration	Site	Treatment	Follow-up
Hamperl 1962[4]	55	M	–	–	Nose	–	–
Briggs and Evans 1967[5]	71	F	–	–	Palate	–	2 mo
Cohen and Batsakis 1968[6]	61	M	Obstruction, epistaxis, rhinorrhea	1 y	Nose	Caldwell-Luc	8 y 2 recurrences
Johns et al 1973[7]	61	M	–	–	Nose	Caldwell-Luc, local excision × 2	Local recurrence at 5 and 7 y No recurrence at 8 y
Handler and Ward 1979[8]	64	M	Pain, paresthesia of left cheek	2 y	Maxilla	Radical maxillectomy	A&W 1 year
Mahmoud 1979[9]	54	M	–	–	Nose	Local excision, radiotherapy, Caldwell-Luc, maxillectomy	Local recurrence at 3 and 13 y No recurrence at 14 y
Chui et al 1985[10]	60	F	Nasal obstruction, epiphora		Ethmoid	Craniofacial and eye	A&W 3 y
Buchanan et al 1988[11]	40	F	–	–	Nasal vestibule	Local excision	Not specified
Mikhail et al 1988[12]	84	F	Swollen cheek with paresthesia, diplopia, epistaxis	–	Maxilla	Radical maxillectomy	Died 1 y of intercurrent disease
Damm et al 1989[13]	73	F	–	–	Alveolus	Local excision	No recurrence at 2 y
Savic et al 1989[14]	45	M	–	–	Nose	Denkers local excision	Local recurrence at 15 mo No recurrence at 4 y
Fayet et al 1990[15]	69	F	–	–	Nose	Lateral rhinotomy	A&W 9 mo
Martin et al 1990[16]	86	M	–	–	Nose	Not specified	Not specified
Klausen et al 1992[17]	66	M	–	–	Nose	Polypectomy	A&W 2 y
Corbridge et al 1996[18]	78	F	Nasal obstruction	2 mo	Nose and bilateral LNs	Lateral rhinotomy	DOD 7 mo, local disease
Comin et al 1997[19]	60	F	Epistaxis	1 mo	Nose (septum)	Surgery: approach not specified	A&W 3 y
Nayak 1999[20]	60	F	Nasal obstruction, nasal discharge	10 years	Nose	Radiotherapy and surgery	A&W 6 mo
Hamdan et al 2002[21]	33	M	Mass, epistaxis	1 y	Nose (septum)	Local excision	–
Lombardi et al 2006[22]	45	M	Swelling of palate	5 mo	Palate	Lateral rhinotomy and radiotherapy	A&W 3 y
Abe et al 2007[23]	47	M	Epistaxis, nasal obstruction	1 y	Nose (inferior turbinate)	Lateral rhinotomy and radiotherapy	DOD 27 mo, local disease

continued ▷

Table 7.2 Oncocytomas of the upper jaw: world literature and personal cases (continued)

Author	Age (y)	Sex	Symptoms	Duration	Site	Treatment	Follow-up
Hu 2010[24]	80	M	–	–	Nasal cavity and LNS	Surgery and radiotherapy (IMRT)	A&W 2 y
Howard and Lund (unpublished)	37	F	Nasal obstruction	3 mo	Nose	Lateral rhinotomy, craniofacial, neck dissection	DOD 2 y, local disease
	70	M	Nasal obstruction		Maxilla and ethmoid	Lateral rhinotomy	A&W 15 y
	79	F	Nasal obstruction		Ethmoid	Lateral rhinotomy	A&W 10 y

Abbreviations: A&W, alive and well; DOD, dead of disease; F, female; IMRT, intensity-modulated radiotherapy; M, male; mo, month(s); y, year(s).

obstruction, nasal discharge, and epistaxis. More extensive and malignant lesions will produce tissue destruction with a visible swelling due to the mass breaking into the orbit or cheek together with associated epiphora, diplopia, proptosis, edema, and paresthesia.

Imaging

There are nonspecific features of a soft tissue mass with additional obstruction of adjacent sinuses and bone destruction depending on the aggressiveness of the lesion.

Histological Features and Differential Diagnosis

Oncocytomas are, as one might expect, composed of oncocytes which are large cuboidal or columnar cells with an abundant eosinophilic cytoplasm. This cytoplasm is particularly rich in mitochondria, which give it a granular appearance, and was first confirmed by electron microscopy.[26] Lymphocytes are very rare within the tumor, which is positive for cytokeratin and epithelial membrane antigen but negative for S100. This must be distinguished from oncocytic metaplasia, which is not uncommon in the upper respiratory tract, oncocytic papillomas, and malignant oncocytomas, which are extremely rare. Oncocytic metaplasia may occur due to trauma or be a degenerative process. The other differential diagnoses include adenocarcinoma and adenoid cystic carcinoma.

There is no true capsule but compression of adjacent tissue may produce a "pseudo-capsule."

In the major salivary glands, the benign forms are described as being papillary or cystic, whereas the more malignant appear solid.

Natural History

It is not known how many, if any, benign oncocytomas transform into a malignancy. However, as a general principle, tumors in minor salivary glands tend to be more aggressive than their counterparts in major glands and half of the reported tumors have acted in an aggressive

fashion with locoregional recurrence[10,18,23,24] and sometimes the demise of the patient.

Treatment and Outcome

Wide local excision is the mainstay of treatment by whatever appropriate route to completely encompass the mass. Lateral rhinotomy, midfacial degloving, and craniofacial routes have all been used in the literature. As in one of our cases, a neck dissection may be required.

The role of radiotherapy and chemotherapy is undetermined in the malignant tumors but may be limited in effect as in adenocarcinoma or adenoid cystic carcinoma. Nonetheless, adjunctive radiotherapy has been used.[9,20,22,24,27]

Long-term surveillance is required as local recurrence has been reported up to 13 years after initial treatment.[9]

References

1. Hamperl H. Oncocytes and the so-called Hurthle cell tumour. Arch Pathol (Chic) 1950;49:536–567
2. Hamperl H. Beitrage zur normalen und pathologischen histologie menschlicher speicheldrusen. Z Mikrosk Anat Forsch 1931;27:1–55
3. Gruenfeld G, Jorsted L. Adenoma of the parotid salivary gland: oncocyte tumor. Am J Cancer 1936;26:571–575
4. Hamperl H. Benign and malignant oncocytoma. Cancer 1962;15:1019–1027
5. Briggs J, Evans JNG. Malignant oxyphilic granular-cell tumor (oncocytoma) of the palate. Review of the recent literature and report of a case. Oral Surg Oral Med Oral Pathol 1967;23(6):796–802
6. Cohen MA, Batsakis JG. Oncocytic tumors (oncocytomas) of minor salivary glands. Arch Otolaryngol 1968;88(1):71–73
7. Johns ME, Batsakis JG, Short CD. Oncocytic and oncocytoid tumors of the salivary glands. Laryngoscope 1973;83(12):1940–1952
8. Handler SD, Ward PH. Oncocytoma of the maxillary sinus. Laryngoscope 1979;89(3):372–376
9. Mahmoud NA. Malignant oncocytoma of the nasal cavity. J Laryngol Otol 1979;93(7):729–734
10. Chui RT, Liao S-Y, Bosworth H. Recurrent oncocytoma of the ethmoid sinus with orbital invasion. Otolaryngol Head Neck Surg 1985;93(2):267–270

11. Buchanan JA, Krolls SO, Sneed WF, Wetzel WJ. Oncocytoma in the nasal vestibule. Otolaryngol Head Neck Surg 1988;99(1):63–65

12. Mikhail RA, Reed DN Jr, Bybee DB, Okoye MI, Dodds ME. Malignant oncocytoma of the maxillary sinus—an ultrastructural study. Head Neck Surg 1988;10(6):427–431

13. Damm DD, White DK, Geissler RH Jr, Drummond JF, Henry BB. Benign solid oncocytoma of intraoral minor salivary glands. Oral Surg Oral Med Oral Pathol 1989;67(1):84–86

14. Savić D, Djerić D, Jasović A. Oncocytoma of the nose and ethmoidal and sphenoidal sinuses. [Article in French] Rev Laryngol Otol Rhinol (Bord) 1989;110(5):481–483

15. Fayet B, Bernard JA, Zachar D, et al. Malignant nasal oncocytoma disclosed by mucocele of the lacrimal sac with hemolacrimia. [Article in French] J Fr Ophtalmol 1990;13(3):153–158

16. Martin H, Janda J, Behrbohm H. Locally invasive oncocytoma of the nasal cavity. [Article in German] Zentralbl Allg Pathol 1990;136(7-8):703–706

17. Klausen OG, Steinsvåg S, Olofsson J. Oncocytoma presenting as a choanal polyp: a case report. J Otolaryngol 1992;21(3):196–198

18. Corbridge RJ, Gallimore AP, Dalton CG, O'Flynn PE. Oncocytomas of the upper jaw. Head Neck 1996;18(4):374–380

19. Comin CE, Dini M, Lo Russo G. Oncocytoma of the nasal cavity: report of a case and review of the literature. J Laryngol Otol 1997;111(7):671–673

20. Nayak DR, Pillai S, Balakrishnan R, Thomas R, Rao R. Malignant oncocytoma of the nasal cavity: a case report. Am J Otolaryngol 1999;20(5):323–327

21. Hamdan AL, Kahwagi G, Farhat F, Tawii A. Oncocytoma of the nasal septum: a rare cause of epistaxis. Otolaryngol Head Neck Surg 2002;126(4):440–441

22. Lombardi D, Piccioni M, Farina D, Morassi ML, Nicolai P. Oncocytic carcinoma of the maxillary sinus: a rare neoplasm. Eur Arch Otorhinolaryngol 2006;263(6):528–531

23. Abe T, Murakami A, Nakajima N, et al. Oncocytic carcinoma of the nasal cavity with widespread lymph node metastases. Auris Nasus Larynx 2007;34(3):393–396

24. Hu YW, Lin CZ, Li WY, Chang CP, Wang LW. Locally advanced oncocytic carcinoma of the nasal cavity treated with surgery and intensity-modulated radiotherapy. J Chin Med Assoc 2010;73(3):166–172

25. Eneroth CM. Oncocytoma of major salivary glands. J Laryngol Otol 1965;79(12):1064–1072

26. Johns ME, Regezi JA, Batsakis JG. Oncocytic neoplasms of salivary glands: an ultrastructural study. Laryngoscope 1977;87(6):862–871

27. DiMaio SJ, DiMaio VJ, DiMaio TM, Nicastri AD, Chen CK. Oncocytic carcinoma of the nasal cavity. South Med J 1980;73(6):803–806

Malignant Epithelial (Nonepidermoid) Tumors

Adenocarcinoma

Definition

Adenocarcinoma is a malignant epithelial tumor characterized by the presence of glandular structures. It may be divided into intestinal (ICD-O 8144/3) and sinonasal nonintestinal (ICD-O 8140/3) types.

Etiology

Considerable research has been conducted on the association with exposure to hardwood dust since the lesion was first noted in furniture makers of Buckinghamshire in the United Kingdom in the 1960s by Hadfield and colleagues.[1,2] Adenocarcinoma became a recognized industrial disease in the United Kingdom in 1969. Exposure to hardwood dust typically gives rise to intestinal-type adenocarcinomas (ITAC) and, since it was described in the United Kingdom, most countries with woodworking industries of note have reported similar findings. In Germany, however, it was not recognized as an occupational disease until 1988.[3] In keeping with other cohort studies in Scandinavia, significant hyperplasia, dysplasia, and carcinoma in situ are found on the middle turbinate in populations of woodworkers[3,4] as compared with controls. However, the exact carcinogen in the dust remains unknown, with suggestions including alkaloids, saponins, stilbenes, aldehydes, quinones, flavinoids, terpenes, tannins, and even fungal particles.

The size of the dust particles is also relevant. For it to be deposited in the middle meatus, it needs to be >5 μm in diameter. Thus relevant exposure is limited to certain jobs such as lath operating and sanding and this puts joiners and cabinet makers at particular risk. Schroeder et al[3] considered a cohort of 246 patients with intestinal-type adenocarcinoma due to exposure to oak and beech wood dust, wood dust exposure was at concentrations between 10 mg/m³ and 500 mg/m³. Around 75% had worked as joiners or cabinet makers and most had worked in small workshops.

It is worth noting that environmental levels of wood dust in excess of 5 mg/m³ are regarded as unsafe.[5]

Other etiological factors include formaldehyde, isopropyl alcohol, nickel, or chrome exposure (particularly to hexavalent chromium[6]), and those working with leather tannins. It is usually considered an occupational pathology but spontaneous cases do occur[7,8] and in our series only 30% had relevant occupational exposure, which in part reflects the mixed histological subtypes.

The importance of duration of exposure and a latency period are also acknowledged between exposure and presentation with the tumor. In the literature the duration of exposure varies from 9 to 40 years and the latency from exposure to presentation with the tumor varies from 22 to 70 years. However, there is a report of much shorter exposure to organic dusts in a subset of ITAC patients (16 out of 148, 4 to 18 years, mean 7.5 years; as compared with 25 to 55 years for the majority)[9] followed by a long interval before presentation, which has also been our observation in some individuals. The increased relative risk is similar to that for bronchial carcinoma in smokers, with a cumulative lifetime risk of 1 in 120 and a 500- to 1000-fold increased risk compared with the normal population.

In the developed world it is increasingly difficult now to estimate the risk because of the rarity of hardwoods, the changes that have occurred in industrial safety regulations, the rarity of individuals remaining in a single occupation throughout their working life, and changes in processes that might expose workers to the potential carcinogens. Nonetheless, their significance should not be underestimated, particularly elsewhere in the world where the situation may be different. Furthermore, there may be genetic predisposition, with one study showing an overrepresentation of CYP1A1 codon 461 polymorphism in patients with ITAC compared with controls.[10]

Incidence

Adenocarcinoma accounts for 10 to 20% of sinonasal malignancies and, with squamous cell carcinoma, is the most common malignancy found in the paranasal sinuses.[8,11–15] In our series it constitutes 12% of our malignant sinonasal tumors.

Males are affected much more commonly than females, reflecting occupational factors, and this inequality is most marked in the ITAC group.[3,8,9,16] In women, the menopause may be responsible for a temporary downturn in incidence around 50 years, which is similar to Clemmesen's hook observed in breast cancer.[17]

Patients' age ranges from 9 to 90 years, though average age of presentation is between 50 and 60 years. In our cohort of 117 primary cases, ages ranged from 27 to 89 years (mean 59.7 years) and the ratio of men to women was 3.6:1. The majority of cases occurred in the 6th to 8th decades (Table 7.3).

Site

Traditionally adenocarcinoma has been regarded as an ethmoidal tumor (40%) but it can be found in other areas of the nasal cavity (27%) and maxillary sinus (20%).[18] In our series the majority (59%) affected the ethmoid,

followed by antroethmoid/maxillary sinus (29%), which largely reflects our interest in craniofacial resection. This distribution of site of origin also reflects the deposition of carcinogens in the middle meatus. It has recently been suggested on the basis of endoscopic findings that many, if not all, adenocarcinomas arise in the olfactory cleft.[19] However, this has not been our experience or that of others.

Late presentation (T3 and T4) has generally negated the relevance of the TNM classification.[20]

Diagnostic Features

Clinical Features

Presentation is usually similar to that of inflammatory sinonasal pathology, so diagnosis may be delayed. As with other sinonasal malignancies the presence of unilateral symptoms, typically obstruction, rhinorrhea, and epistaxis or serosanguinous discharge, should be regarded with suspicion by clinicians. Approximately 40% of cases in one series had symptoms for more than 6 months.[8] Spread to adjacent structures will also produce clinical changes, such as displacement of the eye, epiphora, reduced mobility, and diplopia. Spread anteriorly through the nasal bones can produce a glabellar mass, whereas extension posteriorly into the sphenoethmoidal recess and nasopharynx and superiorly into the anterior cranial fossa is generally silent. However, extension into the pterygopalatine and infratemporal fossae can produce trismus, pain, and paresthesia.

Endoscopic appearances are nonspecific, either a friable or a smooth fleshy mass in the upper nasal cavity (Fig. 7.3a). The surface may be ulcerated. It is usually unilateral but, as both the septum and contralateral ethmoid can be affected, the mass can present on both sides of the nose. It is not particularly vascular and so does not bleed significantly to touch.

Table 7.3 Adenocarcinoma: personal series 1970–2010

	n	Age		M:F	CFR	Maxill	ESS	MFD	LR	No surgery[a]
		Range (y)	Mean (y)							
All	117	27–89	59.7	3.6:1	63	8	23	3	7	13
DXT	69				26	5	17	2	3	13
Chemo	10				6	–	2	–	–	2
Overall actuarial survival										
5 y					58%		83%			
10 y					40%					
15 y					33%					

Abbreviations: CFR, craniofacial resection; Chemo, chemotherapy; DXT, radiotherapy; ESS, endoscopic sinus surgery; F, female; LR, lateral rhinotomy; M, male; Maxill, maxillectomy; MFD, midfacial degloving; y, year(s).
[a] Palliative treatment only in advanced disease at presentation.

Imaging

(See **Figs. 7.3, 7.4, 7.5.**)

The appearances again are rather nonspecific on both CT and MRI. As usual CT provides bony definition whereas MRI is complementary and allows differentiation of retained secretions and inflamed mucosa from the tumor bulk. The relationship of the tumor to the orbit and anterior cranial fossa is also better defined by MRI.[21,22] Interestingly, adenocarcinoma often pushes rather than infiltrates adjacent structures and at surgery a definite plane may be found between tumor and orbital periosteum or dura, so it is not possible to be didactic about extent until after surgery and confirmatory histology.

While the tissue characteristics are not specific, sometimes the pattern of spread may give a clue. The tumor may extend forward from the anterior ethmoids into the glabellar region, as previously mentioned, to produce a soft tissue mass anterior to the nasal bones and/or extend posteriorly into the sphenoethmoidal recess and nasopharynx. Also it will often involve both ethmoid complexes.

Follow-up using standard screening protocols with regular MRI is mandatory over a lifetime due to the potential for late recurrence.

Lymph node involvement occurs in <10%, obviating the need for routine ultrasound/screening of the neck. However, screening for another primary source is worth considering in the ITACs with particular attention to the lower gastrointestinal tract, kidney, and pancreas.

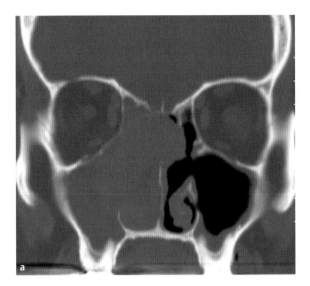

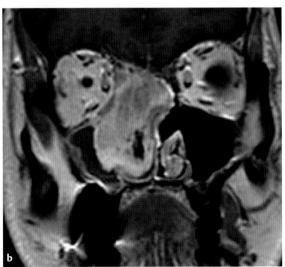

Fig. 7.3a–i

a Adenocarcinoma. Coronal CT showing a unilateral mass with opacification of the maxillary and posterior ethmoids, displacement of the superior septum, but intact skull base and lamina papyracea.

b Coronal MRI (T1W post gadolinium enhancement) of the same patient defining the extent of the mass, which affects the nasal cavity and ethmoids with obstruction of the maxillary sinus.

c Sagittal MRI (T1W post gadolinium enhancement) in the same patient showing the mass abutting the skull base but not grossly extending through it.

Fig. 7.3d–i ▷

◁ continued

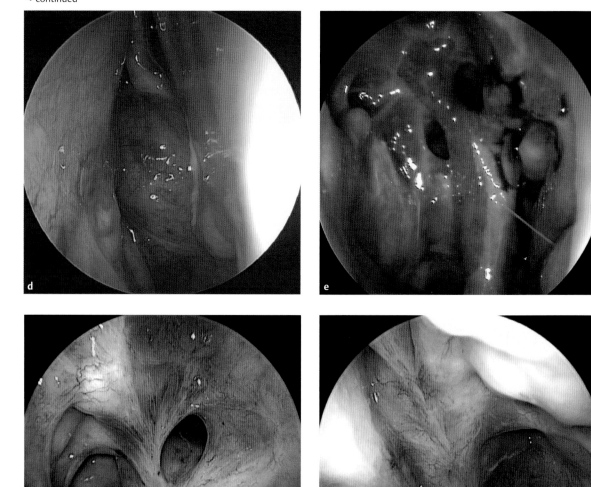

d Endoscopic view of a smooth mass filling the nasal cavity in the same patient.

e Endoscopic view in the same patient 1 month following endoscopic resection of the tumor.

f Endoscopic view in the same patient 4 months following endoscopic resection of the tumor.

g Close-up endoscopic view of skull base repair in the same patient 4 months following endoscopic resection of the tumor.

◁ continued

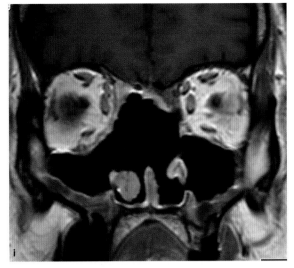

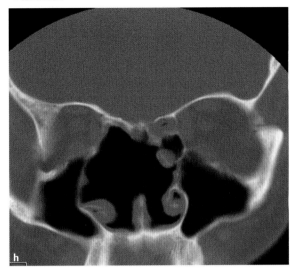

h Coronal CT scan showing the postoperative cavity at 4 months.

i Coronal MRI (T1W post gadolinium enhancement) showing the postoperative cavity at 4 months.

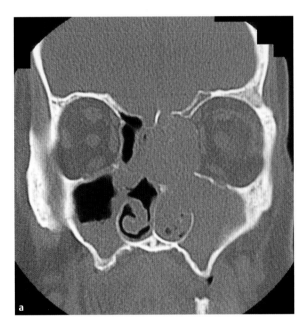

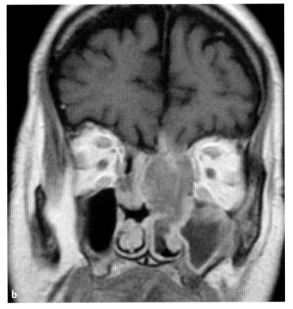

Fig. 7.4a, b

a Adenocarcinoma. Coronal CT showing a mass in the left nasal cavity with opacification of the posterior ethmoids and maxillary sinus and with possible skull base erosion.

b Coronal MRI (T1W post gadolinium enhancement) showing the mass in the left nasal cavity and posterior ethmoids with obstruction of maxillary sinus and confirming extension into the crista galli region and possibly the superior sagittal sinus. Craniofacial resection was undertaken in this case, which confirmed microscopic involvement of the superior sagittal sinus.

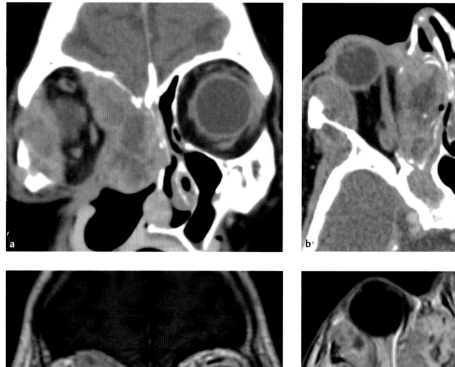

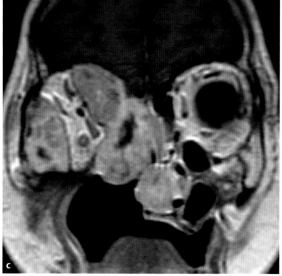

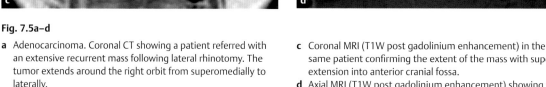

Fig. 7.5a–d

a Adenocarcinoma. Coronal CT showing a patient referred with an extensive recurrent mass following lateral rhinotomy. The tumor extends around the right orbit from superomedially to laterally.

b Axial CT in the same patient; the mass extends lateral to the orbit into the infratemporal fossa.

c Coronal MRI (T1W post gadolinium enhancement) in the same patient confirming the extent of the mass with superior extension into anterior cranial fossa.

d Axial MRI (T1W post gadolinium enhancement) showing the extent of the tumor at the orbital apex, cavernous sinus, and abutting temporal lobe. The patient underwent a craniofacial resection and orbital clearance and is alive with residual disease 2 years later.

Histological Features and Differential Diagnosis

Primary adenocarcinomas of the sinonasal tract are a diverse group of malignancies that can initially be classified as salivary (5–10%) and nonsalivary types.[18] The World Health Organization (WHO) classification of nonsalivary gland type nasal and paranasal adenocarcinomas considers the categories: high- and low-grade adenocarcinoma of nonintestinal type, and the more common intestinal type adenocarcinoma (ITAC) of colonic and mucinous subtypes.[23] This has largely replaced the papillary-tubular cylindrical cell, alveolar-goblet cell, signet-ring cell, and transitional types proposed by Kleinsasser and Schroeder and also the papillary, colonic, solid, mucinous, and mixed subtypes of Barnes.[20,24]

The main differentiation for the nonintestinal form is from *chordoma*, while the lower-grade tumors resemble respiratory epithelioid hamartomas.

Although, as previously discussed, ITAC is classically associated with occupational exposure to wood dust, one should always consider the possibility of the tumor being a metastasis from the gastrointestinal tract, pancreas, or kidney and further imaging should be undertaken if there is any suspicion.

Immunohistochemistry can demonstrate positivity for certain keratins such as CK7 and CK20 and comparative genomic hybridization studies have generally shown gains at 7q, 8q, and 20q with losses at 5q, 17q, and 18q.[25,26] VEGF-C is associated with higher-grade tumors but is not correlated with survival.[27]

Sinonasal nonintestinal adenocarcinomas can be high- or low-grade and are said to be divided on the basis of site, behavior, and prognosis—low-grade and more indolent in the ethmoid and high-grade, more aggressive, in the maxilla.[9,28]

Natural History

ITAC may demonstrate a spectrum of aggressiveness, ranging from indolent to locally aggressive with a recurrence rate of 50% or more. This is the cause of disease-related death in approximately half of cases[29–31] and is most often due to direct intracranial extension. Metastases are relatively uncommon (none in 143 cases in 1 series) but usually quoted as occurring in 20% of cases.[31,32] Nine of our patients are known to have developed secondary disease in the lungs and/or bone. Lymph node spread occurs in ~10% of cases[31] and occurred in only 2 of our 117 cases.

In common with many other sinonasal tumors, adenocarcinoma in its various forms may recur many years later and thus require long-term follow-up.

Treatment

Reports on sinonasal malignancies and their management often consist of retrospective case series of heterogeneous group of histologies, stages, and interventions from single institutions grouped together.[27,33] There is a general consensus in the literature that the optimal treatment of adenocarcinoma is surgery and postoperative radiotherapy,[34] but the evidence for this combined therapy is not strong.[35] The treatment undertaken in our own patients may be seen in **Table 7.3**.

Surgery

Surgery remains the mainstay of treatment. A wide range of open approaches have been used from lateral rhinotomy, to midfacial degloving, to a variety of maxillectomies and craniofacial resections[15] with or without orbital clearance, determined by extent of spread to the eye or through the skull base. Traditionally, if tumor abutted the skull base, a formal "en bloc" resection encompassed the upper septum, entire ethmoids, face of the sphenoid, and cribriform plate together with cranialization of the frontal

sinuses and removal of adjacent structures, depending on extent, via some form of craniofacial approach.[8,9,12,15,36] However, in common with other neoplasms in recent years, endoscopic approaches are increasingly being used in selected cases.[34,37–45] **Whatever approach is chosen, the primary aim is complete and safe complete tumor excision**, the only exception being for individuals in whom the extent of disease is so great that palliation is the only option. That said, even with extensive disease, a low-morbidity operation may still have an important role to play.

The limitations for an endoscopic resection are changing as experience grows in several tertiary centers. The addition of extended frontal sinus procedures and endoscopic medial maxillectomy has considerably improved access and postoperative surveillance. Dural invasion, which was previously regarded as a limitation,[41] can be encompassed safely from below in many cases. However, once the sagittal sinus or frontal lobes are involved, it becomes significantly more difficult to achieve adequate resection from below, although it could be argued that cure is rarely possible in these circumstances irrespective of the approach. The endonasal endoscopic approach can of course be combined with craniotomy.

As the tumor may be associated with widespread field change and has a tendency to cross the midline, whatever the surgical approach, complete extirpation of both lateral walls, including ethmoid complexes and the upper septum is strongly recommended, at the least to provide accurate staging. Specific attention should also be paid to the sphenoethmoidal recess, lateral nasopharynx, and anterior superior nasal cavity. Notwithstanding this, some ostensibly large tumors may arise from quite small areas, for example, pedicled on the middle turbinate, and the endoscopic approach allows one to accurately determine this site of origin.

A plane of cleavage is often present between the tumor and the orbital periosteum even when the lamina has been eroded. It has been our practice for some decades to preserve the eye under these circumstances, having resected the adjacent orbital periosteum and confirmed with frozen section that tumor has not transgressed the periosteum microscopically. Using this approach only 6 eyes have been removed in 117 cases at initial major resection.

Once the skull base has been breached, it has been our practice to resect adjacent bone and dura on a wide front, to adequately assess the frontal lobes. Tumor may on occasion be seen to infiltrate the brain and this can be resected, although from a prognostic perspective the outcome is usually very poor.

As lymphatic involvement is rare, prophylactic treatment of the first-order lymph nodes (which may be retropharyngeal) has not been shown to be warranted.[46] Only one of our patients required a formal neck dissection (<1%).

Radiotherapy

Pre- or postoperative radiotherapy has commonly been used for this disease, although there are no randomized nor even controlled trials of its use. Standard protocols are available for tumor in close proximity to the skull base or eye to minimize collateral damage. Other radiotherapy techniques have also been used for tumors affecting the skull base, such as gamma knife, intensity-modulated radiotherapy (IMRT), and proton beam radiotherapy. These techniques have a higher dose gradient of radiation compared with conventional techniques, which can help spare critical structures near the target such as retina and optic nerve. The tumor can thus be given a higher dose of radiotherapy with the expectation that side effects are reduced, although large long-term studies are lacking. These techniques are not intended to replace surgery and still rely on the radiosensitivity of the target tissue.

Given the overall lack of evidence for radiotherapy, it should not be given for small tumors that are not close to the orbit, skull base, or major vascular structures,[47] nor for those lesions where complete resection with reasonable margins has been achieved. There is no evidence to support prophylactic neck irradiation.[8,47]

Chemotherapy and Other Therapies

Several centers have advocated the use of topical chemotherapy.[48,49] This has involved surgical debulking of sinonasal adenocarcinoma followed by application of topical fluorouracil (5-FU) up to eight times combined with debridement of necrotic tissue on each occasion. Although good results have been reported (see later), they have been difficult to replicate, involve a considerable commitment on the part of the clinician and patient, and have not been widely adopted.

There are several reports of sinonasal adenocarcinoma responding to docetaxel, cisplatin, and 5-fluorouracil.[50] Selective intra-arterial chemotherapy has also been tried but, as with other selective infusion techniques, has not demonstrated a role in clinical medicine.[51]

Some new therapeutic approaches such as the use of monoclonal antibodies for epidermal growth factor receptor (EGFR) inhibitor may be helpful in the future, an approach that is being trialed in some intestinal adenocarcinomas.

Prognostic Factors and Outcome

There are no trials comparing surgery alone with other treatment regimes, but in pooled series of varying types of sinonasal malignancies surgery is more beneficial than other techniques (**Table 7.4**).[27]

In a series of 418 patients with sinonasal adenocarcinoma, the French GETTEC group showed a significant survival advantage with surgery (alone or in combination with radiotherapy) when compared with radiotherapy alone.[8] The surgical approach was transfacial in 274 cases (72.5%), combined in 77 (20%), neurosurgical in 22 (6%), and endoscopic in 6 (1.5%). Postoperative complications included 20 (4.8%) cerebrospinal fluid leakage, 13 (3.1%) meningitis, 7 (1.7%) deaths, and 6 (1.4%) hemorrhage.[8]

In a series of 153 patients with ITAC affecting the ethmoids,[9] the majority of whom underwent craniofacial resection, 5- and 10-year cause-specific mortality was 44% and 53%, respectively (i.e., 56% and 47% survival) compared with 50% and 57% mortality in 36 non-ITACs of the ethmoid or maxillary sinus, but this difference was not significant. Nor was there a difference in mortality between the well-, moderately, and poorly differentiated subsets of ITAC. Disease relapse was 51% and 58% for ITAC at 5 years and 10 years and again there was no statistical difference between the ITAC and non-ITAC nor between the histological subsets of ITAC.

Craniofacial resection was reported by the collaborative group of Ganly et al, considering 334 cases, of which 107 (32%) were adenocarcinomas.[14] They reported 44% overall survival, 52% disease-specific survival, and 46.4% recurrence-free survival in the adenocarcinoma subgroup. These included several (unspecified numbers) of preoperative and adjuvant treatment strategies. In our own series of 62 adenocarcinomas treated by craniofacial resection, the 5-year actuarial survival was 58%, dropping to 40% and 33% at 10 and 15 years, respectively.[15] This of course included tumors of all stages, with the majority either T3 or T4. Specifically, prognosis was directly related to extent of intracranial involvement at craniofacial resection when patients were stratified to involvement of skull base alone, dural infiltration, or involvement of the frontal lobe. Despite the affected areas being cleared macroscopically and microscopically, survival at 5 years was 82%, 20%, and 0%, respectively. However, although our own complication rate was low, in the pooled data on 1,193 patients of Ganly et al[63] there was a postoperative mortality of 4.7% and significant morbidity in at least one-third.

As this disease frequently affects older patients with other comorbidities, it is not surprising that there has been a trend toward endoscopic resection. Several authors[37,40–44,64,65] have reported series of endoscopically resected sinonasal tumors with comparatively good outcomes. Lund et al reported an 83% overall 5-year survival and 72% disease-free survival for adenocarcinomas resected endoscopically.[40] Some of these also received radiotherapy. The Bogaerts et al series of 44 adenocarcinoma patients had an overall survival, disease-specific survival, and local control rate of 81%, 91%, and 73%, respectively.[41] Corresponding rates for the 5-year follow-up were 53%, 83%, and 62%. There will clearly be a bias toward the smaller, lower-staged tumors being more suitable for endoscopic resection but, as the above authors

Table 7.4 Adenocarcinoma: major series 1984–2010

First author	Adenocarcinoma cases	Management	Outcome	Stage at presentation
Klintenberg et al[52]	28	19 received preop RT (40–70 Gy) followed by surgery, 4 surgery alone, 3 deemed inoperable, 2 not treated	76% 2 y survival, 50% 5 y survival (12 cases lost)	
Tran et al[53]	10	Surgery + RT or RT alone	82% overall 5 y survival, 57% at 10 y, 25% at 15 y	
Roux et al[54]	63	Neoadjuvant chemo-therapy (cisplatin, 5-FU) followed by open approach surgery PORT (mean 65 Gy) Only 54 received neoadjuvant chemo 63 operated	Mean 19 month survival Overall actuarial survival: 85% at 1 y 70% at 2 y 53% at 3 y 42.5% at 5 y	T1 = 5 T2 = 5 T3 = 12 T4 = 41 (16 cases = recurrences)
Brasnu et al[55]	22	Neoadjuvant cisplatin and 5-FU followed by craniofacial resection 5 received PORT	68.1% 3 y survival 65.7% 3 y local control 8 (36%) responded to chemo 5 (23%) complete response	T1 = 10 T2 = 1 T3 = 11
Harbo et al[56]	37	Mixture of surgery, RT, neoadjuvant or postop RT	5 y disease-specific survival 65% 10 y disease-specific survival 52%	
Moreau et al[57]	23	Surgery and PORT	68% 3 y survival 48% 5 y survival	T1 = 1 T2 = 6 T3 = 9 T4 = 9
Shah et al[58]	17	Craniofacial resection (76 of 115 cases received RT in pooled series)	57% 5 y survival 29% 10 y survival	
Salvan et al[59]	31	Craniofacial resection and postop RT 20 also received neoadjuvant chemo (cis, 5-FU, epirubicin)	86% 1 y survival 62% 3 y survival 39% 5 y survival	
Cantu et al[12]	50 (out of 91 cases in a pooled series)	Craniofacial resection 72% of the pooled series received RT	47% 5 y overall survival 24% 5 y disease free survival (pooled series)	
Tiwari et al[60]	29	Surgery and PORT (1 = RT only)	59% 5 y survival 50% 10 y survival	
Dulguerov et al[13]	25 (out of a pooled series of 220)	4 surgery, 18 surgery and PORT, 3 RT alone	84%, 69%, and 63% 2 y, 5 y, and 7 y actuarial locoregional control 84% 2 y actuarial locoregional control (69% at 5 y, 63% at 10 y)	T1 = 1 T2 = 10 T3 = 10 T4 = 4 Ethmoid = 16 Maxillary = 4 Nasal cavity = 5

continued ▷

Table 7.4 Adenocarcinoma: major series 1984–2010 (continued)

First author	Adenocarcinoma cases	Management	Outcome	Stage at presentation
Knegt et al[49]	62	Surgery (Caldwell-Luc) and postop topical 5-FU (8 times) (32 patients received 7 × 2 Gy RT; these had no difference in outcome)	79% overall 5 year survival (92% at 2 y, 64% at 10 y) 87% 5 y disease-specific survival (96% at 2 y, 74% at 10 y) 78% 5 y local relapse-free survival (91% at 2 y, 66% at 10 y)	T1 = 3 T2 = 10 T3 = 24 T4 = 25
Claus et al[61]	47	Surgery (80% craniofacial resection) and postoperative RT	71% 3 y overall survival 62% 3 y disease-specific survival 60% overall 5 y survival 36% 5 y disease-specific survival 59% 5 y local control	T1 = 2 T2 = 17 T3 = 11 T4 = 17
Ganly et al[14]	107		44.8% overall 5 y survival 52% disease-specific 5 y survival 46.4% 5 y recurrence-free survival	
Orvidas et al[62]	24	23 surgery, 7 of which with PORT (1 chemoRT) and 2 preop chemoRT	58% 5 y overall survival (SE = 11.5%) 73% 5 y disease-specific survival	
Howard et al[15]	62 (out of 259 malignancies)	Craniofacial resection ± RT	5 y survival 58% 10 y 40% 15 y 33%	
Almeyda et al[32]	14	7 RT 7 RT and debulking	50% 5 y disease-free survival	Stage 2:13 Stage 3:1
	11	11 debulking and topical 5-FU	86% 5 y disease-free survival	Stage 2:11
Choussy et al[8]	418	Surgery alone 55 (13.2%) Radiotherapy alone 33 (7.9%) Surgery and RT 324 (77.7%) No treatment 5 (1.2%)	72% 3 y overall survival 64% 5 y overall survival 49% 10 y overall survival	T1 = 14 T2 = 133 T3 = 95 T4 = 174 (10 out of 416 N+)
Airoldi et al[27]	82	Majority surgery and PORT	47% 5 y overall survival	
De Gabory et al[47]	95	Surgery alone 16% (all T1 and 5 T2 cases) Surgery and PORT 78% (palliative in 5 cases) 1 received no treatment (Surgery: 65% transfacial; 35% CFR)	Median time to recurrence 3 y 78% disease-specific survival at 5 y (64% at 10 y) 61% disease-free survival at 5 y (44% at 10 y)	T1 = 2 T2 = 21 T3 = 35 T4 = 37 N+ = 3 M+= 0

Abbreviations: Chemo, chemotherapy; CFR, craniofacial resection; 5-FU, 5-fluorouracil; PORT, postoperative radiotherapy; RT, radiotherapy; y, year(s).

conclude, the outcome is certainly not adversely affected by endoscopic resection, giving control rates comparable to those of open techniques (**Table 7.5**).[41]

As a single modality, radiotherapy produces poorer results than surgery alone with or without radiotherapy and has a high rate of complications when used on the skull base.[8,13,37,48,52,66–72] It cannot be relied on to deal with residual disease,[57] nor if there is intracranial invasion (all cases relapsing in less than 7 months in one series).[47,61]

Neoadjuvant or primary radiotherapy with salvage surgery has been advocated by some.[71,72] In a pooled series of 29 ethmoid carcinoma cases of varying pathology, 9 of which were adenocarcinomas, 48% were reported to be controlled with radiotherapy alone.[72] The overall 5-year survival for this group was 39% and 5-year disease-specific survival was 58%, which compares poorly with series where surgery was the primary modality.

There are several published series on the use of IMRT in sinonasal malignancies but all include a heterogeneous group of malignancies, of which between 33% and 79% were adenocarcinomas.[73–78] The median radiation dose was 64 to 70 Gy, usually given postoperatively. Overall 5-year survival in these pooled series ranged from 45 to 58.5% with 5-year local control ranging from 58 to 70.7%,[76–78] which is comparable to traditional radiotherapy but may be associated with less morbidity.

Conversely, proton beam used alone in the treatment of primary salivary gland neoplasms affecting the skull base revealed a high risk of local recurrence, whereas it has been reported that gamma knife therapy can enhance local control while adding little additional toxicity.[79]

Topical 5-FU has been reported to produce a 79% overall 5-year survival and 87% 5-year disease-specific survival,[49] an effect that has been attributed to the combination of tumor cytotoxicity and immune stimulation. Interestingly, this outcome was not altered by low-dose radiotherapy used in half the cases. Good results were also reported by Almeyda et al using a similar strategy in a series of 25 cases of ethmoidal intestinal type adenocarcinoma attributed to hardwood exposure.[32] A historical control group of 14 patients receiving primary radiotherapy, 7 of whom went on to have surgical resection, was compared with 11 cases undergoing extended ethmoidectomy with repeated topical 5-FU packing. The 5-year disease-free survival for the radiotherapy ± surgery group was 50% compared with 86% with surgery and 5-FU. The literature is lacking in other series.

With regard to systemic chemotherapy, the outcome combined with surgical resection is, at best, comparable to other series without chemotherapy. Brasnu et al considered cisplatin and 5-FU as neoadjuvant agents in a small group of patients.[55] Overall 36% ($n = 8$) responded, 22.7% showed a complete clinical response, and 13.6% complete histological response. Less encouraging results were reported by Roux et al in a larger series of 54 ethmoid adenocarcinomas given neoadjuvant cisplatin and 5-FU, where 8 (15%) showed complete response, 12 (22%) had a >50% reduction in tumor volume, and 34 (63%) had no response or <50% reduction in tumor volume.[54] However, all those who had a complete response with chemotherapy were alive at 10 years.

As expected several series have shown that a higher tumor T stage is associated with poorer outcome,[27,34,54] it being significantly worse in T4b cases than the lower stages.[74] Invasion of the brain, dura, sphenoid, infratemporal fossa, or orbit all confer a statistically significantly worse prognosis[8,47,80] and, in particular, invasion of brain was not associated with survival beyond a year in our

Table 7.5 Adenocarcinoma: larger published series resected by an entirely endoscopic approach

First author (y)	Adenocarcinoma n	DXT	Outcome
Stammberger (1999)[64]	7	N/A	5 clear of disease at 30 mo
Goffart (2000)[37]	40	87.9%	5 y disease-specific survival 57.6%
Lund (2007)[40]	15	76%	5 y actuarial survival 83%
Nicolai (2008)[42]	44	35%	5 y disease-specific survival 94.4%
Bogaerts (2008)[41a]	44	100%	5 y disease-specific survival 83%
Jardeleza (2009)[44]	12	75%	91.6% disease-specific survival at 30 mo
Villaret (2010)[45b]	36	N/A	2 DOD at 15 mo and 39 mo, 1 recurrence at 12 mo, now A&W

Abbreviations: A&W, alive and well; DOD, dead of disease; DXT, radiotherapy; mo, month(s); N/A, not available; y, year(s)

Source: After and with permission of *Rhinology*: Lund V, Stammberger H, Nicolai P et al. European position paper on endoscopic management of tumours of the nose, paranasal sinuses and skull base. Rhinology Supplement 2010;22: 45.

[a] May include cases already reported by Goffart et al.[37]

[b] May include cases already reported by Nicolai et al.[42]

original craniofacial cohort.[36] The tumor volume itself is inversely proportional to survival.[54] Again as anticipated, positive surgical margins are associated with poorer local control and survival[37] as is positive nodal status, albeit rare. Nonetheless, as long as there is active management, recurrence may not confer a worse outcome than a comparable de novo adenocarcinoma.[54]

Although not supported by all studies,[9] overall histopathological type is related to outcome, with the poorly differentiated subtypes faring worse, which has been our own experience.[20,28] ITACs appear to have a higher recurrence rate than lower-grade tumors in around 50%. Cumulative 5-year survival rates vary from 40 to 60%, with most deaths occurring in the first 3 years.[8] For lower-grade non-ITACs, 5-year survival is better, with figures of up to 85% quoted.[49] However, it should be remembered that local recurrence can occur 10 years or more after treatment of the original tumor.[36] Positive immunostaining for Ki-67, CD31 and microvessel density have also been shown to correlate with survival.[27]

Age and sex may also affect outcome. Those 65 years old or over apparently had a worse outcome, with a 33% 5-year survival compared with 60% in the 55 to 64 year group.[16] Others have suggested that women are more likely to suffer recurrence.[62]

Key Points

- Adenocarcinoma is one of the commoner malignant sinonasal tumors, associated in some cases with occupational exposure to hardwood dust.
- Occupationally induced adenocarcinoma is of the intestinal type and is potentially associated with wide field change.
- Sinonasal adenocarcinoma may sometimes be a metastasis from the kidney or elsewhere, which should be excluded.
- The principal treatment is surgery and the role of radiotherapy is unproven.
- Craniofacial resection significantly improved survival but more recently endonasal endoscopic resection has proved equally successful in selected cases.

References

1. Acheson ED, Hadfield EH, Macbeth RG. Carcinoma of the nasal cavity and accessory sinuses in woodworkers. Lancet 1967;1(7485):311–312
2. Acheson ED, Cowdell RH, Hadfield E, Macbeth RG. Nasal cancer in woodworkers in the furniture industry. BMJ 1968;2(5605):587–596
3. Schroeder H-G, Wolf J, Steinhart H. New aspects of carcinogenesis of occupational sinonasal carcinoma in woodworkers. In: Werner JA, Lippert BM, Rudert HH, eds. Head and Neck Cancer: Advances in Basic Research: Proceedings of the International Symposium, Kiel Germany. Amsterdam: Elsevier Science BV; 1996:47–52
4. Wilhelmsson B, Hellquist H, Olofsson J, Klintenberg C. Nasal cuboidal metaplasia with dysplasia. Precursor to adenocarcinoma in wood-dust-exposed workers? Acta Otolaryngol 1985;99(5–6):641–648
5. Blot WJ, Chow WH, McLaughlin JK. Wood dust and nasal cancer risk. A review of the evidence from North America. J Occup Environ Med 1997;39(2):148–156
6. Industrial Injuries Advisory Council. Chromium and Sinonasal Cancer. Report by the Industrial Injuries Advisory Council in accordance with Section 171 of the Social Security Administration Act 1992. Department of Work & Pensions report Cm 7740. London: The Stationary Office; 2009: 31
7. Luce D, Leclerc A, Bégin D, et al. Sinonasal cancer and occupational exposures: a pooled analysis of 12 case-control studies. Cancer Causes Control 2002;13(2):147–157
8. Choussy O, Ferron C, Védrine PO, et al; GETTEC Study Group. Adenocarcinoma of ethmoid: a GETTEC retrospective multicenter study of 418 cases. Laryngoscope 2008;118(3):437–443
9. Cantu G, Solero CL, Mariani L, et al. Intestinal type adenocarcinoma of the ethmoid sinus in wood and leather workers: a retrospective study of 153 cases. Head Neck 2011;33(4):535–542
10. Pastore E, Perrone F, Orsenigo M, et al. Polymorphisms of metabolizing enzymes and susceptibility to ethmoid intestinal-type adenocarcinoma in professionally exposed patients. Transl Oncol 2009;2(2):84–88
11. Robin PE, Powell DJ, Stansbie JM. Carcinoma of the nasal cavity and paranasal sinuses: incidence and presentation of different histological types. Clin Otolaryngol Allied Sci 1979;4(6):431–456
12. Cantù G, Solero CL, Mariani L, et al. Anterior craniofacial resection for malignant ethmoid tumors—a series of 91 patients. Head Neck 1999;21(3):185–191
13. Dulguerov P, Jacobsen MS, Allal AS, Lehmann W, Calcaterra T. Nasal and paranasal sinus carcinoma: are we making progress? A series of 220 patients and a systematic review. Cancer 2001;92(12):3012–3029
14. Ganly I, Patel SG, Singh B, et al. Craniofacial resection for malignant paranasal sinus tumors: Report of an International Collaborative Study. Head Neck 2005;27(7):575–584
15. Howard DJ, Lund VJ, Wei WI. Craniofacial resection for tumors of the nasal cavity and paranasal sinuses: a 25-year experience. Head Neck 2006;28(10):867–873
16. Gatta G, Bimbi G, Ciccolallo L, Zigon G, Cantú G; EUROCARE Working Group. Survival for ethmoid sinus adenocarcinoma in European populations. Acta Oncol 2009;48(7):992–998
17. Roush GC. Epidemiology of cancer of the nose and paranasal sinuses: current concepts. Head Neck Surg 1979;2(1):3–11
18. Leivo I. Update on sinonasal adenocarcinoma: classification and advances in immunophenotype and molecular genetic make-up. Head Neck Pathol 2007;1(1):38–43
19. Jankowski R, Georgel T, Vignaud JM, et al. Endoscopic surgery reveals that woodworkers' adenocarcinomas originate in the olfactory cleft. Rhinology 2007;45(4):308–314
20. Franchi A, Gallo O, Santucci M. Clinical relevance of the histological classification of sinonasal intestinal-type adenocarcinomas. Hum Pathol 1999;30(10):1140–1145
21. Lloyd G, Lund VJ, Howard D, Savy L. Optimum imaging for sinonasal malignancy. J Laryngol Otol 2000; 114(7):557–562
22. Madani G, Beale TJ, Lund VJ. Imaging of sinonasal tumors. Semin Ultrasound CT MR 2009;30(1):25–38
23. Franchi A, Santucci M, Wenig B. Adenocarcinoma. In: Barnes L, Eveson JW, Reichart P, Sidransky D, eds. World Health Organization Classification of Tumours. Pathology and Genetics of Head and Neck Tumours. Lyon: IARC Press; 2005

24. Barnes L. Intestinal-type adenocarcinoma of the nasal cavity and paranasal sinuses. Am J Surg Pathol 1986;10(3):192–202

25. Ariza M, Llorente JL, Alvarez-Marcas C, et al. Comparative genomic hybridization in primary sinonasal adenocarcinomas. Cancer 2004;100(2):335–341

26. Korinth D, Pacyna-Gengelbach M, Deutschmann N, et al. Chromosomal imbalances in wood dust-related adenocarcinomas of the inner nose and their associations with pathological parameters. J Pathol 2005;207(2):207–215

27. Airoldi M, Garzaro M, Valente G, et al. Clinical and biological prognostic factors in 179 cases with sinonasal carcinoma treated in the Italian Piedmont region. Oncology 2009;76(4):262–269

28. Heffner DK, Hyams VJ, Hauck KW, Lingeman C. Low-grade adenocarcinoma of the nasal cavity and paranasal sinuses. Cancer 1982;50(2):312–322

29. Kraus DH, Sterman BM, Levine HL, Wood BG, Tucker HM, Lavertu P. Factors influencing survival in ethmoid sinus cancer. Arch Otolaryngol Head Neck Surg 1992;118(4):367–372

30. Rosen A, Vokes EE, Scher N, Haraf D, Weichselbaum RR, Panje WR. Locoregionally advanced paranasal sinus carcinoma. Favorable survival with multimodality therapy. Arch Otolaryngol Head Neck Surg 1993;119(7):743–746

31. Lund VJ, Stammberger H, Nicolai P, et al; European Rhinologic Society Advisory Board on Endoscopic Techniques in the Management of Nose, Paranasal Sinus and Skull Base Tumours. European position paper on endoscopic management of tumours of the nose, paranasal sinuses and skull base. Rhinol Suppl 2010; (22):1–143

32. Almeyda R, Capper J. Is surgical debridement and topical 5 fluorouracil the optimum treatment for woodworkers' adenocarcinoma of the ethmoid sinuses? A case-controlled study of a 20-year experience. Clin Otolaryngol 2008;33(5):435–441

33. Allen MW, Schwartz DL, Rana V, et al. Long-term radiotherapy outcomes for nasal cavity and septal cancers. Int J Radiat Oncol Biol Phys 2008;71(2):401–406

34. Nicolai P, Castelnuovo P, Lombardi D, et al. Role of endoscopic surgery in the management of selected malignant epithelial neoplasms of the naso-ethmoidal complex. Head Neck 2007;29(12):1075–1082

35. Lund VJ, Chisholm E, Takes R, et al. Evidence for treatment strategies in sinonasal adenocarcinoma. Head Neck 2012;34:1168–1178

36. Lund VJ, Howard DJ, Wei WI, Cheesman AD. Craniofacial resection for tumors of the nasal cavity and paranasal sinuses—a 17-year experience. Head Neck 1998;20(2):97–105

37. Goffart Y, Jorissen M, Daele J, et al. Minimally invasive endoscopic management of malignant sinonasal tumours. Acta Otorhinolaryngol Belg 2000;54(2):221–232

38. Castelnuovo P, Battaglia P, Locatelli D, Delu G, Sberze F, Bignami M. Endonasal micro-endoscopic treatment of malignant tumors of the paranasal sinuses and anterior skull base. Oper Tech Otolaryngol Head Neck Surg 2006;17:152–167

39. Dave SP, Bared A, Casiano RR. Surgical outcomes and safety of transnasal endoscopic resection for anterior skull tumors. Otolaryngol Head Neck Surg 2007;136(6):920–927

40. Lund V, Howard DJ, Wei WI. Endoscopic resection of malignant tumors of the nose and sinuses. Am J Rhinol 2007;21(1):89–94

41. Bogaerts S, Vander Poorten V, Nuyts S, Van den Bogaert W, Jorissen M. Results of endoscopic resection followed by radiotherapy for primarily diagnosed adenocarcinomas of the paranasal sinuses. Head Neck 2008;30(6):728–736

42. Nicolai P, Battaglia P, Bignami M, et al. Endoscopic surgery for malignant tumors of the sinonasal tract and adjacent skull base: a 10-year experience. Am J Rhinol 2008;22(3):308–316

43. Hanna E, DeMonte F, Ibrahim S, Roberts D, Levine N, Kupferman M. Endoscopic resection of sinonasal cancers with and without craniotomy: oncologic results. Arch Otolaryngol Head Neck Surg 2009;135(12):1219–1224

44. Jardeleza C, Seiberling K, Floreani S, Wormald PJ. Surgical outcomes of endoscopic management of adenocarcinoma of the sinonasal cavity. Rhinology 2009;47(4):354–361

45. Villaret AB, Yakirevitch A, Bizzoni A, et al. Endoscopic transnasal craniectomy in the management of selected sinonasal malignancies. Am J Rhinol Allergy 2010;24(1):60–65

46. Rice DH. Benign and malignant tumors of the ethmoid sinus. Otolaryngol Clin North Am 1985;18(1):113–124

47. de Gabory L, Maunoury A, Maurice-Tison S, et al. Long-term single-center results of management of ethmoid adenocarcinoma: 95 patients over 28 years. Ann Surg Oncol 2010;17(4):1127–1134

48. Sato Y, Morita M, Takahashi HO, Watanabe N, Kirikae I. Combined surgery, radiotherapy, and regional chemotherapy in carcinoma of the paranasal sinuses. Cancer 1970;25(3):571–579

49. Knegt PP, Ah-See KW, vd Velden LA, Kerrebijn J. Adenocarcinoma of the ethmoidal sinus complex: surgical debulking and topical fluorouracil may be the optimal treatment. Arch Otolaryngol Head Neck Surg 2001;127(2):141–146

50. Nagano H, Yoshifuku K, Deguchi K, Kurono Y. Adenocarcinoma of the paranasal sinuses and nasal cavity with lung metastasis showing complete response to combination chemotherapy with docetaxel, cisplatin and 5-fluorouracil (TPF): a case report. Auris Nasus Larynx 2010;37(2):238–243

51. Lee YY, Dimery IW, Van Tassel P, De Pena C, Blacklock JB, Goepfert H. Superselective intra-arterial chemotherapy of advanced paranasal sinus tumors. Arch Otolaryngol Head Neck Surg 1989;115(4):503–511

52. Klintenberg C, Olofsson J, Hellquist H, Sökjer H. Adenocarcinoma of the ethmoid sinuses. A review of 28 cases with special reference to wood dust exposure. Cancer 1984;54(3):482–488

53. Tran L, Sidrys J, Horton D, Sadeghi A, Parker RG. Malignant salivary gland tumors of the paranasal sinuses and nasal cavity. The UCLA experience. Am J Clin Oncol 1989;12(5):387–392

54. Roux FX, Brasnu D, Devaux B, et al. Ethmoid sinus carcinomas: results and prognosis after neoadjuvant chemotherapy and combined surgery—a 10-year experience. Surg Neurol 1994;42(2):98–104

55. Brasnu D, Laccourreye O, Bassot V, Laccourreye L, Naudo P, Roux FX. Cisplatin-based neoadjuvant chemotherapy and combined resection for ethmoid sinus adenocarcinoma reaching and/or invading the skull base. Arch Otolaryngol Head Neck Surg 1996;122(7):765–768

56. Harbo G, Grau C, Bundgaard T, et al. Cancer of the nasal cavity and paranasal sinuses. A clinico-pathological study of 277 patients. Acta Oncol 1997;36(1):45–50

57. Moreau JJ, Bessede JP, Heurtebise F, et al. Adenocarcinoma of the ethmoid sinus in woodworkers. Retrospective study of 25 cases. [Article in French] Neurochirurgie 1997;43(2):111–117

58. Shah JP, Kraus DH, Bilsky MH, Gutin PH, Harrison LH, Strong EW. Craniofacial resection for malignant tumors involving the anterior skull base. Arch Otolaryngol Head Neck Surg 1997;123(12):1312–1317

59. Salvan D, Julieron M, Marandas P, et al. Combined transfacial and neurosurgical approach to malignant tumours of the ethmoid sinus. J Laryngol Otol 1998;112(5):446–450

60. Tiwari R, Hardillo JA, Tobi H, Mehta D, Karim AB, Snow G. Carcinoma of the ethmoid: results of treatment with

conventional surgery and post-operative radiotherapy. Eur J Surg Oncol 1999;25(4):401–405

61. Claus F, Boterberg T, Ost P, et al. Postoperative radiotherapy for adenocarcinoma of the ethmoid sinuses: treatment results for 47 patients. Int J Radiat Oncol Biol Phys 2002;54(4):1089–1094

62. Orvidas LJ, Lewis JE, Weaver AL, Bagniewski SM, Olsen KD. Adenocarcinoma of the nose and paranasal sinuses: a retrospective study of diagnosis, histologic characteristics, and outcomes in 24 patients. Head Neck 2005;27(5):370–375

63. Ganly I, Patel SG, Singh B, et al. Complications of craniofacial resection for malignant tumors of the skull base: report of an International Collaborative Study. Head Neck 2005;27(6):445–451

64. Stammberger H, Anderhuber W, Walch C, Papaefthymiou G. Possibilities and limitations of endoscopic management of nasal and paranasal sinus malignancies. Acta Otorhinolaryngol Belg 1999;53(3):199–205

65. Buchmann L, Larsen C, Pollack A, Tawfik O, Sykes K, Hoover LA. Endoscopic techniques in resection of anterior skull base/paranasal sinus malignancies. Laryngoscope 2006;116(10):1749–1754

66. Ellingwood KE, Million RR. Cancer of the nasal cavity and ethmoid/sphenoid sinuses. Cancer 1979;43(4):1517–1526

67. Bush SE, Bagshaw MA. Carcinoma of the paranasal sinuses. Cancer 1982;50(1):154–158

68. Parsons JT, Mendenhall WM, Mancuso AA, Cassisi NJ, Million RR. Malignant tumors of the nasal cavity and ethmoid and sphenoid sinuses. Int J Radiat Oncol Biol Phys 1988;14(1):11–22

69. Logue JP, Slevin NJ. Carcinoma of the nasal cavity and paranasal sinuses: an analysis of radical radiotherapy. Clin Oncol (R Coll Radiol) 1991;3(2):84–89

70. Roa WH, Hazuka MB, Sandler HM, et al. Results of primary and adjuvant CT-based 3-dimensional radiotherapy for malignant tumors of the paranasal sinuses. Int J Radiat Oncol Biol Phys 1994;28(4):857–865

71. Curran AJ, Gullane PJ, Waldron J, et al. Surgical salvage after failed radiation for paranasal sinus malignancy. Laryngoscope 1998;108(11 Pt 1):1618–1622

72. Waldron JN, O'Sullivan B, Warde P, et al. Ethmoid sinus cancer: twenty-nine cases managed with primary radiation therapy. Int J Radiat Oncol Biol Phys 1998;41(2):361–369

73. Claus F, Mijnheer B, Rasch C, et al. Report of a study on IMRT planning strategies for ethmoid sinus cancer. Strahlenther Onkol 2002;178(10):572–576

74. Duthoy W, Boterberg T, Claus F, et al. Postoperative intensity-modulated radiotherapy in sinonasal carcinoma: clinical results in 39 patients. Cancer 2005;104(1):71–82

75. Combs SE, Konkel S, Schulz-Ertner D, et al. Intensity modulated radiotherapy (IMRT) in patients with carcinomas of the paranasal sinuses: clinical benefit for complex shaped target volumes. Radiat Oncol 2006;1:23

76. Chen AM, Daly ME, Bucci MK, et al. Carcinomas of the paranasal sinuses and nasal cavity treated with radiotherapy at a single institution over five decades: are we making improvement? Int J Radiat Oncol Biol Phys 2007;69(1):141–147

77. Daly ME, Chen AM, Bucci MK, et al. Intensity-modulated radiation therapy for malignancies of the nasal cavity and paranasal sinuses. Int J Radiat Oncol Biol Phys 2007;67(1):151–157

78. Madani I, Bonte K, Vakaet L, Boterberg T, De Neve W. Intensity-modulated radiotherapy for sinonasal tumors: Ghent University Hospital update. Int J Radiat Oncol Biol Phys 2009;73(2):424–432

79. Douglas JG, Goodkin R, Laramore GE. Gamma knife stereotactic radiosurgery for salivary gland neoplasms with base of skull invasion following neutron radiotherapy. Head Neck 2008;30(4):492–496

80. Jansen EP, Keus RB, Hilgers FJ, Haas RL, Tan IB, Bartelink H. Does the combination of radiotherapy and debulking surgery favor survival in paranasal sinus carcinoma? Int J Radiat Oncol Biol Phys 2000;48(1):27–35

Adenoid Cystic Carcinoma

Definition

(ICD-O code 8200/3)

Adenoid cystic carcinoma is an infiltrating malignant tumor, often with a characteristic cribriform appearance, derived from minor seromucinous salivary glands that can be found throughout the mucosa of the nose and paranasal sinuses.

Etiology

Since it was first described by Billroth in 1856, no obvious causative factors have been found.[1]

Synonyms

Synonyms have been numerous and include cylindroma, adenocystic carcinoma, cribriform adenocarcinoma.

Incidence

A common aphorism is that 70% of minor salivary glands tumors are malignant, although the figures vary from 65 to 88% depending on the series as none are especially numerous.[2–5] Nonetheless, adenoid cystic carcinoma (ACC) is rare, constituting <2% of all tumors of the nose and sinuses.[6] In a study of 242 malignant tumors in the nose and sinuses in Denmark between 1995 and 2004, 5% were adenoid cystic carcinoma.[7]

Site

As a consequence of the origin from minor salivary glands, the majority occur in the oral cavity, especially on the palate (~25%) from whence they may involve the nasal cavity and maxillary sinus.[6,8] After the palate, the majority affect the maxillary sinus (57%)[9] and nasal cavity (14–32%).[10–12] From there the tumor invades the skull base and the pterygopalatine and infratemporal fossae. ACC has also been described extending from the sphenoid or nasopharynx into the clivus.[13] Very rarely they may be metastases from elsewhere such as the trachea.[14] For our own series, the distribution is shown in **Table 7.6**.

Diagnostic Features

Clinical Features

In our personal series of 54 patients, their ages range from 34 to 89 years (mean 52.6 years), with a male-to-female ratio of 1.7:1. This is in keeping with other published series[12,15] and no specific ethnic variation has been observed.

Presenting symptoms include the usual unilateral nasal obstruction and serosanguinous discharge, but more specifically patients may have neurological symptoms of facial pain and paresthesia in the terminal branches of the trigeminal nerve due to perineural infiltration.[3,16] Similarly, ACC may present with a cavernous sinus syndrome.[17] Spread to the orbit can produce proptosis, diplopia, and epiphora, or a mass may be found in the adjacent facial tissue such as the medial canthus. A firm or ulcerating mass that displaces a denture may be found on the palate. Unlike torus palatinus, adenoid cystic tumors rarely start in the midline and usually occur posterior to a line drawn between the first molars.

Although a significant number develop systemic disease in the lungs, most are asymptomatic until late in the course of their disease. At least eight of our patients developed pulmonary metastases, the latest being 18 years after her original craniofacial resection.

Imaging

The specific diagnosis of adenoid cystic carcinoma cannot be made on imaging alone other than to say that the features of a locally aggressive infiltrative malignant tumor are seen producing a soft tissue mass and bone erosion on CT and MRI. There may be evidence of submucosal spread and subperiosteal bone invasion resulting in a combination of bone erosion and sclerosis in some cases.[18,19] On MRI an intermediate T2W signal intensity can be seen with high-grade tumors whereas low-grade tumors may show high signal intensity that may be mistaken for inflammatory disease (**Figs. 7.6 and 7.7**).

MRI with contrast may also reveal perineural infiltration which can be contiguous or embolic, resulting in enlargement of the foramen rotundum or ovale when the trigeminal branches are involved.[18,19] Thus middle cranial fossa involvement can result by this route or via the orbital nerve and cavernous sinus.[20]

Although cervical metastases are uncommon at presentation, ACC frequently spreads to the lungs, so regular imaging of the chest should be undertaken (**Fig. 7.8**).

The role of PET/CT remains to be determined.

Histological Features and Differential Diagnosis

Adenoid cystic carcinoma is notorious for its low-key presentation. Macroscopically normal mucosa may yield positive biopsies even in the absence of an obvious mass. Histopathologists have classified the tumor into tubular, cribriform ("Swiss cheese"), and solid in order of increasing aggressiveness, although this has not always been supported and mixed forms frequently occur. The appearance is often rather characteristic, but it must be distinguished from other salivary gland tumors, ameloblastoma, and even basal cell or basaloid squamous cell carcinoma. Immunohistochemistry may be helpful showing myoepithelial and epithelial differentiation with reactions to p63, S100, SMA, and pancytokeratin.[21-23] The cells are sometimes strongly immunoreactive to c-Kit (CD117) which may help distinguish it from other salivary gland tumors[24] and could have therapeutic implications (see later).

Estrogen receptor α was found in 75% of adenoid cystic tumors, while only 17% were positive for estrogen receptor β, the clinical relevance is unknown.[25]

Perineural spread has been attributed to perineural lymphatic infiltration and occurs in many patients.[26,27]

Table 7.6 Adenoid cystic carcinoma: personal series 1976–2010

	n	Age		M:F	CFR	Maxill	LR	MFD	ESS	Other
		Range (y)	Mean (y)							
	54	31–89	52.6	1.7:1	19	11 (2 bilateral)	9	4	2	9
Orbital clearance	19				11	5	3			
DXT	24				10	5	1	2	1	5
Overall actuarial survival										
5 y					61%					
10 y					31%					
15 y					31%					

Abbreviations: CFR, craniofacial resection; Chemo, chemotherapy; DXT, radiotherapy; ESS, endoscopic sinus surgery; F, female; LR, lateral rhinotomy; M, male; Maxill, maxillectomy; MFD, midfacial degloving; y, year(s).

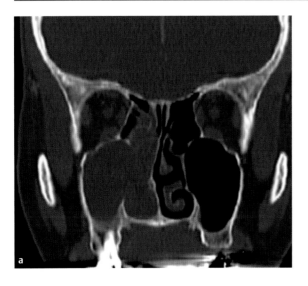

Fig. 7.6a, b

a Adenoid cystic carcinoma. Coronal CT scan showing a mass filling the nasal cavity, maxillary sinus, and adjacent ethmoid.

b Axial CT scan in the same patient showing the mass partially filling the maxillary sinus with extension into the postnasal space.

Furthermore, embolization along nerves has been observed.[20] This propensity compromises complete surgical extirpation.

Natural History

Adenoid cystic carcinoma has a unique natural history that almost invariably results in the demise of the patient unless some other fatal event intervenes. However, this can extend over several decades. Indeed, it is an enormous disappointment for both patient and clinician to find true recurrence occurring 20 years after an ostensible cure. The majority of patients present with advanced disease (77%) though few have lymphatic or metastatic disease (2 to 3%).[12] However, the disease is characterized by frequent local recurrence and early perineural and hematogenous spread (38%). It has one of the highest rates of local recurrence of all sinonasal malignancy (75 to 90% and possibly 100% with long enough follow-up) (**Table 7.7**), but it should be noted that not all patients experience an indolent course. It is unknown why this occurs rather than conventional lymphatic spread, although the latter has been reported in 9 to 16% in some series.[3,27,34,35] Systemic disease may affect 50% or more, including the lungs, brain, bone, liver and even skin, rarely occurring at presentation, sometimes taking decades to appear. Notwithstanding this, patients may survive for significant periods with systemic disease which produce little clinical symptoms, particularly in the lung.[32] This has led to more aggressive management of this problem.[36] In ACC the time to metastasis can range from 13 to 77 months[37] and the disease-free interval can range from 1 month to 19 years.[20,33] Given the often significant time interval, fine needle aspiration of the lung lesion should be undertaken to confirm that it relates to the original ACC.[38]

Treatment

Given the natural history, any treatment aims to prolong the interval to local recurrence balanced against the morbidity of the treatment. Radical surgery has usually been undertaken in the form of craniofacial resection and/or maxillectomy together with orbital clearance. Even bilateral maxillectomies have been undertaken in some cases using a midfacial degloving approach,[39] but there has been an increasing reticence to radically extirpate all cranial nerves in the vicinity to the skull base and beyond as no survival advantage can be shown to justify the resulting complications. Resection of the cavernous sinus contents and internal carotid artery is associated with high morbidity and mortality as might be expected.[40]

Most recently endoscopic techniques have been tentatively undertaken,[41–48] although surgeons should be familiar with the unusual behavior of this tumor and the difficulties in determining extent. There are only a few anecdotal cases in the literature thus far with limited follow-up. Endoscopic techniques may be combined with external approaches in selected cases.

Neck dissection is rarely required and certainly has no prophylactic role. However, resection of pulmonary metastases is increasingly being undertaken either by wedge resection or lobectomy as this may "buy" a reasonable period of survival.[36] Patient selection will be determined by local control and whether there is any other

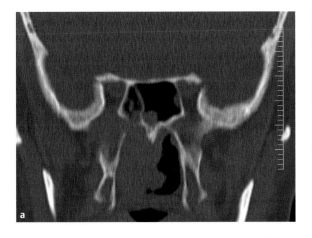
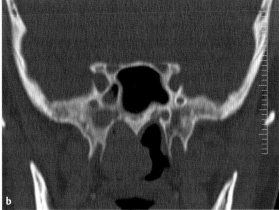
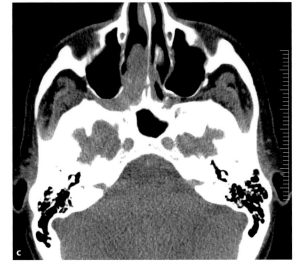
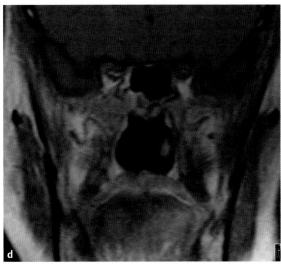

Fig. 7.7a–d

a Adenoid cystic carcinoma. Coronal CT scan showing a mass in the right posterior choana with expansion and erosion of the root of the pterygoid plates, and infiltration of the basisphenoid and orbital apex.

b Coronal CT scan in the same patient showing enlargement of the pterygoid canal due to tumor infiltration.

c Axial CT scan in the same patient showing the mass in the posterior nasal cavity extending laterally with expansion of the pterygomaxillary fissure.

d Coronal MRI (T1W post gadolinium enhancement) in the same patient defining tumor infiltration in the root of the pterygoid plates.

Fig. 7.8 Chest CT showing widespread metastases to the lungs from adenoid cystic carcinoma of the maxilla.

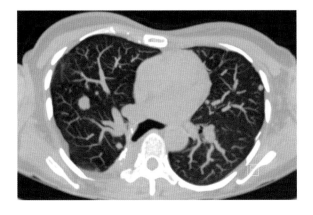

Table 7.7 Percentage incidence of local recurrence and metastatic disease in adenoid cystic carcinoma of the upper jaw in major published series

Author	No.	Local recurrence (%)	Metastatic disease (%)
Moran et al 1961[28]	10	70	41
Tauxe et al 1962[29]	27	92	22
Conley and Dingman 1974[3]	78	42	41
Spiro et al 1974[4]	43	67	42
Osborn 1977[5]	23	50	–
Marsh and Allen 1979[30]	7	71	57
Chilla et al 1980[6]	11	90	18
Matsuba et al 1984[31]	28	N/A	58 (paranasal sinuses) 22 (palate)
Spiro et al 1997[32]	37	N/A	35
Wiseman et al 2002[33]	35	54	31
Rhee et al 2006[11]	35	30 (5 y) 57 (10 y)	25 (5 y) 43 (10 y)
Lupinetti et al[12]	105	31	38
Howard and Lund (unpublished)	54	77	40
Abbreviations: N/A, not available; y, year.			

disseminated disease as well as the individual's cardiopulmonary reserve.

Although radiotherapy is often given, its role is not well determined. It is rarely used as a single primary modality as the tumor is not classically radiosensitive. Combined with surgery it may delay recurrence but cannot be shown to significantly improve "cure." Although there have been recent reports of the use of IMRT,[49,50] determining the field might be problematic and long-term follow-up in reasonable numbers of patients is lacking. In a study by Coombs et al advocating IMRT in 46 patients with sinonasal malignancy, 20 of whom had adenoid cystic carcinoma, median follow-up was only 16 months (range 3–40 months).[49] Even with this short follow-up, local control dropped from 85% at 1 year to 49% at 3 years using this as the primary modality, and distant control was 83% at 1 year and 0% at 2 years in the group as a whole.

Proton beam therapy is also being used in a few centers, but again numbers and follow-up preclude any conclusions.[51,52] Disease-free survival was 56% at 5 years in a series of 23 patients with ACC in the skull base. Stereotactic radiosurgery with the gamma knife has also been reported[53] in 29 of 34 patients with salivary gland malignancy involving the skull base after failed neutron beam therapy.

Chemotherapy has been used for some years to treat both systemic and advanced local disease.[54–57] Regimes generally used cisplatin and/or doxorubicin, 5-FU, mito-

mycin-C, or cyclophosphamide. More recently epirubicin, mitoxantrone, and gemcitabine have been used in Phase II trials[58–60] and there has also been interest in docetaxel–cisplatin and paclitaxel–carboplatin in advanced disease.[61,62] C-Kit expression has led to trials of oral imatinib which has a synergistic interaction with cisplatin[63] but without encouraging results in vivo.[64,65]

The neuropathic pain experienced by patients may be helped by drugs such as carbamazepine and gabapentin.

Outcome

As already stated, this disease can recur throughout a lifetime so 5-year survival figures are particularly deceptive and some patients may surprisingly survive for several years with secondary disease (**Table 7.8**). Spiro et al found a 10-year survival of 7% in their early series of 242 cases[4] but this improved in a later series (1960–1986)[32] with reduction in both treatment failure and local recurrence, which they attributed to the regular addition of postoperative radiotherapy in more recent cases. However, there was no significant improvement in the frequency of distant metastases with or without radiotherapy. Lupinetti et al[11] also showed that surgery with postoperative radiotherapy provided the best overall and disease-specific survival compared with other treatment modalities (p = 0.018 and p = 0.05, respectively), while surgery alone significantly improved survival (p < 0.001) as compared with radiotherapy or chemotherapy, although this may also reflect patient selection.

Table 7.8 Overall survival in adenoid cystic carcinoma of the upper jaw in major published series

Author	No.	Survival (%) after			
		5 y	10 y	15 y	20 y
Tauxe et al 1962[29]	27	73	41	7	0
Conley and Dingman 1974[3]	78	64	34	23	8
Spiro et al 1974[4]	43				
	Nose	–	7	–	–
	Palate	–	16	–	–
Spiro et al 1997[32]	196 (all sites) 37 (sinus)	–	46	34	25
Wiseman et al 2002[33]	35	65	55	28	
Rhee et al 2006[11]	35	86	53		
Lupinetti et al 2007[12]	105	63	28		
Howard and Lund (unpublished)	19	61	31	31	??
Abbreviation: y, year(s).					

In our craniofacial series the patients fared somewhat better, with a 5-year survival that dropped from 61% to 31% at 15 years.[66] As might be expected, skull base invasion is a significant factor in survival in this and other series.[12] In a series of 59 patients of which 13 (22%) were sinonasal, the overall survival rates were 76% and 40%, and 87% and 65% for disease-free survival at respectively 5 and 10 years after combined surgery and radiotherapy, but figures for the sinonasal lesions alone were not given. However, the authors confirmed that clinical nerve involvement was an important prognostic factor.[67] As previously noted, adjunctive radiotherapy may delay recurrence but cannot be shown to improve cure.[11,12,32,33]

Overall, major salivary gland adenoid cystic carcinomas do better than minor salivary gland lesions, and palatal lesions do better than those closer to the skull base.[32] In a large European study of 2,611 cases of adenoid cystic carcinoma at all sites, nasal cavity lesions did worse than oral cavity lesions.[68] The large MD Anderson study[12] showed that cribriform lesions did best and solid forms worst of the histological types.

The numbers treated endoscopically are too few and with too short a follow-up from which to draw any conclusions, usually in single numbers in otherwise small series of mixed malignant tumors.[41–48] However, one could argue that in a disease with a generally poor outcome, wide-field endoscopic resection with its associated low morbidity might offer advantages in a carefully selected group of patients.

Patients may die from local disease, often without secondaries,[33] although they can succumb to metastatic disease alone. Continued treatment of local recurrence can therefore be worthwhile, even in the presence of distant disease. Similarly, the resection of pulmonary metastases is increasingly undertaken. In the short term, pulmonary resection may be helpful. Liu reported 84% 5-year survival in a small group of patients with ACC in the head and neck, too short a follow-up to be meaningful, and all were dead at 14 years.[69] Interestingly, no difference was shown between patients with a single nodule and those with multiple lesions. A more compelling study by Bobbio et al[70] considered 9 patients with pulmonary metastases from ACC without locoregional disease who underwent metastasectomy who had a mean survival of 72 months compared with a mean survival of 62 months in 11 patients with lung secondaries who did not undergo surgery. Unfortunately, the second group may have had more extensive lung involvement, so conclusions are difficult to draw. Overall, distant metastases remain one of the most important factors in determining survival.[11,32,68]

Key Points

- Adenoid cystic carcinoma is a rare malignant tumor of salivary origin.
- The tumor spreads along perineural lymphatics directly and embolically, making complete resection very difficult.
- The tumor recurs locally and can do so throughout the life of the patient, so follow-up is for life and patients die of the tumor unless something else intervenes.
- The tumor rarely spreads to the cervical lymph nodes but often produces pulmonary metastases.
- Pulmonary metastases are not necessarily associated with the rapid demise of the patient, so pulmonary resection is sometimes undertaken.

References

1. Billroth T. Die Cylindergeschwulst (Cylindroma). In: Untersuchungen uber die Entwicklung der Blutgefasse, nebst Beobachtungen aus der Koniglichen Chirurgischen. Reimer, Berlin: Universtas-Klinik zu Berlin; 1856: 55–69
2. Leafstedt SW, Gaeta JF, Sako K, Marchetta FC, Shedd DP. Adenoid cystic carcinoma of major and minor salivary glands. Am J Surg 1971;122(6):756–762
3. Conley J, Dingman DL. Adenoid cystic carcinoma in the head and neck (cylindroma). Arch Otolaryngol 1974;100(2):81–90
4. Spiro RH, Huvos AG, Strong EW. Adenoid cystic carcinoma of salivary origin. A clinicopathologic study of 242 cases. Am J Surg 1974;128(4):512–520
5. Osborn DA. Morphology and the natural history of cribriform adenocarcinoma (adenoid cystic carcinoma). J Clin Pathol 1977;30(3):195–205
6. Chilla R, Schroth R, Eysholdt U, Droese M. Adenoid cystic carcinoma of the head and neck. Controllable and uncontrollable factors in treatment and prognosis. ORL J Otorhinolaryngol Relat Spec 1980;42(6):346–367
7. Thorup C, Sebbesen L, Danø H, et al. Carcinoma of the nasal cavity and paranasal sinuses in Denmark 1995–2004. Acta Oncol 2010;49(3):389–394
8. Eneroth CM. Salivary gland tumors in the parotid gland, submandibular gland, and the palate region. Cancer 1971;27(6):1415–1418
9. Horrée WA. Adenoid cystic carcinoma of the maxilla. Arch Otolaryngol 1974;100(6):469–472
10. Barnes L, Brandwein M, Som PM. Diseases of the nose, paranasal sinuses and nasopharynx. In: Barnes L, ed. Surgical Pathology of the Head and Neck. 2nd ed. New York: Marcel Decker; 2001:439–555
11. Rhee CS, Won TB, Lee CH, et al. Adenoid cystic carcinoma of the sinonasal tract: treatment results. Laryngoscope 2006;116(6):982–986
12. Lupinetti AD, Roberts DB, Williams MD, et al. Sinonasal adenoid cystic carcinoma: the M. D. Anderson Cancer Center experience. Cancer 2007;110(12):2726–2731
13. Solares CA, Fakhri S, Batra PS, Lee J, Lanza DC. Transnasal endoscopic resection of lesions of the clivus: a preliminary report. Laryngoscope 2005;115(11):1917–1922
14. Khorsandi AS, Silberzweig JE, Wenig BM, Urken ML, Holliday RA. Adenoid cystic carcinoma of the trachea metastatic to the nasal cavity: a case report. Ear Nose Throat J 2009;88(12):E9–E11
15. Issing PR, Hemmanouil I, Stöver T, et al. Adenoid cystic carcinoma of the skull base. Skull Base Surg 1999; 9(4):271–275
16. Eby LS, Johnson DS, Baker HW. Adenoid cystic carcinoma of the head and neck. Cancer 1972;29(5):1160–1168
17. Dumitrascu OM, Costa RMS, Kirsch C, Arnold AC, Gordon LK. Cavernous sinus syndrome resulting from contiguous spread of adenoid cystic carcinoma: a systematic analysis of reported cases. Neuro-Ophthalmol 2009;33:300–307
18. Maroldi R, Ravanelli M, Borghesi A, Farina D. Paranasal sinus imaging. Eur J Radiol 2008;66(3):372–386
19. Madani G, Beale TJ, Lund VJ. Imaging of sinonasal tumors. Semin Ultrasound CT MR 2009;30(1):25–38
20. Howard DJ, Lund VJ. Reflections on the management of adenoid cystic carcinoma of the nasal cavity and paranasal sinuses. Otolaryngol Head Neck Surg 1985;93(3):338–341
21. Azumi N, Battifora H. The cellular composition of adenoid cystic carcinoma. An immunohistochemical study. Cancer 1987;60(7):1589–1598
22. Prasad AR, Savera AT, Gown AM, Zarbo RJ. The myoepithelial immunophenotype in 135 benign and malignant salivary gland tumors other than pleomorphic adenoma. Arch Pathol Lab Med 1999;123(9):801–806
23. Edwards PC, Bhuiya T, Kelsch RD. Assessment of p63 expression in the salivary gland neoplasms adenoid cystic carcinoma, polymorphous low-grade adenocarcinoma, and basal cell and canalicular adenomas. Oral Surg Oral Med Oral Pathol Oral Radiol Endod 2004;97(5):613–619
24. Holst VA, Marshall CE, Moskaluk CA, Frierson HF Jr. KIT protein expression and analysis of c-kit gene mutation in adenoid cystic carcinoma. Mod Pathol 1999;12(10):956–960
25. Luo SD, Su CY, Chuang HC, Huang CC, Chen CM, Chien CY. Estrogen receptor overexpression in malignant minor salivary gland tumors of the sinonasal tract. Otolaryngol Head Neck Surg 2009;141(1):108–113
26. Leroux R, Leroux-Robert J. Essai de classification architecturale des tumeurs des glands salivaires. Bull Assoc Fr Etud Cancer 1934;23:304–340
27. Gil Z, Carlson DL, Gupta A, et al. Patterns and incidence of neural invasion in patients with cancers of the paranasal sinuses. Arch Otolaryngol Head Neck Surg 2009;135(2):173–179
28. Moran JJ, Becker SM, Brady LW, Rambo VB. Adenoid cystic carcinoma. A clinicopathological study. Cancer 1961;14:1235–1250
29. Tauxe WN, McDonald JR, Devine KD. A century of cylindromas. Short review and report of 27 adenoid cystic carcinomas arising in the upper respiratory passages. Arch Otolaryngol 1962;75:364–376
30. Marsh WL Jr, Allen MS Jr. Adenoid cystic carcinoma: biologic behavior in 38 patients. Cancer 1979;43(4):1463–1473
31. Matsuba HM, Thawley SE, Simpson JR, Levine LA, Mauney M. Adenoid cystic carcinoma of major and minor salivary gland origin. Laryngoscope 1984;94(10):1316–1318
32. Spiro RH. Distant metastasis in adenoid cystic carcinoma of salivary origin. Am J Surg 1997;174(5):495–498
33. Wiseman SM, Popat SR, Rigual NR, et al. Adenoid cystic carcinoma of the paranasal sinuses or nasal cavity: a 40-year review of 35 cases. Ear Nose Throat J 2002;81(8):510–514, 516–517
34. Allen MS Jr, Marsh WL Jr. Lymph node involvement by direct extension in adenoid cystic carcinoma. Absence of classic embolic lymph node metastasis. Cancer 1976; 38(5):2017–2021
35. Stell PM, Cruickshank AH, Stoney PJ, McCormick MS. Lymph node metastases in adenoid cystic carcinoma. Am J Otolaryngol 1985;6(6):433–436
36. Syed IM, Howard DJ. Should we treat lung metastases from adenoid cystic carcinoma of the head and neck in asymptomatic patients? Ear Nose Throat J 2009;88(6):969–973
37. Takagi D, Fukuda S, Furuta Y, et al. Clinical study of adenoid cystic carcinoma of the head and neck. Auris Nasus Larynx 2001;28(Suppl):S99–S102
38. Pitman MB, Sherman ME, Black-Schaffer WS. The use of fine-needle aspiration in the diagnosis of metastatic pulmonary adenoid cystic carcinoma. Otolaryngol Head Neck Surg 1991;104(4):441–447
39. Howard DJ, Lund VJ. The role of midfacial degloving in modern rhinological practice. J Laryngol Otol 1999;113(10):885–887
40. Saito K, Fukuta K, Takahashi M, Tachibana E, Yoshida J. Management of the cavernous sinus in en bloc resections of malignant skull base tumors. Head Neck 1999;21(8):734–742
41. Poetker DM, Toohill RJ, Loehrl TA, Smith TL. Endoscopic management of sinonasal tumors: a preliminary report. Am J Rhinol 2005;19(3):307–315
42. Buchmann L, Larsen C, Pollack A, Tawfik O, Sykes K, Hoover LA. Endoscopic techniques in resection of anterior skull base/paranasal sinus malignancies. Laryngoscope 2006;116(10):1749–1754
43. Castelnuovo P, Battaglia P, Locatelli D, Delu G, Sberze F, Bignami M. Endonasal micro-endoscopic treatment of

malignant tumors of the paranasal sinuses and anterior skull base. Oper Tech Otolaryngol 2006;17:152–167

44. Dave SP, Bared A, Casiano RR. Surgical outcomes and safety of transnasal endoscopic resection for anterior skull tumors. Otolaryngol Head Neck Surg 2007;136(6):920–927

45. Lund V, Howard DJ, Wei WI. Endoscopic resection of malignant tumors of the nose and sinuses. Am J Rhinol 2007;21(1):89–94

46. Nicolai P, Battaglia P, Bignami M, et al. Endoscopic surgery for malignant tumors of the sinonasal tract and adjacent skull base: a 10-year experience. Am J Rhinol 2008;22(3):308–316

47. Hanna E, DeMonte F, Ibrahim S, Roberts D, Levine N, Kupferman M. Endoscopic resection of sinonasal cancers with and without craniotomy: oncologic results. Arch Otolaryngol Head Neck Surg 2009;135(12):1219–1224

48. Villaret AB, Yakirevitch A, Bizzoni A, et al. Endoscopic transnasal craniectomy in the management of selected sinonasal malignancies. Am J Rhinol Allergy 2010;24(1):60–65

49. Combs SE, Konkel S, Schulz-Ertner D, et al. Intensity modulated radiotherapy (IMRT) in patients with carcinomas of the paranasal sinuses: clinical benefit for complex shaped target volumes. Radiat Oncol 2006;1:3

50. Madani I, Bonte K, Vakaet L, Boterberg T, De Neve W. Intensity-modulated radiotherapy for sinonasal tumors: Ghent University Hospital update. Int J Radiat Oncol Biol Phys 2009;73(2):424–432

51. Pommier P, Liebsch NJ, Deschler DG, et al. Proton beam radiation therapy for skull base adenoid cystic carcinoma. Arch Otolaryngol Head Neck Surg 2006;132(11):1242–1249

52. Malyapa R, Mendenhall W, Yeung D, et al. Proton therapy of cancers of the nasal cavity and paranasal sinuses: the UFPTI experience. J Neurol Surg 2012;73:A034 [Congress Abstract]

53. Douglas JG, Goodkin R, Laramore GE. Gamma knife stereotactic radiosurgery for salivary gland neoplasms with base of skull invasion following neutron radiotherapy. Head Neck 2008;30(4):492–496

54. Schramm VL Jr, Srodes C, Myers EN. Cisplatin therapy for adenoid cystic carcinoma. Arch Otolaryngol 1981;107(12):739–741

55. Budd GT, Groppe CW. Adenoid cystic carcinoma of the salivary gland. Sustained complete response to chemotherapy. Cancer 1983;51(4):589–590

56. Dreyfuss AI, Clark JR, Fallon BG, Posner MR, Norris CM Jr, Miller D. Cyclophosphamide, doxorubicin, and cisplatin combination chemotherapy for advanced carcinomas of salivary gland origin. Cancer 1987;60(12):2869–2872

57. de Haan LD, De Mulder PH, Vermorken JB, Schornagel JH, Vermey A, Verweij J. Cisplatin-based chemotherapy in advanced adenoid cystic carcinoma of the head and neck. Head Neck 1992;14(4):273–277

58. Vermorken JB, Verweij J, de Mulder PH, et al. Epirubicin in patients with advanced or recurrent adenoid cystic carcinoma of the head and neck: a phase II study of the EORTC Head and Neck Cancer Cooperative Group. Ann Oncol 1993;4(9):785–788

59. Verweij J, de Mulder PH, de Graeff A, et al; EORTC Head and Neck Cancer Cooperative Group. Phase II study on mitoxantrone in adenoid cystic carcinomas of the head and neck. Ann Oncol 1996;7(8):867–869

60. van Herpen CM, Locati LD, Buter J, et al. Phase II study on gemcitabine in recurrent and/or metastatic adenoid cystic carcinoma of the head and neck (EORTC 24982). Eur J Cancer 2008;44(17):2542–2545

61. Haddad RI, Posner MR, Busse PM, et al. Chemoradiotherapy for adenoid cystic carcinoma: preliminary results of an organ sparing approach. Am J Clin Oncol 2006;29(2):153–157

62. Handra-Luca A, Planchard D, Fouret P. Docetaxel-cisplatin-radiotherapy in adenoid cystic carcinoma with high-grade transformation. Oral Oncol 2009;45(11):e208–e209

63. Bruce IA, Slevin NJ, Homer JJ, McGown AT, Ward TH. Synergistic effects of imatinib (STI 571) in combination with chemotherapeutic drugs in head and neck cancer. Anticancer Drugs 2005;16(7):719–726

64. Hotte SJ, Winquist EW, Lamont E, et al. Imatinib mesylate in patients with adenoid cystic cancers of the salivary glands expressing c-kit: a Princess Margaret Hospital phase II consortium study. J Clin Oncol 2005;23(3):585–590

65. Pfeffer MR, Talmi Y, Catane R, Symon Z, Yosepovitch A, Levitt M. A phase II study of Imatinib for advanced adenoid cystic carcinoma of head and neck salivary glands. Oral Oncol 2007;43(1):33–36

66. Howard DJ, Lund VJ, Wei WI. Craniofacial resection for tumors of the nasal cavity and paranasal sinuses: a 25-year experience. Head Neck 2006;28(10):867–873

67. Gomez DR, Hoppe BS, Wolden SL, et al. Outcomes and prognostic variables in adenoid cystic carcinoma of the head and neck: a recent experience. Int J Radiat Oncol Biol Phys 2008;70(5):1365–1372

68. Ciccolallo L, Licitra L, Cantú G, Gatta G; EUROCARE Working Group. Survival from salivary glands adenoid cystic carcinoma in European populations. Oral Oncol 2009;45(8):669–674

69. Liu D, Labow DM, Dang N, et al. Pulmonary metastasectomy for head and neck cancers. Ann Surg Oncol 1999;6(6):572–578

70. Bobbio A, Copelli C, Ampollini L, et al. Lung metastasis resection of adenoid cystic carcinoma of salivary glands. Eur J Cardiothorac Surg 2008;33(5):790–793

Mucoepidermoid Carcinoma

Definition

(ICD-O code 8430/3)

A tumor of minor salivary gland origin characterized by the presence of epidermoid, mucus-secreting and intermediate cells.

Etiology

The etiology is unknown but a t(11;19) molecular abnormality has been reported.[1]

Synonyms

Previously described as adenosquamous carcinoma[2] or mucoepidermoid tumor, it was first reported in the parotid by Masson and Berger in 1924[3] and in the nose by Stewart et al.[4]

Incidence

Mucoepidermoid carcinoma (MEC) is rare (<1% of all sinonasal tumors) but is the second commonest malignancy of minor salivary glands. Between 1956 and 1993, of 1,923 reported cases of minor salivary gland tumors, 183 occurred in the upper jaw (0.95%).[5]

Site

While this tumor has been reported in the nasal cavity, it is more often seen on the palate, from where it may involve the nose and maxillary and ethmoid sinuses.[6–8] In the reported literature, 56% affected the palate, 17% the maxillary sinus, and 5% the nasal cavity.[5] It has also been reported on the nasal bridge, from where it can involve the orbits.[9]

Diagnostic Features

Clinical Features

MEC can occur at any age between 10 and 80 years, with a mean around 50 years, and it is one of the commoner malignant salivary gland tumors in children. The male-to-female ratio is more or less equal. Clinical presentation is characterized by nasal obstruction and epistaxis, or a painless mass. The palatal lesions can ulcerate and there may be orbital symptoms. A small number have been reported in the nasopharynx.[10]

Imaging

The features are of a nonspecific mass with a variable degree of bone erosion or destruction on CT and MRI. High signal intensity on T2W MRI sequences is usual. It is also worth examining the neck with ultrasound or other imaging.

Histological Features and Differential Diagnosis

The typical association of epidermoid and mucus-secreting cells is not always seen in the nose, which has led to the suggestion that mucoepidermoid carcinoma is a variant of squamous cell carcinoma.

The tumor is categorized histologically into low, intermediate, and high grade and exhibits a range of aggressiveness. Low-grade[1] tumors have more goblet cells and varying degrees of cyst formation; high-grade[3] tumors are predominantly squamous cell and mainly solid.[11] However, Branwein et al[11] in their study of 85 patients with MEC (only one of which affected the nasal cavity) also found that a careful analysis of tumor grading suggested considerable interobserver variation even among experienced head and neck pathologists, as a consequence of which they proposed various modifications to improve reproducibility.

When biopsying a lesion, it is important to take representative tissue or an erroneous diagnosis of adenocarcinoma or squamous cell carcinoma may be made.

Natural History

Although some lesions may appear well-differentiated, all MEC should be regarded as potentially malignant, having the possibility of metastatic spread and frequent recurrence.

Treatment and Outcome

Wide surgical excision is the primary treatment, which may include some form of maxillectomy and reconstruction. Additional radiotherapy has been employed[6,12] although the tumor was not thought to be particularly radiosensitive; there are reports of single-modality radiotherapy producing good local control with follow-up of 2.5 to 21 years.[13] Unfortunately, of the 14 cases of MEC in this study, only 5 occurred in the nose and sinuses, of these only one patient received radiotherapy alone.

There is a wide range of survival, better in the nasal cavity than the maxilla. This can also be related to the histological grade, with metastases associated with high-grade lesions even when survival exceeds 5 years. In an early series of 76 minor salivary gland MECs, the majority affected the palate and 20 occurred in the nose and sinuses.[14] Overall determinate cure rate was 69% at 10 years, ranging from 79–53% depending on the degree of differentiation. However, the literature is lacking series devoted exclusively to MEC in the nose and sinuses, with small numbers at best included in larger cohorts of sinonasal cancer or mixed in with other cases of MEC occurring in the head and neck. In a cohort of 109 previously untreated sinonasal carcinomas, Mendenhall et al included 4 cases of MEC, 2 treated with surgery and radiotherapy and 2 with radiotherapy alone, from which it is difficult to draw conclusions.[15] Triantafillidou et al[8] considered 16 MECs occurring in minor salivary gland tumors of which only one involved the nose and sinuses, having spread from the hard palate. Pires et al[16] included 7 cases affecting the maxilla and 2 the nasal cavity in their series of 173 cases but were not able to make specific comments about outcome other than to say that maxillary tumors were larger than those on the palate.

In general, low-grade tumors have survival rates of between 90 and 100% with surgery alone; higher-grade lesions may require adjuvant treatment as well as surgery. With nodal spread, 10-year survival may drop to ~50% and in our small series, two presented with extensive local disease for which only palliative radiotherapy was given with inevitable consequences (**Table 7.9**).[17–25]

In general in the head and neck, significant independent prognostic factors are age >40 years, fixed tumors, T and N stage, and histological grade.[16] Expression of proliferating cell nuclear antigen and p53 was correlated with a poor prognosis and improved prognosis was correlated with expression of carcinoembryonic antigen ($p = 0.01$) and bcl-2 expression ($p < 0.001$).

References

1. Tonon G, Modi S, Wu L, et al. t(11;19)(q21;p13) translocation in mucoepidermoid carcinoma creates a novel fusion product that disrupts a Notch signaling pathway. Nat Genet 2003;33(2):208–213
2. Gerughty RM, Hennigar GR, Brown FM. Adenosquamous carcinoma of the nasal, oral and laryngeal cavities. A clini-

Table 7.9 Mucoepidermoid carcinoma of nose and sinuses: reports in the literature and personal cases

Author	No.	Treatment			Outcome					
		Surgery	DXT	Surgery + DXT	A&W	AWR	DOD	DICD	Lost	Metastases
Stuteville and Corley 1967[17]	17	13		4	8 (>5 y)		3		6	
Luna et al 1968[18]	9				4 (>5 y)		3	1	1	
Smith et al 1968[19]	6	5		1	3 (1 at 4 y, 1 at 14 y, 1 at 35 y)		3			
Bergman 1969[20]	2			2	2					50
Rafla 1969[21]	2						1		1	
Eneroth 1971[22]	27									18
Frable and Elzay 1970[23]	11	11			7 (3 >5 y)	1		2	1	
Healey et al 1970[24]	10	4		6	2		6 (5/7 maxilla)	2		20 (cervical lymph nodes)
Tran et al 1987[25]	12	10		2		N/A	N/A	N/A	N/A	N/A
Brandwein et al 2001[11]	1 (out of 78)	N/A	N/A	N/A	N/A	N/A	N/A	N/A	N/A	N/A
Pires et al 2004[16]	9 (out of 173)	N/A	N/A	N/A	N/A	N/A	N/A	N/A	N/A	N/A
Mendenhall et al 2009[15]	4		2	2	N/A	N/A	N/A	N/A	N/A	N/A
Harrison and Lund 1993[5]	5	1	2 (palliative)	2	1 (>13 y)		3 (<1 year)		1	

Abbreviations: A&W, alive and well; AWR, alive with recurrence; DICD, dead of intercurrent disease; DOD, dead of disease; DXT, radiotherapy; N/A, not available; y, year(s).

copathologic survey of ten cases. Cancer 1968;22(6):1140–1155

3. Masson P, Berger L. Epitheliomes a double metaplasie de la parotide. Bull Assoc Fr Etud Cancer 1924;13:366–375

4. Stewart FW, Foote FW, Becker WF. Muco-epidermoid tumors of salivary glands. Ann Surg 1945;122(5):820–844

5. Harrison D, Lund V. Tumours of the Upper Jaw. London: Churchill Livingstone; 1993: 121–123

6. Jiang GL, Ang KK, Peters LJ, Wendt CD, Oswald MJ, Goepfert H. Maxillary sinus carcinomas: natural history and results of postoperative radiotherapy. Radiother Oncol 1991;21(3):193–200

7. Kraus DH, Sterman BM, Levine HL, Wood BG, Tucker HM, Lavertu P. Factors influencing survival in ethmoid sinus cancer. Arch Otolaryngol Head Neck Surg 1992;118(4):367–372

8. Triantafillidou K, Dimitrakopoulos J, Iordanidis F, Koufogiannis D. Mucoepidermoid carcinoma of minor salivary

glands: a clinical study of 16 cases and review of the literature. Oral Dis 2006;12(4):364–370

9. Thomas GR, Regalado JJ, McClinton M. A rare case of mucoepidermoid carcinoma of the nasal cavity. Ear Nose Throat J 2002;81(8):519–522

10. Zhang XM, Cao JZ, Luo JW, et al. Nasopharyngeal mucoepidermoid carcinoma: a review of 13 cases. Oral Oncol 2010;46(8):618–621

11. Brandwein MS, Ivanov K, Wallace DI, et al. Mucoepidermoid carcinoma: a clinicopathologic study of 80 patients with special reference to histological grading. Am J Surg Pathol 2001;25(7):835–845

12. Hosokawa Y, Shirato H, Kagei K, et al. Role of radiotherapy for mucoepidermoid carcinoma of salivary gland. Oral Oncol 1999;35(1):105–111

13. Parsons JT, Mendenhall WM, Stringer SP, Cassisi NJ, Million RR. Management of minor salivary gland carcinomas. Int J Radiat Oncol Biol Phys 1996;35(3):443–454

14. Spiro RH, Koss LG, Hajdu SI, Strong EW. Tumors of minor salivary origin. A clinicopathologic study of 492 cases. Cancer 1973;31(1):117–129
15. Mendenhall WM, Amdur RJ, Morris CG, et al. Carcinoma of the nasal cavity and paranasal sinuses. Laryngoscope 2009;119(5):899–906
16. Pires FR, de Almeida OP, de Araújo VC, Kowalski LP. Prognostic factors in head and neck mucoepidermoid carcinoma. Arch Otolaryngol Head Neck Surg 2004;130(2):174–180
17. Stuteville OH, Corley RD. Surgical management of tumors of intraoral minor salivary glands. Report of eighty cases. Cancer 1967;20(10):1578–1586
18. Luna MA, Stimson PG, Bardwil JM. Minor salivary gland tumors of the oral cavity. A review of sixty-eight cases. Oral Surg Oral Med Oral Pathol 1968;25(1):71–86
19. Smith RL, Dahlin DC, Waite DE. Mucoepidermoid carcinomas of the jawbones. J Oral Surg 1968;26(6):387–393
20. Bergman F. Tumors of the minor salivary glands. A report of 46 cases. Cancer 1969;23(3):538–543
21. Rafla S. Mucous gland tumors of paranasal sinuses. Cancer 1969;24(4):683–691
22. Eneroth CM. Salivary gland tumors in the parotid gland, submandibular gland, and the palate region. Cancer 1971;27(6):1415–1418
23. Frable WJ, Elzay RP. Tumors of minor salivary glands. A report of 73 cases. Cancer 1970;25(4):932–941
24. Healey WV, Perzin KH, Smith L. Mucoepidermoid carcinoma of salivary gland origin. Classification, clinical-pathologic correlation, and results of treatment. Cancer 1970;26(2):368–388
25. Tran L, Sadeghi A, Hanson D, Ellerbroek N, Calcaterra TC, Parker RG. Salivary gland tumors of the palate: the UCLA experience. Laryngoscope 1987;97(11):1343–1345

Acinic Cell Carcinoma

Definition

(ICD-O code 8550/3)
    A rare malignant tumor of minor salivary glands.

Etiology

No etiology is known.

Synonyms

Acinous cell carcinoma, acinar cell carcinoma.

Incidence

Its first report in a major salivary gland was in the parotid in 1892[1] where acinic cell carcinoma (ACC) is now recognized to make up 2.5 to 4% of tumors. Thus 75% of ACC occur in the parotid, 20% in intraoral sites, and it occurs very rarely elsewhere in the head and neck. It is exceptionally rare in the nose and sinuses, with only a few case reports in the literature, none being bilateral, which has been observed in the parotid. In a review of 1,353 cases of ACC collected in the National Cancer Database, 9% occurred in minor salivary glands but were sufficiently rare for no site to be defined.[2]

Site

As with many of the other minor salivary gland tumors, acinic cell carcinomas are more often found in the oral cavity (on the palate, buccal mucosa, and lips) than in the nasal cavity, but since 1961 at least 24 cases have been described on the lateral nasal wall, on the inferior or middle turbinate, in superior meatus, on the septum, or in the antroethmoid region (**Table 7.10**).[3–20] One case report describes an ACC lesion in the nasopharynx presenting with a large sphenoidal mucocele.[21]

Diagnostic Features

Clinical Features and Imaging

Epistaxis is a feature of these tumors as well as nasal obstruction due to a polypoid swelling or nodule. Bony destruction is not a feature. They occur over a wide age range (42–76 years, mean 58 years), but present at an earlier age than other salivary gland cancers and more often in women (1:1.6 M:F).

Histological Features and Differential Diagnosis

Batsakis et al[22] reported that ACC arose from progenitor reserve cells of the terminal tubules and intercalated ducts of salivary tissue and graded it from low to high. ACC displays a wide range of histological patterns including solid, cystic, papillary-cystic, and follicular. However, most of the neoplastic cells should show acinic differentiation and be polyhedral with abundant granular basophilic cytoplasm and small hyperchromatic nuclei.[23] It is sometimes referred to as the "blue dot" tumor because of these zymogenlike blue granules. Ducts are largely absent and an intratumoral lymphocytic infiltrate can be present. Focal atypia and dedifferentiation may occur and correlates with an increased risk of recurrence.[24] The granules are PAS-positive and diastase resistant. On immunohistochemistry the acinic cells are positive for cytokeratins[25] and there is no expression of myoepithelial antigens.[26] A small number react with antibodies to amylase.[27]

    ACC is a difficult diagnosis to make, particularly on cytology,[15] and the solid forms must be distinguished from adenocarcinoma NOS.

Natural History

Although there has been some debate as to whether ACC should really be regarded as a malignant tumor, it is certainly capable of local recurrence and occasionally metastasizes, although the precise incidence is difficult to determine due to the very small numbers and short follow-up. With ACC in general the rate of cervical metastases was 9.9% in 1,353 cases collected between 1985 and 1995 and distant spread occurred in 2.1%.[2] Metastatic spread at presentation occurred more often in the

Table 7.10 Acinic cell carcinoma of the nasal cavity: case reports in literature

Author	No.	Sex	Age (y)	Site	Treatment of minor gland	Follow-up
Chaudhry et al 1961[3]	1	–	–	Palate		N/S
Hjertman and Eneroth 1970[4]	1	–	–	Palate		N/S
Kleinsasser 1970[5]	3	–	–	Nasal cavity		N/S
Manace and Goldman 1971[6]	1	F	47	Antroethmoid	S	A&W 16 mo
Spiro et al 1973[7]	2	–	–	Nasal cavity Gum		N/S
Perzin et al 1981[8]	1	F	75	Nasal cavity: inferior turbinate	S	N/S
Ordonez and Batsakis 1986[9]	1	F	60	Nasal cavity	S	A&W 7 y
Finkelhor and Maves 1987[10]	1	F	45	Nasal cavity: septum	S	N/S
Hanada et al 1988[11]	1	M	68	Nasal cavity: inferior turbinate	S + RT	A&W 3 y
Takimoto et al 1989[12]	1	F	60	Nasal cavity: middle + inferior turbinate	S	A&W 2 y
Dimitrakopoulos et al 1992[13]	1	M	65	Maxillary sinus	S (total maxillectomy)	N/S
Valerdiz-Casasola et al 1993[14]	1	M	47	Nasal cavity	S + RT	A&W 10 months
Schmitt et al 1994[15]	1	M	60	Nasal cavity: inferior turbinate	N/S	N/S
Fujii et al 1998[16]	1	F	71	Maxilla	S	Recurrence after 22 y
Von Biberstein et al 1999[17]	1	F	76	Nasal cavity: middle turbinate	S	A&W 3 y
Sapci et al 2000[18]	1	M	47	Nasal cavity: septum	S	A&W 20 mo
Neto et al 2005[19]	4	2M:2F	42, 50, 60, 65	Nasal cavity: inferior turbinate[2]	S[3] S + RT[1]	A&W 4–17 y 1 recurrence A&W 12 y
Wong et al 2010[20]	1	F	42	Posterior ethmoid	S (ESS)	A&W 1 y

Abbreviations: A&W, alive and well; ESS, endoscopic sinus surgery; F, female; M, male; N/S, not stated; RT, radiotherapy; S, surgery; y, year(s).

high-grade tumors. Local recurrence has been reported in one-third of cases but rarely causes death.

Treatment and Outcome

Wide local excision is mandatory to avoid local "recurrence," which can occur late. Radiotherapy has generally been reserved for positive surgical margins and higher-grade tumors, but it is difficult to demonstrate that radiotherapy improves survival.[2,28] Only three of the reported cases received radiotherapy, one of which developed a recurrence at 12 years.

Overall ACC has the best survival of all carcinomas of salivary origin with 65 to 80% alive at 15 years.[29] In 585 cases (mainly ACC in major salivary glands) 5-year disease-specific survival was 91.4% and observed survival 83.3%. Worse outcome was determined by higher grade, regional or distant metastases at presentation, site in the submandibular gland, and age >30 years.[2] In this group surgery alone was associated with the best outcome, with 5-year survival of 96.8%, whereas those who received combined surgery and radiotherapy had a 5-year survival of 88% due to the selection bias for cases with worse prognostic factors. The numbers of patients were too small for a meaningful independent factor analysis. In addition, two authors have reported what must be regarded as genuine recurrence many years later (12 and 22 years, respectively),[16,19] so lifetime surveillance is recommended.

In the major salivary glands, estimation of proliferation rate by Ki-67 immunostaining has been shown to be an independent prognostic factor for ACC.[30]

References

1. Nasse D. Die Geschwulste der Speicheldrusen und verwandte Tumoren des Kopfes. Archiv Klin Chirurg 1892;44:233–302
2. Hoffman HT, Karnell LH, Robinson RA, Pinkston JA, Menck HR. National Cancer Data Base report on cancer of the head and neck: acinic cell carcinoma. Head Neck 1999;21(4):297–309
3. Chaudhry AP, Vickers RA, Gorlin RJ. Intraoral minor salivary gland tumors. An analysis of 1,414 cases. Oral Surg Oral Med Oral Pathol 1961;14:1194–1226
4. Hjertman L, Eneroth CM. Tumours of the palate. Acta Otolaryngol Suppl 1969;263:179–182
5. Kleinsasser O. Acinic cell tumors of the mucous glands. Mucous acinic cell carcinomas of the nose. [Article in German] Arch Klin Exp Ohren Nasen Kehlkopfheilkd 1970;195(4):345–354
6. Manace ED, Goldman JL. Acinic cell carcinoma of the paranasal sinuses. Laryngoscope 1971;81(7):1074–1082
7. Spiro RH, Koss LG, Hajdu SI, Strong EW. Tumors of minor salivary origin. A clinicopathologic study of 492 cases. Cancer 1973;31(1):117–129
8. Perzin KH, Cantor JO, Johannessen JV. Acinic cell carcinoma arising in nasal cavity: report of a case with ultrastructural observations. Cancer 1981;47(7):1818–1822
9. Ordonez NG, Batsakis JG. Acinic cell carcinoma of the nasal cavity: electron-optic and immunohistochemical observations. J Laryngol Otol 1986;100(3):345–349
10. Finkelhor BK, Maves MD. Pathologic quiz case 1. Acinous cell carcinoma. Arch Otolaryngol Head Neck Surg 1987;113(10):1120–1122
11. Hanada T, Moriyama I, Fukami K. Acinic cell carcinoma originating in the nasal cavity. Arch Otorhinolaryngol 1988;245(6):344–347
12. Takimoto T, Kano M, Umeda R. Acinic cell carcinoma of the nasal cavity: a case report. Rhinology 1989;27(3):191–196
13. Dimitrakopoulos I, Lazaridis N, Triantafillidou E. Acinic cell carcinoma of the maxillary sinus. A case report. Int J Oral Maxillofac Surg 1992;21(6):350–351
14. Valerdiz-Casasola S, Sola J, Pardo-Mindan FJ. Acinic cell carcinoma of the sinonasal cavity with intracytoplasmic crystalloids. Histopathology 1993;23(4):382–384
15. Schmitt FC, Wal R, Santos GdaC. Acinic cell carcinoma arising in nasal cavity: diagnosis by fine-needle aspiration. Diagn Cytopathol 1994;10(1):96–97
16. Fujii M, Kumanomidou H, Ohno Y, Kanzaki J. Acinic cell carcinoma of maxillary sinus. Auris Nasus Larynx 1998;25(4):451–457
17. von Biberstein SE, Spiro JD, Mancoll W. Acinic cell carcinoma of the nasal cavity. Otolaryngol Head Neck Surg 1999;120(5):759–762
18. Sapçi T, Yıldırım G, Peker K, Karavus A, Akbulut UG. Acinic cell carcinoma originating in the nasal septum. Rhinology 2000;38(3):140–143
19. Neto AG, Pineda-Daboin K, Spencer ML, Luna MA. Sinonasal acinic cell carcinoma: a clinicopathologic study of four cases. Head Neck 2005;27(7):603–607
20. Wong A, Leong JL, Ho B. Primary acinic cell carcinoma of the ethmoid sinus. Ear Nose Throat J 2010;89(7):E40–E41
21. Nicolai P, Redaelli de Zinis LO, Tomenzoli D, Maroldi R, Antonelli AR. Sphenoid mucocele with intracranial invasion secondary to nasopharyngeal acinic cell carcinoma. Head Neck 1991;13(6):540–544
22. Batsakis JG, Chinn E, Regezi JA, Repola DA. The pathology of head and neck tumors: salivary glands, part 2. Head Neck Surg 1978;1(2):167–180
23. Stelow E, Mills P. Biopsy Interpretation of the Upper Aerodigestive Tract and Ear. Philadelphia: Lippincott Williams & Wilkins; 2008: 111
24. Lewis JE, Olsen KD, Weiland LH. Acinic cell carcinoma. Clinicopathologic review. Cancer 1991;67(1):172–179
25. Nikitakis NG, Tosios KI, Papanikolaou VS, Rivera H, Papanicolaou SI, Ioffe OB. Immunohistochemical expression of cytokeratins 7 and 20 in malignant salivary gland tumors. Mod Pathol 2004;17(4):407–415
26. Prasad AR, Savera AT, Gown AM, Zarbo RJ. The myoepithelial immunophenotype in 135 benign and malignant salivary gland tumors other than pleomorphic adenoma. Arch Pathol Lab Med 1999;123(9):801–806
27. Childers EL, Ellis GL, Auclair PL. An immunohistochemical analysis of anti-amylase antibody reactivity in acinic cell adenocarcinoma. Oral Surg Oral Med Oral Pathol Oral Radiol Endod 1996;81(6):691–694
28. Spiro RH, Thaler HT, Hicks WF, Kher UA, Huvos AH, Strong EW. The importance of clinical staging of minor salivary gland carcinoma. Am J Surg 1991;162(4):330–336
29. Spiro RH. Salivary neoplasms: overview of a 35-year experience with 2,807 patients. Head Neck Surg 1986;8(3):177–184
30. Hellquist HB, Sundelin K, Di Bacco A, Tytor M, Manzotti M, Viale G. Tumour growth fraction and apoptosis in salivary gland acinic cell carcinomas. Prognostic implications of Ki-67 and bcl-2 expression and of in situ end labelling (TUNEL). J Pathol 1997;181(3):323–329

Clear Cell Carcinoma

This is a rare nonepidermoid epithelial tumor of salivary gland origin (ICD-O 8310/3). The lesion can be locally aggressive but rarely metastasizes.

It may be a variant of acinic cell carcinoma and must be distinguished from secondaries from a renal cell carcinoma to the sinonasal region. It can occur in monomorphic or dimorphic forms (*epithelial-myoepithelial carcinoma*, which is distinguished by a separate ICD code: ICD-O 8562/3).

Histologically the cells are rich in glycogen (hence the problem with renal carcinoma) but negative for S100. We have seen one case, in a 73-year-old woman who underwent a midfacial degloving approach after endoscopic biopsy to a large lesion and who has remained well over 3 years (**Fig. 7.9**).

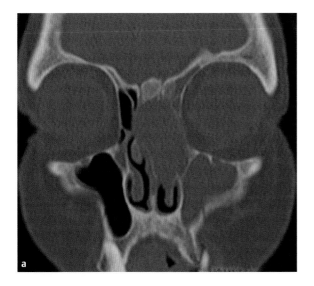

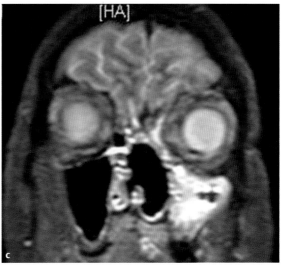

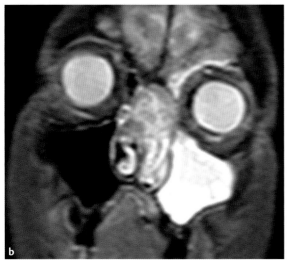

Fig. 7.9a–c

a Clear cell carcinoma. Coronal CT showing a mass in the left nasal cavity with opacification of the maxillary sinus and erosion of adjacent bone.

b Coronal MRI (STIR) in the same patient showing tumor in the nasal cavity with secretion in the maxillary sinus.

c Coronal MRI (STIR) performed 1 year after midfacial degloving showing the surgical cavity without any evidence of recurrence.

Respiratory Epithelial Adenomatoid Hamartoma

This is rare benign hamartomatous proliferation of respiratory epithelium, submucosal glands, and sometimes mesenchymal elements. There is no ICD code.

Originally described by Wenig and Heffner in 1995, the cause of respiratory epithelial adenomatoid hamartomas (REAH) is unknown.[1] Some have suggested a congenital problem, others an association with inflammatory disease. One study considered genetic predisposition and reported a higher loss of heterozygosity at loci on chromosome 9p and 18q than might be anticipated in a benign lesion.[2] In either case, these lesions are exceptionally rare

and usually present with unilateral obstruction with few other nasal symptoms. They can achieve quite large dimensions and present as a mass on endoscopy and CT though without bone destruction. They may occur in the nasal cavity, either in the superior nasal cavity or posteriorly, in the nasopharynx or sinuses (maxillary, ethmoid, and frontal sinus have all been reported) (**Fig. 7.10**). The lesion can be bilateral and has been described as expanding the olfactory clefts on CT[3,4] in comparison with normal controls and nasal polyposis, from which the condition must be distinguished. Calcification can occur rarely, making distinction from an inverted papilloma difficult (chondro-osseous variety).

Classically an REAH consists of a marked submucosal glandular proliferation lined with respiratory ciliated

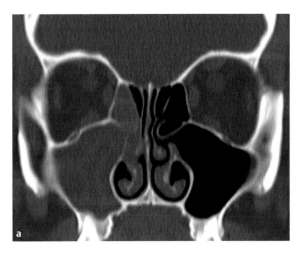
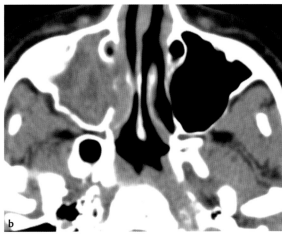

Fig. 7.10a, b

a Respiratory epithelial adenomatoid hamartoma. Coronal CT scan showing opacification of the right maxillary sinus and anterior ethmoids with slight elevation of the orbital floor.

b Axial CT scan in the same patient showing opacification of the maxillary sinus with some heterogeneity of signal and expansion of the medial wall.

epithelium. The differential diagnosis includes inflammatory polyps, inverted papilloma, and low-grade adenocarcinoma.[5]

REAH has a tendency to continue to proliferate and therefore is usually removed by whatever approach is deemed appropriate. Endoscopic resection has been undertaken and indeed was the approach used in our own case of a 41-year-old woman who actually presented to the ophthalmologists with mild proptosis from a lesion in the maxillary sinus. An excisional "biopsy" was undertaken due to apparently ambiguous histology from another institution. If it is completely removed, in common with other benign lesions, one may anticipate cure.

References

1. Wenig BM, Heffner DK. Respiratory epithelial adenomatoid hamartomas of the sinonasal tract and nasopharynx: a clinicopathologic study of 31 cases. Ann Otol Rhinol Laryngol 1995;104(8):639–645
2. Ozolek JA, Hunt JL. Tumor suppressor gene alterations in respiratory epithelial adenomatoid hamartoma (REAH): comparison to sinonasal adenocarcinoma and inflamed sinonasal mucosa. Am J Surg Pathol 2006;30(12):1576–1580
3. Lima NB, Jankowski R, Georgel T, Grignon B, Guillemin F, Vignaud JM. Respiratory adenomatoid hamartoma must be suspected on CT-scan enlargement of the olfactory clefts. Rhinology 2006;44(4):264–269
4. Cao Z, Gu Z, Yang J, Jin M. Respiratory epithelial adenomatoid hamartoma of bilateral olfactory clefts associated with nasal polyposis: three cases report and literature review. Auris Nasus Larynx 2010;37(3):352–356
5. Perez-Ordoñez B. Hamartomas, papillomas and adenocarcinomas of the sinonasal tract and nasopharynx. J Clin Pathol 2009;62(12):1085–1095

8 Mesenchymal Neoplasms and Other Lesions

Eosinophilic Angiocentric Fibrosis

Definition

A rare benign cause of submucosal thickening and fibrosis within the upper respiratory tract.

Etiology

The etiology is unknown. It has been suggested that previous nasal surgery, some form of chronic inflammation, or autoimmune factors may be relevant, but this is largely supposition and, despite the marked eosinophilia, no allergic or parasitic cause has been shown.

Synonyms

First described in 1985, eosinophilic angiocentric fibrosis has been regarded as a possible submucosal variant of granuloma faciale.[1,2]

Incidence

This is an extremely rare condition with around 32 cases reported in the literature, although it is certain that many cases go undiagnosed.[1-21]

Site

This rare condition can affect any part of the upper respiratory tract but is most often seen in the nasal cavity and midfacial soft tissues.

Diagnostic Features

Clinical Features

The patient usually presents with slow onset of nasal obstruction, which can be unilateral or bilateral depending on the area affected. Facial pain and bleeding are not generally present. The septum and anterior columella are most often affected and the abnormal tissue may form a visible swelling. The process can then spread into the external nose and involve the superficial facial tissues so that a diffuse swelling is then seen on the external nose, cheeks, glabella, or frontal region. In some patients, the process spreads into the orbit, producing progressive proptosis and/or hypertelorism.

This condition can very rarely affect the subglottis (two cases) but multisite involvement has not been described. The orbit is also occasionally involved.[22]

Our clinical cohort comprises 7 cases (Table 8.1) comprising 2 men and 5 women, aged 46 to 68 years (mean 54 years). In 28 of the additional cases reported in the literature, there are 13 men and 15 women, age range 19 to 64 years (mean 45 years) (Table 8.2).

Table 8.1 Eosinophilic angiocentric fibrosis: personal series

Age/sex	Presenting lesion	Management	Long-term follow-up
37/F	Frontonasal/intranasal mass 18 y earlier	Surgical excision Lateral rhinotomy ×2 Oral steroids and azathioprine	NSR since 8 y
68/M	Frontonasal/septal mass for 5 y	Surgical excision Extended lateral rhinotomy	NSR 11 y
57/F	Nasal mass extending into midface and orbit for 25 y	Lateral rhinotomy ×2 Dapsone, hydroxychloroquine, azathioprine	Residual disease in orbit
58/F	Septal thickening 1 y	Surgical excision Lateral rhinotomy	NSR 8 y
51/M	Septal thickening 1 y	Surgical excision External rhinoplasty	NSR 4 y
46/F	Septal/lateral wall thickening 2 y	Surgical excision External rhinoplasty	NSR 6 mo
65/F	Submucosal mass over alar cartilage/ septal mass 2 y	Surgical excision Subtotal rhinectomy	NSR 6 mo
Abbreviations: F, female; M, male; mo, month(s); NSR, no sign of recurrence; y, year.			

Table 8.2 Reported cases of sinonasal eosinophilic angiocentric fibrosis

Report	Age/sex	Presenting lesion	Management	Long-term follow-up
Holmes and Panje[1]	49/F	Intranasal mass	Surgical excision	Unknown
Roberts and McCann[2]	27/F	Septal/turbinate thickening	Surgical excisions	Residual disease
	59/F	Septal thickening/mass over nasal bridge	Unavailable	Unavailable
	54/F	Septal thickening	Surgical excisions/ radiotherapy	Unavailable
	50/F	Submucosal mass over alar cartilage	Surgical excisions	Residual disease
Altemani et al[4]	54/F	Septal/lateral wall thickening	Surgical excisions	Residual disease
Matai et al[6]	51/M	Septal thickening	Surgical excision	Residual disease
Burns et al[7]	38/M	Septal thickening/mass from alar cartilage	Surgical excisions	Residual disease
Loane et al[8]	42/M	Septal deviation/nasal adhesions post septoplasty	Surgical excision	Unavailable
Thompson and Heffner[9]	28/M	Septal/maxillary sinus mass	Surgical excision/steroids	Residual disease
	49/F	Septal thickening	Surgical excision/steroids	Residual disease
	64/F	Septal/maxillary sinus mass	Surgical excision/steroids	Residual disease
Pereira et al[10]	52/M	Septum	Surgical excisions	Unavailable
Tabaee et al[11]	79/M	Septum and lateral wall	Surgical resection	Unavailable
Nguyen et al[12]	45/M	Septum/middle meatus	Surgical excision	Unavailable

Abbreviations: F, female; M, male.

Imaging

The changes are nonspecific, a soft tissue infiltrative process that is homogeneous and not encapsulated or delineated (**Figs. 8.1, 8.2, 8.3**). The septum is most frequently affected and appears thickened, especially anteriorly.[15] This swelling then extends to the lateral wall and beyond, although the cavities of the sinuses are generally spared in the early stages of the process. Bone destruction is not regarded as a common feature of this disease,[7] but in several of our cases the lamina papyracea was eroded to involve the orbit.

Histological Features and Differential Diagnosis

Smooth submucosal mass(es) can be seen. Microscopically the tissue shows a marked eosinophilic vasculitis involving the submucosal capillaries and venules.[3,4,6–9] Typically a concentric, perivascular fibrosis ("onion-skin" type) is seen.[2] While eosinophils predominate, plasma cells and T lymphocytes are common in the early stages. However, true granulomas, giant cells, and necrosis are not generally seen.[4,5,9] As other inflammatory cells progressively reduce in number, eosinophils increase further. There are some similarities to granuloma faciale but "onion-skin whorling" is not seen in granuloma faciale.

Due to its rarity, slow and indolent growth, and rather nonspecific findings of inflammation and fibrosis, this condition may not be recognized by the unsuspecting general pathologist and diagnosis is often delayed.

The differential diagnosis includes fibrosing forms of invasive fungal disease, midline granulomatous diseases such as Wegener's granulomatosis and sarcoid, Kimura disease, angiolymphoid hyperplasia, and neurogenic and mesenchymal tumors.

Natural History

Although benign, this process can continue to spread insidiously and produce significant functional and cosmetic deformity. The infiltration of the orbit can eventually lead to visual problems due to the mass effect and corneal exposure. It has most often been diagnosed by accident when septal surgery has been undertaken for nasal obstruction.

Treatment

The only effective treatment is complete surgical excision. This can be difficult due to the extent of infiltration and the poorly defined nature of the process but should be done sooner rather than later. As this may produce significant cosmetic problems, surgeons may be tempted to be conservative but **failure to completely excise the tissue will lead to repeated "recurrences" and multiple operations leading ultimately to problems as**

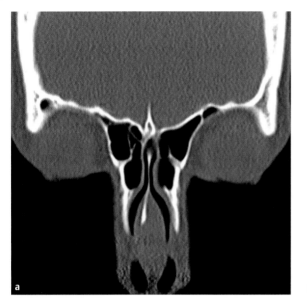

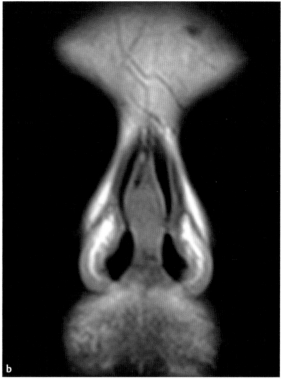

Fig. 8.1a, b

a Coronal CT scan showing expansion of the nasal septum by eosinophilic angiocentric fibrosis.

b Coronal MRI (T1W post-gadolinium enhancement) showing infiltration of the anterior nasal septum in the same patient with an ill-defined plane of cleavage.

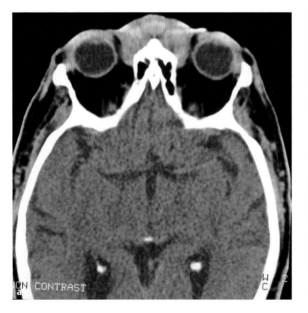

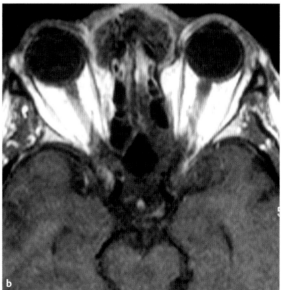

Fig. 8.2a, b

a Axial CT scan showing infiltration of the glabella with eosinophilic angiocentric fibrosis abutting the orbits on both sides.

b Axial MRI (T1W unenhanced) in the same patient showing a defined mass.

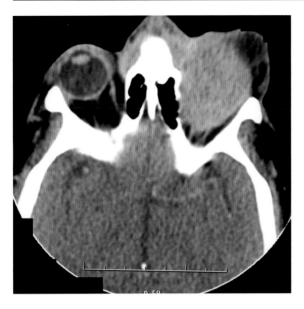

Fig. 8.3 Axial CT showing significant involvement of the superior right orbit by eosinophilic angiocentric fibrosis in addition to infiltration of the glabella.

significant if not worse. Of the 32 cases reported in the literature, over half had residual disease or the outcome was not reported. In our 7 cases, 5 of whom have been under long-term follow-up, only 1 has residual disease and 4 are clear due to radical surgery.

An endoscopic approach may be possible in limited disease but generally an external procedure is required to adequately access the superficial facial tissues and/or orbit. In our cohort, external rhinoplasty,[2] lateral rhinotomy,[3] a coronal approach to the frontal region[1] and a total rhinectomy[1] have been employed.

Medical therapies have included nasal, oral, and intralesional steroids with some limited success, and hydroxychloroquine. Dapsone has been given because it has proved beneficial in granuloma faciale, again with little response in our patients.[23,24] Radiotherapy is not recommended.

Outcome

Untreated, the process will continue inexorably although generally rather slowly over many years. It is not known to undergo malignant transformation.

References

1. Holmes DK, Panje WR. Intranasal granuloma faciale. Am J Otolaryngol 1983;4(3):184–186
2. Roberts PF, McCann BG. Eosinophilic angiocentric fibrosis of the upper respiratory tract: a mucosal variant of granuloma faciale? A report of three cases. Histopathology 1985;9(11):1217–1225
3. Fageeh NA, Mai KT, Odell PF. Eosinophilic angiocentric fibrosis of the subglottic region of the larynx and upper trachea. J Otolaryngol 1996;25(4):276–278
4. Altemani AM, Pilch BZ, Sakano E, Altemani JM. Eosinophilic angiocentric fibrosis of the nasal cavity. Mod Pathol 1997;10(4):391–393
5. Roberts PF, McCann BG. Eosinophilic angiocentric fibrosis of the upper respiratory tract: a postscript. Histopathology 1997;31(4):385–386
6. Matai V, Baer S, Barnes S, Boxer M. Eosinophilic angiocentric fibrosis. J Laryngol Otol 2000;114(7):563–564
7. Burns BV, Roberts PF, De Carpentier J, Zarod AP. Eosinophilic angiocentric fibrosis affecting the nasal cavity. A mucosal variant of the skin lesion granuloma faciale. J Laryngol Otol 2001;115(3):223–226
8. Loane J, Jaramillo M, Young HA, Kerr KM. Eosinophilic angiocentric fibrosis and Wegener's granulomatosis: a case report and literature review. J Clin Pathol 2001;54(8):640–641
9. Thompson LD, Heffner DK. Sinonasal tract eosinophilic angiocentric fibrosis. A report of three cases. Am J Clin Pathol 2001;115(2):243–248
10. Pereira EM, Millas I, Reis-Filho JS, Maeda SA, Franco M. Eosinophilic angiocentric fibrosis of the sinonasal tract: report on the clinicopathologic features of a case and review of the literature. Head Neck 2002;24(3):307–311
11. Tabaee A, Zadeh MH, Proytcheva M, LaBruna A. Eosinophilic angiocentric fibrosis. J Laryngol Otol 2003;117(5):410–413
12. Nguyen DB, Alex JC, Calhoun B. Eosinophilic angiocentric fibrosis in a patient with nasal obstruction. Ear Nose Throat J 2004;83(3):183–184, 186
13. Onder S, Sungur A. Eosinophilic angiocentric fibrosis: an unusual entity of the sinonasal tract. Arch Pathol Lab Med 2004;128(1):90–91
14. Narayan J, Douglas-Jones AG. Eosinophilic angiocentric fibrosis and granuloma faciale: analysis of cellular infiltrate and review of literature. Ann Otol Rhinol Laryngol 2005;114(1 Pt 1):35–42
15. Paun S, Lund VJ, Gallimore A. Nasal fibrosis: long-term follow up of four cases of eosinophilic angiocentric fibrosis. J Laryngol Otol 2005;119(2):119–124
16. Clauser L, Mandrioli S, Polito J, Marchetti E. Eosinophilic angiocentric fibrosis. J Craniofac Surg 2006;17(4):812–814
17. Watanabe N, Moriwaki K. Atypical eosinophilic angiocentric fibrosis on nasal septum. Auris Nasus Larynx 2006;33(3):355–358
18. Jain R, Robblee JV, O'Sullivan-Mejia E, et al. Sinonasal eosinophilic angiocentric fibrosis: a report of four cases and review of literature. Head Neck Pathol 2008;2(4):309–315
19. Kosarac O, Luna MA, Ro JY, Ayala AG. Eosinophilic angiocentric fibrosis of the sinonasal tract. Ann Diagn Pathol 2008;12(4):267–270
20. Fanlo P, Perez C, Ibanez J, Zubimendi K, Arbizu L, Bragado FG. Eosinophilic angiocentric fibrosis: an unusual entity producing saddle nose and nasal septal perforation. APMIS 2009;117(Suppl S127):100
21. Sunde J, Alexander KA, Reddy VV, Woodworth BA. Intranasal eosinophilic angiocentric fibrosis: a case report and review. Head Neck Pathol 2010;4(3):246–248
22. Leibovitch I, James CL, Wormald PJ, Selva D. Orbital eosinophilic angiocentric fibrosis case report and review of the literature. Ophthalmology 2006;113(1):148–152
23. Goldner R, Sina B. Granuloma faciale: the role of dapsone and prior irradiation on the cause of the disease. Cutis 1984;33(5):478–479, 482
24. van de Kerkhof PC. On the efficacy of dapsone in granuloma faciale. Acta Derm Venereol 1994;74(1):61–62

Myxoma

Definition

Myxoma is a benign soft tissue tumor characterized by fibroblasts, myofibroblasts, and scattered vessels that are embedded in a hypovascular myxoid stroma. Usually myxomas contain only minimal amounts of thin collagen fibers within a mucus-rich stroma; where larger amounts of collagen exist they are sometimes referred to as fibromyxomas. Cardiac myxomas and intramuscular myxomas in the extremities are by far the most commonly encountered forms of these tumors (ICD-O 8840/0).

They are rare in the head and neck and comprise three different forms: (1) odontogenic myxoma; (2) soft tissue myxoma, which may occur within muscles; and (3) cutaneous or superficial angiomyxoma.

Etiology

There are no known etiological factors, but cutaneous myxomas may involve the head and neck and, at times, when they are multiple, particularly when they are in the eyelids or external ear, they may be associated with the rare Carney's complex.[1] Odontogenic myxomas, which may become large enough to involve the nasal cavity and paranasal sinuses, are not associated with the Carney's complex or any other genetic lesions.

Incidence and Site

The intraosseous odontogenic myxoma represents over 60% of all noncutaneous myxomas affecting the head and neck, with approximately two-thirds of them involving the mandible and the remainder the maxilla.[2] The most common site of these odontogenic myxomas in the maxilla is the posterior aspect of the alveolar region and they represent a high proportion of odontogenic tumors in children. The slowly growing mass tends to obliterate the maxillary sinus. The origin in the tooth-bearing areas of the gnathic bones, the presence of odontogenic epithelial structures, and the resemblance to dental papillae support the thesis that these tumors arise from odontogenic mesenchyme.[3] (See Chapter 12.)

In contrast, true sinonasal myxomas, while being extremely rare in the literature, appear to arise in the anterior maxillary wall with no evidence of odontogenic origin.[4]

Diagnostic Features

Clinical Features

Heffner[4] presented four cases from the tumor files of the Armed Forces Institute of Pathology, all being children between the ages of 1 and 12 years. The anterior maxillary wall appeared to be involved in all lesions, the main symptoms being cheek and facial swelling accompanied by pain. When these true sinonasal tumors are more advanced, symptoms of nasal block and epistaxis also occur.[5] In contrast to these pediatric cases, rare cases of myxoma developing in the sphenoid sinus have been reported in adults.[6,7]

We have treated one case, a 14-month-old West Indian girl who presented with a large disfiguring mass in the right nasal cavity that was increasing in size in 1985 (**Fig. 8.4**). This was biopsied via a sublabial approach and, following histological confirmation as a myxoma, was excised via a lateral rhinotomy. The lesion appeared to arise within the maxilla and had breached the anterior and superior walls. She remained free of disease for the next 7 years of follow-up. This treatment predated the regular use of the midfacial degloving approach in our unit, and today this lesion would undoubtedly have been biopsied and excised endoscopically. With either approach, a facial incision would have been avoided in a young child.

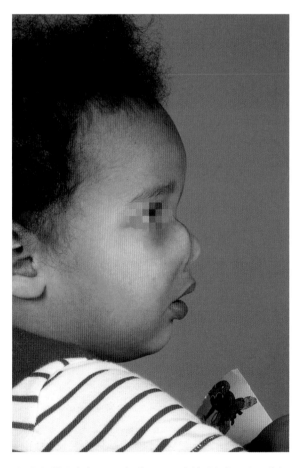

Fig. 8.4 Clinical photograph of a young child with distortion of the right cheek and nose by myxoma.

Histological Features and Differential Diagnosis

Heffner found the tissue in all his sinonasal pediatric cases to be mostly soft and semigelatinous. The myxoid neoplasm contains a relatively uniform distribution of spindled and stellate cells and although the nuclei are slightly enlarged, they are not hypochromatic or anaplastic. Mitoses are rare. There are no cross-striations and no densely cellular areas. Additionally, others have commented on the wispy strands of thin collagen that appear to blend with the delicate cytoplasmic processes on the lesional cells. These sinonasal myxomas appeared more cellular than most myxomas and potentially could be confused with rhabdomyosarcoma in these young patients. However, recent advances in immunohistochemistry and our knowledge of rhabdomyosarcoma make this far less likely.

Treatment

The gelatinous and friable nature of these lesions is associated with infiltrative capacity into surrounding bone and makes complete removal by simple curettage unreliable. Despite the limited literature, they obviously have a propensity to recur and, while radical surgery is not indicated, they do need thorough local removal by endoscopic or open surgical approaches with at least a few millimeters of adjacent bone, cartilage, and mucosa. If this is not done, they may further invade the paranasal sinuses, skull base, and cranial cavity.[4,8]

As with many of the other benign but locally invasive neoplasms within the nose, sinuses, and skull base, the possibility of local recurrence, even years later, requires long-term follow-up, good patient education regarding the possibility of recurrence, and appropriate re-imaging as necessary.

References

1. Carney JA, Gordon H, Carpenter PC, Shenoy BV, Go VL. The complex of myxomas, spotty pigmentation, and endocrine overactivity. Medicine (Baltimore) 1985;64(4):270–283
2. Lo Muzio L, Nocini P, Favia G, Procaccini M, Mignogna MD. Odontogenic myxoma of the jaws: a clinical, radiologic, immunohistochemical, and ultrastructural study. Oral Surg Oral Med Oral Pathol Oral Radiol Endod 1996;82(4):426–433
3. Harrison JD. Odontogenic myxoma: ultrastructural and histochemical studies. J Clin Pathol 1973;26(8):570–582
4. Heffner DK. Sinonasal myxomas and fibromyxomas in children. Ear Nose Throat J 1993;72(5):365–368
5. Prasannan L, Warren L, Herzog CE, Lopez-Camarillo L, Frankel L, Goepfert H. Sinonasal myxoma: a pediatric case. J Pediatr Hematol Oncol 2005;27(2):90–92
6. Andrews T, Kountakis SE, Maillard AA. Myxomas of the head and neck. Am J Otolaryngol 2000;21(3):184–189
7. Sato H, Gyo K, Tomidokoro Y, Honda N. Myxoma of the sphenoidal sinus. Otolaryngol Head Neck Surg 2004;130(3):378–380
8. Fu Y, Perzin K. Non-epithelial tumors of the nasal cavity, paranasal sinuses and nasopharynx: a clinicopathologic study. VII. Myxomas. Cancer 1977;39:195–203

Borderline and Low Malignancy–Potential Tumors of Soft Tissue

The sarcomas described in this book are rare in comparison with the many benign soft tissue tumors that can occur in the head and neck of both children and adults. The benign tumors and tumorlike lesions of the head and neck are often different from their soft tissue counterparts in other sites of the body. Some have an increased potential for recurrence, such as desmoid type fibromatosis, glomangiopericytoma and angiofibroma. They may even require adjuvant treatment to control the local disease, even when they are nonmetastasizing benign lesions. Atypical variants of these low-grade tumors and tumorlike lesions have at times in the past been confused with sarcomas and the names and classification of these lesions have changed considerably over recent years, which unfortunately can be a source of confusion in the literature. **However, increasing evidence from ultrastructural studies, immunohistochemistry, and recently cytogenetics, is helping to clarify the continually evolving classification of these tumors** when added to long-term knowledge of the clinical features and morphology. A good example is glomangiopericytoma (sinonasal hemangiopericytoma), which in the WHO classification is regarded as a soft tissue tumor of borderline malignant potential but which we have included with the vasoform tumors because of its relationship to the pericyte.

Desmoid-Type Fibromatosis

Definition

(ICD-O code 8821/1)

Desmoid-type fibromatosis is a locally aggressive lesion composed of bland cellular spindled cells of the myofibroblastic phenotype. It is comprised of intra-abdominal, abdominal, and extra-abdominal types. It does not metastasize.

Synonyms

The terms infantile fibromatosis, juvenile desmoid-type fibromatosis, aggressive fibromatosis, desmoid tumor, extra-abdominal desmoid, and extra-abdominal fibromatosis have all been commonly used in the literature.

Incidence and Site

Approximately 15% of cases of desmoid-type fibromatosis occur in the head and neck, but it is rare in the sinonasal tract. All ages can be affected but it is more common in children, and the so-called infantile aggressive fibromatosis represents the childhood version of the desmoid tumors seen in adults.[1–3] The lesions are common in patients with familial adenomatous polyposis, an autosomal inherited disease caused by a genetic mutation in the *APC* tumor suppressor gene.[4,5]

We have treated two patients, both children, aged 2 and 4 years. In the 2-year-old girl the condition affected the antrum and the ethmoid and impinged on the orbit. In the 4-year-old boy only the maxilla was involved.

Diagnostic Features

Clinical Features and Imaging

These relatively slow-growing lesions in the sinonasal tract have presented with nasal obstruction, epistaxis, facial swelling, facial pain, proptosis, loosening of teeth, nonhealing tooth sockets following extraction, and swelling of the hard palate.[1–3,6] Both of our patients presented with a mass in the cheek and in one case orbital displacement.

On examination any visible lesions within the nasal cavity often have a glistening quality, but in contrast to simple nasal polyps they are usually rubbery and firm. They may measure up to several centimeters in size with displacement of both the lateral wall of the nose and nasal septum, intraorbital extension, and skull base erosion.[4] Occasionally there may be multiple lesions, particularly when associated with Gardener's syndrome.[7] Imaging by CT usually shows a nonspecific mildly enhancing heterogeneous soft tissue mass.

Histological Features and Differential Diagnosis

On macroscopic examination fibromatosis is usually pinkish-white in color and firm and rubbery in consistency with infiltration into surrounding tissues. It usually comprises of fascicles of bland-looking spindle cells and collagen fibers, frequently arranged in a fairly uniform manner and with elongated blood vessels that tend to run parallel to each other. The spindle cells have a myofibroblastic appearance and the nuclei are usually ovoid with indistinct nucleoli. Normal mitosis may be present but atypical mitosis and necrosis are not features of fibromatosis. The matrix may contain keloidlike collagen and myxoid areas.

The main differential diagnosis in the sinonasal area is between variants of fibrosarcoma and malignant fibrous histiocytoma, and while in classical lesions immunohistochemistry may not be required, the myofibroblasts may be positive for actins and vimentin, but are usually negative for desmin, S100 protein, HMB 45, keratins, and CD 34. Beta-catenin is an important genetic immunohistochemistry marker showing nuclear reactivity in fibromatosis.

It is important to separate the fibromatosis in the head and neck region from a variety of benign and malignant lesions, since although it is locally aggressive and may be difficult to excise, it does not require the same level of treatment as more concerning lesions, such as the fibrosarcoma variants. Fortunately, β-catenin, while being specific to desmoid-type fibromatosis, is either negative or shows only cytoplasmic reactivity in all of the other tumors.

Treatment and Prognosis

Desmoid-type fibromatosis in the sinonasal area may be difficult to excise and can erode bone of the paranasal sinus and skull base area, but with modern approaches by midfacial degloving and craniofacial techniques, prognosis in these rare lesions should be excellent, and it is to be hoped that the quoted 20% recurrence rates from publications derived from the 1980s and 1990s can be further reduced by obtaining adequate surgical margins. As the lesion does not metastasize, total removal to prevent local recurrence is the primary aim. Both radiotherapy and chemotherapy have been advocated for aggressive and recurrent surgically nonresectable lesions. This has potential problems, particularly in the long term, for the children, given that this is a benign nonmetastasizing tumor.[8–10]

Wehl et al[11] reported the results of liposomal doxorubicin in three children with progressive fibromatosis in the nasal cavity, oral cavity, infratemporal fossa, supraclavicular fossa, and abdomen. Tumor response was confirmed by MRI in all children without major short-term complications.

Both our young patients were treated successfully with surgery. The young boy treated in the early 1980s underwent a lateral rhinotomy; the little girl had a midfacial degloving for her extensive lesion.

Extrapleural Solitary Fibrous Tumors

Definition

(ICD-O code 8815/1)

Solitary fibrous tumors are tumors of CD34-positive fibroblasts. This mesenchymal spindle cell neoplasm was originally found in pleural tissue but subsequently numerous extrapleural sites have been described, including the upper respiratory tract.

Etiology, Incidence, and Site

There are no known etiological factors and the tumor is extremely rare. Hicks and Moe reported a nasal case arising from the anterior cranial fossa, estimated to be the fourteenth case in the English literature.[12] Tumors have been reported affecting the nasal cavity, paranasal sinuses, and nasopharynx. We have seen two patients, one a man aged 37 years who underwent removal of a solitary lesion on the lateral nasal wall via a lateral rhinotomy in the late 1960s and was free of disease at the end of 5 years' follow-up. The second, a 53-year-old man, recently underwent surgical removal via an endoscopic approach (**Fig. 8.5**).

Diagnostic Features

Clinical Features and Imaging

A wide range of ages and approximately equal numbers of males and females have been reported. Recorded patients present with the usual nonspecific symptoms of nasal obstruction and epistaxis and in those cases where the tumor can be visualized in the nose it is usually described as polypoid and firm. Substantial hemorrhage is a feature of note on biopsy. Approximately half the tumors recorded have infiltrated the ethmoid sinuses and extend posteriorly into the nasopharynx, but only a single reported case breached the anterior skull base. Imaging features have been nonspecific but obviously essential to accurately delineate the size of the lesion.

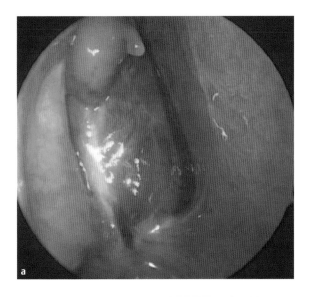

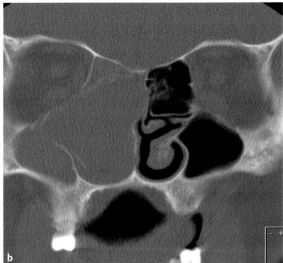

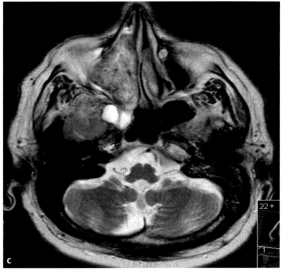

Fig. 8.5a–d

a   Endoscopic view of a solitary fibrous tumor completely filling the right nasal cavity.

b,c   Coronal CT scan (**b**) of the same patient showing the tumor filling the nasal cavity with associated opacification of adjacent sinuses due to retained secretions, confirmed with MRI (T1W post-gadolinium enhancement) (**c**).

d   View of nasal cavity at the end of endoscopic removal of the tumor.

Histological Features, Immunohistochemical Features, and Differential Diagnosis

These tumors are usually well circumscribed but with a variable proliferation of cells with appearances ranging from plump to spindle. A nondescript growth pattern associated with "ropey" keloidal collagen bundles interlaced with thin-walled vascular spaces appears to be the most common element. Vascular spaces may be prominent, exhibiting a hemangiopericytoma-like pattern.

Immunohistochemical testing results in prominent staining for CD34 and variable reactivity for vimentin, and is generally negative for actin. Additionally, staining is usually negative for keratin, epithelial membrane antigen, S100 protein, factor 8-related antigen, carcinoembryonic antigen, desmin, HHF-35, and glial fibrillary acidic protein.

The differential diagnosis includes glomangiopericytoma, fibrous histiocytoma, leiomyoma, schwannoma, synovial sarcoma, and fibrous sarcoma.

Treatment and Prognosis

Total resection is the treatment of choice at present with these rare tumors and this has been obtained by a variety of anterior facial approaches up to and including ethmoidectomy, maxillectomy, and craniofacial resection in case of Hicks and Moe.[12] Their review of the previous 14 cases showed that all have been resected without recurrence. An endoscopic resection may be technically feasible but the vascularity of the lesion should be noted.

Inflammatory Myofibroblastic Tumor

Definition

(ICD-O code 8825/1)

Inflammatory myofibroblastic tumor (IMT) is a lesion composed of myofibroblastic spindle cells with an inflammatory infiltrate of eosinophils, plasma cells, and lymphocytes.

Etiology

Most IMTs occur in the lung and much of the older literature regards this as a nonneoplastic condition, possibly related to trauma or infection. Gomez-Roman et al[13] described human herpes virus-8 DNA sequences and overexpression of interleukin-6 and cyclin D1 in some of these lesions, which supports the possibility of an infectious etiology. However, not all these lesions exhibit benign behavior and those of the sinonasal tract can be particularly destructive and are known to have recurred after excision. Reports of these lesions metastasizing have further added to the possibility that it is a true neoplasm. **However, as is so often the case with these rare lesions,** it may be that our current knowledge is at the stage we were at with fibrosarcomas in the past, in that IMTs may represent a diverse group of lesions of multiple etiologies that only share a common histological stem, that being a tumor mass of inflammatory cells with a variable myofibroblastic fibrous tissue response.

Synonyms

With the difficulties so far inherent in understanding these lesions, it is not surprising that a wide variety of names has been used in the past, including inflammatory pseudo-tumor, plasma cell granuloma, benign myofibroblastoma, and xanthomatous pseudo-tumor, which have added to the confusion. Fortunately, the name inflammatory myofibroblastic tumor has been adopted by WHO and is gaining wider acceptance from its initial proposal in 1990 by Pettinato et al.[14]

Incidence and Site

Soysal et al[15] presented a case in a 10-year-old white girl and in reviewing the previous literature found only six cases of IMT in the nasal cavity. Cho[16] et al presented a single case of a 4-year-old girl with a mass presenting on the nasal dorsum, while others have reported them occurring in the maxillary sinuses in adults.[17–19]

Diagnostic Features

Clinical Features and Imaging

These extremely rare cases have been reported with symptoms of nasal obstruction, epistaxis, nasal discharge, a dorsal nasal mass, and headache. On examination the intranasal mass tends to be red/bluish and may actually protrude from the nostril. Those cases that underwent computed tomography simply showed a mass within the nasal cavity, and in some cases accompanying inflammatory changes in the maxillary and ethmoid sinuses. Interestingly, work-ups for specific infectious etiology have been negative and biopsy material sent for fungal and acid-fast organisms have been clear.

Histological Features and Immunohistochemical Features

The excised lesions have been primarily composed of fibroblasts, lymphocytes, plasma cells, histiocytes and widely varying amounts of eosinophils. Histiocytes are generally bland and the fibroblasts show no atypia. Mitoses are infrequent, although encompassed blood vessels may show obliterative changes. Inflammatory cells in the walls of blood vessels are rare to absent. Immunohistochemically, spindle cells tend to be positive for vimentin and actin (more than 80%).[20]

Differential Diagnosis

The potential different diagnosis for IMT is enormous as they must be distinguished from sinusitis, granulomatous inflammations, collagen vascular diseases, sarcoidosis, and neoplastic disorders. An important clinical difference for those that originate in the head and neck is that they do not produce systemic symptoms, unlike those originating from visceral organs, and all routine blood and laboratory work-ups for an infectious etiology have been negative. Clinical and radiological appearances of these lesions can certainly be misinterpreted as malignancy and there is little doubt that the diagnosis requires ample biopsy material and preferably excision of the entire mass.

The largest study of lesions to date, by Coffin et al,[21] who evaluated 84 extrapulmonary cases of IMT, concluded that the lesions were inflammatory pseudotumors that were benign, nonmetastasizing, proliferations of myofibroblasts with the potential for persistent local growth and recurrence.

Treatment

With so few cases having been recorded from the nasal cavity and paranasal sinuses, definitive treatment advice is difficult to propose; **the main point is not to misinterpret this lesion as a malignant neoplasm**. Complete surgical resection may be possible by endoscopic means or approaches such as midfacial degloving, but radiation would seem inappropriate in these cases unless surgery is not a feasible option.

References

1. Gnepp DR, Henley J, Weiss S, Heffner D. Desmoid fibromatosis of the sinonasal tract and nasopharynx. A clinicopathologic study of 25 cases. Cancer 1996;78(12):2572–2579
2. Abdelkader M, Riad M, Williams A. Aggressive fibromatosis of the head and neck (desmoid tumours). J Laryngol Otol 2001;115(10):772–776
3. Ogunsalu C, Barclay S. Aggressive infantile (desmoid-type) fibromatosis of the maxilla: a case report and new classification. West Indian Med J 2005;54(5):337–340
4. Gurbuz AK, Giardiello FM, Petersen GM, et al. Desmoid tumours in familial adenomatous polyposis. Gut 1994;35(3):377–381
5. Okuno S. The enigma of desmoid tumors. Curr Treat Options Oncol 2006;7(6):438–443
6. Mannan AA, Ray R, Sharma SC, Hatimota P. Infantile fibromatosis of the nose and paranasal sinuses: report of a rare case and brief review of the literature. Ear Nose Throat J 2004;83(7):481–484
7. de Silva DC, Wright MF, Stevenson DA, et al. Cranial desmoid tumor associated with homozygous inactivation of the adenomatous polyposis coli gene in a 2-year-old girl with familial adenomatous polyposis. Cancer 1996;77(5):972–976
8. Ballo MT, Zagars GK, Pollack A. Radiation therapy in the management of desmoid tumors. Int J Radiat Oncol Biol Phys 1998;42(5):1007–1014
9. Ray ME, Lawrence TS. Radiation therapy for aggressive fibromatosis (desmoid tumor). J Clin Oncol 2006;24(22):3714–3715, author reply 3715
10. Lev D, Kotilingam D, Wei C, et al. Optimizing treatment of desmoid tumors. J Clin Oncol 2007;25(13):1785–1791
11. Wehl G, Rossler J, Otten JE, et al. Response of progressive fibromatosis to therapy with liposomal doxorubicin. Onkologie 2004;27(6):552–556
12. Hicks DL, Moe KS. Nasal solitary fibrous tumor arising from the anterior cranial fossa. Skull Base 2004;14(4):203–207
13. Gómez-Román JJ, Sánchez-Velasco P, Ocejo-Vinyals G, Hernández-Nieto E, Leyva-Cobián F, Val-Bernal JF. Human herpesvirus-8 genes are expressed in pulmonary inflammatory myofibroblastic tumor (inflammatory pseudotumor). Am J Surg Pathol 2001;25(5):624–629
14. Pettinato G, Manivel JC, De Rosa N, Dehner LP. Inflammatory myofibroblastic tumor (plasma cell granuloma). Clinicopathologic study of 20 cases with immunohistochemical and ultrastructural observations. Am J Clin Pathol 1990;94(5):538–546
15. Soysal V, Yigitbasi OG, Kontas O, Kahya HA, Guney E. Inflammatory myofibroblastic tumor of the nasal cavity: a case report and review of the literature. Int J Pediatr Otorhinolaryngol 2001;61(2):161–165
16. Cho SI, Choi JY, Do NY, Kang CY. An inflammatory myofibroblastic tumor of the nasal dorsum. J Pediatr Surg 2008;43(12):e35–37
17. Lee H-M, Choi G, Choi CS, Kim CH, Lee SH. Inflammatory pseudotumor of the maxillary sinus. Otolaryngol Head Neck Surg 2001;125(5):565–566
18. Huang W-H, Dai Y-C. Inflammatory pseudotumor of the nasal cavity. Am J Otolaryngol 2006;27(4):275–277
19. Ushio M, Takeuchi N, Kikuchi S, Kaga K. Inflammatory pseudotumour of the paranasal sinuses—a case report. Auris Nasus Larynx 2007;34(4):533–536
20. Coffin CM, Humphrey PA, Dehner LP. Extrapulmonary inflammatory myofibroblastic tumor: a clinical and pathological survey. Semin Diagn Pathol 1998;15(2):85–101
21. Coffin CM, Watterson J, Priest JR, Dehner LP. Extrapulmonary inflammatory myofibroblastic tumor (inflammatory pseudotumor). A clinicopathologic and immunohistochemical study of 84 cases. Am J Surg Pathol 1995;19(8):859–872

Lipoma and Liposarcoma

Tumors of fatty origin are exceptionally rare in the upper aerodigestive tract and particularly so in the sinonasal region (ICD-O codes 8850/0 [lipomas]; 8850/3 [liposarcoma]).

They have been reported more commonly in the larynx and oral cavity, mainly in adult men. In 256 cases of nonepithelial sinonasal tumors reported by Fu and Perzin in 1977, there was one lipoma and one liposarcoma.[1] We also have only one case of each in our cohort of over 1,700 patients with sinonasal neoplasms. There are occasional case reports of sinonasal lipomas in the literature[2–4] and in infants they may be associated with lipoma in the corpus callosum or the encephalocraniocutaneous lipomatosis syndrome, which is a rare disorder comprising seizures, mental deficiency, and unilateral cutaneous, ophthalmic, and cerebral lipomatous malformations.[5]

Similarly a very small number of liposarcomas have been reported, the largest number being 4 sinonasal cases in a series of 48 sarcomas in Chinese patients though no other clinical information is available in English.[6–8] We treated a 14-year-old male patient whose liposarcoma affected the orbit and adjacent ethmoid. He was treated by orbital exenteration and lateral rhinotomy 22 years ago but unfortunately was lost to follow-up after 2 years. From these few cases of both benign and malignant fatty tumors, it can be seen why few conclusions can be drawn on distribution by age, although they do seem to be commoner in men.

Lipomas can occur as an isolated lesion on the septum or within one of the sinuses and have occasionally been reported in the subcutaneous nasal tissues and in the nasal vestibule.[9,10] Thus the patient has a relatively soft mass, with associated nasal obstruction. However, our single case occurred in the maxilla and cheek of a man aged 49 years who was successfully treated 20 years ago by a midfacial degloving approach.

On imaging, both lesions can be anticipated to show a soft tissue mass on both CT and MRI, characterized by a low attenuation on CT due to the high water content, a low signal intensity on T1W MRI, and a high signal on T2W sequences. As might be anticipated, lipomas are well-circumscribed, whereas liposarcomas are said to be more infiltrative. Nonlipomatous components may be seen in the sarcoma, often in the form of septations.

The benign lipoma has been subclassified into spindle cell, pleomorphic and chondroid and must be distinguished from liposarcoma as these are usually well-differentiated with mature adipocytes in lobules divided by fibrous septations, some spindle cells, and lipoblasts. The fat cells surprisingly show immunoreactivity to S100, whereas the spindle cells may be positive to CD34.[11] The clinical differential diagnosis in infants includes glioma, nasal dermoid, teratoma, hemangioma, and nasolacrimal cysts.

As illustrated by our own two cases, both lipomas and liposarcomas are treated with surgical excision.

References

1. Fu Y-S, Perzin KH. Non-epithelial tumors of the nasal cavity, paranasal sinuses and nasopharynx: a clinico-pathologic study. VIII. Adipose tissue tumors (lipoma and liposarcoma). Cancer 1977;40(3):1314–1317
2. Preece JM, Kearns DB, Wickersham JK, Grace AR, Bailey CM. Nasal lipoma. J Laryngol Otol 1988;102(11):1044–1046
3. Takasaki K, Yano H, Hayashi T, Kobayashi T. Nasal lipoma. J Laryngol Otol 2000;114(3):218–220
4. Abdalla WM, da Motta AC, Lin SY, McCarthy EF, Zinreich SJ. Intraosseous lipoma of the left frontoethmoidal sinuses and nasal cavity. AJNR Am J Neuroradiol 2007;28(4):615–617
5. Hollis LJ, Bailey CM, Albert DM, Hosni A. Nasal lipomas presenting as part of a syndromic diagnosis. J Laryngol Otol 1996;110(3):269–271
6. Hameed K, Rajendran V. Liposarcoma of the maxilla. Indian J Otolaryngol Head Neck Surg 1991;43:197–198
7. Yang C, Zhang D. [Clinical analysis of 48 cases sarcoma in nasal cavity and sinuses]. Lin Chuang Er Bi Yan Hou Ke Za Zhi 2004;18(10):597–598
8. Thompson SM, Duque CS, Sheth RN, Casiano RR, Morcos JJ, Gomez-Fernandez CR. Case report: Liposarcoma of the sinonasal tract. Br J Radiol 2009;82(980):e160–e163
9. Abulezz T, Allam K. Nasal subcutaneous lipoma, a case report. Rhinology 2008;46(2):151–152
10. Gulbinowicz-Gowkielewicz MM, Kibiłda B, Gugała K. Spindle cell lipoma of the vestibule of the nose. Otolaryngol Head Neck Surg 2008;139(2):325–326
11. Nascimento AF, McMenamin ME, Fletcher CD. Liposarcomas/atypical lipomatous tumors of the oral cavity: a clinicopathologic study of 23 cases. Ann Diagn Pathol 2002;6(2):83–93

Malignant Mesenchymal or Soft Tissue Tumors

Introduction

The majority of head and neck sarcomas are of the soft tissue type with only ~20% in the past being said to derive from bony, cartilaginous, or other tissue origins. Sarcomas are a biologically diverse group of malignancies with a common stem from mesenchymal cells. Indeed, while traditionally they have always been classified according to their histogenetic origin—for example a fibrosarcoma arising from fibroblasts or an osteosarcoma arising from osteoblasts—the more immunohistochemical and experimental data we acquire the clearer the indication that sarcomas arise from multipotential mesenchymal cells that undergo differentiation along one of several lines.[1]

The past 20 years have seen substantial advances in the histological diagnosis of soft tissue sarcomas since the previous publication from our academic unit by Donald Harrison and Valerie Lund. **There are now more than 50 types and subtypes of sarcoma, which are increasingly diagnosed by genetic and morphological criteria, and discussion continues with regard to optimal forms of tumor classification, which essentially have to be clinically useful. The molecular classification of these malignancies is being increasingly considered as a consequence of the sequencing and annotation of the human genome project, and technical advances in gene transcription profiling.[2]**

The problem at present is that the potentially valuable means of defining various tumor characteristics at a DNA and cellular level have, for the moment, produced controversial and variable results, particularly with regard to novel prognostic markers.[3] Obviously this work will continue to evolve and, hopefully, future studies will enable us to develop specific therapies for individual patients' soft tissue sarcomas.

However, for the present, our clinical parameters for soft tissue sarcomas in the head and neck remain of paramount importance as the anatomical location, precise extent of disease, age of the patient, and patients' medical comorbidities remain extremely important when considering treatment and prognosis.

Table 8.3 FNCLCC system for histological grading of sarcoma (usually performed on all available, previously untreated biopsy material)[7]

Differentiation score	1 = Resembles the cell of origin, such as fibro-, lipo-, chondrosarcoma
	2 = Pleomorphic liposarcoma or malignant fibrous histiocytoma (have a better prognosis than myoid sarcomas)
	3 = Round cell tumor and most tumors of uncertain phenotype or pleomorphic myoid sarcoma (rhabdomyosarcoma or leiomyosarcoma)
Mitotic score	1 = 10 mitoses/10 HPF
	2 = 10–19 mitoses/10 HPF
	3 = >20 mitoses/10 HPF
Necrosis score	0 = No necrosis
	1 = <50% necrosis
	2 = >50% necrosis
Total score (adding together scores for differentiation, mitoses, necrosis)	2 or 3 = low grade (grade1/3)
	4 or 5 = intermediate grade (grade 2/3)
	6 to 8 = high grade (grade 3/3)
Abbreviation: HPF, high-power field.	

Modern imaging, particularly a combination of MRI and CT, has allowed us to realize why local recurrence was a persistent problem in all of the older reported series as a consequence of inadequate removal of what are often extensive tumors at initial presentation. The combination of modern craniofacial surgery and targeted radiotherapy should produce better long-term results in these lesions.

Care has to be taken in comparing results for treatment in the last two decades with earlier literature as there is no doubt that a substantial number of lesions described in the past, notably "fibrosarcoma," had a diagnosis that was far from reliable, with many of these tumors falling into other groups. Among these rare tumors, fibrosarcoma was one of the most common soft tissue diagnoses prior to our increasing knowledge of immunohistochemistry and nowadays the tumors would be placed into other classifications such as malignant peripheral nerve sheath tumor, leiomyosarcoma, or rhabdomyosarcoma. Sarcomas represent <1% of all malignant tumors in humans, with the head and neck sarcomas accounting for ~10% of all sarcomas in the large series reported in the literature.[4] However, in the pediatric population the incidence is significantly higher in the head and neck region, with figures varying between 4% and 20% of total body sarcomas depending on the age range considered to be that of a child, the type of sarcoma, and the site of location. Head and neck sarcomas have generated considerable interest over the years, despite their rarity, not least of all because of the wide difference in their biological behavior and the complex anatomy within which they lie, making their treatment particularly complex. Sarcomas continue to present with minimal clinical signs and symptoms, but extensive disease. **Their rarity**

makes it even more difficult for any primary physician to suspect this type of tumor at presentation, so that delayed diagnosis and advanced disease at presentation remain all too common.

Grading

The grading of head and neck sarcomas is the same as that for sarcomas elsewhere and, among soft tissue pathologists and clinicians, has been the subject of much discussion for more than 30 years.[5,6] In recent times, many centers have adopted the 3-tiered system of the French Federation Nationale des Centres de Lutte Contre le Cancer (FNCLCC),[7] which is based on differentiation, mitotic activity, and necrosis (Table 8.3). **It is extremely important for clinicians to provide adequate tissue at the**

Table 8.4 The Enneking staging system for musculoskeletal sarcoma[8]

Stage	Grade	Site[a]	Metastasis
IA	G1	T1	M0
IB	G1	T2	M0
IIA	G2	T1	M0
IIB	G2	T2	M0
III	G1 or G2	T1 or T2	M0

[a] T1 = intra-articular, superficial to deep fascia, paraosseous, intrafascial compartment. T2 = soft tissue extension from intra-articular, deep fascial extension from superficial lesion, intraosseous or extrafascial extension from paraosseous, extrafascial compartment from intrafascial compartment.

Table 8.5 The American Joint Committee on Cancer sarcoma staging: TNM system[9]

Stage	Tumor extent[a]	Nodal status[b]	Distant metastases[c]	Grade	Differentiation
Stage I	T1a, 1b, 2a, 2b	N0	M0	G1	Low
Stage II	T1a, 1b, 2a	N0	M0	G2–3	High
Stage III	T2b	N0	M0	G2–3	High
Stage IV	Any T	N1	M0	Any G	Low or high
Stage IV	Any T	Any N	M1	Any G	Low or high

[a] T1 = size <5 cm; T2 = size >5 cm; a = superficial; b = deep.
[b] NX = lymph node cannot be assessed; N0 = no regional lymph node metastasis; N1 = regional lymph node metastasis.
[c] MX = distant metastasis cannot be assessed; M0 = no distant metastases; M1 = distant metastases.

original biopsy to aid a scoring of 1, 2, or 3 (out of 3) for differentiation of mitosis and necrosis. Treatment can then be directed in relation to the grade, with low-grade tumors being treated generally with wide complete excision and consideration being given to additional pre- or postoperative radiotherapy ± chemotherapy for the more intermediate and high-grade sarcomas. This statement is a general overview with considerable debate and variation being applied to treatment regimes in different centers.

Staging

Staging of soft tissue sarcomas is an excellent example of the modern multidisciplinary approach, combining the pathologists' grading above with clinical and imaging information. There are currently two systems in use: the Enneking Musculoskeletal Tumor Society Staging System[8] and the American Joint Committee on Cancer system (AJCC) (**Tables 8.4 and 8.5**). The AJCC system is the more helpful for head and neck surgeons as it is a TNM system as has become standard for other tumors in head and neck sites and can be used for both pediatric and adult staging standards, with the exception of angiosarcoma.

References

1. Fernandez Sanroman J, Alonso del Hoyo JR, Diaz FJ, et al. Sarcomas of the head and neck. Br J Oral Maxillofac Surg 1992;30(2):115–118
2. Daugaard S. Current soft-tissue sarcoma classifications. Eur J Cancer 2004;40(4):543–548
3. Mertens F, Strömberg U, Rydholm A, et al. Prognostic significance of chromosome aberrations in high-grade soft tissue sarcomas. J Clin Oncol 2006;24(2):315–320
4. Pollock RE, Karnell LH, Menck HR, Winchester DP. The National Cancer Data Base report on soft tissue sarcoma. Cancer 1996;78(10):2247–2257
5. Myhre-Jensen O, Kaae S, Madsen EH, Sneppen O. Histopathological grading in soft-tissue tumours. Relation to survival in 261 surgically treated patients. Acta Pathol Microbiol Immunol Scand A 1983;91(2):145–150
6. Trojani M, Contesso G, Coindre JM, et al. Soft-tissue sarcomas of adults; study of pathological prognostic variables and definition of a histopathological grading system. Int J Cancer 1984;33(1):37–42
7. Guillou L, Coindre JM, Bonichon F, et al. Comparative study of the National Cancer Institute and French Federation of Cancer Centers Sarcoma Group grading systems in a population of 410 adult patients with soft tissue sarcoma. J Clin Oncol 1997;15(1):350–362
8. Enneking WF, Spanier SS, Goodman MA. A system for the surgical staging of musculoskeletal sarcoma. Clin Orthop Relat Res 1980;153(153):106–120
9. American Joint Committee on Cancer Staging. AJCC Cancer Staging Handbook. 6th ed. New York: Springer Verlag; 2002:193

Fibrosarcoma

Definition

(ICD-O code 8810/3)

Classically the term "fibrosarcoma" was applied to any malignant mesenchymal tumor with cells recapitulating the appearance of normal fibroblasts. Diagnosis of fibrosarcoma was one of the two most common soft tissue diagnoses (the other being rhabdomyosarcoma) in the head and neck, but with modern evaluation we now know that many of these tumors would be currently classified as malignant peripheral nerve sheath tumors, leiomyosarcoma, rhabdomyosarcoma, malignant fibrous histiocytoma, spindle cell carcinoma, monophasic synovial sarcoma, glomangiopericytoma, desmoid-type fibromatosis, and nodular fasciitis, all of which are nowadays considered in any differential diagnosis. **Indeed, the term fibrosarcoma is rarely used now by soft tissue pathologists.**

Etiology

As expected, fibrosarcomas, in common with SNUC, leiomyosarcoma, and so on, have been linked to irradiation in the past, but precise information from these historical references is rarely available. In fact, these are now placed in **a separate group of radiation-induced sarcomas (RIS).**[1] One of our patients had been treated for nasopharyngeal carcinoma 6 years previously and developed a

Table 8.6 Fibrosarcoma: personal series

Age/sex	Site	Management[a]	Long-term follow-up
23/M	Nasal septum	Lateral rhinotomy	DOD 6 y
32/M	Antroethmoid	Radiotherapy	DOD 2 y
36/M	Antroethmoid	Midfacial degloving	Lost
55/M	Upper alveolus	Partial maxillectomy	Lost
52/M	Maxilla	Maxillectomy and orbital clearance, radiotherapy	DOD 2 y
67/M	Maxilla	Maxillectomy	Lost
75/M	Maxilla	Maxillectomy	Lost
23/M	Maxilla	Maxillectomy via midfacial degloving	A&W 6 y
66/M	Maxilla	Maxillectomy	A&W 10 y
45/M	Maxilla	Maxillectomy and orbital clearance	Lost
66/M	Maxilla	Chemoradiotherapy	Lost
27/M	Orbit	Orbital clearance, radiotherapy	A&W 13 y
34/M	Orbit	Orbital clearance, lateral rhinotomy	A&W 10 y
43/M	Ethmoid, orbit	Chemoradiation, craniofacial resection	DOD 6 y
60/M	Ethmoid, orbit	Chemoradiotherapy, craniofacial resection	DOD 3 y
74/F	Maxilla	Maxillectomy and orbital clearance	DICD
44/F	Ethmoid	Lateral rhinotomy, radiotherapy	A&W 22 y
51/F	Antroethmoid	Maxillectomy and orbital clearance	DOD 4 y
62/F	Maxilla	Maxillectomy	DICD postop
41/F	Frontal	Craniofacial resection	A&W 5 y
46/F	Maxilla	Chemoradiotherapy, maxillectomy	DOD 4 y
41/F	Upper alveolus	Partial maxillectomy	A&W 12 y
46/F	Antroethmoid	Chemoradiotherapy	Lost

Abbreviations: A&W, alive and well; DICD, dead of intercurrent disease; DOD, dead of disease; F, female; M, male.
[a] Maxillectomy = total unless otherwise stated.

particularly aggressive fibrosarcoma from which he succumbed despite radical treatment.

Synonyms

Johnston[2] reported 71 cases of lesions described as sarcomas in 1904, some of which were probably fibrosarcomas, and Portela[3] used the term to describe a bilateral sinonasal case in 1927.

The commonest synonyms have been fibromyxosarcoma and chondromyxofibrosarcoma. Indeed, the term fibrosarcoma has almost disappeared from the literature in recent years as it has been replaced by the more detailed subcategories such as low-grade myxofibrosarcoma, fibrosarcoma arising in dermatofibrosarcoma protuberans, and sclerosing epithelioid fibrosarcoma. Infantile fibrosarcoma is still considered to be a distinct clinicopathological entity.

The remaining lesions in this range of tumors exhibit pleomorphism and are composed of myofibroblasts and histioid cells and are now divided into four different forms of malignant fibrous histiocytoma (MFH) according to the predominant cellular configuration, namely: (1) inflammatory MFH (mainly from retroperitoneum), (2) giant cell–rich MFH, (3) storiform pleomorphic type of MFH (pleomorphic sarcoma not otherwise specified), and (4) myxoid MFH.

Incidence

Despite the recent changes outlined above, this group of rare sarcomas are still considered to be the second most common soft tissue sarcoma after rhabdomyosarcoma in the head and neck. They occur in all age groups from infants to the elderly, with an approximate 3:2 female-to-male ratio. The term infantile fibrosarcoma is applied to pediatric patients up to the age of 2 years, whereas older children come under the term adult type fibrosarcoma.[4]

In our series, we have treated 23 patients, 15 men and 8 women, aged between 23 and 75 years, with a mean of 50 years (Table 8.6).

Site

Most fibrosarcomas have been described originating in one or more paranasal sinuses, while presentation in the nasal cavity itself is less common. The infantile type of fibrosarcoma is very rare within the sinonasal area, with only a single case being described from 67 cases evaluated by Heffner and Gnepp from the Armed Forces Institute of Pathology USA in 1991.[5]

The majority of our cases arose in the maxilla or antro-ethmoid region (65%), with a few cases affecting the frontal sinus, ethmoids, nasal septum, and orbit (Table 8.6; Fig. 8.6).

Diagnostic Features

Clinical Features

Almost all patients in the larger series present with nasal obstruction, often associated with epistaxis; and as a consequence of the sinus involvement swelling of the cheek, facial numbness, facial masses, proptosis, orbital cellulitis, palatal swelling, loosening of the teeth, and pain have all been described, although the latter is relatively uncommon. While these tumors can affect any age, their commonest presentation is in the 4th to 6th decades.

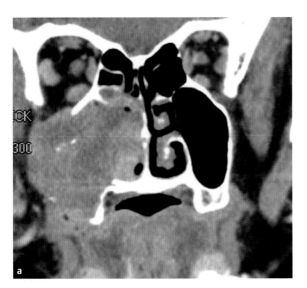

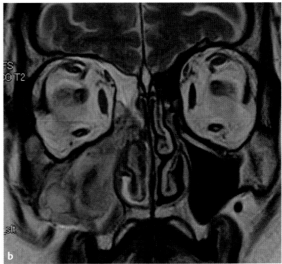

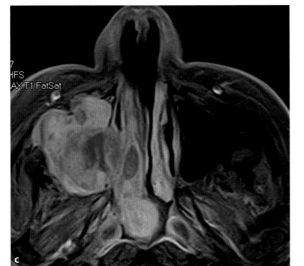

Fig. 8.6a–c

a Fibrosarcoma. Coronal CT scan showing a mass arising in the maxilla and eroding through all adjacent walls.

b Coronal MRI (T1W fat saturation) in the same patient showing a heterogeneous mass with pseudocapsule.

c Axial MRI (T1W fat saturation) in the same patient.

On examination, the tumors vary significantly but can be smooth, nodular, or pedunculated; classically, they have the appearance of a homogeneous, firm, white mass that, although essentially nonencapsulated, may have a pseudo-capsule of compressed surrounding tissues. The larger tumors may fungate or ulcerate with necrotic and hemorrhagic areas. As many fibrosarcoma variants are generally low grade, lymph node metastases are not common at presentation, but the higher-grade sarcomas produce lymph node involvement in up to 15% of cases, with distant metastases varying between 25% and 35% of the cases presented in recent reports (see Malignant Fibrous Histiocytoma below).

Imaging

There are no particular characteristics of either fibrosarcoma or malignant fibrous histiocytoma on CT or MRI imaging, generally showing heterogeneous soft tissue masses with attenuation similar to that of muscle on CT and intermediate in single intensity on T1W MRI. No evidence of adipose tissue is seen and the lesions show heterogeneous enhancement following the administration of intravenous contrast on CT or MRI. The masses may appear relatively well defined with bony expansion and a false capsule (**Fig. 8.6**).

Histological Features

Although they are often well circumscribed, the tumors are nonencapsulated and often infiltrative, depending on their grade. As most sinonasal area fibrosarcomas are low grade, the spindle cells are arranged in compact fascicles that are separated by various amounts of keloidlike collagen. The cell bundles may be arranged in herringbone or chevron patterns with additional areas of fasciculation. Surface epithelium may be invaginated into the tumor, giving rise to the false impression of an inverted papilloma. In the low-grade lesions nuclear pleomorphism is usually minimal, but there is marked variability within and between tumors and mitotic figures vary considerably. Areas of osteocartilage differentiation may occur in addition to areas of myxoid degeneration, hemorrhage, and necrosis. **An important practical point from Heffner and Gnepp's clinicopathological study of 67 cases[5] is that when adjacent normal tissue was present in a biopsy specimen, the tumor often merged gradually with the normal stroma, producing areas of decreased cellularity that would be difficult to discern as neoplastic if these areas were the only ones present in a biopsy. This reminds us yet again that biopsy material must be adequate and representative to assist with these difficult tumors.**

Immunohistochemical Features

Essentially, the formal conventional fibrosarcoma is now a diagnosis of exclusion, as immunohistochemically tumors with myofibroblastic differentiation can display several phenotypes because myofibroblasts share characteristics with both fibroblasts and smooth muscle cells.[6] Fibrosarcomas are stated to be always positive for vimentin and on occasion positive to desmin, muscle-specific actin, and smooth muscle myosin heavy chain.[7]

Differential Diagnosis

The differential diagnosis in this difficult area includes malignant fibrous histiocytoma, spindle cell carcinoma, spindle malignant melanoma, malignant peripheral nerve sheath tumor, monophasic synovial sarcoma, rhabdomyosarcoma, glomangiopericytoma, desmoid-type fibromatosis, and nodular fasciitis.[5,8]

Natural History

As a consequence of the continual and recently expanding classification of these tumors, it is difficult to make precise comments on the widely varying natural history, but certainly the clinical behavior of tumors previously collected under the heading of fibrosarcoma is characterized by a tendency to high local recurrence rates, but with the already stated low incidence of local regional lymph node and distant metastases, particularly in the low-grade lesions. With the higher-grade lesions, distant metastases have been described presenting in the lungs, mediastinum, and bone. The local recurrence rate in the past may have been related to both inadequate imaging and inadequate treatment. Certainly, in the more recent reports, the prognosis has been shown to be more favorable than previously thought, particularly for the lower grade of lesions, as a consequence of improved wide local excision rather than as a consequence of additional radiotherapy and chemotherapy. Four prognostic factors reported to date include male sex, the initial tumor size (which clearly relates to involvement of nasal cavity sinus and multiple adjacent areas), high histological grade, and positive surgical margins.

Treatment

Surgery remains the treatment of choice and not only is modern craniofacial and skull base surgery more effective at removing these lesions, but with bicoronal and midfacial degloving type approaches the morbidity is low and the cosmesis is excellent. Overall long-term survival of 75% has been reported in low-grade and relatively localized tumors. **Local recurrence remains a common finding in the literature and underlines the possibility of incomplete removal as it is essentially residual disease.**[5,9]

The majority of our cases were treated primarily with surgery, which ranged from maxillectomies of varying extent (15 patients, 65%) to craniofacial (4, 17%), and included orbital clearance in 31%. Nine patients (39%) received radiotherapy and 4 (17%) additional chemotherapy (**Table 8.6**). Eight died of disease between 2 and 6 years from treatment, 2 died of intercurrent disease, 7 survived with follow-up between 5 and 22 years (mean 11.1 years), but 6 were lost to follow-up so that statistical analysis is not possible.

Infantile Fibrosarcoma

Most infantile fibrosarcomas present in the extremities and the prognosis appears to be significantly better than that of adult fibrosarcoma because the incidence of local recurrence and overall rate of metastases are lower.[10–13] Isolated sinonasal and nasopharyngeal cases have been treated by total surgical excision via nasal, transpalatal, and intraoral approaches with good long-term cure.[10,12,13]

Key Points

- Many of the tumors previously classified as fibrosarcoma can now be more accurately determined to be a wide range of other benign and malignant lesions.
- Fibrosarcomas linked to previous irradiation are now placed in a separate group.
- The term "infantile fibrosarcoma" applies only to children up to the age of 2 years.
- Although appearing well-circumscribed, the tumors are nonencapsulated and infiltrative.
- Modern skull base surgery gives good long-term survival in low-grade tumors, but local recurrence remains a problem.

References

1. Huber GF, Matthews TW, Dort JC. Soft-tissue sarcomas of the head and neck: a retrospective analysis of the Alberta experience 1974 to 1999. Laryngoscope 2006;116(5):780–785
2. Johnston R. Sarcomata of the nasal septum. Laryngoscope 1904;14:454–473
3. Portela J. Fibrosarcoma envahissant des fosses nasales des deux sinus maxillaires, de l'ethmoide et des deux sinus sphenoidaux. Revue Laryngol 1927;48:530–531
4. Cecchetto G, Carli M, Alaggio R, et al; Italian Cooperative Group. Fibrosarcoma in pediatric patients: results of the Italian Cooperative Group studies (1979–1995). J Surg Oncol 2001;78(4):225–231
5. Heffner DK, Gnepp DR. Sinonasal fibrosarcomas, malignant schwannomas, and "Triton" tumors. A clinicopathologic study of 67 cases. Cancer 1992;70(5):1089–1101
6. Antonescu CR, Baren A. Spectrum of low-grade fibrosarcomas: a comparative ultrastructural analysis of low-grade myxofibrosarcoma and fibromyxoid sarcoma. Ultrastruct Pathol 2004;28(5-6):321–332
7. Hansen T, Katenkamp K, Brodhun M, Katenkamp D. Low-grade fibrosarcoma—report on 39 not otherwise specified cases and comparison with defined low-grade fibrosarcoma types. Histopathology 2006;49(2):152–160
8. Sheng WQ, Hashimoto H, Okamoto S, et al. Expression of COL1A1-PDGFB fusion transcripts in superficial adult fibrosarcoma suggests a close relationship to dermatofibrosarcoma protuberans. J Pathol 2001;194(1):88–94
9. Spiro JD, Soo KC, Spiro RH. Nonsquamous cell malignant neoplasms of the nasal cavities and paranasal sinuses. Head Neck 1995;17(2):114–118
10. Chung EB, Enzinger FM. Infantile fibrosarcoma. Cancer 1976;38(2):729–739
11. Swain RE, Sessions DG, Ogura JH. Fibrosarcoma of the head and neck in children. Laryngoscope 1976;86(1):113–116
12. Smith MC, Soames JV. Fibrosarcoma of the ethmoid. J Laryngol Otol 1989;103(7):686–689
13. Kim KI, Yoo SL. Infantile fibrosarcoma in the nasal cavity. Otolaryngol Head Neck Surg 1996;114(1):98–102

Malignant Fibrous Histiocytoma

Definition

The term "malignant fibrous histiocytoma" (MFH) was introduced in the 1960s to describe a group of lesions with essentially mixed fibroblastic and histiocytic components. It has subsequently been a controversial and difficult area of pathology with the terminology being questioned significantly by the 1980s.[1] Brooks was the first to suggest that MFH was not necessarily a distinct tumor entity but represented a common pathway for tumor progression to other well-defined entities. Subsequently, additional studies by Dehner in 1988,[2] Fletcher in 1992[3] and 2001,[4] Oda in 2002[5] and Nascimento in 2008,[6] seriously called into question whether or not MFH is a distinct clinicopathological entity or whether it should be replaced by the term "pleomorphic sarcoma." **These reports deal with several hundred cases, with up to two-thirds of them being reclassified as other sarcomas; and 13%[3,4] could in fact be reclassified as nonmesenchymal neoplasms.** However, the 2005 WHO[7] classification of malignant soft tissue tumors of the head and neck with reference to the sinonasal area still includes the term malignant fibrous histiocytoma, although it states that it remains in use as a **diagnosis of exclusion** for sarcomas composed largely of myofibroblasts or undifferentiated mesenchymal cells (ICD-O code 8830/3).

Etiology

There is a strong link between both sinonasal and nasopharyngeal malignant fibrous histiocytomas in relation to previous radiation but with a substantial latency period between the treatment and onset of disease.[8,9]

Synonyms

Malignant fibrous xanthoma, fibroxanthosarcoma, myxoid malignant fibrous histiocytoma, myxofibrosarcoma.

Incidence

Initially MFH was thought to be one of the most common soft tissue sarcomas, but with the constant reclassification the oldest studies are somewhat unreliable in terms of figures. Overall, somewhere between 1 and 3% of all MFHs have been reported as occurring in the head and neck and approximately one-third of these arise in the sinonasal area. With the increasing use of the term "pleomorphic sarcoma," these lesions are a group of high-grade sarcomas that at present are not classified elsewhere (see Introduction to mesenchymal tumors', p. 175).

Site

The maxillary sinus appears to be the most commonly affected area, followed by the ethmoid sinuses and nasal cavity. Lesions in the frontal and sphenoid sinuses are comparatively rare. In our series of 6 cases, 5 affected the maxillary sinus together with the ethmoids in 3 cases and the orbit in 2. The nasal septum was the site of only one lesion (Table 8.7).

Diagnostic Features

Clinical Features

The tumors occur more commonly in men than in women and particularly in older age groups; indeed, all the discussed subtypes of MFH generally occur in patients over 50 years of age. This has been our experience with 5 men and 1 woman, their ages ranging from 46 to 81 years with a mean of 59.5 years.

The most common presentation is that of a painless, enlarging mass; with the commonest site of origin being the maxilla, swelling of the cheek, facial pain, and problems with dentition frequently accompany the usual common symptoms of nasal obstruction and epistaxis. As with patients presenting with the variants of fibrosarcoma, tumor masses are generally smooth, pedunculated, or polypoidal but with a fleshy, homogeneous white/yellow/pink mass that tends to have more necrotic and hemorrhagic areas in contradistinction to the lower-grade variants of fibrosarcoma. MFH commonly extends into the orbit, skull base, nasopharynx, and pituitary fossa; and while regional lymph nodes are rarely involved (less than 18% of cases in recent reports), metastatic spread to lungs, bone, and liver are all reported with increasing frequency depending on the grade of tumor.

Imaging

As covered in the section on fibrosarcoma (p. 178), imaging of MFH is indistinguishable from fibrosarcoma, although lesions may be considerably larger in relation to the higher grade of tumor and extension into orbit, skull base, and intracranial fossa. The spread to cervical nodes may be evaluated by CT or ultrasound and, because of the possibility of distant metastases in the larger higher-grade lesions, PET scanning should be considered prior to any biopsy if at all possible, although more commonly this is undertaken prior to definitive treatment following histological diagnosis.

Histological Features and Differential Diagnosis

While MFH can occasionally be circumscribed in a similar fashion to lower-grade fibrosarcomas, MFH is usually infiltrative and often ulcerative. The majority of cases are of the storiform-pleomorphic type or myxoid variants (myxoid malignant fibrous histiocytoma) rather than the inflammatory or giant cell–rich variants that occur elsewhere in the body. The storiform-pleomorphic type is the most common form of MFH to occur in the sinonasal tract and the cells arranged in this pattern have a fusiform shape with multiple, easily identified mitotic figures, including atypical forms. Tumor giant cells with multiple nuclei are often found and there may be significant areas of necrosis.

On immunohistochemistry, while MFH is usually positive for vimentin and focally for actins, it is further differentiated from other tumors by a process of exclusion and is generally negative for specific markers for skeletal muscle, S100 protein, desmin, HMB-45, and

Table 8.7 Malignant fibrous histiocytoma: personal series

Age/sex	Site	Management	Long-term follow-up
46/M	Antroethmoid	Craniofacial resection	A&W 7 y
48/M	Maxilla and orbit	Total maxillectomy 1981, craniofacial resection and orbital clearance, radiotherapy	DOD 37 mo
54/M	Antroethmoid	Partial maxillectomy and orbital clearance 1986, craniofacial resection 1987	A&W 9 y 9 mo
55/M	Maxilla and orbit	Total maxillectomy and orbital clearance	Lost
73/M	Nasal septum	Endoscopic resection	A&W 3 y
81/F	Antroethmoid	Partial maxillectomy	DOD 3 mo
Abbreviations: A&W, alive and well; DOD, dead of disease; F, female; M, male; mo, month(s); y, year(s).			

lymphoid and epithelial markers. This immunohistochemical analysis is important to differentiate between the variants of fibrosarcoma, rhabdomyosarcoma, leiomyosarcoma, monophasic synovial sarcoma, malignant peripheral nerve sheath tumors, spindle cell carcinoma, spindle cell malignant melanoma, and anaplastic large cell lymphoma.

Natural History and Treatments

Reliable figures for the modern treatment of MFH are bedeviled by the numerous recent changes in the histopathological classification of these lesions and the continuing controversy as to whether or not it represents a particular entity. Historically, over the past 40 years, surgery has been considered to be the treatment of choice, with wide resection advocated because of the known fact that the higher-grade lesions have a tendency to spread along facial planes and muscle fascicles well beyond the confines of the presumed edge of the lesion. Radiotherapy and chemotherapy alone are not effective, although both have been used in patients with seemingly higher-grade lesions. Chemotherapeutic agents that have been tried include Adriamycin (doxorubicin hydrochloride),[10] cyclophosphamide, actinomycin D, vincristine, dacarbazine, and ifosfamide. However, neither radiotherapy nor chemotherapy offers significant control if patients have local recurrence after inadequate surgical treatment.[11] In his excellent review of 2008, Rapidis reports survival to be ~60% at 2 years, with a high incidence of recurrent disease (44%) and metastases (44%) for MFH of the head and neck.[12]

In our own small cohort of patients, who were treated between 1981 and 2004, surgery has been the mainstay including maxillectomy (partial or total in 4 cases), craniofacial resection,[3] orbital clearance[2] and most recently endoscopic resection of a relatively small lesion on the nasal septum (**Table 8.7**). Radiotherapy was only given to one individual with very aggressive disease, without effect. Three are alive and well (at 3–9.75 years), 2 have died of disease at 3 and 37 months, and one has been lost to follow-up.

Key Points

- The term "malignant fibrous histiocytoma" remains in use as a diagnosis of exclusion for sarcomas composed largely of myofibroblasts or undifferentiated mesenchymal cells.
- It is doubtful whether it is a distinct tumor entity and may be a common pathway to other better-defined sarcomas.
- Immunohistochemistry is important in the differentiation of this condition from a wide variety of malignant tumors.
- Surgery remains the treatment of choice.

References

1. Brooks JJ. The significance of double phenotypic patterns and markers in human sarcomas. A new model of mesenchymal differentiation. Am J Pathol 1986;125(1):113–123
2. Dehner LP. Malignant fibrous histiocytoma. Nonspecific morphologic pattern, specific pathologic entity, or both? Arch Pathol Lab Med 1988;112(3):236–237
3. Fletcher CD. Pleomorphic malignant fibrous histiocytoma: fact or fiction? A critical reappraisal based on 159 tumors diagnosed as pleomorphic sarcoma. Am J Surg Pathol 1992;16(3):213–228
4. Fletcher CD, Gustafson P, Rydholm A, Willén H, Akerman M. Clinicopathologic re-evaluation of 100 malignant fibrous histiocytomas: prognostic relevance of subclassification. J Clin Oncol 2001;19(12):3045–3050
5. Oda Y, Tamiya S, Oshiro Y, et al. Reassessment and clinicopathological prognostic factors of malignant fibrous histiocytoma of soft parts. Pathol Int 2002;52(9):595–606
6. Nascimento AF, Raut CP. Diagnosis and management of pleomorphic sarcomas (so-called "MFH") in adults. J Surg Oncol 2008;97(4):330–339
7. Barnes L, Eveson J, Reichart P, Sidransky D. Tumours of the nasal cavity and paranasal sinuses. In: Barnes L, Eveson J, Reichart P, Sidransky D, eds. World Health Organization Classification of Tumours. Pathology and Genetics of Head and Neck Tumours. Lyon: IARC Press; 2005:36
8. Ireland AJ, Eveson JW, Leopard PJ. Malignant fibrous histiocytoma: a report of two cases arising in sites of previous irradiation. Br J Oral Maxillofac Surg 1988;26(3):221–227
9. Ko JY, Chen CL, Lui LT, Hsu MM. Radiation-induced malignant fibrous histiocytoma in patients with nasopharyngeal carcinoma. Arch Otolaryngol Head Neck Surg 1996;122(5):535–538
10. Sabesan T, Xuexi W, Yongfa Q, Pingzhang T, Ilankovan V. Malignant fibrous histiocytoma: outcome of tumours in the head and neck compared with those in the trunk and extremities. Br J Oral Maxillofac Surg 2006;44(3):209–212
11. Barnes L, Kanbour A. Malignant fibrous histiocytoma of the head and neck. A report of 12 cases. Arch Otolaryngol Head Neck Surg 1988;114(10):1149–1156
12. Rapidis AD. Sarcomas of the head and neck in adult patients: current concepts and future perspectives. Expert Rev Anticancer Ther 2008;8(8):1271–1297

Synovial Sarcoma

Synovial sarcomas are highly invasive tumors that occur almost exclusively in the extremities of the upper and lower limbs, but ~3% of them have been reported in the head and neck region[1] (ICD-O code 9040/3).

Synovial cell sarcoma is not included in the WHO histological classification of tumors of the nasal cavity and paranasal sinuses (2005),[2] but primary synovial cell sarcomas have been described in maxillofacial sites.[3] These lesions are termed "synovial sarcoma" because of their histological resemblance to the synovium, but as they appear in locations usually unrelated to the synovium they are generally assumed to arise from an undifferentiated mesenchymal stem cell.

Total surgical excision is at present the most appropriate treatment, but postoperative radiation therapy has been advocated for tumors in the head and neck region with large doses of 65 Gy or more being recommended.[4,5]

There does not appear to be any effective chemotherapeutic regime at present, although multidrug chemotherapy using doxorubicin and ifosfamide has been attempted, but distant metastasis remains the predominant cause of death.[6] We have treated one patient, a woman aged 41 years who presented with an ethmoidal lesion that had spread extensively into the infratemporal fossa and who succumbed to her disease despite radical surgical excision.

References

1. Bukawa H, Kawabata A, Murano A, et al. Monophasic epithelial synovial sarcoma arising in the temporomandibular joint. Int J Oral Maxillofac Surg 2007;36(8):762–765
2. Barnes L, Eveson J, Reichert P, Sidransky D, eds. World Health Organization Classification of Tumours. Pathology and Genetics of Head and Neck Tumours. Lyon: IARC Press; 2005
3. Wang H, Zhang J, He X, Niu Y. Synovial sarcoma in the oral and maxillofacial region: report of 4 cases and review of the literature. J Oral Maxillofac Surg 2008;66(1):161–167
4. Guadagnolo BA, Zagars GK, Ballo MT, et al. Long-term outcomes for synovial sarcoma treated with conservation surgery and radiotherapy. Int J Radiat Oncol Biol Phys 2007;69(4):1173–1180
5. Khademi B, Mohammadianpanah M, Ashraf MJ, Yeganeh F. Synovial sarcoma of the parapharyngeal space. Auris Nasus Larynx 2007;34(1):125–129
6. Paulino AC. Synovial sarcoma prognostic factors and patterns of failure. Am J Clin Oncol 2004;27(2):122–127

Alveolar Soft Part Sarcoma

Definition

(ICD-O code 9581/3)

Alveolar soft part sarcoma (ASPS) comprises rare soft tissue malignancies that can occur in the upper respiratory tract and orbit, affecting younger patients.

Incidence and Clinical Features

ASPS is rare even among soft tissue sarcomas, constituting less than 1%.[1] It most often presents between 15 and 35 years but can occur at any age. There is said to be a female preponderance before 30 years of age and a slight male preponderance thereafter. There are a small number of case reports in the literature[2-7] and we have treated 5 patients aged 5 to 23 years, 3 female and 2 male (Table 8.8), so this does not offer any corroboration on this issue.

The tumor may present clinically with a firm and apparently encapsulated mass that is often relatively slow growing. Nasal obstruction may occur in the nasal cavity; in the orbital lesions proptosis and swelling of the lids and face result. **Unfortunately, metastases are an early feature of the disease, with lesions in the brain or lung commonly found**.

The lesion is rather vascular, so in addition to the mass effect and bone erosion of any malignant tumor, contrast-CT and MRI show high signal intensity (Fig. 8.7).[8]

Site

Classically the limbs are affected, in particular the deep tissues of the thigh. In the head and neck the tumor has a predilection for the tongue and orbit, and in our cases four originated in the orbit and one arose on the middle turbinate (Table 8.8).

Diagnostic Features

Histological Features, Immunohistochemical Features, and Differential Diagnosis

Histologically the tumors have a characteristic nested appearance of large epithelioid cells with abundant eosinophilic granular cytoplasm arranged in nests of around 50 cells surrounded by septations of fibrous tissue, which

Table 8.8 Alveolar soft part sarcoma: personal series

Age/sex	Presenting lesion	Site	Management	Long-term follow-up
5/M	Orbital mass	Orbit	Chemotherapy, orbital clearance, radiotherapy	A&W 2 y
15/F	Nasal obstruction	Middle turbinate	Endoscopic resection	A&W 10 y
21/F	Nasal obstruction, proptosis, bilateral lymphadenopathy	Orbit, nasal cavity	Surgical excision and radiotherapy	DOD 18 mo
21/M	Proptosis	Orbit	Orbital clearance	A&W 20 y
23/F	Orbital mass	Orbit	Lateral craniotomy, orbital clearance	A&W 12 y

Abbreviations: A&W, alive and well; DOD, dead of disease; F, female; M, male; mo, month(s); y, year(s).

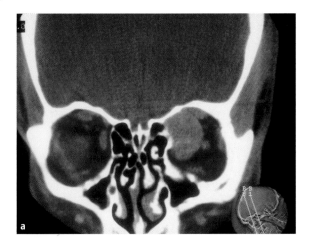

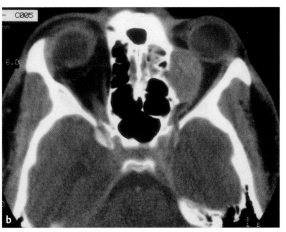

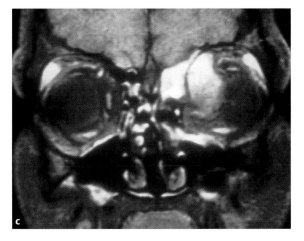

Fig. 8.7a–c

a Alveolar soft part sarcoma. Coronal CT scan showing a mass in the upper medial orbit.

b Axial CT scan in the same patient.

c Coronal MRI (T1W with gadolinium enhancement) in the same patient showing high signal from the mass, and inflamed mucosa in the adjacent ethmoid and lacrimal glands.

creates the "alveolar" appearance. The cells themselves are large and have a granular eosinophilic cytoplasm. They have limited immunoreactivity with antibodies to vimentin, S100 protein, and myogenous antibodies such as desmin, MyoD1, and actins. Electron microscopy is still sometimes used as it shows characteristic crystalloid structures.[9]

The differential diagnosis includes malignant melanoma and clear cell carcinomas such as renal carcinoma metastatic to the ethmoid. Again immunohistochemistry will help make the distinction.[10]

Treatment and Outcome

Treatment has usually consisted of combined surgery with radiotherapy ± chemotherapy depending on the extent of disease and the enthusiasms of the multidisciplinary team. In our small cohort the orbital cases were submitted to orbital clearance and in one case craniofacial resection, whereas the case affecting the middle turbinate was resected endoscopically. Radiotherapy was given in three cases, the youngest patient with the most extensive disease received additional chemotherapy and, as none had metastases at presentation, happily all but the 5-year-old survived long term with follow-up in excess of 8 years (**Table 8.8**).

Sadly, due to the often late presentation, the overall outcome in the literature is frequently poor, although there are a few long-term survivors; this has been associated with a cytogenetic abnormality of t(X;17) (p11.2;q25) that juxtaposes the *TFE3* and *ASPL* genes.[11] Generally, if the tumor is completely excised prior to metastatic spread, cure may be achieved, but unfortunately metastases may appear many years later. Hence, in a study from the Sloan-Kettering Institute in New York, the survival rate for patients without metastases at diagnosis was 60% at 5 years but 38% at 10 years and 15% at 20 years.[12]

Lately, antiangiogenic combinations of monoclonal antibodies, e.g., becacizumab with celecoxib or the use of cedarinib, have been added to conventional regimes,[13,14] although there are no large trials as yet to support this practice.

In addition to metastatic spread, prognosis may be influenced by patient age and tumor size but not by histological features.[12]

References

1. Ordonez N, Ladanyl M. Alveolar soft part sarcoma. In: Fletcher C, Unni K, Mertens F, eds. WHO Classification of Tumours. Tumours of Soft Tissue and Bone. Pathology and Genetics. Lyon: IARC Press; 2002:208–210

2. Chatterji P, Purohit GN, Ramdev IN, Soni NK. Alveolar soft part sarcoma of the nasal cavity and paranasal sinuses. J Laryngol Otol 1977;91(11):1003–1008

3. Font RL, Jurco S III, Zimmerman LE. Alveolar soft-part sarcoma of the orbit: a clinicopathologic analysis of seventeen cases and a review of the literature. Hum Pathol 1982;13(6):569–579

4. Barbareschi M, Ferrero S, Ottaviani F. Alveolar soft part sarcoma of the nasal cavity. Pathologica 1988; 80(1067):363–370

5. Rubinstein MI, Drake AF, McClatchey KD. Alveolar soft part sarcoma of the nasal cavity: report of a case and a review of the literature. Laryngoscope 1988;98(11):1246–1250

6. Yigitbasi OG, Guney E, Kontas O, Somdas MA, Patiroglu T. Alveolar soft part sarcoma: report of a case occurring in the sinonasal region. Int J Pediatr Otorhinolaryngol 2004;68(10):1333–1337

7. Dezanzo P, Lifschitz-Mercer B, Czernobilsky B, Rosai J. Alveolar soft-part sarcoma of paranasal sinuses. Int J Surg Pathol 2010;18(1):66–67

8. Lorigan JG, O'Keeffe FN, Evans HL, Wallace S. The radiologic manifestations of alveolar soft-part sarcoma. AJR Am J Roentgenol 1989;153(2):335–339

9. Welsh RA, Bray DM III, Shipkey FH, Meyer AT. Histogenesis of alveolar soft part sarcoma. Cancer 1972;29(1):191–204

10. Fisher C. Immunohistochemistry in diagnosis of soft tissue tumours. Histopathology 2011;58(7):1001–1012

11. Argani P, Lal P, Hutchinson B, Lui MY, Reuter VE, Ladanyi M. Aberrant nuclear immunoreactivity for TFE3 in neoplasms with TFE3 gene fusions: a sensitive and specific immunohistochemical assay. Am J Surg Pathol 2003;27(6):750–761

12. Lieberman PH, Brennan MF, Kimmel M, Erlandson RA, Garin-Chesa P, Flehinger BY. Alveolar soft-part sarcoma. A clinico-pathologic study of half a century. Cancer 1989;63(1):1–13

13. Conde N, Cruz O, Albert A, Mora J. Antiangiogenic treatment as a pre-operative management of alveolar soft-part sarcoma. Pediatr Blood Cancer 2011;57(6):1071–1073

14. Subbiah V, Kurzrock R. Phase 1 clinical trials for sarcomas: the cutting edge. Curr Opin Oncol 2011;23(4):352–360

9 Vasoform Neoplasms and Other Lesions

Hemangioma and Vascular Malformations

Despite the fact that a sensible biological classification system based on studies correlating physical findings, natural history, and cellular features was described by Mulliken and Glowacki in 1982,[1] the confusion in the literature with regard to these lesions has been considerable and the terminology remains a problem among a whole generation of physicians and surgeons.

There are only two major types of vascular lesions: (1) tumors and (2) malformations. The term "hemangioma" is still all too frequently used indiscriminately and incorrectly and applied to vascular lesions that are completely different in behavior and histopathology. Perhaps the worst "culprit" is the term "cavernous hemangioma," which is usually a venous malformation and only very rarely a deep hemangioma.

Hemangiomas Versus Vascular Malformations

There is continuing controversy between some clinicians and pathologists over the difficult issues involved in separating hemangiomas from vascular malformations. Essentially, **hemangiomas** are composed of excessive amounts of proliferating benign endothelial cells, producing vascular channels that are similar to normal blood vessels. There is a pericyte around each of these endothelium-lined channels but there are simply too many vessels per unit area in comparison with normal tissue. In contrast, **vascular malformations**, which have in the past often had the term hemangioma applied to them, are not proliferative lesions but are due to abnormal developments of blood vessels. While they may hypertrophy over a period of time and thereby enlarge, they are not actually neoplastic. These malformations may comprise a single type of vessel (capillary, arterial, venous, lymphatic) or be a combination. Malformations with an arterial component are usually fast-flow, while the other types are slow-flow.

While hemangioma is by far the most common vascular tumor, with ~60% occurring in the head and neck, almost entirely in infants, other rarities include tufted angioma, glomangiopericytoma, angiofibroma, and angiosarcoma.

Very rarely there are exceptions to this clear classification scheme. For example, a "pyogenic granuloma," which is correctly a small acquired vascular tumor, may occur in an area of capillary or venous malformation.

Papillary Endothelial Hyperplasia

Another vascular variant is endothelial hyperplasia, which may occur as a consequence of stimulation by trauma, ischemia, clotting, embolization, or hormonal influences and can develop in normal vessels anywhere in the body. It has been described in the paranasal sinuses.[2] It is a completely benign process and is essentially a distinct form of organizing thrombus that is covered by a thin layer of benign endothelial cells and contains multiple hyaline nodules. It is treated effectively (if necessary) by simple local excision.

Hemangiomas

While the purpose of this book is to describe conditions of the nose and paranasal sinuses, many hemangiomas and vascular anomalies extensively involve the head and neck, covering many anatomical areas. **History and careful examination of the head and neck can distinguish between vascular tumors and vascular malformations in over 90% of cases. Imprecise and incorrect terminology must be avoided**.

The site, incidence, and clinical features of a particular hemangioma depend on the subtype of hemangioma.
- Capillary hemangioma
  - Hemangioma of infancy
  - Acquired lobular capillary hemangioma
  - Cherry "senile" hemangioma
- Acquired "tufted" angioma
- Intramuscular angioma
- Vascular malformations
  - Venous
  - Lymphatic
  - Capillary

Hemangioma of Infancy

Approximately 60% of these lesions occur in the head and neck and they are up to 3 times more common in females than males.[3] The commonest site in the upper airways is the subglottic portion of the larynx and this may result in stridor and life-threatening airway obstruction.[4] Hemangiomas of infancy have also been reported in the sinonasal tract[5,6] and on the dorsum of the nose.[7]

Diagnostic Features

Clinical Features

These lesions appear at, or shortly after, birth and are the most common tumor in childhood. Single lesions are most common but multiple lesions occur in up to 20% of cases. The lesions progress rapidly, forming prominent, reddish purple nodules that achieve a somewhat rubbery texture as they enlarge ("strawberry" nevus). These lesions begin to regress spontaneously in most cases after the age of 1 year, although this may occur earlier. About half of all patients will have almost complete regression of the lesion by 5 years and virtually all by 12 years of age.[8] The clinical history of these patients is an important aspect in the clinical diagnosis and usually contrasts significantly with other vascular malformations that may be present at birth but have no sex predilection and grow or hypertrophy slowly, without any tendency to involution.

The onset and cause of involution in hemangiomas does not seem to be influenced by the time of onset or duration of the proliferative phase, or by sex, race, site, or overall duration.

Hemangioma of infancy has been associated with multiple cervicofacial hemangiomas.[9] Multiple hemangiomas of infancy may also be associated with visceral hemangiomatosis.[10]

Imaging

Imaging of these hemangiomas does not show any particular features of note other than those of an enhancing soft tissue mass, but it does allow evaluation of the extent of the lesion and some differential from the more typical pathognomonic imaging features of other types of vascular malformations.

Histological Features

Grossly, these lesions vary from tan through red to purple, irregular nodules that are separated from the adjacent dermal and subcutaneous tissues. Initially, during the growth phase, they are composed of cytologically bland, short, spindled cells that are endothelial cells and pericytes forming tight groups of capillaries with minimal lumina. There is obvious mitotic activity and often a prominent, overall "jigsawlike" pattern. There may be associated mast cells within an inflammatory component.

As the lesions mature, the lumen of the vascular channels become more obvious but fibrosis and reduction of the number of vessels commences. Over the long term, with increasing fibrosis, the end result is a fibrofatty residual structure with varying numbers of scattered capillaries.

Immunohistochemical Features

Considerable additional help in diagnosis has been provided by the finding that the cells of hemangioma of infancy characteristically express glucose transporter protein isoform I (GLUT-1).[11] In addition, the pericytes around the endothelium-lined channels are positive for SMA (smooth muscle actin).

Differential Diagnosis

The main area of difficulty with hemangioma of infancy, is where it requires separation from so-called "cavernous hemangiomas," of which the vast majority are venous malformations that clinically do not have the striking appearance of the fully developed hemangioma of infancy and whose dilated large vascular channels with mitotically inactive epithelial cells do not show signs of resolution and do not exhibit expression of GLUT 1. Glomangiopericytomas may occur in infancy but strong GLUT 1 expression would assist with separation of the lesions.

Treatment and Prognosis

Counseling

The value of counseling cannot be overemphasized. Good rapport at a first visit is essential, with adequate time to have a full discussion with the parents. Hemangiomas often present weeks after birth in previously normal, healthy children. Parental fears, frustrations, and misinformation are common. Photographs are essential and accurate information from a coordinated professional team is paramount.

Observation

These rare lesions in the sinonasal tract may not require any treatment as they undergo spontaneous involution. Therefore, most small hemangiomas should simply be observed through their period of proliferation and involution and over 50% will leave normal or only slightly blemished skin of the nose and adjacent face.

Corticosteroids

Corticosteroids, both topical and intralesional, for the smaller lesions are usually the first line of medical therapy, with a response rate of more than 90% of individuals.[12] Systemic corticosteroids may be the first line of treatment for problematic, airway-encroaching lesions. Doses of prednisolone of 2 to 3 mg/kg/day may be required, with gradual tapering of the dose over one year. Rebound growth can occur.

Laser Therapy

Laser therapy has been used but does not seem to have any particularly beneficial effect on reducing the growth rate in the initial phase of the lesions.[13]

Chemotherapy

Interferon alfa therapy has been used in large, extensive lesions involving the face and associated orbital and sinonasal structures. It has a response rate of ~50% but has potential neurological complications limiting its use as a first-line treatment.[14] Vincristine has been used as an alternative.[15]

Irradiation is not indicated.

Propranolol

This nonselective β-blocker appears to have a vasoconstrictive action and downregulates angiogenic factors such as VEGF and bFGF. It also appears to upregulate the apoptosis of capillary endothelial cells and reduces the proliferative phase. It has potential cardiovascular side effects but looks, at present, to be replacing steroids in the management of these infants.[16]

Surgical Treatment of Hemangiomas of Infancy Involving the Nasal Dorsum

This controversial topic requires considerable care in assessing and treating both the child and the parents. The vast majority of hemangiomas involving the nose ± the adjacent cheeks or the interior of the nasal cavity, develop significantly in the weeks following birth. This naturally produces considerable anxiety and the desire to halt the process and achieve normality for the child. Considerable counseling is required for the parents and reassurance with regard to satisfactory regression with conservative treatment. However, even those that resolve may give rise to residual fibrofatty lesions in the cosmetically important area of the nose and degrees of residual deformity of the underlying nasal bones and cartilages.

Profound swelling of the nasal tip producing a bright red bulbous appearance is particularly disconcerting. Pitanguy and colleagues in 1996[7] presented a series of 33 patient with nasal tip hemangioma, with at least 85% of them having at least one surgical procedure commencing at an age as young as 7 months. They discuss the merits of a vertical midline approach on the dorsum of the nose but, while they define their final scars in the older children as giving satisfactory results, that was, to say the least, debatable.

There is no doubt that the major deformity of the large dorsal nasal hemangioma is distressing even for children as young as 3 or 4 years of age, and certainly once they commence any form of schooling. Intralesional or systemic steroids may be used on a monthly basis and laser treatment may be added if the lesion is flat and superficial, but the parents need to understand that it may not provide significant benefit if there is a notable, deeper component. Multiple laser sessions may be required. At present, the majority of experienced surgeons perform any necessary excision in the 3- to 5-year age group prior to them attending schooling. This gives the majority of hemangiomas of infancy time to commence involution and avoids unnecessary excision. Access by external rhinoplasty approaches and even midfacial degloving may remove the need for any notable additional scarring and allow for any augmentation procedures at a later date, particularly after the nose ceases to grow.

Acquired Lobular Capillary Hemangioma

Synonyms

These are many and varied, and a review of the older literature can be very confusing! The terms pyogenic granuloma, granuloma pyogenicum, capillary hemangioma, nasal granuloma gravidarum, epulis gravidarum, and cavernous hemangioma have all been used.

Site, Incidence, and Specific Clinical Features

These lesions commonly occur in the head and neck and the fingers, but in the sinonasal tract the septal mucosa, particularly Little's area, and the tip of the turbinates are the sites most often involved (**Fig. 9.1**). Again, some examples have been reported in the paranasal sinuses.[17] These lesions can occur at almost any age but with peaks noted in males younger than 18 years of age and females during their reproductive years. Many of these women are pregnant at the time of presentation and the lesion is referred to in past literature by a wide variety of names such as granuloma gravidarum. The nasal lesions most commonly present with epistaxis with or without accompanying nasal obstruction; they may additionally be ulcerated, but rarely painful (**Fig. 9.2**).

Histological Features and Differential Diagnosis

The lobular capillary hemangioma is the underlying lesion of virtually all these previously described pathologies named under "synonyms" above. It is an exophytic growth that may have surface ulceration and an inflammatory cell infiltration with lymphocytes, plasma cells, histiocytes, and neutrophils (i.e., granulation tissue–like changes). Beneath any surface ulceration there is a diagnostic lobular arrangement of capillaries at the base. The lobules consist of discrete clusters of endothelial cells

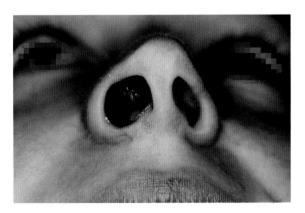

Fig. 9.1 Clinical photograph of acquired lobular capillary hemangioma arising from Little's area of the right nasal septum.

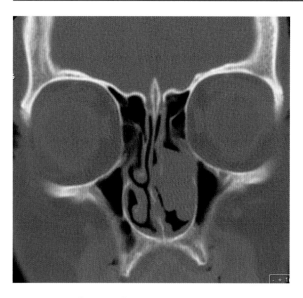

Fig. 9.2 Coronal CT scan showing an acquired lobulated capillary hemangioma of the left nasal cavity arising from the middle turbinate.

and the lumina vary from indistinct to prominent.[18] The lesion may be delineated at its periphery and base by an epithelial collar. With time, the lesion fibroses and the vessels reduce.

These histopathological changes are not observed in the infantile hemangioma and, immunohistochemically, GLUT 1 is not expressed.[11,19] The hemangioma of infancy and acquired lobular capillary hemangioma usually occur in different age groups and are distinguished clinically and histopathologically, but both must be differentiated on rare occasions from the naevus flammeus ("port wine stain") that presents at birth as a large, red, macular lesion. In the Sturge-Weber syndrome (see later), this is located in the distribution of the ophthalmic branch of the trigeminal nerve. In contrast to the two forms of hemangioma, naevus flammeus is a capillary vascular malformation.

Treatment and Prognosis

The marked variation in sex distribution that is seen in the larger reports of these lesions suggests a hormonal factor and certainly both progesterone and estrogen are known to alter the vascularity of the nasal mucosa.[20] Lobular capillary hemangiomas will spontaneously regress in pregnant women following delivery.[21] Trauma has been suggested as playing a role in the past but there is no strong evidence for this and when the lesions are fully excised by a variety of simple nasal surgical or endoscopic procedures, they do not recur. Recurrence is documented, however, with attempted reduction by cautery, electrocoagulation, or cryotherapy. The neodymium-YAG laser has the well-recognized advantages of precision and hemostasis for removing these local vascular lesions, but

the larger lesions on the lateral wall of the nose, involving particularly the anterior end of the turbinate, are still commonly pedunculated and can be excised endoscopically without notable difficulty.

Cherry ("Senile") Hemangioma

These skin lesions are most common on the trunk and upper limbs and usually present following puberty; they are asymptomatic lesions that gradually increase in size to form erythematous papules a few millimeters across. While they may occur in the head and neck, they have not been described in the sinonasal tract.[22]

Acquired "Tufted" Angioma

Acquired "tufted" angiomas present as dull red plaques or nodules that occur in the skin of the head and neck and upper trunk. They grow slowly and most commonly present in children by the age of 5 years. They are asymptomatic lesions that commonly regress, although more slowly than the hemangioma of infancy. They have *not* been described in the sinonasal tract. The histopathology of the nodules showing ectatic, thin-walled vessels forming a cellular tuft, usually in the middle and deep dermis, separates them clearly (along with the clinical history in most cases) from infantile hemangioma and acquired lobular capillary hemangioma.

Intramuscular Hemangioma

These rare vascular lesions arise within skeletal muscle, most commonly in adolescents and young adults of both sexes, and affect the lower extremities most commonly, followed by the head and neck. They have been recorded in the masseter muscle, trapezius, sternocleidomastoid, temporalis, and periorbital muscles.[23] They do not affect the sinonasal tract.

Vascular Malformations

Venous Malformations

Site, Incidence, and Clinical Features

Venous malformations are the most common type of vascular malformation and may be present at birth and in similar areas of the head and neck to the capillary hemangioma of infancy. However, they may become apparent in children and adults of all ages and occur in an almost equal male-to-female ratio. It is likely that **the majority of previously so-called cavernous hemangiomas are congenital venous vascular malformations due to abnormal vessel morphogenesis**. They do not grow and merely hypertrophy, increasing in size only as the individual grows. They show no evidence

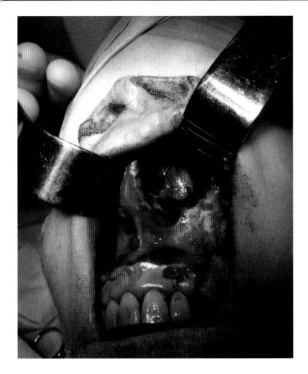

Fig. 9.3 Intraoperative photograph during midfacial degloving showing an intraosseous venous malformation affecting the left maxilla.

of regression with age and indeed may swell at times related to minor degrees of inflammation.

While they principally occur in skin and subcutaneous tissues and thereby involve the dorsum of the nose in some patients, venous malformations can also involve muscle and deeper structures of the larynx, all areas of the neck, oral cavity, skull base, central nervous system, temporal bones, sinonasal area, and orbit (**Figs. 9.3 and 9.4**). Cutaneous lesions appear as variable areas which are usually bluish and sometimes nodular and they blanch and compress with pressure. Equally, they may increase and expand notably during a Valsalva maneuver.

All deep extensive malformations involving the nose, sinuses, oropharynx, and larynx may compress and deviate the upper airway to cause insidious obstructive sleep apnea (**Figs. 9.5 and 9.6**). Cervical facial lesions are often unilateral, resulting in marked facial and neck asymmetry in addition to upper airway obstruction.

Intraorbital venous malformations may expand the orbital cavity and communicate to adjacent areas via the superior and inferior orbital fissures, thereby extending into the nose, sinuses, and adjacent regions. They may result in dependant exophthalmia or occasionally anophthalmia when the patient stands.

Multiple cavernous hemangiomas are associated with the autosomal dominant condition known as blue rubber bleb nevus syndrome.[24] With such an enormous range in the size and involvement of these lesions, adequate imaging is necessary for documenting their nature and extent.

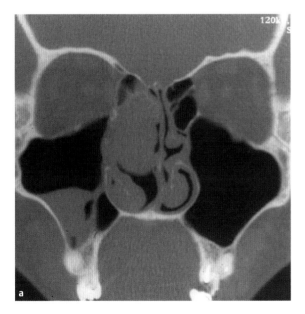

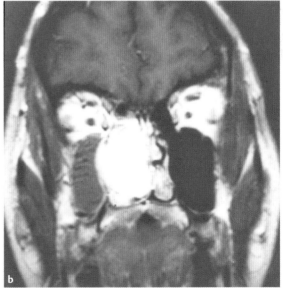

Fig. 9.4a, b

a Coronal CT scan showing a well-defined venous malformation.

b Coronal MRI (T1W unenhanced) in the same patient showing high signal from the lesion and retained secretion in the adjacent maxillary sinus.

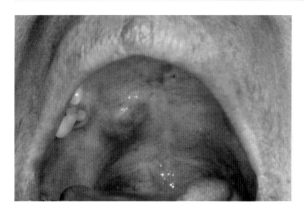

Fig. 9.5 Clinical photograph showing hard palate extension of a maxillary mixed venous/lymphatic malformation.

Imaging

In the head and neck, venous malformations may clinically and histologically resemble lymphatic malformations and may be a mixture of the two elements. Radiologically, the venous lesions frequently demonstrate phlebolith formation (organized calcified thrombi). Plain radiographs may demonstrate these in up to 50% of venous lesions. Both CT and ultrasonography may be useful but MRI is the best imaging modality to identify and characterize these lesions. It is able to distinguish between the slow flow lesion—exhibiting low signal intensity on T1 weighting and high signal intensity on T2 weighting. The lesions may be well defined or infiltrative and their total extent may be significantly underestimated on clinical examination. Angiography is rarely required for these lesions

and many do not have any form of specific feeding vessel (contrary to the accepted clinical view). Angiography may be performed if interventional radiological treatment is envisaged.

Histological Features

Cavernous lesions vary between being poorly circumscribed to rather more definitive lobular masses but contain multiple, dilated vascular spaces with thin walls and surrounding fibrous connective tissue, usually with only minimal amounts of interspersed smooth muscle. The vascular spaces are frequently engorged with blood and thrombosis of these low-flow areas is common, with the resulting formation of a phlebolith. There may additionally be abnormal lymphatic and capillary channels and these lesions may become inflamed at times, displaying chronic inflammatory cells. They are truly vascular malformations rather than hemangiomas if there is no pericyte around each endothelium-lined blood channel and no signs of proliferation. These pericytes will be positive for SMA (smooth muscle actin).

Treatment

Treatment may vary between none at all through a wide range of therapeutic modalities depending on the site, size, and symptoms. Treatment options include elastic compression, sclerotherapy, surgical resection, or combinations thereof, depending on the site. Treatment may be required for cosmetic appearance, functional airway problems, impairment of speech, and, at times, recurrent pain. Low-dose aspirin taken daily does provide some

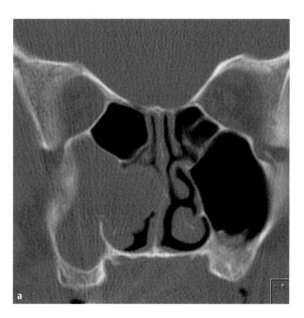

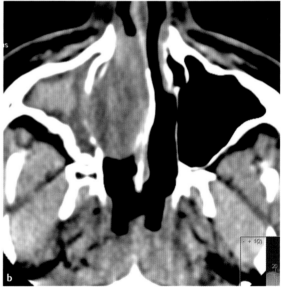

Fig. 9.6a, b

a Coronal CT scan showing a mixed venous/lymphatic malformation.

b Axial view of the same patient showing a nasal cavity lesion with retained secretions in the adjacent maxillary sinus.

prophylaxis against pain associated with thrombosis and phlebolith formation.

Sclerotherapy

Sclerotherapy has been used in various degrees over many years, the main aim of the injection of any agent being to induce inflammation and obliteration of the affected venous channels. It may be effective in small cutaneous and mucosal lesions and for larger lesions in the sinonasal area it may be necessary to undertake this under general anesthesia with an experienced interventional radiologist using real-time fluoroscopic and often ultrasonic monitoring. Unfortunately, multiple treatments may be required to shrink large venous malformations because recanalization of venous channels and local complications such as blistering, necrosis and bleeding, nerve injury, and dissemination of the sclerosing agent are possible. The reported success rates are variable, but up to three-quarters of patients may have marked improvement or cure.[25]

Endoscopic or Open Surgery

Small intranasal lesions may be excised endoscopically but larger lesions involving the nasal cavity and adjacent sinuses may require open approaches such as lateral rhinotomy or midfacial degloving. Large cervicofacial lesions extending to involve the nose, sinuses, and nasopharynx, in addition to multiple other areas of the head and neck, may present a massive surgical challenge either in the child or in the adult and should be reviewed by a multidisciplinary team comprising surgeons from different disciplines with special interest and experience in these problems. Large-scale surgery is occasionally necessary as a consequence of severe upper respiratory tract problems, feeding problems, dental malalignment, visual disturbance, and neurological impairment, but many patients, even with notably deep lesions, may not require any intervention and achieve a normal life span.

Several reports have described endoscopic resection of cavernous hemangiomas in the sinonasal region, notably a study by Song et al in 2009.[26] They described a series of 22 patients, comprising 13 capillary hemangiomas, 8 cavernous (probably venous malformations) and 1 mixed. All were excised endoscopically, with preoperative embolization used in three cases. None recurred with a follow-up of 8 to 48 months (mean 21 months).

Lymphatic Malformations

Lymphatic malformations vary in the same way from small localized lesions to massive lesions of the head and neck and may be microcystic or macrocystic, the latter large macrocystic lesions being given the name "cystic hygroma" for many years and the term "lymphangioma" being used for the microcystic lesions. The management of these lesions follows a similar pattern to the venous malformations and may require sclerotherapy or a wide variety of surgical procedures from the most minor to the most major.

Sclerotherapy

Sclerotherapy has its maximum effect for macrocystic lesions, particularly those with a single compartment in the lesion that can be aspirated, injected with sclerosant, and then compressed. Both intralesional bleomycin and OK-432 (a lyophilized mixture of attenuated group A *Streptococcus pyogenes* of human origin) have been reported to give good results.[27,28]

Lasers

Argon, neodymium-YAG, and carbon dioxide lasers have all been used in an attempt to coagulate both venous and lymphatic anomalies but their use is limited to the more superficial aspects of the lesions and may only be of real use in small lesions.

Open Surgery

Neonates with extensive cervicofacial venous, lymphatic, or mixed malformations may present with respiratory obstruction secondary to involvement of the nose, sinuses, tongue, oral cavity, or pharyngolarynx, and immediate tracheostomy may be required. Subsequent resection may be deferred until infancy or early childhood; certainly the dissection of delicate neurovascular structures is a little easier in the older child, but complete removal of all of the lesion is rarely possible.

Staged excision has been recommended, removing different components from anatomical sites at different times, but previous scarring from an adjacent area may make these procedures more difficult and certainly reoperation on a previously operated area can be particularly complicated. A downside of previous sclerotherapy, particularly if it was inappropriately used in microcystic lesions, can be to make any subsequent operation considerably more difficult as the malformation is more adherent to surrounding structures.

Capillary Malformations

Capillary malformations are usually sporadic but genetic research in the last decade has studied familial cases with an autosomal dominant inheritance pattern due to a gene *RASA1* on chromosome 5q.[29,30] A subgroup of the families with this mutation also have arteriovenous malformations and fistulas. Interestingly, the defect in hereditary benign telangiectasia has also been mapped to the same chromosome.[31]

Capillary malformations can occur anywhere in the body and vary from small areas of minor cutaneous erythema to extensive areas of involved skin—commonly referred to in the past as a port-wine stain. Approximately half of all facial capillary malformations are confined to one of three trigeminal dermatomes but there may be overlapping or crossing of the midline.[32] The sinonasal and oral mucous membranes may be involved.

The lesions are usually evident at birth and generally darken with age; they may develop nodular expansion and underlying maxillary or mandibular expansion. They may be accompanied by nasal and labial hypertrophy and hyperplasia of the gums.

Treatment

Involvement of the nose and sinonasal tract by capillary malformations may require a range of treatments extending from cosmetic camouflage make-up; through multiple applications of laser photocoagulation, resection, and skin grafting; to contour bone resection with orthognathic procedures to correct maxillary overgrowth.

Sturge-Weber Syndrome

This syndrome consists of a facial capillary malformation with ipsilateral leptomeningeal and ocular anomalies (Fig. 9.7). The leptomeningeal abnormalities may be capillary, venous or arteriovenous. Large pial vascular lesions may cause delayed motor and cognitive development with epilepsy and contralateral hemiplegia. Regular ophthalmic assessment in infants and children is necessary as choroidal involvement may result in retinal detachment, glaucoma, and blindness.

Syndromes Associated with Hemangiomas and Vascular Malformations

The numerous syndromes (at least 15 to date) associated with these vascular lesions[33] are beyond the scope of this book but further illustrate the need for all children and young adults to be seen by experienced multidisciplinary teams with specialist expertise to facilitate accurate diagnosis, expert imaging, and good patient and family communication and support. A full overall assessment is frequently essential and patients with large, complex lesions may require combined therapies over long periods.

Treatment of Hemangiomas and Vascular Malformations; Personal Series

We have a series of 21 cases of vascular malformations in adults, two-thirds of which have been venous malformations (Table 9.1). The capillary vascular malformations presented at an earlier age (mean of 37.3 years) compared with a mean of 49.8 years in the venous group; there was no particular sex difference either within the two groups or between them, with men and women equally affected. Eleven patients had lesions affecting the nasal cavity, structures either on the lateral wall or septum, and were mainly capillary vascular malformations. The venous lesions, as expected, tended to be more extensive, involving soft tissues and bone and affecting the midface, skull base, and orbit. However, all were amenable to surgical excision, which was complete and curative in all but two, both of whom had massive mixed venous/lymphatic

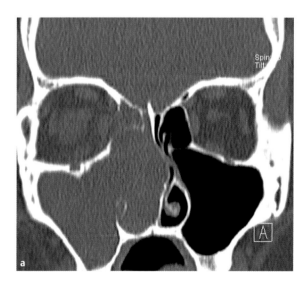

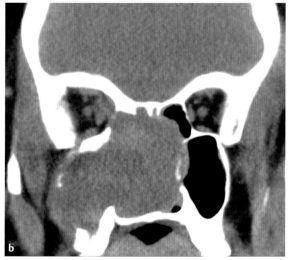

Fig. 9.7a, b
a Coronal CT scan in a patient with Sturge-Weber syndrome who had an extensive facial skin capillary malformation showing an underlying mixed capillary/venous malformation of the ipsilateral paranasal sinuses and orbit.

b Coronal CT scan in the same patient in a more posterior section showing orbital involvement.

Table 9.1 Vascular malformations: personal series

Histology	Sex	Age	Site	Surgical management	Long-term follow-up (y)
Capillary vascular malformations	F	63	Lateral wall	ESS	1
	F	24	Nasal septum	ESS	4
	F	35	Nasal septum	ESS	5
	F	53	Lateral wall	ESS + laser	5.5
	M	31	Nasal septum	ESS	14
	M	11	Nasal septum	ESS + laser	17
	M	44	Nasal septum	ESS	18
Venous malformations	M	68	Lateral nasal wall, orbit	ESS + laser (debulking)	1
	M	23	Maxilla: intra-osseous	MFD	3
	M	23	Lateral wall	ESS	8.5
	F	50	Lateral wall	ESS	10.5
	M	73	Lateral wall	ESS	11
	F	35	Maxilla, orbit	MFD	16
	F	72	Maxilla, orbit	MFD	12
	M	64	Orbit, skull base	CFR	16
	F	42	Frontal	OPF	15
	F	52	Orbit	LR	3
	F	55	Orbit	LR	10
	F	48	Orbit, maxilla	MFD	2
	M	31	Orbit, maxilla	LR	5
	M	61	Orbit, nasal cavity, maxilla, mid face	CFR (debulking)	13

Abbreviations: CFR, craniofacial resection; ESS, endoscopic sinus surgery; F, female; LR, lateral rhinotomy; M, male; MFD, midfacial degloving; OPF, osteoplastic flap; y, years.

malformations and who had had many previous surgical interventions elsewhere. A third patient had had a resection undertaken in our institution 14 years earlier.

Surgery ranged from endoscopic resection in 52% to midfacial degloving (19%), lateral rhinotomy (14%), craniofacial resection (10%), and an osteoplastic flap (5%). Embolization has not been required in any case and to date there have been no recurrences with a follow-up of 12 months to 18 years (mean 9.5 years).

Key Points

- There are essentially two types of vascular lesions, which are either tumors or malformations.
- The term "hemangioma" should not be used indiscriminately.
- Numerous symptoms are associated with these vascular lesions and many children and young adults require review by experienced multidisciplinary teams.

- Large, complex lesions may require combined therapies over a prolonged period.

References

1. Mulliken JB, Glowacki J. Hemangiomas and vascular malformations in infants and children: a classification based on endothelial characteristics. Plast Reconstr Surg 1982;69(3):412–422
2. Lancaster JL, Alderson DJ, Sherman IW, Clark AH. Papillary endothelial hyperplasia (Masson's tumour) of the maxillary sinus. J Laryngol Otol 1998;112(5):500–502
3. Marler JJ, Mulliken JB. Current management of hemangiomas and vascular malformations. Clin Plast Surg 2005;32(1):99–116, ix
4. Brodsky L, Yoshpe N, Ruben RJ. Clinical-pathological correlates of congenital subglottic hemangiomas. Ann Otol Rhinol Laryngol Suppl 1983;105:4–18
5. Fu YS, Perzin KH. Non-epithelial tumors of the nasal cavity, paranasal sinuses, and nasopharynx: A clinicopathologic study. I. General features and vascular tumors. Cancer 1974;33(5):1275–1288

6. Strauss M, Widome MD, Roland PS. Nasopharyngeal hemangioma causing airway obstruction in infancy. Laryngoscope 1981;91(8):1365–1368
7. Pitanguy I, Machado BH, Radwanski HN, Amorim NF. Surgical treatment of hemangiomas of the nose. Ann Plast Surg 1996;36(6):586–592, discussion 592–593
8. Hunt SJ, Santa Cruz DJ. Vascular tumors of the skin: a selective review. Semin Diagn Pathol 2004;21(3):166–218
9. Orlow SJ, Isakoff MS, Blei F. Increased risk of symptomatic hemangiomas of the airway in association with cutaneous hemangiomas in a "beard" distribution. J Pediatr 1997;131(4):643–646
10. Metry D. Update on hemangiomas of infancy. Curr Opin Pediatr 2004;16(4):373–377
11. North PE, Waner M, Mizeracki A, Mihm MC Jr. GLUT1: a newly discovered immunohistochemical marker for juvenile hemangiomas. Hum Pathol 2000;31(1):11–22
12. Gampper TJ, Morgan RF. Vascular anomalies: hemangiomas. Plast Reconstr Surg 2002;110(2):572–585, quiz 586, discussion 587–588
13. Batta K, Goodyear HM, Moss C, Williams HC, Hiller L, Waters R. Randomised controlled study of early pulsed dye laser treatment of uncomplicated childhood haemangiomas: results of a 1-year analysis. Lancet 2002;360(9332):521–527
14. Werner JA, Dünne AA, Folz BJ, et al. Current concepts in the classification, diagnosis and treatment of hemangiomas and vascular malformations of the head and neck. Eur Arch Otorhinolaryngol 2001;258(3):141–149
15. Perez J, Pardo J, Gomez C. Vincristine—an effective treatment of corticoid-resistant life-threatening infantile hemangiomas. Acta Oncol 2002;41(2):197–199
16. Zimmermann AP, Wiegand S, Werner JA, Eivazi B. Propranolol therapy for infantile haemangiomas: review of the literature. Int J Pediatr Otorhinolaryngol 2010; 74(4):338–342
17. Sheppard LM, Mickelson SA. Hemangiomas of the nasal septum and paranasal sinuses. Henry Ford Hosp Med J 1990;38(1):25–27
18. Mills SE, Cooper PH, Fechner RE. Lobular capillary hemangioma: the underlying lesion of pyogenic granuloma. A study of 73 cases from the oral and nasal mucous membranes. Am J Surg Pathol 1980;4(5):470–479
19. Dyduch G, Okoń K, Mierzyński W. Benign vascular proliferations—an immunohistochemical and comparative study. Pol J Pathol 2004;55(2):59–64
20. Harrison DFN. The Effect of Systemic Oestrogen Upon the Nasal Mucous Membrane and Its Application to the Treatment of Familial Haemorrhagic Telangiectasia. MS thesis. London, UK: University of London; 1959
21. Leyden JJ, Master GH. Oral cavity pyogenic granuloma. Arch Dermatol 1973;108(2):226–228
22. Childers EL, Furlong MA, Fanburg-Smith JC. Hemangioma of the salivary gland: a study of ten cases of a rarely biopsied/excised lesion. Ann Diagn Pathol 2002;6(6):339–344
23. Rossiter JL, Hendrix RA, Tom LW, Potsic WP. Intramuscular hemangioma of the head and neck. Otolaryngol Head Neck Surg 1993;108(1):18–26
24. Fine RM, Derbes VJ, Clark WH Jr. Blue rubber bleb nevus. Arch Dermatol 1961;84:802–805
25. Berenguer B, Burrows PE, Zurakowski D, Mulliken JB. Sclerotherapy of craniofacial venous malformations: complications and results. Plast Reconstr Surg 1999;104(1):1–11, discussion 12–15
26. Song CE, Cho JH, Kim SY, Kim SW, Kim BG, Kang JM. Endoscopic resection of haemangiomas in the sinonasal cavity. J Laryngol Otol 2009;123(8):868–872
27. Okada A, Kubota A, Fukuzawa M, Imura K, Kamata S. Injection of bleomycin as a primary therapy of cystic lymphangioma. J Pediatr Surg 1992;27(4):440–443
28. Greinwald JH Jr, Burke DK, Sato Y, et al. Treatment of lymphangiomas in children: an update of Picibanil (OK-432) sclerotherapy. Otolaryngol Head Neck Surg 1999;121(4):381–387
29. Eerola I, Boon LM, Watanabe S, Grynberg H, Mulliken JB, Vikkula M. Locus for susceptibility for familial capillary malformation ("port-wine stain") maps to 5q. Eur J Hum Genet 2002;10(6):375–380
30. Eerola I, Boon LM, Mulliken JB, et al. Capillary malformation-arteriovenous malformation, a new clinical and genetic disorder caused by RASA1 mutations. Am J Hum Genet 2003;73(6):1240–1249
31. Brancati F, Valente EM, Tadini G, et al. Autosomal dominant hereditary benign telangiectasia maps to the CMC1 locus for capillary malformation on chromosome 5q14. J Med Genet 2003;40(11):849–853
32. Enjolras O, Riche MC, Merland JJ. Facial port-wine stains and Sturge-Weber syndrome. Pediatrics 1985;76(1):48–51
33. Hiatt K, Pashaei S, Smoller B. Pathology of selected skin lesions of the head and neck. In: Barnes L, ed. Surgical Pathology of the Head and Neck. 3rd ed. New York: Informa; 2008:523

Angiofibroma

Definition

(ICD-O code 9160/0)

Angiofibroma is a benign but locally aggressive mesenchymal neoplasm with a distinct pattern of an abundant fibrous stroma containing vascular structures ranging from capillary size to large ectatic sinuses.

Synonyms, Incidence, and True Site of Origin

Chaveau introduced the term "juvenile nasopharyngeal angioma" in 1906.[1] Friedburg added the term angiofibroma in his report of 1940 following his histological studies on operative specimens.[2] Historically, ENT examination by head mirror techniques coupled with brain radiology led to the erroneous conclusion that angiofibromas arise within the nasopharynx. However, as we now know, both the terms "juvenile" and "nasopharyngeal" are inaccurate. **Our own series of over 150 patients has an age range of 6 years to 43 years and our detailed imaging and clinical studies over a 30-year period have shown that angiofibromas actually originate in the pterygopalatine fossa at the anterior aspect of the pterygoid (vidian) canal (Fig. 9.8) and initially erode the base of the sphenopalatine foramen and the bone behind, formed by the sphenoidal process of the palatine bone and medial pterygoid lamina. The tumor expands medially into the posterior nasal cavity via the sphenopalatine foramen and subsequently spreads into the nasopharynx.**

Invasion of the sphenoid and extension via the pterygomaxillary fissure into the infratemporal fossa and posterior aspect of the maxilla may follow (**Figs. 9.9 and 9.10**). The lateral extension may result in the mass coming to lie beneath the skin of the cheek by passing

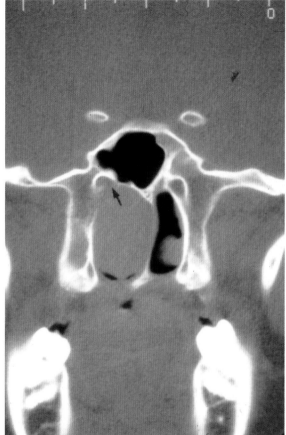

Fig. 9.8 Coronal CT scan showing angiofibroma in the right nasal cavity originating in the pterygopalatine fossa at the anterior aspect of the pterygoid (vidian) canal and initially eroding the base of the sphenopalatine foramen and the bone behind, formed by the sphenoidal process of the palatine bone and medial pterygoid lamina—a pathognomonic sign.

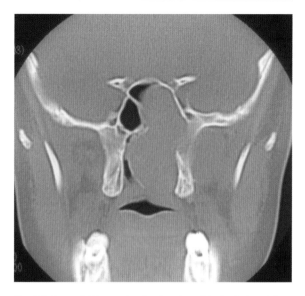

Fig. 9.9 Coronal CT scan showing invasion of the basisphenoid and extension into the sinus by angiofibroma.

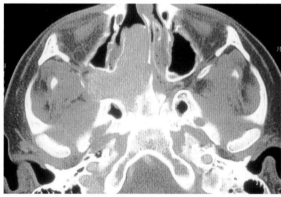

Fig. 9.10 Axial CT scan showing extension of angiofibroma via the pterygomaxillary fissure into the infratemporal fossa and posterior aspect of the maxilla, which may be pushed anteriorly.

between the upper molar teeth and the ascending ramus of the mandible. The orbit may be additionally invaded by the infraorbital fissure and there may be further extension to the middle cranial fossa, although this can also occur by direct lateral extension from the sphenoid (**Fig. 9.11**). **While secondary attachments may occur, it is important to understand the site of origin of angiofibroma and natural history of angiofibroma to provide the best possible treatment.**[3]

These are rare lesions that primarily occur in adolescent males, and are quoted as representing less than 0.05% of all head and neck tumors. The true incidence is speculative, however. While there are multiple small series within the literature, there is no definitive evidence of particular ethnic susceptibility; it may be that the large series that have been reported from countries such as India and Egypt merely reflect local referral patterns to the few centers of expertise. A recently published Danish national study found the incidence rate in Denmark to be 0.4 cases per million inhabitants per year, equating to 3.7 cases per million males (aged 10 to 24 years) per year over the period 1981–2003.

Likewise, the time of presentation of these cases in different countries may give rise to the erroneous impression of variation in natural history in different ethnic groups. While the majority of patients are between 10 and 20 years of age at diagnosis, cases from the first or third decades of life are not uncommon and our own series of over 150 patients has an age range of 6 to 43 years in common with those of colleagues from other countries (**Table 9.2**).[4-8]

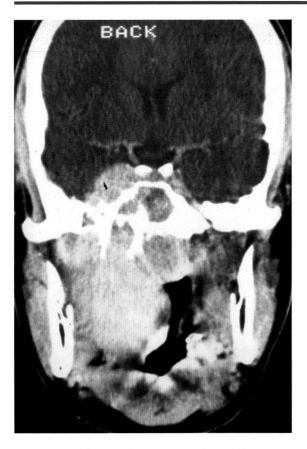

Fig. 9.11 Coronal CT scan showing an extensive angiofibroma involving the middle cranial fossa, although this can also occur by direct lateral extension from the sphenoid.

Etiology

While angiofibroma has occasionally been reported in women, there is no convincing evidence for this and most large series from prominent institutions do not contain any cases. Probably the best-documented case of an angiofibroma in a female patient was described by Osbourne and Sokoloski in 1965 from our own institution.[9] Osbourne was an experienced head and neck pathologist and the sex and histological diagnosis were not in doubt, in contrast to some other case reports in female patients.

As we have now accurately established the site of origin with modern scanning, the reports of Brunner in 1942[10] and Harrison in 1987[11]—which detailed notable endothelium-lined vascular spaces within the region of the basisphenoid, sphenopalatine foramen, and base of the pterygoid plates in both male and female patients—might suggest that some specific genetic or endocrine abnormality in males plays a role in the formation of this tumor. Beham et al[12] performed detailed immunohistochemical and electron-microscopic analysis, looking particularly at the vascular architectural features of 32 angiofibromas. They concluded that all the morphological irregularities that they demonstrated suggested that angiofibroma is a vascular malformation rather than a true neoplasm. Schick et al[13] proposed further that the vascular component of angiofibromas can be explained embryologically as a consequence of incomplete regression of the first branchial arch artery. In the late stages of embryological development, remnants of the subsequent vascular plexus of the former first branchial arch artery are found in the area of the sphenopalatine foramen. The authors proposed that the vascular component of an angiofibroma might arise due to growth stimulation at the time of adolescence.

However, there has been notable disputation over the possibility of sex hormone receptors playing some part in the common presentation of this tumor in adolescent boys. Various immunocytochemical techniques have reported variation in androgen, estrogen, and progesterone receptors in both fibrous and endothelial cells.[14–16]

Table 9.2 Angiofibroma: personal series

	n	Age	
		Mean (y)	Range (y)
Lateral rhinotomy (1968–1988)	42	15.2	8–26
Midfacial degloving (1988–)	97	16.4	8–32
Weber–Fergusson (1979–1987)	3	15(2),16	–
Craniofacial resection (1980, 1982)	1	27	–
Endoscopic resection (2000–)	12	18.5	16–22
Total	155	16.3	8–32
Abbreviations: mo, month(s); y, year(s).			

In contrast to the above findings regarding the vascular component, mounting recent evidence suggests that the fibrous tissue (often termed "stroma" in the past) is, in fact, the neoplastic component of the angiofibroma. Nuclear B-catenin staining of the fibroblastic cells has been definitively demonstrated.[17,18] This is consistent with B-catenin-modulated tumorigenesis, and angiofibromas have also been shown to have a significantly higher incidence in patients with familial adenomatous polyposis where deregulation of the APC/B-catenin/Tcf pathway has been consistently documented.[19-21] Ultrastructural investigations performed in the 1970s and 1980s also support the impression of the fibroblastic cells being the tumor component.[22-24]

Diagnostic Features

Clinical Features

Classically, the patient with angiofibroma presents as a male adolescent with slowly increasing nasal obstruction and recurrent epistaxis, which may be severe, in ~80% of patients at the time of diagnosis. As the tumor enlarges, there may be additional symptoms such as bulging of the soft palate, proptosis, facial swelling, deafness, rhinorrhea, or cranial nerve paresis. The extent of skull base involvement and the severity of epistaxis are both extremely variable and not always a reflection of either the angiomatous content of the lesion or the overall extent. More extensive invasion of the orbit and cavernous sinus may cause diplopia, visual loss, headache, and facial pain.

On examination, a small number of patients may present with a tumor protruding from an anterior narus (**Figs. 9.12 and 9.13**) or easily visible protruding from the nasopharynx into the oropharynx. More commonly, anterior rhinoscopy shows abundant mucopurulent secretions in the nasal cavity that may well obscure the tumor from

vision, and gentle suction of these secretions may be required to visualize the tumor.

On oral examination, the soft palate may be displaced inferiorly by the bulk of the tumor and posterior mirror rhinoscopy may show the pink or reddish mass occluding the nasopharynx if it has not already presented into the oropharynx. Larger tumors that have been in the oropharynx for some time may have a significant coating of metaplastic epithelium such that they appear white rather than pink, red, or purple. This occasionally gives rise to a misdiagnosis of anterochoanal polyp, which is also seen in young males.

Examination of the neck is necessary to rule out any nodal masses that might accompany the extremely rare malignant lesions of the nose, nasopharynx, and paranasal sinuses.

> **Biopsy**
>
> No attempt should be made to biopsy these lesions in outpatients, nor indeed as inpatients, as serious bleeding may result. Diagnosis can now be made with almost complete certainty radiologically, which additionally allows accurate assessment of tumor extent and vascularity.

Imaging

Imaging studies now play a key role in the diagnosis, staging, and management of angiofibroma. They have been sufficiently specific for more than two decades now to render excisional biopsy, with its associated risk of severe bleeding, completely unnecessary. Where available, MRI can also demonstrate the vascular character of these tumors and obviate the need for angiography in many cases unless this is part of preoperative tumor embolization. A combination of CT and MRI adds great

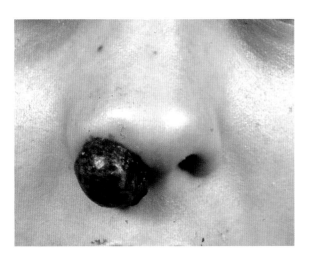

Fig. 9.12 Clinical photograph showing angiofibroma presenting at the anterior nasal vestibule.

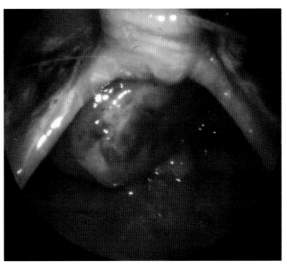

Fig. 9.13 Clinical photograph showing angiofibroma visible in the oropharynx.

refinement and detail to the previously known classical, so-called "antral" sign described by Holman and Miller in 1965 (**Fig. 9.14**).[25] This radiological sign consists of anterior bowing of the posterior wall of the maxillary sinus seen on lateral plain radiographs and more recently on axial CT. Our studies[3] looking at 20 years of modern imaging in angiofibroma found this sign to be present in 81% of 72 consecutive patients. Holman and Miller found it to be 87% in their series of patients.

However, any slow-growing lesion in the infratemporal fossa such as a schwannoma, hemangiopericytoma, or rhabdomyosarcoma can produce anterior bowing of the posterior maxillary wall. Our studies[3] have shown 100% of cases to have a mass in the pterygopalatine fossa with erosion of the bone of the posterior margin of the sphenopalatine foramen extending to the base of the medial pterygoid plate. Ninety-six percent of 72 cases had enlargement or erosion of the vidian canal, 83% extension into the sphenoid sinus, and 64% enlargement of the pterygomaxillary fissure and extension to the infratemporal fossa. These features do not occur with antrochoanal polyps, which may, when squamous metaplasia is present, simulate angiofibromas within the nasopharynx.[3]

Involvement of the sphenoid sinus, infratemporal fossa, orbit or middle cranial fossa is well demonstrated by a combination of CT and MRI (**Figs. 9.11, 9.15, 9.16**); in particular, the MRI will distinguish between the mass and fluid in an obstructed sinus and the vascularity of the lesion can be clearly indicated by signal voids from vessels in the angiofibroma. Gadolinium enhancement aids

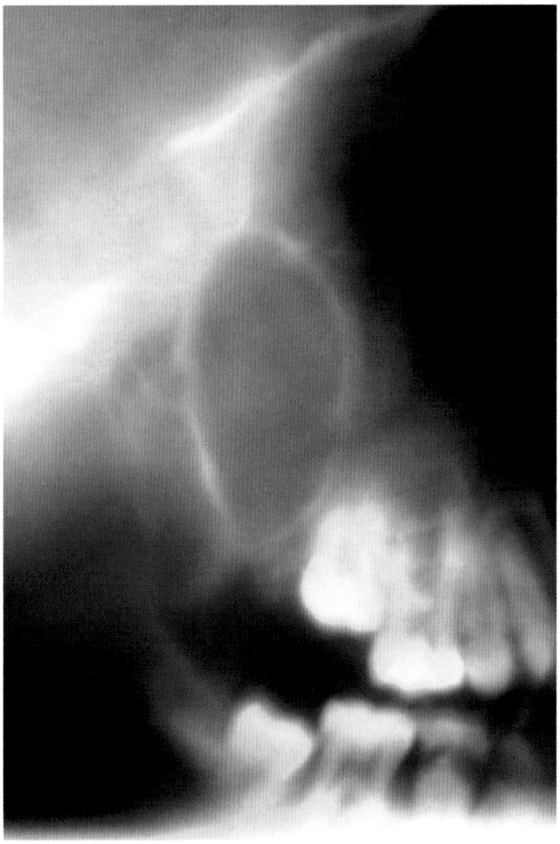

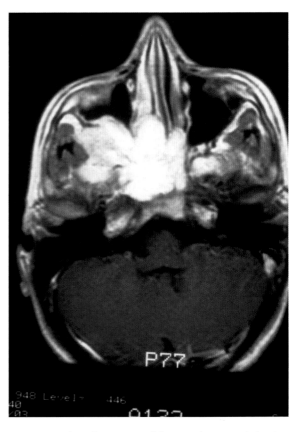

Fig. 9.15 Axial MRI (T1W post gadolinium enhancement) showing high signal with "salt and pepper" appearance in the angiofibroma due to signal voids in high-flow vessels.

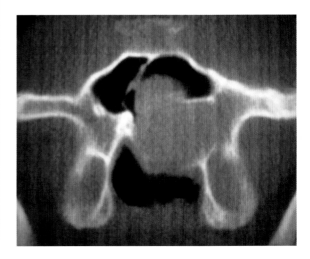

Fig. 9.16 Coronal CT scan showing erosion of the basisphenoid in the region of pterygoid canal.

Fig. 9.14 Lateral hypocycloidal tomography showing bowing of the posterior wall of the maxillary sinus (antral sign).

further with this evaluation. Even the larger lesions with significant skull base erosion may well be **intracranial** but **extradural**.

If there are concerns with the very large lesions, bilateral carotid angiography may be essential to delineate tumor blood supply, but this is by far the exception rather than the rule. Most angiofibromas derive their main blood supply from the internal maxillary artery, but additional supplies may come from the sphenoid and ophthalmic branches of the internal carotid as well as the ascending pharyngeal and palatal branches of the external carotid artery. While any additional supply from the internal carotid artery is usually of no practical consequence in the earlier lesions, allowing them nowadays to be removed endoscopically with a low morbidity, substantial connections with the internal carotid system may be evident in the larger tumors and, particularly, those that are recurrent, when their original predominant blood supply from the internal maxillary artery has been removed. This may also be true with recurrences after radiotherapy and there may be substantial tumor adjacent to the internal carotid arteries and cavernous sinus, making any subsequent treatment considerably more hazardous. Additionally, in larger primary tumors and substantial recurrent lesions, further blood supply may come from the arteries on the contralateral side of the tumor, thus limiting the potential value of embolization or balloon catheterization.

The use of angiography varies tremendously in reports from around the world but has notably increased with the increasing use of endoscopic techniques (**Fig. 9.17**). In our own series of 155 patients, two boys were referred following loss of sight associated with preoperative embolization and the third with a dense hemiplegia, which fortunately resolved over a period of one week following

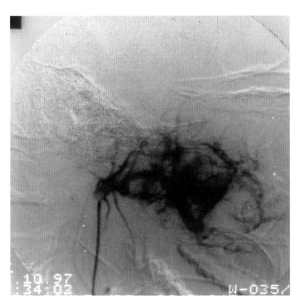

Fig. 9.17 Angiogram showing vascular blush of the angiofibroma.

embolization. It should be emphasized that all three boys were embolized in experienced tertiary interventional radiology centers. The literature contains further isolated reports of morbidity with embolization but we suspect that this is underreported overall. **The role of preoperative embolization, as outlined in the world literature, remains controversial. While many endoscopic surgeons regard it as essential prior to endoscopic surgery, others at the other end of the spectrum use the technique sparingly. There are, of course, all grades in between. There are no detailed prospective studies and certainly there is no doubt that the blood supply to the smaller tumors from the internal maxillary artery can be easily controlled at the time of surgery**. Full angiographic assessment and preoperative embolization prior to surgery is indicated (a) with massive tumors with intracranial, intradural extension, and notably (b) with major recurrences acquiring further blood supply from branches of the internal and external carotid artery. Intraoperative blood loss is generally agreed to be less after embolization.[26]

While less intraoperative bleeding might be thought to improve operative conditions and aid with overall resection and reduce the rate of recurrence, an earlier study from our unit showed in a small number of cases that, in contrast, recurrence rates seem to be increased following preoperative embolization.[27] This was at a time when all operations were by means of open surgery and we concluded that perhaps shrinkage of the tumor makes it more difficult to define its entirety within the operative field.

Staging Systems

Although angiofibroma is not a malignant lesion, these aggressive and difficult tumors have had several classification systems advocated to assist with planning and assessment of treatment. Sessions' system report in 1981 was based on anatomical location and similar to that used for nasopharyngeal carcinoma.[28] However, this system did not take into account the natural history of the lesions and their growth pattern and Chandler in 1984 modified this system but did not allow for the complexities of intracranial extension.[29] Chandler's system has been used by many people but did not have the benefit of the experience of modern radiological techniques. We have favored the system proposed by Andrews and Fish in 1989,[30] which essentially details growth and spread of these lesions and more clearly designates which tumors are potentially resectable by endoscopic techniques and those which necessitate more open midfacial degloving, infratemporal fossa, and combined neurosurgical approaches. Further classification systems have been proposed and are summarized in **Table 9.3**, recently published in the "European position paper on endoscopic management of tumours of the nose, paranasal sinuses and skull base."[31]

Table 9.3 Staging systems for angiofibroma[31]

Sessions[28] 1981 (n = 23)	Fisch[56] 1983 (n = 41)	Chandler[29] 1984 (n = 13)	Bremer[5] 1986 (n = 30)	Antonelli[32] 1987 (n = 23)
IA limited to the posterior nasal cavity and/or choanal border	I limited to the nasopharynx and nasal cavity without bone destruction	I confined to the nasopharynx	IA limited to the posterior nares or nasopharynx vault	I limited to the nasopharynx and/or nasal fossa
IB includes posterior nasal fossa and/or choanal border with involvement of at least one paranasal sinus			IB extension to one or more paranasal sinuses	
IIA minimal lateral extension to the pterygopalatine fossa	II invading the PMF and maxillary, ethmoid, and the sphenoid sinus with bone destruction	II extending into the nasal cavity and/or the sphenoid sinus	IIA minimal lateral extension through the sphenopalatine foramen into the medial PMF	II extending into the sphenoid sinus and/or PMF
IIB full occupation of the pterygopalatine fossa with or without orbital bone erosion			IIB full occupation of the PMF displacing the posterior wall of the antrum forward Superior extension eroding orbital bone	
			IIC extension through the PMF into the cheek and temporal fossa	
IIIA skull base erosion (e.g., middle fossa, pterygoid plates) with minimal intracranial invasion	III invading the ITF, orbit, and parasellar region, remaining lateral to the cavernous sinus	III extending into one or more of the following: antrum, ethmoid sinus, pterygomaxillary and infratemporal fossae, orbit, and/or cheek	III intracranial extension	III beyond stage II, limits extending to one or more of the following structures: maxillary sinus, ethmoid, orbit, ITF, cheek, palate
IIIB extensive intra-cranial extension ± invasion of the cavernous sinus				
	IV massive invasion of cavernous sinus, the optic chiasmal region, or pituitary fossa	IV extending into cranial cavity		IV intracranial extension

Abbreviations: ITF, infratemporal fossa; PMF, pterygomaxillary fissure.

Andrews[30] 1989 (n = 15)	Radkowski[33] 1996 (n = 23)	Önerci[68] 2006 (n = 36)	Carrillo[34] 2008 (n = 54)	Snyderman[35] 2010 (n = 35)
I limited to the naso-pharynx and nasal cavity Bone destruction negligible or limited to the sphenopalatine foramen	IA = Sessions	I extension to the nose, nasopharyngeal vault, and sphenoid sinus	(A) medial, with tumor limited to the nasopharynx, nasal fossae, maxillary antrum, and anterior ethmoid cells	I no significant extension beyond the site of origin and remaining medial to the midpoint of the pterygopalatine space
	IB = Sessions			
II invading the PMF or the maxillary, ethmoid, or sphenoid sinus with bone destruction	IIA = Sessions	II extension to the maxillary sinus or the anterior cranial fossa, full occupation of the PMF, limited extension to the ITF, or the pterygoid plates posteriorly	(B) invasion to the PMF or anterior ITF with tumor <6 cm in diameter	II extension to the paranasal sinuses and lateral to the midpoint of the pterygopalatine space
	IIB = Sessions			
	IIC = Sessions or posterior to pterygoid plates			
IIIA involving the ITF or orbital region without intracranial involvement	IIIA erosion of the skull base; minimally intracranial	III deep extension into the cancellous bone at the base of the pterygoid or the body and the greater wing of the sphenoid; significant extension to the ITF or pterygoid plates posteriorly or orbital region, and obliteration of cavernous sinus	(C) extension to the PMF or anterior ITF with tumor ≥6 cm in diameter	III locally advanced with skull base erosion or extension to additional extracranial spaces, including the orbit and ITF; no residual vascularity following embolization
IIIB invading the ITF or orbit with intracranial extradural (parasellar) involvement	IIIB erosion of skull base; extensive intracranial extension ± cavernous sinus			
IV intracranial intradural tumor with infiltration of the cavernous sinus, pituitary fossa or optic chiasm		IV intracranial extension between the pituitary gland and internal carotid artery, tumor extension posterolateral to the internal carotid artery, and extensive intracranial extension	(D) extension to the posterior ITF or roof of the skull base	IV skull base erosion, orbit, ITF Residual vascularity
			(E) extensive skull base and intracranial invasion	V intracranial extension, residual vascularity M: medial extension L: lateral extension

Abbreviations: ITF, infratemporal fossa; PMF, pterygomaxillary fissure.

Histological Features

Macroscopically, angiofibromas vary from small, smooth, multilobulated masses varying from gray-white to red/purple and from as little as 2 to 3 cm up to 10 cm or more (**Fig. 9.18**). Surface erosion and ulceration may be present with areas of obvious bleeding. Microscopically they show varying degrees of blood vessels and fibrous components with the vascular structures ranging widely from capillaries to compressed slitlike spaces and ectatic sinusoidal areas. Vessels are usually thin-walled, containing only a single layer of flattened endothelium, but thick-walled vessels with smooth muscle may also be seen along with an accompanying layer of pericyte cells.

These findings may be altered by preoperative embolization with obviously accompanying areas of infarction and visible intravascular occlusive material of one form or another. The fibrous tissue is usually composed of stellate spindled fibroblastic or myofibroblastic cells and currently this is thought to be the neoplastic component of the lesion. There is an accompanying coarse or wavy arrangement of collagen bundles that may be quite dense. Lesions may contain binucleate or multinucleate cells or large ganglionlike cells. Mitotic activity is always minimal and, overall, angiofibromas have a moderate to low cellularity. The components of fibrosis and vascularity are generally thought to decrease in long-standing tumors, although our series has shown notably fibrotic tumors in young boys and highly vascular tumors in adults in their twenties and thirties, so that this is not a consistent finding.

Immunohistochemical evaluation is rarely required for the diagnosis, but the fibroblastic tumor cells are consistently positive for vimentin and the endothelial cells are CD31, CD34, and factor 8-related antigen-immunoreactive. As stated previously, the studies for androgen, estrogen, and progesterone receptor staining have yielded variable results, but nuclear β-catenin staining of the fibroblastic cells is consistent with the β-catenin modulated pathogenesis.

Differential Diagnosis

Presentation of the histology along with the classic imaging findings is usually sufficient to provide an accurate diagnosis. The differential diagnosis includes any sinonasal and antrochoanal polyps but these have different radiological characteristics and notable evidence of inflammation on histology. Lobular capillary hemangiomas occur in the nasal cavity but rarely involve the nasopharynx and their classical lobular arrangement of capillary structures with endothelial cells contrasts with angiofibroma.

Spontaneous malignant change has not been clearly identified in angiofibromas although occurrence of sarcomas has been documented following repeated surgical removals and high-dose irradiation. The neoplasm in most cases is fibrosarcoma or one of its variants.[36]

The interval between irradiation and diagnosis of these malignant cases varies from 11 months to 21 years. Among the 55 patients reported by Cummings et al in 1984 treated with primary radiotherapy, 2 later developed malignant tumors within the head and neck. One case with thyroid carcinoma occurred 14 years post treatment and the other, a basal cell carcinoma, was diagnosed 13 years after the initial irradiation.[37]

Natural History

Despite the oft-repeated anecdotal belief that angiofibromas will spontaneously involute, our experience is that this must be a very rare occurrence. Certainly, there is no definitive relationship proven between age and tumor aggressiveness and while there are reports by Jacobsson et al[38] and Stansbie and Phelps,[39] confirmed by radiological follow-up, that even intracranial extensions can cease to grow after cessation of unsuccessful surgery, a long-term follow-up in excess of two decades would be required to make sure that this is not the case as the authors have seen substantial proven lesions in 36- and 43-year-old male adults.

Treatment

The absolutely essential requirement for the treatment of tumors of the skull base is an understanding of their natural history and pathology, and nowhere is this better demonstrated than the necessity of understanding the site of origin of angiofibroma, the pathways of potential extension, and the significant potential for recurrence of this locally aggressive and potentially

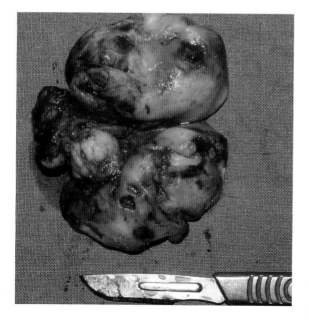

Fig. 9.18 Photograph of a surgical specimen.

destructive tumor. **Failure to appreciate these important points continues to result in a relatively high incidence of incomplete removal together with significant morbidity, even mortality**. These young male patients may die as a result of their treatment and not necessarily from their tumor.[40] As a consequence of our superior diagnostic imaging of the last two decades, surgical techniques have moved away from the earlier transpalatal approach, often with forceps avulsion, poor visualization, and severe bleeding. The operation nowadays can be chosen to fit each individual patient and tumor depending on the extent of involvement of the skull base.

However, excision of these tumors still requires special expertise and the best chance of success lies with the first operation. **The exact technique will also depend on the availability of expertise and equipment in any given center**.

Recurrence

Recurrent tumors, after both surgery and failed radiotherapy, are almost without exception considerably more adherent to the structures of the skull base, and with initial removal of the predominant blood supply from the internal maxillary artery, they have frequently taken on multiple additional connections, notably from the internal carotid artery. **The vast majority of recurrent tumors occur at their originating site in the basisphenoid and both at primary and at secondary revision surgery, irrespective of the type of surgical approach, it is essential for the operating surgeon to understand this point of the natural history (Fig. 9.19)**.[41] **Inspection of the basisphenoid following removal of the tumor is insufficient; it is necessary to meticulously drill out the basisphenoid area enough to be sure that there is no residual angiofibroma within the pterygoid (vidian) canal or cancellous bone of the basisphenoid**.

Historical Note

The *Lancet* of October 1841 carries a case report by the famous surgeon Liston on the removal of a large tumor mass projecting from the left nostril and adjacent cheek of a 21-year-old man from Gibraltar. The patient had a history of more than 3 years of profound intermittent nasal bleeding and several attempts had been made to destroy sections of the tumor by ligation, but with each sloughing there was significant bleeding and when there was involvement of the pharynx, oral cavity, and alveolar process, the patient presented with significant airway obstruction. Liston removed the lesion along with the whole maxilla with preservation of the eye over a period of ~4 hours without the benefit of general anesthesia; the estimated blood loss was 8 to 10 oz [240 to 300 mL]. Twenty-four days postoperatively, the *Lancet* reported a satisfactory recovery with the patient eating a mutton chop daily. Unfortunately, he died three and a half months postoperatively from erysipelas of the scalp! Myhre and Michaels retrieved the operative specimen from the pathology museum at University College School of Medicine in 1987 and confirmed the histological pattern to be that of a typical angiofibroma (**Fig. 9.20**).[42]

Preoperative Embolization

Throughout the 20th century there were many papers detailing treatment strategies, but no uniformity has yet been reached and until this century most tumors were resected through a transpalatal, a Weber–Fergusson, a lateral rhinotomy, a midfacial degloving, or a craniofacial approach. While open approaches have been used for tumors of all stages, a wide variety of teams have used preoperative embolization as part of the surgical management of these tumors, but the subject remains

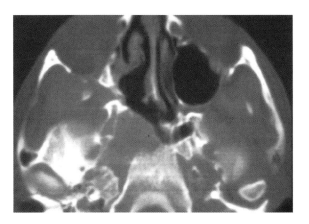

Fig. 9.19 Axial CT scan showing recurrence of angiofibroma in the basisphenoid.

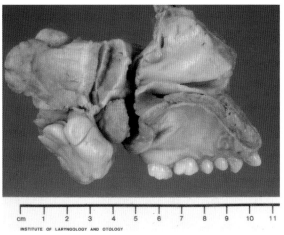

Fig. 9.20 A surgical specimen removed by Liston in 1841.

controversial. With the recent application of endonasal endoscopic techniques, preoperative embolization is almost always undertaken, notwithstanding its controversial benefit.

It seems obvious that when considering the surgical excision of any vascular lesion, it may be beneficial to reduce the blood supply by embolization to minimize intraoperative hemorrhage, facilitate visualization (and hence removal), and minimize operative morbidity. Embolization of the entire vascular bed may be preferable to ligating feeding vessels, many of which may be inaccessible at the commencement of the operation. However, it is certainly possible through open approaches such as lateral rhinotomy and midfacial degloving to gain early access to the predominant supply through the internal maxillary artery and to ligate the main trunk of this vessel laterally to the tumor before commencing any mobilization of the tumor mass.

If substantial intravascular thrombosis is to be obtained preoperatively, the choice of embolic material, accurate angiographic assessment, and the timing of subsequent surgery are important considerations that in themselves remain to be standardized. Anecdotal reports of reduction in the expected amount of bleeding can be related to the different degrees of fibrous tissue within angiofibromas and, as the male patients range from young children to full-grown adults, the percentage of total blood volume lost is a far more accurate assessment of the situation.

Prior to the availability of high-resolution CT and MRI, angiography was used initially to verify diagnosis but now only needs to be employed in the majority of these tumors as a means of embolization prior to surgery. In the tumors presenting primarily, the vascular supply comes mainly from the internal maxillary artery, the ascending pharyngeal artery, and the artery to the vidian canal. Embolization should usually be performed less than 48 hours prior to surgery, and while a wide variety of materials have been advocated, the interval between embolization and surgery for resorbable materials should certainly not exceed this time as the blood supply through the artery can be rapidly reestablished.[43] Recently, onyx has been proposed as a material that produces extensive tumor infarction with improved arterial catheterization.[44]

In primary extracranial tumors notable blood supply from the internal carotid artery is both rare and rarely of significance. However, in recurrent tumors where the cavernous sinus is involved and in the rare advanced tumors that are actually intracranial and intradural, embolization may be undertaken but the risk of complications is higher (**Fig. 9.21**). As described above under "Imaging," the authors, in a series of 155 tumors, have been referred 3 patients from major centers, 2 of whom became blind in one eye following embolization and a third boy with a dense hemiplegia which fortunately resolved after 36 hours. Direct intratumoral embolization under general

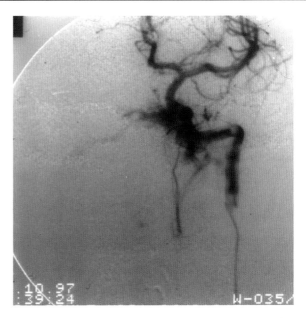

Fig. 9.21 Angiogram showing a feeding vessel from the internal carotid to the angiofibroma.

anesthesia has been advocated for these cases through an intranasal or lateral percutaneous route under imaging control.[45]

Preoperative embolization is certainly not a newly advocated procedure as Robertson et al were the first to recommend its use in 1972.[46] Shrinkage of tumor may result in incomplete removal by allowing small areas of tumor to remain undetected and to rapidly regrow. The current continuing recurrence rate reported in the endoscopic surgical literature gives some cause for concern that this may still be an issue.[31]

As an alternative to preoperative embolization, a senior author utilizing a midfacial degloving approach (D.J.H.) uses the alternative of direct intraoperative identification and ligation/coagulation of the major supplying vessels with the additional aid of hypotensive general anesthesia, rather than preoperative embolization. Preoperative autologous donation and the cell saver systems for immediate re-transfusion of the collected blood are additional techniques which allow for the management of these difficult cases and minimize the need for a blood transfusion. The open approach is frequently considerably shorter in time than an endoscopic approach, particularly during the learning curve for the latter, and for the larger tumors.

Preoperative Hormonal Therapy

The initial proponent of this rationale appears to be Schiff in 1959.[47] This uncontrolled study on just two patients receiving 15 mg of diethylstilbestrol per day for a month was followed by other small, equally variable, studies relating to testosterone and estrogen that did not provide definite conclusions. Naturally, the subject has been viewed with considerable interest as many of the patients are young boys pre and post puberty. Estrogen therapy at this point for adolescent boys can produce secondary feminizing effects and any shrinkage has been reported as extremely variable.[48] The nonsteroidal androgen receptor blocker flutamide was reported to produce shrinkage of up to 44% in a small number of patients by Gates et al,[49] but it is notable that there have not been further long-term reports on its use. Labra et al, reporting on 7 cases in 2004 with extensive stage IV disease, found a mean shrinkage of only 7.5%, which was not considered to be significant.[50]

Radiotherapy

Concerns over the technical surgical aspects and potential severe hemorrhage, particularly with advanced stage angiofibromas, have led several centers, notably in North America, to report radiotherapy as primary or secondary therapy over the past 40 years.[37,51,52] Dosages and regimens have varied from implantation of radon seeds, 270 to 400 kV, to modern-day external beam linear accelerator irradiation. Cummings et al in Toronto, Canada[37] have been the most enthusiastic proponents of primary radiotherapy, but permanent control of symptoms was obtained in only 80% of these patients and regression following radiation is slow, with disease persisting for longer than 2 years and a high incidence of eventual symptomatic regrowth. While all these series report regression in the size of the angiofibromas, these series have not been assessed by interval scanning and long-term recurrence of symptoms in these young patients

is well documented. These results have to be balanced against the hazards and morbidity of surgical excision, particularly in the larger lesions, but the development of late malignant change in these young male patients remains a concern. Two of Cummings's initial 55 patients developed neoplasms, one a capillary thyroid carcinoma 14 years later and the other a basal cell carcinoma 8 years post irradiation. Make et al reported 6 patients who developed fibrosarcoma and malignant fibrous histiocytoma.[36]

Up to one-third of patients in the reported series have had further complications including growth retardation, panhypopituitarism, temporal lobe necrosis, radiation necrosis, cataracts, and radiation keratopathy in the first two decades after treatment (**Fig. 9.22**). Even 30 years after radiotherapy, many of these patients have only just reached middle age and as with any residual disease there is always the risk of further regrowth.[53] Long-term monitoring of these patients with MRI is essential both post radiotherapy and post surgery if residual or recurrent disease is demonstrated.

Chemotherapy

With the potential surgical and radiotherapeutic problems involved in treating recurrent or advanced-stage angiofibromas, Goepfert et al 1985[54] used the chemotherapeutic agents doxorubicin, dacartrazine, vincristine, dactinomycin, cyclophosphamide, and cisplatin in two differing regimes and achieved some regression but this approach for these benign tumors has not been advocated further.

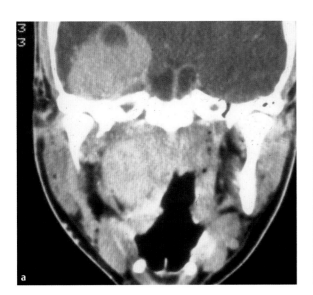
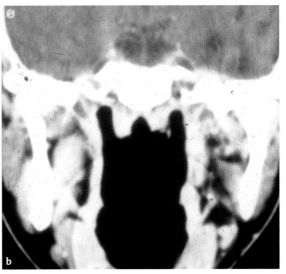

Fig. 9.22a, b

a Coronal CT scan showing significant recurrence in the middle cranial fossa.

b Coronal CT scan in same patient one year following radiotherapy with resolution of the lesion.

Surgical Treatment

The surgical approaches are many and varied and will continue to be so around the world as a consequence of varying availability of modern radiological assessment and surgical instrumentation. No single approach is possible for all stages of tumor and ultimately the approach used will depend on the experience of the surgeon, the tumor size and location, patient's age and physical condition, and the availability of additional procedures such as tumor embolization. Over the last two decades, transnasal endoscopic removal has become the favored technique for many benign tumors limited to the nasal cavity, nasopharynx, and paranasal sinuses, and for none more so than angiofibroma. Endoscopic techniques permit a minimally invasive resection of the entire tumor mass, minimal blood loss, and low morbidity. However, the approach is not applicable for all tumors and in all centers.

Irrespective of the surgical approach and overall technique, the commonest serious complication following the initial surgery remains recurrence of the disease. It is important for the surgical team to understand that, irrespective of the approach, recurrent disease is almost certainly due to inadequate resection leaving behind residual disease within the basisphenoid. This may occur irrespective of preoperative embolization or after any type of surgical approach. The natural history of angiofibroma is that it begins in the pterygopalatine fossa in relation to the sphenopalatine foramen and the anterior aspect of the pterygoid (vidian) canal. It begins its erosion of the upper aspect of the medial pterygoid plate, pterygoid canal, and adjacent basisphenoid from a very early stage.[3] It is essential to undertake a meticulous drilling out of the basisphenoid area to ensure that there is no residual angiofibroma within the pterygoid canal or the cancellous bone of the basisphenoid. Erosion into this area can be substantial in both primary and recurrent cases of disease. Our studies show that 93% of recurrent disease occurs at this site.[41] Increasing use of endoscopic approaches for the removal of angiofibroma is a significant step forward in the treatment but it will only be accompanied by satisfactory long-term results preventing recurrence if this drilling out of the basisphenoid ensures that there is no residual tumor that can give rise to recurrence.

Transpalatal Approach

The transpalatal approach so commonly used in the past allowed removal of angiofibroma involving the nasal cavity, nasopharynx, and sphenoid sinus but gave poor access to tumors passing laterally through the pterygomaxillary fissure and often involved considerable blind dissection and, at times, poor control of bleeding. An underreported complication of this approach, particularly in young boys, was the subsequent alteration of their speech as a consequence of scarring of the palate.

Lateral Rhinotomy and Weber–Fergusson Approaches

While both these approaches have traditionally in the past given good access to many angiofibromas, the resulting facial scar in a predominantly young population of patients is unnecessary nowadays, and although a good cosmetic result can be obtained with a lateral rhinotomy in many instances, this is certainly not always the case. The Weber–Fergusson incision rarely gives a cosmetic result that the patient feels is excellent, and is a lifelong reminder of what can be a serious disease process.

Midfacial Degloving

Midfacial degloving has been our open approach of choice in all patients with angiofibromas treated since 1986,[55] offering as it does, excellent access, control of hemorrhage, and cosmesis when the lesions are too extensive for consideration of endoscopic techniques (**Fig. 9.23**). In our center its use nowadays is confined to those patients whose lesions are IIIA and IIIB on the Andrews-Fisch classification or Radkowski IIC and IIIA (**Table 9.3**).

The approach allows removal of the medial, posterior, and lateral aspects of the maxilla to mobilize even large tumors in the infratemporal fossa and buccal area, bringing them medially with clipping, ligation, and diathermy of the internal maxillary supply before any degree of tumor mobilization is necessary. Both the operating microscope and additional endoscopic visualization can of course be added to the technique, particularly when drilling out the basisphenoid following removal of all macroscopic tumor (**Fig. 9.24**). An excellent view of the skull base can be achieved even with notable intracranial but extradural disease. The commonest reported complication after this procedure is paresthesia of the infraorbital nerve and this can be lessened by careful retraction on either side of the nerve by the assistant. The other notable complication of vestibular stenosis can be lessened by creating an irregular circumvestibular incision, notably by turning the intercartilaginous incision downward to the piriform aperture in a right angle and then a further right angle to

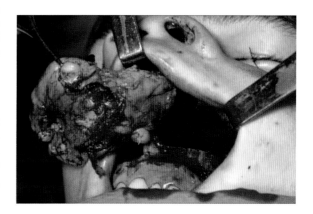

Fig. 9.23 Removal of angiofibroma during a midfacial degloving approach.

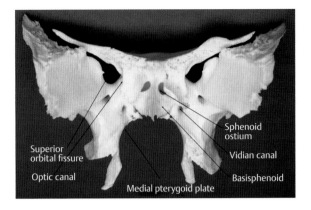

Fig. 9.24 Photograph of disarticulated sphenoid.

follow the inferior aspect of the piriform aperture. This produces an incision which is almost z-shaped in the lateral aspect of the circumvestibular incision and with careful suturing postoperatively, vestibular stenosis can be avoided (**Fig. 9.25**).

The Infratemporal Fossa Approach

While this approach has been used for stages IIIA, IIIB, and IV of the Andrews-Fisch classification, as stated previously, many IIIA and IIIB tumors can be removed through a midfacial degloving bearing in mind that the most important area of note is the basisphenoid. However, extensive IIIB and stage IV tumors may have notable expansion through the basisphenoid, particularly in the triangular region between the foramen ovale, rotundum, and lacerum to involve the middle cranial fossa and hence the parasellar region. While these tumors usually remain extradural and lateral to the cavernous sinus, previous surgery or radiotherapy may have promoted both extensive new vascular connections and adherence of the tumor mass to surrounding structures, making the infratemporal fossa route a better approach. This is particularly the case if the tumor has destroyed the posterior wall of the sphenoid sinus and is infiltrating the cavernous sinus, pituitary fossa, and optic chiasm. In addition it may be adherent to, or surrounding, the internal carotid artery. The rare patients with preoperative angiographic assessment showing a major blood supply to the angiofibroma

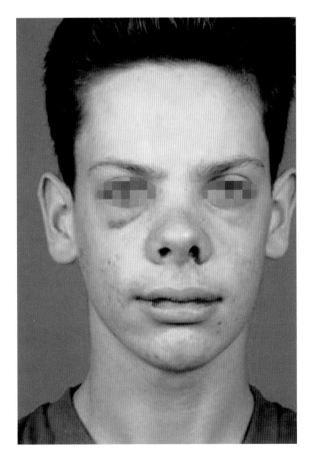

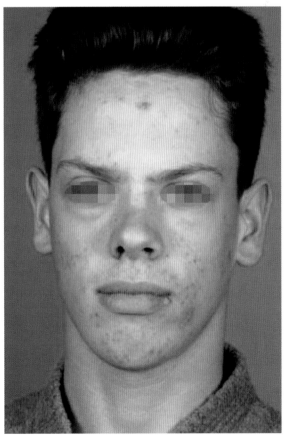

Fig. 9.25a, b

a Postoperative photograph 4 days following midfacial degloving.

b Postoperative photograph 2 months following midfacial degloving.

from the internal carotid artery will need an assessment to consider preoperative closure of the vessel by a balloon occlusion technique.

The operative details of the Fisch infratemporal fossa type C approach are well described via a retroauricular dissection, mastoidectomy, subtotal petrosectomy, and mobilization of the dura of the middle cranial fossa medially and anteriorly.[56,57] To augment the exposure, it is necessary to open the glenoid fossa and excise the articular tubercle of the temporal bone. This is followed by transection of the mandibular branch of the trigeminal nerve and middle meningeal artery to allow for inferior retraction of the mandible. To dissect along the internal carotid artery in its horizontal course up to the foramen lacerum, it is necessary to resect a portion of the eustachian tube.

If this procedure is only used in those extensive tumors that really justify it, the pterygoid base and lateral lamina are usually already eroded by tumor and do not require much in the way of additional removal prior to exposure of the sphenoid sinus and parasellar region. Additionally, the maxillary branch of the trigeminal nerve is divided to allow extradural elevation of the temporal lobe. The medial pterygoid plate is drilled away if necessary, giving access to the nasal cavity part of the tumor, and operative microscopic control then allows removal of the tumor with good visualization of the internal carotid artery.

It is often necessary to divide the tumor and remove the extracranial component to provide improved mobilization of any intracranial, intradural extension. Most commonly even significant intracranial involvement will remain extradural and only gentle retraction of the tumor is usually required to separate it from the dura unless there has been notable previous surgery or radiotherapy. Even a tumor that has grown through the dura often remains external to the arachnoid, but once it has infiltrated the cavernous sinus it may be better to leave a small portion of the tumor in place to avoid any injury to the abducens-oculomotor or trochlear nerves. In very rare cases, the infratemporal fossa approach may be combined with a modified middle fossa craniectomy.[58]

The resulting surgical defect may be filled with a temporalis muscle flap whose blood supply has been maintained by its insertion into the coronoid process and ramus of the mandible. This extensive procedure is appropriate for some stage IIIB and stage IV tumors, but as it involves permanent closure of the external auditory canal with a permanent conductive hearing loss, resection of the glenoid fossa, and usually division of both mandibular and maxillary divisions of the trigeminal nerve, it is not recommended for smaller lesions. Additionally, combined intra- and extracranial approaches using frontotemporal craniotomy are rarely required and total maxillectomy gives an unnecessary degree of debility and is contra-indicated.[59–61]

The major benefit of the infratemporal fossa type C approach is the fact that it allows safe management of any intracranial tumor extension as the internal carotid artery is exposed in its vertical and horizontal course, up to and including the foramen lacerum, and the cavernous sinus can be optimally approached as well. However, the important point emphasized by Andrews and Fisch, in their well-known report describing this approach in 51 patients treated during the 1970s and 1980s,[30] is that even large intracranial tumor extensions are usually found to remain **extradural** and can be resected without the necessity to open the dura. Even in those cases with intradural invasion, the arachnoid layer remains intact. **In primary cases, many of these lesions can be treated endoscopically or by means of midfacial degloving or a combination of the two, which avoids the greater morbidity encountered after the infratemporal fossa approach**.

Endoscopic Management of Angiofibromas

Many teams around the world now undertake removal of Andrews-Fisch tumor stage I, II, and IIIA using a one- or two-surgeon technique (**Fig. 9.26**). The advantages of the nasal endoscopic approach are potentially reduced intraoperative blood loss, fewer postoperative complications, and a reduced length of hospital stay. However, there is notable bias in the literature as there are no prospective studies and comparison of the endoscopic technique with open techniques in terms of such factors as blood loss is often inappropriate because the comparison is commonly between smaller and somewhat larger lesions. In general, one would expect the main blood loss to be lower in endoscopic procedures[62,63] and in the early staged tumors.[62]

Additionally, the KTP (potassium titanyl phosphate) laser[64,65] and ultrasonic scalpel[66] have been advocated to try to further reduce bleeding during the endoscopic approach. Blood loss during endoscopic removal may also be variable depending on the quality and extent of preoperative embolization and the overall tumor volume.[67,68]

In contrast to some potential advantages of the endoscopic procedure, a relative disadvantage may be the length of the endonasal procedure and, additionally, the learning curve required for the surgeon undertaking these procedures. **An inexperienced surgeon carrying out an incomplete removal of an angiofibroma with rapid recurrence of the disease is certainly not assisting the progress of the patient and this must be avoided under all circumstances**. Again, the point must be stressed that complete removal of this aggressive benign tumor is required and all residual angiofibroma must be removed from the area of the pterygoid (vidian canal) and the invaded cancellous bone of the basisphenoid, which may indeed extend out into the greater wing of the sphenoid.

In summary, while the endoscopic approach for excision of stage I and stage II angiofibromas has been associated with good results from several published series, recurrence rates are unfortunately comparable to those with classical external approaches (**Table 9.4**).[31]

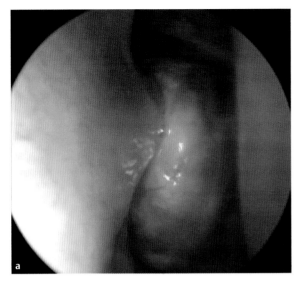

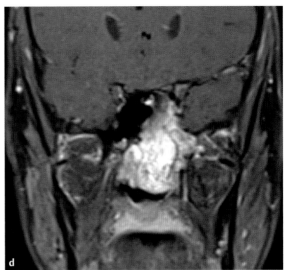

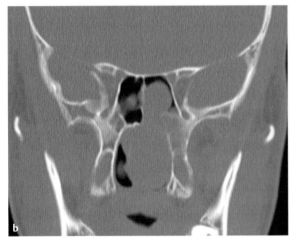

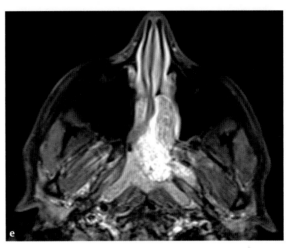

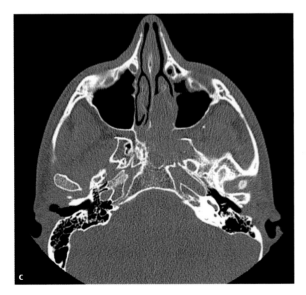

Fig. 9.26a–e

a Endoscopic view of angiofibroma in the left nasal cavity.

b Coronal CT scan showing angiofibroma in the nasal cavity with erosion of the superior medial pterygoid plate with extension into the sphenoid.

c Axial CT scan in the same patient.

d Coronal MRI (T1W post gadolinium enhancement with fat saturation) in the same patient.

e Axial MRI (T1W post gadolinium enhancement with fat saturation) in the same patient.

Table 9.4 Results after endoscopic removal of angiofibromas

Author[a] (year of publication)	Total n	Classification	n + stage	Mean follow-up (mo) (range)	Recurrence/residual
Schick (1999)[69]	5	Fisch	5 type II	(5–39)	No (0%)
Jorissen (2000)[70]	13	Radkowski/ Chandler/ Andrews/ Sessions[b]	2 stage IA 2 stage IB 2 stage IIA 2 stage IIB 4 stage IIC 1 stage IIIA	35.3 (12–72) (f-u available for 11 patients)	1 recurrence after 6 mo of a stage IIC (cured by ESS) 1 recurrence of a stage IIIA after 4 mo. Regression after embolization of ICA
Roger (2002)[71]	20	Radkowski	4 stage I 7 stage II 9 stage IIIA (Including 7 recurrences after open surgery)	22	2 residual of stage IIIA were asymptomatic 30 and 36 mo after surgery
Önerci (2003)[68]	12	Radkowski	8 stage IIC 4 stage IIIA	Min. 6	No recurrence in stage IIC 2 residual asymptomatic in stage IIIA with no progression after 24 mo f-u
Nicolai (2003)[67]	15	Andrews	2 type I 9 type II 3 type IIIA 1 type IIIB	50 (24–93) [SD 19.9])	1 residual (24 mo postop)
Naragi (2003)[72]	12	Bremer	2 stage IA 2 stage IB 3 stage IIA 5 stage IIB	15	2 (endosc.-C-L) Recurrence rate 18%
Wormald (2003)[73]	7	Radkowski	1 stage I 2 stage IIA 3 stage 1 stage IIC	45 (SD 23)	No
Munoz del Castillo (2004)[74]	11	Andrews	8 type II		36.3% recurrence
Mann (2004)[75]	15	Fisch	Stages I–III (number of cases not specified)	(12–240) (referred to a total of 30 patients with JA)	1 (stage not mentioned)
Pryor (2005)[76]	6	–	–	14	No recurrences 1 patient underwent endoscopic removal secondarily after prior treatment elsewhere
Hofmann (2005)[77]	21	Andrews	1 type I 15 type II 5 type IIIA	51.7 (5–120)	3 (14.3%) recurrences (2 underwent endoscopic resection, one gamma-knife) + 3 asymptomatic[c]
Sciaretta (2006)[78]	9	Radkowski/ Andrews[b]	1 stage IA 4 stage IIA 1 stage IIB 2 stage IIC 1 stage IIIA	18.1 (6–75)	1 recurrence of a stage IIB 20 mo postop, now staged IIA: reoperated by ESS, 25 mo disease-free
Tosun (2006)[79]	9	Radkowski	2 stage IA 2 stage IB 3 stage IIA 2 stage IIIA	20.6 (12–55)	No recurrence 2 endoscopically assessed were recurrent tumors

Author[a] (year of publication)	Total n	Classifica-tion	n + stage	Mean follow-up (mo) (range)	Recurrence/residual
Borghei (2006)[62]	23	Radkowski	5 stage IA 9 stage IB 4 stage IIA 5 stage IIB	33.1 (14–57)	1 recurrence (4.3%) of a stage IIB 19 mo postop. Endoscopic re-operation, now 28 mo disease-free
Eloy (2007)[80]	6	Radkowski	1 stage I 1 stage IB 4 stage IIB	67	1 recurrence cured by ESS. 1 residual nonsymptomatic nodule in the pterygopalatine fossa, regressing on MRI 4 y postop)
Andrade (2007)[81]	12	Andrews	8 stage I 4 stage II	5–42[e] 24 (12–60)[f]	No
Yiotakis (2008)[82]	9	Radkowski	Stages between I and IIB	10.5 (6–36)	1 recurrence[g]
Gupta (2008)[83]	28	Radkowski	6 stage I 14 stage IIA 6 stage IIB 2 stag IIC	Min.12 mo (12–65)	No recurrence 1 residual (prior recurrence of stage IIC) 7 had prior external approaches, the recurrences being approached now endoscopically
Hackmann (2009)[84]	15	–	4 had prior surgery	48 (12–120) (including 16 cases with combined/open surgery)	1 (not specified)
Bleier (2009)[63]	10	Andrews	1 stage I 8 stage II 1 stage IIA	24.4 (3.6–88.4) (including 8 cases with open surgery)	No
Ardehali (2010)[85]	47[d]	Radkowski	21 stages IA to IIB 22 stage IIC 3 stage IIIA 1 stage IIIB	33.1 (8–74)	6/31 recurrences of primary treated patients (1 stage IA, 1 stage IB 2 stage IIA; 1 stage IIIA and 1 stage IIC) 3/16 recurrences in secondarily treated (1 stage IIIA, 2 stage IIC) 5 patients embolized before surgery. 4 patients combined approach

Abbreviations: C-L, Caldwell Luc; endosc., endoscopy; ESS, endoscopic sinus surgery; f-u, follow-up; ICA = internal carotid artery; JA, juvenile angiofibroma; mo = months; Rec.-rate: recurrence rate; SD = standard deviation; y, year(s).

Source: Al-Deen S, Bachmann-Harilstad G. Rhinology 2008;46(4):281[31] with permission of *Rhinology.*

[a] Only first author mentioned, in chronological order.

[b] Radkowski chosen among the staging systems used in the paper.

[c] MRI enhancement without symptoms or growth during follow-up of 3, 5, and 10 years, respectively.

[d] 31 (66%) cases were primarily treated, the remaining 16 (34%) cases were treated secondarily, having been previously operated by conventional or endoscopic methods; 43 cases were approached endoscopically and 4 cases by combined approaches.

[e] In the abstract.

[f] In the text.

[g] 2 recurrences attributed to transpalatal approach in the text, but one found for endoscopic approach.

Key Points

- This aggressive benign tumor occurs almost exclusively in young male patients and has attracted considerable attention in the literature over the past 50 years.
- A tertiary care referral center that specializes in tumors of the nose, paranasal sinuses, and skull base is preferred for the treatment of these rare and difficult cases.
- Late presentation with extensive tumors remains a common situation around the world and recurrence rates for a benign lesion remain unacceptably high.
- A thorough understanding of the natural history of this lesion and the availability of all surgical approaches is to be preferred.
- High-quality skull base imaging, preoperative embolization, and the occasional need for modern, targeted radiotherapy are additional requirements for the satisfactory treatment of this lesion.

References

1. Chaveau C. Histoire des maladies du pharynx. Paris: Barriere; 1906
2. Friedberg P. Vascular fibromas of the nasopharynx. Arch Otolaryngol 1940;41:313–326
3. Lloyd G, Howard D, Phelps P, Cheesman A. Juvenile angiofibroma: the lessons of 20 years of modern imaging. J Laryngol Otol 1999;113(2):127–134
4. Neel HB III, Whicker JH, Devine KD, Weiland LH. Juvenile angiofibroma. Review of 120 cases. Am J Surg 1973;126(4):547–556
5. Bremer JW, Neel HB III, DeSanto LW, Jones GC. Angiofibroma: treatment trends in 150 patients during 40 years. Laryngoscope 1986;96(12):1321–1329
6. Rao BN, Shewalkar BK. Clinical profile and multimodality approach in the management of juvenile nasopharyngeal angiofibroma. Indian J Cancer 2000;37(4):133–139
7. Paris J, Guelfucci B, Moulin G, Zanaret M, Triglia JM. Diagnosis and treatment of juvenile nasopharyngeal angiofibroma. Eur Arch Otorhinolaryngol 2001;258(3):120–124
8. Glad H, Vainer B, Buchwald C, et al. Juvenile nasopharyngeal angiofibromas in Denmark 1981-2003: diagnosis, incidence, and treatment. Acta Otolaryngol 2007;127(3):292–299
9. Osborn DA, Sokolovski A. Juvenile nasopharyngeal angiofibroma in a female. Report of a case. Arch Otolaryngol 1965;82(6):629–632
10. Brunner H. Nasopharyngeal fibroma. Ann Otol Rhinol Laryngol 1942;51:29–63
11. Harrison DF. The natural history, pathogenesis, and treatment of juvenile angiofibroma. Personal experience with 44 patients. Arch Otolaryngol Head Neck Surg 1987;113(9):936–942
12. Beham A, Beham-Schmid C, Regauer S, Auböck L, Stammberger H. Nasopharyngeal angiofibroma: true neoplasm or vascular malformation? Adv Anat Pathol 2000;7(1):36–46
13. Schick B, Plinkert PK, Prescher A. Aetiology of angiofibromas:reflection on their specific vascular component. [Article in German] Laryngorhinootologie 2002; 81(4):280–284
14. Hwang HC, Mills SE, Patterson K, Gown AM. Expression of androgen receptors in nasopharyngeal angiofibroma: an immunohistochemical study of 24 cases. Mod Pathol 1998;11(11):1122–1126
15. Schick B, Rippel C, Brunner C, Jung V, Plinkert PK, Urbschat S. Numerical sex chromosome aberrations in juvenile angiofibromas: genetic evidence for an androgen-dependent tumor? Oncol Rep 2003;10(5):1251–1255
16. Montag AG, Tretiakova M, Richardson M. Steroid hormone receptor expression in nasopharyngeal angiofibromas. Consistent expression of estrogen receptor beta. Am J Clin Pathol 2006;125(6):832–837
17. Abraham SC, Montgomery EA, Giardiello FM, Wu TT. Frequent beta-catenin mutations in juvenile nasopharyngeal angiofibromas. Am J Pathol 2001;158(3):1073–1078
18. Zhang PJ, Weber R, Liang HH, Pasha TL, LiVolsi VA. Growth factors and receptors in juvenile nasopharyngeal angiofibroma and nasal polyps: an immunohistochemical study. Arch Pathol Lab Med 2003;127(11):1480–1484
19. Giardiello FM, Hamilton SR, Krush AJ, Offerhaus JA, Booker SV, Petersen GM. Nasopharyngeal angiofibroma in patients with familial adenomatous polyposis. Gastroenterology 1993;105(5):1550–1552
20. Ferouz AS, Mohr RM, Paul P. Juvenile nasopharyngeal angiofibroma and familial adenomatous polyposis: an association? Otolaryngol Head Neck Surg 1995;113(4):435–439
21. Guertl B, Beham A, Zechner R, Stammberger H, Hoefler G. Nasopharyngeal angiofibroma: an APC-gene-associated tumor? Hum Pathol 2000;31(11):1411–1413
22. Stiller D, Katenkamp D, Küttner K. Cellular differentiations and structural characteristics in nasopharyngeal angiofibromas. An electron-microscopic study. Virchows Arch A Pathol Anat Histol 1976;371(3):273–282
23. Taxy JB. Juvenile nasopharyngeal angiofibroma: an ultrastructural study. Cancer 1977;39(3):1044–1054
24. Hill DL. Morphology of nasopharyngeal angiofibroma. An electron microscope study. J Submicrosc Cytol 1985;17(3):443–448
25. Holman C, Miller W. Juvenile nasopharyngeal angiofibroma. AJR Am J Roentgenol 1965;94:292–298
26. Petruson K, Rodriguez-Catarino M, Petruson B, Finizia C. Juvenile nasopharyngeal angiofibroma: long-term results in preoperative embolized and non-embolized patients. Acta Otolaryngol 2002;122(1):96–100
27. McCombe A, Lund VJ, Howard DJ. Recurrence in juvenile angiofibroma. Rhinology 1990;28(2):97–102
28. Sessions RB, Bryan RN, Naclerio RM, Alford BR. Radiographic staging of juvenile angiofibroma. Head Neck Surg 1981;3(4):279–283
29. Chandler JR, Goulding R, Moskowitz L, Quencer RM. Nasopharyngeal angiofibromas: staging and management. Ann Otol Rhinol Laryngol 1984;93(4 Pt 1):322–329
30. Andrews JC, Fisch U, Valavanis A, Aeppli U, Makek MS. The surgical management of extensive nasopharyngeal angiofibromas with the infratemporal fossa approach. Laryngoscope 1989;99(4):429–437
31. Lund VJ, Stammberger H, Nicolai P, et al. European position paper on endoscopic management of tumours of the nose, paranasal sinuses and skull base. Rhinol Suppl 2010;(22):1–143
32. Antonelli AR, Cappiello J, Di Lorenzo D, Donajo CA, Nicolai P, Orlandini A. Diagnosis, staging, and treatment of juvenile nasopharyngeal angiofibroma (JNA). Laryngoscope 1987;97(11):1319–1325
33. Radkowski D, McGill T, Healy GB, Ohlms L, Jones DT. Angiofibroma. Changes in staging and treatment. Arch Otolaryngol Head Neck Surg 1996;122(2):122–129
34. Carrillo JF, Maldonado F, Albores O, Ramírez-Ortega MC, Oñate-Ocaña LF. Juvenile nasopharyngeal angiofibroma: clinical factors associated with recurrence, and proposal of a staging system. J Surg Oncol 2008;98(2):75–80

35. Snyderman CH, Pant H, Carrau RL, Gardner P. A new endoscopic staging system for angiofibromas. Arch Otolaryngol Head Neck Surg 2010;136(6):588–594
36. Makek MS, Andrews JC, Fisch U. Malignant transformation of a nasopharyngeal angiofibroma. Laryngoscope 1989;99(10 Pt 1):1088–1092
37. Cummings BJ, Blend R, Keane T, et al. Primary radiation therapy for juvenile nasopharyngeal angiofibroma. Laryngoscope 1984;94(12 Pt 1):1599–1605
38. Jacobsson M, Petruson B, Ruth M, Svendsen P. Involution of juvenile nasopharyngeal angiofibroma with intracranial extension. A case report with computed tomographic assessment. Arch Otolaryngol Head Neck Surg 1989;115(2):238–239
39. Stansbie JM, Phelps PD. Involution of residual juvenile nasopharyngeal angiofibroma (a case report). J Laryngol Otol 1986;100(5):599–603
40. Sellars SL. Juvenile nasopharyngeal angiofibroma. S Afr Med J 1980;58(24):961–964
41. Howard DJ, Lloyd G, Lund V. Recurrence and its avoidance in juvenile angiofibroma. Laryngoscope 2001;111(9):1509–1511
42. Myhre M, Michaels L. Nasopharyngeal angiofibroma treated in 1841 by maxillectomy. J Otolaryngol 1987;16(6):390–392
43. De Vincentiis M, Gallo A, Minni A, Torri E, Tomassi R, Della Rocca C. Preoperative embolization in the treatment protocol for rhinopharyngeal angiofibroma: comparison of the effectiveness of various materials. [Article in Italian] Acta Otorhinolaryngol Ital 1997;17(3):225–232
44. Gore P, Theodore N, Brasiliense L, et al. The utility of onyx for preoperative embolization of cranial and spinal tumors. Neurosurgery 2008;62(6):1204–1211, discussion 1211–1212
45. Tranbahuy P, Borsik M, Herman P, Wassef M, Casasco A. Direct intratumoral embolization of juvenile angiofibroma. Am J Otolaryngol 1994;15(6):429–435
46. Roberson GH, Biller H, Sessions DG, Ogura JH. Presurgical internal maxillary artery embolization in juvenile angiofibroma. Laryngoscope 1972;82(8):1524–1532
47. Schiff M. Juvenile nasopharyngeal angiofibroma. a theory of pathogenesis. Laryngoscope 1959;69:981–1016
48. Johnsen S, Kloster JH, Schiff M. The action of hormones on juvenile nasopharyngeal angiofibroma. A case report. Acta Otolaryngol 1966;61(1):153–160
49. Gates GA, Rice DH, Koopmann CF Jr, Schuller DE. Flutamide-induced regression of angiofibroma. Laryngoscope 1992;102(6):641–644
50. Labra A, Chavolla-Magaña R, Lopez-Ugalde A, Alanis-Calderon J, Huerta-Delgado A. Flutamide as a preoperative treatment in juvenile angiofibroma (JA) with intracranial invasion: report of 7 cases. Otolaryngol Head Neck Surg 2004;130(4):466–469
51. Reddy KA, Mendenhall WM, Amdur RJ, Stringer SP, Cassisi NJ. Long-term results of radiation therapy for juvenile nasopharyngeal angiofibroma. Am J Otolaryngol 2001;22(3):172–175
52. Lee JT, Chen P, Safa A, Juillard G, Calcaterra TC. The role of radiation in the treatment of advanced juvenile angiofibroma. Laryngoscope 2002;112(7 Pt 1):1213–1220
53. Gold DG, Neglia JP, Potish RA, Dusenbery KE. Second neoplasms following megavoltage radiation for pediatric tumors. Cancer 2004;100(1):212–213
54. Goepfert H, Cangir A, Lee YY. Chemotherapy for aggressive juvenile nasopharyngeal angiofibroma. Arch Otolaryngol 1985;111(5):285–289
55. Howard DJ, Lund VJ. The role of midfacial degloving in modern rhinological practice. J Laryngol Otol 1999;113(10):885–887
56. Fisch U. The infratemporal fossa approach for nasopharyngeal tumors. Laryngoscope 1983;93(1):36–44
57. Fisch U, Fagan P, Valavanis A. The infratemporal fossa approach for the lateral skull base. Otolaryngol Clin North Am 1984;17(3):513–552
58. Donald PJ, Enepikedes D, Boggan J. Giant juvenile nasopharyngeal angiofibroma: management by skull-base surgery. Arch Otolaryngol Head Neck Surg 2004;130(7):882–886
59. Krekorian EA, Kato RH. Surgical management of nasopharyngeal angiofibroma with intracranial extension. Laryngoscope 1977;87(2):154–164
60. Jafek BW, Krekorian EA, Kirsch WM, Wood RP. Juvenile nasopharyngeal angiofibroma: management of intracranial extension. Head Neck Surg 1979;2(2):119–128
61. Cummings BJ. Relative risk factors in the treatment of juvenile nasopharyngeal angiofibroma. Head Neck Surg 1980;3(1):21–26
62. Borghei P, Baradaranfar MH, Borghei SH, Sokhandon F. Transnasal endoscopic resection of juvenile nasopharyngeal angiofibroma without preoperative embolization. Ear Nose Throat J 2006;85(11):740–743, 746
63. Bleier BS, Kennedy DW, Palmer JN, Chiu AG, Bloom JD, O'Malley BW Jr. Current management of juvenile nasopharyngeal angiofibroma: a tertiary center experience 1999–2007. Am J Rhinol Allergy 2009;23(3):328–330
64. Nakamura H, Kawasaki M, Higuchi Y, Seki S, Takahashi S. Transnasal endoscopic resection of juvenile nasopharyngeal angiofibroma with KTP laser. Eur Arch Otorhinolaryngol 1999;256(4):212–214
65. Mair EA, Battiata A, Casler JD. Endoscopic laser-assisted excision of juvenile nasopharyngeal angiofibromas. Arch Otolaryngol Head Neck Surg 2003;129(4):454–459
66. Ochi K, Watanabe S, Miyabe S. Endoscopic transnasal resection of a juvenile angiofibroma using an ultrasonically activated scalpel. ORL J Otorhinolaryngol Relat Spec 2002;64(4):290–293
67. Nicolai P, Berlucchi M, Tomenzoli D, et al. Endoscopic surgery for juvenile angiofibroma: when and how. Laryngoscope 2003;113(5):775–782
68. Önerci TM, Yücel OT, Oğretmenoğlu O. Endoscopic surgery in treatment of juvenile nasopharyngeal angiofibroma. Int J Pediatr Otorhinolaryngol 2003;67(11):1219–1225
69. Schick B, el Rahman el Tahan A, Brors D, Kahle G, Draf W. Experiences with endonasal surgery in angiofibroma. Rhinology 1999;37(2):80–85
70. Jorissen M, Eloy P, Rombaux P, Bachert C, Daele J. Endoscopic sinus surgery for juvenile nasopharyngeal angiofibroma. Acta Otorhinolaryngol Belg 2000;54(2):201–219
71. Roger G, Tran Ba Huy P, Froehlich P, et al. Exclusively endoscopic removal of juvenile nasopharyngeal angiofibroma: trends and limits. Arch Otolaryngol Head Neck Surg 2002;128(8):928–935
72. Naraghi M, Kashfi A. Endoscopic resection of nasopharyngeal angiofibromas by combined transnasal and transoral routes. Am J Otolaryngol 2003;24(3):149–154
73. Wormald PJ, Van Hasselt A. Endoscopic removal of juvenile angiofibromas. Otolaryngol Head Neck Surg 2003;129(6):684–691
74. Muñoz del Castillo F, Jurado Ramos A, Bravo-Rodríguez F, Delgado Acosta F, López Villarejo P. Endoscopic surgery of nasopharyngeal angiofibroma. [Article in Spanish] Acta Otorrinolaringol Esp 2004;55(8):369–375
75. Mann WJ, Jecker P, Amedee RG. Juvenile angiofibromas: changing surgical concept over the last 20 years. Laryngoscope 2004;114(2):291–293
76. Pryor SG, Moore EJ, Kasperbauer JL. Endoscopic versus traditional approaches for excision of juvenile nasopharyngeal angiofibroma. Laryngoscope 2005;115(7):1201–1207
77. Hofmann T, Bernal-Sprekelsen M, Koele W, Reittner P, Klein E, Stammberger H. Endoscopic resection of

juvenile angiofibromas—long term results. Rhinology 2005; 43(4):282–289

78. Sciarretta V, Pasquini E, Frank G, et al. Endoscopic treatment of benign tumors of the nose and paranasal sinuses: a report of 33 cases. Am J Rhinol 2006;20(1):64–71

79. Tosun F, Ozer C, Gerek M, Yetiser S. Surgical approaches for nasopharyngeal angiofibroma: comparative analysis and current trends. J Craniofac Surg 2006;17(1):15–20

80. Eloy P, Watelet JB, Hatert AS, de Wispelaere J, Bertrand B. Endonasal endoscopic resection of juvenile nasopharyngeal angiofibroma. Rhinology 2007;45(1):24–30

81. Andrade NA, Pinto JA, Nóbrega MdeO, Aguiar JE, Aguiar TF, Vinhaes ES. Exclusively endoscopic surgery for juvenile nasopharyngeal angiofibroma. Otolaryngol Head Neck Surg 2007;137(3):492–496

82. Yiotakis I, Eleftheriadou A, Davilis D, et al. Juvenile nasopharyngeal angiofibroma stages I and II: a comparative study of surgical approaches. Int J Pediatr Otorhinolaryngol 2008;72(6):793–800

83. Gupta AK, Rajiniganth MG, Gupta AK. Endoscopic approach to juvenile nasopharyngeal angiofibroma: our experience at a tertiary care centre. J Laryngol Otol 2008; 122(11):1185–1189

84. Hackman T, Snyderman CH, Carrau R, Vescan A, Kassam A. Juvenile nasopharyngeal angiofibroma: the expanded endonasal approach. Am J Rhinol Allergy 2009; 23(1):95–99

85. Ardehali MM, Samimi Ardestani SH, Yazdani N, Goodarzi H, Bastaninejad S. Endoscopic approach for excision of juvenile nasopharyngeal angiofibroma: complications and outcomes. Am J Otolaryngol 2010;31(5):343–349

Glomangiopericytoma (Sinonasal Type Hemangiopericytoma)

Introduction

Throughout our ENT surgical careers, we have listened to the tale of the highly controversial pericyte contractile cell adjacent to capillaries from our original pathology mentor, Professor Leslie Michaels, and subsequently from the next generation of pathologists, Dr. Andrew Gallimore and Dr. Ann Sandison. The addition of the solitary extrapleural fibrous tumor to the debate in the 1980s, which was originally thought to be a primary neoplasm of the pleura (first reported in 1931),[1] has on many occasions during combined clinical pathology and radiology meetings caused us some confusion and has certainly been associated with considerable humor on occasions! We have fortunately worked long enough to see some clarification of these matters, and in 2005 the WHO classification of tumors[2] finally allocated the term "glomangiopericytoma" to the sinonasal form of hemangiopericytoma. This tumor at present appears to be specific to the head and neck. In contrast to hemangiopericytomas and solitary fibrous tumors occurring elsewhere in the body (which now are recognized to have considerable overlap of their histological features and which are strongly CD34 positive, probably representing a specialist fibroblast),

the glomangiopericytoma is negative for CD34 and positive for SMA, indicating a myopericytoma phenotype.

Definition

(ICD-O code 9150/1)

A sinonasal tumor demonstrating a perivascular myopericytoma phenotype.

Synonyms

As indicated above, the term sinonasal hemangiopericytoma has long been in use, but additionally hemangiopericytoma-like tumor, sinonasal glomus tumor, and simply hemangiopericytoma have all been used within the literature.

Etiology

There are no defined etiological factors.

Site and Incidence

Glomangiopericytomas have a predilection for the nasal cavity and paranasal sinuses but they remain a rare lesion comprising less than 0.5% of all neoplasms in this area. Catalano et al,[3] presenting seven of their own patients in 1996, undertook a thorough review of the available literature and ascertained a total of 119 cases with sufficient evidence for sinonasal hemangiopericytoma. Over 150 cases have now been reported in the literature and we have treated 13 cases.

The majority of reported cases appeared to arise in the nasal cavity and many were noted to arise from the inferior or middle turbinate (**Fig. 9.27**). However, involvement of the ethmoids, sphenoid, maxillary, frontal sinuses, and nasopharynx have all been noted. The ethmoids and sphenoid are commoner than the maxillary or frontal sinuses. A small proportion of the tumors are bilateral. Extension through the cribriform plate into the intracranial structures can occur. Two of Catalano's own seven cases had involved the cribriform plate.[3] In our group, 7 arose in the nasal cavity, 2 the ethmoid sinuses (one breaching the skull base), and 4 originated in the orbit, specifically affecting the nasolacrimal sac. Within the nasal cavity both the lateral wall and septum were affected (**Table 9.5**).

Diagnostic Features

Clinical Features

The reported ages ranged from 4 to 80 years with an approximately equal distribution of males to females, although Catalano's own series of seven cases had a female predominance of 6:1,[3] as does ours with 9 women versus 4 men. Our patients also had a wide age range from 20 to 82 years, mean 59.6 years.

Table 9.5 Glomangiopericytoma: personal series

Age/sex	Site	Management	Long-term follow-up
33 F	Ethmoid	INE	Lost
69 F	Nasal cavity	Lateral rhinotomy	A&W 2 y then lost
82 F	Nasal cavity	Lateral rhinotomy	DICD
54 F	Nasal cavity	Lateral rhinotomy	A&W 2 y then lost
69 F	Posterior ethmoid	Craniofacial resection	A&W 22 y
54 F	Nasal cavity–ethmoid	ESS	A&W 5 y
50 M	Nasal cavity–frontonasal recess	ESS	A&W 7 y 4 mo
49 M	Nasal cavity–septum	ESS	A&W 10 y 4 mo
79 M	Nasal cavity–septum	ESS	A&W 4 y
20 F	Orbit–nasolacrimal sac	DCR via lateral rhinotomy	A&W 10 y
68 F	Orbit–nasolacrimal sac	DCR via lateral rhinotomy	A&W 10 y
68 M	Orbit–nasolacrimal sac	Orbital clearance, radiotherapy	AWR 2 y
80 F	Orbit–nasolacrimal sac	Orbital clearance	A&W 8 y

Abbreviations: A&W, alive and well; AWR, alive with recurrence; DCR, dacryocystorhinectomy; ESS, endoscopic sinus surgery; F, female; INE, intranasal ethmoidectomy; M, male; mo, month(s); y, year(s).

Nasal obstruction and epistaxis are the commonest non-specific presenting symptoms. Others include rhinorrhea, serous otitis media, proptosis, facial pain, and infraorbital paresthesia. On examination those tumors visible in the nasal cavity generally appear to be tan or gray colored polypoidal lesions that bleed briskly on manipulation.

Imaging

Imaging features are nonspecific showing nasal cavity or paranasal sinus lesions, which often have a significant polypoidal appearance with associated inflammatory changes in the dependant sinuses, bone erosion, and sclerosis (**Fig. 9.27**).

Histological Features and Differential Diagnosis

On histological evaluation, these lesions are subepithelial and well delineated but they are nonencapsulated cellular tumors that may surround other normal structures. Most tumors are highly cellular with short to medium-sized spindle cells that are tapered and without much cytoplasm, which helps to distinguish them from higher-grade lesions such as leiomyosarcoma and fibrosarcoma. The nucleoli are usually single and not prominent and chromatin is finely dispersed. The pattern is generally one of short fascicles, small whorls, and perpendicular orientation around vessels. Vascular channels vary from capillary size to large patchoulis spaces that may have a "stag horn" or antlerlike configuration. A prominent periepitheliomatous hyalinization is characteristic. Occasional mitotic figures may be present but necrosis is not found in these lesions. Associated extravasated erythrocytes, mast cells, and eosinophils are frequently present and occasionally giant cells may be seen.

Immunohistochemistry

As noted in the introduction to this section, glomangiopericytoma of the sinonasal tract is distinctly different from soft tissue hemangiopericytoma in the rest of the body and lacks the strong diffuse staining for CD34. Glomangiopericytomas usually have diffuse reactivity for actins, factor XIIIa, and vimentin. While for many years this lesion was known as a sinonasal hemangiopericytoma, it is clinically, morphologically and biologically distinct from other soft tissue type hemangiopericytomas.

Differential diagnosis includes hemangioma, solitary fibrous tumor, glomus tumor, leiomyoma, synovial sarcoma, leiomyosarcoma, fibrosarcoma, and malignant fibrous histiocytoma. Additionally, olfactory neuroblastoma, solid adenoid cystic carcinoma, angiofibroma, and carcinomas have been mentioned as possible areas of confusion in the past, but with modern immunohistochemistry and our increased understanding of this lesion, they should not present a problem in the future.

Treatment and Prognosis

Both the large reviews of cases by Catalano et al[3] and Thompson et al[4] stress that surgery was the treatment of choice for the majority of these patients. Provided that complete surgical excision appears to be achieved, they have greater than 90% 5-year survival. Recurrence has been reported in up to 30% of cases, but in the 104 cases reported from the files of the Armed Forces Institute of

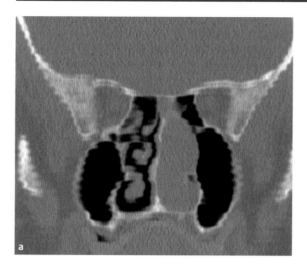

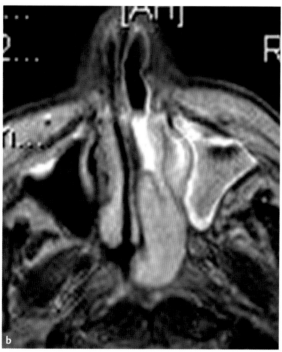

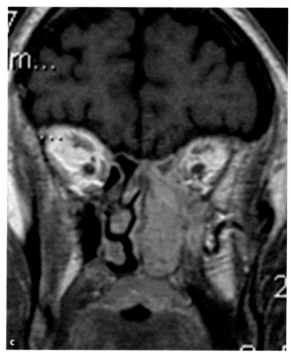

Fig. 9.27a–c

a Glomangiopericytoma. Coronal CT scan (reconstructed) showing a polypoid mass filling the left nasal cavity without obvious bone erosion, subsequently excised endoscopically.

b Coronal MRI (T1W post gadolinium enhancement) in the same patient taken several weeks later and showing a nasal mass with secretions in the obstructed adjacent maxillary and posterior ethmoid sinuses.

c Axial MRI (T1W post gadolinium enhancement) in the same patient.

Pathology between 1970 and 1995 by Thompson and colleagues,[4] the 18 recurrences developed over periods of between 1 and 12 years. Recurrent tumor can be managed by additional surgery and only 4 of their 104 cases were given additional radiotherapy. Of interest in this particular paper by three internationally eminent pathologists—Lester Thompson, Markkus Miettinen, and Bruce Wenig—is the considerable debate that they undertake in this paper over the biological behavior of these sinonasal tract lesions, and their statement that their preferred terminology for this tumor was sinonasal type hemangiopericytoma. Less than 2 years later it was listed in the WHO classification as glomangiopericytoma! Their detailed histopathological and immunohistochemistry studies did

not shed light on the small number of recurrences but did confirm the relatively indolent behavior with a potential for local recurrence but not metastatic disease. They concluded that the evaluation demonstrated a kinship to glomus tumors, reporting the contention that sinonasal type hemangiopericytoma is a perivascular tumor with myoid or glomus-like differentiation distinctly contrasting with the hemangiopericytoma of soft tissues.

As might be expected, endoscopic resection has been undertaken for this lesion and small numbers appear as single case reports[5,6] or in the various series appearing in the literature,[7] the largest of which is a retrospective review of 10 cases treated between 1997 and 2008.[8] This comprised 5 men and 5 women with an average age of 59 years, one of whom had a stroke related to the surgery. However, only one patient had a recurrence that required combined external and endoscopic surgery together with orbital exenteration, and died of disease at 138 months.

In our series of 13 patients, treatment was surgical in all cases, only one receiving additional radiotherapy for recurrent disease. The surgical procedures ranged from intranasal ethmoidectomy in 1970 to endoscopic surgery for the four most recent cases (post 2000). One patient had a craniofacial resection for skull base involvement early in the series and five had lateral rhinotomy approaches to access either nasal or medial orbital lesions. In the orbit complete resection of the nasolacrimal system has been required together with the adjacent orbital periosteum and/or orbital clearance for the two most extensive lesions (**Table 9.5**).

Overall the results have been excellent, irrespective of the surgical approach, with 10 patients alive and well with long-term follow-up ranging from 2 to 22 years, one is alive with recurrence, one died of "old age" and the earliest patient was not followed up, having come from abroad. Our series concurs with the reported literature.

Key Points

- The WHO classification now uses the term "glomangiopericytoma" instead of sinonasal hemangiopericytoma as it is clinically, morphologically and biologically distinct from hemangiopericytomas in the rest of the body.
- On immunohistochemistry glomangiopericytoma lacks the strong diffuse staining for CD34.
- Complete surgical excision is treatment of choice by whatever approach is appropriate.

References

1. Klemperer P, Rabin C. Primary neoplasms of the pleura: A report of five cases. Arch Pathol (Chic) 1931;11:385–412
2. Barnes L, Everson J, Reicchart P, Sidransky D, eds. World Health Organization Classification of Tumours. Pathology and Genetics of Head and Neck Tumours. Lyon: IARC Press; 2005
3. Catalano PJ, Brandwein M, Shah DK, Urken ML, Lawson W, Biller HF. Sinonasal hemangiopericytomas: a clinicopathologic and immunohistochemical study of seven cases. Head Neck 1996;18(1):42–53
4. Thompson LD, Miettinen M, Wenig BM. Sinonasal-type hemangiopericytoma: a clinicopathologic and immunophenotypic analysis of 104 cases showing perivascular myoid differentiation. Am J Surg Pathol 2003; 27(6):737–749
5. Serrano E, Coste A, Percodani J, Hervé S, Brugel L. Endoscopic sinus surgery for sinonasal haemangiopericytomas. J Laryngol Otol 2002;116(11):951–954
6. Schatton R, Golusinski W, Wielgosz R, Lamprecht J. Endonasal resection of a sinonasal haemangiopericytoma. Rep Pract Oncol Radiother 2005;10:261–264
7. Kassam AB, Prevedello DM, Carrau RL, et al. Endoscopic endonasal skull base surgery: analysis of complications in the authors' initial 800 patients. J Neurosurg 2011; 114(6):1544–1568
8. Bignami M, Dallan I, Battaglia P, Lenzi R, Pistochini A, Castelnuovo P. Endoscopic, endonasal management of sinonasal haemangiopericytoma: 12-year experience. J Laryngol Otol 2010;124(11):1178–1182

Angiosarcoma

Definition

(ICD-O code 9120/3)

Angiosarcomas are rare, highly malignant tumors of vascular phenotype with anastomosing vascular channels lined with remarkably atypical endothelial cells.

Synonyms

Alternative names for these tumors include malignant hemangioendothelioma, malignant angioendothelioma, hemangiosarcoma, and lymphangiosarcoma.

Etiology

It is now generally accepted that there are five variants of angiosarcoma: (1) lymphedema angiosarcoma, first reported by Stewart and Treves in 1948[1]; (2) post-mastectomy angiosarcoma[2,3]; (3) breast angiosarcoma; (4) deep soft tissue angiosarcoma; and (5) cutaneous angiosarcoma. Only the last two forms of angiosarcoma occur in the head and neck, and the scalp is by far the most common site for cutaneous angiosarcoma although the tongue, oral cavity, oropharynx, nasopharynx, sinonasal tract, and larynx may all be involved.[4–7] While no specific etiological factors are known at a cellular level, angiosarcoma has also been reported to occur following administration of Thorotrast and following radiotherapy.[8,9] Cytogenetic studies of angiosarcoma have not shown any consistent recurrent chromosomal abnormalities but typically complex karyotypes. TP53 mutational inactivation and an increase of MDM2 expression have been reported to lead to upregulation of VEGF expression in up to 80% of angiosarcomas.[10,11]

Site and Incidence

Angiosarcomas most commonly arise in the skin and superficial soft tissues of the head and neck but the disease is rare, accounting for less than 2% of all sarcomas. More than half of all angiosarcomas occur in the head and neck. The scalp, forehead, and face—in descending order—are by far the commonest sites in the larger reported series.[6,12]

In the sinonasal tract, the maxillary sinus is the most frequently reported site of origin, although as the nasal cavity and other paranasal sinuses are frequently involved as well at the time of presentation, the exact site of origin is not always clearly defined. Of the combined total of 43 cases from two reports emanating from major head and neck centers in the United States, only two cases involved the nose and sinuses, one each involving the ethmoid and maxilla. A recent report by Nelson and Thompson presented 10 cases of sinonasal tract angiosarcoma that were retrospectively retrieved from the Otorhinolaryngologic Registry of the Armed Forces Institute of Pathology.[13]

Diagnostic Features

Clinical Features

Angiosarcomas can occur at all ages, from infants to the elderly, but predominate in the latter group. Those reported from the sinonasal tract appear to have a peak in the fifth decade and a notable male predilection of between 2:1 and 3:1. The female patients tend to be approximately a decade younger in the reported cases.[14–16] This said, our single case of angiosarcoma occurred in a 58-year-old woman from Cyprus whose tumor arose in the middle meatus, affecting the middle turbinate and anterior ethmoids without obvious orbital involvement.

Elderly male patients predominate in reports with lesions presenting in the sinonasal tract in the same way as the much commoner presentation of the skin and soft tissues of the scalp and face. The duration of symptoms reported in the sinonasal cases seems to vary from weeks to months but is generally shorter than many of the cases affecting areas of skin. The latter often remain incorrectly diagnosed for long periods of time and have been reported to be confused with diagnosis such as rhinophyma, arteriovenous malformations, lymphoma, sarcoidosis, or facial granuloma. Sinonasal cases, however, commonly present with recurrent epistaxis and an intranasal/sinus mass lesion, nasal obstruction, nasal discharge (which has often been described as foul smelling and blood tinged), paresthesia, facial pain, and dental symptoms. In contrast again to the commoner skin lesions, lymph node involvement and distant metastases are not common at presentation of the sinonasal lesions.

Tumors present with a mean size of around 4 cm in the sinonasal area but may be considerably larger and have been described as red to purple, soft and friable, but additionally nodular or polypoidal and often ulcerated with associated hemorrhage, blood clot, and notable areas of necrosis.

Imaging

Angiosarcomas presenting in the sinonasal tract have nonspecific imaging appearances and, despite being highly anaplastic vasoformative lesions, they do not usually have sufficiently large vascular channels or spaces for them to be clearly demonstrated either on CT or MRI. The value of imaging is related more to defining the extent of the lesion, although the lesions may be diffuse and infiltrative, giving rise to an underevaluation of their true extent.

Histological Features

Nelson and Thompson's study of 10 cases of sinonasal tract angiosarcomas showed that all tumors had anastomosing vascular channels lined with notably atypical endothelial cells that protrude into the lumen.[13] The vascular channels appear to dissect the stroma and there are both capillary-sized vessels and more cavernous vascular spaces. The endothelial cells vary considerably from being somewhat flattened to spindle and epithelioid types that may form papillary tufts. Neolumen formation is common and there are often considerable numbers of atypical mitotic figures. There are notable areas of necrosis and hemorrhage, and immunohistochemistry shows them to be immunoreactive for CD34, CD31, factor VIII, R-Ag, and smooth muscle actin. They are generally nonreactive for keratin and S100 protein.

Differential Diagnosis

The rarity of these lesions has presented considerable problems in the past as the differential diagnosis includes a wide range of possibilities ranging from granulation tissue through intravascular capillary endothelial hyperplasia, hemangioma, angiofibroma, and glomangiopericytoma, to poorly differentiated neoplasms including malignant melanoma, carcinoma, large cell lymphoma, and Kaposi's sarcoma.

CD31 reactivity and negativity for epithelial membrane antigen, S100 protein, and melanoma markers help to distinguish angiosarcoma from other tumor types and the infiltrative growth pattern, mitotic activity, and marked atypia help to distinguish angiosarcoma from benign vascular tumors. Unfortunately, the reports of these rare lesions confirm the difficulties experienced with the differential diagnosis in many cases and the consequences of this are inadequate or inappropriate treatment. **As angiosarcomas have a poor prognosis, it is particularly appropriate to distinguish them from other possible conditions**.

Treatment and Prognosis

Virtually all reported patients have been treated by surgical resection with postoperative radiation and, more recently, variable amounts of additional chemotherapy. Nelson and Thompson's 10 sinonasal cases were all treated by surgery with postoperative radiation, but 6 died from disease with a mean survival of 28.8 months.[13] Two further patients died without evidence of disease with a mean of 267 months and 2 remained alive with no evidence of disease at last follow-up with a mean of 254 months. So while recurrences appear to occur in more than 50% of patients, most likely due to incomplete excision or possibly multifocal areas of the lesions, several authors have stated that nasal angiosarcoma appears to have a better prognosis than the commoner scalp and facial skin lesions. There is insufficient literature to know whether this is due to most sinonasal angiosarcomas being described as histologically relatively low grade or a consequence of a shorter interval between diagnosis and treatment. Different survival rates may be related to different treatment, although most reports agree that the outcome is more favorable with the smaller-sized cutaneous and soft tissue lesions.[17,18] Lymph node and distant metastases seem to be uncommon in the reports of sinonasal cases, supporting the potential for a better prognosis.[19] Our patient underwent a wide-field clearance via a lateral rhinotomy in 1995 following failed chemoradiotherapy in Cyprus. She remained disease-free for 3 years until lost to follow-up.

Kaposi's sarcoma

Definition

(ICD-O code 9140/3)

Kaposi's sarcoma (KS) is an angioproliferative lesion that is regarded as one of the commonest variants of angiosarcoma. It was first recognized by Moritz Kaposi in 1872[20] and reported in Africa in the 1940s.[21] In 1972 it was described after renal transplantation and in the early 1980s was reported in New York and Los Angeles in association with HIV infection.[21]

Thus Kaposi's sarcoma is classified into four main forms: (1) classic, (2) African endemic, (3) immunosuppression- or transplantation-associated, and (4) AIDS-associated[22] of which type 4 is most commonly encountered in the upper respiratory tract. A further variant has been recently described in HIV-negative men.[23]

Etiology

Kaposi's sarcoma is now known to occur secondarily to infection with human herpes virus (HHV)-8[24,25] and the mode of transmission is mainly via saliva.[26] HHV-8 has been found in 49 to 100% of KS-affected patients. HHV-8 has been shown to replicate in oropharyngeal cells.

Incidence and Site

The AIDS-associated form is commonly found in the upper respiratory tract, especially in the oral cavity, although the other forms are rather rare in the head and neck.[27]

Where antiretroviral therapy has been available there has been a decrease in KS in Europe and the United States but it is increasing in Africa.[28] A 20-fold increase has been reported, composed of both African endemic and HIV-associated KS and is affecting men, women, and children.[29] In Zimbabwe, KS is the commonest cancer in men, with the age-standardized rate of KS between 1993 and 1995 being 47.2/100,000 for men and 17.3/100,000 for women.[28]

Diagnostic Features

Clinical Features and Histology

While classic KS typically affects elderly men, as a consequence of the association with HIV the demographic of KS in the head and neck is most often young to middle-aged males. However, as mentioned above, **women and children can also be affected**.

A wide variety of presentations have been described but the commonest appearances are of a patch (early) or nodular violaceous (late) lesion on the skin or mucosa. These are most often seen in the oral cavity, particularly on the hard palate and gingivae. The lesions may occasionally affect the nasal cavity and maxilla with or without AIDS and often in cases of disseminated disease.[30–33] The lesions may be single or multiple and are not painful. As they are superficial lesions, the imaging appearances are minor.

At the outset they are nonspecific proliferations of vascular tissue but become more infiltrative with time, developing nodularity. At this stage they are composed of spindle cells together with evidence of neoangiogenesis, inflammation, and edema. KS must therefore be differentiated from other tumors such as fibrosarcoma and kaposiform hemangioendothelioma, a lesion that is more typically seen in the retroperitoneum and limbs in children.[34] However, an array of immunohistochemistry markers are needed to show positivity to endothelial antigens (CD31, CD34) and factor VIII-related antigen as well as immunoreactivity to HHV-8.[22] The lesions are also usually positive to vimentin, LYVE-1, VEGFR-2 and -3 (vascular endothelial growth factor), angiopoietin-2, and D2–40.

Natural History

There is some debate whether KS is actually a malignancy or rather a reactive change or a combination of both. This is because, unlike most cancer cells, in KS the cells do not show autonomous growth and are dependent on exogenous cytokines for in vitro growth.[21] The latest evidence suggests that eventually a true neoplastic monoclonal component develops[31] and it is therefore generally regarded as a lesion of intermediate malignancy that can act in a locally aggressive fashion in the immunosuppressed.

Treatment and Outcome

This depends on the variant of KS. In the classic form, the slow process may require no treatment, although surgical excision and radiotherapy may also be used. With more aggressive forms, chemotherapy such as liposomal doxorubicin may be used.[25]

In AIDS-KS, antiretroviral drugs use alone may control the problem but again systemic chemotherapy may be used for more aggressive later forms. This can include liposomal daunorubicin, doxorubicin, and taxane/paclitaxel. Radiotherapy, laser therapy, and cryotherapy are also employed. For many patients a combination of antiretrovirals and doxorubicin provides complete or partial response rates of >70% and a low rate of relapse.[35,36]

The emerging profile of cytokines, growth factors, monoclonal antibodies, and transforming genes is opening up the possibility of specific therapies. This includes targeting the herpes virus and using thalidomide, interleukin-12, and monoclonal antibodies such as bevacizumab and sorafenib, both targeting VEGF.[21,37,38]

References

1. Stewart FW, Treves N. Lymphangiosarcoma in postmastectomy lymphedema; a report of six cases in elephantiasis chirurgica. Cancer 1948;1(1):64–81
2. Miettinen M, Lehto VP, Virtanen I. Postmastectomy angiosarcoma (Stewart-Treves syndrome). Light-microscopic, immunohistological, and ultrastructural characteristics of two cases. Am J Surg Pathol 1983;7(4):329–339
3. d'Amore ES, Wick MR, Geisinger KR, Frizzera G. Primary malignant lymphoma arising in postmastectomy lymphedema. Another facet of the Stewart-Treves syndrome. Am J Surg Pathol 1990;14(5):456–463
4. Kurien M, Nair S, Thomas S. Angiosarcoma of the nasal cavity and maxillary antrum. J Laryngol Otol 1989;103(9):874–876
5. Kimura Y, Tanaka S, Furukawa M. Angiosarcoma of the nasal cavity. J Laryngol Otol 1992;106(4):368–369
6. Aust MR, Olsen KD, Lewis JE, et al. Angiosarcomas of the head and neck: clinical and pathologic characteristics. Ann Otol Rhinol Laryngol 1997;106(11):943–951
7. Di Tommaso L, Colombo G, Miceli S, et al. Angiosarcoma of the nasal cavity. Report of a case and review of the literature. [Article in Italian] Pathologica 2007;99(3):76–80
8. Cafiero F, Gipponi M, Peressini A, et al. Radiation-associated angiosarcoma: diagnostic and therapeutic implications—two case reports and a review of the literature. Cancer 1996;77(12):2496–2502
9. Lipshutz GS, Brennan TV, Warren RS. Thorotrast-induced liver neoplasia: a collective review. J Am Coll Surg 2002;195(5):713–718
10. Naka N, Tomita Y, Nakanishi H, et al. Mutations of p53 tumor-suppressor gene in angiosarcoma. Int J Cancer 1997;71(6):952–955
11. Zietz C, Rössle M, Haas C, et al. MDM-2 oncoprotein overexpression, p53 gene mutation, and VEGF up-regulation in angiosarcomas. Am J Pathol 1998;153(5):1425–1433
12. Panje WR, Moran WJ, Bostwick DG, Kitt VV. Angiosarcoma of the head and neck: review of 11 cases. Laryngoscope 1986;96(12):1381–1384
13. Nelson BL, Thompson LD. Sinonasal tract angiosarcoma: a clinicopathologic and immunophenotypic study of 10 cases with a review of the literature. Head Neck Pathol 2007;1(1):1–12
14. Fu YS, Perzin KH. Non-epithelial tumors of the nasal cavity, paranasal sinuses, and nasopharynx: A clinicopathologic study. I. General features and vascular tumors. Cancer 1974;33(5):1275–1288
15. Narula AA, Vallis MP, el-Silimy OE, Dowling F, Bradley PJ. Radiation induced angiosarcomas of the nasopharynx. Eur J Surg Oncol 1986;12(2):147–152
16. Triantafillidou K, Lazaridis N, Zaramboukas T. Epithelioid angiosarcoma of the maxillary sinus and the maxilla: a case report and review of the literature. Oral Surg Oral Med Oral Pathol Oral Radiol Endod 2002;94(3):333–337
17. Rich AL, Berman P. Cutaneous angiosarcoma presenting as an unusual facial bruise. Age Ageing 2004;33(5):512–514
18. Hanke CW, Sterling JB. Prolonged survival of angiosarcoma on the nose: a report of 3 cases. J Am Acad Dermatol 2006;54(5):883–885
19. Bankaci M, Myers EN, Barnes L, DuBois P. Angiosarcoma of the maxillary sinus: literature review and case report. Head Neck Surg 1979;1(3):274–280
20. Kaposi M. Idiopathisches multiples Pigmentsarkon der Haut. Arch Derm Syphilol 1872;4:265–273
21. Mesri EA, Cesarman E, Boshoff C. Kaposi's sarcoma and its associated herpesvirus. Nat Rev Cancer 2010;10(10):707–719
22. Lamovec J, Knuutila P. Kaposi sarcoma. In: Fletcher C, Unni K, Mertens F, eds. Pathology and Genetics of Tumours of Soft Tissue and Bone. Lyon: IARC Press; 2002;170–172
23. Lanternier F, Lebbé C, Schartz N, et al. Kaposi's sarcoma in HIV-negative men having sex with men. AIDS 2008;22(10):1163–1168
24. Chang Y, Cesarman E, Pessin MS, et al. Identification of herpesvirus-like DNA sequences in AIDS-associated Kaposi's sarcoma. Science 1994;266(5192):1865–1869
25. Uldrick TS, Whitby D. Update on KSHV epidemiology, Kaposi sarcoma pathogenesis, and treatment of Kaposi sarcoma. Cancer Lett 2011;305(2):150–162
26. Pica F, Volpi A. Transmission of human herpesvirus 8: an update. Curr Opin Infect Dis 2007;20(2):152–156
27. Ramírez-Amador V, Anaya-Saavedra G, Martínez-Mata G. Kaposi's sarcoma of the head and neck: a review. Oral Oncol 2010;46(3):135–145
28. Chokunonga E, Levy LM, Bassett MT, Mauchaza BG, Thomas DB, Parkin DM. Cancer incidence in the African population of Harare, Zimbabwe: second results from the cancer registry 1993–1995. Int J Cancer 2000;85(1):54–59
29. Mwanda OW, Fu P, Collea R, Whalen C, Remick SC. Kaposi's sarcoma in patients with and without human immunodeficiency virus infection, in a tertiary referral centre in Kenya. Ann Trop Med Parasitol 2005;99(1):81–91
30. Fliss DM, Parikh J, Freeman JL. AIDS-related Kaposi's sarcoma of the sphenoid sinus. J Otolaryngol 1992;21(4):235–237
31. Ziegler JL, Katongole-Mbidde E. Kaposi's sarcoma in childhood: an analysis of 100 cases from Uganda and relationship to HIV infection. Int J Cancer 1996;65(2):200–203
32. Wyatt ME, Finlayson CJ, Moore-Gillon V. Kaposi's sarcoma masquerading as pyogenic granuloma of the nasal mucosa. J Laryngol Otol 1998;112(3):280–282
33. Venizelos I, Andreadis C, Tatsiou Z. Primary Kaposi's sarcoma of the nasal cavity not associated with AIDS. Eur Arch Otorhinolaryngol 2008;265(6):717–720
34. Lyons LL, North PE, Mac-Moune Lai F, Stoler MH, Folpe AL, Weiss SW. Kaposiform hemangioendothelioma: a study of 33 cases emphasizing its pathologic, immunophenotypic, and biologic uniqueness from juvenile hemangioma. Am J Surg Pathol 2004;28(5):559–568
35. Di Lorenzo G, Konstantinopoulos PA, Pantanowitz L, Di Trolio R, De Placido S, Dezube BJ. Management of AIDS-related Kaposi's sarcoma. Lancet Oncol 2007;8(2):167–176
36. Martín-Carbonero L, Palacios R, Valencia E, et al; Caelyx/Kaposi's Sarcoma Spanish Group. Long-term prognosis of HIV-infected patients with Kaposi sarcoma treated with pegylated liposomal doxorubicin. Clin Infect Dis 2008;47(3):410–417

37. Dezube BJ, Sullivan R, Koon HB. Emerging targets and novel strategies in the treatment of AIDS-related Kaposi's sarcoma: bidirectional translational science. J Cell Physiol 2006;209(3):659–662
38. Casper C. New approaches to the treatment of human herpesvirus 8-associated disease. Rev Med Virol 2008; 18(5):321–329

Hereditary Hemorrhagic Telangiectasia

Definition

An inherited disorder characterized by telangiectasia with endothelium deficient in muscle or elastic tissue.[1]

Etiology

Hereditary hemorrhagic telangiectasia (HHT) is an autosomal dominant non–sex-linked condition. Genetic mutation in Cr9,12,5 with signal transforming growth factor (TGF-β) causes abnormal development of blood vessels.[2] There are three types of mutation:

- Type 1: in the gene Endoglin, located on bands 9q33-q3
- Type 2: in the gene Activin-like receptor kinase (*ALK1*), located on band 12q13
- Type 3: involving the long arm of Cr 5 (5q31.1–32)

Synonyms

The names of Osler (1901),[3] Rendu (1896),[4] and Weber (1907)[5] are associated with this condition but, as is so often the case with eponyms, it was described earlier by Sutton (1864)[6] and Babington (1865).[7] Sutton described "curious cases of recurrent epistaxis associated with internal hemorrhages and telangiectases of the skin" and Babington reported habitual epistaxis in five generations in one of the earliest issues of the *Lancet*.

Incidence

HHT overall affects between 12.5 and 15.6/100,000 of the population but there are significant geographical variations, for example, 1:2,351 in certain parts of France, 1:39,000 in the north of England.[2,8]

Site

The telangiectasia can occur throughout the body, on skin, lips, fingertips and nailbeds, and any mucosal surface, and in organs such as the liver, lung, and brain where larger arteriovenous malformations are also found. They are particularly common in the nasal cavity, being principally found on the septum and lateral wall, and tend to be confined to the anterior half of the nasal cavity.

Diagnostic Features

Clinical Features

These clinical findings have been formulated into a table of criteria that assist diagnosis (**Table 9.6**)[9] and have been recently validated[10] and an international guideline has been developed.[11] An individual has a "definite" diagnosis if three criteria are present, "suspected" if two are present, and "unlikely" if only one is present.

Telangiectasia can potentially cause problems wherever it occurs in the body, but the symptom that is the most common and most troublesome is epistaxis.[12] This can vary from slight spotting to repeated life-threatening hemorrhage. There is a tendency for the nosebleeds to get worse with age, but this might simply reflect other age-related comorbidities. Most patients start with their nosebleeds in childhood.[13] In our cohort of 298 patients 54% started then and 17% in their teens to early twenties. However, the age range at presentation was from 2 to 70 years (**Fig. 9.28**). About half experience daily nosebleeds (51%), and 59% had more than three bleeds a day on most days. Extremes of temperature and dryness increased bleeding, as did activities such as bending over, exercise, and coughing or sneezing; but for nearly a third the bleeding was spontaneous and unpredictable. A recent survey considered factors that might precipitate bleeding: for example, environmental temperature and humidity, eating and drinking, and physical activities, all

Table 9.6 The Curaçao criteria for hereditary hemorrhagic telangiectasia[9]

The HHT diagnosis is:
• "Definite" if 3 criteria are present
• "Possible" or "suspected" if 2 criteria are present
• "Unlikely" if only 1 criterion is present
Criteria
Epistaxis: spontaneous, recurrent nosebleeds
Telangiectases multiple, at characteristic sites:
• Lips
• Oral cavity
• Fingers
• Nose
Visceral lesions such as:
• Gastrointestinal telangiectasia (with or without bleeding)
• Pulmonary AVM
• Hepatic AVM
• Cerebral AVM
• Spinal AVM
Family history of a first-degree relative with HHT according to these criteria

Abbreviations: AVM, arteriovenous malformation; HHT, hereditary hemorrhagic telangiectasia.

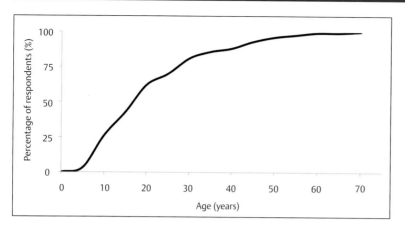

Fig. 9.28 Graph showing the ages of 127 of our HHT patients at presentation.

of which can cause a bleed, but emotion and stress were also regarded as important precipitants.

Examination of the skin of the face, pinna, hands, lips, and oral cavity will usually reveal some telangiectasia (**Fig. 9.29**). Examination of the nose must be done with great care to avoid precipitating a bleed. This can be done endoscopically (**Fig. 9.30**) but the nasal cavity is often full of old clot and crust, which should not be disturbed. Any attempt to anesthetize the nose in outpatients is also unrewarding, but it is worth a gentle view into the nose if only to assess whether the septum is intact as this will have some bearing on treatment options.

Bleeding can also occur from any part of the gastrointestinal tract, causing chronic anemia or overt hemorrhage. Hepatic arterivenous malformations (AVMs) are asymptomatic in >90% but can cause cardiac failure and portal hypertension.[14,15]

Many women complain of menorrhagia, which may have led them to undergo a hysterectomy.

Cerebrovascular accidents are more frequent in HHT patients, who may also experience migraine, headaches, and epilepsy. Around 23% of patients have cerebral vascular malformations and 3.7 to 11% of these are high flow AVMs.[2]

Pulmonary Arteriovenous Malformations

Pulmonary arteriovenous malformations (PAVMs) are more frequent with HHT1 than with HHT2 (75% versus 44%). Patients may experience hemoptysis (which can be massive), dyspnea, cyanosis, headaches, or clubbing or may exhibit none of these.[13,16] Mortality rates of untreated symptomatic patients vary in historical reviews from 4 to 22% and up to 40% in severe cases.[17]

Between 30 and 40% of HHT patients have PAVMs, which can produce significant right-to-left shunting; work at the Hammersmith Hospital, London, UK, has shown that this in turn may be associated with ischemic stroke and brain abscesses, which are particularly likely in patients with PAVMs who become pregnant.

Embolization reduces these risks.[2] **PAVMs rarely regress with time and tend to increase in size, especially if multiple.[18,19] Consequently, screening and treatment are recommended for all adults with HHT.[20]** Detection methods vary but the most sensitive are contrast echocardiography and thoracic CT, the latter being our method of choice. In a study of 127 patients, 57.5% had undergone investigation for PAVMs of which 40% have been positive. **Thirty-eight percent were unsuspected. If the main feeding vessel is >3 mm, patients are offered interventional embolization and in our group this was undertaken in 59% of those found to have them.** The rest remain under observation but should receive antibiotic prophylaxis for any dental work as this may be the source of bacterial emboli to the brain through the shunts.

Using a severity assessment, the more severe the nosebleeds, the more likely patients are to be investigated for PAVMs and the more likely they were to have them (51.5% compared with 27% of moderate and 35.5% of mild epistaxis sufferers).

Imaging

Imaging of the sinuses is rarely required unless concomitant disease is suspected or embolization is contemplated.

However, imaging of the chest is now routinely performed to screen for PAVMs (see above) (**Fig. 9.31**). Post embolization, a chest CT at 6 to 12 months and then 3-yearly is recommended.[11] If the PAVMs are too small to need treatment, follow-up scans are suggested 1- to 5-yearly.

How far screening should extend in asymptomatic individuals is open to debate, particularly with respect to the brain lesions where the potential problems associated with the investigations and treatment may outweigh the possibility of problems from the AVM. Attitudes to this vary from country to country but screening for brain lesions is not routinely recommended in the United Kingdom at present in contrast to the USA.

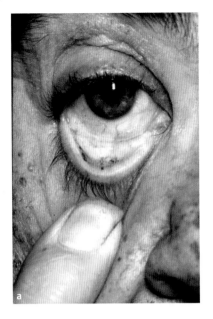

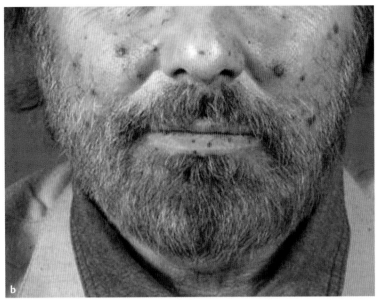

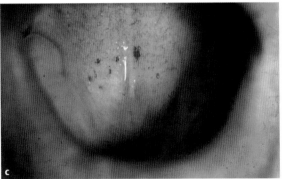

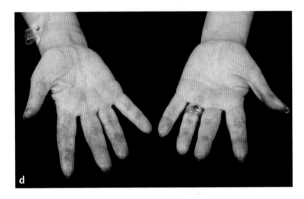

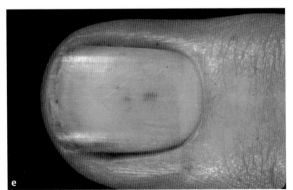

Fig. 9.29a–e Clinical appearances of HHT.
a Conjunctival lesions.
b Lesions on face and lips.
c Tongue lesions.
d Lesions on hands.
e Subungual lesions.

Histological Features and Differential Diagnosis

The smallest HHT lesion is a focal dilatation of a postcapillary venule (**Fig. 9.32**).[21] When these enlarge and connect with dilated arterioles with loss of the intervening capillary bed, arteriovenous communications form. **Vascular remodeling leads to large AVMs. The walls of all these lesions are thinned, with loss of smooth muscle in the tunica media and a disorganized adventitia so that any trauma, however slight, results in bleeding and** **an inability to vasoconstrict normally. Thus, bleeding continues until clotting intervenes which is generally normal in HHT.** However, HHT should be distinguished from von Willebrand's disease, which is also an autosomal dominant trait, often associated with nosebleeds and may exhibit telangiectasia on the skin, mucosa, and gastrointestinal tract.

Diagnosis can be confirmed by genetic testing if there is significant doubt but is not necessary in the "definite"

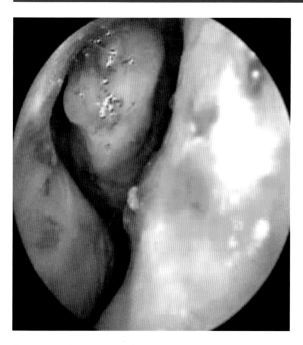

Fig. 9.30 Endoscopic view of nasal telangiectasia.

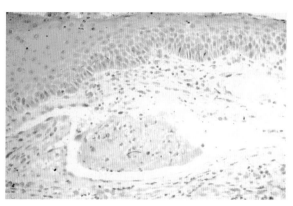

Fig. 9.32 Histological specimen showing HHT lesions in nasal mucosa.

cases. However, an estimated 10 to 20% of families have genetic variation of uncertain significance that can lead to confusion.

Natural History and Staging

Nasal bleeding seems to worsen with age and this, combined with chronic anemia and frequent hospitalizations, can have a profound effect on quality of life that has been demonstrated in several recent studies.[22-25] In a study of 127 of our patients, 42.5% felt that HHT severely affected their lives, 37% felt moderately affected, and 20.5% mildly.

Studies considering HHT life expectancy have not shown any increase in mortality overall[26] but have shown an excess mortality in HHT patients who presented at a younger age, mainly due to cerebral AVM bleeds in childhood or pregnancy-related maternal deaths.[2] Others have suggested that the severity of nasal or gastrointestinal bleeding is the strongest predictor of early mortality.[8]

Patients are particularly at risk during pregnancy due to life-threatening hemorrhage and thrombotic effects.[27]

Several authors have considered stratification of HHT patients to assist in determining the best treatment options.[28-32] We[29] have relied on the need for regular blood

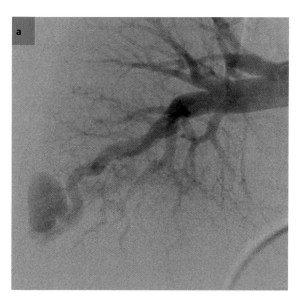

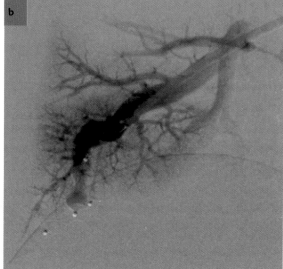

Fig. 9.31 Pulmonary angiogram of thorax showing a right basal pulmonary arteriovenous malformation (PAVM) before (**a**) and after (**b**) embolization with Amplatzer vascular plugs. (Courtesy of Dr. C. Shovlin and reproduced with permission of the author and *Rhinology*.[6]

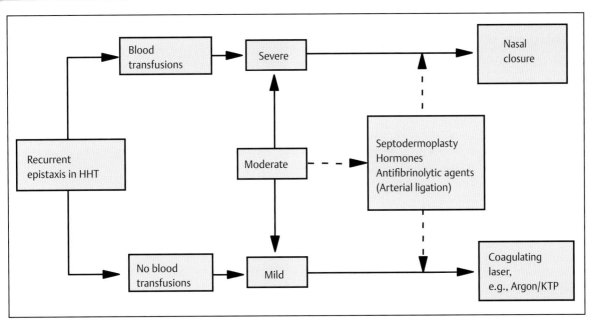

Fig. 9.33 Algorithm for HHT management.

transfusions due to epistaxis as a simple way of dividing patients into mild/moderate and severe (**Fig. 9.33**). Others have considered simple quantification of bleeding and frequency. Al-Deen and Bachmann-Harildstad[31] have combined these aspects into an epistaxis grading scale (**Table 9.7**).

Treatment

Treatment strategies can be divided into general groups to deal with the acute situation or more chronic supportive measures. These include iron supplements, blood transfusion, and local measures for the various bleeding sites.

A long list of therapies have been proposed for the nosebleeds, all of which are designed to reduce both the frequency and severity of the bleeding (**Table 9.8; Fig. 9.33**).

Laser Therapy

Cautery, both electric and chemical, has been used in the past but with very limited success as the effect of burning is often to make the bleeding worse. Coagulation is more successful, particularly if there is limited collateral damage to surrounding tissue, and several types of lasers may be used including KTP532 (potassium titanyl phosphate), argon, and neodymium–YAG.[33–38] "Cutting" lasers such as carbon dioxide (CO_2) and holmium–YAG are not recommended. The energy is absorbed within the red-green spectrum by the telangiectasias, which are effectively "cooked," shrinking and appearing blanched. Charring should be avoided if possible. Lasering rarely produces much postoperative bleeding but fibrin sealant has been used post laser in one study.[39]

Table 9.7 Epistaxis grading scale

Observation of intensity, frequency, and blood transfusion during a period of 4 weeks					
Intensity of the bleeding (I)		**Frequency of the bleeding (F)**		**Blood transfusion (T)**	
0	None	0	None	0	None
1	Slight stains on the handkerchief	1	1–5 times	1	Once
2	Soaked handkerchief	2	6–10 times	2	More than once
3	Soaked towel	3	11–29 times		
4	Bowl or similar vessel is necessary	4	Daily bleeding		
Source: Al-Deen S, Bachmann-Harilstad G. Rhinology 2008;46(4):281[31] with permission of *Rhinology*.					

Table 9.8 Treatment options for epistaxis in HHT

Treatment	Features
Laser	Coagulating, e.g., KTP, argon, neodymium-YAG
Septodermoplasty	
Hormonal	Topical
	Systemic, e.g., ethinylestradiol, medroxyprogesterone, tamoxifen
Antifibrinolytic agents	Tranexamic acid, aminocaproic acid
Closure of nostril	
In extremis	Interventional radiology—embolization
	Arterial ligation—sphenopalatine, ethmoidal, maxillary, external carotid
Under investigation	Bevacizumab
	Thalidomide
	N-acetylcysteine

This therapy is most successful in the mild to moderate cases that do not require regular blood transfusions as the laser deals less well with larger lesions of diameter >2 to 3 mm (**Fig. 9.34**). New lesions will also form on the adjacent mucosa so that, in time, further treatment is required. No complications have been observed with this treatment. We have developed a protocol in which laser treatment is offered every 3 to 4 months initially and then on an as-required basis. This can be combined with other treatments such as septodermoplasty.

Lasers can also be used to improve the cosmetic appearance and reduce pain in the fingertip lesions.

Septodermoplasty

Removing the HHT-bearing mucosa from the septum and grafting the area with split skin was first described by Saunders in 1960.[40] Other tissues have been used including buccal mucosa and amniotic membrane but unfortunately none of these is respiratory ciliated epithelium so the grafted area often crusts. Although both sides of the septum can be grafted, it is better to have an interval of ~3 months between one side and the other to reduce the chances of septal perforation due to damage of the blood supply.

The majority of the lesions are in the anterior septum so it is not usually necessary to extend the graft more posteriorly than the anterior end of the middle turbinate. The dissection is ideally performed in the submucosal plane, leaving behind the perichondrium on which the fenestrated skin graft is placed. This can be held in position with biological glues, gelatin sponge, and/or packing soaked in Whitehead's varnish.[41] Recently a

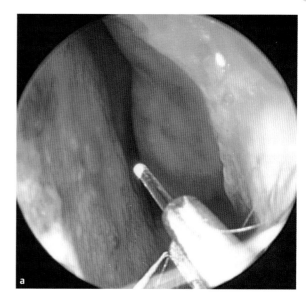
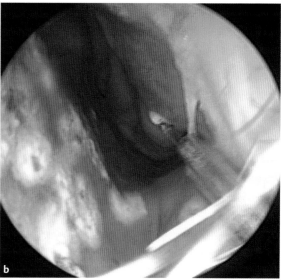

Fig. 9.34a, b Endoscopic view of nasal telangiectasia.
a Before KTP laser treatment.
b After KTP laser treatment.

microdebrider has been successfully used to remove the mucosa. If there is already a large septal perforation, it is obviously technically difficult to perform the grafting and in these circumstances a silastic septal button can be helpful.

The lower half of the lateral wall can also be grafted but is technically more difficult; it requires removal of the inferior turbinates, but preservation of the nasolacrimal opening.[42]

Over 80% of patients noted an improvement in bleeding, but this deteriorates with time as the graft shrinks (**Fig. 9.35**). However, it can be repeated if necessary. In a 5-year period, 131 HHT patients underwent 268 KTP

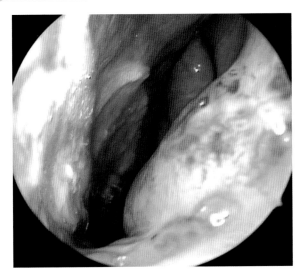

Fig. 9.35 Endoscopic view after septodermoplasty showing contracted graft on left septum and HHT lesions on inferior turbinate.

laser procedures and 33 septodermoplasties. Following septodermoplasty, there was a 57% reduction in the need for subsequent lasering within the 5-year study period, so the procedure is certainly worth considering in selected patients.[43] This benefit has also been shown by others.[44]

Hormones

The use of oral hormones in HHT was based on the observation that epistaxis can increase at the end of the menstrual cycle[45] or may decrease when patients take the contraceptive pill or hormone replacement therapy. This has been attributed to squamous metaplasia in the nasal mucosa, protecting the lesions from trauma,[46] although the exact mechanism is not clear. This translated into the use of oral ethinylestradiol at dose of 0.25 to 1 mg/day.[47] While this proved effective and popular with postmenopausal women, the use of high-dose unopposed estrogen can have potential adverse effects on other organs such as the breast, so Van Cutsem and colleagues[48] recommended that a daily dose of 0.5 mg of ethinylestradiol be combined with 1 mg/day of norethisterone. Even so there are still potential side effects such as breakthrough bleeding or menorrhagia in women who have not undergone a hysterectomy. In men, loss of libido, gynecomastia, and cardiovascular issues are notable problems.

In men another option is medroxyprogesterone (15 to 25 mg/day), which is much less feminizing than the estrogens but can be associated with water retention and bloating sensation. It is generally reserved for older male patients.

An alternative approach has been to use topical estrogen either in combination with other treatments[49] or as creams, although these probably work as lubricants rather than having any specific action on hormone receptors or

the mucosa. This is supported by the positive response experienced by some patients using three different antibiotic ointments in rotation, each a week at a time.

A recent alternative that has been shown to be effective is the anti-estrogen, tamoxifen.[50] This was given in a dose of 20 mg/day versus placebo for between 3 and 50 months (mean 24 months) to 38 patients, who showed significant improvement in both bleeding and quality of life in the active arm without major side effects, although potentially there is an increased risk of deep vein thrombosis, stroke, uterine cancer, and cataracts. Another possible therapy is raloxifene, a selective estrogen modulator.[51]

Antifibrinolytic Agents

In most patients with HHT, the clotting is normal. Tranexamic acid has been used both topically and systemically in doses of 1 to 2 g three times a day[52] to enhance clotting, but again cannot be used where there is a risk of thrombosis. Aminocaproic acid (EACA) has also been used as a topical intranasal spray.[53]

Nasal Closure

As the fundamental problem in HHT is the incapacity of the delicate lesions to constrict, the slightest trauma can provoke a nosebleed. Even the drying effect of airflow through the nose is potentially a problem. Consequently, complete cessation of airflow generally results in complete cessation of bleeding as evidenced by closure of the nasal cavity at the vestibules. This procedure was first described by Young in 1967[54] for atrophic rhinitis and was first applied to HHT patients by Gluckman and Portugal in 1993.[55] Since that time, a modification of the original Young's procedure has been undertaken in a series of 60 patients (54 bilaterally) (**Figs. 9.36 and 9.37**). **If complete airtight closure is achieved, it is exceptional for the patients to bleed from the nose again.** Revision surgery has occasionally been required, using either primary closure or a nasolabial flap and three patients have needed laser treatment to oral lesions

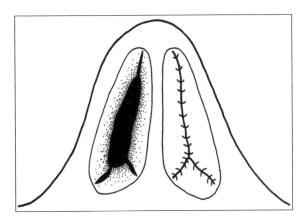

Fig. 9.36 Diagram showing incisions for flaps in nasal closure.

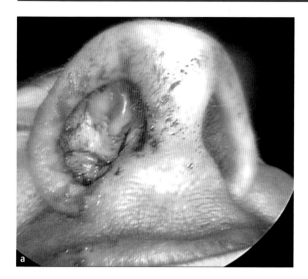
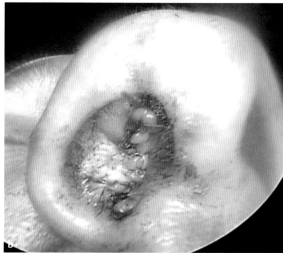
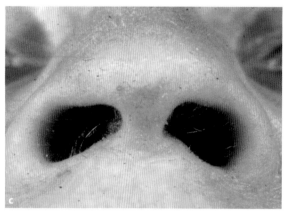

Fig. 9.37a–c Peroperative images of nasal closure.
a Flaps raised retrogradely and sitting in position.
b Flaps sutured with fine dissolvable sutures.
c Nasal view some months after bilateral closure with retraction of flaps into nose.

subsequent to closure.[56] **Nasal closure is reserved for the most severely incapacitated patients who are prepared to sacrifice breathing through the nose (often already compromised by clot and crust) for a more normal lifestyle.**

New Treatments

Bevacizumab (Avastin)

Bevacizumab is a recombinant full-length humanized antibody active against all forms of VEGF and TGF-β and was introduced after a chance observation in an HHT patient undergoing treatment with this agent for cancer.[57] Although this has provoked considerable interest, thus far only anecdotal improvement has been reported[58–60] and there are substantial potential side effects when it is used intravenously, including hemorrhage, hypertension, proteinuria, thromboembolic events, and gastrointestinal perforation. Consequently, topical delivery is being considered and Simonds et al[61] have applied it after KTP laser treatment ($n = 10$) and compared it to KTP treatment alone. Outcomes include frequency and severity of epistaxis, need for blood transfusion and/or iron, and quality of life at 1-month and 1-year follow-up. Significant benefits were reported in frequency of bleeding, need for blood transfusion, disability, and effect on social life (80% vs. 56% overall benefit).

Thalidomide

This drug was also "discovered" as a possible treatment for HHT coincidentally when being used for cancer treatment,[62] possibly because it has an effect on immature blood vessel networks. It has been shown to normalize excessive retinal vessel sprouting in the $Eng^{+/-}$ mouse model and rectified inadequate coverage by α-smooth muscle actin-containing mural cells.[63] Trials in HHT are awaited cautiously, given the known side effects of this drug.

Antioxidants

De Gussem et al have shown benefit, at least in the short term, in an uncontrolled study of oral N-acetylcysteine in 43 patients.[64]

Emergency Treatment

When patients present acutely with significant nasal bleeding, they may need some form of packing to arrest the flow; conventional materials will generally traumatize the fragile telangiectasia further, so atraumatic gelatin sponge or other dissolvable packs are advisable.[65] If more permanent packing is required, a pack soaked in Whitehead's solution has proved successful as it can be left for a week or more.[41]

Interventional radiology to embolize branches of the sphenopalatine artery,[66] or surgical ligation of this and maxillary and/or ethmoidal and even external carotid arteries can be successful in arresting an acute bleed. However, as this is an "end-organ" problem and it is not possible to stop all blood flow to the nose, eventually the effects will wear off.

Outcome

A treatment algorithm has been developed that depends on the severity of the bleeding and the need for blood transfusion. Although anemia can result from other sites of bleeding, epistaxis is the main source of blood loss for most patients. With the exception of nasal closure, the various treatments aim to reduce the frequency and severity of bleeding, improve hemoglobin levels, and reduce the need for iron supplements and transfusion. Success can be measured in terms of the severity and frequency of the bleeding, which can be assessed with diary cards and visual analog scores. In addition, quality of life assessments can be undertaken to show benefit for the various treatments. Of all therapies currently undertaken, **nasal closure provides the most significant improvement in quality of life**.[23]

Most patients have more than one type of treatment and, as bleeding may worsen with age, the treatments may escalate, but only 20% have required nasal closure (**Tables 9.9 and 9.10**).

Table 9.9 Main treatment modalities: personal series[a]

Treatment	Success
Argon/KTP laser	238 (78%)
Hormones	31 (10%)
• Progesterone	15
• Estrogen	8
• Tamoxifen	5
Septodermoplasty	57 (19%)
Nasal closure	60 (20%)

[a] Multiple therapies in some patients n = 298.

Table 9.10 Success of main treatment modalities: personal series

Outcome	Laser	SDP	Oral hormones	Nasal closure
Successful (%)	86	83	72	93
VAS increase (%)	35–90	25–90	50–80	80–100
Mean (%)	65	55	60	88

SDP, septodermoplasty; VAS, visual analog score 0–100%.

Key Points

- Always check the family history in any patient with epistaxis, irrespective of the patient's age.
- Always check for telangiectasia in the nose, mouth, skin, hands, and nailbeds in any patient with epistaxis.
- Treat the nose as gently as possible and avoid packing with conventional materials, which traumatize the lesions.
- Screen patients for pulmonary arteriovenous malformations irrespective of the severity of epistaxis and lack of pulmonary symptoms.
- Of all therapies, nasal closure provides the most significant improvement in quality of life.

References

1. Siegel MB, Keane WM, Atkins JF Jr, Rosen MR. Control of epistaxis in patients with hereditary hemorrhagic telangiectasia. Otolaryngol Head Neck Surg 1991;105(5):675–679
2. Shovlin CL. Hereditary haemorrhagic telangiectasia: pathophysiology, diagnosis and treatment. Blood Rev 2010;24(6):203–219
3. Osler W. On a family form of recurring epistaxis associated with multiple telangiectases of skin and mucous membrane. John Hopkins Med Bulletin 1901;12:333–337
4. Rendu M. Epistaxis repetees chez un sujet postuer de petits angiones cutanes et murqueux. Bull Mem Soc Med Hop Paris 1896;13:731–733
5. Weber F. Multiple hereditary developmental angiomata of the skin and mucous membranes with recurrent haemorrhage. Lancet 1907;2:160–162
6. Sutton H. Epistaxis as an indicator of impaired nutrition and degeneration of the vascular system. Med Mirror 1864;1:769–771
7. Babington B. Hereditary epistaxis. Letter to the Editor of the Lancet. Lancet 1865;2:362–363
8. Kjeldsen AD, Vase P, Green A. Hereditary haemorrhagic telangiectasia: a population-based study of prevalence and mortality in Danish patients. J Intern Med 1999;245(1):31–39
9. Shovlin CL, Guttmacher AE, Buscarini E, et al. Diagnostic criteria for hereditary hemorrhagic telangiectasia (Rendu-Osler-Weber syndrome). Am J Med Genet 2000;91(1):66–67
10. Van Gent M, Post M, Mager J, et al. Diagnostic Curacao Criteria for HHT: are they still valid? Hematol Meeting Rep 2009;3:13
11. Faughnan ME, Palda VA, Garcia-Tsao G, et al; HHT Foundation International - Guidelines Working Group. International guidelines for the diagnosis and management of hereditary haemorrhagic telangiectasia. J Med Genet 2011;48(2):73–87

12. AAssar OS, Friedman CM, White RI Jr. The natural history of epistaxis in hereditary hemorrhagic telangiectasia. Laryngoscope 1991;101(9):977–980
13. Govani FS, Shovlin CL. Hereditary haemorrhagic telangiectasia: a clinical and scientific review. Eur J Hum Genet 2009;17(7):860–871
14. Begbie ME, Wallace GMF, Shovlin CL. Hereditary haemorrhagic telangiectasia (Osler-Weber-Rendu syndrome): a view from the 21st century. Postgrad Med J 2003; 79(927):18–24
15. Byahatti SV, Rebeiz EE, Shapshay SM. Hereditary hemorrhagic telangiectasia: what the otolaryngologist should know. Am J Rhinol 1997;11(1):55–62
16. Folz BJ, Wollstein AC, Alfke H, et al. The value of screening for multiple arterio-venous malformations in hereditary hemorrhagic arteriologic telangiectasia: a diagnostic study. Eur Arch Otorhinolaryngol 2004;261(9):509–516
17. Shovlin CL, Letarte M. Hereditary haemorrhagic telangiectasia and pulmonary arteriovenous malformations: issues in clinical management and review of pathogenic mechanisms. Thorax 1999;54(8):714–729
18. Sluiter-Eringa H, Orie NGM, Sluiter HJ. Pulmonary arteriovenous fistula. Diagnosis and prognosis in noncomplainant patients. Am Rev Respir Dis 1969;100(2):177–188
19. Vase P, Holm M, Arendrup H. Pulmonary arteriovenous fistulas in hereditary hemorrhagic telangiectasia. Acta Med Scand 1985;218(1):105–109
20. Shovlin CL, Jackson JE, Bamford KB, et al. Primary determinants of ischaemic stroke/brain abscess risks are independent of severity of pulmonary arteriovenous malformations in hereditary haemorrhagic telangiectasia. Thorax 2008;63(3):259–266
21. Braverman IM, Keh A, Jacobson BS. Ultrastructure and three-dimensional organization of the telangiectases of hereditary hemorrhagic telangiectasia. J Invest Dermatol 1990;95(4):422–427
22. Pasculli G, Resta F, Guastamacchia E, Di Gennaro L, Suppressa P, Sabbà C. Health-related quality of life in a rare disease: hereditary hemorrhagic telangiectasia (HHT) or Rendu-Osler-Weber disease. Qual Life Res 2004; 13(10):1715–1723
23. Hitchings AE, Lennox PA, Lund VJ, Howard DJ. The effect of treatment for epistaxis secondary to hereditary hemorrhagic telangiectasia. Am J Rhinol 2005;19(1):75–78
24. Lennox PA, Hitchings AE, Lund VJ, Howard DJ. The SF-36 health status questionnaire in assessing patients with epistaxis secondary to hereditary hemorrhagic telangiectasia. Am J Rhinol 2005;19(1):71–74
25. Ingrand I, Ingrand P, Gilbert-Dussardier B, et al. Altered quality of life in Rendu-Osler-Weber disease related to recurrent epistaxis. Rhinology 2011;49(2):155–162
26. Sabbà C, Pasculli G, Suppressa P, et al. Life expectancy in patients with hereditary haemorrhagic telangiectasia. QJM 2006;99(5):327–334
27. Shovlin CL, Sodhi V, McCarthy A, Lasjaunias P, Jackson JE, Sheppard MN. Estimates of maternal risks of pregnancy for women with hereditary haemorrhagic telangiectasia (Osler-Weber-Rendu syndrome): suggested approach for obstetric services. BJOG 2008;115(9):1108–1115
28. Rebeiz EE, Bryan DJ, Ehrlichman RJ, Shapshay SM. Surgical management of life-threatening epistaxis in Osler-Weber-Rendu disease. Ann Plast Surg 1995;35(2):208–213
29. Lund VJ, Howard DJ. A treatment algorithm for the management of epistaxis in hereditary hemorrhagic telangiectasia. Am J Rhinol 1999;13(4):319–322
30. Bergler W, Sadick H, Gotte K, Riedel F, Hörmann K. Topical estrogens combined with argon plasma coagulation in the management of epistaxis in hereditary hemorrhagic telangiectasia. Ann Otol Rhinol Laryngol 2002;111(3 Pt 1):222–228
31. Al-Deen S, Bachmann-Harildstad G. A grading scale for epistaxis in hereditary haemorrhagic teleangectasia. Rhinology 2008;46(4):281–284
32. Pagella F, Colombo A, Matti E, et al. Correlation of severity of epistaxis with nasal telangiectasias in hereditary hemorrhagic telangiectasia (HHT) patients. Am J Rhinol Allergy 2009;23(1):52–58
33. Levine HL. Endoscopy and the KTP/532 laser for nasal sinus disease. Ann Otol Rhinol Laryngol 1989;98(1 Pt 1):46–51
34. Haye R, Austad J. Hereditary hemorrhagic teleangiectasia—argon laser. Rhinology 1991;29(1):5–9
35. Harries PG, Brockbank MJ, Shakespeare PG, Carruth JA. Treatment of hereditary haemorrhagic telangiectasia by the pulsed dye laser. J Laryngol Otol 1997;111(11):1038–1041
36. Lennox PA, Harries M, Lund VJ, Howard DJ. A retrospective study of the role of the argon laser in the management of epistaxis secondary to hereditary haemorrhagic telangiectasia. J Laryngol Otol 1997;111(1):34–37
37. Shah RK, Dhingra JK, Shapshay SM. Hereditary hemorrhagic telangiectasia: a review of 76 cases. Laryngoscope 2002;112(5):767–773
38. Pagella F, Semino L, Olivieri C, et al. Treatment of epistaxis in hereditary hemorrhagic telangiectasia patients by argon plasma coagulation with local anesthesia. Am J Rhinol 2006;20(4):421–425
39. Richmon JD, Tian Y, Husseman J, Davidson TM. Use of a sprayed fibrin hemostatic sealant after laser therapy for hereditary hemorrhagic telangiectasia epistaxis. Am J Rhinol 2007;21(2):187–191
40. Saunders W. Hereditary hemorrhagic telengiectasia: effective treatment of epistaxis by septal dermoplasty. Acta Otolaryngol 1964;58:497–502
41. Lim M, Lew-Gor S, Sandhu G, Howard D, Lund VJ. Whitehead's varnish nasal pack. J Laryngol Otol 2007; 121(6):592–594
42. Ross DA, Nguyen DB. Inferior turbinectomy in conjunction with septodermoplasty for patients with hereditary hemorrhagic telangiectasia. Laryngoscope 2004;114(4):779–781
43. Lund VJ, Harvey R, Kanagalingam J. The impact of septodermoplasty and potassium-titanyl-phosphate (KTP) laser therapy in the treatment of hereditary hemorrhagic telangiectasia-related epistaxis. Am J Rhinol 2008;22:182–187
44. Fiorella ML, Ross D, Henderson KJ, White RI Jr. Outcome of septal dermoplasty in patients with hereditary hemorrhagic telangiectasia. Laryngoscope 2005;115(2):301–305
45. Koch HJ Jr, Escher GC, Lewis JS. Hormonal management of hereditary hemorrhagic telangiectasia. J Am Med Assoc 1952;149(15):1376–1380
46. Harrison DF. Use of estrogen in treatment of familial hemorrhagic telangiectasia. Laryngoscope 1982;92(3):314–320
47. Harrison D. Familial haemorrhagic telangiectases. 20 cases treated with systemic oestrogen. Q J Med 1963;33:25–38
48. van Cutsem E, Rutgeerts P, Vantrappen G. Treatment of bleeding gastrointestinal vascular malformations with oestrogen-progesterone. Lancet 1990;335(8695):953–955
49. Sadick H, Naim R, Oulmi J, Hörmann K, Bergler W. Plasma surgery and topical estriol: effects on the nasal mucosa and long-term results in patients with Osler's disease. Otolaryngol Head Neck Surg 2003;129(3):233–238
50. Yaniv E, Preis M, Hadar T, Shvero J, Haddad M. Antiestrogen therapy for hereditary hemorrhagic telangiectasia: a double-blind placebo-controlled clinical trial. Laryngoscope 2009;119(2):284–288
51. Albiñana V, Bernabeu-Herrero ME, Zarrabeitia R, Bernabéu C, Botella LM. Estrogen therapy for hereditary haemorrhagic telangiectasia (HHT): Effects of raloxifene, on Endoglin and ALK1 expression in endothelial cells. Thromb Haemost 2010;103(3):525–534

52. Fernandez-L A, Garrido-Martin EM, Sanz-Rodriguez F, et al. Therapeutic action of tranexamic acid in hereditary haemorrhagic telangiectasia (HHT): regulation of ALK-1/endoglin pathway in endothelial cells. Thromb Haemost 2007;97(2):254–262

53. Saba HI, Morelli GA, Logrono LA. Brief report: treatment of bleeding in hereditary hemorrhagic telangiectasia with aminocaproic acid. N Engl J Med 1994;330(25):1789–1790

54. Young A. Closure of the nostrils in atrophic rhinitis. J Laryngol Otol 1967;81(5):515–524

55. Gluckman JL, Portugal LG. Modified Young's procedure for refractory epistaxis due to hereditary hemorrhagic telangiectasia. Laryngoscope 1994;104(9):1174–1177

56. Lund VJ, Howard DJ. Closure of the nasal cavities in the treatment of refractory hereditary haemorrhagic telangiectasia. J Laryngol Otol 1997;111(1):30–33

57. Flieger D, Hainke S, Fischbach W. Dramatic improvement in hereditary hemorrhagic telangiectasia after treatment with the vascular endothelial growth factor (VEGF) antagonist bevacizumab. Ann Hematol 2006;85(9):631–632

58. Mitchell A, Adams LA, MacQuillan G, Tibballs J, vanden Driesen R, Delriviere L. Bevacizumab reverses need for liver transplantation in hereditary hemorrhagic telangiectasia. Liver Transpl 2008;14(2):210–213

59. Bose P, Holter JL, Selby GB. Bevacizumab in hereditary hemorrhagic telangiectasia. N Engl J Med 2009; 360(20):2143–2144

60. Oosting S, Nagengast W, de Vries E. More on bevacizumab in hereditary hemorrhagic telangiectasia. N Engl J Med 2009;361(9):931

61. Simonds J, Miller F, Mandel J, Davidson TM. The effect of bevacizumab (Avastin) treatment on epistaxis in hereditary hemorrhagic telangiectasia. Laryngoscope 2009;119(5):988–992

62. Kurstin R. Using thalidomide in a patient with epithelioid leiomyosarcoma and Osler-Weber-Rendu disease. Oncology (Williston Park) 2002;16(1):21–24

63. Lebrin F, Srun S, Raymond K, et al. Thalidomide stimulates vessel maturation and reduces epistaxis in individuals with hereditary hemorrhagic telangiectasia. Nat Med 2010;16(4):420–428

64. de Gussem EM, Snijder RJ, Disch FJ, Zanen P, Westermann CJ, Mager JJ. The effect of N-acetylcysteine on epistaxis and quality of life in patients with HHT: a pilot study. Rhinology 2009;47(1):85–88

65. Gallitelli M, Pasculli G, Fiore T, Carella A, Sabbà C. Emergencies in hereditary haemorrhagic telangiectasia. QJM 2006;99(1):15–22

66. Braak SJ, de Witt CA, Disch FJ, Overtoom TT, Westermann JJ. Percutaneous embolization on hereditary hemorrhagic telangiectasia patients with severe epistaxis. Rhinology 2009;47(2):166–171

10 Neoplasms of Muscle

Leiomyoma

Definition

(ICD-O code 8890/0)

Leiomyomas are benign, smooth muscle tumors which show varying degrees of differentiation.

Etiology

There is little in the way of smooth muscle within the sinonasal tract and the most likely source of smooth muscle is the vasculature of the region, although it is possible that the tumors may arise from pluripotential mesenchymal cells. There have been reports linking radiotherapy and cyclophosphamide treatment with the onset of leiomyosarcoma[1,2] but there is no satisfactory evidence for factors predisposing to leiomyoma. Likewise, there is little evidence to suggest that benign leiomyomas predispose to leiomyosarcoma, although the literature (as is so common with rare benign tumors) contains conflicting evidence on this possibility.

Fu and Perzin described an area with the pattern of leiomyoma existing in a single case of leiomyosarcoma.[3] Huang and Antonescu reported a clinicopathological and immunohistochemical analysis of 12 cases of sinonasal smooth muscle tumors, looking in particular at the histological parameters of circumscription, mucosal ulceration, cellularity, nuclear atypia, mitotic count, necrosis, and destruction of adjacent bony structures.[4] They ultimately grouped them into 7 leiomyomas, 2 smooth muscle tumors with uncertain malignant potential, and 3 low-grade leiomyosarcomas. While this makes for interesting academic discussion with regard to the histopathology, the important clinical point was that all 12 patients were treated by surgical excision and only one patient with definitive leiomyosarcoma received postoperative irradiation. In all 12 cases, there was no evidence of local recurrence or metastases after a follow-up period that averaged over 7 years.

Synonyms

Angiomyoma, angioleiomyoma, vascular leiomyoma, nonvascular leiomyoma, epithelioid leiomyoma, leiomyoblastoma.

Incidence

While the head and neck is not an uncommon site for superficial smooth muscle tumors, primary leiomyomas of the sinonasal tract are very rare.[4,5] Leiomyosarcomas appear to be slightly more common than benign leiomyomas in the literature and overall there is a female predilection of cases with a ratio of ~3:1. Leiomyomas are common in the uterus and the alimentary tract, in contrast to their rarity in the nose and sinuses. Enzinger and Weiss reported 7,748 leiomyomas, with 95% of them occurring in the female genital system, 3% in the skin, and 1.5% in the gastrointestinal tract.[6] We have treated 3 patients in our cohort of >1,700 sinonasal tumors, all female.

Site

In the nose and sinuses, the tumor has been most commonly reported as arising from the turbinates with an additional smaller number of cases throughout the nasal cavity and sinuses.[4,5,7–10] The alveolus and palate may be involved with spread into the nasal cavity and sinuses, and this simple fact accounts for some confusion in the literature as to the exact number of cases of this rare tumor, depending on whether the whole of the upper jaw is included in the overall count. In all of our 3 patients, the lesions arose on the lateral wall, either middle (2 cases) or inferior turbinate (1 case).

Diagnostic Features

Clinical Features and Imaging

Age at presentation varies from childhood to elderly (mean of 48 years in the literature). Our patients were respectively 5, 41, and 55 years old when first seen. By far the most common presenting symptom is nasal obstruction, although associated rhinorrhea, epistaxis, facial pain, facial swelling, and proptosis have all been reported.[4,5,7,10] The most common clinical problem is that, as the lesions are well circumscribed and pale gray or pink in color, they are commonly thought initially to be simple nasal polyps being removed to relieve nasal obstruction. This is particularly the case when the lesion arises from the middle meatus, but the fact that they are unilateral should always give cause for concern. The average size reported in the literature is around 2 cm. Long-standing lesions as large as 10 cm have been reported. They are commonly polypoidal, but remain well circumscribed, even when considerably larger.

There are no specific features on imaging, with the majority of preoperative scans showing a unilateral mass within the nasal cavity, with no direct invasion of adjacent structures. Most commonly the mass will appear to arise from one of the turbinates.

Histological Features

Under light microscopy, leiomyomas are noted to be in the submucosa, usually covered by an intact respiratory mucosa that may be modified by nonspecific inflammation. The lesions exhibit varying degrees of vascularity, with vascular leiomyoma being by far the commonest type. The lesion may contain capillary, cavernous, or venous vascular spaces with highly differentiated smooth muscle cells exhibiting little or no atypia. Smooth muscle cells may be clearly associated with the vessel walls and are generally spindled and arranged in longitudinal and cross-sectional bundles surrounded by bipolar fibrillar eosinophilic cytoplasm. In larger lesions, mucinous degeneration, fibrosis, or hyalinization may be seen in focal areas, but necrosis and invasion are absent. In true leiomyomas, mitotic activity is scarce or absent with 0 or <4 mitoses per high-power field (HPF). More than 4 mitotic figures (MF) per 10 high-power fields (4 MF/10 HPF) is indicative of low-grade malignant potential and >10 MF/10 HPF is generally accepted as confirmation of a leiomyosarcoma. Electron microscopy demonstrates the myofibrils in their characteristic focal condensations and immunohistochemistry usually confirms that the tumor cells are strongly immunoreactive for desmin, h-caldesmon, and vimentin, confirming their differentiation. The KI67 index is usually <5%.

Differential Diagnosis

These benign smooth muscle tumors must be distinguished from leiomyosarcoma and other spindle cell tumors such as sinonasal glomangiopericytoma, peripheral nerve sheath tumors, hemangiomas, and fibrosarcoma.

Natural History

While leiomyomas can achieve a large size and extend throughout the maxilla, ethmoid, and sphenoid areas, they can be completely cured by total excision. The excision must be complete because recurrence is well documented, but is most likely to be residual disease as a consequence of inadequate resection.

Treatment

With the average size of these lesions being around 2 cm and their commonest site being the turbinate, they are ideally removed by modern endoscopic sinus surgery, as was the case in our patient. In the past and in countries where this is not available, lateral rhinotomy or midfacial degloving usually provide excellent access to allow complete removal of the tumor. This latter point cannot be overemphasized as these tumors may recur many years later and require more extensive procedures such as craniofacial resection. In younger patients and those in whom there is concern about adequacy of complete removal, long-term follow-up is advised with careful examination at approximately yearly intervals

and appropriate imaging if symptoms and signs suggest residual disease.

Our youngest patient dramatically demonstrates the problems of undertreatment, having had a polypectomy at 5 years of age, followed by three lateral rhinotomies elsewhere and ultimately requiring a craniofacial resection at the age of 15 years in 1989 to remove the lesion from the skull base and nasal bones. She subsequently has had to have a reconstructive rhinoplasty, but happily has not had any further "recurrence" to date.

References

1. Lalwani AK, Kaplan MJ. Paranasal sinus leiomyosarcoma after cyclophosphamide and irradiation. Otolaryngol Head Neck Surg 1990;103(6):1039–1042
2. Reich DS, Palmer CA, Peters GE. Ethmoid sinus leiomyosarcoma after cyclophosphamide treatment. Otolaryngol Head Neck Surg 1995;113(4):495–498
3. Fu YS, Perzin KH. Nonepithelial tumors of the nasal cavity, paranasal sinuses, and nasopharynx: a clinicopathologic study. IV. Smooth muscle tumors (leiomyoma, leiomyosarcoma). Cancer 1975;35(5):1300–1308
4. Huang HY, Antonescu CR. Sinonasal smooth muscle cell tumors: a clinicopathologic and immunohistochemical analysis of 12 cases with emphasis on the low-grade end of the spectrum. Arch Pathol Lab Med 2003;127(3):297–304
5. Tsobanidou CH. Leiomyoma of the nasal cavity. Report of 2 cases and review of the literature. Oral Oncol Extra 2006;42:255–257
6. Enzinger F, Weiss P. In: Soft Tissue Tumours. 2nd ed. St Louis: Mosby; 1988:383–401
7. Trott MS, Gewirtz A, Lavertu P, Wood BG, Sebek BA. Sinonasal leiomyomas. Otolaryngol Head Neck Surg 1994;111(5):660–664
8. Llorente JL, Suárez C, Seco M, Garcia A. Leiomyoma of the nasal septum: report of a case and review of the literature. J Laryngol Otol 1996;110(1):65–68
9. Murono S, Ohmura T, Sugimori S, Furukawa M. Vascular leiomyoma with abundant adipose cells of the nasal cavity. Am J Otolaryngol 1998;19(1):50–53
10. Vincenzi A, Rossi G, Monzani D, Longo L, Rivasi F. Atypical (bizarre) leiomyoma of the nasal cavity with prominent myxoid change. J Clin Pathol 2002;55(11):872–875

Leiomyosarcoma

Definition

(ICD-O code 8890/3)

Leiomyosarcoma is a rare, malignant, mesenchymal tumor of smooth muscle phenotype that most frequently occurs in the uterine myometrium, the gastrointestinal (GI) tract, the retroperitoneum, and the skin. It is a rare tumor in the head and neck.

Etiology

Leiomyosarcoma, in common with other rare sarcomas, has been reported to occur following previous radiotherapy and, in a small number of cases, following treatment with cyclophosphamide. A total of 10 cases had been reported in the literature by 1990.[1] Patients presented in these series had received radiation with or without systemic chemotherapy between 6 and 40 years previously. Unfortunately, as we have consistently pointed out in the sections on soft tissue tumors, the unreliability of these reports prior to the modern developments in immunohistochemistry and genetics makes it doubtful whether these lesions were always leiomyosarcomas. These radiation induced-tumors had been reported after orbital radiation for retinoblastoma, mediastinal and neck irradiation for ganglioneuroblastoma, and pelvic irradiation and treatment for Wilms tumor. The case of Lalwani and Kaplan was said to have occurred after radiation and cyclophosphamide treatment for Wegener's granulomatosis, but it is quite likely that their case actually represented a T cell lymphoma and this raises the question whether or not the subsequent disease was indeed a leiomyosarcoma.[1] The WHO classification 2005 now places radiation-induced sarcomas in a separate group.

Smooth muscle tumors are extraordinarily rare in the head and neck, probably because of the paucity of smooth muscle tissue; the most likely source is thought to be the arterial tunica media but it is also possible that they arise from pluripotential mesenchymal cells in common with other forms of sarcomas. Primary head and neck cutaneous leiomyosarcomas are thought to arise either from the muscular walls of blood vessels or from the erector pili muscles.

Incidence and Site

Leiomyosarcomas of the head and neck are essentially adult tumors with a peak incidence in the 5th decade of life and have an approximately equal sex distribution.[2,3] Kuruvilla et al[2] found only 9 examples of leiomyosarcoma out of 602 sinonasal tract sarcomas (1.5%) extracted from the files of the Armed Forces Institute of Pathology.

Leiomyosarcoma of the oral cavity has a particular predilection for the mandible and maxilla; ~70% of reported cases arise in the jaws with the remainder originating in the tongue, hard and soft palate, floor of mouth, buccal mucosa, gingiva, and upper lip. Those arising in the hard and soft palate and maxilla may further involve the paranasal sinuses and nasal cavity and this simple fact again complicates the figures for incidence in the sinonasal tract within the literature.[4,5] Cutaneous leiomyosarcoma is not uncommon in the head and neck, usually presenting in older, male patients and varies in appearance between small plaques or nodules to extensive, ulcerating masses that may involve the nose and underlying paranasal sinuses.[6]

We have treated five patients with leiomyosarcoma. In the two earlier cases, there was extensive involvement of the maxillary sinuses and orbit. In the three more recent cases the disease involved the ethmoid and nasal cavity.

Diagnostic Features

Clinical Features

Sinonasal leiomyosarcomas have a similar age range as their benign counterparts, from 18 to 75 years in the literature (mean 52 years) and are said to affect men and women equally. Our cases comprised 2 men and 3 women, aged 47, 73, 38, 39, and 54 years, respectively. These lesions most commonly present with unilateral nasal obstruction and epistaxis. Other later symptoms clearly depend on the site of origin and spread of the lesion and include facial swelling, facial pain, and oral and orbital signs and symptoms.[2]

On examination, tumors visible within the nasal cavity have been described as polypoidal, nodular, and bulky but with no features to differentiate them from any other lesions. They vary from soft and gelatinous to firm and rubbery with a cut surface that varies from white to tan. Necrotic areas may be seen, and clearly these changes may vary with the grade of the lesion as in other sarcomas.

Imaging

Tanaka, Westesson, and Wilbur reviewed the imaging of leiomyosarcoma in their own case arising in the maxillary sinus in 1998.[7] They reviewed 38 previous articles on oral and sinonasal leiomyosarcomas from which CT images were shown in 9 cases only. Six of these showed frank, bony destruction as in their own case, with no particular points of note. They noted that MRI of leiomyosarcomas in other locations shows an intermediate signal intensity on T1W images with moderate enhancement after gadolinium injection and intermediate to high signal intensity on T2W images. These are nonspecific characteristics and in addition the heterogeneity often seen simply reflects areas of hemorrhage and necrosis that do not enhance with contrast. The value of the imaging, as in other sarcomas, is to accurately detect the size and extent of the tumor as well as osseous invasion (**Fig. 10.1**).

Histological Features and Differential Diagnosis

The rapidly increasing literature on the complexity of diagnosis surrounding leiomyosarcomas, as with many other rare sarcomas, is an excellent demonstration of an increasing understanding of the subject, but although recent cytogenetic studies of leiomyosarcomas in particular have shown highly complex genetic aberrations, as yet no specific abnormalities within leiomyosarcomas have been identified.[8,9] Depending on their grade, leiomyosarcomas are more or less infiltrative, with bone and cartilage invasion being more frequent than surface or seromucinous gland invasion. Tumors are generally hypercellular, but necrosis and hemorrhage can lessen this appearance. They are usually composed of right-angle intersecting bundles of spindle cells with elongated

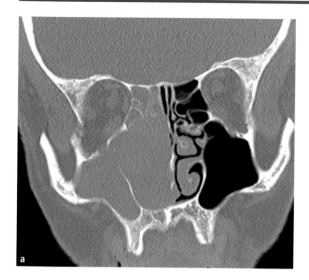
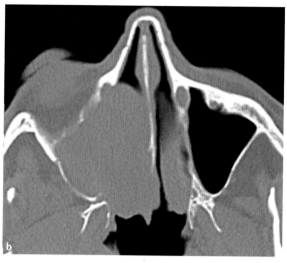
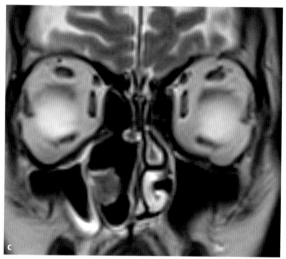

Fig. 10.1a–c

a Coronal CT showing opacification of the right nasal cavity and maxilla, although the lateral wall appears partially intact.
b Axial CT scan in the same patient.
c Coronal MRI scan in the patient after chemoradiotherapy and prior to endoscopic surgical clearance, which showed a small amount of residual disease in the inferior turbinate.

fascicular to hyperchromatic lobulated or indented nuclei with blunt ends (so-called cigar shape). Various patterns of the tumor cells may occur including palisading storiform and so-called hemangiopericytoma patterns, which of course give rise to a variety of difficulties in the differential diagnosis. Mitoses, both typical and atypical, are present in varying degrees as documented by Huang and Antonescu in their excellent review of 12 sinonasal smooth muscle tumors in 2003.[10] They based the classification of these tumors on the guidelines for smooth muscle tumors of deep tissues using more than 4 mitotic figures per 10 high-power fields to separate leiomyomas from intermediate lesions with malignant potential, and those which were frank sarcomas. The latter group with more than 4 mitotic figures per 10 high-power fields were clearly what most would consider to be low-grade sarcomas. In contrast Kuruvilla et al concluded that the only significant prognostic indicator in sinonasal leiomyosarcomas was the extent of tumor involvement at

presentation and not its histological grading.[2] Huang and Antonescu[10] suggested that histological grading still plays a role in the clinical behavior of sinonasal smooth muscle tumors as 2 of their 3 leiomyosarcomas, treated only with excision, were free of recurrence even when they had extensively involved both nasal cavity and paranasal sinuses. This latter report would certainly fit with the grading of soft tissue sarcomas in general, which helps to predict clinical aggressiveness.

Unfortunately, variations in histological appearances of leiomyosarcoma are not uncommon; they may be either focal or quite widespread and have led to considerable diagnostic dilemmas. Variable granularity may mimic a true granular cell tumor and osteoclastlike giant cells may lead to a diagnosis of giant cell malignant fibrous histiocytoma. There are myxoid variants of leiomyosarcoma and occasionally they may contain additional sarcomatous components with foci of apparent osteosarcoma and chondrosarcoma.

Immunohistochemistry

Immunohistochemistry has accordingly proved to be invaluable with regard to these rare tumors and usually they exhibit strong and diffuse expression of vimentin and actin (smooth muscle or muscle specific) and desmin (variable, but most cases), calponin, h-caldesmon, and smooth muscle myosin expression. In general, most pathologists prefer to see at least two myogenic markers to support the diagnosis. This is particularly relevant with the differentiation from malignant fibrous histiocytoma (pleomorphic sarcoma), which tends to have a marked reduction in myogenic markers. There is generally no reactivity with keratin markers but, again, rare examples of leiomyosarcoma may exhibit focal expression of keratin, giving rise to further difficulties. Electron microscopy, when available, aids by revealing variable features of smooth muscle cells with longitudinally arrayed myofilaments and dense bodies within the filaments, cell junctions, pinocytotic vesicles, and basal lamina. Unfortunately, again, poorly differentiated examples may have very few or absent smooth muscle features. As mentioned above, cytogenetic studies have shown complexity of genetic changes in these tumors but as yet no specific abnormalities. Differential diagnosis in this difficult area is therefore considerable and includes malignant fibrous histiocytoma (pleomorphic sarcoma), sinonasal glomangiopericytoma, malignant peripheral nerve sheath tumor, spindle cell melanoma, spindle cell sarcoma, low-grade myxofibrosarcoma, monophasic synovial sarcoma, and myoepithelioma. References 11 to 18 are recommended for a comprehensive review of this difficult area.[11–18]

Treatment

When reviewing the literature for details of treatment and prognosis, there is the recurring problem of the rarity of these lesions and the lack of certainty with regard to the accuracy of tissue diagnosis in the older publications. There remains general agreement from the more recent publications from the 1990s onward that favorable long-term outcome in these patients is attributable to a radical surgical approach, with a variety of operations being necessary for total removal of the tumor. As we ourselves have found with a 30-year experience of craniofacial surgery, the areas of recurrence in leiomyosarcomas are principally the orbit, skull base, anterior cranial fossa, and pterygomaxillary fissure. These local recurrences seem to be responsible for the majority of deaths, particularly in the lower grade of lesions, and Ulrich et al[3] in a detailed review of the literature in 2005 noted a recurrence rate for leiomyosarcoma of ~30% and a rate of distant metastases of around 8%. That most recurrences were diagnosed in the first 2 years after treatment makes it likely that these are all cases of residual disease. Patients are more likely to die from the effects of this direct residual disease than from metastases, but this will clearly relate to the proportion of low- or high-grade tumors in any given series, all of which are small in sinonasal reports. Aside from the comments by Huang and Antonescu, the majority of authors agree that the poor prognosis for sinonasal leiomyosarcoma is related to large tumor size, and extension beyond the nasal cavity, particularly to the orbit pterygomaxillary fissure, or skull base.[10]

Leiomyosarcomas are generally considered to be radioresistant with a uniformly poor response to radiotherapy used as either primary or adjuvant treatment; until recently, both radiotherapy and chemotherapy have been generally advocated as palliative measures. However, Fusconi et al presented a single case of a 57-year-old woman with sinonasal leiomyosarcoma that recurred after approach by palatal fenestration[19] and Caldwell-Luc in 1995 (this would certainly be considered as an inadequate surgical approach). She had recurrence in the nasal cavity within 6 months and was commenced on ifosfamide, epirubicin, dacarbazine, and adriamycin in three different courses. She then received additional radiotherapy over a 2-month period, although details of dosage were not included in the publication. The tumor mass resolved and examination and extensive imaging (including for metastases) were clear 4 years post treatment. They make the point that in gynecology, where the results of chemotherapy are still controversial, the gynecological-oncologic group in the United States has recognized the effectiveness of ifosfamide and mesna in the treatment of patients with advanced or recurrent uterine sarcomas and, while they are unable to express a favorable or unfavorable opinion based on a single case, the quadruple chemotherapy that this patient received certainly appears to have contributed to her cure. Bearing in mind the results obtained in other disciplines dealing with oncology, it is to be hoped that progress in chemotherapy will eventually assist with these rare and variable sarcomas.

In our small group of patients, the two cases presenting in the 1980s with more advanced disease both underwent maxillectomy and orbital clearance. One was followed up for 5 years without recurrence; the other died 4 months after the operation of disseminated disease. Of the three patients presenting between 2002 and 2008 (38, 39, and 73 years old), two were treated with wide-field endoscopic resection following chemoradiation and one required craniofacial resection. All are alive and well and subject to regular imaging and endoscopic examination.

References

1. Lalwani AK, Kaplan MJ. Paranasal sinus leiomyosarcoma after cyclophosphamide and irradiation. Otolaryngol Head Neck Surg 1990;103(6):1039–1042
2. Kuruvilla A, Wenig BM, Humphrey DM, Heffner DK. Leiomyosarcoma of the sinonasal tract. A clinicopathologic study of nine cases. Arch Otolaryngol Head Neck Surg 1990;116(11):1278–1286

3. Ulrich CT, Feiz-Erfan I, Spetzler RF, et al. Sinonasal leio-myosarcoma: review of literature and case report. Laryn-goscope 2005;115(12):2242–2248
4. Wertheimer-Hatch L, Hatch GF III, HatchB S KF, et al. Tumors of the oral cavity and pharynx. World J Surg 2000;24(4):395–400
5. Vilos GA, Rapidis AD, Lagogiannis GD, Apostolidis C. Leio-myosarcomas of the oral tissues: clinicopathologic analysis of 50 cases. J Oral Maxillofac Surg 2005;63(10):1461–1477
6. Kaddu S, Beham A, Cerroni L, et al. Cutaneous leiomyosar-coma. Am J Surg Pathol 1997;21(9):979–987
7. Tanaka H, Westesson PL, Wilbur DC. Leiomyosarcoma of the maxillary sinus: CT and MRI findings. Br J Radiol 1998;71(842):221–224
8. El-Rifai W, Sarlomo-Rikala M, Knuutila S, Miettinen M. DNA copy number changes in development and progres-sion in leiomyosarcomas of soft tissues. Am J Pathol 1998;153(3):985–990
9. Mandahl N, Fletcher CD, Dal Cin P, et al. Comparative cyto-genetic study of spindle cell and pleomorphic leiomyo-sarcomas of soft tissues: a report from the CHAMP Study Group. Cancer Genet Cytogenet 2000;116(1):66–73
10. Huang HY, Antonescu CR. Sinonasal smooth muscle cell tumors: a clinicopathologic and immunohistochemical analysis of 12 cases with emphasis on the low-grade end of the spectrum. Arch Pathol Lab Med 2003;127(3):297–304
11. Cavazzana AO, Schmidt D, Ninfo V, et al. Spindle cell rhab-domyosarcoma. A prognostically favorable variant of rhab-domyosarcoma. Am J Surg Pathol 1992;16(3):229–235
12. Nakhleh R, Zarbo R, Ewing S, et al. Myogenic differentiation in spindle cell (sarcomatoid) carcinomas of the upper aero digestive tract. Appl Immunohistochem 1993;1:58–68
13. Mentzel T, Dry S, Katenkamp D, Fletcher CD. Low-grade myofibroblastic sarcoma: analysis of 18 cases in the spectrum of myofibroblastic tumors. Am J Surg Pathol 1998;22(10):1228–1238
14. Coffin C. Fletcher J. Inflammatory myofibroblastic tumour. In: Fletcher CDM, Unni K, Mertens F, eds. Tumours of the Soft Tissue and Bone. Lyon: IARC Press; 2002:91–93
15. Fisher C, Montgomery E, Healy V. Calponin and h-caldes-mon expression in synovial sarcoma; the use of calponin in diagnosis. Histopathology 2003;42(6):588–593
16. Hornick JL, Fletcher CD. Myoepithelial tumors of soft tissue: a clinicopathologic and immunohistochemical study of 101 cases with evaluation of prognostic param-eters. Am J Surg Pathol 2003;27(9):1183–1196
17. Cardesa A, Zidar N. Spindle cell carcinoma. In: Barnes L, Eveson J, Reichart P, Sidransky D, eds.World health Organization Classification of Tumours. Pathology and Genetics of Head and Neck Tumours. Lyon: IARC Press; 2005:127–128
18. Miettinen M, Fetsch JF. Evaluation of biological potential of smooth muscle tumours. Histopathology 2006;48(1):97–105
19. Fusconi M, Magliulo G, Della Rocca C, Marcotullio D, Suri-ano M, de Vincentiis M. Leiomyosarcoma of the sinonasal tract: a case report and literature review. Am J Otolaryngol 2002;23(2):108–111

Rhabdomyoma

Definition

(ICD-O code 8904/0)

This is a benign mesenchymal tumor that shows skel-etal muscle differentiation.

Incidence and Site

Rhabdomyomas are rare tumors that account for only ~2% of all skeletal muscle tumors. They have a propensity for the head and neck and are divided by means of their histology (rather than age of the patient), into fetal, juve-nile or adult subtypes, all of which may be diagnosed at any patient age, although the fetal and juvenile types are more common in younger patients. They may be termed extracardiac rhabdomyomas to distinguish them from the cardiac rhabdomyomas arising from the heart. These rare tumors occur most commonly in the skin of the head and neck, the oral cavity, and the laryngopharynx. Occasional cases have been described involving the nasopharynx and the skin of the nose.[1–5]

Diagnostic Features

Clinical and Histological Features

These lesions present as a nonspecific mass in the affected area, often with a long history. While they differ to some degree on histological evaluation, all three types of rhabdomyoma consistently express markers associated with skeletal muscle differentiation including desmin, myoglobin, and muscle-specific actin. The desmin reac-tivity is usually particularly strong. Fetal rhabdomyomas require distinction from embryonal rhabdomyosarcomas. Lack of significant infiltration and the absence of mitosis, necrosis, and cellular pleomorphism assist in this, and the recognition of muscle maturation in the lesion indicates rhabdomyoma.

Treatment and Prognosis

Conservative but complete removal of these lesions is required and a small proportion of the adult type may be multifocal, either asynchronous or synchronous. This fact may explain some of the recurrences described with this lesion, which may occur at a period ranging from months to decades later. There are no reported cases of malignant change.

References

1. Di Sant'Agnese PA, Knowles DM II. Extracardiac rhabdo-myoma: a clinicopathologic study and review of the litera-ture. Cancer 1980;46(4):780–789
2. Gale N, Rott T, Kambic V. Nasopharyngeal rhabdo-myoma. Report of case (light and electron microscopic studies) and review of the literature. Pathol Res Pract 1984;178(5):454–460
3. Kapadia SB, Meis JM, Frisman DM, Ellis GL, Heffner DK, Hyams VJ. Adult rhabdomyoma of the head and neck: a clinicopathologic and immunophenotypic study. Hum Pathol 1993;24(6):608–617
4. Kapadia SB, Meis JM, Frisman DM, Ellis GL, Heffner DK. Fetal rhabdomyoma of the head and neck: a clinicopatho-logic and immunophenotypic study of 24 cases. Hum Pathol 1993;24(7):754–765

5.   Hansen T, Katenkamp D. Rhabdomyoma of the head and neck: morphology and differential diagnosis. Virchows Arch 2005;447(5):849–854

Rhabdomyosarcoma

Definition

Rhabdomyosarcoma is a malignant tumor derived from primitive mesenchymal tissue expressing myogenic differentiation. It probably arises from satellite cells associated with skeletal muscle embryogenesis.

Etiology

Rhabdomyosarcomas are subdivided into three major groups: embryonal, alveolar, and pleomorphic.

Embryonal rhabdomyosarcoma is associated with a consistent loss of heterozygosity or loss of imprinting at a specific locus on the short arm of chromosome 11p15. This cytogenetic abnormality is also found with other early childhood malignant tumors, such as hepatoblastoma and Wilms tumor.[1]

Synonyms

The terms myosarcoma, embryonal sarcoma, malignant rhabdomyoma, rhabdosarcoma, rhabdomyoblastoma, and botryoidsarcoma have all been used to various degrees in the literature.

Incidence and Site

Rhabdomyosarcoma represents between 2% and 5% of all soft tissue sarcomas in adults, but in distinct contrast, this tumor represents ~60% of all soft tissue sarcomas in children, with ~35% of all rhabdomyosarcomas arising in the head and neck region.[2]

The embryonal subtype predominates in children, while the alveolar subtype is more common in adults and the pleomorphic subtype is rare overall.[3,4] The exact figures for the various subtypes differ from different series, but ~20% of rhabdomyosarcomas of the head and neck occur in the nasal cavity, nasopharynx, and paranasal sinuses.[5] The nasopharynx is more commonly involved than the sinonasal tract overall, and in adults rhabdomyosarcoma appears to be most common in the ethmoid sinuses, in contrast to the maxillary sinuses. In the study by Nayar et al of 26 adult patients reported in 1993, the commonest sinonasal site was the ethmoid followed by the maxilla.[6]

In our cohort of 26 cases, 8 arose in the orbit and in a further 5 the orbit was involved from the adjacent sinuses. Of those cases arising in the sinuses, 9 affected the maxilla and ethmoids at presentation, 5 were confined to the ethmoids, 1 the maxillary sinus, and 3 the nasal cavity. Three presented with widespread metastases.

Diagnostic Features

Clinical Features

As a consequence of their rapid growth and extensive nature, particularly in the more aggressive tumors, rhabdomyosarcoma in the sinonasal tract can present with a wide variety of signs and symptoms, including nasal obstruction, epistaxis, pain, facial swelling, paresthesia, proptosis, headache, toothache, visual problems, and decreased hearing as a consequence of serous otitis media. The majority of cases occur in children above the age of 1 year up to 15 years. Approximately 10% occur between the ages of 15 and 25 years.[7] Rhabdomyosarcomas are rare in adults above 30 years. In our group the male-to-female ratio was almost equal (1.2:1) and the ages ranged from 4 to 70 years (mean 26.8 years) with 46% 20 years old or younger at presentation (Fig. 10.2a).

Rhabdomyosarcomas of the sinonasal area frequently invade the adjacent orbit, skull base, and pterygomaxillary region, and as rhabdomyosarcoma is the most frequent malignant orbital neoplasm in children, they may extend medially from the orbit to give rise to nasal obstruction and bleeding once the tumor has entered the nasal airway, as occurred in 8 of our cases. Most ocular rhabdomyosarcomas arise in the soft tissues of the orbit but also in the conjunctiva, the eyelid, and the uveal tract.[8] Most adult sinonasal and nasopharyngeal rhabdomyosarcomas are staged as group III or IV, according to the intergroup rhabdomyosarcoma study.[7]

Approximately 40% metastasize to lymph nodes, bones, and lungs. Unfortunately, although rare, additional metastases to bone marrow, soft tissues, liver, and brain can occur.[6]

Imaging

Hoon Lee et al, reviewing imaging findings of rhabdomyosarcoma in 11 adult patients, found poorly defined homogeneous masses destroying adjacent bony structures on CT and MRI.[9] On CT scans the masses enhanced to the same degree as adjacent muscle and showed some heterogeneous pattern in four cases. On MRI there was intermediate signal intensity on T1W and intermediate to high signal intensity on T2W images (Fig. 10.2b and Fig. 10.3a–d). Hagiwara et al presented the results of CT and MRI on 9 patients with rhabdomyosarcoma between 6 and 53 years of age. Only three of these tumors originated in the paranasal sinuses;[10] the others originated in the cheeks, soft palate, orbit, sternoclavicular muscle, and parapharyngeal space. In four tumors there was multiple ring enhancement on MRI resembling bunches of grapes. This sign had not been previously described and they speculated that this "botryoid sign" represented thin layers of tumor around mucoid stroma, characteristic of botryoid rhabdomyosarcoma. Unfortunately, one-to-one comparison was not possible between the contrast-enhanced MRI and pathological specimens because the latter were small and this sign only occurred in three of the patients who were less than 15 years old.

Histological Features

Embryonal rhabdomyosarcomas make up the majority of rhabdomyosarcomas in the head and neck and generally exhibit round to spindle cells with hyperchromatic nuclei. The round and differentiated cells are similar to rhabdomyoblasts seen in embryonal muscle. These are the most primitive cells and can also be spindled. Larger rhabdomyoblasts with eosinophilic cytoplasm are seen but cross-striations are often difficult to recognize and are reported in varied numbers in up to about one-third of cases. Following chemotherapy with further differentiation, strap cells and cross-striations may become more prominent. The stroma in embryonal rhabdomyosarcoma can vary considerably between myxoid, fibrotic, or edematous.

Botryoid rhabdomyosarcoma differs from embryonal sarcomas by generally having an abundant myxoid stroma with grapelike polypoid growth pattern and a cambium layer.

Alveolar rhabdomyosarcoma is usually characterized by fibrous septa separating groups of small to medium, round tumor cells with hyperchromatic nuclei and scant eosinophilic cytoplasm. Multinucleated giant cells with overlapping peripheral nuclei are often seen. There is a solid variant in which the cells grow in sheets and lack septa, and a third type with a mixed alveolar and embryonal pattern.

Pleomorphic rhabdomyosarcoma is almost entirely confined to adults and overall makes up less than 5% of cases of rhabdomyosarcoma. It is extremely uncommon in the sinonasal tract.

Immunohistochemical Features

Immunohistochemistry has been invaluable in the improving diagnosis of rhabdomyosarcomas and generally they are positive for muscle-specific actin, desmin, and nuclear skeletal muscle-specific myoregulatory proteins, including MyoD1 and myogenin. Morotti et al evaluated 956 rhabdomyosarcomas, showing that MyoD1 and myogenin were equally sensitive, positive in 97% of cases, and highly specific.[11]

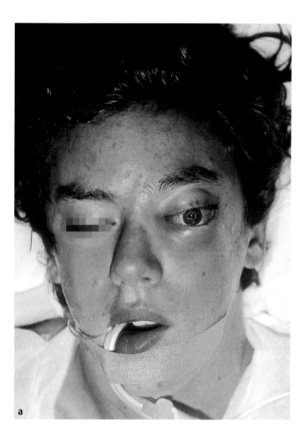
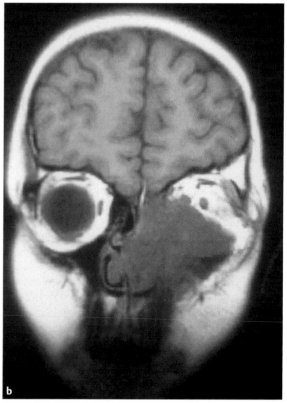

Fig. 10.2a, b

a Peroperative clinical photograph of a patient with proptosis due to a large embryonal rhabdomyosarcoma affecting the left maxilla.

b Coronal MRI in the same patient (T1W with gadolinium enhancement) showing the tumor mass filling the left maxilla and infiltrating the orbit.

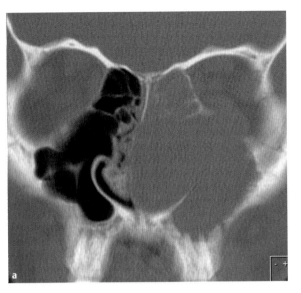

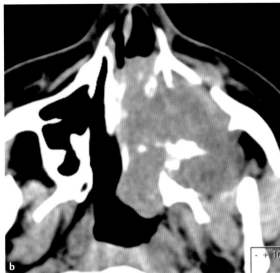

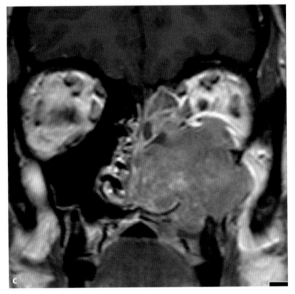

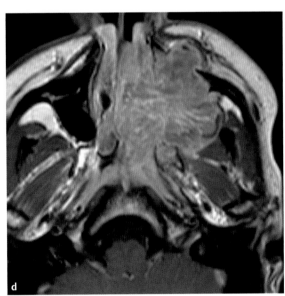

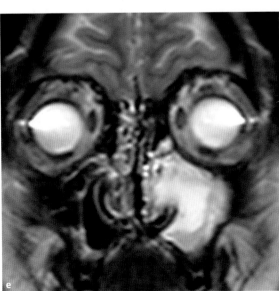

Fig. 10.3a–e

a Coronal CT scan of a patient with embryonal rhabdomyosarcoma showing opacification of the nasal cavity, maxillary sinus, and posterior ethmoids with marked bony destruction of the floor of the orbit and lateral wall of the nose.

b Axial CT in the same patient showing in addition bone erosion of the anterior and posterior maxillary walls.

c Coronal MRI scan (sequence) in the same patient showing the soft tissue mass more clearly.

d Axial MRI scan in the same patient.

e Coronal MRI scan 15 months after chemoradiotherapy showing resolution of the mass with inflammatory change in the maxillary sinus, confirmed by endoscopic surgery.

Electron microscopy generally shows some degree of skeletal muscle differentiation.

In our 26 cases, embryonal rhabdomyosarcoma accounted for 61% (16 cases), alveolar for 23% (6 cases), and pleomorphic for 16% (4 cases).

Differential Diagnosis

Differential diagnosis for rhabdomyosarcoma is an extensive subject with considerable potential for error, but the immunohistochemistry details outlined above have aided diagnosis considerably. Differential diagnosis includes other tumors exhibiting "rhabdoid features," and small round cell tumors. Possibilities therefore include sarcomas, carcinomas, and melanomas. Extrarenal rhabdoid tumor is a malignancy of infants and children that can arise in the head and neck; it is negative for myoregulatory skeletal muscle-specific markers and desmin but often expresses neural markers and keratins. Both fetal rhabdomyoma and adult rhabdomyoma can mimic rhabdomyosarcoma, but the former does not usually display significant cytological atypia, mitotic figures, or necrosis. Cross-striations are more easily seen.

Sinonasal polyps may contain histiocytes and fibroblasts that are particularly pleomorphic, and because botryoid rhabdomyosarcoma cannot macroscopically mimic benign polyps, these atypical polyps can be mistaken for sarcomas, although they are still completely benign. However, these polyps lack a cambian layer and usually have abundant inflammatory cells, including eosinophils, plasma cells, and neutrophils, and are positive to histiocyte markers, such as CD68 and CD163.[12]

Many small round cell tumors, notably lymphoma, olfactory neuroblastoma, nasopharyngeal carcinoma, malignant melanoma, and Ewing's sarcoma can also occur in the head and neck; and while they can often be distinguished by their particular classic cellular and growth patterns, these frequently merge and overlap in a typical form. Histochemistry and cytogenetics now assist with the clarification of these issues and this is of extreme importance when one considers the different treatments necessary for olfactory neuroblastoma, lymphoma, rhabdomyosarcoma, lymphoepithelial carcinoma, and malignant melanoma. An excellent example here would be that in the past a poorly differentiated malignant melanoma, at times amelanotic, could be confused with rhabdomyosarcoma in older patients. Immunohistochemistry now easily separates the two with a variety of melanocytic markers, which are expressed in melanoma and not in rhabdomyosarcoma.

Other soft tissue tumors such as leiomyosarcoma and malignant fibrous histiocytoma may also be confused with spindle cell rhabdomyosarcoma in adults, but they are extremely rare tumors. Details of their specific immunohistochemistry are found in the respective chapters.

Treatment and Prognosis

The treatment of rhabdomyosarcoma, particularly in children, has dramatically improved since the 1980s. In the classical paper of Fu and Perzin, presenting 16 cases of rhabdomyosarcoma involving the nasal cavity, paranasal sinuses, and nasopharynx, there were 14 children and 2 adults.[13] They were treated with different regimes of local excision. Nine received varying amounts of vincristine, actinomycin D, methotrexate, or cytoxan, but 11 patients died of disease within 2 years of diagnosis and only 3 have survived more than 5 years, with one patient succumbing at 7 years to generalized metastasis. These and other early studies using single-modality chemotherapy showed 5-year survival rates varying between 8% and 20%.[13,14] Following the introduction of triple therapy (i.e., chemotherapy, radiotherapy, and improved surgery), disease-free survival now exceeds 70% overall.

There has been considerable debate with regard to prognostic factors over the years, but there is general agreement now that the patients' age, tumor size, stage, location, histology, and the presence of metastasis are important factors. Younger patients and those with head and neck tumors have a better prognosis than adults, and orbital tumors have the best outcomes in head and neck.

Staging is done by two methods—clinical staging (IRSV stage)[15] and pathological staging (IRSG group).[16] A recent excellent report from Japan reviewed 331 cases treated between 1991 and 2002[17] and showed 10-year survival rates for low-risk groups of 80% and for the higher-risk groups of 38%. The 10-year results are, of course, particularly relevant to children and their prognosis is significantly better than that of adults. Botryoid and spindle cell rhabdomyosarcoma have a notably better prognosis in children.[16] In contrast, in adults prognosis unfortunately remains generally poor regardless of morphology, even with the spindle cell variants of rhabdomyosarcoma.[18]

Surgery

With the substantial improvements in prognosis following the introduction of triple therapy, there is an increasing tendency among some oncologists to consider that surgery now functions purely to provide tissue diagnosis or to "debulk" the tumor. However, in the same way that the chemotherapeutic regimes and the introduction of IMRT (*intensity-modulated radiation therapy*) have pushed forward the boundaries of chemotherapy and radiotherapy, there is a tendency to overlook the fact that modern craniofacial surgery, via approaches such as midfacial degloving and bicoronal incisions, can provide comprehensive removal of residual rhabdomyosarcoma that may have not fully resolved with chemo- and radiotherapeutic treatments. Residual sinonasal and orbital disease may be totally resectable by these approaches with low morbidity. While no one would advocate orbital exenteration in a child without consideration of all options, if there is residual disease following primary treatment, orbital exenteration is a rapid and effective procedure, provided that the orbital apex is fully cleared, and with modern osseointegrated techniques, excellent orbital implants provide a subsequent excellent standard of cosmesis for the child. This situation is preferable to allowing the disease to escape posteriorly via the apex of the orbit into the intracranial compartment, making the situation all but incurable. Multidisciplinary discussion between all treating physicians and surgeons remains essential in the management of this still potentially lethal disease.

Our cohort gathered over more than four decades shows the evolution that has occurred in this disease with increasing use of chemoradiation as initial therapy (Table 10.1). However, it is clear that two-thirds of our patients still required radical surgery, be it craniofacial resection (5 cases), orbital clearance (alone or combined with craniofacial surgery), or maxillectomy (5 cases). One approach that may be of value in the future is the possibility of a wide-field endoscopic resection post chemoradiotherapy, which offers accurate staging of response with low morbidity (Fig. 10.3e).

The numbers in our cohort preclude detailed statistical analysis, but we can report that 10 patients are alive with no evidence of disease between 6 months and 13 years after treatment (mean 4.6 years), 6 have died of disease (2–47 months), 2 have died of intercurrent disease, and 7 have been lost to follow-up, generally coming from abroad.

Key Points

- Rhabdomyosarcoma, although rare in the nose and sinuses, is one of the commoner malignant tumors occurring in the head and neck in children, most often affecting the orbit.
- The embryonal subtype is commonest in children, while in adults the alveolar form is more frequent.
- There has been a significant improvement in survival as a result of triple therapy (chemotherapy, radiotherapy, and surgery).

References

1. Parham DM, Ellison DA. Rhabdomyosarcomas in adults and children: an update. Arch Pathol Lab Med 2006;130(10):1454–1465
2. Pappo AS, Meza JL, Donaldson SS, et al. Treatment of localized nonorbital, nonparameningeal head and neck rhabdomyosarcoma: lessons learned from intergroup rhabdomyosarcoma studies III and IV. J Clin Oncol 2003;21(4):638–645
3. Furlong MA, Fanburg-Smith JC. Pleomorphic rhabdomyosarcoma in children: four cases in the pediatric age group. Ann Diagn Pathol 2001;5(4):199–206
4. Furlong MA, Mentzel T, Fanburg-Smith JC. Pleomorphic rhabdomyosarcoma in adults: a clinicopathologic study of 38 cases with emphasis on morphologic variants and recent skeletal muscle-specific markers. Mod Pathol 2001;14(6):595–603
5. Weiss S, Goldblum J. In: Enzinger and Weiss's Soft Tissue Tumors. 4th ed. St Louis: Mosby; 2001
6. Nayar RC, Prudhomme F, Parise O Jr, Gandia D, Luboinski B, Schwaab G. Rhabdomyosarcoma of the head and neck in adults: a study of 26 patients. Laryngoscope 1993;103(12):1362–1366
7. Crist W, Gehan EA, Ragab AH, et al. The Third Intergroup Rhabdomyosarcoma Study. J Clin Oncol 1995; 13(3):610–630
8. Sheilds C, Sheilds J, Honavar S, Demirci H. Primary ophthalmic rhabdomyosarcoma in thirty-three patients. Trans Am Ophthalmol Soc 2001;99:133–143
9. Lee JH, Lee MS, Lee BH, et al. Rhabdomyosarcoma of the head and neck in adults: MR and CT findings. AJNR Am J Neuroradiol 1996;17(10):1923–1928
10. Hagiwara A, Inoue Y, Nakayama T, et al. The 'botryoid sign': a characteristic feature of rhabdomyosarcomas in the head and neck. Neuroradiology 2001;43(4):331–335
11. Morotti RA, Nicol KK, Parham DM, et al; Children's Oncology Group. An immunohistochemical algorithm to facilitate diagnosis and subtyping of rhabdomyosarcoma: the Children's Oncology Group experience. Am J Surg Pathol 2006;30(8):962–968
12. Nakayama M, Wenig BM, Heffner DK. Atypical stromal cells in inflammatory nasal polyps: immunohistochemical and ultrastructural analysis in defining histogenesis. Laryngoscope 1995;105(2):127–134
13. Fu Y-S, Perzin KH. Nonepithelial tumors of the nasal cavity paranasal sinuses, and nasopharynx: a clinicopathologic study. V. Skeletal muscle tumors (rhabdomyoma and rhabdomyosarcoma). Cancer 1976;37(1):364–376
14. Meza JL, Anderson J, Pappo AS, Meyer WH; Children's Oncology Group. Analysis of prognostic factors in patients with nonmetastatic rhabdomyosarcoma treated on intergroup

Table 10.1 Rhabdomyosarcoma: treatment in personal series[a]

	n	Age		M:F	CFR	Maxill	ESS	Orbit	No Surgery
		Range (y)	Mean (y)						
	26	4–70	26.8	1.2:1	5	5	2	7	9
Radiotherapy alone	2					1		1	
Chemotherapy alone	1							1	
Chemoradiotherapy	19								9

Abbreviations: CFR, craniofacial resection; ESS, endoscopic sinus surgery; F, female; M, male; Maxill, maxillectomy; Orbit, orbital clearance; y, year(s).
[a] Multiple operations in some cases.

rhabdomyosarcoma studies III and IV: the Children's Oncology Group. J Clin Oncol 2006;24(24):3844–3851

15. Raney RB, Anderson JR, Barr FG, et al. Rhabdomyosarcoma and undifferentiated sarcoma in the first two decades of life: a selective review of intergroup rhabdomyosarcoma study group experience and rationale for Intergroup Rhabdomyosarcoma Study V. J Pediatr Hematol Oncol 2001;23(4):215–220

16. Asmar L, Gehan EA, Newton WA, et al. Agreement among and within groups of pathologists in the classification of rhabdomyosarcoma and related childhood sarcomas. Report of an international study of four pathology classifications. Cancer 1994;74(9):2579–2588

17. Hosoi H, Teramukai S, Matsumoto Y, et al. A review of 331 rhabdomyosarcoma cases in patients treated between 1991 and 2002 in Japan. Int J Clin Oncol 2007;12(2):137–145

18. Rubin BP, Hasserjian RP, Singer S, Janecka I, Fletcher JA, Fletcher CD. Spindle cell rhabdomyosarcoma (so-called) in adults: report of two cases with emphasis on differential diagnosis. Am J Surg Pathol 1998;22(4):459–464

11 Cartilaginous Tumors

A range of cartilaginous tumors can occur in this region, exhibiting a spectrum of histological aggressiveness. However, all should be regarded as having malignant potential. Even those that never metastasize are capable of insidious local infiltration which, in the skull base, can ultimately cause the demise of the patient. Thus, radical treatment from the outset is recommended.

Chondroma

(ICD-O code 9220/0)

True benign cartilaginous tumors are extremely rare and distinction between this and a well-differentiated chondrosarcoma can be difficult.[1,2] Thus early cases such as that described by Muller in 1836 must be regarded with some circumspection.[3]

Sometimes referred to as ecchondromas, they are surprisingly rare in the cartilaginous septum, more often affecting the ethmoid and maxilla, suggesting that they may arise from focal hypertrophy of heterotopic nests of cartilage within the mucosa.

A well-circumscribed lesion, without mitoses, which can be completely excised may qualify as a true chondroma but is rarely encountered.

References

1. Fu YS, Perzin KH. Non-epithelial tumors of the nasal cavity, paranasal sinuses, and nasopharynx: a clinicopathologic study. 3. Cartilaginous tumors (chondroma, chondrosarcoma). Cancer 1974;34(2):453–463
2. Michaels L, Hellquist H. Ear, Nose and Throat Histopathology. 2nd ed. New York: Springer; 2000:236–237
3. Muller M. Die Chondrom. Arch Klin Exp Ohren Nasen Kehlkopfheilkde (Berlin) 1870;12:323

Chondroblastoma

(ICD-O code 9230/0)

Chondroblastoma typically affects the epiphyseal end of long bones such as the distal femur and occurs in young people less than 20 years old. The tumor is composed of chondroblasts in a chondroid matrix with foci of calcification. This may give it a similar appearance on imaging to a well-differentiated chondrosarcoma. The presence of giant cells may also make histological differentiation from a giant cell tumor difficult.

There are a very small number of case reports of chondroblastoma affecting the upper jaw,[1,2] though the lesion is somewhat more common in the temporal bone.

Although curettage has been used, ideally a complete resection should be undertaken by whatever surgical approach is possible. Radiotherapy is not recommended because of the potential risk of provoking malignant change.

References

1. Al-Dewachi HS, Al-Naib N, Sangal BC. Benign chondroblastoma of the maxilla: a case report and review of chondroblastomas in cranial bones. Br J Oral Surg 1980;18(2):150–156
2. Madhup R, Srivastava M, Srivastava A, Bhatt M, Kirti S. Chondroblastoma of maxilla. Oral Oncol Extra 2005; 41:159–161

Chondromyxoid Fibroma

(ICD-O code 9241/0)

Chondromyxoid fibroma is a rare benign tumor of cartilaginous origin.

It is most often seen in adolescents and young adults, in whom it affects the long bones such as the tibia.[1,2] It is extremely rare in the sinonasal region, where the maxilla is the most frequently affected. From there, adjacent structures such as the nasal bones, ethmoid, sphenoid, clivus, and orbit may be involved.[3–5]

Macroscopically it forms a discrete mass that causes nasal obstruction, facial swelling, and/or displacement of the orbital contents.

Imaging shows a circumscribed expansile lesion with a sharply delineated lobulated margin (**Fig. 11.1a** and **Fig. 11.2**).[6] Microscopically it is also lobulated, composed of spindle or stellate cells in a myxochondroid stroma. It can be aggressive and so must be distinguished from chordoma and chondrosarcoma.[7]

Complete surgical excision is curative by whatever approach is appropriate, otherwise "recurrence" can be anticipated.[8] One of our cases occurred in an Italian boy of 7 years of age who underwent a craniofacial resection in 1990 without recurrence over 10.5 years follow-up, although it is almost certain that if he presented today an endoscopic excision would be undertaken (**Fig. 11.1b**).[9] A second case is that of a 30-year-old woman who had had surgery performed abroad and was left with residual disease in the nasal cavity. After histological confirmation, she has recently undergone an endoscopic resection (**Fig. 11.2**).

References

1. Rahimi A, Beabout JW, Ivins JC, Dahlin DC. Chondromyxoid fibroma: a clinicopathologic study of 76 cases. Cancer 1972;30(3):726–736
2. Wu CT, Inwards CY, O'Laughlin S, Rock MG, Beabout JW, Unni KK. Chondromyxoid fibroma of bone: a clinicopathologic review of 278 cases. Hum Pathol 1998;29(5):438–446

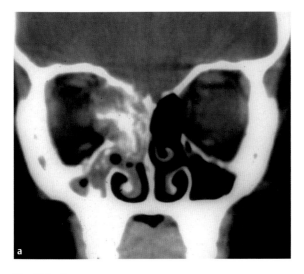

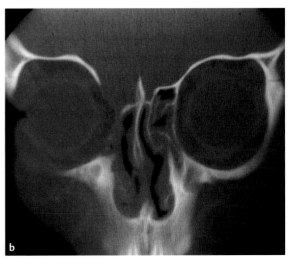

Fig. 11.1a, b

a Coronal CT scan showing chondromyxoid fibroma affecting the right ethmoids and adjacent skull base, treated by craniofacial resection in 1990.

b Coronal CT scan in the same patient 10.5 years later.

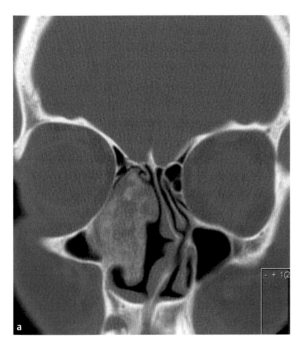

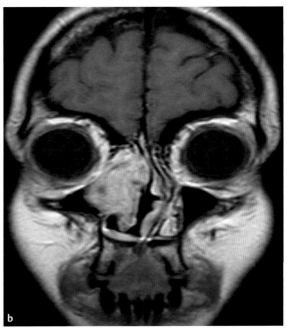

Fig. 11.2a, b

a Coronal CT showing chondromyxoid fibroma in the nasal cavity following partial removal via Caldwell-Luc approach 15 years earlier when the patient was 9 years old.

b Coronal MRI (T2W sequence) in the same patient.

3. Baujat B, Attal P, Racy E, et al. Chondromyxoid fibroma of the nasal bone with extension into the frontal and ethmoidal sinuses: report of one case and a review of the literature. Am J Otolaryngol 2001;22(2):150–153

4. Koay CB, Freeland AP, Athanasou NA. Chondromyxoid fibroma of the nasal bone with extension into the frontal and ethmoidal sinuses. J Laryngol Otol 1995;109(3):258–261

5. Nazeer T, Ro JY, Varma DG, de la Hermosa JR, Ayala AG. Chondromyxoid fibroma of paranasal sinuses: report of two cases presenting with nasal obstruction. Skeletal Radiol 1996;25(8):779–782

6. Curtin H, Rabinov J, Som P. Central skull base: embryology, anatomy and pathology. In: Som P, Curtin H, eds. Head and Neck Imaging. 4th ed. St Louis: Mosby; 2003:821

7. Keel SB, Bhan AK, Liebsch NJ, Rosenberg AE. Chondromyxoid fibroma of the skull base: a tumor which may be confused with chordoma and chondrosarcoma. A report of three cases and review of the literature. Am J Surg Pathol 1997;21(5):577–582

8. Shek TW, Peh WC, Leung G. Chondromyxoid fibroma of skull base: a tumour prone to local recurrence. J Laryngol Otol 1999;113(4):380–385

9. Isenberg SF. Endoscopic removal of chondromyxoid fibroma of the ethmoid sinus. Am J Otolaryngol 1995;16(3):205–208

Chondrosarcoma

Definition

(ICD-O code 9220/3)

Chondrosarcoma is a rare malignant tumor of hyaline cartilage.

Etiology

Previous trauma (accidental or surgical) has been implicated in the development of chondrosarcoma, as has inhalation of hydrocarbons, although these theories are generally discredited.[1,2] Chondrosarcomas have been reported to occur in association with other malignant conditions such as osteosarcoma, malignant melanoma, fibrosarcoma, and leukemia, as well as benign conditions such as Paget's disease and fibrous dysplasia.[3,4] They have also been associated with Maffucci's syndrome,[5] multiple hereditary exostosis, previous irradiation, and previous use of intravenous thorium dioxide contrast.[6]

Mutational inactivation of tumor suppressor genes $p16$, Rb, and $p53$ has been implicated in tumor development. Inactivation of $p53$ has been associated with higher-grade tumors with a worse prognosis, and both Rb and $p53$ mutations have been linked to chondrosarcoma and osteosarcoma.[7]

Synonyms

Aggressive cartilaginous tumors were described by Morgan in 1836 and Heath in 1887.[8,9] Mollison reported the first chondrosarcoma in the paranasal sinuses in 1916, but it was not until 1939 that Ewing identified chondrosarcoma as a separate entity from osteogenic sarcoma.[10,11]

Incidence

Chondrosarcomas constitute ~10 to 20% of all malignant bone tumors, and most commonly arise in long bones and the pelvis.[2,6,12] Between 3% and 10% of all chondrosarcomas arise in the head and neck[6,13,14]; skull base chondrosarcomas constitute 0.15% of all intracranial and 6% of all skull base tumors.[15] Chondrosarcomas account for less than 16% of all sarcomas of the nasal cavity, paranasal sinuses, and nasopharynx and comprise 3 to 5% of nonepithelial sinonasal tumors. In our own series, chondrosarcomas comprise 34 of 1,063 malignant sinonasal tumors (3.2%).

Site

In 1979, Myers and Thawley classified chondrosarcomas into primary, secondary, and mesenchymal subtypes.[16] Primary chondrosarcomas arise de novo from undifferentiated perichondrial cells; secondary ones arise within a preexisting cartilaginous lesion such as a chondroma or exostosis; and mesenchymal ones arise from primitive mesenchymal cells.[16] Primary chondrosarcomas may arise within cartilage or in bone that ossified in cartilage such as the sphenoid. However, they can also arise in soft tissues with no obvious cartilaginous source, and this has been suggested to be the result of embryonal cell rests that have escaped resorption, from ectopic chondroid precursor cells or from cartilaginous differentiation of primitive mesenchymal cells.[2,14,17,18] This may also account for apparent multisite origins.

Classical chondrosarcomas involve the alveolar portion of the maxilla, the maxillary sinus, the nasal septum, the sphenopetrous area, and the clivus, where the disease may be multifocal. Indeed clinical experience suggests that many sinonasal cases are multifocal. From the nasal septum, the tumor can infiltrate superiorly into the skull base or inferiorly into the palate. They also occur in the larynx and cervical vertebrae.[4,6,13,19,20]

Diagnostic Features

Clinical Features

In the literature patients' ages range from 16 months to 89 years,[21,22] but the majority of patents are in their fourth and fifth decades with a mean of 46 years,[4,13,19,22–25] making this a younger group than for some other sinonasal tumors and chondrosarcomas elsewhere. This has also been the experience in our series, where in 38 individuals the age ranged from 5 to 76 years, with a mean of 42 years. When chondrosarcoma is reported in children[20] it must be distinguished from the mesenchymal variant (see below).

The male-to-female ratio varies widely from series to series. The American College of Surgeons' National Cancer Database reported that 64.5% of sinonasal chondrosarcomas occurred in women,[2] which is in keeping with an analysis of 125 cases done by Harrison and Lund in 1993[26] that showed a ratio of 1:1.2 of men to women. In our own series, a similar male-to-female ratio of 1:1.5 was found. A racial predilection for chondrosarcomas has not been generally found, but the same American Cancer Database reported that mesenchymal and myxoid subtypes are more common in Hispanic (44.9%) and African-American (31.8%) patients than in white patients (17.1%).[2]

Initially a mass effect produces nasal obstruction and/or epistaxis, which may be bilateral when the septum is affected (68% in our series).[22,27,28] Endoscopic examination of the nose can show a smooth swelling covered by normal mucosa (Fig. 11.3). Pain has been reported in less than 50%; swelling of the face and palate may be evident particularly if the tumor is located in the anterior maxilla;[13,29] and loosening of teeth can occur.

Once the tumor involves the skull base, various neurologic sequelae can occur, especially with recurrences.[6,14,22] The orbit may be involved, producing proptosis and sometimes diplopia; and there can be substantial space-occupying intracranial lesions and cranial nerve palsies.[4,6,22,28] Notably, the optic nerve may be compressed, leading to visual loss; and it is not uncommon for the chiasm and both optic nerves to be affected, leading to bilateral blindness. This has occurred in 2 of our patients (6%) (Figs. 11.4, 11.5a,b).

Imaging

Contrast-enhanced CT typically shows a lobulated mass with an irregular matrix containing areas of calcification in ~75%.[4,30] The calcification may be punctate, dystrophic, or in a ring and arc pattern.[31] There is often bony expansion and erosion.[4] The majority of cases involve the naso-ethmoid area and are often centrally located. Two-thirds affect the orbit and two-thirds show intracranial extension in our series (Fig. 11.6a and Fig. 11.7a).

Magnetic resonance imaging typically shows a heterogeneous enhancing mass of low intensity on T1W images and high intensity on T2 weighting due to the high water content of the chondroid matrix.[6,14] After gadolinium enhancement, T1W images show diagnostic contrast enhancement at the periphery and along fibrovascular septa within an otherwise nonenhancing chondromatous core (Figs. 11.5b, 11.6b, 11.7b).[4,30] This can produce a cystic appearance that may be overlooked by the unwary, particularly if MRI alone is being used for follow-up (Fig. 11.5c). It has been our practice to use regular MRI for routine postoperative surveillance but to perform a baseline CT after the initial surgery in cases of chondrosarcoma and to repeat this if the MRI shows any suspicious change (Fig. 11.6c, 11.7c).

Chondrosarcoma must be distinguished from chondroma, meningioma, osteoma, osteosarcoma, osteoblastoma, fibro-osseous lesions, and chordoma.[6,32] Occasionally the tumor may be densely calcified with a "sunray" effect, more commonly seen in osteosarcoma.[6,14,33]

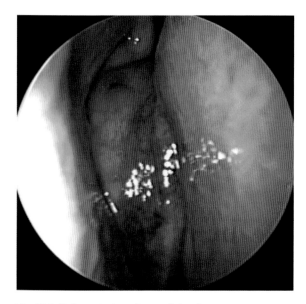

Fig. 11.3 Endoscopic view of a septal chondrosarcoma.

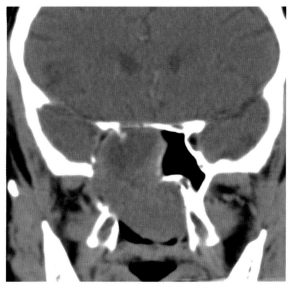

Fig. 11.4 Coronal CT scan showing a chondrosarcoma involving the posterior nasal septum and basisphenoid, extending into the orbital apex and roof of the sphenoid.

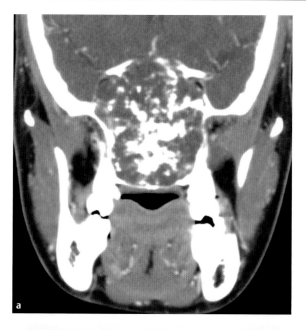

Fig. 11.5a–c

a Coronal CT scan showing a more extensive chondrosarcoma occupying the sphenoid and extending into the middle cranial fossa with typical heterogeneous signal from areas of calcification.

b Coronal MRI (T1W post gadolinium enhancement) in the same patient showing a large central septal tumor mass with compression and obstruction of the maxillary sinuses. Calcification shows as signal voids.

c Coronal MRI (T1W post gadolinium enhancement) in the same patient 2 years following midfacial degloving showing a small cystic recurrence in the right orbital apex, successfully removed endoscopically.

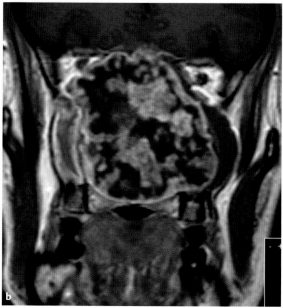

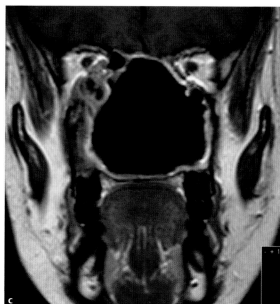

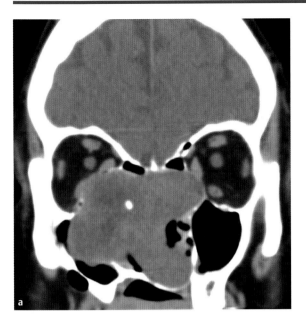

Fig. 11.6a–c

a Coronal CT scan showing a large lobulated chondrosarcoma arising from the septum and extending from the skull base to the palate and laterally to both orbits.

b Coronal MRI in the same patient showing peripheral enhancement with irregular heterogeneous signal.

c Coronal MRI (T1W post gadolinium enhancement) showing the surgical cavity 3 years after midfacial degloving, with no sign of recurrence.

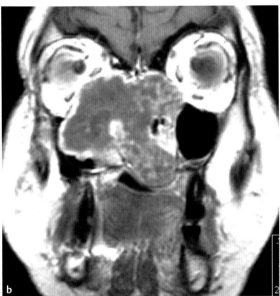

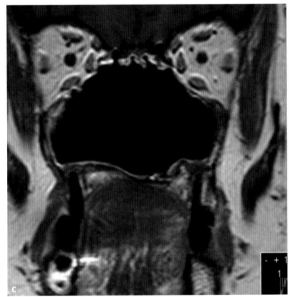

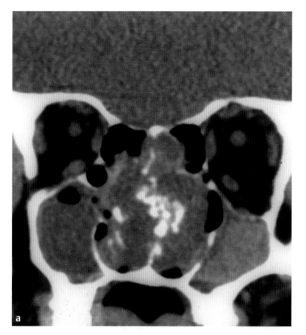

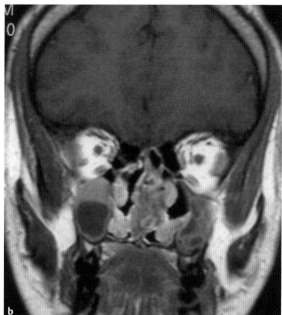

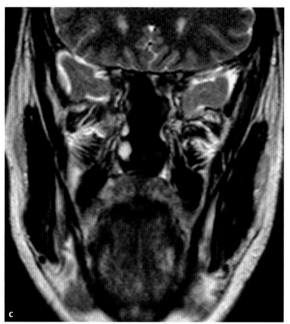

Fig. 11.7a–c

a Coronal CT scan showing a septal mass with calcification, suitable for endoscopic resection.

b Coronal MRI (T1W post gadolinium enhancement) in the same patient showing peripheral enhancement.

c Coronal MRI (T2W) at 4-year follow-up showing the cavity with no sign of recurrence.

Chondrosarcoma of the nasal septum has also been reported as an incidental finding on CT scanning.[32]

Histological Features and Differential Diagnosis

The tumors are usually lobulated and firm with a gray-pink glistening granular or "ripe pear" surface. It can be quite difficult to distinguish tumor from normal cartilage, so microscopic criteria were defined by Lichtenstein and Jaffe in 1942: namely, hypercellularity, hyperchromatism or irregularity of nuclei, double or multiple nuclei, areas of differentiation compatible with nonspecific sarcoma, marked enlargement of the chondrocytes, or mitotic figures.[34]

Classification criteria have been described, primarily relating to the degree of cellularity, the nuclear size, and the number of mitoses (grades 1 to 3, or well to poorly differentiated).[23] Grade 1 tumors are well differentiated with abundant pale chondroid matrix, clusters of chondrocytes with normal or slightly enlarged nuclei, absent mitoses, and occasional double nuclei. Grade 2 (moderately differentiated) tumors have less matrix and more chondrocytes, with occasional mitoses and slightly enlarged hyperchromatic, multiple nuclei. Grade 3, poorly differentiated chondrosarcomas have a myxoid matrix with irregular chondrocytes and increased cellularity, nuclear pleomorphism, and mitoses.[6]

Rare histological variants have been described, including mesenchymal chondrosarcoma (see below) and clear cell chondrosarcoma, which accounts for less than 2% of all chondrosarcomas; metastatic renal cell carcinoma should obviously be excluded in these cases.[32] Myxoid chondrosarcoma is a more aggressive subtype affecting children with more bony destruction and a t(9;22) translocation not seen in typical chondrosarcoma.[35] Dedifferentiated chondrosarcoma is a highly malignant variant.[36]

Because differentiating chondrosarcoma from chordoma, osteogenic sarcoma, and salivary gland tumors can be difficult, as large a biopsy specimen as possible should be provided. It is worth noting that chondrosarcomas stain positive for S100 protein, while chordomas are positive for S100 and cytokeratin.[6] Others have undertaken complex tissue microarray-based comparative analysis to differentiate between chordoma and chondrosarcoma but of the newer markers (brachyury, SOX-9, and podoplanin) have shown only podoplanin to be positive for chondrosarcoma.[37]

As previously stated all cartilaginous tumors in this area should be regarded as having malignant potential.[23,32,38,39] However, these lesions must be distinguished from Ollier disease, which is characterized by benign growths in the metaphyses of bones, some of which may contain atypical cells. We have encountered one patient with this condition, who presented with extensive involvement of the ethmosphenoid and skull base and who underwent craniofacial resection. Four years later she went on to develop multiple systemic lesions when the diagnosis of Ollier disease was confirmed.

Natural History

Sinonasal chondrosarcoma is normally a rather indolent tumor, although less so than in the larynx.[2] Nonetheless, its progress locally is inexorable even though metastatic spread to regional lymph nodes is exceptional.

However, late distant metastases have been reported in up to 20% of cases,[6,21,32,40] and are being seen more since the advent of surgical techniques such as combined craniofacial resection, which has dramatically improved local control of disease, prolonging survival.[41] Metastases tend to be to the lungs, but late bony metastasis has also been reported.[25,42]

Thus the history is one of multiple local recurrences, and local spread throughout the skull base is the most common cause of death for these patients (in up to 88%)[25] and can occur after many years, so that lifelong follow-up is needed.[27]

Table 11.1 Chondrosarcoma: personal series

	n	M:F ratio	Age		Follow-up (mo)	Outcome
			Mean (y)	Range (y)		
Endoscopic resection	5	2:3	49	42–76	12–100	A&W 100%
Craniofacial resection	23	11:12	42.8	19–71	60–232	5-year 94% 10-year 56% 15-year 37%
Other: Midfacial degloving[5] Maxillectomy[3] Lateral rhinotomy[2]	10	8:2	37.6	5–68	6–120	5-year 60% 10-year 35%
Total	38	21:17	47.2	5–76	6–232	
Abbreviations: F, female; M, male; mo, month(s); y, year(s).						

Treatment

Surgery is the principal treatment and one should never be tempted to undertreat this disease because anything less than radical resection will leave residual disease. However, achieving clear margins is often difficult when tumors involve the skull base.[2,25] Craniofacial resection is regarded as the gold standard for sinonasal and skull base tumors of this sort and there are well-documented cohorts reported that include chondrosarcoma.[43,44]

It is also recognized that en bloc resection in the skull base can be technically difficult due to the infiltrative nature of the tumor around vital structures in the skull base. Thus, while endoscopic resection has been and is being undertaken, careful case selection is essential.[32,45–47]

In our series, the majority have undergone craniofacial resection (63%) (**Table 11.1**), but maxillectomy via open or more often a midfacial degloving approach, lateral rhinotomy, and more recently endoscopic resection have been utilized. In 8 patients further surgery was undertaken, in some cases multiple times. Three patients underwent removal of an eye; in 6 individuals orbital apex/canal decompression was successfully undertaken. Only 10% received conventional radiotherapy, which had been given in all cases prior to referral to our unit.

Whatever surgical approach is employed, careful scrutiny of the residual bone is needed, particularly in the basisphenoid where distinguishing the nests of chondrosarcoma from diploic bone can be difficult. Thus the addition of endoscopy during open techniques is recommended. These suspicious areas should be drilled out meticulously.

Conventional transcranial/transfacial skull base approaches are often associated with postoperative cranial neuropathies due to the need to obtain an adequate surgical exposure.[48] Gay et al reported a series of 60 patients with either chordomas or chondrosarcomas, in which only 28 patients (47%) had total resection based on postoperative imaging.[49] However, 48 patients (80%) suffered new cranial neuropathies. In a review of 64 patients by Sekhar et al, only 50% of patients had total resection but 41% of patients incurred additional neurologic deficits.[50] Oghalai et al reported a series of 33 patients in whom only 8 patients (28%) had total resection and 6 patients (18%) suffered surgical complications.[48]

Tzortzidis et al reviewed 47 patients who underwent microsurgical resection over a 20-year period.[51] A gross total resection was obtained in 61.7% of patients and subtotal resection was obtained in 38.3% of patients. A postoperative complication rate, including CSF leaks and new cranial nerve palsies, of 18% was reported. Patients who underwent a gross total resection, especially as a primary procedure, demonstrated better local control and quality of life.[51]

By contrast, after craniofacial resection,[43] complication rates were low in our series despite some patients

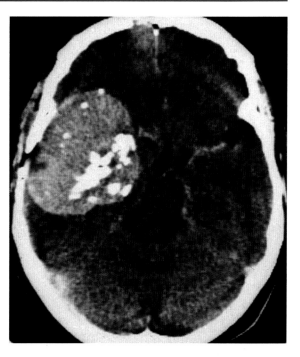

Fig. 11.8 A large intracranial recurrence in a patient who had undergone multiple previous craniofacial resection over a 14-year period.

undergoing multiple revision craniofacial procedures, in one case 6 times (**Fig. 11.8**).

With careful case selection, lesions without significant skull base or orbital involvement, especially if located at the level of the nasal septum, are amenable to an endoscopic resection (**Table 11.2**). In addition chondrosarcoma arising in the sphenoid sinus,[52–54] clivus,[45,55,56] petrous apex,[57] and pterygopalatine fossa[58] may also be dealt with endoscopically. A short hospital stay and lack of perioperative complications, including CSF leaks or neurologic deficits, have been noted following endoscopic transnasal approach.

Traditionally chondrosarcoma has been regarded as radioresistant,[14,19] and chemotherapy is ineffective.[59] Radiotherapy has been used when resection margins are positive, if the location prevents wide tumor resection, and in recurrent or high-grade tumors.[32] There have been a few reports of a good response to standard photon radiotherapy when combined with surgical excision.[60–62]

Proton beam therapy has been used with some success. Protons are subatomic particles (nuclei of hydrogen atoms) that have a higher relative biological efficacy than standard photon radiotherapy and better spatial selectivity with improved dose distribution, resulting in improved sparing of adjacent critical organs.[63,64] **The advantages of proton beam radiotherapy are that it is better able to kill hypoxic cells, the damage inflicted is less readily repaired, and there is less variation in radiosensitivity across the cell cycle.**[65] **It seems to be most effective in slow-growing tumors with reduced**

cell recovery. Chondrosarcomas tend to be slowly pro-liferating and so are ideal targets.

Outcome

Head and neck chondrosarcomas and, in particular, sino-nasal chondrosarcomas have a worse prognosis than chondrosarcomas elsewhere in the body,[6,23,25,66] so one should be wary of discussing "cure." Local recurrence rates vary from 40% to 85% overall for chondrosarcomas in the head and neck, whereas chondrosarcomas else-where in the body have much lower rates of recurrence, ~15%.[14,32,67]

Three factors have been reported to affect prognosis: the location and extent of the tumor; the adequacy of surgery with negative margins; and the degree of dif-ferentiation of the tumor.[23,48,68] The more posterior the tumor, the worse the outcome, so tumors in the naso-pharynx, posterior nasal cavity, and sphenoid sinus have a worse prognosis than more anterior tumor. Disease that involves the skull base is more likely to recur,[6,23] as it is more difficult to achieve clear resection margins, which obviously give a significant survival advantage.[25] The grade of the tumor does not seem to correlate with the likelihood of local recurrence but it is related to distant metastases and overall survival. Five-year survival has been reported as 80 to 90% for grade 1 tumors, 71 to 81% for grade 2, and 38 to 43% for grade 3 tumors. Survival rates at 10 years are lower: 71 to 83% in grade 1 tumors, 40 to 64% in grade 2, and 29 to 36% for grade 3 disease.[66]

Initial results of surgical treatment are generally encouraging. Overall survival for all grades has variously been reported from 44% to 81% at 5 years.[6,14,69–72] **How-ever, the infiltrative nature and possible multisite origin mean that "recurrences" are common and may occur over a lifetime.** Thus in our craniofacial series of 22 patients, 5-year survival was 94%, dropping to 56% at 10 years and 37% at 15 years (**Table 11.1**).[43] The large series from the American National Cancer Database reviewed 400 head and neck chondrosarcomas and found disease-specific survival rates of 87.2% at 5 years and 70.6% at 10 years. Although this series included laryngeal chondro-sarcomas, which may have favorably skewed the results, it also contained mesenchymal and myxoid subtypes, which do worse.[2]

To date there are only sporadic cases managed endo-scopically (**Table 11.2**),[12,32,72–78] but with careful case selec-tion the extent of resection was ostensibly complete without any morbidity, albeit with a relatively short follow-up. In our own series, all five patients are alive and well with between 1 and 8 years of follow-up but

Table 11.2 Chondrosarcomas (CS) removed via an endonasal endoscopic approach in the literature

Location	Series[a]	Study design	Total number of patients	CS (number)	Extent of resection	Follow-up period	Morbidity	Recurrence
Septum	Matthews[74]	Case series	1	1	Complete		None	
Septum	Giger[73]	Case series	1	1	Complete	3 y	None	
Septum	Coppit[12]	Case series	2	2	Complete		None	
Septum	Betz[75]	Case series	2	1	Incomplete	1 y	None	Early recurrence removed
Septum	Jenny[76]	Case series	1	1	Complete		None	
Sphenoid	Carrau[32]	Case series	1	1	Complete		None	
Sphenoid	Castelnuovo[52]	Case series	41	1				
Sphenoid	Tami[54]	Case series	8	1				
Clivus and sphenopetrous	Frank[45]	Case series	11	2				
Clivus	Zhang[55]	Case series	9	2	Complete/ subtotal	3–39 mo		
Pterygopalatine area	Hu[58]	Case series	1	1				

Abbreviations: CS, chondrosarcoma; mo, month; y, year.

Source: Modified with permission from Lund V, Stammberger H, Nicolai P, et al. European position paper on endoscopic manage-ment of tumours of the nose, paranasal sinuses and skull base. Rhinol Suppl 2010;(22):1–143.

[a] First author only given for each series.

remain under close life-long review. In addition, small recurrences after any form of surgery may be undertaken endoscopically (**Fig. 11.5c**).

Currently proton beam radiotherapy is available in only a few centers as it is 2 to 3 times more expensive than photon radiotherapy, and is more complex to deliver, but results are very promising for skull base chondrosarcomas[64,79] and for chordomas and for ocular melanomas.[63] A large series of 229 patients treated with proton beam radiotherapy showed recurrence-free survival of 98% at 5 years and 94% at 10 years.[80] The increased local control is reflected in a trend toward increased overall survival.[81]

Stereotactic radiosurgery has also been proposed as an adjunct in the treatment of skull base chondrosarcomas, particularly if proton beam radiotherapy is not available. Five-year local control rates in a series of 10 patients were 80%[82] but the use of the treatment is limited by the size of the tumor, with mean volumes of 9.8 to 20 cm³ being included.[82,83]

Key Points

- Surgical resection provides the best long-term results.
- Tumor recurrence rate is directly proportional to the degree of resection as well as the histological grade.
- Craniofacial resection remains the "gold standard" but a total resection can be achieved with endoscopic endonasal approaches in selected cases.
- Skull base lesions are often adjacent to critical neurovascular structures; therefore, their removal is achieved in a piecemeal fashion regardless of the approach.
- Proton therapy may be of value, if available.
- Local recurrence can occur after many years, so life-long follow-up is required.

Mesenchymal Chondrosarcoma

(ICD-O code 9240/3)

First described in 1959 by Lichtenstein and Bernstein, mesenchymal chondrosarcoma (MCS) is a rare and highly malignant tumor that can occur in bone or extraosseous sites, generally in children, teenagers, and young adults, more commonly in women.[84–86] It accounts for 2% of all chondrosarcomas[87] and is most common in the ribs and jaws, affecting the maxilla or mandible in 22 to 27% of cases.[84,88] In the sinonasal region, they produce nasal obstruction and epistaxis initially.[88,89] We have treated 4 patients, 2 male and 2 female whose ages ranged from 15 to 23 years (mean 18.75 years). All four lesions affected the maxilla and also involved the ethmoid sinuses in two of the cases (**Table 11.3**).

Radiologically MCSs are less well circumscribed than other chondrosarcomas, with local infiltration, and lack the heterogeneous calcification seen with other chondrosarcomas (**Fig. 11.9**). MCS is characterized by a biphasic pattern of undifferentiated small, round cells around islands of undifferentiated cartilage.[89–94] The latter may be less obvious, leading to confusion with hemangiopericytoma. Positivity to CD99 (MIC-2) and neuron specific enolase (NSE) can also make difficult the distinction from Ewing's sarcoma and primitive neuroectodermal tumor.[95] There can also be positivity to S100 in the more cartilaginous areas.[96]

In contrast to chondrosarcomas, MCSs metastasize and are extremely aggressive with few, if any, long-term survivors.[2,68,97,98] This has led to aggressive triple therapy using surgery and chemoradiotherapy, despite which prognosis remains poor.[25,85,89,93,99,100] The majority recur locally and, if patients do survive, cervical lymph node and distant metastases to lung and bone may appear many years later.[98,101]

Table 11.3 Mesenchymal chondrosarcoma: personal series

Age	Sex	Site	Treatment			Subsequent treatment	Outcome
			Surgery	CT	RT		
15	F	Maxilla	MFD		Yes	–	DOD
18	M	Maxilla/ethmoid	MFD	Yes	Yes	–	DOD
19	F	Maxilla/ethmoid	MFD	Yes	Yes	MFD × 4 CT	AWR
23	M	Maxilla	MFD/removal of eye	Yes		CFR/ND	DOD

Abbreviations: AWR, alive with recurrence; CFR, craniofacial resection; CT, chemotherapy; DOD, dead of disease; F, female; M, male; MFD, midfacial degloving; ND, neck dissection; RT, radiotherapy.

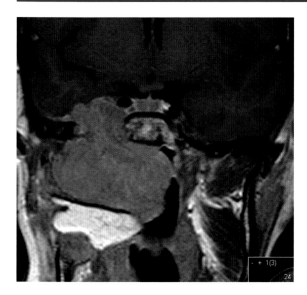

Fig. 11.9 Coronal MRI (T1W post gadolinium enhancement) showing recurrent mesenchymal chondrosarcoma in the right nasal cavity, maxilla, pterygoid region, infratemporal fossa, and middle cranial fossa. Inferiorly, high signal from the fat of the free flap used for previous reconstruction can be seen.

Survival rates have been reported as 42% at 5 years, falling to 28% at 10 years.[102] A more recent series of 13 patients with sinonasal mesenchymal chondrosarcoma had disease-free survival rates of 64% at 5 years and 55% at 10 years, after treatment with surgery, and in some cases postoperative chemotherapy and/or radiotherapy.[89] The American Cancer Database found that survival rates for mesenchymal chondrosarcoma were significantly worse than for conventional chondrosarcoma, 53.2% at 5 years versus 91.4% respectively.

Of our four patients, all were treated with maxillectomy via a midfacial degloving combined with both radiotherapy and/or chemotherapy (**Table 11.3**). Two patients went on to have further radical surgery (on several occasions in one case) including a neck dissection (one case). Despite this, three of the patients are dead of disease and the fourth is alive with recurrence, albeit 13 years later, but sadly undergoing chemotherapy for local and metastatic spread as the disease is too extensive to be considered for proton beam therapy.

References

1. Coates HL, Pearson BW, Devine KD, Unni KK. Chondrosarcoma of the nasal cavity, paranasal sinuses, and nasopharynx. Trans Sect Otolaryngol Am Acad Ophthalmol Otolaryngol 1977;84(5):ORL919–926
2. Koch BB, Karnell LH, Hoffman HT, et al. National cancer database report on chondrosarcoma of the head and neck. Head Neck 2000;22(4):408–425
3. Barton RP. Metachranous chondrosarcoma and malignant melanoma of the nose. J Laryngol Otol 1985;99(5):497–500
4. Chen CC, Hsu L, Hecht JL, Janecka I. Bimaxillary chondrosarcoma: clinical, radiologic, and histologic correlation. AJNR Am J Neuroradiol 2002;23(4):667–670
5. Hyde GE, Yarington CT Jr, Chu FW. Head and neck manifestations of Maffucci's syndrome: chondrosarcoma of the nasal septum. Am J Otolaryngol 1995;16(4):272–275
6. Downey TJ, Clark SK, Moore DW. Chondrosarcoma of the nasal septum. Otolaryngol Head Neck Surg 2001;125(1):98–100
7. Mohammadinezhad C. Chondrosarcoma of the jaw. J Craniofac Surg 2009;20(6):2097–2100
8. Morgan N. Exostoses of the bones of the face. Guys Hosp Rep 1836;1:403–406
9. Heath C. Lectures on disease of the jaws. Br J Dental Sci 1887;30:756–761
10. Mollison W. Some cases of growth of the upper jaw and ethmoidal region. Dent Rec (London) 1916;36:44–47
11. Ewing J. A review of the classification of bone tumors. Surg Gynecol Obstet 1939;68:971–976
12. Coppit GL, Eusterman VD, Bartels J, Downey TJ. Endoscopic resection of chondrosarcomas of the nasal septum: a report of 2 cases. Otolaryngol Head Neck Surg 2002; 127(6):569–571
13. Saito K, Unni KK, Wollan PC, Lund BA. Chondrosarcoma of the jaw and facial bones. Cancer 1995;76(9):1550–1558
14. Rassekh CH, Nuss DW, Kapadia SB, Curtin HD, Weissman JL, Janecka IP. Chondrosarcoma of the nasal septum: skull base imaging and clinicopathologic correlation. Otolaryngol Head Neck Surg 1996;115(1):29–37
15. Berkmen YM, Blatt ES. Cranial and intracranial cartilaginous tumours. Clin Radiol 1968;19(3):327–333
16. Myers EM, Thawley SE. Maxillary chondrosarcoma. Arch Otolaryngol 1979;105(3):116–118
17. Ringetz N. Pathology of malignant tumors arising in the nasal and paranasal cavities and maxilla. Acta Otolaryngol 1938;(Suppl 27):31–42
18. El Ghazali AM. Chondrosarcoma of the paranasal sinuses and nasal septum. J Laryngol Otol 1983;97(6):543–547
19. Koka V, Vericel R, Lartigau E, Lusinchi A, Schwaab G. Sarcomas of nasal cavity and paranasal sinuses: chondrosarcoma, osteosarcoma and fibrosarcoma. J Laryngol Otol 1994;108(11):947–953
20. Gadwal SR, Fanburg-Smith JC, Gannon FH, Thompson LD. Primary chondrosarcoma of the head and neck in pediatric patients: a clinicopathologic study of 14 cases with a review of the literature. Cancer 2000;88(9):2181–2188
21. Gallagher TM, Strome M. Chondrosarcomas of the facial region. Laryngoscope 1972;82(6):978–984
22. Beneck D, Seidman I, Jacobs J. Chondrosarcoma of the nasal septum: a case report. Head Neck Surg 1984;7(2):162–167
23. Fu Y-S, Perzin KH. Non-epithelial tumors of the nasal cavity, paranasal sinuses, and nasopharynx: a clinicopathologic study. 3. Cartilaginous tumors (chondroma, chondrosarcoma). Cancer 1974;34(2):453–463
24. Ajagbe HA, Daramola JO, Junaid TA. Chondrosarcoma of the jaw: review of fourteen cases. J Oral Maxillofac Surg 1985;43(10):763–766
25. Ruark DS, Schlehaider UK, Shah JP. Chondrosarcomas of the head and neck. World J Surg 1992;16(5):1010–1015, discussion 1015–1016
26. Harrison D, Lund V. Tumours of the Upper Jaw. London: Churchill Livingstone; 1990:204
27. Vener J, Rice DH, Newman AN. Osteosarcoma and chondrosarcoma of the head and neck. Laryngoscope 1984;94(2 Pt 1):240–242
28. Lund VJ, Howard DJ, Wei WI, Cheesman AD. Craniofacial resection for tumors of the nasal cavity and paranasal sinuses—a 17-year experience. Head Neck 1998;20(2):97–105

29. Anwar R, Ruddy J, Ghosh S, Lavery KM, Wilson F. Chondrosarcoma of the maxilla. J Laryngol Otol 1992;106(1):53–55

30. Lloyd G, Lund VJ, Howard D, Savy L. Optimum imaging for sinonasal malignancy. J Laryngol Otol 2000; 114(7):557–562

31. Dass AN, Peh WC, Shek TW, Ho WK. Case 139: nasal septum low-grade chondrosarcoma. Radiology 2008; 249(2):714–717

32. Carrau RL, Aydogan B, Hunt JL. Chondrosarcoma of the sphenoid sinus resected by an endoscopic approach. Am J Otolaryngol 2004;25(4):274–277

33. Sato K, Nukaga H, Horikoshi T. Chondrosarcoma of the jaws and facial skeleton: a review of the Japanese literature. J Oral Surg 1977;35(11):892–897

34. Lichenstein L, Jaffe H. Chondrosarcoma of bone. Am J Pathol 1942;19:553–589

35. Kim YJ, Im SA, Lim GY, et al. Myxoid chondrosarcoma of the sinonasal cavity in a child: a case report. Korean J Radiol 2007;8(5):452–455

36. Munshi A, Atri SK, Pandey KC, Sharma MC. Dedifferentiated chondrosarcoma of the maxilla. J Cancer Res Ther 2007;3(1):53–55

37. Oakley GJ, Fuhrer K, Seethala RR. Brachyury, SOX-9, and podoplanin, new markers in the skull base chordoma vs chondrosarcoma differential: a tissue microarray-based comparative analysis. Mod Pathol 2008;21(12):1461–1469

38. Buchner A, Ramon Y, Begleiter A. Chondrosarcoma of the maxilla: report of case. J Oral Surg 1979;37(11):822–825

39. Michaels L, Hellquist H. Ear, Nose and Throat Histopathology, 2nd ed. Springer; 2001:236–237

40. Hug EB, Loredo LN, Slater JD, et al. Proton radiation therapy for chordomas and chondrosarcomas of the skull base. J Neurosurg 1999;91(3):432–439

41. Lund V. Distant metastases from sinonasal cancer. ORL J Otorhinolaryngol Relat Spec 2001;63(4):212–213. [Ferlito A, guest ed. Distant Metastases from Head and Neck Cancer: a Multi-Institutional View]

42. el-Silimy OE, Harvey L, Bradley PJ. Chondrogenic neoplasms of the nasal cavity. J Laryngol Otol 1987;101(5):500–505

43. Howard DJ, Lund VJ, Wei WI. Craniofacial resection for tumors of the nasal cavity and paranasal sinuses: a 25-year experience. Head Neck 2006;28(10):867–873

44. Wong LY, Lam LK, Fan YW, Yuen AP, Wei WI. Outcome analysis of patients with craniofacial resection: Hong Kong experience. ANZ J Surg 2006;76(5):313–317

45. Frank G, Sciarretta V, Calbucci F, Farneti G, Mazzatenta D, Pasquini E. The endoscopic transnasal transsphenoidal approach for the treatment of cranial base chordomas and chondrosarcomas. Neurosurgery 2006; 59(1, Suppl 1) ONS50–ONS57, discussion ONS50–ONS57

46. Lund V, Howard DJ, Wei WI. Endoscopic resection of malignant tumors of the nose and sinuses. Am J Rhinol 2007;21(1):89–94

47. Nicolai P, Battaglia P, Bignami M, et al. Endoscopic surgery for malignant tumors of the sinonasal tract and adjacent skull base: a 10-year experience. Am J Rhinol 2008;22(3):308–316

48. Oghalai JS, Buxbaum JL, Jackler RK, McDermott MW. Skull base chondrosarcoma originating from the petroclival junction. Otol Neurotol 2005;26(5):1052–1060

49. Gay E, Sekhar LN, Rubinstein E, et al. Chordomas and chondrosarcomas of the cranial base: results and follow-up of 60 patients. Neurosurgery 1995;36(5):887–896, discussion 896–897

50. Sekhar LN, Pranatartiharan R, Chanda A, Wright DC. Chordomas and chondrosarcomas of the skull base: results and complications of surgical management. Neurosurg Focus 2001;10(3):E2

51. Tzortzidis F, Elahi F, Wright DC, Temkin N, Natarajan SK, Sekhar LN. Patient outcome at long-term follow-up after aggressive microsurgical resection of cranial base chondrosarcomas. Neurosurgery 2006;58(6):1090–1098, discussion 1090–1098

52. Castelnuovo P, Pagella F, Semino L, De Bernardi F, Delù G. Endoscopic treatment of the isolated sphenoid sinus lesions. Eur Arch Otorhinolaryngol 2005;262(2):142–147

53. Podboj J, Smid L. Endoscopic surgery with curative intent for malignant tumors of the nose and paranasal sinuses. Eur J Surg Oncol 2007;33(9):1081–1086

54. Tami TA. Surgical management of lesions of the sphenoid lateral recess. Am J Rhinol 2006;20(4):412–416

55. Zhang Q, Kong F, Yan B, Ni Z, Liu H. Endoscopic endonasal surgery for clival chordoma and chondrosarcoma. ORL J Otorhinolaryngol Relat Spec 2008;70(2):124–129

56. Ceylan S, Koc K, Anik I. Extended endoscopic approaches for midline skull-base lesions. Neurosurg Rev 2009; 32(3):309–319, discussion 318–319

57. Zanation AM, Snyderman CH, Carrau RL, Gardner PA, Prevedello DM, Kassam AB. Endoscopic endonasal surgery for petrous apex lesions. Laryngoscope 2009;119(1):19–25

58. Hu A, Thomas P, Franklin J, Rotenberg B. Endoscopic resection of pterygopalatine chondrosarcoma. J Otolaryngol Head Neck Surg 2009;38(3):E100–E103

59. Smith TS, Schaberg SJ, Pierce GL, Collins JT. Case 42, part II: Chondrosarcoma of the maxilla. J Oral Maxillofac Surg 1982;40(12):803–805

60. Paddison GM, Hanks GE. Chondrosarcoma of the maxilla. Report of a case responding to supervoltage irradiation and review of the literature. Cancer 1971;28(3):616–619

61. Lott S, Bordley JE. A radiosensitive chondrosarcoma of the sphenoid sinus and base of the skull. Report of a case. Laryngoscope 1972;82(1):57–60

62. Noël G, Feuvret L, Ferrand R, Boisserie G, Mazeron JJ, Habrand JL. Radiotherapeutic factors in the management of cervical-basal chordomas and chondrosarcomas. Neurosurgery 2004;55(6):1252–1260, discussion 1260–1262

63. Jereczek-Fossa BA, Krengli M, Orecchia R. Particle beam radiotherapy for head and neck tumors: radiobiological basis and clinical experience. Head Neck 2006; 28(8):750–760

64. Ares C, Hug EB, Lomax AJ, et al. Effectiveness and safety of spot scanning proton radiation therapy for chordomas and chondrosarcomas of the skull base: first long-term report. Int J Radiat Oncol Biol Phys 2009;75(4):1111–1118

65. Laramore GE, Griffith JT, Boespflug M, et al. Fast neutron radiotherapy for sarcomas of soft tissue, bone, and cartilage. Am J Clin Oncol 1989;12(4):320–326 (CCT)

66. Waga S, Tochio H, Yamagiwa M, Nishioka H. Chondrosarcoma of the ethmoid sinus extending to the anterior fossa. Surg Neurol 1981;16(5):324–328

67. Ertefai P, Moghimi M. Chondrosarcoma of the nasal septum. Eur Arch Otorhinolaryngol 1997;254(5):259–260

68. Bloch OG, Jian BJ, Yang I, et al. A systematic review of intracranial chondrosarcoma and survival. J Clin Neurosci 2009;16(12):1547–1551

69. Crockard HA, Cheeseman A, Steel T, et al. A multidisciplinary team approach to skull base chondrosarcomas. J Neurosurg 2001;95(2):184–189

70. Wanebo JE, Bristol RE, Porter RR, Coons SW, Spetzler RF. Management of cranial base chondrosarcomas. Neurosurgery 2006;58(2):249–255, discussion 249–255

71. Almefty K, Pravdenkova S, Colli BO, Al-Mefty O, Gokden M. Chordoma and chondrosarcoma: similar, but quite different, skull base tumors. Cancer 2007;110(11):2457–2467

72. Cho YH, Kim JH, Khang SK, Lee JK, Kim CJ. Chordomas and chondrosarcomas of the skull base: comparative analysis of clinical results in 30 patients. Neurosurg Rev 2008;31(1):35–43, discussion 43

73. Giger R, Kurt AM, Lacroix JS. Endoscopic removal of a nasal septum chondrosarcoma. Rhinology 2002;40(2):96–99

74. Matthews B, Whang C, Smith S. Endoscopic resection of a nasal septal chondrosarcoma: first report of a case. Ear Nose Throat J 2002;81(5):327–329

75. Betz CS, Janda P, Arbogast S, Leunig A. [Myxoma and myxoid chondrosarcoma of the nasal septum: two case reports]. HNO 2007;55(1):51–55

76. Jenny L, Harvinder S, Gurdeep S. Endoscopic resection of primary nasoseptal chondrosarcoma. Med J Malaysia 2008;63(4):335–336

77. Kainuma K, Netsu K, Asamura K, et al. Chondrosarcoma of the nasal septum: a case report. Auris Nasus Larynx 2009;36(5):601–605

78. Lund V, Stammberger H, Nicolai P, et al. European position paper on endoscopic management of tumours of the nose, paranasal sinuses and skull base. Rhinol Suppl 2010;(22):1–143

79. Amichetti M, Amelio D, Cianchetti M, Enrici RM, Minniti G. A systematic review of proton therapy in the treatment of chondrosarcoma of the skull base. Neurosurg Rev 2010;33(2):155–165

80. Hug EB, Slater JD. Proton radiation therapy for chordomas and chondrosarcomas of the skull base. Neurosurg Clin N Am 2000;11(4):627–638

81. Nguyen Q-N, Chang EL. Emerging role of proton beam radiation therapy for chordoma and chondrosarcoma of the skull base. Curr Oncol Rep 2008;10(4):338–343

82. Martin JJ, Niranjan A, Kondziolka D, Flickinger JC, Lozanne KA, Lunsford LD. Radiosurgery for chordomas and chondrosarcomas of the skull base. J Neurosurg 2007;107(4):758–764

83. Hasegawa T, Ishii D, Kida Y, Yoshimoto M, Koike J, Iizuka H. Gamma Knife surgery for skull base chordomas and chondrosarcomas. J Neurosurg 2007;107(4):752–757

84. Lightenstein L, Bernstein D. Unusual benign and malignant chondroid tumors of bone. A survey of some mesenchymal cartilage tumors and malignant chondroblastic tumors, including a few multicentric ones, as well as many atypical benign chondroblastomas and chondromyxoid fibromas. Cancer 1959;12:1142–1157

85. Bottrill ID, Wood S, Barrett-Lee P, Howard DJ. Mesenchymal chondrosarcoma of the maxilla. J Laryngol Otol 1994;108(9):785–787

86. Pellitteri PK, Ferlito A, Fagan JJ, Suárez C, Devaney KO, Rinaldo A. Mesenchymal chondrosarcoma of the head and neck. Oral Oncol 2007;43(10):970–975

87. Ly JQ. Mesenchymal chondrosarcoma of the maxilla. AJR Am J Roentgenol 2002;179(4):1077–1078

88. Vencio EF, Reeve CM, Unni KK, Nascimento AG. Mesenchymal chondrosarcoma of the jaw bones: clinicopathologic study of 19 cases. Cancer 1998;82(12):2350–2355

89. Knott PD, Gannon FH, Thompson LD. Mesenchymal chondrosarcoma of the sinonasal tract: a clinicopathological study of 13 cases with a review of the literature. Laryngoscope 2003;113(5):783–790

90. Dahlin DC, Henderson ED. Mesenchymal chondrosarcoma. Further observations on a new entity. Cancer 1962;15:410–417

91. Bertoni F, Picci P, Bacchini P, et al. Mesenchymal chondrosarcoma of bone and soft tissues. Cancer 1983;52(3):533–541

92. Ito T, Hiratsuka H, Kohama G. Mesenchymal chondrosarcoma of the maxilla. Report of a case. Int J Oral Maxillofac Surg 1991;20(1):44–45

93. Lockhart R, Menard P, Martin JP, Auriol M, Vaillant JM, Bertrand JC. Mesenchymal chondrosarcoma of the jaws. Report of four cases. Int J Oral Maxillofac Surg 1998;27(5):358–362

94. Iezzoni JC, Mills SE. "Undifferentiated" small round cell tumors of the sinonasal tract: differential diagnosis update. Am J Clin Pathol 2005;124(Suppl):S110–S121

95. Granter SR, Renshaw AA, Fletcher CD, Bhan AK, Rosenberg AE. CD99 reactivity in mesenchymal chondrosarcoma. Hum Pathol 1996;27(12):1273–1276

96. Devoe K, Weidner N. Immunohistochemistry of small round-cell tumors. Semin Diagn Pathol 2000;17(3):216–224

97. Ariyoshi Y, Shimahara M. Mesenchymal chondrosarcoma of the maxilla: report of a case. J Oral Maxillofac Surg 1999;57(6):733–737

98. Tien N, Chaisuparat R, Fernandes R, et al. Mesenchymal chondrosarcoma of the maxilla: case report and literature review. J Oral Maxillofac Surg 2007;65(6):1260–1266

99. Aziz SR, Miremadi AR, McCabe JC. Mesenchymal chondrosarcoma of the maxilla with diffuse metastasis: case report and literature review. J Oral Maxillofac Surg 2002;60(8):931–935

100. Gelderblom H, Hogendoorn PC, Dijkstra SD, et al. The clinical approach towards chondrosarcoma. Oncologist 2008;13(3):320–329

101. Chidambaram A, Sanville P. Mesenchymal chondrosarcoma of the maxilla. J Laryngol Otol 2000;114(7):536–539

102. Huvos AG, Rosen G, Dabska M, Marcove RC. Mesenchymal chondrosarcoma. A clinicopathologic analysis of 35 patients with emphasis on treatment. Cancer 1983;51(7):1230–1237

Nasal Chondromesenchymal Hamartoma

Definition

Nasal chondromesenchymal hamartoma is the current name for a lesion of which the pathogenesis has not been entirely established. It is a tumefactive process of the nasal cavity and/or the adjacent paranasal sinuses with a variety of chondroid, stromal, and cystic features that have distinct similarities to the so-called mesenchymal hamartoma of the chest wall.[1–3]

Some of the most complex developmental sequences occur in the head and neck region in the embryo, with extremely intricate changes within the three germ layers. Some resulting malformations may be hamartomatous in nature and may be composed of different elements of muscle, neural tissue, fat, salivary gland, and so on.

Incidence and Site

To date there are only 15 reported cases in the literature, with by far the largest majority being neonates and infants under 3 months of age. The lesion is more common in males than in females with an approximate ratio of 3:1. There is a single case in a 16-year-old (sex not stated) which was thought to have been present for many years.[4] The authors concluded that this lesion had probably been present and undetected for many years. McDermott et al presented a series of seven cases in 1998 which included a single patient of 7 years of age at diagnosis but the remaining six were less than 3 months of age at diagnosis.[5]

Diagnostic Features

Clinical Features

All patients presented with a nasal mass and approximately half had associated respiratory difficulty; prenatal ultrasonography had disclosed an abnormality in the anterior cranial fossa associated with hydrocephalus in one patient. The 7-year-old patient had a prior history of a right chest wall tumor at 2 years of age.

Imaging

CT and MRI confirm the presence of a nasal mass varying from 2 to 6 cm in size; in the majority of cases the lesions extend to involve the ethmoid and frontal sinuses. Four out of the seven cases in McDermott's series showed intracranial extension through the cribriform plate into the anterior cranial fossa. The lesions usually produce a heterogeneous appearance, occasionally with calcification and cystic features, but while there is associated bone erosion, cortical thinning, and displacement of the septum and turbinates, there is not usually any overt bony destruction.

Histological Features

Macroscopically the lesions are usually well circumscribed, with both solid and cystic areas, some with obvious faucial cartilage. McDermott et al[5] noted that the exact origin of the mass was difficult to determine but the upper nasal cavity, nasal septum, sphenoid, and floor of the anterior cranial fossa were all possibilities. Histologically all these lesions demonstrated nodules of cartilage of various sizes, shapes, and degrees of differentiation. While some nodules are well-differentiated cartilaginous structures, others are similar to the chondromyxomatous nodules of a chondromyxoid fibroma. Around the nodules there is usually a loose spindle cell or hypocellular fibrous stroma, but the pattern varies considerably as there may be a cellular stroma with hyalinized nodules with or without perivascular stromal cells or a prominent cellular stromal component and small areas of immature woven bone that can resemble fibrous dysplasia. Osteoclast-like multinucleated giant cells may be present in association with areas similar to the appearance of an aneurysmal bone cyst.

Immunohistochemistry can be helpful in these lesions as the cartilage, mature or immature, is immunoreactive for S100 protein. There is strong vimentin positivity in the stromal-mesenchymal elements of the lesion. The spindle/mononuclear cell population may be positive for CD68, smooth muscle actin, and muscle-specific actin in the majority of cases.

Differential Diagnosis

As this lesion is extremely rare there is a possibility of it being confused with other cartilaginous tumors, such as chondromyxoid fibroma, chondroblastoma, and even chondrosarcoma, although this latter in the pediatric age group would be extremely unusual, particularly as it rarely involves patients under 21 years of age. Confusion may arise with aneurysmal bone cysts, fibrous dysplasia, and another rare congenital lesion, osteochondromyxoma. This latter lesion is associated with the Carney's complex.[6] In contrast, nasal chondromesenchymal hamartoma has not been associated with the Carney's complex.[6]

Treatment and Prognosis

McDermott et al reported in 1998 that complete resection was difficult to achieve by an intranasal approach alone and the combined intranasal surgical approach with craniotomy was used, but precise details were not made available.[5] They felt that excision was incomplete in five cases and four patients underwent subsequent procedures with gross total excision of the residual mass; one of these areas of recurrence continued to enlarge after the primary surgery judged on serial CT scans, requiring a second procedure at 16 months of age. Full details of the surgical approaches were not available, and therefore it remains possible that these lesions could have been treated by endoscopic surgery or a midfacial degloving approach.

No long-term follow-up details have been reported despite the known recurrences following incomplete excision.

References

1. MacLeod R, Dahling D. Hamartoma (mesenchymoma) of the chest wall in infancy. Radiology 1979;131:625–661
2. Odell JM, Benjamin DR. Mesenchymal hamartoma of chest wall in infancy: natural history of two cases. Pediatr Pathol 1986;5(2):135–146
3. Cohen MC, Drut R, Garcia C, Kaschula RO. Mesenchymal hamartoma of the chest wall: a cooperative study with review of the literature. Pediatr Pathol 1992;12(4):525–534
4. Alrawi M, McDermott M, Orr D, Russell J. Nasal chondromesynchymal hamartoma presenting in an adolescent. Int J Pediatr Otorhinolaryngol 2003;67(6):669–672
5. McDermott MB, Ponder TB, Dehner LP. Nasal chondromesenchymal hamartoma: an upper respiratory tract analogue of the chest wall mesenchymal hamartoma. Am J Surg Pathol 1998;22(4):425–433
6. Carney JA, Boccon-Gibod L, Jarka DE, et al. Osteochondromyxoma of bone: a congenital tumor associated with lentigines and other unusual disorders. Am J Surg Pathol 2001;25(2):164–176

12 Odontogenic Tumors and Other Lesions

Humans have suffered from odontogenic tumors and cysts for thousands of years (**Fig. 12.1**). Tumors arising in relation to the teeth were described in the 18th century[1] and the first attempt at classification was by Broca in 1868.[2] Thoma and Goldman 1946 classified them according to their tissue of origin: epithelial, mesenchymal, and mixed odontogenic.[3] These tumors are renowned for their variation in growth, behavior, and histology and debate continues to this day with regard to their classification.

The name "odontogenic tumor" covers a group of neoplasms and hamartomatous lesions originating from cells involved in the formation of teeth or remnants of tissues that had been implicated in odontogenesis. Very few of these lesions actually have formed dental hard tissue in them; most are rare and many exceedingly rare. Recent use of electron microscopy, immunohistochemistry, and molecular biological techniques has considerably increased our knowledge of these tumors and their classification becomes ever more complex.

The tumors occur in three locations: (1) intraosseous (centrally) within the jaws, (2) extraosseous (peripherally) in the alveolar mucosa or gingiva adjacent to tooth-bearing areas, and (3) in the cranial base as one of the variants of the craniopharyngioma.

Philipsen and Reichart[4] have published an excellent review of the history of classification of odontogenic tumors and reading of this is highly recommended if you wish to evaluate the matter further. For the purposes of the remainder of this chapter, the WHO 2005 classification will be used, see **Table 12.1**.[5]

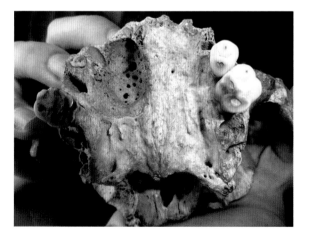

Fig. 12.1 Photograph of a neolithic skull ca. 2,500 BC showing a palatal lesion excavating the hard palate in a female aged between 35 and 40 years, found in the Tomb of the Eagles, South Ronaldsay, Orkney. Photograph courtesy of E Chevretton.

Table 12.1 Odontogenic tumors affecting the nose and paranasal sinuses

Benign odontogenic tumors
Ameloblastoma (ICD-O 9310/0)
Squamous odontogenic tumor (ICD-O 9312/0)
Calcifying epithelial odontogenic tumor (CEOT) (ICD-O 9340/0)
Adenomatoid odontogenic tumor (AOT) (ICD-O 9300/0)
Keratocystic odontogenic tumor (KCOT) (ICD-O 9270/0)
Tumors of odontogenic epithelium with odontogenic ectomesenchyme with or without hard-tissue formation
Ameloblastic fibroma (AF) (ICD-O 9330/0)
Ameloblastic fibrodentinoma (AFD) (ICD-O 9271/0)
Ameloblastic fibro-odontoma (AFOD) (ICD-O 9290/0)
Odontomas (ICD-O 9280/0)   • Complex (ODTx) (ICD-O 9282/0)   • Compound (ODTp) (ICD-O 9281/0)
Odontoameloblastoma (ICD-O 9311/0)
Odontogenic ghost cell lesions
Calcifying cystic odontogenic tumor (CCOT) (ICD-O 9301/0)
Calcifying cystic odontogenic tumors associated with other types of odontogenic tumors
Dentinogenic ghost cell tumor (ICD-O 9302/0)
Tumors of odontogenic ectomesenchyme with or without included odontogenic epithelium
Odontogenic fibroma
Odontogenic myxoma and myxofibroma (ODOMYX)
Cementoblastoma
Malignant odontogenic tumors
Metastasizing ameloblastoma (METAM) (ICD-O 9310/3)
Ameloblastic carcinoma–primary type (ICD-O 9270/3)
Ameloblastic carcinoma–secondary type (dedifferentiated), intraosseous (ICD-O 9270/3)
Ameloblastic carcinoma-secondary type (dedifferentiated), peripheral (ICD-O 9270/3)
Primary intraosseous squamous cell carcinomas (PIOSCC) (ICD-O 9270/3)
Clear cell odontogenic carcinoma (ICD-O 9341/3)
Ghost cell odontogenic carcinoma (GCOC) (ICD-O 9302/3)
Odontogenic sarcomas (ICD-O 9330/0 & 9290/3)
Source: Modified from Barnes et al.[5]

Etiology

The etiology of odontogenic tumors remains unknown apart from some recent indications suggesting genetic factors playing a role in some cases. The overall pathogenesis is only partially understood and the reader is referred again to the excellent 2004 review by Philipsen and Reichart.[4]

Despite the WHO histological classification of odontogenic tumors commencing with a list of malignant tumors, it seems more appropriate to initiate the discussion of these lesions with a review of benign tumors. As a consequence of a close working relationship with dental and maxillofacial colleagues from every aspect of the discipline at the Eastman Dental Hospital and Institute of Oral Pathology, London, UK, we are fortunately able to base some of this chapter on personal experience, although our knowledge of the exceedingly rare tumors is based on literature reports of cases that often amount to only a single description.

While the majority of small odontogenic lesions will present to dental and oral surgeons, those lesions expanding into the maxillary sinuses, orbit, and skull base may well present to maxillofacial, ENT, and occasionally ophthalmological colleagues. In this chapter, we have endeavored to cover both the commoner and rarer lesions that can involve the sinonasal and skull base areas in contrast to the mandibular sites.

Benign Odontogenic Tumors

This group of tumors comprises those of essentially odontogenic epithelium without evidence of odontogenic ectomesenchyme and with a mature fibrous stroma.

Ameloblastoma

(ICD-O code 9310/0)

Ameloblastomas are currently classified into four different types by WHO, although a variety of additional names have been used in the literature in the past.
1. Ameloblastoma, solid/multicystic
2. Ameloblastoma, extraosseous/peripheral type
3. Ameloblastoma—desmoplastic type (DESAM)
4. Ameloblastoma—unicystic type

Ameloblastoma, Solid/Multicystic

This central, solid/multicystic ameloblastoma is a histologically benign tumor originating from epithelial components of the embryonic tooth. It is a locally invasive neoplasm of the jaws with potentially a high rate of recurrence, but a low tendency to metastasize.

Etiology

The etiology essentially remains unknown, although studies of cytokeratins[6] support the hypothesis that ameloblastomas are of odontogenic origin and not, as has been suggested by other authors, derivatives of basal cells of the oral epithelium.

Synonyms

Many names have been used in the older literature, including the following examples: conventional ameloblastoma, classical intraosseous ameloblastoma, multicystic jaw tumor, epithelial odontoma, epithelioma ameloblastoides, cystoma, adamantinoma.

Incidence

While numerous publications in the past have produced figures for the incidence of these lesions, few contain any subdivisions in ameloblastoma variants and there has been much confusion with other odontogenic tumors. However, overall, ameloblastoma is probably the second most common odontogenic tumor after the odontomas. The well-known report by Shear et al evaluating the incidence rates in South Africa between 1965 and 1974 shows that ameloblastoma is much more common in black than white Africans.[7] Larsson et al in 1978 reported on all cases of ameloblastoma from the Swedish Cancer Registry in the period 1958–1971.[8] They estimated a true incidence of 0.6 cases per year per million people. This provides a reasonable baseline estimate for the incidence of ameloblastoma in the worldwide white population.

The largest review of ameloblastomas was published by Reichart et al in 1995, profiling 3,677 cases published in many languages between 1960 and 1993.[9] There were 693 case reports and the rest from reviews. As Gardner pointed out in 1999, numbers from reports do not necessarily reflect the occurrence of ameloblastomas in any particular racial group but rather the number of published cases in those groups.[10] It does not necessarily indicate the actual prevalence in a population. Cases reported from Africa are an outstanding example in that, anecdotally, they are thought to be even more common than the literature implies.

Site

The Reichart et al review[9] showed the ratio between maxillary and mandibular tumors (of all variants of ameloblastoma) to be 1:5.8. The maxillary sinus was more often affected in males than females. While there are numerous studies showing the presence of ameloblastomas within the sinonasal cavity, particularly the maxilla, there are rarer reports that document true, primary sinonasal ameloblastomas without connection to gnathic sites[11–17] and there is a particularly useful review by Schafer et al of 24 cases published in 1998.[18]

Those ameloblastomas arising from the gnathic maxilla and extending into the sinuses have a mean age of occurrence between 35 and 45 years,[19] whereas those tumors reported as originating from the sinonasal tract have a distinct predilection for older men, aged between the sixth and eighth decades of life. The gnathic tumors frequently present as a painless expansion of the upper jaw, most commonly posterior to the canine tooth with approximately half being sited in the molar region. **Approximately 15% of them progress to involve the antrum and nasal floor.** Ameloblastomas arising in the posterior aspect of the maxilla can reach a large size before diagnosis as a consequence of expanding in the antrum, cheek, or palate. Those tumors reported as arising from the sinonasal tract, present with unilateral nasal obstruction with or without symptoms of sinusitis. Seven out the 24 cases of primary ameloblastoma of the sinonasal tract reported by Schafer additionally presented with epistaxis.[18] In contrast to the overall published literature on ameloblastoma, 19 of 21 of these cases where the patient's race was documented were white and only 2 were African American. The duration of symptoms ranged from one month to several years. **On examination, 9 of these 24 sinonasal ameloblastomas involved the nasal cavity alone. Six were confined to the paranasal sinuses (maxillary, frontal, ethmoid or sphenoid) and 9 involved both the nasal cavity and paranasal sinuses at presentation.**

Diagnostic Features

Clinical Features

The mean ages from case reports can also be misleading as there are significant differences between the variants of ameloblastoma with solid/multicystic and central ameloblastoma having a mean age at presentation of around 40 years, whereas unicystic ameloblastoma (UNAM) has a mean age at presentation of between 14 and 26 years in the literature. Again, there appear to be racial differences with the majority of ameloblastomas in white children being of the unicystic variety whereas the pattern in African children seems to resemble more that of adults.[20,21]

Notable in the review by Reichart et al[9] was that they found the mean age of patients with tumors involving the maxilla to be 47.0 years in contrast to those with tumors arising in the mandible, who had a mean age of 35.2 years. This again, however, may be explained by the fact that UNAMs are rare in the maxilla. Approximately 30% of solid/multicystic ameloblastomas and extraosseous, peripheral type ameloblastomas occur in the maxilla. There is approximately equal male-to-female distribution.

As might be expected, these patients present with a painless swelling of the cheek, gingiva, or palate, occasionally nasal obstruction, and sometimes distortion of the dentition with malocclusion, ill-fitting dentures, or loosening of teeth. In our small cohort of 6 patients, comprising 5 males and 1 female, aged 16 to 80 years (mean 50.8 years) all had some degree of facial swelling, 2 had nasal obstruction, and 2 had oroantral fistula (**Table 12.2**).

Imaging

In contrast to the characteristic multilocular and radiolucent presentation of ameloblastomas within the jaws ("soap bubble appearance"), sinonasal lesions have been most often described radiographically as solid masses filling the nasal cavity and sinuses with bone destruction and remodeling in some cases. Primary origin in or continuity with the maxillary alveolar area is not demonstrated in any of the true sinonasal cases. **On examination, the lesions ranged from a size of several millimeters to 9 cm in the sinonasal lesions reported by Schafer et al.[18] In contrast, Reichart et al noted a mean size of 4.6 cm for maxillary tumors with many in excess of 10 cm.[9]** In this latter group, embedded teeth were detected in 8.7% and root resorption of neighboring teeth in 3.8%.

Table 12.2 Maxillary ameloblastomas: personal series

Age/sex	Presenting lesion	Management	Long-term follow-up
16/M	Mass in posterior alveolus	Partial maxillectomy, radiotherapy	A&W 30 y
35/F	Facial swelling, fistula after multiple previous operations	Radical extended maxillectomy	Lost to follow-up after 3 y
45/M	Nasal obstruction, mass	Midfacial degloving	A&W 5 y
60/M	Oroantral fistula, facial swelling. Previous Caldwell-Luc	Total maxillectomy	A&W 10 y
69/M	Facial swelling	Midfacial degloving	A&W 7 y
82/M	Nasal blockage, swelling over zygoma, fungating mass upper alveolus	Radiotherapy, maxillectomy	DOD 3 y
Abbreviations: A&W, alive and well; DOD, dead of disease; F, female; M, male; y, year(s).			

Histological Features

Microscopically, these tumors are usually solid in appearance with a glistening gray-white or yellow-tan coloration. The consistency varies from solid to cystic, although the sinonasal lesions rarely appear cystic on gross examination.

Microscopically, these tumors consist of odontogenic epithelium contained in a relatively cell-poor collagenous stroma. Two predominant growth patterns—follicular and plexiform—are recognized with four main cell types: stellate reticulum-like cell type, acanthomatous (squamous cell) cell type, granular cell type, and basal cell type. Interestingly, the plexiform pattern comprising of a network of long anastomosing cords of odontogenic epithelium was the sole or predominant histological pattern in 22 out of the 24 sinonasal cases (92%) studied by Schafer et al.[18] Both patterns may be present in the same tumor and there is no general consensus whether growth pattern is related to the clinical behavior of the tumor. Both the stellate reticulum-like component and the acanthomatous pattern, characterized by squamous metaplasia and keratin formation of the central portions of the epithelial islands, made up only a small secondary or focal component of the sinonasal plexiform pattern ameloblastomas. In 15 of Schafer's 24 sinonasal cases, the ameloblastomatous proliferation could be observed arising in direct continuity with the intact sinonasal surface mucosal epithelium.[18] They conclude from this that this form of peripheral ameloblastoma most likely originates from pluripotential cells in the mucosal surface epithelium. Alternatively, the ameloblastomatous epithelium could have originated in the submucosa and secondarily extended to involve the surface epithelium, but certainly no odontogenic dental lamina within the submucosa was observed in any of the cases.

Immunohistochemical Features

There has been considerable interest in ameloblastoma, as it is one of the commonest odontogenic tumors, and there are numerous publications on immunohistochemistry and with molecular biological investigations. In addition to electron microscopy, studies have looked at oncogenes, gene modifications, tumor suppressor genes, DNA repair genes, oncovirus growth factors, telomerase, cell cycle regulators, apoptosis-related factors, regulators of tooth development, cell adhesion molecules, matrix-degrading proteinases, angiogenic factors, and osteolytic cytokines. The reader is referred to two comprehensive reviews by Kumamoto in 2006[22] and Praetorius in 2009[23] (see ref. 23: p. 1208).

Differential Diagnosis

Ameloblastomas with a plexiform growth pattern have to be distinguished from hyperplastic odontogenic epithelium, which is commonly seen in the walls of odontogenic cysts. The granular cell type of solid/multicystic ameloblastoma may be confused with the granular cell odontogenic tumor (GCOT), but while the ameloblastoma is an epithelial tumor, the granular cell tumor is ectomesenchymal; and while cords and islands of odontogenic epithelium are seen, they are different from the proliferating epithelium of ameloblastoma.

Treatment and Prognosis

There continues to be a difference of opinion in the world literature about the preferable methods of treatment of the solid/multicystic variant of ameloblastoma either in the maxilla or in the mandible. What is not in doubt is that recurrence rates of approximately one-third of the cases are not unusual even in recent times.[24] Some centers have strongly advocated radical surgical procedures and Carson in 2006 reported that conservative treatment was unpredictable and that recurrent or persistent disease could not then always be treated adequately. They studied 82 cases of resected solid/multicystic ameloblastomas showing that tumor extends up to 8 mm beyond its radiographic demarcation (mean 4.5 mm) and they recommended resection with a 1 to 1.5 cm linear bone margin whenever possible. Ghandhi et al 2006[25] showed that primary care by conservative treatment (comparing cases from West Scotland with those in San Francisco) led to recurrence in ~80% of cases. Recurrence rates following local enucleation and curettage seem unacceptably high.

Much of the older literature with regard to maxillary and sinonasal tract lesions demonstrates inadequate surgery by means of intranasal polypectomy type procedures, limited Caldwell-Luc approaches, minimal excision and curettage, and inadequate partial maxillectomy. Reluctance to consider a facial incision, particularly in children, such as lateral rhinotomy or a Weber–Fergusson incision, can now be completely discarded. **Modern, high-quality and thorough endoscopic techniques, external rhinoplasty type approaches, and midfacial degloving procedures allow radical removal of these lesions with magnification and additional frozen section control with further endoscopic removal in the sinonasal cases should there be any concerns following definitive histopathology. It is therefore to be hoped that in future the high level of recurrence within the literature, and both early and late recurrence of disease (in the latter often several years after surgical treatment), will not continue to be widely reported**.

Schafer et al[18] found that 5 of the 24 patients (21%) experienced at least one recurrence, generally within a period of 1 to 2 years after the initial treatment, but one patient did not experience recurrence until 13 years after initial surgery. Recurrences of gnathic ameloblastomas have been reported up to 30 years after primary surgery.[26] Schafer's 24 cases of sinonasal ameloblastoma had follow-up periods ranging from 1 year to 44 years (average 9.5 years) and all were alive without evidence of disease, or had died of unrelated causes without evidence of recurrence.[18] One case was lost to follow-up.

In our group, two had already undergone inadequate surgery and all required some form of maxillectomy. In the two more recent cases this was successfully achieved via a midfacial degloving approach. All but one have survived long-term follow-up but unfortunately one has been lost to follow-up and an elderly man with the most advanced lesion treated in 1963 died of his disease after 3 years, having initially refused treatment.

Key Points

- Approximately 15% of these lesions progress to involve the maxillary antrum and nasal floor.
- Duration of symptoms may extend over years.
- Sinonasal lesions may be several centimeters in diameter.
- A high rate of local recurrence has been common in the past.

Ameloblastoma, Extraosseous/Peripheral Type

Peripheral ameloblastoma (PERAM) is a rare benign, slowly growing, exophytic lesion occurring on the gingiva or the attached alveolar ridge mucosa in edentulous areas. **Philipsen et al,[27] reviewing the literature of 160 cases, found 46 (29.1%) located in the maxilla.** The most common area was the soft palatal tissue of the tuberosity area. Lesions are generally painless with a long history beyond a year. **None were associated with any significant invasion of bone or the sinonasal area.** Treatment was by local excision.

Ameloblastoma, Desmoplastic Type

Definition

Ameloblastoma, desmoplastic type (DESAM) is a rare, benign, locally infiltrative tumor that is considered a variant of ameloblastoma.

Diagnostic Features

Clinical Features

Philipsen et al[27] reviewed 100 cases from the literature and their own files showing that this rare tumor occurs in females in the fourth and fifth decades but with a male peak in the sixth decade. It is rare outside of the 30 to 60 age group and, in contrast to the much more common solid/multicystic ameloblastoma, **it had an almost equal distribution of cases within the maxilla and mandible. Notably, 7 cases involved the entire maxilla and 3 of these maxillary cases involved the nasal cavity and crossed the midline.** Again, in contrast to the solid/multicystic ameloblastoma, the majority of cases were in the anterior aspect of the upper jaw. The most common clinical presentation was a painless hard swelling often present for years prior to presentation.

Imaging

Of the cases reviewed by Philipsen et al,[27] 53% showed a mixed radiolucent/radiopaque pattern with ill-defined margins making the lesion look more suggestive of fibro-osseous disease than of ameloblastoma. Thompson et al,[28] in an excellent paper, demonstrated the value of CT and MRI, in particular the details of the margins of the lesion and the detection of the mixed fine and coarse trabecular pattern at the periphery of the lesion.

Histological Features

This was described in detail by Eversole et al in their early defining paper of 1984.[29]

DESAM is composed of strands and islands of tumor epithelium with a high cellular density. The epithelium lacks stellate reticulum cells and columnar basal cells and the epithelial cells are small, spindle-shaped, or polygonal. There is abundant stroma with pronounced collagen formation and moderate cellularity. Myxomatous changes may be seen around the epithelial islands in addition to a cellular amorphous eosinic material. Invasion of tumor tissue into surrounding bone has been noted in some cases, but a mixture of bone and trabecular resorption and new bone production may be found at the periphery of the tumor. Debate continues about whether DESAM should be considered as a separate lesion from conventional ameloblastomas. Lesions with the histopathological features of both occurring simultaneously have been described.[30]

Immunohistochemical Features

Multiple studies have been undertaken to differentiate desmoplastic ameloblastoma from solid/multicystic ameloblastoma, perhaps the most notable being the Takata et al study[31] comparing 7 cases of DESAM with 10 cases of conventional ameloblastoma showing a marked immunoexpression in both peripheral and central cells in the tumor nests of DESAMs but none in conventional ameloblastoma. The TGF-β produced by the tumor cells is believed to play a part in the desmoplastic matrix formation. Philipsen et al[32] detected marked staining or collagen type VI in the stroma adjacent to tumor islands in DESAMs. Conventional ameloblastomas were negative.

Treatment and Prognosis

The treatment of desmoplastic ameloblastoma is essentially the same as that advocated for solid/multicystic ameloblastoma: resection with at least 1 cm of bony margin; and in the maxilla it may be necessary to under-take hemi or total maxillectomy to achieve this. Again, there are cases reported recurring years after excision.[33]

Ameloblastoma, Unicystic Type

Unicystic ameloblastoma (UNAM) is an odontogenic cystic neoplasm with a single, often large lumen and development of an initial intralining, intraluminal, or intramural ameloblastoma or combinations of these. **The pathologist requires the entire specimen to make an exact diagnosis of the tumor**.

Synonyms

Cystogenic ameloblastoma, plexiform unicystic amelo-blastoma, intracystic ameloblastoma, cystic ameloblas-toma, unilocular ameloblastoma, extensive dentigerous cyst, and intracystic ameloblastic papilloma.

Diagnosis and Specific Features

Clinical Features

All series report more than 90% of these lesions occur-ring in the mandible with only small numbers of tumors in the maxilla.[34] Most patients present with an incidental swelling that on imaging is a well-defined uni-locular radiolucency.

Treatment and Prognosis

These lesions are rarely suspected to be an ameloblas-toma preoperatively and are usually removed by enucle-ation and curettage as a nonneoplastic odontogenic cyst. When the final diagnosis is made following histopathol-ogy, the risk of recurrence is related to the histological type and if the diagnosis is UNAM grade III (intramural), an additional marginal segmental resection of the upper jaw or partial maxillectomy may be required to prevent recurrence.

Key Points

- These lesions are very rare in the maxilla.
- The pathologist requires the entire specimen to make an exact diagnosis of the tumor.

Squamous Odontogenic Tumor

Definition

(ICD-O code 9312/0)

Squamous odontogenic tumor is a locally infiltrative neoplasm consisting of islands of well-differentiated squamous epithelium in a fibrous stroma. It usually

occurs intraosseously, properly developing in the peri-odontal ligaments between the roots of vital erupted permanent teeth. Approximately 50 cases have been published, of which 36 were reviewed by Philipsen and Reichart.[35] Patients may present with simple swelling, local pain, or mobility of teeth. Imaging shows unilocular or triangular radiolucency between the roots of adjacent teeth.

Treatment and Prognosis

None have been recorded to involve the nose and sinuses and conservative surgical procedures in terms of enucleation and curettage or minimal local incision are considered to be adequate, although recurrence has been documented.[36]

Calcifying Epithelial Odontogenic Tumor

Definition

(ICD-O code 9340/0)

Calcifying epithelial odontogenic tumor (CEOT) is a benign, slow-growing, nonencapsulated and locally invasive lesion. It has a distinctive histomorphological pattern characterized by variable sheets and islands of eosinophilic, polyhedral, and often pleomorphic cells, which merge into an eosinophilic, amorphous substance that stains with amyloid marker and tends to calcify, although not in all cases. The tumor was first described by Pindborg in 1955 and its most common synonym is Pindborg tumor.[37,38]

Incidence and Site

This tumor is rare, with ~200 cases at present published in the literature. Franklin and Pindborg reviewed 113 cases and Philipsen and Reichart reviewed 181 cases.[39,40] CEOT occurs as an intraosseous and a less aggressive extraos-seous variant with a roughly equal male-to-female ratio and an age range of 8 to 92 years. The extraosseous cases are more likely to occur in the anterior segment of the jaw and the mandible-to-maxillary ratio is 2:1. Multifocal examples are extremely rare but have been described.[41]

Diagnostic Features

Clinical Features

These tumors grow slowly and are often symptomless, presenting as a firm swelling from either jaw **but there are examples of extensive lesions involving the nasal cavity and maxillary sinus** to a degree where they pres-ent with unilateral nasal obstruction, epistaxis, pain, and proptosis.[39] Bridle et al in 2006 published an extensive case involving the whole maxilla causing significant displacement of the eye in a 30-year-old woman.[42]

Imaging

Imaging is essentially unhelpful as there is considerable variation in these lesions, with findings ranging from a well-circumscribed unilocular radiolucency to a diffuse, poorly demarcated lesion with small intralesional septa producing a multiloculated pattern. Additionally, there may be flecks of calcification and overall these lesions may resemble an ameloblastoma or a dentigerous cyst. With increasing calcification, the radiological differential diagnosis starts to include ossifying fibroma and odontogenic fibroma.[43]

Histological Features

Microscopically these lesions appear to be a solid tumor; cystic changes are not seen. The tumor consists of islands and sheets of polyhedral epithelial cells with abundant eosinophilic cytoplasm, sharply defined cell borders, and well-developed intercellular bridges, all within a fibrous stroma. Mitotic figures are rarely encountered; indeed, if they are, frequent malignant transformation must be suspected. Nuclei are usually pleomorphic. Giant nuclei are quite common. Concentric rings of calcification may be present either within or around the tumor cells, which lie in a homogeneous hyaline material that is amyloid. The amount of amyloid varies, with some tumors being predominantly epithelial. Calcification is more commonly absent in extraosseous tumors and clear cells containing glycogen may be present within the epithelial nests and make up a significant proportion of the tumor.[40]

Differential Diagnosis

As a consequence of cytonuclear pleomorphism and intercellular bridges, it is important to avoid mistaking CEOT for an intraosseous squamous carcinoma. A clear cell variant of the CEOT has been described as having a more aggressive behavior.[44]

Treatment and Prognosis

The size of lesions at the time of surgery varies between a few millimeters and as much as 10 cm within the reported literature and hence treatment has varied from simple enucleation and curettage to hemi and total maxillectomy. Treatment will clearly be dictated by the extent and site of the tumor. All publications are agreed that complete removal is necessary with a tumor-free surgical margin if at all possible, and long-term follow-up is advised.[45] The older surgical series, as with other tumors in this group, report notable recurrence rates; for example, Franklin and Pindborg in 1976[39] reviewing 17 cases with a follow-up of 10 years or more, reported a recurrence rate of 14%. It is likely that

this is due to inadequate treatment, and modern surgical approaches and pathology evaluation could reduce this. Occasional cases of malignant transformation have been reported.[46]

Key Point

- The size of lesions varies from a few millimeters to 10 cm with substantial involvement of the nasal cavity, maxillary sinus, and orbital floor.

Adenomatoid Odontogenic Tumor

Definition

(ICD-O code 9300/0)

Adenomatoid odontogenic tumor (AOT) is a slow-growing, encapsulated epithelial odontogenic tumor that has a single histomorphological pattern with whirled nodules of spindle cells, plexiform double cell strands, and microcystic or ductlike spaces. It has a limited growth potential and debate continues whether or not it is a neoplasm.[47]

Etiology

The pathogenesis of AOT is not known but it is thought to develop from residues of the dental lamina and proliferations of odontogenic epithelium adjacent to the reduced enamel epithelium of unerupted teeth.

Synonyms

Adenoameloblastoma.

Incidence and Site

Although AOT is an uncommon lesion, Philipsen et al[48] found a total of 1,082 cases published from 12 different countries and **it is generally regarded as the third or fourth most common odontogenic tumor.** More than 95% of all cases are interosseous, occurring within the bone, and **the maxilla is affected twice as often as the mandible.** The commonest site is adjacent to the upper canine area and the peripheral extraosseous type of lesion has been described, almost all of which have occurred in the anterior part of the maxilla.[49]

Diagnostic Features

Clinical Features

Females are affected approximately twice as commonly as males; few patients have been reported older than 30 years[48] and ~50% of patients are teenagers. Intraosseous AOTs are usually diagnosed during dental radiographic imaging to evaluate the cause of any disturbance in tooth eruption. The growth rate is known to be slow and **larger lesions which may involve the entire maxillary sinus reaching the orbital floor and impacting on the nasal cavity** may be painless or only associated with slight pain.

Imaging

As a consequence of the majority of these lesions developing at an early age and often in the canine area, the eruption of the permanent canines is disturbed and the AOT wraps around the crown of the tooth and sometimes the entire tooth. This so-called "follicular" AOT simulates a dentigerous cyst unless the radiolucency extends apically along the root past the cement–enamel junction. The lesions are usually well defined and unilocular and the intraoral film commonly shows scattered, fine radiopacities within the radiolucent area.[50] Follicular type is by far the commonest form of AOT, but intraosseous AOTs that are unrelated to an erupted tooth ("extrafollicular type") present as well-delineated radiolucent lesions. This extrafollicular type can simulate a residual, a periapical radicular, a lateral radicular, or a lateral periodontal cyst, but sizable lesions within the upper jaw have been described that invade the maxillary sinus.[51–53]

Leon et al[53] found a range in the size of these lesions between 1 cm and 7 cm, with an average of 2.9 cm.

Histological Features

Microscopically, the tumors are usually well circumscribed and vary from solid to cystic, and may be situated around the crown of a tooth. Interestingly, the histopathology shows a consistent pattern irrespective of the location of the lesion in the jaws. The solid lesions show variably sized, solid nodules of columnar or cuboidal cells of odontogenic epithelium that may form small nests ("rosettes"). Between the epithelial cells and in the center of the rosette is eosinophilic amorphous material ("tumor droplets").

Cystic spaces of variable size may be seen between the nodules ("ductlike spaces"). These are not present in all tumors. These ductlike spaces are lined by single rows of columnar epithelial cells and actually represent pseudolumina formed by the secretion of the columnar epithelial cells. The cytoplasm of these cells is usually lightly stained and the oval nuclei are polarized away from the lumen. Larger cystic spaces are usually lined with cuboidal epithelium without polarization of the nuclei. Some of the cystic spaces may show invagination. Additionally, there may be scattered foci of polyhedral squamous cells in the tumor.

An additional, well-recognized, cellular pattern is found in some tumors where long, narrow epithelial strands of cubic cells are seen that may be in single or double layers and form large loops in a plexiform pattern. Loose stroma inside these loops may sometimes be missing and this pattern is more common toward the

periphery of the lesion. There may be a hyaline, dysplastic material or calcified osteodentin in AOTs. This is thought to be due to a metaplastic process as odontogenic ectomesenchyme is absent. In rare cases, dentinlike material containing dentinal tubules may occur. AOTs may have areas with a similar pattern to calcifying epithelial odontogenic tumor (CEOT) but these are considered as a histological variant of AOT and do not appear to change the behavior of the AOT. AOTs may also contain areas that mimic calcifying ghost cell odontogenic cysts or other odontogenic tumors or hamartomas. None have been shown to alter the situation.

Treatment and Prognosis

In contrast to other odontogenic tumors, published reports agree that enucleation of a tumor followed by curettage is all that is necessary and the thick connective tissue capsule facilitates the enucleation. The risk of recurrence is extremely low and malignant transformation has never been described. This agrees with the fact that many authors consider the AOT to be a hamartoma, but certainly there is no evidence that these lesions stop growing. **As they are known to achieve a size of several centimeters and to involve the whole maxillary sinus and even the skull base, the removal does need to be thorough along with any significantly involved teeth.**[47,52,53]

Keratocystic Odontogenic Tumor

Definition

(ICD-O code 9270/0)

A benign intraosseous tumor of odontogenic origin, keratocystic odontogenic tumor (KCOT) may be unicystic or multicystic. It is a potentially aggressive, infiltrative lesion composed of parakeratinized stratified squamous epithelium. The multiple lesions may be associated with nevoid basal cell carcinoma syndrome (NBCCS).

Etiology

Recent studies have described the role of the human homologue of the *Drosophila* patched gene (*PTCH*) tumor suppressor gene in KCOT. Somatic mutations of the *PTCH* gene have been reported in sporadic odontogenic keratocysts as well as those associated with the nevoid basal cell carcinoma syndrome.[54–56]

Synonyms

An important and long-standing synonym is odontogenic keratocyst (OKC), a term introduced by Philipsen in 1956.[54] This widely used synonym suggests a benign process, but the WHO working group reclassified this lesion as KCOT in 2005 as that better reflects its neoplastic aggressive nature.[5] Other synonyms include primordial cyst, epidermoid cyst of the jaws, cholesteatoma of the jaw, and odontogenic keratocystoma.

Incidence and Site

There is a ratio of ~2:1 of keratocysts occurring more frequently in the mandible than maxilla. The prevalence within all odontogenic lesions varies considerably depending on the age of the literature and the understanding at the time of these different entities. Figures up to 16.5% have been noted.[57] In the maxilla, the commonest site appears to be in the region of the canine tooth. Bearing in mind the time at which this substantial publication was written, Brannon (1976) reported 312 cases with the age of the patients ranging from 7 years to 93 years.[58]

The mean age of patients with multiple KCOTs, with or without the NBCCS, is lower than that of those with single KCOTs. There appears to be a slight preponderance in males. Briefly, the NBCCS was first described by Gorlin and Goltz in1960[59] and is characterized by (1) basal cell carcinoma at an early stage, (2) multiple odontogenic keratocysts in the jaws, (3) broad nasal base, (4) frontal and parietal bossing, (5) calcification of the falx cerebri, (6) bifid ribs and other skeletal abnormalities, (7) palmar and plantar pits. It is of autosomal dominant inheritance with marked penetration and **odontogenic keratocysts are present in over 65% of these patients**. Multiplicity of the cysts is common and, within the upper jaw, the second molar region is the commonest site of occurrence. Recurrence in the older literature is extremely common, with figures of up to 85%.[60]

Multiple odontogenic keratocysts have also been reported in association with Marfan's and Noonan's syndromes.[61,62]

Diagnostic Features

Clinical Features

As with other odontogenic lesions, presentation within the maxilla is often a painless swelling that may enlarge to involve the face and produce nasal obstruction if the tumor enlarges further. **Cases have been described displacing the lateral wall of the nose, destroying the anterior wall of the maxilla, and extending as a soft tissue cystic swelling up to the medial canthus.** Lesions may be associated with loosening of the teeth and may reach a large size prior to presentation.[62] If these larger cysts are opened then they are found to contain foul-smelling cheesy material not unlike cholesteatoma, hence some of the previous synonyms.

Imaging

KCOTs are generally well defined with sclerosis around mono- or multicystic areas. They may be related to an impacted tooth or root apex with considerable adjacent expansion of the upper jaw. Radiographically, they may be indistinguishable from a dentigerous cyst, a lateral periodontal cyst may cause divergence of tooth roots but rarely resorption (**Fig. 12.2**).

Histological Features

The KCOT has a distinct histological appearance, the cyst being lined with a thin layer of parakeratinized stratified squamous epithelium usually around 5 to 7 cells thick. The lumen is usually filled with keratin. Because of the lack of rete ridges, the cyst's lining frequently separates from the underlying cyst wall and this overall structure is one of the explanations for the recurrence of this lesion because **as the cyst's lining is extremely thin, it is readily torn at the time of surgery**. The basal layer is hypochromatic and exhibits prominent palisading of the basal cells. Secondary inflammatory changes may be present and, importantly, "daughter cysts" and proliferative odontogenic epithelium may be seen in the wall, suggesting the possibility of the NBCCS. **These daughter and satellite cysts are another reason why the lesion may be incompletely removed**. Cellular atypia and mitosis are said to be uncommon, but **cyst lining left in situ will rapidly regrow.**[63]

Differential Diagnosis

Some odontogenic cysts may demonstrate surface and luminal keratin but they do not exhibit the hyperchromatic basal cell layer and should not be confused with the KCOT. This is important as they do not exhibit the aggressive behavior associated with KCOT.

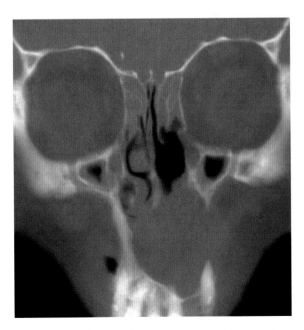

Fig. 12.2 Coronal CT scan showing an odontogenic keratocyst.

Treatment and Prognosis

While, in the past, enucleation and curettage have been recommended as treatment for these patients, as outlined in the clinical features and histopathology sections the thin lining, multiplicity, and daughter cysts make complete removal by these limited techniques difficult. Removal of surrounding bone and chemical cauterization may be added but the overall propensity to recur ranges between 3% and 62% in reported series. **Even in large series from notable centers, recurrence rates of around 30%[64] remain common and careful consideration should be given to achieving clearance with a single procedure, particularly in the case of single isolated lesions where adequate partial maxillectomy may cure the patient in a single procedure rather than multiple recurrences over many years, which are all too common in the literature.**

Long-term follow-up of these cases is certainly recommended and the yearly review would seem appropriate; if that is not the case, an information sheet should be provided instructing the patient to return with new symptoms as the cysts may recur decades later. Patients with multiple KCOT should be evaluated for the NBCCS if this has not already been diagnosed.

Our own unit has several outstanding examples of patients who have had multiple recurrences of these lesions; the most notable was a 64-year-old woman first seen in November 1983 with a 44-year history of a recurrent KCOT involving her maxillary sinus and orbit. Despite a partial maxillectomy and excision of a generous portion of her malar bone, the lesion recurred 4 years later in the left lateral wall of the orbit, firmly attached to the orbital periosteum and requiring further resection. This patient therefore had a total history of recurrence over a 48-year period (**Fig. 12.3**).[65] Two more recent cases have been treated by us primarily in 2003 and 2007 with a midfacial degloving and endoscopic resection, respectively, with apparent success to date.

Key Points

- The lining of the cyst is extremely thin and easily torn at the time of surgery. Cyst lining remaining in situ will lead to regrowth.

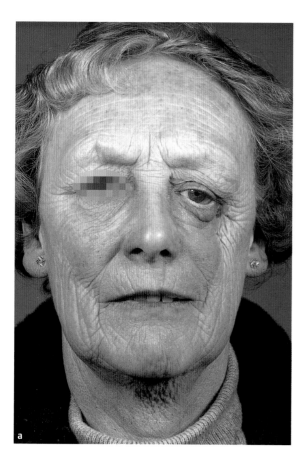

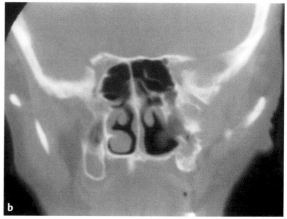

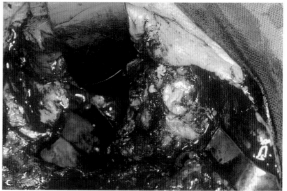

Fig. 12.3a–c Recurrent odontogenic keratocyst.

a Clinical photograph of a patient after multiple operations.
b Coronal CT scan of the same patient showing residual disease in the posterior maxilla and pterygoid.

c Operative photograph showing the view from below during midfacial degloving with a molar tooth embedded in residual KCOT.

- Daughter and satellite cysts may also cause incomplete removal.
- Multiple recurrences over many years may necessitate major surgical resection.

Tumors of Odontogenic Epithelium with Odontogenic Ectomesenchyme with or without Hard Tissue Formation

Introduction

This group of tumors is composed of tumors and some lesions that are hamartomatous. They are believed to be truly odontogenic in that they are composed of odontogenic ectomesenchyme and odontogenic epithelium that, under certain conditions, can produce the dental hard tissues similar to the process of normal odontogenesis. A better understanding is obtained if the mechanisms of odontogenesis are understood and the reviews of Sharpe and Cobourne and Sharpe[66,67] are recommended.

Ameloblastic Fibroma

Definition

(ICD-O code 9330/0)

Ameloblastic fibroma (AMF) is a rare, benign odontogenic neoplasm with odontogenic epithelium growing in an abundant and cell-rich ectomesenchymal tissue which resembles the dental papilla. No formation of dental hard tissue is present. If there is dentin present, the lesion is referred to as an ameloblastic fibrodentinoma.

Site and Incidence

The total number of published cases is ~200 at the time of writing and the comprehensive review of Philipsen et al 1997 is to be recommended.[68] The ratio of cases reported between the mandible and the maxilla varies from 2.7:1 to 5:1 in favor of the mandible. The majority of mandibular tumors occur in the posterior part. While the growth rate is slow, **many tumors in both the upper and lower jaws reach a considerable size** varying between 0.5 cm and 16 cm in the reports **with an average of around 4 cm**.[69]

Diagnosis and Specific Features

Clinical Features

Most cases of AMF present as a painless swelling or are diagnosed following investigation for disturbance of tooth eruption. Facial swelling and nasal blockage are reported with the larger maxillary lesions and this was the case in our group of 5 patients with this condition, ranging in age from 12 to 78 years (mean 49.3 years) (**Fig. 12.4a**). There were 2 men and 3 women, which again is in keeping with the reported cases indicating an approximately equal male and female incidence with a mean age of around 15 years, but an age range of between 6 months and 60 years.

Imaging

Radiologically, these tumors appear as a well-defined uni- or multilocular radiolucency usually with a radiopaque border. The multilocular appearance is particularly seen in larger lesions. Approximately 75% of cases are related to an unerupted tooth, and in the maxilla the **AMF may encroach upon the entire maxillary sinus and lateral wall of the nose**. CT scanning is particularly recommended for definition of the tumor (**Fig. 12.4b, c**).[69]

Histological Features

Microscopically, these tumors usually present as a white-gray rounded or oval mass with a smooth surface covered by a thin capsule. Cystic changes are rare and the cut surface is uniform. Microscopically, the epithelial component of AMF consists of branching and anastomosing epithelial strands of varying density, growing in a cell-rich mesenchymal tissue with a histomorphology similar to that of the dental papilla. These strands may form into knotlike arrangements of varying size. These have a rim of columnar cells similar to the inner enamel epithelium. In some areas, the strands may be broader and the central area occupied by stellate cells. Buds of varying size arise from the epithelial strands and these buds are composed of stellate cells bordered by a basal layer of cylindrical cells with a reverse nuclear polarity. These thickenings resemble the early stages of enamel organs.

Dental hard tissues do not form part of the histological picture of AMF. The epithelial component, at times, resembles ameloblastoma but the stromal content differs significantly in that it is an immature cell–rich myxoid tissue with an embryonic appearance. Some AMFs may contain granular cells.

If there are significant numbers of mitotic figures in either the epithelial or mesenchymal component, they should raise doubts about the benign nature of the case, particularly together with nuclear atypia and a high cellularity.

Differential Diagnosis

The main differential diagnoses are from ameloblastoma, ameloblastic fibro-odontoma (AFOD), ameloblastic fibrodentinoma (AFD), developing odontomes, and odontogenic fibroma (OF). Briefly, in contrast to ameloblastomas, the epithelium in the AMF forms bilaminar

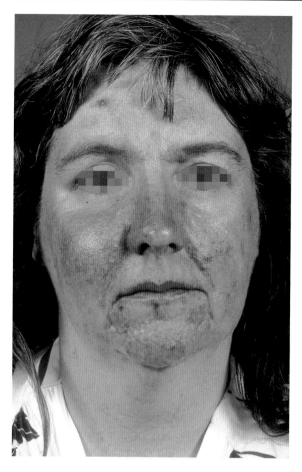

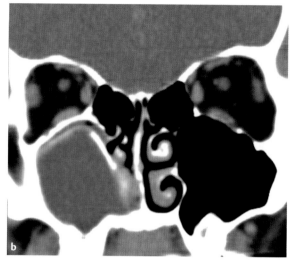

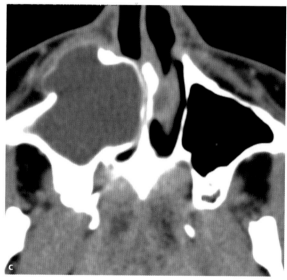

Fig. 12.4a–c

a Clinical photograph of a patient with a large odontogenic myxoma.
b Coronal CT scan in the same patient.
c Axial CT scan in the same patient.

strands with buds in contrast to broad strands, large islands with a tendency for acanthomatous changes, and cysts. The amount of stellate reticulumlike epithelium is usually more pronounced in the ameloblastoma. The connective tissue component is very different as in the AMF there is no stroma and usually the connective tissue is an equal component of the neoplasm with histomorphology like the dental papilla. In contrast to AFD and the AFOD, the AMF does not contain the dental hard tissue dentin and enamel. Debate continues with regard to these lesions with histochemical and molecular genetic studies ongoing.

Treatment and Prognosis

As for many odontogenic tumors, ameloblastic fibroma has been treated with conservative surgery consisting of enucleation and curettage as well as more radical surgery. Variable recurrence rates have been recorded but the exact histopathology in the older papers is at times doubtful. Chen et al 2007,[70] in a superb review of the English literature of the last century, found 123 cases of AMF with quality clinicopathological and follow-up data. Details of the surgical treatment were available in 118 cases, of which only 10 were treated by radical surgery (due to their significant size at presentation). Radical surgery was marginal resection, segmental resection, or semiresection of mandible or maxilla. Conservative surgery (108 patients) involved enucleation, curettage, or simple local excision. Recurrence was reported in 41 of the 118 cases (33.3%). The recurrence-free period ranged from 1 month to 96 months with a mean of 33 months. The recurrence-free interval was significantly longer in patients treated with radical procedures even allowing for the fact that only the largest lesions were treated radically.

Malignant transformation was reported in 14 recurrent cases (11.4%) with an increasing tendency to malignant transformation over increasing lengths of time. The 5-year malignant transformation rate was 10.2% and the 10-year rate 22.2%. Follow-up of 11 cases treated for malignancy by further surgery showed recurrence in 6 cases but only one case was detailed with extensive distal metastases.

Statistical analysis of the data showed that patients older than 22 years were significantly more likely to develop malignant transformation and the authors concluded that, on this data, patients younger than 22 years could be treated by conservative surgery but with more radical procedures should they recur. **In patients older than 22 years, particularly with the larger tumors, radical surgery should be considered as a primary treatment and certainly if these tumors recur subsequently.**

In our cohort, 4 underwent midfacial degloving and 1 endoscopic surgery with an anterior antrostomy for benign ameloblastic fibroma, with no evidence of malignant change or recurrence with between 4 and 10 years of follow-up.

Key Points

- AMF may encroach upon the entire maxillary sinus and nasal cavity.
- Patients older than 22 years should be considered for radical surgery.

Ameloblastic Fibrodentinoma

Definition

(ICD-O code 9271/0)

Ameloblastic fibrodentinoma (AFD) is an odontogenic tumor that has the histological features of ameloblastic fibroma (AMF) but the odontogenic ectomesenchyme resembles the dental papillae and the epithelial strands and nests resemble dental lamina and enamel organ. Dentinoid formation is usually seen, and more rarely tubular dentine.

Synonyms

The terms dentinoma and immature dentinoma have been used in the past and Takeda in 1994 discussed the differences between cases published as AFD and "immature dentinoma."[71]

Etiology, Incidence, and Site

The etiology is unknown and AFD is an exceedingly rare tumor, the subject of considerable debate in the literature.

Reichart and Philipsen 2004 reviewed 28 cases.[72] More than 70% of AFDs have been located in the posterior part of the mandible and **only 7 have been diagnosed in the maxilla**: 4 anterior and 3 posterior.

Diagnostic Features

Clinical Features and Imaging

These rare cases have been described as slow-growing, painless tumors but quite large on presentation, and in some cases, have been associated with unerupted teeth. On imaging, they are usually well delineated with scalloped borders and a multilocular radiolucency. In those cases where the tumor is associated with a tooth, it has been usually adjacent to the crown of the tooth.

Histological Features

The soft tissue component of AFD is similar to that of AMF, with embryonic pulplike ectomesenchyme, usually with notable cellularity, although some cases are less cell rich, in which strands of odontogenic epithelium with bulbous extensions are seen. Adjacent to the odontogenic epithelium, there are varying amounts of dentinoid and tubular dentin is seen in some cases. This dentin may be mineralized, giving rise to the varying degrees of irregular radiopacity seen on imaging. Mitoses are not seen in this lesion.

Treatment and Prognosis

This lesion is a good example where both the long-term biological behavior of the tumor and the histopathology require close correlation.[73] Because, in contrast to AMF, simple surgical excision of this lesion is sufficient and given the limited number of cases published, no recurrences or malignant transformation have been reported.

Ameloblastic Fibro-Odontoma

Definition

(ICD-O code 9290/0)

The ameloblastic fibro-odontoma (AFOD) is a rare, benign tumor composed of all the components seen in odontogenesis; namely, embryonic pulplike ectomesenchyme, odontogenic epithelium, dentin, enamel, and occasionally cementum.

Etiology

There has been much controversy in past literature and ameloblastic fibro-odontoma has often been included among odontomas, which are essentially hamartomas. The differentiation can be particularly difficult in the early stages of both forms of lesion as they share many features, but AFOD is a continuously growing neoplasm. Odontomas may achieve a considerable size but they eventually stop growing.

Synonyms

The confusing term ameloblastic odontoma has been used in the past.

Incidence and Site

Incidence is difficult to assess from the older literature but Philipsen et al 1997[68] reviewing the literature found a total of 86 cases including those previously described by Slootweg.[74] Philipsen et al found the age range to be between 1 year and 22 years, with a mean of 9 years, and just over half the cases were located in the posterior part of the mandible but **30 cases were diagnosed in the maxilla** (18 posterior, 12 anterior, and 1 large lesion involving both aspects of the maxilla).

Diagnostic Features

Clinical Features and Imaging

In common with other odontogenic tumors, this rare lesion usually presents as a painless, slow-growing mass that expands the jaw, causing swelling, and may be associated with an unerupted tooth. These smaller spherical tumors with little formation of dentin and enamel may be extremely difficult to differentiate from immature odontomas, but this has no clinical significance as the treatment is identical. The larger lesions may cause considerable expansion of the maxilla, impinging on the maxillary sinus, but there is no bony infiltration.

AFODs may be unilocular or multilocular radiolucencies on imaging, with well-defined hyperostotic borders.[68] Larger lesions may have scattered radiopacities in contrast to smaller immature odontomas, which may present with a rounded, regular radiopaque center with a surrounding area of radiolucency. Additionally, small spherical lesions located at the occlusal surface of an unerupted molar are more likely to be immature odontomas. **Large tumors in the maxilla may encroach on the maxillary sinus** and CT scanning will define the details of these lesions to facilitate treatment planning.[75]

Histological Features

Microscopically, AFOD has a smooth surface varying from white to tan. The cut surface is granular and contains hard nodules depending on the amount of dental hard tissue within the lesion. The soft tissue component may be identical to ameloblastic fibroma and the two hard and soft components may be present in varying proportions. The cell-rich myxoid connective tissue of ectomesenchymal origin is similar to the embryonic dental papilla. In

examples where there is limited dental hard tissue formation, extensive sampling may be necessary.

Differential Diagnosis

Distinguishing these lesions from ameloblastoma should be straightforward, but in the early stages of AFOD they look very similar to AMF and later in their course, there are similarities to AFD. **While confusion with an AFD has no particular clinical consequences, AMF—as detailed earlier—has a high tendency to recur and it is an example where clinical information coupled with histopathology findings is important in the differential diagnosis.** For instance, a tumor with features of an AMF recurring in a person older than 20 years, even in these rare lesions, is certainly likely to be an AMF.

Treatment and Prognosis

Enucleation followed by thorough curettage is the accepted treatment for most cases, but clearly the larger lesions that have encroached upon the maxillary sinus may require partial maxillary resection, which is not always an easy decision in small children. The tendency is therefore for initial conservative treatment, but in the rare cases of recurrence more aggressive resection must be considered. There have been two reports of lesions in teenagers undergoing malignant transformation but neither had the benefit of the recently increased histopathological understanding.[76,77]

Key point

- These rare tumors may involve the whole maxilla.

Odontomas, Complex and Compound

Definition

(ICD-O code 9280/0)

Odontomas are tumorlike but nonneoplastic developmental anomalies (hamartomas). They are the most highly differentiated lesion among those arising from odontogenic epithelium and odontogenic ectomesenchyme. Complex odontomas (ODTx) show a complex pattern of dentin and enamel, whereas compound odontomas (ODTp) consist of toothlike structures (odontoids). Distinction between these lesions can, at times, be difficult as they may show elements of both patterns, but from a clinical point of view this is not of great concern.

Etiology

The etiology of both these types of odontomas is unknown but there is evidence that genetic factors are involved as odontomas occur as part of Gardner's syndrome and other hereditary syndromes.[78]

Synonyms

Both these odontomas have been described with the addition of the descriptive term "composite," i.e., complex composite odontomas and compound composite odontoma.

Incidence and Site

Both of these lesions are common and ODTp is reported in many series to be the most common of all odontogenic neoplasms and tumorlike lesions. The exact incidence in different countries is imprecise owing to the relative frequency with which these lesions are sent to pathology departments for evaluation. The lesions are often diagnosed microscopically by oral surgeons and not submitted for histological examination. It is not surprising therefore that the incidence of material received by pathology departments in various countries ranges from as little as 1.2% in China[79] to 36.7% in the United States[80] in studies comprising more than 300 samples of odontogenic tumors.

Both types of lesion occur in tooth-bearing regions but the ODTx is said to occur more commonly in the maxilla in some reports and in the mandible in others. In the maxilla it occurs primarily in the anterior region; within the mandible it is most common in the posterior region.[81] In contrast to this, reviews of substantial numbers of ODTp have consistently found a predominant occurrence in the maxilla, particularly in the anterior region. Again, in contrast to the ODTx, the ODTp occurs in the anterior region of the mandible.[82]

Peripheral (extraosseous) odontomas are very rare but have been reported in the maxillary sinus[83,84] and the nasopharynx.[85]

Diagnostic Features

Clinical Features

There is no obvious sex predilection for either of these odontomas and both are primarily diagnosed in children and adolescents, although the complex type has also been reported in young adults.

The growth rate of both these lesions is very low; sequential orthopantomograms taken in children suggest that these lesions take at least 5 years to mature, and in many instances the patients reach the late mixed-dentition stage by the time the diagnosis is made.[86]

The lesions usually present as a painless swelling, but pain may occur in association with inflammation. Impaction and alterations of tooth eruption are common symptoms, and swelling of the cheek and upper lip may occur if the lesion in the maxilla attains sufficient size.[87]

Imaging

Findings on imaging vary and depend on the stage of development and degree of mineralization of the lesions. Complex odontomas vary from a radiolucent, well-demarcated lesion to those that have a central core of densely opaque masses with a peripheral zone of varying radiolucency, ultimately progressing to a radiopaque mass of hard dental tissue with only a thin surrounding radiolucent zone. They are usually located above an unerupted tooth. Resorption of neighboring teeth is very unusual with these lesions, in contrast to the odontoma-associated calcifying cystic odontogenic tumor.[88] **The size of these lesions varies from a few millimeters to several centimeters and they may occupy the whole of the maxilla, which means their presentation to maxillofacial surgeons, ENT surgeons, plastic surgeons, and head and neck surgeons depends on the symptoms, the country, and the facilities available.[89,90]**

The ODT usually presents as a dense mass of small toothlike opacities (odontoids) with a surrounding thin radiolucent area and a hyperostotic border. Unerupted teeth are often seen and initially small lesions may arise between the roots of erupted teeth.[87] As with ODTx, ODTp is not associated with resorption of neighboring tooth roots.

Histological Features and Differential Diagnosis

The essential difference between complex and compound odontomas is mainly based on the presence of toothlike structures in the compound odontomas. The compound lesion can be seen to contain toothlike structures in a thin fibrous capsule, particularly if the lesion has matured. Even the immature compound lesions show several dysmorphic tooth germs within loose connective tissue but with surrounding cords and islands of odontogenic epithelium as is seen in the complex lesions. The enamel matrix in the compound lesion may still be present after decalcification.

In the developing odontoma, the outer part of the lesion shows a cell-rich zone of soft tissue with formation of enamel and dentin, but this does not resemble tooth morphology. The massive, primarily tubular, dentin encloses oval or circular hollow structures and an enamel matrix producing epithelium with connective tissue. The differential diagnosis between a developing complex odontoma and an ameloblastic fibro-odontoma can be very difficult. In mature complex odontomas, the surrounding capsule consists of loose connective tissue with islands and strands of odontogenic epithelium. **It is essential that the pathologist reporting intraosseous jaw lesions either has access to the imaging or, preferably, conducts a thorough discussion with radiological colleagues and the clinicians involved with these cases, as the differential diagnosis between these various odontogenic lesions can be difficult. In particular,** differentially diagnosing an immature odontoma from AMF, AFD, and AFOD without this additional knowledge is inappropriate. The value of regular multidisciplinary team meetings at which all team members are present with the maximum amount of information allows for more accurate diagnosis and careful consideration of the most appropriate treatment.

Treatment and Prognosis

Both types of odontoma are generally treated by conservative enucleation and minimal curettage as they separate easily from the smooth surface of the surrounding bony tissue in which they arise. Prognosis is excellent; recurrences are rare and these are felt to occur only in cases of incomplete removal or incorrect histopathology.[91,92]

This conservative treatment frequently allows associated impacted teeth to erupt satisfactorily or to be aided by additional orthodontic management.

Large odontomas of the maxilla and mandible obviously require further special surgical considerations, but bearing in mind that these lesions are frequently in children or adolescents, partial maxillary and mandibular procedures or intraoral approaches should be sufficient to remove the entire lesion without the need for facial incisions. Additional considerations for prostheses or soft tissue and bone reconstruction will be necessary only in very rare cases.

Key Point

- It is essential that the pathologist reporting intraosseous jaw lesions either has access to the imaging or, preferably, conducts a thorough discussion with radiological colleagues and the clinicians involved with these cases, as the differential diagnosis between these various odontogenic lesions can be difficult. In particular, differentially diagnosing an immature odontoma from AMF, AFD, and AFOD without this additional knowledge is inappropriate. The value of a regular multidisciplinary team meeting where all team members are present with the maximum amount of information allows for more accurate diagnosis and careful consideration of the most appropriate treatment.

Odontoameloblastoma

Definition

(ICD-O code 9311/0)

This rare composite tumor, as the name implies, includes areas that on histopathological evaluation resemble an ameloblastoma together with areas that correspond to an immature odontoma or AFOD.

Synonyms

The terms ameloblastic odontoma and odontoblastoma have also been used to describe these lesions.

Etiology, Incidence, and Site

The etiology of these extremely rare tumors is unknown and only 12 published cases had sufficient accepted diagnostic criteria for the WHO working group of 2005.[93-99] **Only 6 cases have been described in the maxilla but 4 were large, between 4 and 6 cm.**

Diagnostic Features

Clinical Features and Imaging

Patients have presented with painless swelling that in some cases was long-standing, tooth displacement, and occasional pain. Imaging has shown a well-defined lesion that may be unilocular or multilocular, usually associated with some irregular radiopacities whether centrally or peripherally, but, in contrast to ameloblastomas, no honeycombing pattern has been described. Displacement and resorption of tooth roots has been described.[94-99] Most have occurred before the age of 25 years.

Histological Features

The epithelial component of this tumor is essentially typical of ameloblastoma, with islands and cords of odontogenic epithelium that may demonstrate both follicular and flexible patterns. However, these tumors also contain varying amounts of mineralized dental tissues, as seen in odontomas, among the cellular myxoid tissue adjacent to the epithelium. Small areas containing ghost cells may also be found.[98]

Treatment and Prognosis

In the few published cases the patients have been treated by curettage for the small lesion, but wider surgical and en bloc resection up to and including hemi-maxillectomy has also been undertaken. Unfortunately, only a single publication gives follow-up for 5 years or longer[93] but this patient's cystic lesion, treated by curettage, recurred twice with increasing histopathological appearances of ameloblastoma. The second time it was treated by en bloc resection and, although the literature on the subject is minimal, it would appear that these lesions would be more appropriately treated by wide resection and long-term follow-up, as would be appropriate for the far more common ameloblastomas.

Odontogenic Ghost Cell Lesions

Definition

The term odontogenic ghost cell lesions covers a heterogeneous group of odontogenic lesions that range from cysts through solid benign neoplasms to solid malignant neoplasms and at times a combination of these. Lesions may be intraosseous or extraosseous in the upper and lower jaws. A wide variety of names have been used in the past 80 years and considerable change has taken place since the first WHO classification of odontogenic tumors and cysts published in 1971.[100]

These ghost cell lesions share histological features similar to ameloblastomas but additionally have notable areas of ghost cells, which tend to calcify and show formation of dysplastic dentin in the connective tissue adjacent to the epithelial areas. Multiple different classification systems have been suggested and the reader is referred to Praetorius 2009 for a full discussion of this complex debate (see ref. 23: p. 1260). In the WHO classification of head and neck tumors of 2005,[5] dentinogenic ghost cell tumor is the name given to the benign neoplasm and ghost cell odontogenic carcinoma that given to the malignant form. Cysts with a neoplastic potential were grouped together under the term calcifying cystic odontogenic tumor. In the past these have been most commonly described and published under the names calcifying odontogenic cysts and calcifying ghost cell odontogenic tumor. The situation becomes even more complicated in that many cystic odontogenic lesions are nonneoplastic.

Calcifying Cystic Odontogenic Tumor

Definition

(ICD-O code 9301/0)

Calcifying cystic odontogenic tumor (CCOT) is a benign cystic neoplasm of odontogenic origin with a particular lining that resembles that of a unicystic ameloblastoma, with a basal layer of columnar cells but with groups of epithelial ghost cells either in the lining or in the epithelial strands and islands in the fibrous capsule. These may calcify. Dysplastic dentin is commonly seen adjacent to the basal layer of the cystic lining or the epithelial islands in the fibrous capsule.

Etiology

The etiology of CCOTs is unknown but the intraosseous cysts probably arise from reduced enamel epithelium of unerupted teeth or remnants of the dental lamina.

Synonyms

The terms keratinizing and calcifying odontogenic cyst have been used for more than 50 years and, following the recognition by Gorlin et al in 1962 that the lesion was a separate entity, it has also been called Gorlin cyst.[101] The somewhat more precise term of calcifying ghost cell odontogenic cyst has also been used.

Incidence and Site

It is simply not possible to give accurate figures for the incidence of these lesions because of the considerable debate in the literature over the years, but recent studies suggest they are commonest in the second decade and rare in patients older than 40 years of age. There is no particular sex predilection and they may present as intra- or extraosseous lesions. There is an **even distribution between the maxilla and mandible**, with a preference for the anterior aspects. While the majority of reports quote size ranges of 0.5 to 4 cm at diagnosis, **maxillary lesions may involve the antrum even to the point of complete obliteration**.

Diagnostic Features

Clinical Features and Imaging

Both extraosseous and intraosseous lesions present as a painless swelling, and while imaging may show some saucerization and displacement of adjacent teeth in the extraosseous lesions, the intraosseous lesions are usually unilocular with a well-circumscribed border and approximately half of them contain radiopaque areas. Both root divergence and root resorption are common with CCOTs but an unerupted tooth is seen in only approximately one-third of cases.[102,103]

Histological Features and Differential Diagnosis

These lesions are usually unicystic but multicystic examples have been described. While the morphology of the epithelial lining may vary, in some areas it resembles that of an ameloblastoma. Mitoses are rare. Clusters of ghost cells are present in the epithelium, as large, pale eosinophilic cells with a distinct outline and these cells are larger than the epithelial cells. Some may contain remnants of the nucleus but most show a central empty space, hence the term ghost cell. These cells may calcify. Tubular dentinoid is often found adjacent to the epithelial lining and may contain entrapped cells.

Ghost cells have been described in a variety of other lesions including simple eruption cysts, ameloblastomas, AMFs, AOFDs and particularly in odontomas. Ghost cells are therefore an insufficient criterion for the diagnosis and stellate reticulumlike areas and elongated basal cells must also been seen. **Sufficient histological sampling together with clinical information and imaging help with the borderline cases**. While mitoses are rare in CCOTs, they are numerous in ghost cell odontogenic carcinoma.

Treatment and Prognosis

There is general agreement that enucleation is the most appropriate treatment for these lesions when they are of a small size. However, recurrences have been reported for the intraosseous type and **lesions of several centimeters in size involving the maxilla, adjacent lateral wall of the nose, and nasal cavities will require considerably larger resection to avoid recurrence and the possibility of long-term malignant transformation**, which has been reported in a few cases. Indeed there is continuing controversy with regard to the more benign cystic lesions arising in association with malignant ghost cell–containing tumor.[104]

Calcifying Cystic Odontogenic Tumors Associated with Other Types of Odontogenic Tumors

In rare cases these cysts have been described in association with malignant epithelial odontogenic tumors, solid/multicystic ameloblastoma, unicystic ameloblastoma, adenomatoid odontogenic tumor, ameloblastic fibroma, ameloblastic fibro-odontoma, odontoameloblastoma, odontogenic fibromyxoma, and odontomas. The last combination, where there is an association between calcifying cystic odontogenic tumor and odontoma, is much more common than any of the other CCOT variants.

Dentinogenic Ghost Cell Tumor

Definition

(ICD-O code 9302/0)

This is a benign but nonencapsulated and locally invasive epithelial odontogenic tumor that has ameloblastoma-like islands in a mature fibrous connective tissue stroma. Groups of ghost cells are seen in the epithelial islands and occasionally in the connective tissue. Various amounts of dentinoid lie adjacent to the epithelium.

Etiology

Etiology is unknown but both extraosseous and intraosseous variants have been described.

Synonyms

These are many and varied but previously these lesions were often described as the solid variant of the calcifying odontogenic cyst. The terms dentinoameloblastoma, calcifying ghost cell odontogenic tumor, odontogenic ghost cell tumor, and epithelial odontogenic ghost cell tumor have all been used.

Incidence and Site

These tumors are extremely rare, with just over 30 extraosseous cases having been published and 14 intraosseous cases (see ref. 23: p. 1272). **Only 8 tumors have been located in the maxilla**, 7 in the anterior region.

Diagnostic Features

Clinical Features

The tumor usually presents as an asymptomatic swelling but intraosseous lesions have been reported up to 10 cm in diameter with displacement and loosening of adjacent teeth. **The whole maxillary antrum may be obliterated**. There is a wide age range at presentation from 10 years to 92 years of age.

Imaging

Imaging has not been particularly helpful in this rare disease. Intraosseous lesions may be uni- or multilocular radiolucent but with both well-defined and ill-defined borders. Varying amounts of scattered radiopaque material have been seen and teeth adjacent to the lesions may show root absorption or impaction. Substantial maxillary tumors may invade the sinus.[105,106] CT scanning will further define borders of the tumor, particularly in larger cases with significant erosion.

Histological Features

There are no significant differences between the intra- and extraosseous variants and notably these tumors infiltrate the surrounding tissues. Sheets and rounded islands of odontogenic epithelium resembling that of ameloblastoma are seen. Mitoses are absent, however. The significant feature is the transformation of the epithelial cells into ghost cells and large accumulations of ghost cells may be seen in addition to individual cells. The ghost cells extruding into the fibrous connective tissue evoke a foreign body reaction and some undergo calcification. As the name suggests, the tumor forms dysplastic dentin, although in small amounts. Ghost cells may be trapped within this dysplastic dentin. It is the large number of ghost cells that distinguishes this lesion from ameloblastoma, but it may be difficult to distinguish this lesion from a multicystic calcifying cystic odontogenic tumor.

Treatment and Prognosis

While simple excision may be sufficient for extraosseous lesions, an important point with regard to intraosseous dentinogenic ghost cell tumors is that they are known to recur in the long term and it would appear that wide local resection is the appropriate treatment particularly if, on imaging, the lesion is ill defined. In the limited number of cases reported, long-term follow-up details are not available but it would seem appropriate to recommend a long-term postsurgical follow-up time of up to 20 years.

Tumors of Odontogenic Ectomesenchyme with or without Included Odontogenic Epithelium

Odontogenic Fibroma

Definition

(ICD-O code 9321/0)

The odontogenic fibroma is a rare, benign, noninfiltrating odontogenic tumor composed of proliferating fibrous tissue which contains various quantities of "inactive looking" odontogenic epithelium. As with other odontogenic lesions, debate continues with regard to this particular lesion to an even greater degree than some of its counterparts. In the WHO classification of 2005, the tumor has been divided into an epithelium-poor type and an epithelium-rich type. The tumor occurs as an extraosseous/peripheral variant and an intraosseous/central variant.

Synonyms

Odontogenic fibroma simple type (without epithelium) and odontogenic fibroma complex type (with epithelium).

Incidence and Site

These are rare lesions but with two notable reviews in 1991 and 1994 describing 39 and 51 cases, respectively.[107,108] Although the tumors may occur at any age, they are most common in the second to fourth decades and are more common in the female. The distribution between maxilla and mandible appears to be approximately equal.

Diagnosis and Specific Features

Clinical Features and Imaging

These tumors present as slow-growing, progressive but painless swellings with great variation in the imaging appearances. They vary from small and unilocular to large and multilocular and can resemble ameloblastomas or myxomas.[109] The borders may be well defined but vary considerably through to diffuse lesions. Tooth displacement, resorption, and root changes are too variable to be of use. **Multilocular lesions tend to be larger with most of them greater than 3 cm at presentation**.

Histological Features

Debate continues with regard to the histopathology, and variants of odontogenic fibromas have been described. Histopathology of the epithelium-poor type resembles that of a dental follicle with moderate cellularity with dispersed, delicate collagen fibers. There is a substantial amount of ground substance producing a fibromyxoid quality. There are irregular islands and cords of inactive-looking odontogenic epithelium with variable amounts of calcification. The epithelium-rich type is more cellular with fibroblastic connective tissue interwoven in less cellular and vascular areas. The islands and strands of inactive-looking odontogenic epithelium may be sparse but are usually conspicuous. There is no mitotic activity. Calcified material is often seen in these lesions with varying histomorphology that may resemble dysplastic cementum, osteoid, or dentinoid. The differential diagnosis of these lesions may be difficult and depends in the main on exclusion of other lesions.[110] **As with other difficult odontogenic lesions, the diagnosis requires a knowledge of the histopathology combined with imaging and the clinical features**.

Treatment and Prognosis

Both types of odontogenic fibroma are benign lesions and the recommended treatment has been enucleation but with vigorous curettage, particularly for those lesions with a diffuse border on imaging. Recurrence has been reported in a few cases but long-term follow-up details are virtually absent from the literature. It is highly likely that considerable debate will continue with regard to this particular lesion.

Odontogenic Myxoma and Myxofibroma

Definition

(ICD-O code 9320/0)

Odontogenic myxoma (ODOMYX) is a benign, intraosseous neoplasm **with potential for significant local invasion**. The lesion is composed of spindle-shaped, stellate, or rounded cells that are contained within a prominent myxoid or mucoid extracellular matrix. Some lesions have substantial amounts of collagen within them and the name myxofibroma is then used.

Etiology

No etiological factors are known but the tissue of origin is thought to be the odontogenic ectomesenchyme of a developing tooth or undifferentiated mesenchymal cells of the periodontal ligament. This view is supported by histological similarities to embryonic pulpal ectomesenchyme and the dental follicle. The lesions are rare in non–tooth-bearing areas; several cases of infantile extraosseous paranasal myxomas have been published, but the question whether they are of odontogenic origin remains debatable.[111–115]

Incidence and Site

The frequency of the odontogenic myxoma varies considerably in studies published from different parts of the world, **but it would appear to be the third most reported tumor after the odontomas and ameloblastomas in the majority of publications**. Excluding the infantile extraosseous paranasal myxomas,[116] the age range of these lesions extends from children to patients in their seventies. The majority occur in the second and third decades with no particular sex bias. In most studies, the majority of these lesions appear to have arisen in the posterior part of the maxilla or mandible with an approximately equal distribution, although this does vary considerably between reports. **The larger lesions of the maxilla which involve the antrum often appear to have a more rapid growth pattern and may involve both posterior and anterior aspects.**[110]

Diagnostic Features

Clinical Features

Most series report a generally slow growth of these lesions, with small lesions being essentially asymptomatic other than the noted swelling. Pain is unusual and displacement and loosening of teeth are more common forms of presentation. **The larger maxillary sinus tumors may impinge on the nasal cavity, causing nasal obstruction, and expand into the floor of the orbit, causing exophthalmos** (Fig. 12.4a).

Imaging

The imaging features are variable and odontogenic myxomas may appear as either unilocular or multilocular radiolucencies with usually well-defined limits, but they can also show a diffuse edge. Occasionally, the presence of trabeculations can be accompanied by a "honeycomb soap bubble," "tennis racket," or "ground glass" appearance.[117] Both root displacement and root resorption may be present along with significant periosteal reaction with larger lesions. In 11 of the maxillary cases of Noffke et al,[117] there was significant invasion of the maxillary sinus and 2 additionally invaded the nasal cavity. Peltola et al describing a radiographic study of 21 odontogenic

myxomas also demonstrated a "sun ray" or "sun burst" appearance mimicking that seen in osteosarcoma.[118] As the larger tumors can cause significant bone erosion, cortical perforation, and involvement of adjacent soft tissues, they are best imaged by a combination of CT and MRI.

Histological Features

Microscopically, these lesions are usually white-gray masses and vary from firm to gelatinous depending on the extent of collagen. Microscopically, they are nonencapsulated and characteristically have randomly orientated stellate, spindle-shaped, and round cells with lengthy, slender, anastomosing processes that extend to the centrally placed nucleus. The cells are generally evenly distributed in the abundant myxoid or mucoid stroma that contains sparse, fine collagen fibers.[119]

Mild pleomorphism, binucleate cells, and mitotic figures may be evident. Those lesions with a greater degree of collagen, which are therefore designated as myxofibromas, appear to have the same natural history as the myxomas.

Differential Diagnosis

Small odontogenic myxomas may have a similar histopathology to myxoid enlarged or hyperplastic dental follicles and the dental papillae of a developing tooth. Some lesions may appear to permeate into the marrow spaces of adjacent bone, giving rise to concerns of malignancy. Additionally, the larger lesions that impinge on the nasal cavity from the maxilla may give rise to some confusion with nasal polyposis. **All these potential misdiagnoses can, as with other odontogenic tumors, be avoided by knowledge of the clinical history and radiology in addition to the histopathology**. The overall differential diagnosis also includes other myxoid types of tumor such as myxoid fibrosarcoma, myxoid nerve sheath tumors, and chondromyxoid fibroma. **As ever, adequate amounts of good quality biopsy material are essential to aid the diagnosis**.

Treatment

It is important to stress that these lesions, while initially small and slow-growing in many cases, are nonencapsulated and have an infiltrative and sometimes aggressive growth pattern. The tendency of odontogenic myxoma to permeate into marrow spaces alone makes conservative treatment by enucleation and curettage fraught with the likelihood of recurrence, and average recurrence rates, even in recently reported literature, are as high as 25%. In an excellent report in 2006, Li et al[120] presented the details of 25 cases of which 17 were treated by relatively radical procedures such as segmental resection or partial or complete maxillectomy. One patient with a maxillary tumor had recurrence 6 months after surgery, but details on 12 patients available for follow-up over a decade showed no further recurrences. Only four cases of possible malignant transformation to odontogenic myxosarcoma have been reported.[121]

Cementoblastoma

Definition

(ICD-O code 9273/0)

Cementoblastomas are benign tumors composed of irregular cementumlike trabeculae with multiple basophilic reversal lines. This hard tissue is attached to the resorbed surface of the root of an associated tooth, which is usually significantly shortened by resorption.

Etiology, Incidence, and Site

The etiology is unknown and these are extremely rare tumors with only ~120 cases having been published, of which ~80% are located in the mandible, particularly adjacent to the permanent first molar tooth.[122]

Diagnostic Features

Clinical Features and Imaging

These usually present as a painful swelling of the alveolar region and imaging shows a well-defined radiopaque or mixed-density lesion surrounded by a thin radiolucent zone. There is notable root absorption and obliteration of the periodontal ligament space.

Histological Features and Differential Diagnosis

Cementoblastomas consist of dense masses of acellular cementumlike material in a fibrous stroma that may contain multinucleated cells and vascular elements. The associated tooth has root resorption and this is important to differentiate the cementoblastoma from osteoblastoma and osteosarcoma. Osteoblastomas do not fuse with the surface of the tooth roots and remain separated from bone. On occasions, the cementoblastoma may exhibit some pleomorphism, which may give rise to concern that it is an osteosarcoma, again emphasizing the important point that **the diagnosis of many of these lesions cannot simply be made on the biopsy material. The patient's clinical history and imaging studies have to be considered alongside the histopathology** and here the definitive relationship to the root of the tooth is unique to the cementoblastoma. These lesions **do not significantly involve the maxillary antrum** and as such are rarely seen by ENT surgeons.

Treatment

Brannon et al 2002[122] reported a recurrence rate of 37% in 44 of their own cases following incomplete removal of tumor tissue. While these slow-growing neoplasms are readily enucleated, they do require removal of the affected tooth or teeth, followed by thorough curettage or a peripheral ostectomy.[123]

Malignant Odontogenic Tumors

Metastasizing Ameloblastoma

Definition

(ICD-O code 9310/3)

Metastasizing ameloblastoma (METAM) has histological features identical to those of ameloblastomas that do not metastasize. Diagnosis is made subsequently by the clinical behavior of the lesion.

Synonyms

The terms metastasizing malignant ameloblastoma and atypical ameloblastoma have also been used.

Ameloblastomas which, at presentation, have histological signs of malignancy should be classified as ameloblastic carcinomas (AMCA). It is only the long-term clinical behavior of an apparently benign ameloblastoma that determines its malignant potential. More than 80% of ameloblastomas occur in the mandible; **these lesions are extremely rare in the literature of the upper jaw and adjacent sinuses**. The most common site of metastases is the lung.[124]

There are no differences in the clinical signs, imaging, pathology, or immunohistochemistry detected so far to differentiate the apparently benign ameloblastomas that will metastasize.

As a consequence of this rare occurrence, it is important that all ameloblastomas are resected adequately, if at all possible, in their location in the maxilla and adjacent nasal cavity, and paranasal sinuses. Metastases can occur many years after removal of the primary tumor, all ameloblastoma patients should be followed up for many years with annual chest imaging, as long-term survival with resection of lung lesions has been documented.[125,126]

Key Point

- There are currently no particular methods of evaluation of ameloblastoma at presentation that can predict their long-term malignant potential.

Ameloblastic Carcinoma

Primary Type

Definition

(ICD-O code 9270/3)

The term primary type ameloblastic carcinoma covers an extremely rare variant of malignant odontogenic tumor that has the histological appearance of ameloblastoma with additional cytological atypia. The term is used even without the presence of metastases.

These rare lesions involve the mandible in more than two-thirds of cases and Dhir et al 2003 reported **only 19 cases in the maxilla.**[127]

The pattern of histology is that of an ameloblastoma but with additional malignant cytological features usually comprising tall, columnar cellular morphology with notable mitoses, focal necrosis, nuclear hyperchromatism, and perineural invasion. The lesions overall show a high proliferation index compared with benign ameloblastomas. In the Laughlin et al series, over one-third of patients died from pulmonary metastases.[124]

Ameloblastic Carcinoma–Secondary Type (Dedifferentiated), Intraosseous

Definition

(ICD-O code 9270/3)

This term is used for these lesions where ameloblastic carcinoma is known to arise in a preexisting benign ameloblastoma. The term "dedifferentiated ameloblastoma" has also been used when morphological features of typical ameloblastoma were noted. This helps to separate this extremely rare lesion from metastasizing ameloblastoma since there is no evidence of cytological atypia in this previously described lesion.

To further complicate matters, the term carcinoma ex intraosseous ameloblastoma has also been used to describe these rare lesions, but to date only 7 cases of this lesion have been described, all in the mandible.[128]

Ameloblastic Carcinoma–Secondary Type (Dedifferentiated), Peripheral

Definition

(ICD-O code 9270/3)

Only 6 cases of ameloblastic carcinoma arising within a preexisting peripheral ameloblastoma have been reported but they required wide local excision with en bloc resection of the involved segment of the maxilla.[129,130]

Primary Intraosseous Squamous Cell Carcinoma

Definition

(ICD-O code 9270/3)

Primary intraosseous squamous cell carcinomas (PIOSCCs) are central jaw carcinomas that are derived from odontogenic epithelial remnants; three different subcategories are currently recognized. **They are all extremely rare lesions, occurring far less frequently in the maxilla than in the mandible.** The three types are:
1. **A solid type** that invades the marrow spaces of the bone producing resorption but having no connection to the upper aerodigestive tract mucosa.
2. **A cystogenic type** arising from an odontogenic keratocyst.
3. **A keratocystic odontogenic tumor. When these tumors enlarge and involve the surface mucosa of the maxilla or nasal cavity, it may become impossible to distinguish between them and a true antral or nasal primary tumor. The extensive cases may show significant cortical bone expansion and destruction and require radical surgical treatment such as partial or complete maxillectomy along with radiotherapy or chemoradiation.** Owing to the small numbers of cases in the literature and the considerable confusion with regard to their histological origin, exact prognosis is difficult to provide, but metastases at the time of presentation of around 30% and 5-year survival between 30% and 50% have been reported.[131–134]

Clear Cell Odontogenic Carcinoma

(ICD-O code 9341/3)

Clear cell odontogenic carcinoma is a relatively new diagnosis and was first described by Hansen et al in 1985 using the term clear cell odontogenic tumor.

Waldron et al in 1985 used the term clear cell ameloblastoma. Both were considered to be benign tumors in the WHO classification of 1992.[135,136] **Only 5 cases of these malignant lesions have been described in the maxilla** but they are aggressive lesions and require radical resection plus postoperative radiotherapy with long-term follow-up.[137,138]

Ghost Cell Odontogenic Carcinoma

Definition

(ICD-O code 9302/3)

Ghost cell odontogenic carcinoma (GCOC) is the malignant counterpart of the calcifying odontogenic cyst and is characterized by large, cell-rich islands of small, round epithelial cells with numerous mitoses and hyperchromatic nuclei that are mixed in with ghost cells, and occasionally areas of calcification.[139]

Synonyms

Synonyms are many, varied, and confusing! The terms malignant calcifying ghost cell odontogenic tumor, calcifying ghost cell odontogenic carcinoma, malignant epithelial odontogenic ghost cell tumor, malignant calcifying odontogenic cyst, carcinoma arising in a calcifying odontogenic cyst, and aggressive epithelial ghost cell odontogenic tumor have all been used.

Incidence, Site, and Clinical Features

The number of names for this tumor almost equals the number of cases in the English literature. Takata reported 19 cases in 2005.[139] It is of importance that **this tumor occurs primarily in the maxilla** with a ~3:1 male-to-female ratio and that **those reported have frequently been large, extending to involve the entire maxilla and adjacent nasal cavity orbit, and crossing the midline and invading soft tissues**. While these tumors may initially present as a painless swelling, the growth rate is obviously high; and even though a small number of patients have been reported, several symptoms were related to the invasion of tumor into the nasal cavities, maxillary sinus, and orbit. There are no specific features on imaging but these tumors may be extensive and MRI and CT are required for their site evaluation.

Histological Features

For precise identification of this rare tumor, the malignant epithelial tumor has to contain the classic benign features of calcifying cystic odontogenic tumor. The malignant component consists of small, round, dark cells in a fibrous stroma with multiple mitoses. Variously sized islands of ghost cells are seen, which are large, polygonal cells with homogeneous, pale eosinophilic cytoplasm. There are round empty spaces where the nuclei have disintegrated, although some remnants of chromatin may be seen. There may be a foreign body giant cell reaction where the ghost cell masses are in contact with the connective tissue stroma, and additionally there may be a varying degree of calcification in the ghost cells. Necrosis is often seen in the middle of tumor islands but the malignant epithelial component may be mixed in with the classical benign lesion or it may be separated; this is a significant point as these rapidly growing lesions may be quite large at diagnosis and **it is important that substantial amounts of good quality biopsy material are obtained to identify the malignant component of the lesion**.

Treatment and Prognosis

The literature records a considerable spectrum of growth patterns with some lesions slowly growing but others that appear to be highly aggressive. Approximately half of the published cases have recurrence, often despite aggressive surgery. Of 26 patients described by Praetorius in 2009 (see ref. 23: p. 1306) from the published cases, 12 had recurrence after operation, often multiple, and often despite radical surgery. Death from recurrent local tumor extension and metastases was reported in those patients not lost to follow-up. Only 2 patients were reported to be tumor free beyond 5 years. **While this lesion is extremely rare, it is obviously an aggressive tumor and appropriate radical surgery with additional radiotherapy appears to be indicated** (see ref. 23: p. 1306).

Odontogenic Sarcomas

(ICD-O codes 9330/0 & 9290/3)

This group of rare, malignant ectomesenchymal odontogenic neoplasms comprises ameloblastic fibrosarcoma, ameloblastic fibrodentinosarcoma, and ameloblastic fibro-odontosarcoma. The term "ameloblastic sarcoma" has also been used as a collective name for these lesions, causing considerable confusion in the literature. From a therapeutic point of view, these rare lesions have similar clinical features with ~80% of the cases being confined to the mandible.[140] They have an age range extending from children to old age and in the small number of cases in the literature there is a male-to-female ratio of 3:1.

They present as **painful** swellings that, on imaging, show expansile intraosseous radiolucency with ill-defined borders.[141]

Diagnosis

Histological Features

These sarcomas all contain benign odontogenic epithelium, but the ameloblastic fibrosarcoma resembles an ameloblastic fibroma in which **the epithelial tissue is benign but the connective tissue is malignant**. The ameloblastic fibrodentinosarcomas and fibro-odontosarcomas contain additional hard tissue in terms of dentin or dentinoid, or enamel or enamaloid, respectively.

Treatment and Prognosis

The biological behavior of these lesions is extremely aggressive locally but they have a low potential for regional or distant metastases. They require adequate surgical resection.[141,142]

Key Points

- While the majority of small odontogenic lesions will present to dental and oral surgeons, it is important that colleagues in maxillofacial, ENT, plastics, and ophthalmology are aware that these lesions may expand substantially into the paranasal sinuses, nasal cavity, orbit, and skull base.
- The pathologist requires the entire specimen to make an exact diagnosis of the tumor, supported by imaging and full clinical information to distinguish between the many odontogenic lesions.
- The natural history of most of these lesions can extend over many years and they can achieve impressive size. Rapid growth should, therefore, raise suspicion of malignancy.

References

1. Toller P. Origin and growth of cysts of the jaws. Ann R Coll Surg Engl 1967;40(5):306–336
2. Broca P. Recherches sur une nouveau groupe de tumeurs designees sous le nom d'odontames. Gazette Hebdomadaire de Médecine et de Chirurgie 1868;8:113–115
3. Thoma KH, Goldman HM. Odontogenic tumors: classification based on observations of the epithelial, mesenchymal, and mixed varieties. Am J Pathol 1946;22:433–471
4. Philipsen H, Reichart P. The development and fate of epithelial residues after completion of the human odontogenesis with special reference to the origins of epithelial odontogenic neoplasms, hamartomas and cysts. Oral Biosci Med 2004;1:171–179
5. Barnes L, Eveson J, Reichart P, Sidransky D, eds. World Health Organization Classification of Tumours. Pathology and Genetics of Head and Neck Tumours. Lyon: IARC Press; 2005:1–430
6. Heikinheimo K, Hormia M, Stenman G, Virtanen I, Happonen RP. Patterns of expression of intermediate filaments in ameloblastoma and human fetal tooth germ. J Oral Pathol Med 1989;18(5):264–273
7. Shear M, Singh S. Age-standardized incidence rates of ameloblastoma and dentigerous cyst on the Witwatersrand, South Africa. Community Dent Oral Epidemiol 1978;6(4):195–199
8. Larsson A, Almerén H. Ameloblastoma of the jaws. An analysis of a consecutive series of all cases reported to the Swedish Cancer Registry during 1958–1971. Acta Pathol Microbiol Scand A 1978;86A(5):337–349
9. Reichart PA, Philipsen HP, Sonner S. Ameloblastoma: biological profile of 3677 cases. Eur J Cancer B Oral Oncol 1995;31B(2):86–99
10. Gardner DG. Critique of the 1995 review by Reichart et al. of the biologic profile of 3677 ameloblastomas. Oral Oncol 1999;35(4):443–449
11. De Gandt J-B, Gerard M. Ameloblastoma of the maxillary sinus. [Article in French] Acta Otorhinolaryngol Belg 1974;28(3):365–368
12. Pantoja E, Kopp EA, Beecher TS. Maxillary ameloblastoma: report of a tumor originating in the antrum. Ear Nose Throat J 1976;55(11):358–361
13. Reaume C, Wesley RK, Jung B, Grammer FC. Clinical-pathological conference. Case 31, part 1. J Oral Surg 1980;38(6):435–437
14. Reaume C, Wesley RK, Jung B, Grammer FC. Clinico-pathological conference. Case 31, part 2. Ameloblastoma of the maxillary sinus. J Oral Surg 1980;38(7):520–521
15. Gaillard J, Haguenauer JP, Pignal JL, Dubreuil C. Ameloblastoma of the maxillary sinus. [Article in French] J Fr Otorhinolaryngol Audiophonol Chir Maxillofac 1981;30(2):107–110
16. Wenig BL, Sciubba JJ, Cohen A, Goldstein A, Abramson AL. An unusual cause of unilateral nasal obstruction: ameloblastoma. Otolaryngol Head Neck Surg 1985;93(3):426–432
17. Seabaugh JL, Templer JW, Havey A, Goodman D. Ameloblastoma presenting as a nasopharyngeal tumor. Otolaryngol Head Neck Surg 1986;94(2):265–267
18. Schafer DR, Thompson LD, Smith BC, Wenig BM. Primary ameloblastoma of the sinonasal tract: a clinicopathologic study of 24 cases. Cancer 1998;82(4):667–674
19. Regezi J, Sciubba J. Odontogenic tumours. Oral Pathology: Clinical Pathologic Correlations. 2nd ed. Philadelphia: WB Sanders; 1993:362–397
20. Ord RA, Blanchaert RH Jr, Nikitakis NG, Sauk JJ. Ameloblastoma in children. J Oral Maxillofac Surg 2002;60(7):762–770, discussion, 770–771
21. Arotiba GT, Ladeinde AL, Arotiba JT, Ajike SO, Ugboko VI, Ajayi OF. Ameloblastoma in Nigerian children and adolescents: a review of 79 cases. J Oral Maxillofac Surg 2005;63(6):747–751
22. Kumamoto H. Molecular pathology of odontogenic tumors. J Oral Pathol Med 2006;35(2):65–74
23. Praetorius F. Odontogenic tumours. In: Barnes L, ed. Surgical Pathology of the Head and Neck. 3rd ed. New York: Informa Healthcare; 2009:1208–1214, 1260–1261, 1272, 1306
24. Nakamura N, Higuchi Y, Mitsuyasu T, Sandra F, Ohishi M. Comparison of long-term results between different approaches to ameloblastoma. Oral Surg Oral Med Oral Pathol Oral Radiol Endod 2002;93(1):13–20
25. Ghandhi D, Ayoub AF, Pogrel MA, MacDonald G, Brocklebank LM, Moos KF. Ameloblastoma: a surgeon's dilemma. J Oral Maxillofac Surg 2006;64(7):1010–1014
26. Hayward JR. Recurrent ameloblastoma 30 years after surgical treatment. J Oral Surg 1973;31(5):368–370
27. Philipsen HP, Reichart PA, Takata T. Desmoplastic ameloblastoma (including "hybrid" lesion of ameloblastoma). Biological profile based on 100 cases from the literature and own files. Oral Oncol 2001;37(5):455–460
28. Thompson IO, van Rensburg LJ, Phillips VM. Desmoplastic ameloblastoma: correlative histopathology, radiology and CT-MR imaging. J Oral Pathol Med 1996;25(7):405–410
29. Eversole LR, Leider AS, Hansen LS. Ameloblastomas with pronounced desmoplasia. J Oral Maxillofac Surg 1984;42(11):735–740
30. Waldron CA, el-Mofty SK. A histopathologic study of 116 ameloblastomas with special reference to the desmoplastic variant. Oral Surg Oral Med Oral Pathol 1987;63(4):441–451
31. Takata T, Miyauchi M, Ogawa I, et al. Immunoexpression of transforming growth factor beta in desmoplastic ameloblastoma. Virchows Arch 2000;436(4):319–323
32. Philipsen HP, Ormiston IW, Reichart PA. The desmo- and osteoplastic ameloblastoma. Histologic variant or clinicopathologic entity? Case reports. Int J Oral Maxillofac Surg 1992;21(6):352–357
33. Ng KH, Siar CH. Desmoplastic variant of ameloblastoma in Malaysians. Br J Oral Maxillofac Surg 1993;31(5):299–303
34. Li TJ, Wu YT, Yu SF, Yu GY. Unicystic ameloblastoma: a clinicopathologic study of 33 Chinese patients. Am J Surg Pathol 2000;24(10):1385–1392
35. Philipsen HP, Reichart PA. Squamous odontogenic tumor (SOT): a benign neoplasm of the periodontium. A review of 36 reported cases. J Clin Periodontol 1996;23(10):922–926

36. Haghighat K, Kalmar JR, Mariotti AJ. Squamous odontogenic tumor: diagnosis and management. J Periodontol 2002;73(6):653–656

37. Pindborg J. Calcifying epithelial odontogenic tumours. Acta Pathol Microbiol Scand 1955;(Suppl 111):71

38. Pindborg JJ. A calcifying epithelial odontogenic tumor. Cancer 1958;11(4):838–843

39. Franklin CD, Pindborg JJ. The calcifying epithelial odontogenic tumor. A review and analysis of 113 cases. Oral Surg Oral Med Oral Pathol 1976;42(6):753–765

40. Philipsen HP, Reichart PA. Calcifying epithelial odontogenic tumour: biological profile based on 181 cases from the literature. Oral Oncol 2000;36(1):17–26

41. Sedghizadeh PP, Wong D, Shuler CF, Linz V, Kalmar JR, Allen CM. Multifocal calcifying epithelial odontogenic tumor. Oral Surg Oral Med Oral Pathol Oral Radiol Endod 2007;104(2):e30–e34

42. Bridle C, Visram K, Piper K, Ali N. Maxillary calcifying epithelial odontogenic (Pindborg) tumor presenting with abnormal eye signs: case report and literature review. Oral Surg Oral Med Oral Pathol Oral Radiol Endod 2006; 102(4):e12–e15

43. Kaplan I, Buchner A, Calderon S, Kaffe I. Radiological and clinical features of calcifying epithelial odontogenic tumour. Dentomaxillofac Radiol 2001;30(1):22–28

44. Anavi Y, Kaplan I, Citir M, Calderon S. Clear-cell variant of calcifying epithelial odontogenic tumor: clinical and radiographic characteristics. Oral Surg Oral Med Oral Pathol Oral Radiol Endod 2003;95(3):332–339

45. Sciubba J, Fantasia J, Kahn L. Tumors and Cysts of the Jaws. 3rd series. Washington, DC: Armed Forces Institute of Pathology; 2001:1–275

46. Kawano K, Ono K, Yada N, et al. Malignant calcifying epithelial odontogenic tumor of the mandible: report of a case with pulmonary metastasis showing remarkable response to platinum derivatives. Oral Surg Oral Med Oral Pathol Oral Radiol Endod 2007;104(1):76–81

47. Reichart P, Philipsen H. Adenomatoid odontogenic tumor. Odontogenic Tumors and Allied Lesions. London: Quintessence; 2004:105–155

48. Philipsen HP, Reichart PA, Siar CH, et al. An updated clinical and epidemiological profile of the adenomatoid odontogenic tumour: a collaborative retrospective study. J Oral Pathol Med 2007;36(7):383–393

49. Philipsen HP, Reichart PA. Adenomatoid odontogenic tumour: facts and figures. Oral Oncol 1999;35(2):125–131

50. Philipsen HP, Reichart PA, Zhang KH, Nikai H, Yu QX. Adenomatoid odontogenic tumor: biologic profile based on 499 cases. J Oral Pathol Med 1991;20(4):149–158

51. Giansanti JS, Someren A, Waldron CA. Odontogenic adenomatoid tumor (adenoameloblastoma). Survey of 3 cases. Oral Surg Oral Med Oral Pathol 1970;30(1):69–88

52. Takahashi K, Yoshino T, Hashimoto S. Unusually large cystic adenomatoid odontogenic tumour of the maxilla: case report. Int J Oral Maxillofac Surg 2001;30(2):173–175

53. Leon JE, Mata GM, Fregnani ER, et al. Clinicopathological and immunohistochemical study of 39 cases of adenomatoid odontogenic tumour: a multicentric study. Oral Oncol 2005;41(8):835–842

54. Philipsen H. Om Keratoyster (kolesteatomer) Kalberne. Tandlaegebladet 1956;60:936–969

55. Barreto DC, Gomez RS, Bale AE, Boson WL, De Marco L. PTCH gene mutations in odontogenic keratocysts. J Dent Res 2000;79(6):1418–1422

56. Gu XM, Zhao HS, Sun LS, Li TJ. PTCH mutations in sporadic and Gorlin-syndrome-related odontogenic keratocysts. J Dent Res 2006;85(9):859–863

57. Radden BG, Reade PC. Odontogenic keratocysts. Pathology 1973;5(4):325–334

58. Brannon RB. The odontogenic keratocyst. A clinicopathologic study of 312 cases. Part I. Clinical features. Oral Surg Oral Med Oral Pathol 1976;42(1):54–72

59. Gorlin RJ, Goltz RW. Multiple nevoid basal-cell epithelioma, jaw cysts and bifid rib. A syndrome. N Engl J Med 1960;262:908–912

60. Donatsky O, Hjörting-Hansen E, Philipsen HP, Fejerskov O. Clinical, radiologic, and histopathologic aspects of 13 cases of nevoid basal cell carcinoma syndrome. Int J Oral Surg 1976;5(1):19–28

61. Connor JM, Evans DA, Goose DH. Multiple odontogenic keratocysts in a case of the Noonan syndrome. Br J Oral Surg 1982;20(3):213–216

62. Shenoy P, Paulose KO, Al Khalifa S, Sharma RK. Odontogenic keratocyst involving the maxillary antrum. J Laryngol Otol 1988;102(12):1168–1171

63. Chuong R, Donoff RB, Guralnick W. The odontogenic keratocyst. J Oral Maxillofac Surg 1982;40(12):797–802

64. Myoung H, Hong SP, Hong SD, et al. Odontogenic keratocyst: Review of 256 cases for recurrence and clinicopathologic parameters. Oral Surg Oral Med Oral Pathol Oral Radiol Endod 2001;91(3):328–333

65. Lund VJ. Odontogenic keratocyst of the maxilla: a case report. Br J Oral Maxillofac Surg 1985;23(3):210–215

66. Sharpe PT. Neural crest and tooth morphogenesis. Adv Dent Res 2001;15:4–7

67. Cobourne MT, Sharpe PT. Tooth and jaw: molecular mechanisms of patterning in the first branchial arch. Arch Oral Biol 2003;48(1):1–14

68. Philipsen HP, Reichart PA, Praetorius F. Mixed odontogenic tumours and odontomas. Considerations on interrelationship. Review of the literature and presentation of 134 new cases of odontomas. Oral Oncol 1997;33(2):86–99

69. Chen Y, Li TJ, Gao Y, Yu SF. Ameloblastic fibroma and related lesions: a clinicopathologic study with reference to their nature and interrelationship. J Oral Pathol Med 2005;34(10):588–595

70. Chen Y, Wang JM, Li TJ. Ameloblastic fibroma: a review of published studies with special reference to its nature and biological behavior. Oral Oncol 2007;43(10):960–969

71. Takeda Y. So-called "immature dentinoma": a case presentation and histological comparison with ameloblastic fibrodentinoma. J Oral Pathol Med 1994;23(2):92–96

72. Reichart P, Philipsen H. Odontogenic Tumours and Allied Lesions. London: Quintessence; 2004

73. Gardner DG. The mixed odontogenic tumors. Oral Surg Oral Med Oral Pathol 1984;58(2):166–168

74. Slootweg P. Ameloblastic fibroma/fibrodentinoma. In: Barnes L, Everson J, Reichart P, Sidransky D, eds. World Health Oorganization Classification of Tumours. Pathology and Genetics of Head and Neck Tumours. Lyon: IARC Press; 2005:308

75. Favia GF, Di Alberti L, Scarano A, Piattelli A. Ameloblastic fibro-odontoma: report of two cases. Oral Oncol 1997; 33(6):444–446

76. Howell RM, Burkes EJ Jr. Malignant transformation of ameloblastic fibro-odontoma to ameloblastic fibrosarcoma. Oral Surg Oral Med Oral Pathol 1977;43(3):391–401

77. Herzog U, Putzke HP, Bienengräber V, Radke C. The ameloblastic fibro-odontoma—an odontogenic mixed tumor progressing into an odontogenic sarcoma. [Article in German] Dtsch Z Mund Kiefer Gesichtschir 1991;15(2):90–93

78. Gardner DG, Farquhar DA. A classification of dysplastic forms of dentin. J Oral Pathol 1979;8(1):28–46

79. Jing W, Xuan M, Lin Y, et al. Odontogenic tumours: a retrospective study of 1642 cases in a Chinese population. Int J Oral Maxillofac Surg 2007;36(1):20–25

80. Regezi JA, Kerr DA, Courtney RM. Odontogenic tumors: analysis of 706 cases. J Oral Surg 1978;36(10):771–778

81. Olgac V, Koseoglu BG, Aksakalli N. Odontogenic tumours in Istanbul: 527 cases. Br J Oral Maxillofac Surg 2006; 44(5):386–388

82. O'Grady JF, Radden BG, Reade PC. Odontomes in an Australian population. Aust Dent J 1987;32(3):196–199

83. Zachariades N, Koundouris J, Angelopoulous AP. Odontoma of the maxillary sinus: report of case. J Oral Surg 1981;39(9):697–698

84. Castro GW, Houston G, Weyrauch C. Peripheral odontoma: report of case and review of literature. ASDC J Dent Child 1994;61(3):209–213

85. McClure G. Odontoma of the nasopharynx. Arch Otolaryngol 1946;44:51–60

86. Jacobs HG. The period of hard substance formation in compound composite odontomas. A clinical/radiographic documentation. [Article in German] Dtsch Z Mund Kiefer Gesichtschir 1988;12(3):201–204

87. Hisatomi M, Asaumi JI, Konouchi H, Honda Y, Wakasa T, Kishi K. A case of complex odontoma associated with an impacted lower deciduous second molar and analysis of the 107 odontomas. Oral Dis 2002;8(2):100–105

88. Or S, Yücetaş S. Compound and complex odontomas. Int J Oral Maxillofac Surg 1987;16(5):596–599

89. Salama N, Hilmy A. Extensive complex composite odontome occupying the whole of the left maxilla. Br Dent J 1950;89(3):68–70

90. De Visscher JG, Güven O, Elias AG. Complex odontoma in the maxillary sinus. Report of 2 cases. Int J Oral Surg 1982;11(4):276–280

91. Friedrich RE, Siegert J, Donath K, Jäkel KT. Recurrent ameloblastic fibro-odontoma in a 10-year-old boy. J Oral Maxillofac Surg 2001;59(11):1362–1366

92. Tomizawa M, Otsuka Y, Noda T. Clinical observations of odontomas in Japanese children: 39 cases including one recurrent case. Int J Paediatr Dent 2005;15(1):37–43

93. Frissell CT, Shafer WG. Ameloblastic odontoma; report of a case. Oral Surg Oral Med Oral Pathol 1953;6(9):1129–1133

94. Silva CA. Odontoameloblastoma. Oral Surg Oral Med Oral Pathol 1956;9(5):545–552

95. Jacobsohn PH, Quinn JH. Ameloblastic odontomas. Report of three cases. Oral Surg Oral Med Oral Pathol 1968;26(6):829–836

96. LaBbiola JD, Steiner M, Bernstein ML, Verdi GD, Stannard PF. Odontoameloblastoma. J Oral Surg 1980;38(2):139–143

97. Kaugars GE, Zussmann HW. Ameloblastic odontoma (odonto-ameloblastoma). Oral Surg Oral Med Oral Pathol 1991;71(3):371–373

98. Mosqueda-Taylor A, Carlos-Bregni R, Ramírez-Amador V, Palma-Guzmán JM, Esquivel-Bonilla D, Hernández-Rojase LA. Odontoameloblastoma. Clinico-pathologic study of three cases and critical review of the literature. Oral Oncol 2002;38(8):800–805

99. Mosqueda-Taylor A. Odontoameloblastoma. In: Barnes L, Everson J, Reichart P, Sidransky D, eds. World Health Organization Classification of Tumours. Pathology and Genetics of Head and Neck Tumours. Lyon: IARC Press; 2005:312

100. Pindborg J, Kramer I. Histological Typing of Odontogenic Tumours, Jaw Cysts and Allied Lesions. Geneva: World Health Organization; 1971

101. Gorlin RJ, Pindborg JJ, Odont, Clausen FP, Vickers RA. The calcifying odontogenic cyst—a possible analogue of the cutaneous calcifying epithelioma of Malherbe. An analysis of fifteen cases. Oral Surg Oral Med Oral Pathol 1962;15:1235–1243

102. Buchner A. The central (intraosseous) calcifying odontogenic cyst: an analysis of 215 cases. J Oral Maxillofac Surg 1991;49(4):330–339

103. Ellis GL. Odontogenic ghost cell tumor. Semin Diagn Pathol 1999;16(4):288–292

104. Ikemura K, Horie A, Tashiro H, Nandate M. Simultaneous occurrence of a calcifying odontogenic cyst and its malignant transformation. Cancer 1985;56(12):2861–2864

105. Hong SP, Ellis GL, Hartman KS. Calcifying odontogenic cyst. A review of ninety-two cases with reevaluation of their nature as cysts or neoplasms, the nature of ghost cells, and subclassification. Oral Surg Oral Med Oral Pathol 1991;72(1):56–64

106. Castro V, Knezevic MR, Barrero MV, Diaz JM, Baez O, Castellano JJ. The central (intraosseus) epithelial odontogenic ghost cell tumor: Report of a case. Med Oral 1998;3(2):101–106

107. Handlers JP, Abrams AM, Melrose RJ, Danforth R. Central odontogenic fibroma: clinicopathologic features of 19 cases and review of the literature. J Oral Maxillofac Surg 1991;49(1):46–54

108. Kaffe I, Buchner A. Radiologic features of central odontogenic fibroma. Oral Surg Oral Med Oral Pathol 1994;78(6):811–818

109. Dahl EC, Wolfson SH, Haugen JC. Central odontogenic fibroma: review of literature and report of cases. J Oral Surg 1981;39(2):120–124

110. Odell E, Morgan P. Odontogenic tumours. Biopsy, Pathology of the Oral Tissues. London: Chapman and Hall Medical; 1998:365–439

111. James DR, Lucas VS. Maxillary myxoma in a child of 11 months. A case report. J Craniomaxillofac Surg 1987; 15(1):42–44

112. Leiberman A, Forte V, Thorner P, Crysdale W. Maxillary myxoma in children. Int J Pediatr Otorhinolaryngol 1990;18(3):277–284

113. Fenton S, Slootweg PJ, Dunnebier EA, Mourits MP. Odontogenic myxoma in a 17-month-old child: a case report. J Oral Maxillofac Surg 2003;61(6):734–736

114. Wachter BG, Steinberg MJ, Darrow DH, McGinn JD, Park AH. Odontogenic myxoma of the maxilla: a report of two pediatric cases. Int J Pediatr Otorhinolaryngol 2003;67(4):389–393

115. Boussault P, Boralevi F, Raux-Rakotomalala F, Chauvel A, Taïeb A, Léauté-Labrèze C. Odontogenic myxoma: a diagnosis to add to the list of facial tumours in infants. J Eur Acad Dermatol Venereol 2006;20(7):864–867

116. Slater LJ. Infantile lateral nasal myxoma: is it odontogenic? J Oral Maxillofac Surg 2004;62(3):391

117. Noffke CE, Raubenheimer EJ, Chabikuli NJ, Bouckaert MM. Odontogenic myxoma: review of the literature and report of 30 cases from South Africa. Oral Surg Oral Med Oral Pathol Oral Radiol Endod 2007;104(1):101–109

118. Peltola J, Magnusson B, Happonen RP, Borrman H. Odontogenic myxoma—a radiographic study of 21 tumours. Br J Oral Maxillofac Surg 1994;32(5):298–302

119. Buchner A, Odell E. Odontogenic myxoma/myxofibroma. In: Barnes L, Everson J, Reichart P, Sidransky D, eds. World Health Organization Classification of Tumours. Pathology and Genetics of Head and Neck Tumours. Lyon: IARC Press; 2005: 316–317

120. Li TJ, Sun LS, Luo HY. Odontogenic myxoma: a clinicopathologic study of 25 cases. Arch Pathol Lab Med 2006;130(12):1799–1806

121. Pahl S, Henn W, Binger T, Stein U, Remberger K. Malignant odontogenic myxoma of the maxilla: case with cytogenetic confirmation. J Laryngol Otol 2000;114(7):533–535

122. Brannon RB, Fowler CB, Carpenter WM, Corio RL. Cementoblastoma: an innocuous neoplasm? A clinicopathologic study of 44 cases and review of the literature with special emphasis on recurrence. Oral Surg Oral Med Oral Pathol Oral Radiol Endod 2002;93(3):311–320

123. Williams T. Aggressive odontogenic cysts and tumours. Oral Maxillofac Surg Clin North Am 1997;9:329–338

124. Laughlin EH. Metastasizing ameloblastoma. Cancer 1989;64(3):776–780

125. Ciment LM, Ciment AJ. Malignant ameloblastoma metastatic to the lungs 29 years after primary resection: a case report. Chest 2002;121(4):1359–1361

126. Goldenberg D, Sciubba J, Koch W, Tufano RP. Malignant odontogenic tumors: a 22-year experience. Laryngoscope 2004;114(10):1770–1774

127. Dhir K, Sciubba J, Tufano RP. Ameloblastic carcinoma of the maxilla. Oral Oncol 2003;39(7):736–741

128. Abiko Y, Nagayasu H, Takeshima M, et al. Ameloblastic carcinoma ex ameloblastoma: report of a case-possible involvement of CpG island hypermethylation of the p16 gene in malignant transformation. Oral Surg Oral Med Oral Pathol Oral Radiol Endod 2007;103(1):72–76

129. Philipsen HP, Reichart PA, Nikai H, Takata T, Kudo Y. Peripheral ameloblastoma: biological profile based on 160 cases from the literature. Oral Oncol 2001;37(1):17–27

130. Wettan HL, Patella PA, Freedman PD. Peripheral ameloblastoma: review of the literature and report of recurrence as severe dysplasia. J Oral Maxillofac Surg 2001;59(7):811–815

131. Shear M. Primary intra-alveolar epidermoid carcinoma of the jaw. J Pathol 1969;97(4):645–651

132. Eversole LR, Sabes WR, Rovin S. Aggressive growth and neoplastic potential of odontogenic cysts: with special reference to central epidermoid and mucoepidermoid carcinomas. Cancer 1975;35(1):270–282

133. To EH, Brown JS, Avery BS, Ward-Booth RP. Primary intraosseous carcinoma of the jaws. Three new cases and a review of the literature. Br J Oral Maxillofac Surg 1991;29(1):19–25

134. Thomas G, Pandey M, Mathew A, et al. Primary intraosseous carcinoma of the jaw: pooled analysis of world literature and report of two new cases. Int J Oral Maxillofac Surg 2001;30(4):349–355

135. Hansen LS, Eversole LR, Green TL, Powell NB. Clear cell odontogenic tumor—a new histologic variant with aggressive potential. Head Neck Surg 1985;8(2):115–123

136. Waldron CA, Small IA, Silverman H. Clear cell ameloblastoma—an odontogenic carcinoma. J Oral Maxillofac Surg 1985;43(9):707–717

137. Maiorano E, Altini M, Viale G, Piattelli A, Favia G. Clear cell odontogenic carcinoma. Report of two cases and review of the literature. Am J Clin Pathol 2001;116(1):107–114

138. Braunshtein E, Vered M, Taicher S, Buchner A. Clear cell odontogenic carcinoma and clear cell ameloblastoma: a single clinicopathologic entity? A new case and comparative analysis of the literature. J Oral Maxillofac Surg 2003;61(9):1004–1010

139. Takata T, Lu Y. Ghost cell odontogenic carcinoma. In: Barnes L, Everson J, Reichart P, Sidransky D, eds. World Health Organization Classification of Tumours. Pathology and Genetics of Head and Neck Tumours. Lyon: IARC Press; 2005:293

140. Bregni RC, Taylor AM, García AM. Ameloblastic fibrosarcoma of the mandible: report of two cases and review of the literature. J Oral Pathol Med 2001;30(5):316–320

141. Altini M, Thompson SH, Lownie JF, Berezowski BB. Ameloblastic sarcoma of the mandible. J Oral Maxillofac Surg 1985;43(10):789–794

142. Slater LJ. Odontogenic sarcoma and carcinosarcoma. Semin Diagn Pathol 1999;16(4):325–332

13 Tumors and Other Lesions of Bone

This section includes the following conditions:
- Fibrous dysplasia; no ICD-O code
- Ossifying fibroma; no ICD-O code
- Osteoma; ICD-O 9180
- Osteoblastoma; ICD-O 9200/0
- Osteoid osteoma; ICD-O 9191/0
- Aneurysmal bone cyst; no ICD-O code
- Giant cell lesion; no ICD-O code
- Giant cell tumor of bone; ICD-O 9250/1
- Cherubism; no ICD-O code
- "Brown tumor" of hyperparathyroidism; no ICD-O code
- Osseous metaplasia; no ICD-O code
- Paget's disease; no ICD-O code
- Osteosarcoma; ICD-O 9200/0

Benign Fibro-Osseous Lesions

Definition

This grouping comprises tumors and proliferative disorders that can affect the jaws in which the common denominator is replacement of normal bone architecture by collagen, fibroblasts, and varying amounts of bone or osteoid. They can range from incidental findings on imaging to massive disfiguring lesions and can affect all regions of the paranasal sinuses.[1-3] The commonest fibro-osseous lesions of the sinonasal tract are fibrous dysplasia and ossifying fibroma. Other lesions that are sometimes considered in this group include giant cell tumors and osteoblastoma, but it is an area subject to much change in pathological nomenclature to the extent that ossifying fibroma, as such, no longer features in the latest WHO classification (see pp. 42–44). A simpler classification of the conditions is shown in **Table 13.1** and the most important features of fibrous dysplasia, ossifying fibroma, and osteoma are shown in **Table 13.2**.

Given the considerable overlap in histological composition, the diagnosis can certainly be difficult for the histopathologist, who will often require clinical and

Table 13.1 Benign fibro-osseous disease

Fibromatosis	Ossifying fibroma
Developmental	Fibrous dysplasia
Reactive/reparative	Giant cell tumor
	"Brown tumor"
	Paget's disease
Neoplasms	Osteoma
	Osteoblastoma

radiological information in addition to the tissue and recourse to a dedicated bone pathologist may be necessary in some instances.

In our series of 112 cases of benign fibro-osseous conditions (**Table 13.3**), patients' age range was 2 to 80 years, mean 27 years, the ratio of men to women was 2.2:1 and the patients were referred by ophthalmologists (44%), or ENT colleagues (56%), most often with proptosis, diplopia, visual loss, and/or epiphora.

Key Points

Benign fibro-osseous disease:
- Exhibits a spectrum of disease.
- Is difficult to diagnose on histology alone.
- Requires clinical history, histology, and imaging to make diagnosis.
- Does not always require treatment!
- Requires an appropriate surgical approach to be chosen to encompass the lesion.

Fibrous Dysplasia

Definition

Fibrous dysplasia (FD) was first described by Lichtenstein in 1938 and later by Lichtenstein and Jaffe as a monostotic or polyostotic tumorlike lesion that is composed of fibrous stroma and osseous tissue.[1,5-7]

Etiology

Pensler et al[8] investigated cultures derived from the involved bone in two children with monostotic disease and in one child with McCune-Albright syndrome and showed a 2- to 3-fold increased level of estrogen and progesterone receptors by radioimmunoassay and immunocytochemical assay. From their results they concluded that estrogen may play a major role in the bony metabolism of FD. The actual cause of fibrous dysplasia and related disorders, including McCune-Albright syndrome, has recently been defined as a set of mutations in the *GNAS1* gene, located on chromosome 20q13.2, which normally codes for the α subunit of the G-protein.[9-11] It should, therefore, be regarded as a genetically based developmental anomaly and probably as a hamartomatous process.

Synonyms

Over 33 different terms have been used for this condition, ranging from focal fibrosis of bone through osteitis fibrosis localis to fibrosis chondroficans.

Table 13.2 Main characteristics of fibro-osseous lesions of the nose and paranasal sinuses

	Fibrous dysplasia	Ossifying fibroma	Osteoma
Incidence	Not known	Not known	0.43–3%
Most frequent site of origin	Mandible and maxilla	Mandible	Frontal sinus
Histology	Replacement of bone by fibrous tissue	Fibrous tissue, calcification	Ivory, mature, and mixed type
	Nonencapsulated	Capsulated	No separate capsule
	Bone nonlamellar and immature	Bone lamellar and surrounded by fibroblasts	
Age of presentation	First to second decade	Second to fourth decade	Third to fourth decade
Male-to-female ratio	1:1	1:5	1.5–3.1:1
Radiology	"Ground glass" appearance on CT	Expansile mass with sharp demarcation	Homogeneous, dense, well-circumscribed
Symptoms	Facial asymmetry	Painless swelling, nasal obstruction	Frontal headache
Growth	Slow, progressive but finite	Can be locally aggressive and continues after cessation of skeletal growth	Slow, progressive but may slow or stop with age
Malignant transformation	0.5% in polyostotic form	Not known	No reports
Treatment	Observation; surgery only in symptomatic cases	Observation; if possible complete surgical resection in extended cases	Observation in asymptomatic cases; surgery in symptomatic patients and complications

Source: From reference 4 with permission of *Rhinology*.

Table 13.3 Histopathology in our personal series (*n* = 112)

Osteoma	55
Ossifying fibroma	31
Fibrous dysplasia	18
Other, e.g., osteoblastoma	8
Total	**112**

Incidence

The incidence of FD involving the sinonasal system is not known.[12]

Site

Fibrous dysplasia can be polyostotic (15–30%), involving more than one bone, or monostotic (70–85%), involving only one bone.[13] The femur and other long bones are often involved as well as the jaws, skull, and ribs. Twenty-five percent of monostotic cases arise in the facial skeleton.[14] The maxilla and mandible are the most common sites in the head and neck, although it has been reported throughout the maxillofacial skeleton, including all the other paranasal sinuses.[13,15–17] In our cohort of 18 cases, 8 involved the sphenoid and orbital apex (**Figs. 13.1 and 13.2**). A third rare disseminated form, McCune-Albright

syndrome, has been described that is part of the polyostotic group.[12,18]

Diagnostic Features

Clinical Features

Fibrous dysplasia is variously described as more common in females than in males,[19,20] usually in the polyostotic forms, having a ratio of 1:1[19] in monostotic forms, or, as in our group of 18 cases, 2:1 (male-to-female ratio) (**Table 13.4**).

The condition usually presents in the first two decades.[1,12,21,22] The condition tends to stabilize after puberty and may burn out in the patient's thirties.[12,19] Our patient group ranged from 20 to 66 years with a mean age of 37 years. McCune-Albright syndrome, a polyostotic form of fibrous dysplasia characterized by precocious puberty and café au lait spots, is the rarest form and preferentially involves young girls.[23] Asymptomatic fibrous dysplasia is often an incidental finding on radiographs obtained for other reasons (trauma or evaluation of hearing loss). The sphenoid bone and central skull base are frequently involved in such cases.

Cosmetic changes due to facial swelling and asymmetry are the most common clinical signs.[14,17,22,24] These are

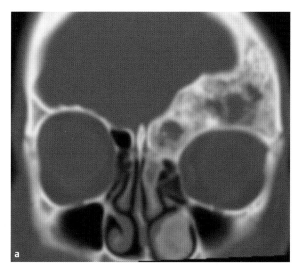

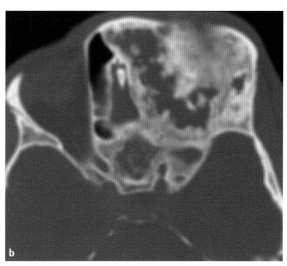

Fig. 13.1a,b

a Coronal CT scan showing fibrous dysplasia affecting the left frontal bone and middle and inferior turbinates in a 40-year-old man.

b Axial CT scan in the same patient showing extension into the sphenoid and ethmoid roof.

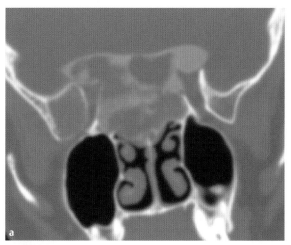

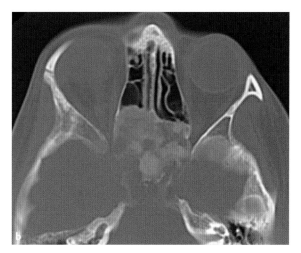

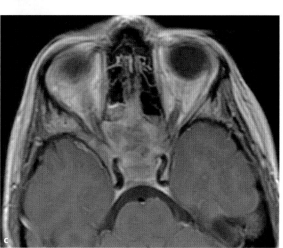

Fig. 13.2a–c

a Coronal CT showing fibrous dysplasia affecting the sphenoid with areas of cystic and ground glass appearance in a 28-year-old woman.

b Axial CT scan in the same patient showing compression of the orbital apices, for which an endoscopic decompression was undertaken on the right with improvement in visual acuity.

c Axial MRI (T1W post gadolinium enhancement) in the same patient showing fibrous dysplasia encroaching on the orbital apices and encasing the carotid arteries on each side.

Table 13.4 Major benign tumors of bone: personal series

	n	Age		M:F	CFR	MFD	OPF	LR	EFE	ESS	WW	Recurrence
		Range (y)	Mean (y)									
Osteoma	55	15–85	42	2:1	10	–	16	3	10	13	3	0%
Ossifying fibroma	31	7–59	24	21:10	6	13	4	1	3	4	–	11.5% (treated MFD (×2), ESS
Juvenile	20	6–20	11.3	9:1								
Nonjuvenile	11	22–59	40.5	2:3								
Fibrous dysplasia	18	20–66	37	2:1	2	–	–	–	3	10	3	N/A as all had residual disease

Abbreviations: CFR, craniofacial resection; EFE, external frontoethmoidectomy; ESS, endoscopic sinus surgery; F, female; LR, lateral rhinotomy; M, male; MFD, midfacial degloving; N/A, not applicable; OPF, osteoplastic flap; WW, watchful waiting; y, year(s).

most often painless but some patients may complain of pain, ocular symptoms, and neurological changes.[12,19,25,26] Proptosis is not uncommon and ultimately visual loss may occur but the nerve can withstand an impressive degree and duration of compromise when it occurs slowly (**Fig. 13.2**).

Imaging

For the diagnosis of FD the "ground glass" bone appearance on CT scans[27] with bone window is the most useful radiographic sign.[28] However, the lesion changes with time. Early lesions can be radiolucent or cystic, radiopaque in mid-stage lesions, and a mixture of radiolucent and radiopaque in late-stage lesions (**Figs. 13.1 and 13.2**). The lesion is not encapsulated and infiltrates the bone widely, sometimes spreading to adjacent bones (e.g., maxilla and zygoma).

FD is sometimes associated with expansion of the adjacent sinus or pneumosinus dilatans, a condition that has been described in association with meningioma, with FD, or spontaneously. It was first described by Benjamin in 1918[29] and more recently by Lloyd in 1985.[30]

Histological Features and Differential Diagnosis

The World Health Organization defined FD as "a nonencapsulated lesion showing replacement of normal bone by fibrous connective tissue of varying cellularity and containing islands of trabecular or immature nonlamellar metaplastic bone. Osteoblastic rimming is inconspicuous or absent."[31]

Histology shows slow replacement of medullary bone by abnormal fibrous tissue with different stages of bone metaplasia.[1,12] It must be distinguished from the "brown tumor" of hyperparathyroidism, from osseous metaplasia, and from osteosarcoma.[7]

Natural History

Growth is variable and usually slows after puberty, but this is not invariable.[32] However, in most cases the condition burns out in the patient's thirties. Fibrous dysplasia has a low rate of malignant transformation into osteosarcoma.[13,14,33] Transformation occurs in 0.5% of polyostotic forms and in 4% of lesions in patients with McCune-Albright syndrome.[13,34]

Treatment and Outcome

As the condition is eventually self-limiting in most cases, it may be best to adopt a policy of "watchful waiting," particularly as neither medical therapy nor surgery can readily cure the problem. Follow-up imaging every one or two years until there is no sign of change on sequential scans is recommended, but because the process is best shown on CT, there is an issue with regard to radiation, which should be considered and discussed with the patient. Radiotherapy is contraindicated in the treatment of the condition.

Medical therapy for FD is restricted to symptomatic relief. Bisphosphonates such as disodium pamidronate have been shown to decrease the incidence of fractures and bony pain[35–37] but also carry potential complications of their own such as osteonecrosis of the jaw.[38] The endocrinological effects of McCune-Albright syndrome can also be treated medically: octreotide can decrease growth hormone secretion; radioactive iodine, methimazole, and propylthiouracil can be applied for hyperthyroidism; spironolactone and ketoconazole can be used as antiandrogens.[27]

The decision to operate depends on the patient's symptoms, the extent of the disease, and the patient's age.[12,18,19,25,39] It is not possible to generalize as no large series exist in the literature. Remodeling of the facial contour may be considered but is probably best left until the disease has burnt out. Some authors have reported endonasal endoscopic treatment of FD, especially for the relief of ocular symptoms (optic nerve decompression) or chronic rhinosinusitis.[22,25,33,39–43] However, the bone is by definition abnormal and bleeds freely, so the procedure can be technically challenging and should only be contemplated by an experienced surgeon. Nonetheless, it is possible to remove involved bone in the medial half on the orbital apex extending to the canal and thus achieve space while the condition runs its course. This has been undertaken in 10 of our 18 cases with good effect, but the objective of the surgery is not cure. It is not normally necessary to incise the orbital periosteum/perineurium in these circumstances.

Key Points

- FD is a genetically based developmental anomaly.
- There is benign monostotic (80%) or polyostotic (20%) unencapsulated proliferation of fibrous tissue and woven bone.
- FD often starts when the patient is <20 years old and eventually stops growing in the majority but may continue into the late thirties or forties.
- Medical treatment is with bisphosphonates; if surgical treatment is needed, it should if possible be deferred until the condition is burnt out.

Ossifying Fibroma

Definition

Ossifying fibroma (OF) is a true benign encapsulated tumor composed of bone, fibrous tissue, calcification, and cementum.[1,44–46] The World Health Organization defined OF as "consisting of spindle-shaped fibroblastic cells usually arranged in a whorled pattern and containing small islands and spicules of metaplastic bone and mineralized masses. It may appear encapsulated. The bony spicules may rarely show a lamellar structure peripherally and are frequently rimmed by osteoblasts."

Etiology

The etiology of OF has so far not been clarified. Trauma has been reported to play a major role in the development of OF, especially of the cemento-ossifying fibroma.[47] It seems from studies on a small number of cases that there may also be a genetic basis.[48]

Synonyms

Ossifying fibroma was first described by Montgomery in 1927[49] and has its origin mostly in the mandibular bone.[45,50] A multiplicity of terms have been applied to this condition, including cemento-ossifying fibroma,

cementifying fibroma, and psammomatoid OF, although it has been suggested that these all relate to and should be replaced by juvenile active OF.[51]

Incidence

Terminological and histopathological confusion has made an accurate assessment of true incidence difficult. Eversole et al,[21] albeit 30 years ago, examined 841 cases of fibro-osseous disease, of whom 309 were diagnosed as having fibrous dysplasia and 225 ossifying fibroma. In our own series of 112 patients, 28% had ossifying fibroma (Table 13.4).

Site

OF can be found in any bones ossified in membrane and is most commonly located in the facial skeleton where it most often affects the mandible (~75% of cases) and where it can be clinically silent for a long period. However, OF can occasionally occur in other areas such as the maxilla (10–15%), and rarely the ethmoid bone including the middle turbinate and nasal cavity (Figs. 13.3, 13.4, 13.5).[20,45] The maxilla was the commonest area in our series of 31 cases (38%), although the nasal cavity, ethmoid, and frontal were also affected.

Diagnostic Features

Clinical Features

The literature suggests that OF is more frequent in women than men[8] with a male-to-female ratio of 1:5.[52] This has also been our experience in 11 cases affecting older patients (Table 13.4). Patients usually present between the second and fourth decades of life, somewhat older than those with fibrous dysplasia. The mean age of our patients was 40.5 years.

Depending on its extent, it can lead to swelling, facial pain, nasal obstruction, rhinosinusitis, and ocular symptoms such as proptosis, diplopia, and epiphora.[44,47,53,54] There may be changes to dentition if the alveolus is involved and distortion of the mid-face and external nose.

An aggressive variant of OF is termed "juvenile OF," which starts at an earlier age and was defined by Reed and Hagy[55] as "a localized actively growing destructive lesion occurring predominantly in children and teenagers." The terms "active" or "aggressive" are also included in the name by some authors. We have a group of 20 patients with age range 6 to 20 years, mean 11.3 years (Fig. 13.4). This condition predominantly affects male subjects (in our group 18:2) and is clinically more aggressive with extension of the tumor to the skull base and orbit.[56] The condition has been studied in 112 cases by Johnson et al[57] and appears to favor the ethmoid and frontal with maxillary lesions constituting 20%.

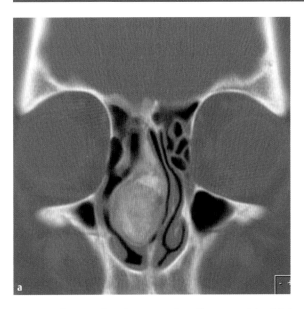
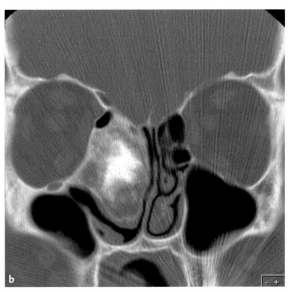

Fig. 13.3a, b Coronal CT showing ossifying fibroma involving (**a**) the middle turbinate and (**b**) the posterior ethmoid with attachment to the lamina papyracea and skull base in a 38-year-old man. Tumor was removed endoscopically with repair of the exposed dura.

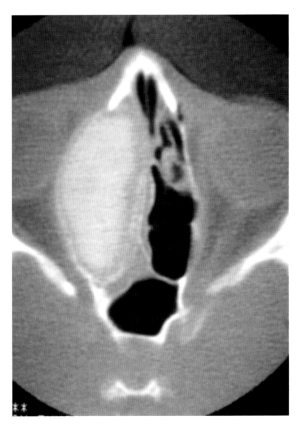

Fig. 13.4 Axial CT showing juvenile ossifying fibroma as a typical circumscribed lesion in the left ethmoids in a 15-year-old boy.

Imaging

CT images show a characteristic well-demarcated benign expansile mass covered by a thick shell of bone, sometimes with a multiloculated internal appearance and a content of varying density,[45,58] and as a consequence is sometimes mistaken for a mucocele. There may be areas of low density or scattered calcification. The mass expands, thins, and destroys adjacent bone, displacing structures such as teeth, nasal septum, the orbital contents, and the skull base (**Figs. 13.4, 13.5a**).

The MRI appearances will vary depending on the cystic change and calcification. However, the bony walls present signal voids or low density on T2W images and are isointense with gray matter on T1W scans. The contents are isointense with muscle on T1W and T2W scans and gadolinium contrast usually produces only mild homogeneous enhancement on T1W images (**Fig. 13.5c**).[59]

Histological Features and Differential Diagnosis

Macroscopically OF presents a circumscribed lesion with defined margins consisting of homogeneous pinkish gray granular/gritty material with a firm consistency. Microscopically it is composed of fibrous tissue with varying amounts of mineralized or calcified psammomatoid bodies.[60] This has led to the term "cementifying ossifying fibroma."

The juvenile OF is characteristically composed of "ossicles," a stroma, and "chondricles" in myxomatous areas. Some believe that this tumor derives from myxoid tissue, the precursor of cartilage and bone found in

Fig. 13.5a–c

a Coronal CT scan showing a lobulated mass of ossifying fibroma originating from the left ethmoidal roof and filling the nasal cavity in a 35-year-old woman.

b Axial CT in the same patient showing ossifying fibroma arising in the right nasal cavity but also extending into the left nasal cavity.

c Axial MRI (STIR) in the same patient showing heterogeneous signal from the ossifying fibroma.

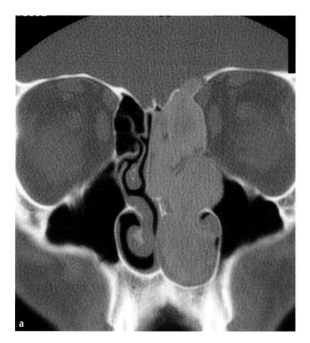

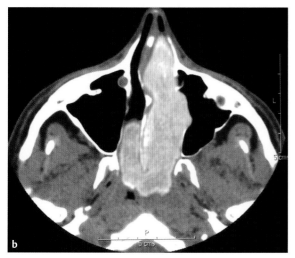

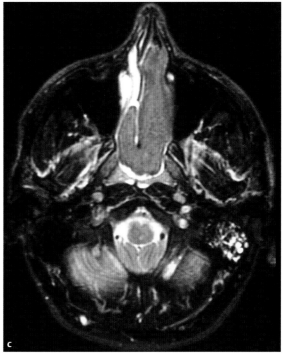

the septations of the paranasal sinuses where it forms the mucoperiosteum. In some individuals a completely myxomatous tumor can result (See Myxoma, p. 169).

As previously stated, distinguishing this lesion from fibrous dysplasia (and other fibro-osseous lesions) can be difficult on histology alone and clinical and radiological information must be provided to the histopathologist (Table 13.2).

Natural History

OF continues to grow throughout life and is therefore regarded as having a more aggressive behavior than fibrous dysplasia due to local destruction.

Treatment and Outcome

The treatment depends on the location but in general requires complete surgical resection. The lesion will regrow if not completely removed, so total extirpation should be undertaken whenever possible.[52,61] Due to its rarity, there are few large series in the literature that include a wide range of surgical approaches including craniofacial resection, midfacial degloving, and lateral rhinotomy as well as some case reports of entirely endoscopic resection.[45,47,62] Draf et al[63] reported on endonasal microendoscopic resection of four OFs without any complications. In two cases the surgery was done for optic nerve decompression. In OF with significant intracranial extension, most authors recommend a combined approach including craniofacial resection.[20,61,64] All 31 cases in our series underwent surgery (Table 13.4) which comprised midfacial degloving in 42%, craniofacial or osteoplastic flap approaches in 32%, and endoscopic resection in 13%.

Recurrence after surgery is directly related to the thoroughness of excision, but up to one-third of patients with the juvenile OF have recurrence despite repeated operations. In our series 10% (3 cases) recurred and were dealt with either by another midfacial degloving (2 cases) or endoscopic resection (1 case). Recurrence manifested itself 3, 6, and 10 years later and in one patient recurred again 18 years after the previous surgery, suggesting lifelong surveillance may be needed in selected cases.

Radiotherapy is not effective and could induce sarcomatous transformation.

Key Points

- OF is an encapsulated true benign neoplasm at one end of the benign fibro-osseous disease spectrum.
- There is proliferation of fibrous tissue and woven bone, sometimes with scattered cementum-like or psammomatoid spherules leading to the description of cementifying ossifying fibroma or the "juvenile" form which is more aggressive.
- It manifests as an often painless swelling that continues to grow slowly and is locally destructive.
- Treatment is by complete surgical excision by whatever approach appropriate.

References

1. Fu YS, Perzin KH. Non-epithelial tumors of the nasal cavity, paranasal sinuses, and nasopharynx. A clinicopathologic study. II. Osseous and fibro-osseous lesions, including osteoma, fibrous dysplasia, ossifying fibroma, osteoblastoma, giant cell tumor, and osteosarcoma. Cancer 1974;33(5):1289–1305
2. Senior BA, Lanza DC. Benign lesions of the frontal sinus. Otolaryngol Clin North Am 2001;34(1):253–267
3. Eller R, Sillers M. Common fibro-osseous lesions of the paranasal sinuses. Otolaryngol Clin North Am 2006;39(3):585–600, x
4. Lund VJ, Stammberger H, Nicolai P, et al. European position paper on endoscopic management of the nose, paranasal sinuses and skull base. Rhinol Suppl 2010;(22):1–143
5. Lichtenstein L. Polyostotic fibrous dysplasia. Arch Surg 1938;36:874–898
6. Lichenstein L, Jaffe H. Fibrous dysplasia of bone. Arch Pathol (Chic) 1942;33:777–816
7. Alawi F. Benign fibro-osseous diseases of the maxillofacial bones. A review and differential diagnosis. Am J Clin Pathol 2002;118(Suppl):S50–S70
8. Pensler JM, Langman CB, Radosevich JA, et al. Sex steroid hormone receptors in normal and dysplastic bone disorders in children. J Bone Miner Res 1990;5(5):493–498
9. Shenker A, Weinstein LS, Moran A, et al. Severe endocrine and nonendocrine manifestations of the McCune-Albright syndrome associated with activating mutations of stimulatory G protein GS. J Pediatr 1993;123(4):509–518
10. Ringel MD, Schwindinger WF, Levine MA. Clinical implications of genetic defects in G proteins. The molecular basis of McCune-Albright syndrome and Albright hereditary osteodystrophy. Medicine (Baltimore) 1996; 75(4):171–184
11. Levine MA. Clinical implications of genetic defects in G proteins: oncogenic mutations in G alpha s as the molecular basis for the McCune-Albright syndrome. Arch Med Res 1999;30(6):522–531
12. Ferguson BJ. Fibrous dysplasia of the paranasal sinuses. Am J Otolaryngol 1994;15(3):227–230
13. MacDonald-Jankowski DS. Fibro-osseous lesions of the face and jaws. Clin Radiol 2004;59(1):11–25
14. Tsai TL, Ho CY, Guo YC, Chen W, Lin CZ. Fibrous dysplasia of the ethmoid sinus. J Chin Med Assoc 2003;66(2):131–133
15. Waldron CA. Fibro-osseous lesions of the jaws. J Oral Maxillofac Surg 1993;51(8):828–835
16. Lustig LR, Holliday MJ, McCarthy EF, Nager GT. Fibrous dysplasia involving the skull base and temporal bone. Arch Otolaryngol Head Neck Surg 2001;127(10):1239–1247
17. Chan EK. Ethmoid fibrous dysplasia with anterior skull base and intraorbital extension. Ear Nose Throat J 2005;84(10):627–628
18. Ramsey HE, Strong EW, Frazell EL. Fibrous dysplasia of the craniofacial bones. Am J Surg 1968;116(4):542–547
19. Rojas R, Palacios E, Kaplan J, Wong LK. Fibrous dysplasia of the frontal sinus. Ear Nose Throat J 2004;83(1):14–15
20. Mehta D, Clifton N, McClelland L, Jones NS. Paediatric fibro-osseous lesions of the nose and paranasal sinuses. Int J Pediatr Otorhinolaryngol 2006;70(2):193–199
21. Eversole LR, Sabes WR, Rovin S. Fibrous dysplasia: a nosologic problem in the diagnosis of fibro-osseous lesions of the jaws. J Oral Pathol 1972;1(5):189–220

22. Mladina R, Manojlovic S, Markov-Glavas D, Heinrich Z. Isolated unilateral fibrous dysplasia of the sphenoid sinus. Ann Otol Rhinol Laryngol 1999;108(12):1181–1184

23. Pacini F, Perri G, Bagnolesi P, Cilotti A, Pinchera A. McCune-Albright syndrome with gigantism and hyperprolactinemia. J Endocrinol Invest 1987;10(4):417–420

24. Ozcan KM, Akdogan O, Gedikli Y, Ozcan I, Dere H, Unal T. Fibrous dysplasia of inferior turbinate, middle turbinate, and frontal sinus. B-ENT 2007;3(1):35–38

25. Ikeda K, Suzuki H, Oshima T, Shimomura A, Nakabayashi S, Takasaka T. Endonasal endoscopic management in fibrous dysplasia of the paranasal sinuses. Am J Otolaryngol 1997;18(6):415–418

26. Kim SW, Kim DW, Kong IG, et al. Isolated sphenoid sinus diseases: report of 76 cases. Acta Otolaryngol 2008;128(4):455–459

27. Hullar TE, Lustig LR. Paget's disease and fibrous dysplasia. Otolaryngol Clin North Am 2003;36(4):707–732

28. Tehranzadeh J, Fung Y, Donohue M, Anavim A, Pribram HW. Computed tomography of Paget disease of the skull versus fibrous dysplasia. Skeletal Radiol 1998;27(12):664–672

29. Benjamin C. Pneumosinus frontalis dilatans. Acta Otolaryngol 1918;1:412–422

30. Lloyd GA. Orbital pneumosinus dilatans. Clin Radiol 1985;36(4):381–386

31. Slootweg PJ. Maxillofacial fibro-osseous lesions: classification and differential diagnosis. Semin Diagn Pathol 1996;13(2):104–112

32. Chen YR, Fairholm D. Fronto-orbito-sphenoidal fibrous dysplasia. Ann Plast Surg 1985;15(3):190–203

33. London SD, Schlosser RJ, Gross CW. Endoscopic management of benign sinonasal tumors: a decade of experience. Am J Rhinol 2002;16(4):221–227

34. Schwartz DT, Alpert M. The malignant transformation of fibrous dysplasia. Am J Med Sci 1964;247:1–20

35. Liens D, Delmas PD, Meunier PJ. Long-term effects of intravenous pamidronate in fibrous dysplasia of bone. Lancet 1994;343(8903):953–954

36. Lala R, Matarazzo P, Bertelloni S, Buzi F, Rigon F, de Sanctis C. Pamidronate treatment of bone fibrous dysplasia in nine children with McCune-Albright syndrome. Acta Paediatr 2000;89(2):188–193

37. Zacharin M, O'Sullivan M. Intravenous pamidronate treatment of polyostotic fibrous dysplasia associated with the McCune Albright syndrome. J Pediatr 2000; 137(3):403–409

38. Crépin S, Laroche M-L, Sarry B, Merle L. Osteonecrosis of the jaw induced by clodronate, an alkylbiphosphonate: case report and literature review. Eur J Clin Pharmacol 2010;66(6):547–554

39. Kessler A, Berenholz LP, Segal S. Use of intranasal endoscopic surgery to relieve ostiomeatal complex obstruction in fibrous dysplasia of the paranasal sinuses. Eur Arch Otorhinolaryngol 1998;255(9):454–456

40. Brodish BN, Morgan CE, Sillers MJ. Endoscopic resection of fibro-osseous lesions of the paranasal sinuses. Am J Rhinol 1999;13(1):11–16

41. Kingdom TT, Delgaudio JM. Endoscopic approach to lesions of the sphenoid sinus, orbital apex, and clivus. Am J Otolaryngol 2003;24(5):317–322

42. Eviatar E, Vaiman M, Shlamkovitch N, Segal S, Kessler A, Katzenell U. Removal of sinonasal tumors by the endonasal endoscopic approach. Isr Med Assoc J 2004;6(6):346–349

43. Socher JA, Cassano M, Filheiro CA, Cassano P, Felippu A. Diagnosis and treatment of isolated sphenoid sinus disease: a review of 109 cases. Acta Otolaryngol 2008;128(9):1004–1010

44. Chong VF, Tan LH. Maxillary sinus ossifying fibroma. Am J Otolaryngol 1997;18(6):419–424

45. Choi YC, Jeon EJ, Park YS. Ossifying fibroma arising in the right ethmoid sinus and nasal cavity. Int J Pediatr Otorhinolaryngol 2000;54(2-3):159–162

46. Granados R, Carrillo R, Nájera L, García-Villanueva M, Patrón M. Psammomatoid ossifying fibromas: immunohistochemical analysis and differential diagnosis with psammomatous meningiomas of craniofacial bones. Oral Surg Oral Med Oral Pathol Oral Radiol Endod 2006;101(5):614–619

47. Yilmaz I, Bal N, Ozluoglu LN. Isolated cementoossifying fibroma of the ethmoid bulla: a case report. Ear Nose Throat J 2006;85(5):322–324

48. Sawyer JR, Tryka AF, Bell JM, Boop FA. Nonrandom chromosome breakpoints at Xq26 and 2q33 characterize cemento-ossifying fibromas of the orbit. Cancer 1995;76(10):1853–1859

49. Montgomery AH. Ossifying fibromas of the jaw. Arch Surg 1927;15:30–44

50. Kendi AT, Kara S, Altinok D, Keskil S. Sinonasal ossifying fibroma with fluid-fluid levels on MR images. AJNR Am J Neuroradiol 2003;24(8):1639–1641

51. Robinson R. Head and Neck Pathology: Atlas for Histologic and Cytologic Diagnosis. Philadelphia: Wolters Kluwer, Lippincott Williams and Wilkins; 2010:102

52. Commins DJ, Tolley NS, Milford CA. Fibrous dysplasia and ossifying fibroma of the paranasal sinuses. J Laryngol Otol 1998;112(10):964–968

53. Hauser MS, Freije S, Payne RW, Timen S. Bilateral ossifying fibroma of the maxillary sinus. Oral Surg Oral Med Oral Pathol 1989;68(6):759–763

54. Cheng C, Takahashi H, Yao K, et al. Cemento-ossifying fibroma of maxillary and sphenoid sinuses: case report and literature review. Acta Otolaryngol Suppl 2002; 547(547, Suppl)118–122

55. Reed RJ, Hagy DM. Benign nonodontogenic fibro-osseous lesions of the skull; Report of two cases. Oral Surg Oral Med Oral Pathol 1965;19:214–227

56. Khoury NJ, Naffaa LN, Shabb NS, Haddad MC. Juvenile ossifying fibroma: CT and MR findings. Eur Radiol 2002;12(Suppl 3):S109–S113

57. Johnson LC, Yousefi M, Vinh TN, Heffner DK, Hyams VJ, Hartman KS. Juvenile active ossifying fibroma. Its nature, dynamics and origin. Acta Otolaryngol Suppl 1991;488(Suppl):1–40

58. Levine PA, Wiggins R, Archibald RW, Britt R. Ossifying fibroma of the head and neck: involvement of the temporal bone- and unusual and challenging site. Laryngoscope 1981;91(5):720–725

59. Bendet E, Bakon M, Talmi YP, Tadmor R, Kronenberg J. Juvenile cemento-ossifying fibroma of the maxilla. Ann Otol Rhinol Laryngol 1997;106(1):75–78

60. Wenig BM, Vinh TN, Smirniotopoulos JG, Fowler CB, Houston GD, Heffner DK. Aggressive psammomatoid ossifying fibromas of the sinonasal region: a clinicopathologic study of a distinct group of fibro-osseous lesions. Cancer 1995;76(7):1155–1165

61. Lund VJ, Howard DJ, Wei WI, Cheesman AD. Craniofacial resection for tumors of the nasal cavity and paranasal sinuses—a 17-year experience. Head Neck 1998;20(2):97–105

62. Post G, Kountakis SE. Endoscopic resection of large sinonasal ossifying fibroma. Am J Otolaryngol 2005;26(1):54–56

63. Draf W, Schick B, Weber R, Keerl R, Saha A. Endonasal micro-endoscopic surgery of nasal and paranasal-sinuses tumors. In: Stamm AC, Draf W, eds. Micro-Endoscopic Surgery of the Paranasal Sinuses and the Skull Base. Berlin: Springer; 2000:481–8

64. Howard DJ, Lund VJ, Wei WI. Craniofacial resection for tumors of the nasal cavity and paranasal sinuses: a 25-year experience. Head Neck 2006;28(10):867–873

Osteoma

Definition

(ICD-O code 9180)

A slow-growing benign bony tumor.

Etiology

There is some debate whether osteomas are tumors or merely reactive bone hyperplasia due to some irritant stimulus. There are three main theories: developmental, traumatic, and infectious. In the developmental theory, previously silent embryonic stem cells become activated later in life and lead to uncontrolled bone formation. In the traumatic and infectious theories, an inflammatory process is regarded as the inciting factor for the osteoma formation.[1–4]

The predilection for osteomas to occur in the sinuses near the junction between the skull vault (formed in membrane) and skull base (formed in cartilage) suggests an area of instability and supports the developmental theory.

Gardner's syndrome is a rare autosomal dominant condition of multiple osteomas in the skull associated with colonic polyps, which may become malignant, and other soft tissue tumors.[5]

History and Synonyms

Viega is credited as being the first physician who reported a sinus osteoma case, which was successfully removed by him in 1506.[6,7] Vallisnieri described the true bony origin of sinonasal osteoma in 1733, and in 1857 Bickersteth reported an antral osteoma that he had to saw in half to remove.[8–10]

Incidence

Osteoma is the most common bone tumor of the facial region.[11] The incidence of osteoma ranges from 0.43%[12] (skull radiographic study) to 3% in an analysis of CT scans.[13] This figure of 3% was confirmed in a more recent prospective study of 1,889 CT scans done for chronic sinus disease.[14] It has been suggested that there were some geographic/ethnic variations with large series being reported from Egypt,[15] but this may have simply reflected local patterns of referral.

Site

Osteoma is a benign, slowly growing neoplasm and arises mostly from the frontal sinus (57%) followed by the ethmoid, maxillary sinus, and sphenoid sinus.[8,13,16–20] A number cross the midline, especially in the frontal region, and can become markedly bilateral (**Figs. 13.6, 13.7, 13.8**).

Diagnostic Features

Clinical Features

The male-to-female ratio ranges from 1.5:1 to 3.1:1 with a male predominance in most series.[3,4,7,8,20,21] Osteomas may be diagnosed at any age but mostly between the third and fourth decades of life.[8,21,22] In our series of 55 cases, the age ranged from 15 to 85 years (mean 42 years) with a male-to-female ratio of 2:1 (**Table 13.4**).

The most common clinical symptom of osteoma is frontal headache or facial pain, and as many as 60% of patients with frontal sinus osteoma complain of headaches.[8,11,19–21,23,24] However, it should be noted that patients with headache are frequently scanned, which brings to light the bony lesion. It is doubtful whether the osteoma per se is responsible for pain; if it is associated at all, it is most probably due to obstruction of the sinuses leading to retention of secretions and possible chronic rhinosinusitis or mucocele formation (see pp. 403–404).[8,25,26] This is supported by the fact that in many patients with an osteoma, the diagnosis is made incidentally on radiological imaging obtained for other reasons and are otherwise asymptomatic.[27]

With time, however, large osteomas may lead to orbital and/or intracranial complications. Several authors have reported osteomas causing orbital symptoms such as diplopia, epiphora, facial distortion, and even blindness.[1,20,28–36] Intracranial complications occur when osteomas impinge on the dura. This may lead to CSF leakage, meningitis, brain abscess, or pneumatocele as a first symptom.[7,17,37–57] Strong nose-blowing can also force air into the orbit, producing emphysema there, as well as into the intracranial compartment.[58]

Imaging

Osteomas are an incidental finding on 0.1 to 1% of radiographs and scans. On CT scans osteomas appear as homogeneous, very dense and well-circumscribed lesions (**Figs. 13.6, 13.7, 13.8**). Osteomas are often lobulated and invaginate into the contours of the sinus, so it can be difficult to determine the exact site of origin. MRI can be helpful[11,18] in more complex cases that have encroached on the intracranial compartment or in patients who present with proptosis while pregnant (**Fig. 13.9**).

Histological Features and Differential Diagnosis

Histologically, three different types of osteoma can be distinguished. The eburnated type is composed of dense cortical bone and is also known as the ivory or compact osteoma. The mature type, also called osteoma spongiosum, contains cancellous bone separated by moderately cellular fibrous tissue.[59] These must be distinguished

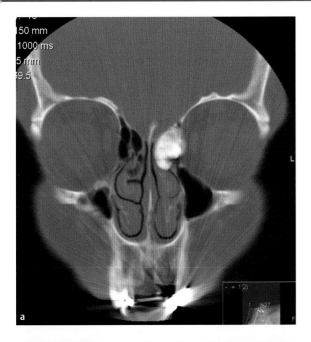

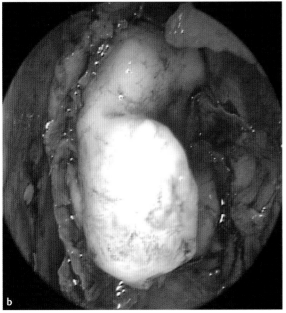

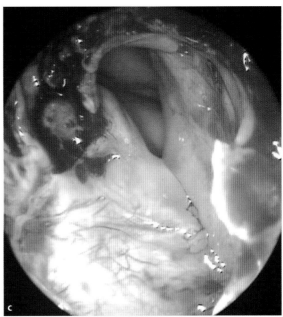

Fig. 13.6a–c

a Coronal CT scan showing a small osteoma arising in the superior middle meatus and originating from lamina papyracea.

b Endoscopic photograph during removal of the osteoma.

c Endoscopic photograph after removal of the osteoma, allowing a view into the previously obstructed frontal sinus.

from ossifying fibromas. The mixed form contains elements of both ivory and mature types.[7,8,21,23,32,33] The ivory osteomas are so dense that one or two months of decalcification can be required before they can be sectioned for histology.

Natural History

The growth rate of osteomas ranges from 0.44 to 6.0 mm/year.[60] Malignant transformation of osteomas has never been described.[25]

Treatment and Outcome

The only treatment is surgical resection but most authors agree that small, asymptomatic lesions can be left with a "wait and scan" policy involving a couple of sequential scans over several years.[8,20,25] Rapid growth of the tumor and those with the symptoms of chronic rhinosinusitis, significant headaches or facial deformity should be offered surgery.[8,20,21,52] Smith and Calcaterra[27] recommended surgery if the tumor occupies more than 50% of the frontal sinus.

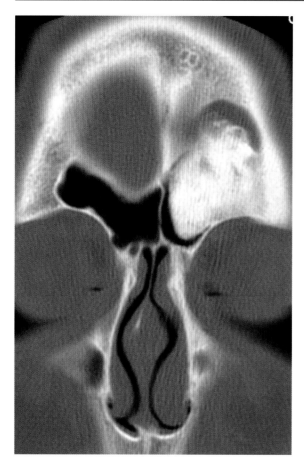

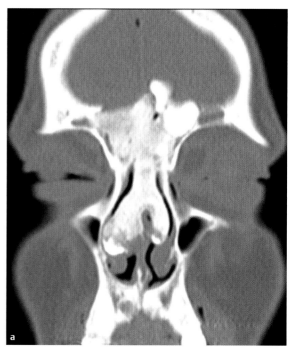

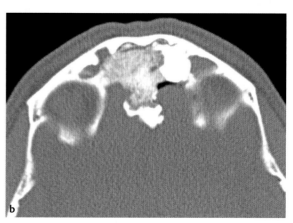

Fig. 13.7 Coronal CT scan showing osteoma in the left frontal sinus with opacification in the lateral sinus, requiring an osteoplastic flap approach for removal.

In general the surgical approaches can be classified as endonasal/endoscopic, external, or combined procedures. External or combined procedures are required for large frontal and frontoethmoidal osteomas; these can be an external frontoethmoidectomy, an osteoplastic flap via a coronal incision, or even a craniofacial resection.[11,20,61,62] Large series on endoscopic removal of paranasal sinus osteomas are rare (**Fig. 13.6b, c**).[19,23,63] Table 13.5 shows series ($n > 8$) where osteomas have been treated by an entirely endonasal/endoscopic approach.

Sometimes the osteoma grows from a small origin from which it can be easily detached or it may be a more diffuse area where it is less easy to distinguish between the osteoma and the underlying bone, particularly the diploic bone in the frontal region. By following the mucosa around the osteoma it is often possible to define the margin of the lesion, but it should always be borne in mind that the underlying bone of the sinus wall can be very thinned or dehiscent. Even with external approaches it may be necessary to divide up the osteoma with a fissure or small rose-head bur to facilitate removal. The overlying bone, particularly in the frontal region, can be

Fig. 13.8a, b

a Coronal CT scan showing a large osteoma involving both frontal sinuses and the septum and extending into both nasal cavities.

b Axial CT scan of the same patient showing extension of the osteoma posteriorly into the anterior cranial fossa with opacification of both lateral frontal sinuses. The lesion was removed via a craniofacial approach.

distorted and attempts may be made to recontour it, but with time it will often remodel. On the posterior wall, if there is a large area of bone dehiscence and the dura is thinned, it is advisable to reinforce the area with fascia lata or similar tissue to avoid frontal lobe prolapse, which we have encountered on a couple of occasions.

Displacement of the eye will resolve after removal of the osteoma as the lamina is generally very thinned or dehiscent, and the patient should be warned that this rapid repositioning of the eye may be associated with diplopia, which is usually temporary.

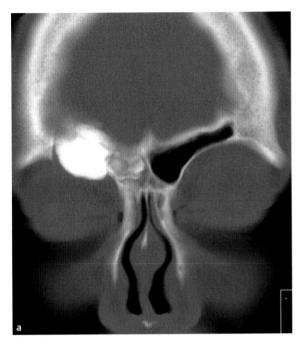
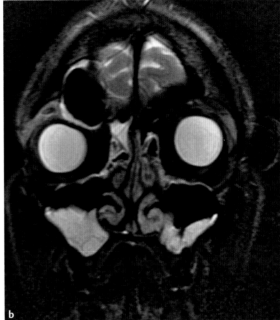

Fig. 13.9a, b

a Coronal CT scan showing an osteoma in the right frontal sinus impinging on the right eye.

b Coronal MRI (T2W fat saturation) in the same patient showing the osteoma as a signal void with inflammatory change in the sinus mucosa.

Table 13.5 Endonasal endoscopic resection of paranasal sinus osteomas

Author	No. of patients	Most common location	Follow-up (mo)	Recurrence
Bignami et al[64]	11	FS	40	0
Brodish et al[19]	9	Eth	1–17	0
Castelnuovo et al[65]	22	Eth	53	0
Schick et al[20]	23	FS	11	3 residual
Seiberling et al[66]	23	FS	36	0
Lund	13	Eth	6–60	0

Abbreviations: FS, frontal sinus; Eth, ethmoid cells; mo, month(s).
Source: Modified from Lund VJ, Stammberger H, Nicolai P, et al. European position paper on endoscopic management of tumours of the nose, paranasal sinuses and skull base. Rhinol Suppl 2010;(22):1–143 with permission from *Rhinology*.

With endoscopic excision, except for small lesions that can be removed in their entirety, it is often necessary to drill out the lesion from within so that the residual outer layer can be dissected free of the soft tissues and in-fractured prior to removal. This has been described as "cavitation." Image guidance may facilitate this process.[67] The lateral limitation of an endoscopic excision is one that extends or arises lateral to the midpoint of the eye. Combined external and endoscopic surgery will be needed when the frontal sinus has an anteroposterior diameter of less than 10 mm. There may be thinning of the dura and the patient should be forewarned about possible CSF leakage following removal of the osteoma. Thinned areas

and any leaks should be repaired at the time of surgery by whatever method the surgeon prefers.

In our series of 55 cases, the commonest operation was an osteoplastic flap followed by endoscopic surgery, external frontoethmoidectomy, and craniofacial resection. In 3 patients (6%) they remain simply under observation.

For the rarer maxillary osteomas, the same debate pertains—open versus endoscopic or combinations thereof. A midfacial degloving avoids facial scars of a lateral rhinotomy, or worse a conventional maxillectomy incision, while affording wide access for larger lesions. Smaller osteomas can be excised via an endonasal endoscopic approach extended to an endoscopic medial maxillectomy or combined with an anterior antrostomy. A comparison of the open versus endoscopic philosophy for maxillofacial osteomas is nicely considered by Castelnuovo and colleagues.[65]

Key Points

- Osteoma is the most common bone tumor of the facial region.
- Osteomas are frequent incidental findings and on CT scans appear as homogeneous, very dense and well-circumscribed lesions.
- Osteomas may be asymptomatic but can be associated with symptoms due to obstruction of a paranasal sinus or by spread into the orbit and skull base.
- Osteomas only cause headache by secondary obstruction of a paranasal sinus.
- Treatment is complete surgical excision if required.

References

1. Sayan NB, Uçok C, Karasu HA, Günhan O. Peripheral osteoma of the oral and maxillofacial region: a study of 35 new cases. J Oral Maxillofac Surg 2002;60(11):1299–1301
2. Naraghi M, Kashfi A. Endonasal endoscopic resection of ethmoido-orbital osteoma compressing the optic nerve. Am J Otolaryngol 2003;24(6):408–412
3. Moretti A, Croce A, Leone O, D'Agostino L. Osteoma of maxillary sinus: case report. Acta Otorhinolaryngol Ital 2004;24(4):219–222
4. Larrea-Oyarbide N, Valmaseda-Castellón E, Berini-Aytés L, Gay-Escoda C. Osteomas of the craniofacial region. Review of 106 cases. J Oral Pathol Med 2008;37(1):38–42
5. Gardner EJ, Richards RC. Multiple cutaneous and subcutaneous lesions occurring simultaneously with hereditary polyposis and osteomatosis. Am J Hum Genet 1953; 5(2):139–147
6. Teed RW. Primary osteoma of the frontal sinus. Arch Otolaryngol 1941;33:255–292
7. Summers LE, Mascott CR, Tompkins JR, Richardson DE. Frontal sinus osteoma associated with cerebral abscess formation: a case report. Surg Neurol 2001;55(4):235–239
8. Broniatowski M. Osteomas of the frontal sinus. Ear Nose Throat J 1984;63(6):267–271
9. Senior BA, Lanza DC. Benign lesions of the frontal sinus. Otolaryngol Clin North Am 2001;34(1):253–267
10. Eller R, Sillers M. Common fibro-osseous lesions of the paranasal sinuses. Otolaryngol Clin North Am 2006; 39(3):585–600, x
11. Strek P, Zagólski O, Składzień J, Kurzyński M, Dyduch G. Osteomas of the paranasal sinuses: surgical treatment options. Med Sci Monit 2007;13(5):CR244–CR250
12. Childrey JH. Osteoma of the sinuses, the frontal and the sphenoid bone: report of fifteen cases. Arch Otolaryngol 1939;30:63–72
13. Earwaker J. Paranasal sinus osteomas: a review of 46 cases. Skeletal Radiol 1993;22(6):417–423
14. Erdogan N, Demir U, Songu M, Ozenler NK, Uluç E, Dirim B. A prospective study of paranasal sinus osteomas in 1,889 cases: changing patterns of localization. Laryngoscope 2009;119(12):2355–2359
15. Handousa A. Nasal osteomata. J Laryngol Otol 1940; 55:197–211
16. Soboroff BJ, Nykiel F. Surgical treatment of large osteomas of the ethmo-frontal region. Laryngoscope 1966;76(6):1068–1081
17. Mendelsohn DB, Hertzanu Y, Friedman R. Frontal osteoma with spontaneous subdural and intracerebral pneumatocele. J Laryngol Otol 1984;98(5):543–545
18. Namdar I, Edelstein DR, Huo J, Lazar A, Kimmelman CP, Soletic R. Management of osteomas of the paranasal sinuses. Am J Rhinol 1998;12(6):393–398
19. Brodish BN, Morgan CE, Sillers MJ. Endoscopic resection of fibro-osseous lesions of the paranasal sinuses. Am J Rhinol 1999;13(1):11–16
20. Schick B, Steigerwald C, el Rahman el Tahan A, Draf W. The role of endonasal surgery in the management of fronto-ethmoidal osteomas. Rhinology 2001;39(2):66–70
21. Atallah N, Jay MM. Osteomas of the paranasal sinuses. J Laryngol Otol 1981;95(3):291–304
22. Samy LL, Mostafa H. Osteomata of the nose and paranasal sinuses with a report of twenty one cases. J Laryngol Otol 1971;85(5):449–469
23. Seiden AM, el Hefny YI. Endoscopic trephination for the removal of frontal sinus osteoma. Otolaryngol Head Neck Surg 1995;112(4):607–611
24. Boysen M. Osteomas of the paranasal sinuses. J Otolaryngol 1978;7(4):366–370
25. Schick B, Dlugaiczyk J. Benign tumors of the nasal cavity and paranasal sinuses. In: Stucker FJ, Souza C, Kenyon GS, Lian TS, Draf W, Schick B, eds. Rhinology and Facial Plastic Surgery. Heidelberg: Springer; 2009:377–386
26. Lund VJ. Anatomical considerations in the aetiology of fronto-ethmoidal mucoceles. Rhinology 1987;25(2):83–88
27. Smith ME, Calcaterra TC. Frontal sinus osteoma. Ann Otol Rhinol Laryngol 1989;98(11):896–900
28. Ataman M, Ayas K, Gürsel B. Giant osteoma of the frontal sinus. Rhinology 1993;31(4):185–187
29. Mansour AM, Salti H, Uwaydat S, Dakroub R, Bashshour Z. Ethmoid sinus osteoma presenting as epiphora and orbital cellulitis: case report and literature review. Surv Ophthalmol 1999;43(5):413–426
30. Kim AW, Foster JA, Papay FA, Wright KW. Orbital extension of a frontal sinus osteoma in a thirteen-year-old girl. J AAPOS 2000;4(2):122–124
31. Huang HM, Liu CM, Lin KN, Chen HT. Giant ethmoid osteoma with orbital extension, a nasoendoscopic approach using an intranasal drill. Laryngoscope 2001;111(3):430–432
32. Naraghi M, Kashfi A. Endonasal endoscopic resection of ethmoido-orbital osteoma compressing the optic nerve. Am J Otolaryngol 2003;24(6):408–412
33. Osma U, Yaldiz M, Tekin M, Topcu I. Giant ethmoid osteoma with orbital extension presenting with epiphora. Rhinology 2003;41(2):122–124
34. Tsai CJ, Ho CY, Lin CZ. A huge osteoma of paranasal sinuses with intraorbital extension presenting as diplopia. J Chin Med Assoc 2003;66(7):433–435
35. Dispenza C, Martines F, Dispenza F, Caramanna C, Saraniti C. Frontal sinus osteoma complicated by palpebral abscess: case report. Acta Otorhinolaryngol Ital 2004;24(6):357–360
36. Karapantzos I, Detorakis ET, Drakonaki EE, Ganasouli DL, Danielides V, Kozobolis VP. Ethmoidal osteoma with intraorbital extension: excision through a transcutaneous paranasal incision. Acta Ophthalmol Scand 2005;83(3):392–394
37. Hardwidge C, Varma TR. Intracranial aeroceles as a complication of frontal sinus osteoma. Surg Neurol 1985; 24(4):401–404
38. Ferlito A, Pesavento G, Recher G, et al. Intracranial pneumocephalus (secondary to frontoethmoidal osteoma). J Laryngol Otol 1989;103(6):634–637

39. Huneidi AH, Afshar F. Chronic spontaneous tension pneumocephalus due to benign frontal sinus osteoma. Br J Neurosurg 1989;3(3):389–392
40. Jackson WA, Bell KA. Pneumocephalus associated with a frontoethmoidal osteoma. J La State Med Soc 1989;141(12):33–34, 37
41. George J, Merry GS, Jellett LB, Baker JG. Frontal sinus osteoma with complicating intracranial aerocele. Aust N Z J Surg 1990;60(1):66–68
42. Lunardi P, Missori P, Di Lorenzo N, Fortuna A. Giant intracranial mucocele secondary to osteoma of the frontal sinuses: report of two cases and review of the literature. Surg Neurol 1993;39(1):46–48
43. Rappaport JM, Attia EL. Pneumocephalus in frontal sinus osteoma: a case report. J Otolaryngol 1994;23(6):430–436
44. Brunori A, Bruni P, Delitala A, Greco R, Chiappetta F. Frontoethmoidal osteoma complicated by intracranial mucocele and hypertensive pneumocephalus: case report. Neurosurgery 1995;36(6):1237–1238
45. Brunori A, de Santis S, Bruni P, Delitala A, Giuffre R, Chiappetta F. Life threatening intracranial complications of frontal sinus osteomas: report of two cases. Acta Neurochir (Wien) 1996;138(12):1426–1430
46. Maiuri F, Iaconetta G, Giamundo A, Stella L, Lamaida E. Fronto-ethmoidal and orbital osteomas with intracranial extension. Report of two cases. J Neurosurg Sci 1996;40(1):65–70
47. Marras LC, Kalaparambath TP, Black SE, Rowed DW. Severe tension pneumocephalus complicating frontal sinus osteoma. Can J Neurol Sci 1998;25(1):79–81
48. Koyuncu M, Belet U, Seşen T, Tanyeri Y, Simşek M. Huge osteoma of the frontoethmoidal sinus with secondary brain abscess. Auris Nasus Larynx 2000;27(3):285–287
49. Nakajima Y, Yoshimine T, Ogawa M, et al. A giant intracranial mucocele associated with an orbitoethmoidal osteoma. Case report. J Neurosurg 2000;92(4):697–701
50. Johnson D, Tan L. Intraparenchymal tension pneumatocele complicating frontal sinus osteoma: case report. Neurosurgery 2002;50(4):878–879, discussion 880
51. Nabeshima K, Marutsuka K, Shimao Y, Uehara H, Kodama T. Osteoma of the frontal sinus complicated by intracranial mucocele. Pathol Int 2003;53(4):227–230
52. Akay KM, Ongürü O, Sirin S, Celasun B, Gönül E, Timurkaynak E. Association of paranasal sinus osteoma and intracranial mucocele—two case reports. Neurol Med Chir (Tokyo) 2004;44(4):201–204
53. Gezici AR, Okay O, Ergün R, Dağlioğlu E, Ergüngör F. Rare intracranial manifestations of frontal osteomas. Acta Neurochir (Wien) 2004;146(4):393–396, discussion 396
54. Roca B, Casado O, Borras JM, Gonzalez-Darder JM. Frontal brain abscess due to Streptococcus pneumoniae associated with an osteoma. Int J Infect Dis 2004;8(3):193
55. Panagiotopoulos V, Tzortzidis F, Partheni M, Iliadis H, Fratzoglou M. Giant osteoma of the frontoethmoidal sinus associated with two cerebral abscesses. Br J Oral Maxillofac Surg 2005;43(6):523–525
56. Onal B, Kaymaz M, Araç M, Doğulu F. Frontal sinus osteoma associated with pneumocephalus. Diagn Interv Radiol 2006;12(4):174–176
57. Umur AS, Gunhan K, Songu M, Temiz C, Yuceturk AV. Frontal sinus osteoma complicated with intracranial inflammatory polyp: a case report and review of the literature. Rev Laryngol Otol Rhinol (Bord) 2008;129(4-5):333–336
58. Jack LS, Smith TL, Ng JD. Frontal sinus osteoma presenting with orbital emphysema. Ophthal Plast Reconstr Surg 2009;25(2):155–157
59. Fu YS, Perzin KH. Non-epithelial tumors of the nasal cavity, paranasal sinuses, and nasopharynx. A clinicopathologic study. II. Osseous and fibro-osseous lesions, including osteoma, fibrous dysplasia, ossifying fibroma, osteoblastoma, giant cell tumor, and osteosarcoma. Cancer 1974;33(5):1289–1305
60. Koivunen P, Löppönen H, Fors AP, Jokinen K. The growth rate of osteomas of the paranasal sinuses. Clin Otolaryngol Allied Sci 1997;22(2):111–114
61. Savić DL, Djerić DR. Indications for the surgical treatment of osteomas of the frontal and ethmoid sinuses. Clin Otolaryngol Allied Sci 1990;15(5):397–404
62. Howard DJ, Lund VJ, Wei WI. Craniofacial resection for tumors of the nasal cavity and paranasal sinuses: a 25-year experience. Head Neck 2006;28(10):867–873
63. Akmansu H, Eryilmaz A, Dagli M, Korkmaz H. Endoscopic removal of paranasal sinus osteoma: a case report. J Oral Maxillofac Surg 2002;60(2):230–232
64. Bignami M, Dallan I, Terranova P, Battaglia P, Miceli S, Castelnuovo P. Frontal sinus osteomas: the window of endonasal endoscopic approach. Rhinology 2007;45(4):315–320
65. Castelnuovo P, Valentini V, Giovannetti F, Bignami M, Cassoni A, Iannetti G. Osteomas of the maxillofacial district: endoscopic surgery versus open surgery. J Craniofac Surg 2008;19(6):1446–1452
66. Seiberling K, Floreani S, Robinson S, Wormald PJ. Endoscopic management of frontal sinus osteomas revisited. Am J Rhinol Allergy 2009;23(3):331–336
67. Samaha M, Metson R. Image-guided resection of fibroosseous lesions of the skull base. Am J Rhinol 2003;17(2):115–118

Osteoblastoma

Definition

(ICD-O code 9200/0)

Osteoblastoma (OB) is a benign tumor consisting of a vascular fibrous stroma containing irregular trabeculae of woven bone and osteoid, surrounded by proliferating osteoblasts.

Synonyms

In the past it was sometimes referred to as osteoblastic osteoid tissue forming tumor or even giant osteoid osteoma. The term "osteoblastoma" was coined by Jaffe and Lichtenstein independently in 1956.[1,2]

Incidence

OB is a relatively rare bone tumor in general, accounting for 1% of bone tumors.[3] It is rare in the sinuses, even though 15 to 20% of osteoblastomas occur in the skull.[4]

Site

OB is most often found in the vertebral column including the sacrum (34%) and long bones of the extremities (30%), small bones of the hands and feet (13%), and the skull as noted above (15–20%).[5] There are a small number of reported cases in the nasal cavity and sinuses, including ethmoid,[6–9] maxilla,[10–13] frontal,[14,15] and sphenoid.[16] Sometimes the size at presentation makes the exact site of origin difficult to determine.[17]

Diagnostic Features

Clinical Features

Clinical presentation can be similar to that of other fibro-osseous lesions,[18,19] with a generally painless swelling of variable speed of growth. Seventy-five percent occur in patients under 20 years of age, most often in childhood, and the male-to-female ratio is 2:1.[12] In our 4 patients, the age ranged from 7 to 22 years (mean 10 years), with 2 males and 2 females. The effect of the mass may be to compress and distort the orbit, leading to proptosis and diplopia, expansion of nasal bones, midfacial swelling, dental distortion and loss, and involvement of the skull base and anterior cranial fossa.

Imaging

CT is the primary imaging modality and demonstrates an expansile lesion usually with an intact bony shell, which may cause compression of adjacent structures such as the orbit (**Fig. 13.10a**). A mixture of ground-glass opacity and dense bone can be present. The less dense portions of the lesion show intense enhancement on MRI; a signal void will be seen on all sequences in the densely sclerotic areas and bony rim.[15,20]

Histological Features and Differential Diagnosis

The histology shows a thin cortical shell around a rich vascular, fibrous stroma with irregular calcified osteoid of proliferating osteoblasts along with small trabeculae of woven bone.

Differential diagnosis includes ossifying fibroma, monostotic fibrous dysplasia, giant cell tumors, chon-drosarcoma, osteosarcoma, and aneurysmal bone cysts as well as eosinophilic fungal rhinosinusitis and inverted papilloma on imaging and also on histology from other cartilaginous and bony tumors.

Natural History

Although the name implies a benign lesion, the increasing size itself may lead to clinical problems. In addition, some OBs exhibit more aggressive behavior and actually invade adjacent structures, but true malignant transformation has only been described following radiotherapy.[5]

Treatment and Outcome

The lesions need to be removed surgically by whatever approach is suitable to encompass the lesion, ranging from craniofacial and midfacial degloving (**Fig. 13.10b**) to endoscopic resection if appropriate. A combination of these techniques should make it possible to avoid facial incisions in the young. As there are only anecdotal case reports, all one can conclude is that with total removal the tumor does not recur and this has been our experience with the patients treated by lateral rhinotomy (one case), craniofacial resection (one case), midfacial degloving (one case), and endoscopic resection (one case), none of whom have had recurrence with between 1 year and 15 years follow-up.

References

1. Jaffe HL. Benign osteoblastoma. Bull Hosp Jt Dis 1956; 17(2):141–151
2. Lichtenstein L. Benign osteoblastoma; a category of oste-oid-and bone-forming tumors other than classical osteoid

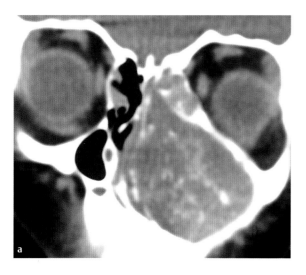
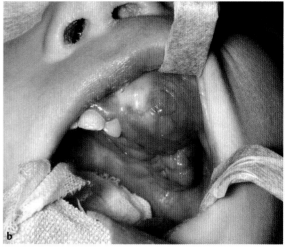

Fig. 13.10a, b

a Coronal CT showing a mass filling the left maxillary sinus with expansion of bone and heterogeneous density within the osteoblastoma in an 8-year-old child.

b Operative photograph in the same patient about to undergo a midfacial degloving approach to the mass, which is producing significant swelling of the gingival sulcus and midface.

osteoma, which may be mistaken for giant-cell tumor or osteogenic sarcoma. Cancer 1956;9(5):1044–1052

3. Capodiferro S, Maiorano E, Giardina C, Lacaita MG, Lo Muzio L, Favia G. Osteoblastoma of the mandible: clinico-pathologic study of four cases and literature review. Head Neck 2005;27(7):616–621

4. Bilkay U, Erdem O, Ozek C, et al. A rare location of benign osteoblastoma: review of the literature and report of a case. J Craniofac Surg 2004;15(2):222–225

5. Clutter DJ, Leopold DA, Gould LV. Benign osteoblastoma. Report of a case and review of the literature. Arch Otolaryngol 1984;110(5):334–336

6. Freedman SR. Benign osteoblastoma of the ethmoid bone. Report of a case. Am J Clin Pathol 1975;63(3):391–396

7. Som PM, Bellot P, Blitzer A, Som ML, Geller SA. Osteoblastoma of the ethmoid sinus: the fourth reported case. Arch Otolaryngol 1979;105(10):623–625

8. Velegrakis GA, Prokopakis EP, Papadakis CE, Karampekios SK, Koutsoubi KG, Helidonis ES. Osteoblastoma of the nasal cavity arising from the perpendicular plate of the ethmoid bone. J Laryngol Otol 1997;111(9):865–868

9. Park Y-K, Kim EJ, Kim SW. Osteoblastoma of the ethmoid sinus. Skeletal Radiol 2007;36(5):463–467

10. Tom LW, Lowry LD, Quinn-Bogard A. Benign osteoblastoma of the maxillary sinus. Otolaryngol Head Neck Surg 1980;88(4):397–402

11. Osguthorpe JD, Hungerford GD. Benign osteoblastoma of the maxillary sinus. Head Neck Surg 1983;6(1):605–609

12. Jones AC, Prihoda TJ, Kacher JE, Odingo NA, Freedman PD. Osteoblastoma of the maxilla and mandible: a report of 24 cases, review of the literature, and discussion of its relationship to osteoid osteoma of the jaws. Oral Surg Oral Med Oral Pathol Oral Radiol Endod 2006;102(5):639–650

13. Mahajan S, Srikant N, Boaz K, George T. Osteoblastoma of maxilla with cartilaginous matrix: review of literature and report of a case. Singapore Dent J 2007;29(1):12–18

14. Meli GA, Meli L, Chiaramonte R, Riva G, Pero G. Osteoblastoma of the orbit: A case report and review of the literature. Neuroradiol J 2008;21:71–76

15. Sidani CA, Karam AR, Bruce JH, Sklar E. Osteoblastoma of the frontal sinuses presenting with headache and blurred vision: case report and review of the literature. J Radiol Case Rep 2010;4(6):1–7

16. Kukwa W, Oziębło A, Oecińska A, Czarnecka AM, Włodarski K, Kukwa A. Aggressive osteoblastoma of the sphenoid bone. Oncol Lett 2010;1(2):367–371

17. Imai K, Tsujiguchi K, Toda C, et al. Osteoblastoma of the nasal cavity invading the anterior skull base in a young child. Case report. J Neurosurg 1997;87(4):625–628

18. Ungkanont K, Chanyavanich V, Benjarasamerote S, Tantinikorn W, Vitavasiri A. Osteoblastoma of the ethmoid sinus in a nine-year-old child—an unusual occurrence. Int J Pediatr Otorhinolaryngol 1996;38(1):89–95

19. Mehta D, Clifton N, McClelland L, Jones NS. Paediatric fibro-osseous lesions of the nose and paranasal sinuses. Int J Pediatr Otorhinolaryngol 2006;70(2):193–199

20. Yang B-T, Wang Z-C, Liu S, Xian J-F, Liu Z-L, Lan B-P. CT and MRI diagnosis of osteoblastoma in paranasal sinus and temporal bone. Zhonghua Fang She Xue Za Zhi 2006;40:365–366

Aneurysmal Bone Cysts

(See **Fig. 13.11**.)

Aneurysmal bone cysts are rare lesions and <5% occur in the craniofacial bones.[1] The long bones and vertebral column are the more common locations. The mandible is involved in approximately two-thirds of the cases and the maxilla in around one-third of cases. Aneurysmal bone cyst in the orbitoethmoid complex is very rare.[2,3] Aneurysmal bone cyst is slightly more frequent in females and develops in ~90% of patients during the first two decades of life.[4-6] The cysts may arise in response to previous trauma and present as an asymptomatic mass or with pain, proptosis, and nasal obstruction.

Histologically the lesion is characterized by multilocular cystlike spaces filled with erythrocytes and separated by connective septa but lacking the smooth muscle walls and endothelial lining of normal vessels. They must be distinguished from osteosarcoma, fibrous dysplasia, and giant cell tumor. Surgical excision is usually offered to limit the cosmetic as well as functional effects of the lesion. Our one case occurred in an 8-year-old boy who underwent a lateral orbitocraniotomy in 1989 with no sign of recurrence after 8 years of follow-up.

References

1. Mehta D, Clifton N, McClelland L, Jones NS. Paediatric fibro-osseous lesions of the nose and paranasal sinuses. Int J Pediatr Otorhinolaryngol 2006;70(2):193–199

2. Citardi MJ, Janjua T, Abrahams JJ, Sasaki CT. Orbitoethmoid aneurysmal bone cyst. Otolaryngol Head Neck Surg 1996;114(3):466–470

3. Chateil JF, Dousset V, Meyer P, et al. Cranial aneurysmal bone cysts presenting with raised intracranial pressure: report of two cases. Neuroradiology 1997;39(7):490–494

4. Jaffe H, Lichtenstein L. Solitary unicameral bone cyst: with emphasis on the roentgen picture, the pathologic appearance and the pathogenesis. Arch Surg 1942;44:1004–1025

5. Calliauw L, Roels H, Caemaert J. Aneurysmal bone cysts in the cranial vault and base of skull. Surg Neurol 1985;23(2):193–198

6. Segall L, Cohen-Kerem R, Ngan B-Y, Forte V. Aneurysmal bone cysts of the head and neck in pediatric patients: a case series. Int J Pediatr Otorhinolaryngol 2008;72(7):977–983

Giant Cell Granulomas and Tumors

Giant cell granulomas and tumors of the craniofacial bones are rare benign lesions but have potentially destructive growth. They occur in a broad age range but tend to affect the under-thirties. They are composed of large multinucleated osteoclastlike cells and mononuclear cells and may have fibrous septa as well as having a vascular stroma.[1] These lesions are extremely rare in the sinonasal region, with only a few cases reported in the sphenoid and ethmoid.[2,3] They have been reported to arise in association with other fibro-osseous lesions such as ossifying fibroma, cherubism and Paget's disease as described by Penfold and colleagues[4] where they may be a reaction to a stromal change within the original lesion. Histologically they must be differentiated from the more common "brown tumor" of hyperparathyroidism and from giant cell reparative granuloma.

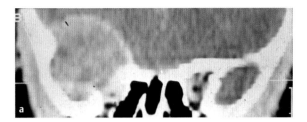

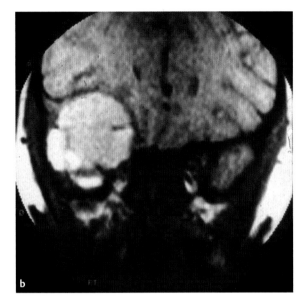

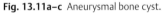

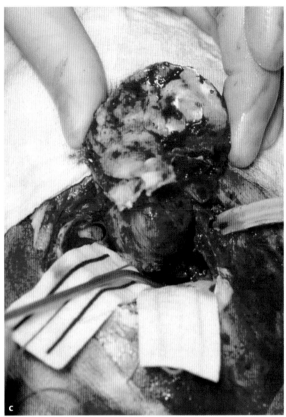

Fig. 13.11a–c Aneurysmal bone cyst.

a Coronal CT scan showing a large lesion in the lateral skull base impinging on the orbit.

b Coronal MRI (STIR) scan of the same patient.

c Peroperative photograph showing lateral craniotomy to remove the lesion.

Treatment with calcitonin changes the histology of giant cell granuloma, causing first giant cells and then the highly cellular stroma to disappear, leaving trabeculae of partially organized woven bone and uninflamed fibrous tissue.[5,6] Some authors have advocated curettage as appropriate in well-localized lesions, claiming a low recurrence rate, but radical excision is almost certainly to be preferred whenever possible[3,7] and additional radiotherapy has also been advocated.[3]

References

1. Auclair PL, Cuenin P, Kratochvil FJ, Slater LJ, Ellis GL. A clinical and histomorphologic comparison of the central giant cell granuloma and the giant cell tumor. Oral Surg Oral Med Oral Pathol 1988;66(2):197–208
2. Gupta OP, Samant HC, Bhatia PL, Agarwal AK, Pant GC. Giant cell tumor of the spenoid bone. Ann Otol Rhinol Laryngol 1975;84(3 Pt 1):359–363
3. Bertoni F, Unni KK, Beabout JW, Ebersold MJ. Giant cell tumor of the skull. Cancer 1992;70(5):1124–1132
4. Penfold CN, McCullagh P, Eveson JW, Ramsay A. Giant cell lesions complicating fibro-osseous conditions of the jaws. Int J Oral Maxillofac Surg 1993;22(3):158–162
5. Harris M. Central giant cell granulomas of the jaws regress with calcitonin theraphy. Br J Oral Maxillofac Surg 1993;31:89–94
6. de Lange J, Rosenberg AJ, van den Akker HP, Koole R, Wirds JJ, van den Berg H. Treatment of central giant cell granuloma of the jaw with calcitonin. Int J Oral Maxillofac Surg 1999;28(5):372–376
7. Chuong R, Kaban LB, Kozakewich H, Perez-Atayde A. Central giant cell lesions of the jaws: a clinicopathologic study. J Oral Maxillofac Surg 1986;44(9):708–713

Cherubism

Definition and Etiology

This rare inherited condition was first described by Jones in 1933[1] as a "familial multilocular cystic disease of the jaws," which he later called "cherubism."[2] This was in recognition of the "raised to heaven" look due to the enlargement of the lower half of the face and retraction of the lower eyelids. It has been suggested that it is an autosomal dominant condition but opinions differ on the degree of penetrance in males and females (from 80 to100% in men; 50 to 80% in women) and variable expressivity.[3,4] Other possible causative factors include latent hyperparathyroidism, trauma, and aberrant ossification in membranous bone.

Synonyms

Familial fibrous dysplasia of the jaws, hereditary fibrous dysplasia of the jaws, bilateral giant cell tumor, fibroosseous dysplasia of the jaws, familial intraosseous fibrous swelling of the jaws.[5,6]

Incidence

By 1978, 145 cases had been reported, which included several affected families although no ethnic predilection has been shown.

Site

The process usually affects the maxilla and mandible and is ultimately symmetrical even if it starts on one side. In the maxilla, change starts posteriorly in the maxillary tuberosity and moves forward to involve the floor of the orbit, the infraorbital area, and ultimately the anterior maxilla. In the mandible the retromolar trigone and ascending rami are affected first, but the condyle is rarely affected, so jaw opening is not usually compromised.

Diagnostic Features

Clinical Features

Children are normal at birth but by the second or third year may show signs of the disease. The age range at presentation is 2 to 12 years with a mean of 7 years.[4] With time, usually in the late teens, the process begins to involute, often starting in the maxilla.[5] Males are twice as commonly affected as females.[7] The one 12-year-old female case we have treated had a severe form of the condition and had undergone multiple procedures prior to referral (**Fig. 13.12**).

Apart from the cosmetic change due to painless swelling, which can have severe psychological effects in the young, there can be disturbance of speech, eating, and breathing. There is fullness of the face; upturned eyes, exposing a rim of sclera below the pupil; orbital problems due to lower lid ectropion; and sometimes reduced visual acuity.[8,9]

Another characteristic is submandibular swelling due to Level 1 lymphadenopathy. This chronic swelling of the nodes begins at the onset of the disease but then regresses with time and so has usually disappeared by 11 to 12 years.[5] The teeth are badly affected, being painful, loose, or missing. Hard painless swelling of the palate produces a V shape. There is no intellectual impairment.

Not surprisingly, alkaline phosphatase levels are raised, although calcium and phosphorus levels are normal.[6] Occasionally other bones are affected—ribs, humerus, or zygoma.[5,6,10]

Imaging

CT shows multiple multiloculated areas of rarefaction and expansion of the bony cortex without bone destruction,[11] giving a soap bubble appearance. The dentition is irregular and displaced. With time the cystic spaces are gradually but not completely replaced by dense granular material giving it the "ground glass" appearance of fibrous dysplasia and even thick trabecular bone. Despite clinical regression, changes are still evident on imaging.

Histological Features and Differential Diagnosis

Macroscopically the lesions are red to red-gray in color, firm, and gritty when dissected.[5] McClendon et al[12] examined 67 cases and showed that the microscopic appearance is one of multinucleated giant cells surrounded by chronic inflammation, proliferating fibrous tissue, and irregular trabecular bone formation, similar to that seen in giant cell reparative granuloma.

Diagnosis is based on the age of onset, the family history, the characteristic appearance, absence of other bony pathology, and the histopathology. The condition has

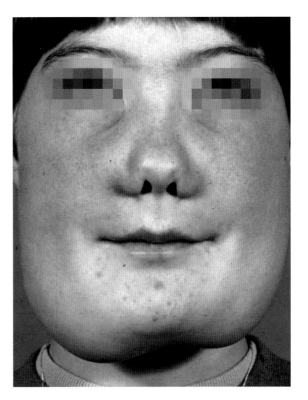

Fig. 13.12 Clinical photograph of a 14-year-old patient with cherubism.

been reported in association with other fibro-osseous lesions such as fibrous dysplasia.[13] However, fibrous dysplasia itself; giant cell granuloma; various dentigerous, odontogenic and aneurysmal cysts; ameloblastomas; and the "brown tumor" of hyperparathyroidism may all pose diagnostic difficulty if histology alone is considered. The diagnosis is clarified by the age of onset, bilaterality, distribution, hereditary nature, and normal calcium and phosphorus levels.

Natural History

As noted above, the disease is not present at birth but appears around 2 or 3 years then generally slows in childhood and involutes in the teens. The maxilla shows regression before the mandible but ultimately both will remodel in the patient's twenties to thirties. However, some deformity may remain.

Treatment and Outcome

There are no agreed protocols, due to the rarity of the condition, but the familial nature leads to some concentration of cases and expertise. As involution occurs to a greater or lesser degree, there has been a tendency to wait until puberty before offering surgery, which usually involves some forms of recontouring. If surgery is undertaken at that time, it does not recur.[14] Unfortunately this is not the case if it is undertaken during the active phase of the process[15] and our patient had undergone multiple operations throughout her childhood that had left her both physically and emotionally scarred. Nonetheless, if the vision is at risk, intervention may be indicated to decompress the orbits.[8,9] It should be noted however, that in young patients the lesion is very vascular, resulting in marked intraoperative blood loss.[7,16]

Radiotherapy should not be used as it may induce malignant change and osteoradionecrosis.[4,14]

References

1. Jones W. Familial multilocular cystic disease of the jaws. Am J Cancer 1933;17:946
2. Jones WA, Gerrie J, Pritchard J. Cherubism—familial fibrous dysplasia of the jaws. J Bone Joint Surg Br 1950; 32-B(3):334–347
3. Anderson B, McClendon J. Cherubism – hereditary fibrous dysplasia of the jaws. I. Genetic considerations. Oral Surg 1962;15(Suppl 2):5–16
4. Peters WJ. Cherubism: a study of twenty cases from one family. Oral Surg Oral Med Oral Pathol 1979;47(4):307–311
5. Thompson N. Cherubism: familial fibrous dysplasia of the jaws. Br J Plast Surg 1959;12:89
6. Topazian RG, Costich ER. Familial fibrous dysplasia of the jaws (cherubism). Report of a case. J Oral Surg 1965;23:559–568
7. Zachariades N, Papanicolaou S, Xypolyta A, Constantinidis I. Cherubism. Int J Oral Surg 1985;14(2):138–145
8. Hawes MJ. Cherubism and its orbital manifestations. Ophthal Plast Reconstr Surg 1989;5(2):133–140
9. Marck PA, Kudryk WH. Cherubism. J Otolaryngol 1992; 21(2):84–87
10. Wayman JB. Cherubism: a report on three cases. Br J Oral Surg 1978;16(1):47–56
11. Bianchi SD, Boccardi A, Mela F, Romagnoli R. The computed tomographic appearances of cherubism. Skeletal Radiol 1987;16(1):6–10
12. McClendon J, Anderson D, Cornelius E. Cherubism—hereditary fibrous dysplasia of the jaws (pathologic considerations). Oral Surg Oral Med Oral Pathol 1962;15(Suppl 2):17–42
13. Zohar Y, Grausbord R, Shabtai F, Talmi Y. Fibrous dysplasia and cherubism as an hereditary familial disease. Follow-up of four generations. J Craniomaxillofac Surg 1989;17(8):340–344
14. Hamner JE III, Ketcham AS. Cherubism: an analysis of treatment. Cancer 1969;23(5):1133–1143
15. Riefkohl R, Georgiade GS, Georgiade NG. Cherubism. Ann Plast Surg 1985;14(1):85–90
16. Koury ME, Stella JP, Epker BN. Vascular transformation in cherubism. Oral Surg Oral Med Oral Pathol 1993;76(1):20–27

"Brown Tumor" of Hyperparathyroidism

Definition

Brown tumors are rare erosive bony lesions caused by osteoclastic activity and peritrabecular fibrosis due to hyperparathyroidism (HPT), resulting in a local destruction.

Etiology

In the mid-1920s HPT began to be recognized around the world, characterized by renal stones.[1] With time it became apparent that both primary and secondary HPT are the principal causes of a specific bone lesion, the "brown tumor." Primary HPT arises from adenomas of the parathyroid gland, whereas secondary HPT may follow chronic renal failure.

Synonyms

The term "osteoclastoma" is sometimes applied and histologically the lesion is identical to giant cell granulomas.

Incidence

Although primary HPT is relatively common (~25/100,000 population/year) and increases with age, brown tumors are a rare phenomenon as the underlying HPT is more often detected these days before the lesions have a chance to develop.[2] In a series of 115 patients with chronic kidney disease, 10 (8.7%) had brown tumors in different bones of the skeleton, 5 of whom had lesions in the craniofacial bones.[3]

Site

The lesion more commonly affects the mandible but may involve the maxilla[4-8] and occasionally the ethmoid[9] or sphenoid[10-12] and thence the orbit.[3] Multiple lesions are possible.[13]

Diagnostic Features

Clinical Features

This condition mainly affects adults >30 years old, with a female preponderance of 2:1. The lesion may be found incidentally or present as a slow-growing mass that produces nasal obstruction, epistaxis, pain, swelling of the face or palate, and dental disruption.[14,15] Sphenoidal lesions may be associated with headache and cranial symptoms and signs. However, not all lesions are slow growing and some pursue an aggressive course suggesting a more malignant pathology.[16]

No difference was found by Cecchetti and colleagues[3] between the age and duration of renal failure of those patients who developed brown tumors and those who did not.

Imaging

The appearances are those of a giant cell lesion with lytic areas. When this appearance is encountered, calcium and other bone markers (alkaline phosphatase, phosphate) must be checked even if the patient is asymptomatic and imaging of the parathyroid region undertaken with CT. A skeletal survey may reveal other lesions and also reveal bone demineralization, particularly in the spine and hands.[17]

More specifically, CT shows an expansile soft tissue attenuation mass and, on bone window settings, lytic change and remodeling of the surrounding bone is seen.[12] On MRI the lesion shows intense enhancement, isointensity on T1W images, and heterogeneous hyperintensity on T2W images.

Histological Features and Differential Diagnosis

Brown tumors are made up of a cell population consisting of rounded or spindlelike mononucleate elements, mixed with a certain number of multinucleate giant cells, resembling osteoclastic cells, among which recent hemorrhagic infiltrates and hemosiderin deposits are often found, hence the brown color. As increased parathyroid hormone and renal failure both adversely affect bone density, it has been suggested that the brown tumor might be an attempt at reparative scarring.[18]

This condition must be considered whenever giant cell lesions are encountered in the sinonasal region. Thus the differential diagnosis includes giant cell tumors and granulomas, aneurysmal bone cysts, and cherubism, but the combination of the clinical, radiological, and biochemical findings of hypercalcemia and elevated parathyroid hormone levels confirms the diagnosis. Fine needle aspiration may have a role in confirming the diagnosis in these circumstances.[19] Other causes of hypercalcemia such as bone metastases from other malignancies, sarcoidosis, and so on also need to be considered.

Natural History

It has been reported that brown tumors resolve after removal of the parathyroid adenoma and/or correction of the HPT but this can take some time to occur.

Treatment and Outcome

Correction of the biochemical disturbance alone will lead to regression of the lesion. Therefore, these patients require endocrine management and removal of any parathyroid tumor. The sinonasal lesion may then regress but if this does not occur, surgical removal/remodeling of the bone lesion can be undertaken by whatever approach is appropriate depending on the size of the lesion.[5] It should be noted that they can be moderately vascular.

Failure to correct the underlying biochemical problem may be associated with further lesions[8] and long-term renal dialysis;[20] and even post renal transplantation, patients have been reported to develop these lesions.[21]

References

1. Albright F. A page out of the history of parathyroidism. J Clin Endocrinol 1948;8:637–642
2. Diamanti-Kandarakis E, Livadas S, Tseleni-Balafouta S, et al. Brown tumor of the fibula: unusual presentation of an uncommon manifestation. Report of a case and review of the literature. Endocrine 2007;32(3):345–349
3. Cecchetti DF, Paula SA, Cruz AA, et al. Orbital involvement in craniofacial brown tumors. Ophthal Plast Reconstr Surg 2010;26(2):106–111
4. Pecovnik Balon B, Kavalar R. Brown tumor in association with secondary hyperparathyroidism. A case report and review of the literature. Am J Nephrol 1998;18(5):460–463
5. Taskapan H, Taskapan C, Baysal T, et al. Maxillary brown tumor and uremic leontiasis ossea in a patient with chronic renal insufficiency. Clin Nephrol 2004;61(5):360–363
6. Lessa MM, Sakae FA, Tsuji RK, Filho BC, Voegels RL, Butugan O. Brown tumor of the facial bones: case report and literature review. Ear Nose Throat J 2005;84(7):432–434
7. Triantafillidou K, Zouloumis L, Karakinaris G, Kalimeras E, Iordanidis F. Brown tumors of the jaws associated with primary or secondary hyperparathyroidism. A clinical study and review of the literature. Am J Otolaryngol 2006;27(4):281–286
8. Proimos E, Chimona TS, Tamiolakis D, Tzanakakis MG, Papadakis CE. Brown tumor of the maxillary sinus in a patient with primary hyperparathyroidism: a case report. J Med Case Reports 2009;3:7495
9. Al-Ghantany M, Cusimano M, Singer W, Bilbao J, Kovacs K, Marotta T. Brown tumors of the skull base. Case report and review of the literature. J Neurosurg 2003;98(2):417–420
10. Kanaan I, Ahmed M, Rifai A, Alwatban J. Sphenoid sinus brown tumor of secondary hyperparathyroidism: case report. Neurosurgery 1998;42(6):1374–1377

11. Erem C, Hacihasanoglu A, Cinel A, et al. Sphenoid sinus brown tumor, a mass lesion of occipital bone and hypercalcemia: an unusual presentation of primary hyperparathyroidism. J Endocrinol Invest 2004;27(4):366–369

12. Takeshita T, Tanaka H, Harasawa A, Kaminaga T, Imamura T, Furui S. Brown tumor of the sphenoid sinus in a patient with secondary hyperparathyroidism: CT and MR imaging findings. Radiat Med 2004;22(4):265–268

13. Duran C, Ersoy C, Bolca N, et al. Brown tumors of the maxillary sinus and patella in a patient with primary hyperparathyroidism. Endocrinologist 2005;15:351–354

14. Antonelli JR, Hottel TL. Oral manifestations of renal osteodystrophy: case report and review of the literature. Spec Care Dentist 2003;23(1):28–34

15. Daniels JS. Primary hyperparathyroidism presenting as a palatal brown tumor. Oral Surg Oral Med Oral Pathol Oral Radiol Endod 2004;98(4):409–413

16. Martínez-Gavidia EM, Bagán JV, Milián-Masanet MA, Lloria de Miguel E, Pérez-Vallés A. Highly aggressive brown tumour of the maxilla as first manifestation of primary hyperparathyroidism. Int J Oral Maxillofac Surg 2000;29(6):447–449

17. Leppla DC, Snyder W, Pak CY. Sequential changes in bone density before and after parathyroidectomy in primary hyperparathyroidism. Invest Radiol 1982;17(6):604–606

18. Hellquist H. Pathology of the Nose and Paranasal Sinuses. Cambridge: Cambridge University Press; 1990:77

19. Galed Placed I, Patiño-Seijas B, Pombo-Otero J, Alvarez-Rodríguez R. Fine needle aspiration diagnosis of brown tumor of the maxilla. Acta Cytol 2010; 54(5, Suppl)1076–1078

20. Masutani K, Katafuchi R, Uenoyama K, Saito S, Fujimi S, Hirakata H. Brown tumor of the thoracic spine in a patient on long-term hemodialysis. Clin Nephrol 2001;55(5):419–423

21. Lee S, Lerer DB, Dorfman HD, Coco M. Brown tumors developing in renal transplant recipients with persistent hyperparathyroidism: two case reports and review of literature. Clin Nephrol 2004;61(4):289–294

Osseous Metaplasia

Metaplasia is the conversion of one fully differentiated cell type into another fully differentiated cell type and can be found in epithelial and connective tissue. Areas of chondromatous and osseous metaplasia are found throughout the upper aerodigestive tract and must be distinguished from neoplasia.[1] The metaplasia can occur rarely in response to chronic inflammation[2] or previous surgery[3,4] but it is important to exclude a concomitant malignancy. Essentially new bone formation is encountered with a well-developed haversian system and bone marrow where one would not normally encounter it. It is not necessary to operate but if the process pushes through the mucosa or impinges on adjacent structures such as the orbit, the process can be debulked and/or completely excised (**Fig. 13.13**). We have seen one case in a 41-year-old woman of Afro-Caribbean origin who had a combined lateral rhinotomy and endoscopic approach to remove an extensive lesion affecting the nasal cavity, sinuses, and orbit. To date, with one year follow-up including imaging, there has been no recurrence.

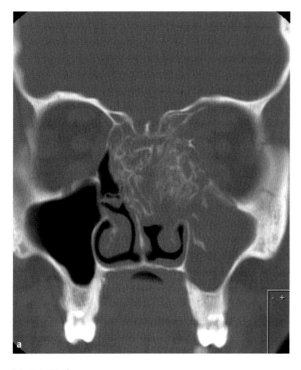
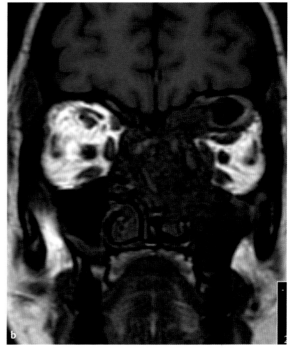

Fig. 13.13a, b

a Coronal CT scan showing extensive osseous metaplasia affecting the left nasal cavity, septum, and ethmoids and extending into the maxillary sinus.

b Coronal MRI scan (T1W unenhanced) in the same patient showing heterogeneous signal from the mass with scattered signal voids and areas of high signal.

References

1. Macdonald-Jankowski DS. Focal cemento-osseous dysplasia: a systematic review. Dentomaxillofac Radiol 2008; 37(6):350–360
2. Daley TD, Damm DD, Wysocki GP, Weir JC. Atypical cartilage in reactive osteocartilagenous metaplasia of the traumatized edentulous mandibular ridge. Oral Surg Oral Med Oral Pathol Oral Radiol Endod 1997;83(1):26–29
3. Lundgren S, Andersson S, Sennerby L. Spontaneous bone formation in the maxillary sinus after removal of a cyst: coincidence or consequence? Clin Implant Dent Relat Res 2003;5(2):78–81
4. Maitra S, Gupta D, Radojkovic M, Sood S. Osseous metaplasia of the maxillary sinus with formation of a well-developed haversian system and bone marrow. Ear Nose Throat J 2009;88(9):1115–1120

Paget's disease

Definition

A disease of unknown etiology characterized by a disordered pattern of bone formation and resorption.

Synonyms

Otherwise referred to as osteitis deformans, this condition was first described by Paget in 1877;[1] it was initially not recognized as a condition affecting the sinonasal region but rather as affecting the skull, pelvis, vertebral column, and femur. It was known to involve the temporal bone but the maxilla and other sinuses have been rather rarely reported, even though it must occur as part of polyostotic disease. Historically it is also a cause of *leontiasis ossea*, or leonine features.[2]

Incidence

Estimations of the incidence vary with age from 1% in the 5th decade to 10% in the 10th decade, but because many do not seek help it is a difficult figure to estimate. However, it is the second most common bone disorder after osteoporosis.[3] A very rare form has been described in young children.[4]

Site

Paget's disease can affect any of the sinuses secondarily to skull involvement. The jaw bones are affected in at least 17% of cases.

Diagnostic Features

Clinical Features

Many patients are asymptomatic and the condition may only come to light as an incidental finding on imaging for some other problem or when the condition produces bone pain or neurological problems.[5,6] In fact it is more often encountered by ENT surgeons as a cause of tinnitus or hearing loss when the temporal bone is involved. It is slightly more common in men.

Ill-fitting dentures, loosening of the teeth, nasal obstruction or facial swelling can all occur or, as in one memorable patient, bilateral frontal mucoceles with fistulas into the upper eyelids. However, rapid growth accompanied by pain and epistaxis in a known case of sinonasal Paget's disease should raise the suspicion of malignant transformation.

Imaging

(See **Fig. 13.14.**)

The appearances vary with the stage of the disease, from radiolucency to sclerosis. It may be a chance finding and may be mistaken for fibrous dysplasia, but a checklist of differences, including the symmetry of Paget's disease and the thickness of the cranial cortices, usually resolves the diagnosis.[7] Further skeletal investigation reveals other involvement—for example, in the spine, pelvis, or long bones.

Histological Features and Differential Diagnosis

The histology features active bone formation coincident with active bone destruction. In the initial osteoporotic phase, there are large amounts of new bone in a loose vascular connective tissue stroma. In the fully developed disease there is obvious osteoclastic and osteoblastic activity producing a characteristic mosaic appearance.

The process is rather diffuse but early lesions must be distinguished from brown tumors of hyperparathyroidism, osteosarcoma, myeloma, and metastases, whereas more mature lesions must be differentiated from the range of fibro-osseous lesions to which this chapter is devoted.

Treatment and Outcome

Apart from a biopsy (which may not even be required), surgery has little role to play in the management of the condition per se but may be required to deal with its consequences—for example, drainage of the mucoceles or occasionally decompression of nerves. It certainly should be deferred until the sclerotic phase if possible because of the vascularity of the process and its diffuse nature.

Generally patients are managed medically. Initially calcitonin[8] was used, which can be delivered intranasally and rectally as well as parenterally,[9,10] but this has been replaced by newer agents such as the bisphosphonates.[11,12] Oral etidronate and intravenous pamidronate have been used extensively with good effect but are being replaced by oral formulation of the new bisphosphonates, including tiludronate, risedronate, and dimethylpamidronate.

Sinonasal involvement is generally part of extensive disease that puts the patient at risk from high-output

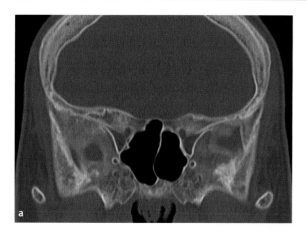
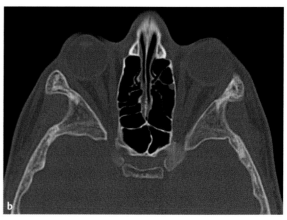

Fig. 13.14a, b

a Coronal CT scan showing widespread Paget's disease affecting the skull base and vault.

b Axial CT scan in the same patient.

cardiac failure due to the multiple arteriovenous shunts within the diseased bone. As previously noted, a small number may also go on to develop osteosarcoma.[13]

References

1. Paget J. On a form of chronic inflammation of the bone (osteitis deformans). Med Chirurg Transact 1877;60:37–42
2. Knaggs RL. Leontiasis ossea. Br J Surg 1923;11:347–348
3. Ankrom MA, Shapiro JR. Paget's disease of bone (osteitis deformans). J Am Geriatr Soc 1998;46(8):1025–1033
4. Bae KB, Kwon JH, Kim YH, Jung TY, Cho JH. Juvenile Paget's disease with paranasal sinus aplasia. Clin Exp Otorhinolaryngol 2008;1(4):224–226
5. Fuller AP. Paget's disease of the ethmoids. J Laryngol Otol 1961;75:860–863
6. Drury BJ. Paget's disease of the skull and facial bones. J Bone Joint Surg Am 1962;44:174–178
7. Tehranzadeh J, Fung Y, Donohue M, Anavim A, Pribram HW. Computed tomography of Paget disease of the skull versus fibrous dysplasia. Skeletal Radiol 1998;27(12):664–672
8. Chesnut CH III, Azria M, Silverman S, Engelhardt M, Olson M, Mindeholm L. Salmon calcitonin: a review of current and future therapeutic indications. Osteoporos Int 2008;19(4):479–491
9. Torres-Lugo M, Peppas NA. Transmucosal delivery systems for calcitonin: a review. Biomaterials 2000; 21(12):1191–1196
10. Ubhi K. Intranasal calcitonin: for postmenopausal osteoporosis. Can Pharm J 2001;134:41–44
11. Reginster JY, Lecart MP. Efficacy and safety of drugs for Paget's disease of bone. Bone 1995; 17(5, Suppl)485S–488S
12. Ezra A, Golomb G. Administration routes and delivery systems of bisphosphonates for the treatment of bone resorption. Adv Drug Deliv Rev 2000;42(3):175–195
13. Epley KD, Lasky JB, Karesh JW. Osteosarcoma of the orbit associated with Paget disease. Ophthal Plast Reconstr Surg 1998;14(1):62–66

Osteosarcoma

Definition

(ICD-O code 9200/0)

Osteosarcoma (OS) is a malignant tumor of bone that is thought to arise from a primitive mesenchymal bone-forming cell and is characterized by the production of osteoid.

Etiology

The exact cause of osteosarcoma is unknown. However, numerous risk factors have been identified. Rapid bone growth appears to predispose patients to osteosarcoma, as suggested by the increased incidence during adolescence and the typical location of osteosarcomas near the metaphyseal growth plate of long bones.

Exposure to radiation is the only known environmental risk factor as evidenced by cases occurring after the Chernobyl nuclear accident.[1] Bone dysplasias, including Paget's disease, fibrous dysplasia, enchondromatosis, and hereditary multiple exostoses, also increase the risk for osteosarcoma, particularly if they have also been irradiated.[2] The latency from radiation exposure to presentation with OS varies from 3 to 38 years and depends on whether normal or abnormal bone was involved and over what period the radiation was given.[1]

A genetic predisposition may be present. Presence of a constitutional mutation of the retinoblastoma *RB* gene (germline retinoblastoma) combined with radiation therapy, is associated with a particularly high risk of developing an osteosarcoma.[3] Of note, the genetic locus retinoblastoma at band 13q14 has also been implicated in the pathogenesis of sporadic osteosarcoma. In addition, the Li-Fraumeni syndrome (germline *TP53* mutation) and Rothmund-Thomson syndrome (i.e., autosomal recessive association of congenital bone defects, hair and skin dysplasias, hypogonadism, cataracts) are associated with an increased risk.

Synonyms

Osteogenic sarcoma or osteoid sarcoma; this tumor has long been recognized as a highly malignant tumor of mesenchymal origin.[4]

Incidence

In the United States, the incidence of OS is 400 cases per year (4.8 cases per million persons <20 years old) and it is the third most common cancer in adolescence. The incidence is slightly higher in African Americans than in whites.[5] The incidence of osteosarcoma of the limbs increases steadily with age and a relatively dramatic increase in adolescence has been observed to coincide with the growth spurt.

Site

Osteosarcoma can occur in any bone but it most commonly occurs in the long bones of the extremities near metaphyseal growth plates.[5] Skull or jaw bones are rarely involved and only 1 to 5% are said to involve the maxilla. Rarely, the ethmoid and sphenoid are primary sites.[6] Only 6.5% of all osteosarcomas were reported to arise in the maxilla and mandible by Garrington et al in 1967.[7] Between 1925 and 1996 out of 4,399 reported cases of OS, 378 (8.5%) affected the head and neck and of these 101 (2.3%) occurred in the maxilla.[1] OS is even less common in the nasal cavity itself.

Diagnostic Features

Clinical Features

Head and neck osteosarcomas differ from other localizations in that patients' mean age ranges between 26 and 40 years; thus, these OSs affect patients that are 10 or 15 years older than those with osteosarcomas of long bones.[8,9] In the large series of sinonasal OS described by Unni and Dahlin,[10] ages ranged from 15 to 50 years with a median of 28 years and there was a sharp peak between 20 and 29 years. OS patients reported from our own institution were even older with a mean of 51 years.[2] The male-to-female ratio in this group of seven patients was 2:5 (**Table 13.6**), although overall there is no sex variation in the literature.

The most obvious clinical feature is a rapidly enlarging bony mass often associated with pain and all the appurtenances of local invasion of the nasal cavity, palate, and orbit. Maxillary OSs often start in the alveolar ridge and from there involve the sinus.[9] There may be pain since nerves are involved, loosening of the teeth, or a malignant oroantral fistula after dental extraction, proptosis, nasal obstruction, and epistaxis.

Imaging

Imaging shows marked destruction by an irregular and often calcified mass.[6] Thus there is a heterogeneous density depending on the amount of bone formation, varying from "cloudlike" to spicules, further altered by any other underlying and previously benign fibro-osseous lesion (**Figs. 13.15 and 13.16**). Postcontrast enhancement will similarly vary. The classical "sunburst" pattern is not so common in sinonasal OSs.

MRI T1W images are iso- or hypointense and this is mirrored in postcontrast scans where moderate to

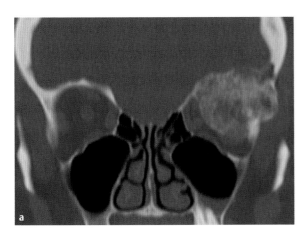
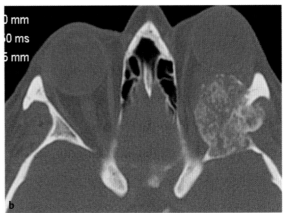

Fig. 13.15a, b

a Coronal CT scan showing osteosarcoma affecting the lateral orbit arising from the greater wing of the sphenoid.

b Axial CT in the same patient.

Table 13.6 Osteosarcoma of upper jaw: personal series

Sex	Age at diagnosis (y)	Year	Primary condition	Previous radiotherapy	Treatment	Follow-up
F	60	1962	Maxilla	220 kV, 5060 cGy (1957)	220 kV and telecesium 5000 R Radical maxillectomy and orbital clearance Recurrence 1963: IA chemotherapy	DOD 18 mo
F	69	1966	Pre-maxilla involving antrum		Partial maxillectomy	DOD 11 mo
M	30	1970	Maxilla–nasal passage–middle fossa	Cobalt 60 5200 cGy (hyperbaric O$_2$)	Radical maxillectomy and orbital clearance; cyclophosphamide	DOD 3 mo
F	30	1971	Lateral wall nose and antrum		Cobalt 60 6100 cGy and lateral rhinotomy	A&W 16 y
F	58	1972	Paget's disease: maxilla and orbit		Cyclophosphamide IA	DOD 3 mo
M	62	1974	Maxilla		Radical maxillectomy and orbital clearance and doxorubicin (Adriamycin)	DICD 14 y, trauma
F	45	1976	Maxilla–orbit, middle cranial fossa		Radical maxillectomy and orbital clearance and doxorubicin (Adriamycin)	A&W 10 y
F	43	1985	Maxilla–orbit	5250 cGy 4 MeV and vincristine and methotrexate (1984)	Radical maxillectomy and orbital clearance. Recurrence 3 mo: cryosurgery	DOD 7 mo
M	40	1985	Maxilla	7000 cGy and cis-platinum (1984)	Radical maxillectomy and orbital clearance	DOD 30 mo
M	22	1987	Ethmoid + sphenoid		Craniofacial resection	Palliative op. DOD 4 mo
F	64	1999	Ethmoid + nasal cavity		Craniofacial resection	A&W at 6 y
M	35	2000	Ethmoid + maxilla		Radical maxillectomy + orbital clearance + DXT	DOD 6 mo

Abbreviations: A&W, alive and well; DICD, dead of intercurrent disease; DOD, dead of disease; DXT, radiotherapy; F, female; M, male; mo, month(s); y, year(s).

marked heterogeneity is seen. A combination of both CT and MRI is required to show the extent of invasion.

In all cases a staging protocol is required to consider metastatic disease. This may include CT of thorax and abdomen and a skeletal survey ± PET scanning.

Histological Features and Differential Diagnosis

Osteosarcoma is an irregularly calcified destructive tumor composed of sarcoma cells mixed with foci of malignant osteoid/bone. The tumor may be quite vascular with dilated capillaries and cavernous structures. Other tissues such as cartilage, or fibrous or myxomatous material can be found, so numerous variants of osteosarcoma are named according to the cellular pattern of differentiation, conventional types (i.e., osteoblastic, chondroblastic, fibroblastic types), and telangiectatic, multifocal, parosteal, and periosteal types. There is no correlation, however, between histological subtype and prognosis.[11]

Differentiation between OSs and other "undifferentiated" small round cell tumors requires histological expertise including immunohistochemistry and information on clinical and imaging findings.[12] The situation is complicated by coincident benign fibro-osseous disease, so providing representative material is, as ever, paramount.

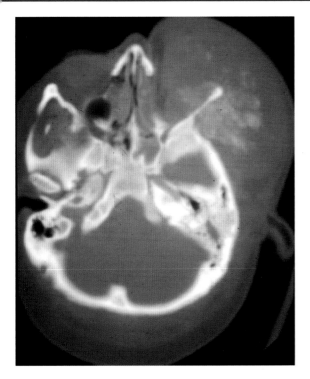

Fig. 13.16 Axial CT scan showing more extensive osteosarcoma arising from the greater wing of the sphenoid and widely infiltrating the orbit.

Natural History

OS of the head and neck behaves differently from osteosarcoma of the trunk and extremity. Local extension occurs rapidly, leading to poor local surgical control of the disease,[11] a phenomenon that is observed with most sarcomas in the head and neck area where wide margins are often impossible and positive margins around critical neurovascular structures are common.

Hematogenous metastases are less frequent than with OS in the long bone, but a search for systemic spread is required as these together with skull base and intracranial disease contribute to the demise of the patient.

Treatment and Outcome

Most sarcomas come within the purview of a multidisciplinary sarcoma oncology team, but it should not be forgotten that the mainstay of therapy remains removal of the lesion. This may take many forms from the full range of maxillectomies via external or midfacial degloving approaches and craniofacial resection with or without removal of the eye. The role of endoscopic surgery is limited but may be a useful adjunct, especially on the skull base, and have a role in recurrence.

Chemotherapy is also recommended to treat micrometastatic disease, which at the time of diagnosis may be present but not detectable in most patients. Before the use of chemotherapy, osteosarcoma was primarily treated with surgical resection alone. However, despite good local control of the disease, more than 80% of patients subsequently developed pulmonary metastases. This triggered the use of adjuvant (postoperative) systemic chemotherapy for the treatment of patients with osteosarcoma of the limbs.[13]

The most useful chemotherapeutic drugs in osteosarcoma are doxorubicin, cisplatin, and high-dose methotrexate. Other therapies are also being studied, such as anthracycline escalation using a cardioprotectant, muramyl tripeptide phosphatidylethanolamine (MTP-PE) and other immune enhancers (e.g., interferon), and monoclonal antibody against the Her2/neu antigen, which is overexpressed in some osteosarcomas.[14,15]

The role of radiotherapy is debated as some tumors are radiation induced. However, it is recommended by some authors alone or in combination with chemotherapy. The use of proton beam therapy remains to be determined due to the lack of numbers but is based on the utility of this therapy in chondrosarcoma.[16]

Traditional predictors of treatment failure for soft tissue sarcomas include larger tumor size, high-grade histology, and positive surgical margins.[17] However, it is noteworthy that resection of metastatic pulmonary nodules is now widely advocated in OS. If OS recurs as a solitary lung lesion more than 1 year after completion of therapy, surgical resection alone can be curative, as the likelihood of metastases to other sites is low.[18] Conversely, if the OS recurs sooner than one year after therapy, chemotherapy is warranted, as the risk of other micrometastatic disease is high.

Carrau et al examined the role of skull base resection in 15 patients presenting with various sarcomas of the sinonasal tract.[19] Although their results were not statistically significant, the authors suggested that resection of the skull base provides an additional margin that aims to achieve an adequate surgical resection and improve the prognosis in patients with sinonasal sarcomas that invade or approach the anterior skull base. Kassir et al examined the role of adjunctive therapy in 173 patients with osteosarcoma of the head and neck.[20] The overall 5-year survival was 37%. Survival of patients with extragnathic tumors was significantly worse than that of patients with mandibular and maxillary lesions ($p < 0.001$). Interestingly, surgery alone was associated with significantly longer survival rates ($p < 0.03$) than surgery with adjuvant therapy, but this may simply signify a significant bias toward the use of adjunctive therapy for advanced tumors or those with positive surgical margins.

Laskar et al[21] also showed in 50 cases of osteosarcoma in the head and neck region that surgery was the mainstay of treatment. They reported 16 cases affecting the maxilla and 5 affecting the paranasal sinuses, finding that the maxilla cases had better overall survival than the sinuses (median 57 months versus 17 months), although the distinction between these sites is unclear and median disease-free survival was only 4 and 2 months, respectively. The addition of radiotherapy was too random in both application and protocols used for any robust conclusions to be drawn.

For patients with uncertain or positive margins following surgical resection, the addition of radiotherapy improved local control and disease-specific and overall survival. In a series of 119 patients, overall survival (OS) rates at 5 years and 10 years were 63% and 55%, respectively.[22] Corresponding disease-specific survival (DSS) rates were 67% and 61%, respectively. Stratified analysis by resection margin status demonstrated that the addition of radiotherapy compared with surgery alone improved OS and DSS for patients with positive/uncertain resection margins. A total of 44 patients (37%) experienced local disease recurrence (LR) and 25 (21%) developed distant metastases.[22] These outcomes are similar to those reported by Patel et al[23] and much improved over those reported in the past of ~25%.[6,24,25]

Key Points

- Osteosarcomas of the sinonasal tract are extremely rare as they typically involve the outer face skeleton and/or maxilla.
- In general, surgery combined with chemotherapy is the treatment of choice with radiotherapy used in selected cases.
- An endonasal endoscopic approach can be used to complement open traditional approaches but is rarely, if ever, appropriate for this tumor as the only approach.

References

1. Harvey RT, Donald PJ, Weinstein GS. Osteogenic sarcoma of the maxillary alveolus occurring five years following the Chernobyl nuclear accident. Am J Otolaryngol 1996;17(3):210–214
2. Windle-Taylor PC. Osteosarcoma of the upper jaw. J Maxillofac Surg 1977;5(1):62–68
3. Schefler A, Kleinerman R, Abramson D. Genes and environment: Effects on the development of second malignancies in retinoblastoma survivors. Expert Rev Ophthalmol 2008;3:51–61
4. Budd J, McDonald J. Osteogenic sarcoma. A modified nomenclature and a review of 118 five-year cures. Surg Gynecol Obstet 1943;77:413–421
5. Ries L, Smith M, Smith M, et al. Cancer Incidence and Survival Among Children and Adolescents: United States SEER Program 1975–1995. Bethseda MD: National Cancer Institute; 1999. NIH Pub. No. 99-4649
6. Yang B-T, Wang Z-C, Liu S, et al. CT and MRI diagnosis of osteosarcoma in paranasal sinus. Zhonghua Fang She Xue Za Zhi 2007;41:1062–1065
7. Garrington GE, Scofield HH, Cornyn J, Hooker SP. Osteosarcoma of the jaws. Analysis of 56 cases. Cancer 1967;20(3):377–391
8. Ha PK, Eisele DW, Frassica FJ, Zahurak ML, McCarthy EF. Osteosarcoma of the head and neck: a review of the Johns Hopkins experience. Laryngoscope 1999;109(6):964–969
9. Mardinger O, Givol N, Talmi YP, Taicher S. Osteosarcoma of the jaw. The Chaim Sheba Medical Center experience. Oral Surg Oral Med Oral Pathol Oral Radiol Endod 2001;91(4):445–451
10. Unni K. Dahlin's Bone Tumours: General Aspects and Data on 11,087 Cases. 5th ed. Philadelphia: Lippincott Williams and Wilkins; 1996
11. Dahlin D, Unni K. Osteosarcoma. Bone Tumors: General Aspects and Data on 8,542 Cases, 4th ed. Springfield, IL: Charles C Thomas; 1986:269–307
12. Iezzoni JC, Mills SE. "Undifferentiated" small round cell tumors of the sinonasal tract: differential diagnosis update. Am J Clin Pathol 2005;124(Suppl):S110–S121
13. Link MP, Goorin AM, Horowitz M, et al. Adjuvant chemotherapy of high-grade osteosarcoma of the extremity. Updated results of the Multi-Institutional Osteosarcoma Study. Clin Orthop Relat Res 1991;270(270):8–14
14. Nagarajan R, Clohisy D, Weigel B. New paradigms for therapy for osteosarcoma. Curr Oncol Rep 2005;7(6):410–414
15. Meyers PA, Schwartz CL, Krailo MD, et al; Children's Oncology Group. Osteosarcoma: the addition of muramyl tripeptide to chemotherapy improves overall survival—a report from the Children's Oncology Group. J Clin Oncol 2008;26(4):633–638
16. Jereczek-Fossa BA, Krengli M, Orecchia R. Particle beam radiotherapy for head and neck tumors: radiobiological basis and clinical experience. Head Neck 2006; 28(8):750–760
17. Potter BO, Sturgis EM. Sarcomas of the head and neck. Surg Oncol Clin N Am 2003;12(2):379–417
18. Briccoli A, Rocca M, Salone M, et al. Resection of recurrent pulmonary metastases in patients with osteosarcoma. Cancer 2005;104(8):1721–1725
19. Carrau RL, Segas J, Nuss DW, Snyderman CH, Johnson JT. Role of skull base surgery for local control of sarcoma of the nasal cavity and paranasal sinuses. Eur Arch Otorhinolaryngol 1994;251(6):350–356
20. Kassir RR, Rassekh CH, Kinsella JB, Segas J, Carrau RL, Hokanson JA. Osteosarcoma of the head and neck: meta-analysis of nonrandomized studies. Laryngoscope 1997;107(1):56–61
21. Laskar S, Basu A, Muckaden MA, et al. Osteosarcoma of the head and neck region: lessons learned from a single-institution experience of 50 patients. Head Neck 2008;30(8):1020–1026
22. Guadagnolo BA, Zagars GK, Raymond AK, Benjamin RS, Sturgis EM. Osteosarcoma of the jaw/craniofacial region: outcomes after multimodality treatment. Cancer 2009;115(14):3262–3270
23. Patel SG, Meyers P, Huvos AG, et al. Improved outcomes in patients with osteogenic sarcoma of the head and neck. Cancer 2002;95(7):1495–1503
24. Clark JL, Unni KK, Dahlin DC, Devine KD. Osteosarcoma of the jaw. Cancer 1983;51(12):2311–2316
25. Mark RJ, Sercarz JA, Tran L, Dodd LG, Selch M, Calcaterra TC. Osteogenic sarcoma of the head and neck. The UCLA experience. Arch Otolaryngol Head Neck Surg 1991;117(7):761–766

14 Lymphoreticular Neoplasia and Other Lesions

Although there is abundant lymphoid tissue in the upper aerodigestive tract, the sinonasal area, unlike the nasopharynx, is surprisingly lacking in both mucosa-associated lymphoid deposits and lymph nodes. This in turn is reflected in the relative paucity of regional lymphadenopathy from most malignant sinonasal tumors. However, the sinonasal area can be the site of a range of lymphoid disorders, from site-specific conditions such as NK/T-cell lymphoma to disseminating tumors that can start there, such as B-cell lymphomas, or more generalized neoplasia which may be associated with deposits in the sinuses—for example, chloroma.

Lymphomas account for <5% of all malignant neoplasms of the head and neck and the nose and sinuses account for ~13% of upper aerodigestive tract lymphomas in general. In our series of malignant sinonasal tumors, they accounted for 12% (Table 14.1).

The classification of hematopoietic and lymphoid tumors has also undergone significant changes in the last few decades in response to a better understanding of genetic predisposition and cellular origin. This has been greatly improved by immunohistochemistry, flow cytometry, cytogenetics and molecular studies, the ability to check T-cell receptor rearrangements, and fusion transcripts. A vast array of conditions are covered in the WHO classification[1] and it is beyond the scope of this book to cover all of these in any detail. In its simplest form, the classification relates to cell of origin and is divided into three: myeloid, lymphoid, and histiocytic/dendritic.

We have chosen to concentrate on the lesions that we have encountered, albeit including some rarities. However, **several *key points* emerge that are applicable to all these conditions**:

1. Always have a low threshold of suspicion when confronted by a patient with a condition that is not quite right for simple chronic rhinosinusitis even in the absence of an obvious mass or ulceration.
2. When taking tissue for biopsy, always provide the pathologist with adequate and representative tissue, avoiding areas of necrosis.
3. If in any doubt, always ask for tissue to be referred to a center with a special interest in lymphoma and/or sinonasal pathology.
4. Once the diagnosis is made, the management is primarily medical but should be conducted by oncologists with a special interest in these conditions to obtain the best results and minimize morbidity.

Immunodeficiency-Associated Lymphoproliferative Disorders

Lymphoid Hyperplasia in HIV

Infection with the human immunodeficiency virus puts the individual at a significant risk of developing a range of malignancies in the head and neck from squamous cell carcinoma through Kaposi's sarcoma to lymphomas, including Burkitt's lymphoma and diffuse large B-cell lymphoma. As a precursor of the latter, marked lymphoid hyperplasia may be encountered in any part of Waldeyer's ring, including the nasopharynx where adenoidal enlargement may impinge on the posterior choana, causing nasal obstruction, either bilateral or unilateral. These

Table 14.1 Lymphoreticular tumors: personal series

	n	Age		M:F	Site[a]				
		Range (y)	Mean (y)		Maxilla	Frontoethmoid	Nasal cavity	Orbit	Other
Myeloid sarcoma	3	38, 52, 74	–	0:3	–	2	–	1	–
DLBCL	60	20–89	58	2:1	10	18	22	18	4
NK/T-cell lymphoma	33	17–87	53.5	7:4	1	6	25	1	–
Burkitt's lymphoma	1	60		1:0	1	1	1	1	1
Extramedullary plasmacytoma	13	28–85	43	11:2	4	4	3	2	–
Langerhans histiocytosis	2	8, 40	–	1:1	1			1	

Abbreviations: DLBCL, diffuse large B-cell lymphoma; F, female; M, male; y, year.
[a] Multiple sites affected in some cases.

lesions are characterized by a marked follicular hyperplasia with enlarged germinal centers that are irregular in shape or "serpentine."[2] An HIV test should be considered, with appropriate counseling, in cases of unexplained or new-onset adenoidal hyperplasia.

References

1. Swerdlow S, Camp E, Harris N, et al, eds. World Health Organization Classification of Tumours of Haematopoietic and Lymphoid Tissues. 4th ed. Lyon: IARC Press; 2008:10–13
2. Stelow E, Mills P. Biopsy Interpretation of the Upper Aerodigestive Tract and Ear. Philadelphia: Wolters Kluwer, Lippincott, Williams and Wilkins; 2008:258–260

Myeloid Malignancies

Myeloid Sarcomas

Definition

(ICD-O code 9930/3)

A myeloid sarcoma is a tumor composed of myeloid blasts with or without maturation at an anatomical site other than in the bone marrow.[1]

Synonyms

Extramedullary myeloid tumor, granulocytic sarcoma, chloroma.

Site

These malignancies can occur anywhere in the body but are very rare in the nose and sinuses. They are more often part of a systemic disease (acute myeloid leukemia or other myeloproliferative neoplasms)[2,3] but can occur as isolated lesions when they may be overlooked by the unwary. Orbital lesions are commoner than the paranasal sinuses.

Diagnostic Features

Clinical Features

In general most of the case reports, when part of a disseminated leukemia, have been in children or young people, whereas isolated deposits can affect an older age group. Although said to be commoner in men, we have seen three patients, all women (38, 52, and 74 years old) who presented with pain and mild swelling that was mistaken as chronic frontal rhinosinusitis (2 cases) and dacrocystitis (1 case) and in two cases had undergone surgery without improvement. In neither of these cases was tissue taken at the initial surgery, although both patients had abnormal material in the frontal sinus and lacrimal sac, respectively. Once diagnosed, full staging did not reveal disease elsewhere and the patients were all treated apparently successfully with radiotherapy (1, 4, and 8 years follow-up, respectively).

Case reports of sinus deposits may describe headache[4] or pain as in our two cases.

Imaging

There are no specific features, as the deposit may initially be confined to the sinus cavity (or sac) but with time will expand and erode the adjacent structures. These are among a small number of malignant tumors that will produce an isolated lesion in the frontal or sphenoid.[5] Both CT and MRI, as usual, are helpful and the MRI signal is generally isointense to the brain on both T1W and T2W images.

Histological Features and Differential Diagnosis

Immunohistochemistry with or without flow cytometry will generally confirm the diagnosis when one is confronted by a tumor composed of sheets of neoplastic cells of varying differentiation and phenotype. Most will react with myeloperoxidase, and CD68/KP1 is the most commonly expressed marker, although there are a host of others.[6] FISH and other cytogenetics investigations can demonstrate chromosomal abnormalities in around 55% of cases; for example, monosomy 7 or trisomy 8.

The tumor must be mainly distinguished from lymphomas such as lymphoblastic, diffuse large B-cell, and Burkitt's lymphoma as treatment protocols will differ. Few if any prognostic factors have been determined, although those undergoing bone marrow transplantation as part of their treatment have a higher probability of long-term survival.[7,8]

References

1. Pileri S, Orazi A, Falini B. Myeloid sarcoma. In: Swerdlow S, Camp E, Harris N, et al, eds. World Health Organization Classification of Tumours of Haematopoietic and Lymphoid Tissues. 4th ed. Lyon: IARC Press; 2008:140–141
2. Barker GR, Sloan P. Maxillary chloroma: a myeloid leukaemic deposit. Br J Oral Maxillofac Surg 1988;26(2):124–128
3. Ferri E, Minotto C, Ianniello F, Cavaleri S, Armato E, Capuzzo P. Maxillo-ethmoidal chloroma in acute myeloid leukaemia: case report. Acta Otorhinolaryngol Ital 2005; 25(3):195–199
4. O'Brien J, Buckley O, Murphy C, Torreggiani WC. An unusual cause of persistent headache: chloroma (2008: 2b). Eur Radiol 2008;18(5):1071–1072
5. Freedy RM, Miller KD Jr. Granulocytic sarcoma (chloroma): sphenoidal sinus and paraspinal involvement as evaluated by CT and MR. AJNR Am J Neuroradiol 1991;12(2):259–262
6. Quintanilla-Martínez L, Zukerberg LR, Ferry JA, Harris NL. Extramedullary tumors of lymphoid or myeloid blasts. The role of immunohistology in diagnosis and classification. Am J Clin Pathol 1995;104(4):431–443

7. Breccia M, Mandelli F, Petti MC, et al. Clinico-pathological characteristics of myeloid sarcoma at diagnosis and during follow-up: report of 12 cases from a single institution. Leuk Res 2004;28(11):1165–1169
8. Pileri SA, Ascani S, Cox MC, et al. Myeloid sarcoma: clinico-pathologic, phenotypic and cytogenetic analysis of 92 adult patients. Leukemia 2007;21(2):340–350

Lymphoid Malignancies

Non-Hodgkin's lymphomas

Diffuse Large B-Cell Lymphoma

Definition

(ICD-O code 9680/3)

Diffuse large B-cell lymphoma (DLBCL) is a neoplasm of large B lymphoid cells with nuclear size equal to or exceeding that of normal macrophage nuclei or more than twice the size of a normal lymphocyte that has a diffuse growth pattern.[1]

Etiology

While the Epstein-Barr virus (EBV) can be found in association with this lymphoma, it is more common in those affecting the immunocompromised.[2] Several molecular and cytogenetic abnormalities may be found as well as chromosomal rearrangements of 3q27 in up to 30% of cases.[3] Gene-expression profiling has been used to subdivide DLCBL into two subtypes, one with a profile of germinal center B cells (GCB-like in 45 to 50%) and one of activated peripheral B cells (ABC-like).

Synonyms

In the past the terms malignant lymphoma and lymphosarcoma were used.

Incidence

DLBCL is the most common form of non-Hodgkin's lymphoma encountered in adults in the West.

Site

Extranodal DLBCL can occur anywhere in the upper aerodigestive tract and throughout the nose and sinuses (and nasopharynx). In our own series of 60 cases, the nasal cavity, followed by maxillary and ethmoid areas, were most often affected, although the orbit was also frequently involved either primarily or by secondary extension.

Diagnostic Features

Clinical Features

DLBCL is generally a disease of older adults. In our series of 60 cases, the patients' ages ranged from 20 to 89 years with a mean of 58 years. The male-to-female ratio was 2:1 in accord with the literature.[4] The patients generally present with a rapidly growing mass, which often involves the adjacent soft tissues and may initially be mistaken for cellulitis. As a consequence patients are often given antibiotics on the presumption of an acute bacterial rhinosinusitis or soft tissue infection. They may also present with orbital symptoms due to a mass effect, or due to infiltration of the apex, or due to the neurologic effects of cavernous sinus involvement.

Imaging

The lesion appears as a soft tissue mass associated with bone remodeling, erosion, or infiltration that shows intermediate enhancement on both CT and MRI, increased by contrast administration (**Figs. 14.1, 14.2, 14.3**).[5]

Full staging should be undertaken in all patients, including imaging of the thorax and abdomen, FDG-PET if available, a skeletal survey together with bone marrow aspiration, and full hematological work-up.

Histological Features and Differential Diagnosis

The tumor mass is usually isolated and referred to as "primary" or it can evolve from lower-grade lymphoid tumors such as chronic lymphocytic leukemia/small lymphocytic lymphoma, follicular lymphoma, or extranodal marginal zone lymphomas (secondary). It can also occur following treatment of lymphoma elsewhere in the body as it did in two of our patients (from disease in the testes and shoulder). In the orbit—a condition that in the past was called "pseudotumor," it is now recognized as a precursor of lymphoma and should be treated as such. These may infiltrate the sinuses and infratemporal fossa, thereby coming within the ambit of the ENT surgeon.

Histologically DLCBLs have large neoplastic cells mixed with smaller more normal-looking lymphocytes. Variants are recognized such as T cell rich and plasmablastic.

This latter more aggressive variety is most often seen in association with HIV infection.[2] However, on immunohistochemistry the cells are positive for B cell markers such as CD19, CD20, CD22, and CD79a.[6] They do not express cyclin D1, which distinguishes them from mantle cell lymphomas.

Diagnosis can be confused by the accompanying inflammatory infiltrate. Other conditions such as Wegener's granulomatosis must be excluded.

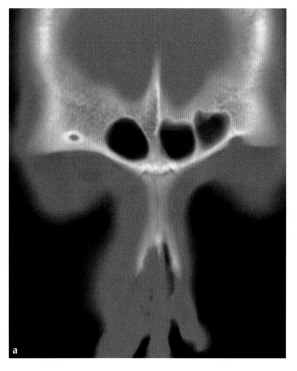

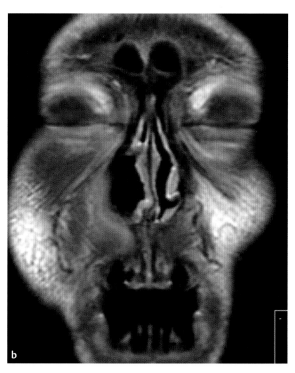

Fig. 14.1a, b

a Coronal CT showing a case of diffuse large B-cell lymphoma affecting soft tissues of the anterior nasal cavity with swelling of the cheek.

b Coronal MRI (T1W post gadolinium enhancement) in the same patient showing the extent of soft tissue involvement and loss of structure on the anterior lateral nasal wall.

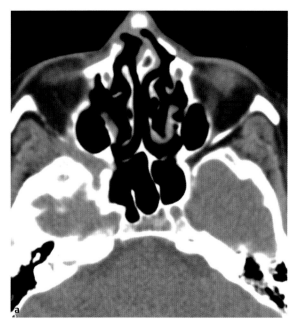

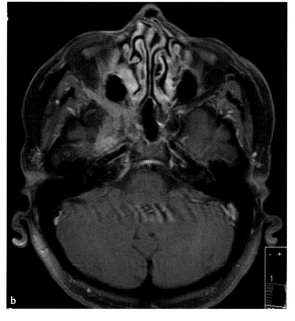

Fig. 14.2a, b

a Axial CT showing a diffuse large B-cell lymphoma affecting the pterygopalatine region with widening of the fissure.

b Axial MRI (T1W post gadolinium enhancement, fat saturation) in the same patient showing the extent of soft tissue involvement with infiltration of the infratemporal fossa, cavernous sinus, and middle cranial fossa.

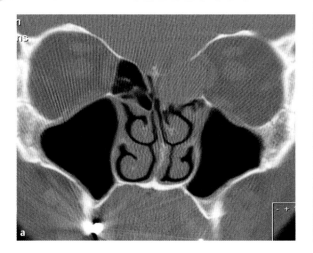

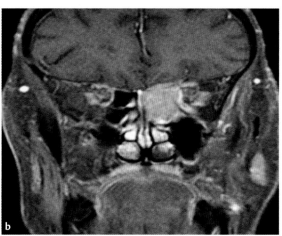

Fig. 14.3a, b

a Coronal CT showing a case of diffuse large B-cell lymphoma affecting the left posterior ethmoid with erosion of the adjacent skull base and lamina papyracea.

b Coronal MRI (T1W post gadolinium enhancement, fat saturation) in the same patient showing the extent of the mass with infiltration of the adjacent dura.

Natural History

Although DLCBL is quite often an isolated lesion, between 11 and 27% are reported to have bone marrow involvement[7] and one-third of these show malignant cells in the peripheral blood.[8]

Treatment and Outcome

Chemotherapy, in particular CHOP (cyclophosphamide, doxorubicin, vincristine, and prednisone), has been used as the primary treatment, to which radiotherapy may be added. The International Prognostic Index (**Table 14.2**) proved reliable for aggressive lymphoma[4] in the past, before rituximab was available. At that time long-term remission rate was between 50% and 60%. The addition of the anti-CD20 antibody, rituximab to conventional CHOP regimes has improved outcome significantly, particularly in those over 60 years old,[9,10] and it is also used as monotherapy for maintenance and relapse.[11] Immunoblastic features and a wide range of immunohistochemical markers have been investigated as prognostic markers, although evidence for their significance is conflicting and has been diminished by the use of rituximab.

Sinonasal NK/T-Cell Lymphoma

Definition

(ICD-O code 9719/3)

This is a slowly progressive, unrelenting ulceration and necrosis of the midline facial tissues. It is a rare form of extranodal non-Hodgkin's lymphoma and has been designated "NK/T" instead of "NK" because, while most cases appear to be genuine natural killer (NK)-cell tumors, some cases show a cytotoxic T cell phenotype.[12]

Table 14.2 International Prognostic Index for aggressive lymphomas

Unfavorable variables		
Age >60 years		
Poor performance status		
Advanced Ann Arbor stage (III–IV)		
Extranodal involvement >2 sites		
High serum LDH (>normal)		

Risk group	Unfavorable variables	
	All patients	*Patients <60 years[a]*
Low	0–1	0
Low/intermediate	2	1
High/intermediate	3	2
High	4 or 5	3

Abbreviation: LDH, lactate dehydrogenase.

Source: Reference 4.

[a] In patients 60 years old or less the age-adjusted international prognostic index (aaIPI) is calculated with three unfavorable variables that include poor performance status, advanced Ann Arbor stage, and high serum LDH.

Etiology

An association with Epstein-Barr virus has been reported. Both EBV DNA and RNA have been found in tumor cells associated with high titers of EBV antibodies, but the exact role of the virus remains to be determined.[13,14] This may account for these tumors being more common in Asia.

The most common cytogenetic abnormality is deletion of the long arm of chromosome 6[15,16] and a low frequency of HLA-A *0201 allele has been reported in patients with EBV-positive tumors.[17]

Synonyms

No neoplastic condition in the nose and sinuses has been the subject of more confusion than granulomatous neoplasia. Terminology such as "midline destructive granuloma," while descriptive, did nothing to assist the understanding of a condition that requires appropriate oncological treatment if patients are to survive. First described by McBride in 1897[18] with a subsequent comprehensive account of the clinical and histological features by Stewart,[19] it has variously been called midline malignant reticulosis, polymorphic reticulosis, osteomyelitis necroticans, lethal midline granuloma, NACE (a malignant neoplasm of histiocytic lymphoma type), and angiocentric immunoproliferative lesion.[20] Modern histopathology techniques confirm that in virtually all cases, these were misnomers for NK/T-cell lymphoma.[21]

Site

Classically the condition starts in the nasal cavity, usually affecting the septum, which perforates, and then spreads inexorably to the surrounding tissue of the midface, palate, and orbits. However, clinicians should be aware that the lesion does not always arise strictly in the midline.

Diagnostic Features

Clinical Features

NK/T-cell lymphoma can occur at any age though the median age is in the fifth or sixth decades. Some series have suggested either a male or female preponderance though this has not been *markedly* so in our experience (Table 14.1).

This condition is rare in Western populations but much more common in Asia and South America.[22]

Classically the disease can be divided into three phases:

1. **Prodromal.** This phase may last for years as the patient experiences common symptoms such as nasal obstruction and discharge. ENT referral at this point may well result in some form of nasal surgery as this is often regarded as a nonspecific chronic rhinitis or rhinosinusitis.[23]
2. **Active.** As the condition progresses, areas of necrosis in and around the nasal cavity develop with increasing discharge, and crusting resulting in tissue loss. There is progressive loss of midline structure with erosion of the septum, erosion of the palate to form oroantral fistulas, and extension into adjacent structures such as the skull base, nasopharynx, and orbit with associated cranial nerve palsies. Secondary infection and inflammation result in pyrexia and malaise.

3. **Terminal.** As the process affects vital structures, overwhelming infection, hemorrhage, and general fatigue lead to death, often in association with disseminated systemic lymphoma. Night sweats and febrile episodes commonly occur. At this point there may be an overlap with NK-cell leukemia with involvement of marrow and peripheral blood.

The speed of the process can vary and may take several years, again lulling clinicians into a false sense of security.

Imaging

The progressive loss of midline structure can be seen on both CT and MRI, involving both soft tissue and bone, but is not pathognomonic (**Fig. 14.4**).[5,24] The lack of a tumor mass frequently delays diagnosis.

The possibility of systemic disease and other conditions in the differential diagnosis may indicate imaging of the chest and abdomen and bone scans.

Histological Features and Differential Diagnosis

Expert histopathology is paramount in this condition as the atypical cellular infiltrates may be missed with a marked nonspecific inflammatory process and widespread necrosis. It is vital to provide representative tissue as superficial biopsies will fail to provide a diagnosis. Modern immunohistochemistry has greatly improved the situation and reveals characteristic phenotypic expression with both NK cells and T cells. A panel of monoclonal antibodies against T cell differentiation antigens are required as aberrant phenotypes are common. Positivity to CD45 and CD56, but not to CD57,[25,26] is common but **the distinction of this condition from the many**

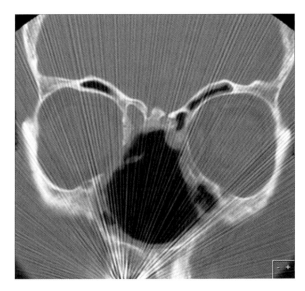

Fig. 14.4 Coronal CT showing a case of NK/T-cell lymphoma.

lymphoproliferative disorders that can occur is the realm of the specialist pathologist and there should be a low threshold for referring all ambiguous cases for a second opinion.

The infiltrates can be monoclonal or polymorphic, consisting of atypical T lymphocytes, plasma cells, small lymphocytes, histiocytes, and eosinophils, which tend to arrange themselves in a necrotizing angiocentric/angio-infiltrative growth pattern. Thrombosis and necrosis are seen, but not granulomas per se. Specific tests for EBV can be helpful in some cases.

A condition that has recently caused considerable diagnostic difficulties is the midline destruction that can be associated with cocaine abuse.[27,28] Although more often confused with Wegener's (C-ANCA-positive) granuloma, it should also be considered in the differential diagnosis for NK/T-cell lymphoma. Similarly, midline necrotizing infections, both bacterial and fungal, can produce similar clinical and radiological appearances (**Fig. 14.4**) (**Table 14.3**).

Thus, laboratory tests should include FBC (full blood count), ESR (erythrocyte sedimentation rate), CRP (C-reactive protein), ANCA (antineutrophilic cytoplasmic antibodies), ACE (angiotensin-converting enzyme) as well as tests for tuberculosis and syphilis and bone marrow evaluation in selected cases.

Table 14.3 Main conditions in differential diagnosis of NK/T-cell lymphoma

Inflammatory	C-ANCA-positive granulomas (Wegener's or GPA)
	Cocaine abuse
	Sarcoid
	Systemic lupus erythematosus
	Polyarteritis nodosum
Repeated trauma	
Infection	Necrotizing fasciitis
	Invasive fungal infections
	Rhinoscleroma
	Tuberculosis
	Syphilis
Neoplastic	Other lymphomas
	Squamous cell carcinoma
	Basal cell carcinoma

Abbreviations: C-ANCA, cytoplasmic antineutrophilic cytoplasmic antibodies; GPA, granulomatosis with polyangiitis.

Natural History

Because of the failure to understand the true nature of this condition, many patients in the past had advanced disease when diagnosed, and death resulted from overwhelming secondary infection, hemorrhage, or disseminated lymphoma.

Treatment and Outcome

A full course of radiotherapy should be given covering all affected areas in the midline combined with chemotherapy. The anthracycline-based CHOP regime (cyclophosphamide, doxorubicin hydrochloride, vincristine sulfate, and prednisone) is generally favored, but small sample sizes make standardization of any protocol difficult and this may vary depending on the stage of the disease.

Unless the disease is correctly staged and treated aggressively, the outcome is poor. In the past, low-dose radiotherapy often produced initially good results but was almost inevitably followed by fatal relapse.[29-31] If disease has spread, prognosis is inevitably worse, although there are few large series with long-term follow-up. In the literature, 5-year survival ranges from 46% to 63% but **early and late relapse is often encountered so lifetime surveillance is recommended** and some authors have quoted 5-year survival rates as low as 20%.[32] However, it appears that more aggressive combined medical oncologic therapy has resulted in better outcomes in recent years, although some individuals express multidrug resistance genes that render chemotherapy less effective.[33] Thus, additional chemotherapy in a series of 25 patients was not shown to be of benefit,[34] but the rarity of the condition means that these cohorts may have been accrued over many years and are generally considered retrospectively, during a period when therapy delivery may have changed.

In our own series of 33 patients, the majority have been treated with a full course of radiotherapy, beginning with cobalt 60 in the 1970s through to more modern regimes. Twenty-one survived (follow-up 6 months to 23 years, mean 4.9 years), 7 died of disease (follow-up 3 months to 12 years, mean 2.7 years), 2 died of intercurrent disease, and 3 were lost to follow-up (**Table 14.1**).

The presence of high titers of circulating EBV DNA correlates with extensive disease, unfavorable response to therapy, and poorer survival.[35] A study of 32 Japanese patients showed that p53 missense mutation was significantly related to worse cause-specific survival.[36] Overall, as might be expected, extent of disease, especially invasion of bone or skin, and high levels of EBV DNA in the circulation and bone marrow are associated with poorer outcome. This is often expressed in the International Prognostic Index (IPI) with higher values equating to poorer prognosis (**Table 14.2**).[37]

Other Lymphomas

Other non-Hodgkin's lymphomas, such as mantle cell, follicular, and extranodal marginal zone, occur in the upper aerodigestive tract and mainly affect the Waldeyer's ring. The mantle cell and follicular lymphomas are exceptionally rare in the sinonasal region, but are usually at an advanced stage at presentation, affecting the bone marrow and highly malignant with few long-term survivors. Recently high-dose chemotherapy with peripheral blood stem cell transplantation has been used with some success[38] and the addition of rituximab to chemotherapy has significantly improved overall survival and disease control.[10,11] Extranodal marginal zone lymphomas or mucosa-associated lymphoid tissue lymphomas (MALTomas) are more indolent and can be associated with Sjögren's syndrome when they involve the seromucinous glands. There are a few case reports in the literature.[39] Some transform into diffuse large B-cell lymphomas.

Burkitt's lymphoma

Definition

(ICD-O code 9687/3)

Burkitt's lymphoma (BL) is a B-cell lymphoma with a very short doubling time that presents at extranodal sites or as an acute leukemia.[40]

Etiology

Three variants of BL are described: endemic, sporadic, and immunodeficiency-associated, usually with human immunodeficiency virus (HIV) infection.

The endemic form occurs in equatorial Africa (Kenya, Ghana, Nigeria, Uganda) with an incidence peak of 4 to 7 years and a male-to-female ratio of 2:1. It was first described by Denis Burkitt in 1958,[41] who also demonstrated that the geographical distribution exactly mirrored that of certain mosquitoes, suggesting an insect vector.[42] Epstein-Barr virus DNA was subsequently shown to be present in most BL cells and the impact of malarial infection on immunity and EBV persistence supports an important etiological relationship. However, this alone does not entirely explain the distribution of the disease and other cofactors are also most likely at work.[43]

The sporadic form also affects children and young adults and is commoner in males. About 30% of these cases show EBV infection, as do cases associated with HIV infection.

Incidence

While endemic BL is the most common childhood malignancy in equatorial Africa, sporadic forms represent only 1 to 2% of all lymphomas in the Western world, but 30 to 50% of childhood lymphomas generally. It often occurs as one of the early indicators of acquired immunodeficiency syndrome (AIDS).

Site

In the endemic form there is a predilection for extranodal disease to affect the upper and lower jaws, orbit, and other facial bones in ~50% of cases,[40] although this is not seen in the sporadic type. The disease often affects the central nervous system and in adults the lymph nodes are frequently involved, as they were in one 60-year-old man from North Africa who presented with a large mass affecting the orbit and midface.

Diagnostic Features

Clinical Features

The disease is characterized by the dramatic speed of growth over a matter of days or weeks. Thus most patients present with advanced disease, which has been the experience of one author (D.H.) in Ghana.

Imaging

BL is characterized by rapidly developing widespread bony destruction that is otherwise indistinguishable from other aggressive malignant tumors (**Fig. 14.5**). Generally isointense to muscle on CT, the tumors may show marked areas of necrosis within the tumor mass. On T1W images, the tumor enhancement is generally low, but has variable intensity on T2W images and with gadolinium-DTPA contrast.[44]

Histological Features and Differential Diagnosis

The tumor cells of BL are medium-sized and show a diffuse monotonous pattern of growth. They exhibit many mitotic figures and a high number of apoptotic cells, which are ingested by macrophages to produce a typical "starry sky" appearance. The tumor cells express moderate to high levels of membrane IgM with light chain restriction and B-cell-associated antigens (CD19, CD20, CD22). Virtually all are Ki67 positive[6] and most show MYC translocations. Gene profiling studies have shown a specific gene expression signature for BL, distinct from that for DLBCL.[45]

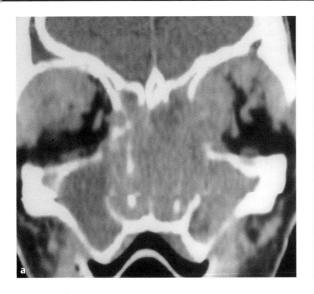

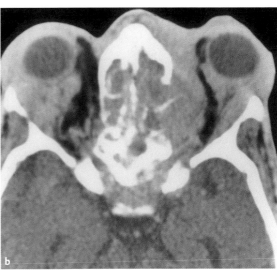

Fig. 14.5a, b

a Burkitt's lymphoma. Coronal CT scan showing widespread disease affecting the midface including the nasal cavity, all paranasal sinuses, both orbits and soft tissues of the face.

b Burkitt's lymphoma. Axial CT scan of the same patient showing extensive infiltration of the orbits and skull base.

Natural History, Treatment, and Outcome

Both endemic and sporadic forms of BL will rapidly overwhelm the patient unless treated. However, BL—particularly the endemic form—is exquisitely sensitive to chemotherapy and both forms are potentially curable when less extensive. Up to 90% may be cured in these circumstances[46] and figures of 60 to 80% cure are reported for later-stage disease[47]; and the addition of rituximab is also proving of benefit.[48] However, due to the tumor bulk, patients may develop a tumor lysis syndrome that can cause death from impaired organ function, particularly renal failure.

Hodgkin's lymphoma

Hodgkin's lymphoma is rarely extranodal but may affect the upper aerodigestive tract, including Waldeyer's ring, where it is much less common than non-Hodgkin's types and exceptionally rare in the nose and sinuses. A wide age range is affected. Mixed cellularity and nodular sclerosis patterns are commonest and diagnosis requires the presence of Reed-Sternberg cells, which are immunoreactive to antibodies to CD15 and CD30 but not CD45. A Cochrane review that considered the treatment of early Hodgkin's lymphoma in general showed that additional radiotherapy with chemotherapy improves tumor control and overall survival.[49] Outcome is similar to that of nodal disease of a similar stage.

References

1. Stein H, Chan J, Warnke R, et al. Diffuse large B cell lymphoma: not otherwise specified. In: Swerdlow S, Camp E, Harris N et al, eds. World Health Organization Classification of Tumours of Haematopoietic and Lymphoid Tissues. 4th ed. Lyon: IARC Press; 2008:233
2. Dong HY, Scadden DT, de Leval L, Tang Z, Isaacson PG, Harris NL. Plasmablastic lymphoma in HIV-positive patients: an aggressive Epstein-Barr virus-associated extramedullary plasmacytic neoplasm. Am J Surg Pathol 2005;29(12):1633–1641
3. Kawasaki C, Ohshim K, Suzumiya J, et al. Rearrangements of bcl-1, bcl-2, bcl-6, and c-myc in diffuse large B-cell lymphomas. Leuk Lymphoma 2001;42(5):1099–1106
4. Armitage JO, Weisenburger DD. New approach to classifying non-Hodgkin's lymphomas: clinical features of the major histologic subtypes. Non-Hodgkin's Lymphoma Classification Project. J Clin Oncol 1998;16(8):2780–2795
5. Madani G, Beale TJ, Lund VJ. Imaging of sinonasal tumors. Semin Ultrasound CT MR 2009;30(1):25–38
6. Harris NL, Jaffe ES, Stein H, et al. A revised European-American classification of lymphoid neoplasms: a proposal from the International Lymphoma Study Group. Blood 1994;84(5):1361–1392
7. Campbell J, Seymour JF, Matthews J, Wolf M, Stone J, Juneja S. The prognostic impact of bone marrow involvement in patients with diffuse large cell lymphoma varies according to the degree of infiltration and presence of discordant marrow involvement. Eur J Haematol 2006;76(6):473–480
8. Arber DA, George TI. Bone marrow biopsy involvement by non-Hodgkin's lymphoma: frequency of lymphoma types, patterns, blood involvement, and discordance with other sites in 450 specimens. Am J Surg Pathol 2005;29(12):1549–1557
9. Coiffier B. Rituximab therapy in malignant lymphoma. Oncogene 2007;26(25):3603–3613

10. Schulz H, Bohlius J, Skoetz N, et al. Chemotherapy plus Rituximab versus chemotherapy alone for B-cell non-Hodgkin's lymphoma. Cochrane Database Syst Rev 2007;4(4):CD003805

11. Keating GM. Rituximab: a review of its use in chronic lymphocytic leukaemia, low-grade or follicular lymphoma and diffuse large B-cell lymphoma. Drugs 2010; 70(11):1445–1476

12. Chan J, Quintanilla-Martinez L, Ferry J, Peh P. Extranodal NK/T-cell lymphoma, nasal type. In: Swerdlow S, Camp E, Harris N et al, eds. World Health Organization Classification of Tumours of Haematopoietic and Lymphoid Tissues. 4th ed. Lyon: IARC Press; 2008:285–288

13. Kanavaros P, Lescs MC, Brière J, et al. Nasal T-cell lymphoma: a clinicopathologic entity associated with peculiar phenotype and with Epstein-Barr virus. Blood 1993; 81(10):2688–2695

14. Dictor M, Cervin A, Kalm O, Rambech E. Sinonasal T-cell lymphoma in the differential diagnosis of lethal midline granuloma using in situ hybridization for Epstein-Barr virus RNA. Mod Pathol 1996;9(1):7–14

15. Strickler JG, Meneses MF, Habermann TM, et al. Polymorphic reticulosis: a reappraisal. Hum Pathol 1994;25(7):659–665

16. Nava VE, Jaffe ES. The pathology of NK-cell lymphomas and leukemias. Adv Anat Pathol 2005;12(1):27–34

17. Kanno H, Kojya S, Li T, et al. Low frequency of HLA-A*0201 allele in patients with Epstein-Barr virus-positive nasal lymphomas with polymorphic reticulosis morphology. Int J Cancer 2000;87(2):195–199

18. McBride P. Photographs of a case of rapid destruction of the nose and face. 1897. J Laryngol Otol 1991;105(12):1120

19. Stewart JP. Progressive lethal granulomatous ulceration of the nose. J Laryngol Otol 1933;48:657–701

20. Michaels L, Gregory MM. Pathology of 'non-healing (midline) granuloma'. J Clin Pathol 1977;30(4):317–327

21. Rodrigo JP, Suárez C, Rinaldo A, et al. Idiopathic midline destructive disease: fact or fiction. Oral Oncol 2005;41(4):340–348

22. Vidal RW, Devaney K, Ferlito A, Rinaldo A, Carbone A. Sinonasal malignant lymphomas: a distinct clinicopathological category. Ann Otol Rhinol Laryngol 1999;108(4):411–419

23. Paik YS, Liess BD, Scheidt TD, Ingram EA, Zitsch RP III. Extranodal nasal-type natural killer/T-cell lymphoma masquerading as recalcitrant sinusitis. Head Neck 2010; 32(2):268–273

24. Ooi GC, Chim CS, Liang R, Tsang KW, Kwong YL. Nasal T-cell/natural killer cell lymphoma: CT and MR imaging features of a new clinicopathologic entity. AJR Am J Roentgenol 2000;174(4):1141–1145

25. Emile JF, Boulland ML, Haioun C, et al. CD5⁻CD56⁺ T-cell receptor silent peripheral T-cell lymphomas are natural killer cell lymphomas. Blood 1996;87(4):1466–1473

26. Jaffe ES, Chan JK, Su IJ, et al. Report of the Workshop on Nasal and Related Extranodal Angiocentric T/Natural Killer Cell Lymphomas. Definitions, differential diagnosis, and epidemiology. Am J Surg Pathol 1996;20(1):103–111

27. Trimarchi M, Gregorini G, Facchetti F, et al. Cocaine-induced midline destructive lesions: clinical, radiographic, histopathologic, and serologic features and their differentiation from Wegener granulomatosis. Medicine (Baltimore) 2001;80(6):391–404

28. Peikert T, Finkielman JD, Hummel AM, et al. Functional characterization of antineutrophil cytoplasmic antibodies in patients with cocaine-induced midline destructive lesions. Arthritis Rheum 2008;58(5):1546–1551

29. Harrison DFN. Midline destructive granuloma: fact or fiction. Laryngoscope 1987;97(9):1049–1053

30. Sheahan P, Donnelly M, O'Reilly S, Murphy M. T/NK cell non-Hodgkin's lymphoma of the sinonasal tract. J Laryngol Otol 2001;115(12):1032–1035

31. Seok JK, Byung SK, Chul WC, et al. Treatment outcome of front-line systemic chemotheraphy for localized extranodal NK/T cell lymphoma in nasal and upper aerodigestive tract. Leuk Lymphoma 2006;47:1265–1273

32. Mendenhall WM, Olivier KR, Lynch JW Jr, Mendenhall NP. Lethal midline granuloma-nasal natural killer/T-cell lymphoma. Am J Clin Oncol 2006;29(2):202–206

33. Drénou B, Lamy T, Amiot L, et al. CD3⁻CD56⁺ non-Hodgkin's lymphomas with an aggressive behavior related to multidrug resistance. Blood 1997;89(8):2966–2974

34. Chen HH, Fong L, Su IJ, et al. Experience of radiotherapy in lethal midline granuloma with special emphasis on centrofacial T-cell lymphoma: a retrospective analysis covering a 34-year period. Radiother Oncol 1996;38(1):1–6

35. Au WY, Pang A, Choy C, Chim CS, Kwong YL. Quantification of circulating Epstein-Barr virus (EBV) DNA in the diagnosis and monitoring of natural killer cell and EBV-positive lymphomas in immunocompetent patients. Blood 2004;104(1):243–249

36. Takahara M, Kishibe K, Bandoh N, Nonaka S, Harabuchi Y. P53, N- and K-Ras, and beta-catenin gene mutations and prognostic factors in nasal NK/T-cell lymphoma from Hokkaido, Japan. Hum Pathol 2004;35(1):86–95

37. Chor-Sang C, Shin-Yan M, Wing-Yan A, et al. Primary nasal natural killer cell lymphoma: long-term outcome and relationship with the International Prognostic Index. Neoplasia 2004;103:216–221

38. Fagnoni P, Milpied N, Limat S, et al; Groupe Ouest-Est des Leucémies et des Autres Maladies du Sang. Cost effectiveness of high-dose chemotherapy with autologous stem cell support as initial treatment of aggressive non-Hodgkin's lymphoma. Pharmacoeconomics 2009;27(1):55–68

39. Babb MJ, Cruz RM, Puligandla B. Sinonasal mucosa-associated lymphoid tissue lymphoma. Arch Otolaryngol Head Neck Surg 1999;125(5):585–588

40. Leoncini L, Raphael M, Stein H, Harris N, Jaffe E, Kluin P. Burkitt lymphoma. In: Swerdlow S, Camp E, Harris N et al, eds. World Health Organization Classification of Tumours of Haematopoietic and Lymphoid Tissues. 4th ed. Lyon: IARC Press; 2008:262–264

41. Burkitt D. A sarcoma involving the jaws in African children. Br J Surg 1958;46(197):218–223

42. Burkitt D, Wright D. Geographical and tribal distribution of the African lymphoma in Uganda. BMJ 1966; 1(5487):569–573

43. van den Bosch CA. Is endemic Burkitt's lymphoma an alliance between three infections and a tumour promoter? Lancet Oncol 2004;5(12):738–746

44. Weber AL, Rahemtullah A, Ferry JA. Hodgkin and non-Hodgkin lymphoma of the head and neck: clinical, pathologic, and imaging evaluation. Neuroimaging Clin N Am 2003;13(3):371–392

45. Dave SS, Fu K, Wright GW, et al; Lymphoma/Leukemia Molecular Profiling Project. Molecular diagnosis of Burkitt's lymphoma. N Engl J Med 2006;354(23):2431–2442

46. Patte C, Auperin A, Gerrard M, et al; FAB/LMB96 International Study Committee. Results of the randomized international FAB/LMB96 trial for intermediate risk B-cell non-Hodgkin lymphoma in children and adolescents: it is possible to reduce treatment for the early responding patients. Blood 2007;109(7):2773–2780

47. Magrath IT, Janus C, Edwards BK, et al. An effective therapy for both undifferentiated (including Burkitt's) lymphomas and lymphoblastic lymphomas in children and young adults. Blood 1984;63(5):1102–1111

48. Thomas DA, Faderl S, O'Brien S, et al. Chemoimmuno-therapy with hyper-CVAD plus rituximab for the treatment of adult Burkitt and Burkitt-type lymphoma or acute lymphoblastic leukemia. Cancer 2006;106(7):1569–1580
49. Herbst C, Rehan FA, Skoetz N, et al. Chemotherapy alone versus chemotherapy plus radiotherapy for early stage Hodgkin lymphoma. Cochrane Database Syst Rev 2011;2(2):CD007110

Extraosseous Plasmacytoma

Definition

(ICD-O code 9734/3)

One of several plasma cell neoplasms, extraosseous plasmacytoma is a monoclonal proliferation of plasma cells that occurs at extraosseous sites without concomitant bone marrow involvement.

Synonyms

Extramedullary plasmacytoma.

Incidence

Rare.

Site

Extraosseous plasmacytoma (EOP) has a predilection for the upper aerodigestive tract mucosa,[1,2] particularly the sinonasal region.[3–5] In our small cohort of 13 patients, 4 affected the maxillary sinus, 4 the frontoethmoid region, 3 the nasal cavity, and 2 the orbit.

Elsewhere in the head and neck, EOP is found in the oropharynx and nasopharynx and in the larynx.[6]

Diagnostic Features

Clinical Features

EOP is said to occur in older patients, usually in the sixth decade. Our patients were somewhat younger, with an age range of 28 to 85 years, mean 43 years. Eleven (85%) were men compared with 66% reported in the literature.

A mass effect depending on the site includes nasal obstruction, rhinorrhea, and epistaxis.

Imaging

Imaging shows a nonspecific mass occupying the nasal cavity or paranasal sinus with or without bone erosion (**Fig. 14.6a**), with CT the most appropriate imaging mode.

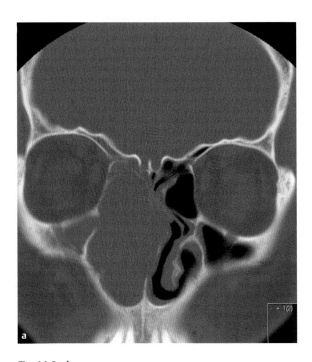
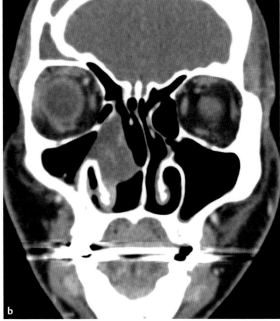

Fig. 14.6a, b

a Plasmacytoma of the right nasal cavity. Coronal CT scan showing unilateral opacification and expansion of the right nasal cavity due to a mass in the nose obstructing the adjacent maxillary, frontal, and ethmoid sinuses.

b Coronal CT scan in the same patient showing a residual mass in the right middle meatus after chemoradiotherapy 6 months earlier. It was subjected to endoscopic excision but contained no viable disease.

Histological Features and Differential Diagnosis

EOP is another of the "undifferentiated" small cell tumors that require immunohistochemical investigation and expert interpretation.[7] Sheets of plasma cells characteristically with eccentrically placed nuclei with granular or clock-faced chromatin are found. Russell bodies are often found.

By definition the bone marrow is not involved but ~20% have a small M-protein, mostly IgA.[8]

The differential diagnosis includes some lymphomas, especially extranodal marginal zone lymphomas (MALT) that have undergone plasma cell differentiation.[9]

Natural History

Up to 1 in 4 is said to recur locally (2/13 in our series) and ~15 to 25% go on to develop cervical lymph node involvement, distant extraosseous sites, and/or myeloma (see below).

Treatment and Outcome

With localized radiotherapy, the outlook for patients with EOP is good, with the majority cured. It is estimated that around 70% of patients are disease free at 10 years, which is the overall survival in our patients available for long-term follow-up (mean 8.6 years, range 4–17 years).[10]

Surgery has little to offer for most patients other than initial biopsy but it is occasionally required if radiotherapy fails. Three of our patients underwent surgical clearance of residual abnormal tissue, including craniofacial resection, orbital clearance, and endoscopic sinus surgery, although in the latter case no residual tumor was demonstrated (**Fig. 14.6b**).

Myelomatosis

Plasma cell myeloma is a bone marrow–based, multifocal plasma cell neoplasm associated with an M-protein in the serum and/or urine, otherwise known as multiple myeloma. It has a spectrum of clinical activity from asymptomatic to aggressive forms and can occasionally be deposited in the sinonasal region. Diagnosis is made by the presence of lytic lesions on imaging, hypercalcemia, a serum M protein, and Bence Jones protein in the urine, and confirmed by bone marrow examination. Staging is based on the Durie and Salmon classification[11] and overall it can be difficult to cure, with a median survival of 3 to 4 years and a range of <6 months to >10 years.[12] We have seen two patients, a 58-year-old man and an 80-year-old woman, who both presented with symptoms suggestive of chronic rhinosinusitis but with other systemic symptoms such as malaise. Biopsy and urinalysis provided the diagnosis.

References

1. Batsakis JG, Medeiros JL, Luna MA, El-Naggar AK. Plasma cell dyscrasias and the head and neck. Ann Diagn Pathol 2002;6(2):129–140
2. Alexiou C, Kau RJ, Dietzfelbinger H, et al. Extramedullary plasmacytoma: tumor occurrence and therapeutic concepts. Cancer 1999;85(11):2305–2314
3. Ampil FL, Borski TG, Nathan CO, et al. Cavernous sinus involvement by extramedullary plasmacytoma of the sphenoid sinus. An argument for the use of adjuvant chemotherapy. Leuk Lymphoma 2002;43(10):2037–2040
4. Ersoy O, Sanlier T, Yigit O, Halefoglu AM, Ucak S, Altuntas Y. Extramedullary plasmacytoma of the maxillary sinus. Acta Otolaryngol 2004;124(5):642–644
5. Anil S. Solitary plasmacytoma of the maxilla—a case report and review of the literature. Gen Dent 2007;55(1):39–43
6. Manganaris A, Conn B, Connor S, Simo R. Uncommon presentation of nasopharyngeal extramedullary plasmacytoma: a case report and literature review. B-ENT 2010;6(2):143–146
7. Iezzoni JC, Mills SE. "Undifferentiated" small round cell tumors of the sinonasal tract: differential diagnosis update. Am J Clin Pathol 2005;124(Suppl):S110–S121
8. Anon.; International Myeloma Working Group. Criteria for the classification of monoclonal gammopathies, multiple myeloma and related disorders: a report of the International Myeloma Working Group. Br J Haematol 2003;121(5):749–757
9. Dimopoulos MA, Kiamouris C, Moulopoulos LA. Solitary plasmacytoma of bone and extramedullary plasmacytoma. Hematol Oncol Clin North Am 1999;13(6):1249–1257
10. Dimopoulos MA, Hamilos G. Solitary bone plasmacytoma and extramedullary plasmacytoma. Curr Treat Options Oncol 2002;3(3):255–259
11. Durie BG, Salmon SE. A clinical staging system for multiple myeloma. Correlation of measured myeloma cell mass with presenting clinical features, response to treatment, and survival. Cancer 1975;36(3):842–854
12. Greipp PR, San Miguel J, Durie BG, et al. International staging system for multiple myeloma. J Clin Oncol 2005;23(15):3412–3420

Histiocytic and Dendritic Cell Malignancies

(ICD-O code 9751/3)

There is a group of rare neoplasms composed of cells resembling macrophages or dendritic cells: histiocytic sarcoma, Langerhans histiocytosis, and dendritic cell sarcomas. Of these, Langerhans cell histiocytosis (LCH) may be encountered in the sinonasal region where it has otherwise been known as histiocytosis X, eosinophilic granuloma (if an isolated lesion), Hand-Schuller-Christian disease (if multiple lesions), and Letterer-Siwe disease (if disseminated or there is visceral involvement).[1,2] There is also an association between T lymphoblastic leukemia and LCH.

Thus bone and adjacent soft tissues (e.g., skull) may be involved in one or many areas, as may the skin, lung,

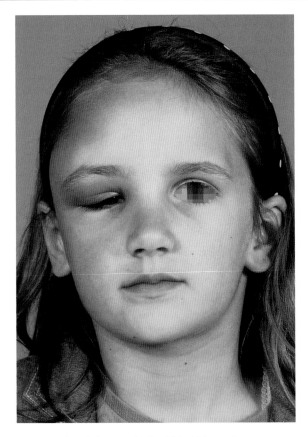

Fig. 14.7 Clinical photograph of a child with Langerhans histiocytosis presenting with "acute" orbital cellulitis.

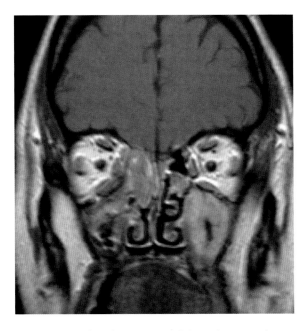

Fig. 14.8 Coronal MRI (T1W post gadolinium enhancement) showing involvement of the right and left maxillary sinuses with deposits of Langerhans histiocytosis.

liver, and spleen. A lytic bone lesion, associated soft tissue mass, or lymphadenopathy may be encountered that may mimic acute infection, such as mastoiditis or sinusitis. There may be systemic morbidity in the form of fever and malaise, together with cytopenia. Generally patients are children, teenagers, or young adults.

We have seen two cases, a girl of 8 years and a man of 40 years. The child presented with an acute orbital mass, initially thought to be orbital cellulitis (**Fig. 14.7**), the man with a maxillary mass thought to be a squamous cell carcinoma, for which he underwent a partial maxillectomy prior to referral (**Fig. 14.8**).

LCH is a clonal neoplastic proliferation of Langerhans-type cells that express CD1a, langerin, and S100 protein. On ultrastructural examination they show Birbeck granules that are described as tennis racquet–shaped.

As with all lymphoreticular lesions, full staging is required because treatment and outcome relate directly to whether the disease is unifocal or multifocal. Poor prognostic factors are involvement of the bone marrow, liver, and lung, but with unifocal disease appropriately treated, nearly all patients can expect to survive. This can be anticipated in only one-third with multifocal disease.[3,4] One of our patients had unifocal disease, the other bilateral involvement of the maxillary sinuses; both have survived long term (5 and 17 years, respectively).

When sinus histiocytosis occurs in association with massive lymphadenopathy, it has been termed Rosai-Dorfman syndrome, which most often affects the skin, upper respiratory tract, and bone, although any area of the body may be involved.[5]

In juvenile xanthogranuloma, a proliferation of histiocytes may be seen in deposits affecting the skin, bone, or viscera. Very rarely the orbit or facial skeleton may be involved.

References

1. Jaffe R, Weiss L, Facchetti F. Tumours derived from Langerhans cells. In: Swerdlow S, Camp E, Harris N et al, eds. World Health Organization Classification of Tumours of Haematopoietic and Lymphoid Tissues. 4th ed. Lyon: IARC Press; 2008:358–360
2. Satter EK, High WA. Langerhans cell histiocytosis: a review of the current recommendations of the Histiocyte Society. Pediatr Dermatol 2008;25(3):291–295
3. Titgemeyer C, Grois N, Minkov M, Flucher-Wolfram B, Gatterer-Menz I, Gadner H. Pattern and course of single-system disease in Langerhans cell histiocytosis data from the DAL-HX 83- and 90-study. Med Pediatr Oncol 2001;37(2):108–114
4. Minkov M, Pötschger U, Grois N, Gadner H, Dworzak MN. Bone marrow assessment in Langerhans cell histiocytosis. Pediatr Blood Cancer 2007;49(5):694–698
5. Foucar E, Rosai J, Dorfman R. Sinus histiocytosis with massive lymphadenopathy (Rosai-Dorfman disease): review of the entity. Semin Diagn Pathol 1990;7(1):19–73

15 Neuroectodermal Lesions

Primary neurogenic lesions presenting in the nose and sinuses are relatively rare but they increasingly come within the ambit of the ENT surgeon who has an interest in the skull base. The following conditions are considered in this section.

- Meningoencephaloceles
- Heterotopic central nervous system tissue (nasal gliomas); no ICD-O code
- Schwannoma (neurolemmoma); ICD-O 9560/0
- Neurofibroma; ICD-O 9540/0
- Extracranial meningioma; ICD-O 9530/0
- Neuroendocrine (small cell) carcinoma; ICD-O 8240/3; 8249/3;8041/3
- Sinonasal undifferentiated carcinoma; ICD-O 8020/3
- Olfactory neuroblastoma; ICD-O 9522/3
- Primitive neuroectodermal tumor; ICD-O 9364/3
- Mucosal malignant melanoma; ICD-O 8720/3
- Melanotic neuroectodermal tumor of infancy; ICD-O 9363/0

Histological differentiation can be particularly challenging in this area and often relies on an array of immunohistochemistry to confirm the diagnosis (**Table 15.1**).[1]

Meningoencephaloceles and Heterotopic Central Nervous System Tissue (Nasal Gliomas)

Definition

These lesions are protrusions of brain contents through a congenital (or traumatic) defect in the skull base. A meningocele contains meninges and cerebrospinal fluid (CSF) alone, a meningoencephalocele contains brain tissue as well and rarely a ventricle may also be involved (meningoencephalocystocele). If no bony defect is present, then the mass containing heterotopic brain is termed a glioma.

Etiology

Several theories have been proposed but in general the frontonasal lesions probably result from a failure of the foramen cecum to close,[2] allowing extrusion of intracranial contents (**Fig. 15.1**). In general it may be regarded as a form of neural tube defect and the frequency of these defects might therefore be anticipated to reduce with folic acid supplementation.[3]

Even when glial tissue is apparently isolated from intracranial structures, a fibrous stalk may be found in 15% of cases.[4]

In the lateral sphenoid, it has been suggested that an embryological failure of Sternberg's canal to close leads to the bone deficiency, which is usually associated with an extensively pneumatized sinus.[5] Here the temporal lobe prolapses, as opposed to frontal lobe, through the anterior defects. A range of other congenital anomalies and syndromes has been described in association with these defects, but usually they occur alone.

Synonyms

A variety of terms may be found for gliomas including glial ectopia, encephaloma, and—perhaps most appropriately—vestigial encephalocele.[6] **However, these lesions should not be regarded as tumors as they are nonneoplastic in origin and behavior**.

Incidence

Initially described by Berger in 1890,[7] these lesions were reported in increasing numbers in the 1960s and 1970s,[8,9] making this a well-recognized condition. However, the incidence has now been shown to range from 1:10,000 live births in the United States to as high as 1:3,000 in South-East Asia. The reason for this geographical distribution is not known. No sexual predilection has been described.

Site

Encephaloceles are generally classified according to their site (**Table 15.2**).[10] Anterior (or sincipital) defects are less common than those found in the occipital region (15% vs. 85%) but more common in Asia. In a series of 257 patients from Cambodia who presented in a 5-year period, the nasoethmoid region was most commonly affected (69%) and there were associated ophthalmological problems in 46% of cases.[11] In the European literature the two common sites for congenital defects are at the vertical attachment of the middle turbinate and within the sphenoid. Multiple encephaloceles, although rare, can also occur.[12]

It has been estimated that ~25% of gliomas occur posterior to the nasal bone as intranasal lesions, 60% as subcutaneous lesions anterior to the nasal bone, and the rest as combinations of the two. Isolated glial tissue has also been reported elsewhere in the upper respiratory tract, including the nasopharynx, paranasal sinuses, and palate.

Diagnostic Features

Clinical Features

The majority of lesions are diagnosed at birth or during early childhood they but may occasionally remain

Table 15.1 Differential diagnosis of undifferentiated/poorly differentiated neoplasia of the sinonasal tract with immunophenotype

Tumor	CK	NSE	SYN	CHR	S100	HMB45ᵃ	LCA	Desmin	MYO	FLI	CD99	EBVᵇ
SNUC	+	+ᶜ	+ᶜ	+ᶜ	−	−	−	−	−	−	−	−
SCC	+	+	+ᵈ	+ᵈ	−	−	−	−	−	−	−	−
NPUCᵉ	+	−	−	−	−	−	−	−	−	−	−	+
ONB	−ᶠ	+	+	+	+ᵍ	−	−	−	−	−	−	−
Melanoma	−	−	−	−	+	+	−	−	−	−	−	−
Lymphomaʰ	−	−	−	−	−	−	+	−	−	−ⁱ	−ⁱ	−ʲ
RMS	−	−	−	−	−	−	−	+	+	−	−	−
PNET	+ᵏ / −	+	+ / −	−	+ / −	−	−	−	−	+	+	−
PA	+	+	+	+	−	−	−	−	−	−	−	−
MC	−	+	−	−	+	−	−	+ / −	−	−	+	−

Abbreviations: CHR, chromogranin; CK, cytokeratin; EBV, Epstein-Barr virus; LCA, leukocyte common antigen; MC, mesenchymal chondrosarcoma; MYO, myogenin; NPUC, nasopharyngeal undifferentiated carcinoma (lymphoepithelioma, etc.); NSE, neuron specific enolase; ONB, olfactory neuroblastoma; PA, pituitary adenoma; PNET, peripheral neuroectodermal tumor; RMS, rhabdomyosarcoma (embryonic and alveolar); SNUC, sinonasal undifferentiated carcinoma; SCC, small cell carcinoma; SYN, synaptophysin.

Source: From Strelow and Mills, reference 1 with permission from Lippin Cott, Williams & Wilkins.

ᵃ Or other specific melanocytic markers.

ᵇ EBV status may be assessed by a variety of means including in situ hybridization.

ᶜ Markers for neuroendocrine differentiation tend to stain SNUCs focally.

ᵈ SCCs may frequently lack staining for more specific endocrine markers.

ᵉ Also known as nonkeratinizing squamous cell carcinoma.

ᶠ ONBs may show focal immunoreactivity with antibodies to CKs.

ᵍ S100 immunoreactivity in ONBs is limited primarily to peripheral staining of the sustentacular cells.

ʰ Including most of the hematological malignancies that may be found throughout this area (e.g., extranodal natural killer/T-cell lymphoma, nasal type, plasmacytoma).

ⁱ Lymphoblastic lymphomas often react with antibodies to CD99 and FLI1.

ʲ Most lymphomas will not show diffuse, strong in situ hybridization for EBV-related nucleic acids or immunoreactivity with antibodies to EBV-related proteins. The notable exceptions include posttransplant lymphoproliferative disorders and extranodal natural killer/T-cell lymphoma, nasal type. In such patients, other markers may be needed.

ᵏ PNETs can sometimes show limited immunoreactivity with antibodies to low–molecular weight keratins.

undetected until adulthood, when they may present with a "spontaneous" cerebrospinal fluid leak.

Classically the child presents with a visible mass in the glabellar region which, if it is an encephalocele, commonly enlarges with crying or jugular compression (positive Furstenberg sign)[4] or may be compressible or pulsatile (Table 15.3). An extranasal glioma simply presents as a mass, which can be covered with normal skin or have a bluish tinge. It does not change with crying or increased intracranial pressure.

Intranasal lesions produce unilateral obstruction (or bilateral depending on the size and site) and the visible mass on endoscopy, or even anterior rhinoscopy, may be pulsatile. Such lesions should never be biopsied without prior imaging as this will risk a CSF leak and/or meningitis. A CSF leak may of course be present ab initio.

The mass may expand the nasal bridge and in extreme cases, at birth, the size of the mass may necessitate emergency intervention to secure the airway in a facultative nose breather.

A mass may be seen on endoscopic examination but the mass may be fused with the septum and/or lateral wall of the nasal cavity and covered with mucosa and so not necessarily appear as a circumscribed "polyp." Sometimes the lesion is too small to be seen easily or is hidden within a sinus (Figs. 15.2a, 15.3a).

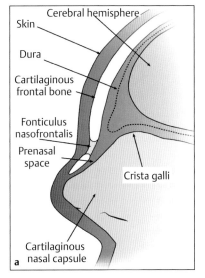

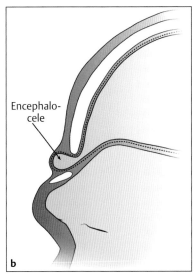

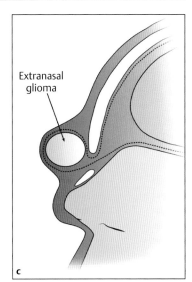

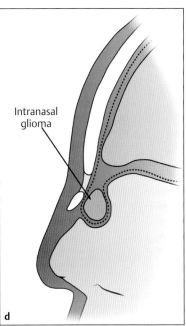

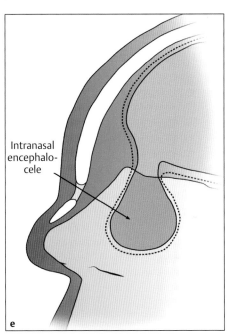

Fig. 15.1a–e

a Diagram showing the normal situation during development of the anterior cranial fossa and glabellar region.

b Formation of an encephalocele.

c Formation of extranasal glioma.

d Formation of intranasal glioma.

e Formation of intranasal encephalocele.

Table 15.2 Classification of encephaloceles

Classification	Site of herniation	Location of mass
I. Frontal		
Sincipital		
1. Nasofrontal	Fonticulus nasofrontalis	Forehead: nasal bridge
2. Nasoethmoidal	Foramen cecum	Nasal bridge
3. Naso-orbital	Medial orbital wall	Orbit
Basal		
1. Transethmoidal	Cribriform plate	Intranasal
2. Sphenoethmoidal	Between ethmoid and sphenoid	Nasopharynx/ethmoid/sphenoid
3. Transsphenoidal	Craniopharyngeal canal	Nasopharynx/sphenoid
4. Sphenomaxillary	Superior and inferior orbital fissure	Pterygopalatine fossa
II. Occipital		
Source: After reference 10.		

Table 15.3 Differential between glioma, meningoencephalocele, and dermoid cysts

	Glioma	Meningoencephalocele	Dermoid
Age	<5	<5 though can present as adult	Any age
Pulsation	No	Yes	No
Variable size, e.g., with crying	No	Yes	No
Texture	Firm	Soft	Variable
Patent intracranial connection	No	Yes	Possible
Neurons	No	Yes	No
Skin adnexal structures	No	No	Yes
Source: After reference 26.			

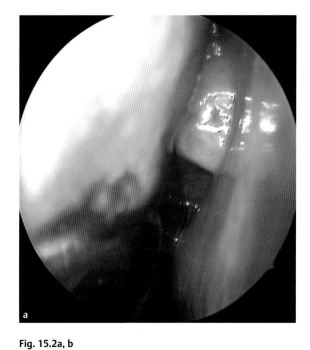
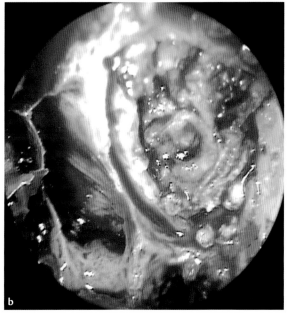

Fig. 15.2a, b

a Endoscopic view of a meningocele in the superior left nasal cavity.

b Endoscopic view of the skull base in the same patient after removal of the meningocele.

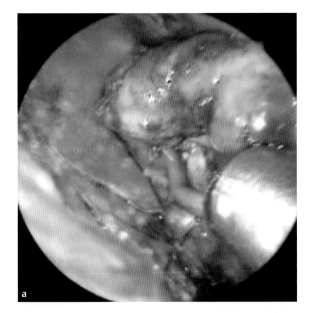

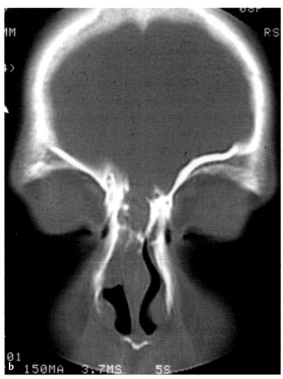

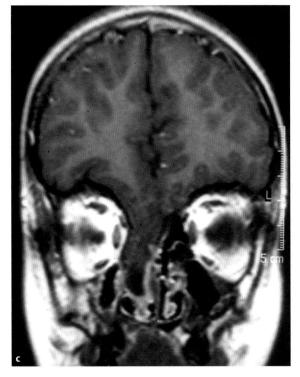

Fig. 15.3a–c

a Endoscopic view during reduction of a meningoencephalocele with endoscopic diathermy at the right skull base.

b Coronal CT scan in same patient showing a meningoencephalocele through the right skull base defect.

c Coronal MRI (T1W post gadolinium enhancement) in the same patient showing the contents of the meningoencephalocele.

337

Other clinical findings may be present as part of a more generalized skull base deformity, for example, optic nerve or endocrine disturbances.[13,14] In later life, the individual may present with meningitis and/or with unilateral watery rhinorrhea due to the CSF leak. These "spontaneous" leaks are most often seen in obese individuals, most often women,[15] and are frequently high flow. They can be multiple, making them difficult to manage.

Several protocols have been developed to assess suspected CSF leaks (**Fig. 15.4**); these consider confirmation of CSF rhinorrhea by the presence of β_2-transferrin or beta-trace protein (prostaglandin D$_2$ synthase) and determination of the site(s) of leakage by imaging.[16–19] β_2-Transferrin analysis has been available since 1979 using electrophoresis by immunofixation or immunoblotting. A minimum volume of 2 µL is required and the test takes 2 to 4 hours. Beta-trace protein has been detectable by laser nephelometry since 2001 and requires a slightly greater volume (5 µL) but is a quicker test[20] with a somewhat higher sensitivity and specificity.

In difficult cases intrathecal sodium fluorescein can be employed intraoperatively.[21] Certain maneuvers and precautions are required such as a blue light and a blocking filter, but the dye can be detected at 1 in 10 million parts

and complications are extremely rare. It can also help to visualize whether or not a CSF-tight closure has been achieved intraoperatively.[22] The intrathecal fluorescein test can give a *false-negative* result, when for instance the defect site is blocked by edema of the mucosa, hematoma, or brain herniation; also, the injection technique can be faulty, timing and patient positioning may be inadequate, or the CSF circulation may be interrupted. However, *intrathecal fluorescein cannot yield false-positive results.*

Only a 5% aqueous sodium fluorescein solution, sterile and free of pyrogens, should be used. No other potentially neurotoxic substances like stabilizers and/or preservatives must be added. Intrathecal application is an off-label use of fluorescein for which informed consent must be obtained from the patient. Recommendations are to inject 0.05 to maximally 0.1 mL per 10 kg body weight; in no case, however, should more than 1.0 mL be given, even in a massively overweight patient. Fluorescein is injected via a standard lumbar puncture. In cases with evident CSF flow, it is administered a few hours or immediately prior to surgical intervention; in unclear or intermittently leaking cases, usually the evening before an intervention (**Table 15.4**). These techniques have superseded the use of radioactive dyes.

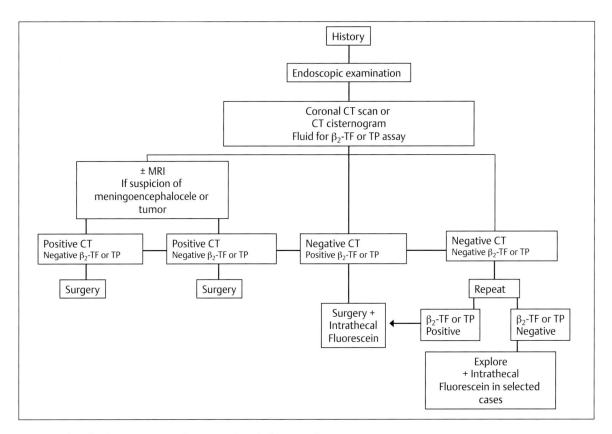

Fig. 15.4 Algorithm for management of a suspected CSF leak. TF, transferrin; TP, trace protein.

Table 15.4 Fluorescein protocol for CSF leaks

Day before operation	Skin test patient with fluorescein (Minims eye drops 2%)
Informed consent	Grand mal seizures, cranial nerve palsies, opisthotonus
Day of operation	10 mg IM Piriton (chlorpheniramine/ chlorphenamine) followed 5 min later by IV 10% fluorescein 0.25 mL diluted to 0.5 mL with water for injection
	Approx. 20 min later intrathecal injection of 0.2 mL 10% fluorescein made up to 7.5 mL with CSF (25G spinal needle)
	Patient goes to recovery (or ward) with head of bed down for approx. 90 min
	Patient undergoes normal anesthetic as for endoscopic sinus surgery
Postoperatively	If required, spinal drain inserted lumbar ¾ 16G epidural catheter. Drainage 5–10 mL per hour plus neurologic observations for 24–48 hours

While the diagnosis is being established, immunization against *Meningococcus*, *Pneumococcus*, and *Haemophilus* spp. is often recommended if not already given.

Imaging

(See **Figs. 15.3b, c, 15.5, 15.6a, b.**)

Detailed imaging should always be undertaken prior to any surgical intervention. CT and MRI are ideally required to demonstrate both the bony defect, the contents and intracranial connections, and any other anomalies. Both CT and MRI should be thin cut and three-planar and, depending on the age[23] and cooperation of a young patient, may require an anesthetic.

When a CSF leak or meningitis occurs later in life, additional imaging may be required. If the individual is leaking on a regular basis, CT cisternography will confirm both the presence and site of leakage.[23] However, many patients leak intermittently and in these circumstances other imaging techniques are required.

Histological Features and Differential Diagnosis

True encephaloceles consist of mature glial tissue with a variable amount of dura and leptomeninges, whereas gliomas are circumscribed but unencapsulated collections of astrocytes in a loose fibrous stroma. Neurons, in contrast to encephaloceles, are rarely if ever seen.

Gliomas may be bluish or reddish in color and may be misdiagnosed as capillary hemangiomas.[24,25] They must also be distinguished from a dermoid cyst (**Table 15.3**) and, albeit they are rare at birth, the whole range of unilateral masses including antrochoanal polyp and benign and malignant tumors.[26] Immunohistochemistry with S100 protein or glial fibrillary acidic protein can be helpful in equivocal cases.

Natural History

Apart from the cosmetic and functional issues posed by these lesions, left untreated the patient remains at risk of meningitis (and CSF leakage) so treatment is recommended in the absence of any confounding factors.

Treatment

In the past, a neurosurgical approach was undertaken but endonasal endoscopic techniques are usually first choice for the majority of lesions. Exceptions would be when they are part of other more complex cranial base anomalies, in the case of extremely large defects, and when there is an extranasal component. Endonasal endoscopic surgery allows complete removal of the redundant tissue, accurate delineation of the defect, and a range of choices for repair materials.

The neural contents of the cele are regarded as redundant and the sac can be shrunk down considerably with endoscopic diathermy and then removed flush with the defect in the anterior skull base (**Fig. 15.3a**). Considerable care is required, however, in the sphenoid where the sac is often intimately related to the optic nerve and carotid artery and other vital structures in some congenital anomalies. The area of the defect needs to be well exposed and denuded of mucosa, which may require skeletonization of quite a large area of the skull base, including a complete ethmoidecomy and removal of the middle turbinate (which is a useful source of graft mucosa). In lesions of the sphenoid and pterygoid region wide exposure is the key to success, so a far-lateral removal of the face of the sphenoid and transpterygoid approach can be required (**Figs. 15.2b, 15.6d**).[27,28]

The endoscopic repair of skull base defects has generated a large literature, but in summary the choice of material is largely determined by the size and site of the defect and surgical preference.[29] A meta-analysis of 35 of the major publications on this topic covering 1,123 patients[30] failed to show any advantage for one material over another from a long list of possible choices, although free grafts of fascia and cartilage in combination with mucosa are most often used. Pinna cartilage will often slot into the funnel shape of some congenital defects, and fat as a "bath plug" can also be very useful in certain circumstances.[31] Larger defects may benefit from a vascularized flap such as that described by Haddad and colleagues

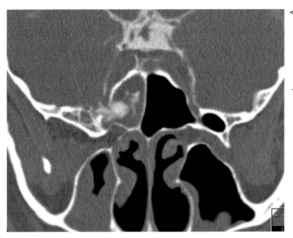

◁ **Fig. 15.5** Coronal CT cisternogram showing a meningoencephalocele through a defect in the lateral wall of the right sphenoid sinus.

▽ **Fig. 15.6a–d**

a Coronal CT scan showing a meningoencephalocele through a defect in the lateral wall of the right sphenoid sinus.

b Coronal MRI (T2W) in same patient showing the contents of the meningoencephalocele and fluid filling the left sphenoid.

c Endoscopic view showing a meningoencephalocele in the lateral compartment of the sphenoid.

d Endoscopic view showing three-layer repair with pinna cartilage, fascia, and mucosa after reduction of a meningoencephalocele in the lateral compartment of the sphenoid.

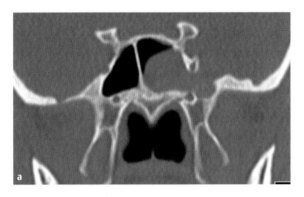

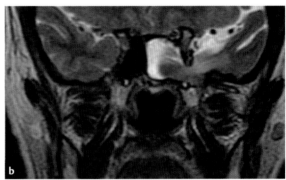

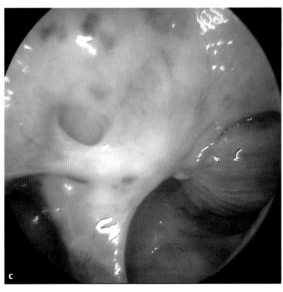

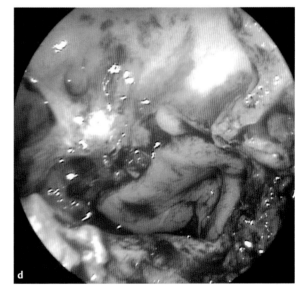

in 2006 that enables larger areas of septal mucosa to be utilized and is based on branches of the sphenopalatine artery.[32]

The technique may be underlay, onlay, or combination thereof; all have been used and there is general agreement that a two- or three-layer closure is required for congenital defects. The use of packing, postoperative medication, and bed rest varies from center to center and might also include antibiotics, antiemetics, and diuretics (e.g., acetazolamide) in the presence of raised intracranial pressure. Similarly, there is no consensus about the use of lumbar drains, although generally they are not used in primary cases unless the CSF leak is high-flow and well established. Occasionally in these cases—often the "spontaneous" leaks—a more permanent lumbar-peritoneal drain may be needed.

Subcranial or transcranial approaches are sometimes needed for extensive lesions or those also involving the orbits.

External glial lesions can sometimes be accessed via an external rhinoplasty or midfacial degloving approach in young children, but sometimes an accompanying external incision/excision may be required.

Outcome

Outcome will depend on many factors, including the size and site of the lesion, the presence of other abnormalities, and whether the aberrant CSF metabolism rectifies itself without additional intervention. Some very extensive encephaloceles may threaten survival and others have long-term mental or neurological deficit. Overall, the results for the anterior lesions are better than for occipital lesions and those within the anterior skull base; the sphenoid lesions are the most difficult, particularly in the adult "spontaneous" group.

Most series of endoscopic repairs include a heterogeneous group of congenital and acquired lesions of different extents, sites, and durations, but in general results are good, with primary closure rates of 90% and better. Follow-up ranged from 1 to 162 months and recurrence occurred between 2 days and 18 months, although it tended to occur within the first few weeks and months.[30] However, 50% success was reported specifically for sphenoid sinus defects and 50% of "spontaneous" leaks overall.[33] In cases of primary failure, a second endoscopic attempt was definitely worthwhile, with success rates of 93 to 100%. External craniotomy remains an option for the most difficult cases but this also cannot guarantee success and carries a somewhat higher morbidity due to frontal lobe retraction and anosmia.[34,35]

In contrast, gliomas by their nature do not recur after complete excision. Rahbar et al[10] reported 10 patients with nasal glioma, mean age 9 months, who were successfully treated without complication and a mean follow-up of 3.5 years.

Key Points

1. Consider these lesions in any infant or child with unilateral nasal obstruction.
2. Do not biopsy such a mass without imaging.
3. Spontaneous unilateral, watery rhinorrhea should be considered as CSF leakage until proven otherwise.
4. Meningoencephaloceles can present in adult life and may be associated with spontaneous CSF leaks, especially in the overweight patient.
5. Most of these lesions can be approached endoscopically with similar rates of success as in conventional craniotomy and with minimal morbidity.

References

1. Stelow E, Mills S. Biopsy Interpretation of the Upper Aerodigestive Tract and Ear. Philadelphia: Wolters Kluwer, Lippincott, Williams & Wilkins; 2008:150
2. Michaels L, Hellquist H. Encephalocoeles. Ear, Nose and Throat Histopathology, 2nd ed. London: Springer; 2001:103
3. MRC Vitamin Study Research Group. Prevention of neural tube defects: results of the Medical Research Council Vitamin Study. Lancet 1991;338(8760):131–137
4. Hedlund G. Congenital frontonasal masses: developmental anatomy, malformations, and MR imaging. Pediatr Radiol 2006;36(7):647–662, quiz 726–727
5. Tomazic PV, Stammberger H. Spontaneous CSF-leaks and meningoencephaloceles in sphenoid sinus by persisting Sternberg's canal. Rhinology 2009;47(4):369–374
6. Macomber WB, Wang MK. Congenital neoplasms of the nose. Plast Reconstr Surg (1946) 1953;11(3):215–229
7. Berger P. Considerations sur l'origine et le mode de la development et le traitement de certaines encephalocoeles. Rev Chir 1890;10:269–321
8. Karma P, Räsänen O, Kärjä J. Nasal gliomas. A review and report of two cases. Laryngoscope 1977;87(7):1169–1179
9. Walker EA Jr, Resler DR. Nasal glioma. Laryngoscope 1963;73:93–107
10. Rahbar R, Resto VA, Robson CD, et al. Nasal glioma and encephalocele: diagnosis and management. Laryngoscope 2003;113(12):2069–2077
11. Oucheng N, Lauwers F, Gollogly J, Draper L, Joly B, Roux F-E. Frontoethmoidal meningoencephalocele: appraisal of 200 operated cases. J Neurosurg Pediatr 2010;6(6):541–549
12. Schlosser RJ, Bolger WE. Management of multiple spontaneous nasal meningoencephaloceles. Laryngoscope 2002;112(6):980–985
13. Pollack IF. Management of encephaloceles and craniofacial problems in the neonatal period. Neurosurg Clin N Am 1998;9(1):121–139
14. Tsutsumi K, Asano T, Shigeno T, Matsui T, Ito S, Kaizu H. Transcranial approach for transsphenoidal encephalocele: report of two cases. Surg Neurol 1999;51(3):252–257
15. Badia L, Loughran S, Lund V. Primary spontaneous cerebrospinal fluid rhinorrhea and obesity. Am J Rhinol 2001;15(2):117–119
16. Sloman AJ, Kelly RH. Transferrin allelic variants may cause false positives in the detection of cerebrospinal fluid fistulae. Clin Chem 1993;39(7):1444–1445
17. Roelandse FW, van der Zwart N, Didden JH, van Loon J, Souverijn JH. Detection of CSF leakage by isoelectric focusing on polyacrylamide gel, direct immunofixation of transferrins, and silver staining. Clin Chem 1998;44(2):351–353

18. Arrer E, Meco C, Oberascher G, Piotrowski W, Albegger K, Patsch W. beta-Trace protein as a marker for cerebrospinal fluid rhinorrhea. Clin Chem 2002;48(6 Pt 1):939–941
19. Scadding G, Lund V. Investigative Rhinology. London: Taylor and Francis; 2004:111
20. Bachmann-Harildstad G. Diagnostic values of beta-2 transferrin and beta-trace protein as markers for cerebrospinal fluid fistula. Rhinology 2008;46(2):82–85
21. Messerklinger W. [Nasal endoscopy: demonstration, localization and differential diagnosis of nasal liquorrhea]. HNO 1972;20(9):268–270
22. Stammberger H, Greistorfer K, Wolf G, Luxenberger W. [Surgical occlusion of cerebrospinal fistulas of the anterior skull base using intrathecal sodium fluorescein]. Laryngorhinootologie 1997;76(10):595–607
23. Lund VJ, Savy L, Lloyd G, Howard D. Optimum imaging and diagnosis of cerebrospinal fluid rhinorrhoea. J Laryngol Otol 2000;114(12):988–992
24. Hoeger PH, Schaefer H, Ussmueller J, Helmke K. Nasal glioma presenting as capillary haemangioma. Eur J Pediatr 2001;160(2):84–87
25. Oddone M, Granata C, Dalmonte P, Biscaldi E, Rossi U, Toma P. Nasal glioma in an infant. Pediatr Radiol 2002; 32(2):104–105
26. Robinson RA, ed. Head and Neck Pathology. Wolters Kluwer; 2010:140
27. Lai SY, Kennedy DW, Bolger WE. Sphenoid encephaloceles: disease management and identification of lesions within the lateral recess of the sphenoid sinus. Laryngoscope 2002;112(10):1800–1805
28. Tabaee A, Anand VK, Cappabianca P, Stamm A, Esposito F, Schwartz TH. Endoscopic management of spontaneous meningoencephalocele of the lateral sphenoid sinus. J Neurosurg 2010;112(5):1070–1077
29. Lund VJ. Endoscopic management of cerebrospinal fluid leaks. Am J Rhinol 2002;16(1):17–23
30. Lund VJ, Stammberger H, Nicolai P, et al. European position paper on endoscopic management of the nose, paranasal sinuses and skull base. Rhinology Suppl 2010(22):1–143
31. Wormald PJ, McDonogh M. 'Bath-plug' technique for the endoscopic management of cerebrospinal fluid leaks. J Laryngol Otol 1997;111(11):1042–1046
32. Hadad G, Bassagasteguy L, Carrau RL, et al. A novel reconstructive technique after endoscopic expanded endonasal approaches: vascular pedicle nasoseptal flap. Laryngoscope 2006;116(10):1882–1886
33. Mirza S, Thaper A, McClelland L, Jones NS. Sinonasal cerebrospinal fluid leaks: management of 97 patients over 10 years. Laryngoscope 2005;115(10):1774–1777
34. Aarabi B, Leibrock LG. Neurosurgical approaches to cerebrospinal fluid rhinorrhea. Ear Nose Throat J 1992;71(7):300–305
35. Hughes RG, Jones NS, Robertson IJ. The endoscopic treatment of cerebrospinal fluid rhinorrhoea: the Nottingham experience. J Laryngol Otol 1997;111(2):125–128

Benign Schwannoma and Malignant Peripheral Nerve Sheath Tumors

Definition

(ICD-O codes 9560/0 & 9540/3)

A tumor of nerve sheath origin, derived from Schwann cells surrounding the neural tissue (ICD-O 9560/0). When malignant, they are referred to as malignant peripheral nerve sheath tumors (MPNSTs) (ICD-O 9540/3).

Etiology

These tumors probably originate from the ophthalmic and maxillary branches of the trigeminal nerve but have been reported arising from the autonomic fibers of the carotid plexus or sphenopalatine ganglion.[1] Schwannomas have been reported in relation to all the cranial nerves with the possible exception of the optic nerve. However, often the exact nerve and/or fiber of origin can be difficult to determine.

The neurosurgical literature also contains several case reports of these lesions arising in the subfrontal region and involving both the anterior cranial fossa and sinonasal region. These often arise from the trigeminal nerve/ganglion.

Synonyms

Verocay first described a nerve sheath tumor in 1910, which he believed to derive from the Schwann cell.[2] Antoni described the two characteristic forms in 1920 and the first case of a "neuroma" in the nose was reported in 1926.[3] In 1935 Stout used the term "neurilemmoma."[4]

Malignant schwannomas, or MPNSTs, have also been described as neurogenic sarcomas or neurosarcomas

Incidence

Schwannomas are found throughout the upper aerodigestive tract; 25 to 40% of schwannomas occur in the head and neck and, after the ear, the nose and sinuses are the commonest site.[5] Notwithstanding this, it has been estimated that overall only 4% of schwannomas affect this area.[6,7] They almost always occur as solitary lesions, unassociated with any genetic disorders.[8]

MPNSTs are exceptionally rare with only 30 to 40 cases reported in the literature.[9] They are said to develop from benign peripheral nerve sheath tumors in between 2.5% and 16.5% of cases.[10] There have been few large studies but in 1973 Ghosh reported out of a total of 115 that 16 malignant schwannomas had occurred in the head and neck.[11]

Site

The ethmoid is said to be the most common site, followed by the maxillary sinus, nasal cavity, and sphenoid.[12] In our series of 13 benign and 4 malignant schwannomas, the benign tumors mainly arose in the nasal cavity on the lateral wall or on the septum, whereas the malignant lesions affected either the ethmoids or maxillary sinuses.

In the nasal cavity the lesions can affect the lateral wall, being one of the few tumors to arise on the inferior turbinate[13] or they may involve the septum.[14–20]

Diagnostic Features

Clinical Features

Benign schwannomas tend to occur in older individuals although they have been reported from childhood to old age. They present as a polypoid mass with nasal obstruction. There is no obvious predilection for sex or age,[15] as exemplified by our group. The nasal lesions tend to present earlier by virtue of their position. Epistaxis is said to result from necrosis. Pain has sometimes been described when the pterygomaxillary region or sphenoid is affected and those arising from the trigeminal system may present with trigeminal neuralgia. Olfactory loss, perhaps surprisingly, is not a specific feature.

Some schwannomas achieve an impressive size with minimal clinical symptoms.[21–24]

MPNSTs also present with a mass effect but they are more infiltrative and destructive, with a high tendency to recur despite radical resection and also manifest their capacity to metastasize.[9]

Imaging

The benign schwannomas grow slowly and usually present as a circumscribed lesion, although some local infiltration may be seen as well as bone remodeling or erosion.[1] CT is the primary tool but MRI, as always, may help in delineating tumor from surrounding inflammation or secretion (**Figs. 15.7 and 15.8**).[25] CT with contrast may show central hypodensities with peripheral enhancement due to areas of increased vascularity versus areas of cystic degeneration or necrosis.[20] Schwannomas vary from isodense to hypodense on T1W MRI, enhance after contrast, and are rarely calcified.[26]

Histological Features and Differential Diagnosis

Classically the tumor is composed of mixed cellular areas—Antoni A, cellular; and Antoni B, less cellular. Cellular palisading or Verocay bodies can sometimes be seen. Some tumors undergo cystic degeneration. Others show significant nuclear pleomorphism, when they are termed "ancient schwannomas."[27]

Diagnosis may be aided by strong immunoreactivity to S100. Occasional reactivity can also be demonstrated to CD34 but less so than in neurofibromas.[5,27] These lesions must be distinguished from neurofibromas and a wide range of fibromatous lesions.

MPNSTs must be distinguished from other sarcomas and can be confused with fibrosarcomas although they are generally less cellular and rarely show nuclear palisading. Again, S100 positivity is exhibited but there are more mitoses compared with their benign counterparts.[28] They typically have bundles of spindle cells with high mitotic rates and irregular cellular borders.[29,30]

Natural History

Slow insidious growth may result in large lesions, depending on their site of origin. Extension into the orbit or anterior skull base may ultimately result and there are

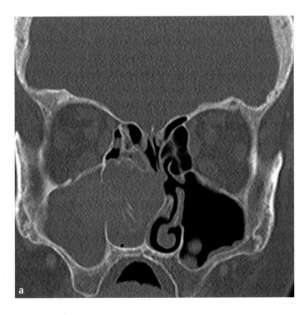
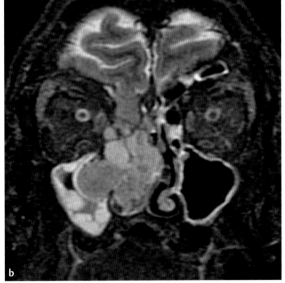

Fig. 15.7a, b

a Schwannoma. Coronal CT showing a soft tissue mass in the right nasal cavity with opacification of the maxillary sinus and displacement of the nasal septum.

b Coronal MRI (STIR) in the same patient showing a lobulated mass with heterogeneous signal in the nasal cavity, invaginating into and obstructing the maxillary sinus.

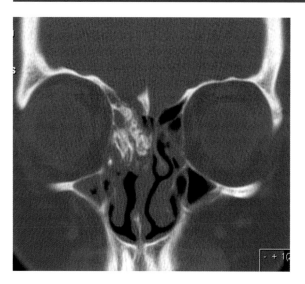

Fig. 15.8 Coronal CT scan showing malignant PNST in patient with associated neo-osteogenesis. The mass was removed entirely by endoscopic surgery including the skull base and lamina papyracea.

several cases that arise in the anterior cranial cavity and appear to spread inferiorly.

There seems to be some debate whether the malignant lesions result from malignant transformation of a benign schwannoma or a neurofibroma,[14] but in a large cohort of 120 cases of MPNSTs occurring throughout the body collected at the Mayo Clinic over 71 years, at least half arose in patients with neurofibromatosis 1 (NF1).[31] Distant metastatic spread can occur even 5 to 10 years later despite local cure, a phenomenon seen with other neuroectodermal tumors, although cervical spread was not seen in a series of 27 cases occurring in the head and neck[32] whereas 18% developed distant spread to the lungs and liver.

Treatment and Outcome

The ability of the tumors, both benign and malignant, to achieve quite large proportions and to involve the anterior cranial cavity has led to the use of lateral rhinotomy, midfacial degloving, and craniofacial resection in some cases.[33–35] Depending on the location and extent of those lesions that originate intracranially, a range of surgical approaches may be required including transmaxillary, presigmoid, retrosigmoid, frontotemporal, transsylvian, and transtentorial, and subfrontal.[36,37]

An endoscopic approach could be and has been employed[38,39] for both the sinonasal and skull base schwannomas. Whereas the earlier cases in our series underwent open procedures, after 1994 they largely had endoscopic resections (**Tables 15.5 and 15.6**).[40–43]

If completely excised, the benign schwannoma does not recur, although technically this may prove a challenge with some skull base lesions such as the intrasellar tumor

described by Esposito et al[40] and a very rare lesion affecting the olfactory nerve subtotally removed by Kurshel and colleagues.[43] Only one of our benign sinonasal schwannomas recurred, where the tumor had extended into the lateral compartment of the frontal sinus and required a further excision by a limited external approach 4 months later, since when no further disease has been observed (4 years follow-up).

MPSNTs, by contrast, frequently "recur" due to their infiltrative behavior and patients often undergo progressively more radical excisions, which may ultimately fail.[44] Two of our four patients experienced further problems within a year of their original open surgery and went on to more extensive resections including orbital clearance in both cases and additional radiotherapy in one. Unfortunately, neither survived longer than 2 years.

Those that arise in neurofibromas associated with NF1 are highly malignant, with recurrence rates of up to 80% and 5-year survival of 15 to 30% irrespective of treatment. In a series of 27 cases, of which 6 occurred in the nose and sinuses, Vege et al[32] described a 33% 5-year survival with 15% of patients dead due to advanced local disease within 18 months, despite radical excision. Distant metastases were seen in 18.5% and, at the end of 5 years, only 15% remained disease free. The main prognostic factor related to size, patients with tumors >5 cm diameter doing worse. There was no significant correlation between grade of tumor and survival.

MPSNTs are not particularly radiosensitive, but this modality has been used more in hope than expectation[1,32] as adjuvant therapy to surgery and for recurrence. Chemotherapy in the form of vincristine, endoxan, and mitomycin D has also been used for recurrence.[32]

References

1. Mey KH, Buchwald C, Daugaard S, Prause JU. Sinonasal schwannoma—a clinicopathological analysis of five rare cases. Rhinology 2006;44(1):46–52
2. Verocay J. Zur Kenntnis der Neurofibrome. Beitrage Pathol Anat Allergy 1910;48:1–6
3. Antoni N. Uber Ruckenmarkstumoven und Neurofibrome. Munich: Bergmann-Verlag; 1920:413–423
4. Stout A. Peripheral manifestations of specific nerve sheath tumours. Am J Cancer 1935;24:751–796
5. Buob D, Wacrenier A, Chevalier D, et al. Schwannoma of the sinonasal tract: a clinicopathologic and immunohistochemical study of 5 cases. Arch Pathol Lab Med 2003;127(9):1196–1199
6. Younis RT, Gross CW, Lazar RH. Schwannomas of the paranasal sinuses. Case report and clinicopathologic analysis. Arch Otolaryngol Head Neck Surg 1991;117(6):677–680
7. Braunschweig F, Kramer MF, Assmann G, Arbogast S, Leunig A. Schwannoma of the nasal cavity: a case report. [Article in German] HNO 2007;55(13):1013–1016
8. Karaman E, Yilmaz S, Ozçora E, Ozek H, Korkut N, Sar M. Schwannoma of the lateral nasal wall:two case reports and a review of the literature. J Otolaryngol 2007;36(3):E1–4
9. Mannan AA, Singh MK, Bahadur S, Hatimota P, Sharma MC. Solitary malignant schwannoma of the nasal cavity and paranasal sinuses: report of two rare cases. Ear Nose Throat J 2003;82(8):634–636, 638, 640

Table 15.5 Benign and malignant schwannomas: personal series 1986–2010

	n	Age Range (y)	Age Mean (y)	M:F	ESS	LR	MFD	CFR	Outcome	Follow-up
Benign	13	26–64	39.3	7:6	8	1	2	2	1 "recurrence" at 4 mo 12 A&W (93%)	2–12 y
Malignant	4	41–53	46.7	2:2	2	2	48	11	50% recurrence at 6 mo 2: DOD 2 y 2: AEW	1 & 26 y

Abbreviations: A&W, alive and well; CFR: craniofacial resection; DOD, dead of disease; ESS, endoscopic sinus surgery; F, female; LR, lateral rhinotomy; M, male; MFD, midfacial degloving; mo, month(s); y, year(s).

Table 15.6 Schwannomas treated via an endonasal endoscopic transsphenoidal approach

Series	Total no. of patients	No. of schwannomas	Histological diagnosis (localization/origin)	Extent of resection	Complications	Follow-up range
Esposito et al[40]	Case report	1	Schwannoma (intrasellar)	Subtotal removal	None	12 mo
Kanaan et al[41]	Case report	1	Schwannoma (olfactory)	Subtotal removal	None	NA
Kassam et al[42]	40	6	Schwannoma (trigeminal)	Total removal 5 Subtotal removal 1	Transient sixth nerve palsy 1	NA
Kurschel et al[43]	58	2	Schwannoma[a] Schwannoma (trigeminal)	Partial removal 1 Total removal 1	None	35–37 mo

Abbreviations: mo, month(s); NA, not available.

[a] Schwannoma extending from the left posterior fossa to the ipsilateral maxillary sinus involving the left middle and infratemporal fossa, and the inter- and intrasellar areas.

10. Leslie MD, Cheung KY. Malignant transformation of neurofibromas at multiple sites in a case of neurofibromatosis. Postgrad Med J 1987;63(736):131–133

11. Ghosh BC, Ghosh L, Huvos AG, Fortner JG. Malignant schwannoma. A clinicopathologic study. Cancer 1973; 31(1):184–190

12. Sheikh HY, Chakravarthy RP, Slevin NJ, Sykes AJ, Banerjee SS. Benign schwannoma in paranasal sinuses: a clinicopathological study of five cases, emphasising diagnostic difficulties. J Laryngol Otol 2008;122(6):598–602

13. Khnifies R, Fradis M, Brodsky A, Bajar J, Luntz M. Inferior turbinate schwannoma: report of a case. Ear Nose Throat J 2006;85(6):384–385

14. Butugan O, Grasel SS, de Almeida ER, Miniti A. Schwannoma of the nasal septum. Apropos of 2 cases. Rev Laryngol Otol Rhinol (Bord) 1993;114(1):33–36

15. Berlucchi M, Piazza C, Blanzuoli L, Battaglia G, Nicolai P. Schwannoma of the nasal septum: a case report with review of the literature. Eur Arch Otorhinolaryngol 2000;257(7):402–405

16. Wada A, Matsuda H, Matsuoka K, Kawano T, Furukawa S, Tsukuda M. A case of schwannoma on the nasal septum. Auris Nasus Larynx 2001;28(2):173–175

17. Cakmak O, Yavuz H, Yucel T. Nasal and paranasal sinus schwannomas. Eur Arch Otorhinolaryngol 2003; 260(4):195–197

18. Facon F, Forman C, Paris J, Chapon F, Moulin G, Dessi P. [A case of nasal septum schwannoma: endoscopic resection]. Ann Otolaryngol Chir Cervicofac 2004;121(3):179–183

19. Wang LF, Tai CF, Chai CY, Ho KY, Kuo WR. Schwannoma of the nasal septum: a case report. Kaohsiung J Med Sci 2004;20(3):142–145

20. Rajagopal S, Kaushik V, Irion K, Herd ME, Bhatnagar RK. Schwannoma of the nasal septum. Br J Radiol 2006; 79(943):e16–e18

21. Schwartz TH, Bruce JN. Extended frontal approach with bilateral orbitofrontoethmoidal osteotomies for removal of a giant extracranial schwannoma in the nasopharynx, sphenoid sinus, and parapharyngeal space. Surg Neurol 2001;55(5):270–274

22. Bezircioğlu H, Sucu HK, Rezanko T, Minoğlu M. Nasal-subfrontal giant schwannoma. Turk Neurosurg 2008;18(4):412–414

23. George KJ, Price R. Nasoethmoid schwannoma with intracranial extension. Case report and review of literature. Br J Neurosurg 2009;23(1):83–85

24. Zheng K, Jiang S, Xu JG, Mao BY. Giant cranionasal schwannoma. J Clin Neurosci 2010;17(4):520–522

25. Dublin AB, Dedo HH, Bridger WH. Intranasal schwannoma: magnetic resonance and computed tomography appearance. Am J Otolaryngol 1995;16(4):251–254

26. Osborn A. Diagnostic Neuroradiology. St Louis: Mosby; 1994

27. Hasegawa SL, Mentzel T, Fletcher CD. Schwannomas of the sinonasal tract and nasopharynx. Mod Pathol 1997;10(8):777–784

28. Hellquist HB, Lundgren J. Neurogenic sarcoma of the sinonasal tract. J Laryngol Otol 1991;105(3):186–190

29. Wanamaker J, Wanamaker H, Kotton B, et al. Schwannomas of the nose and paranasal sinuses. Am J Rhinol 1993;7:59–65

30. Gillman G, Bryson PC. Ethmoid schwannoma. Otolaryngol Head Neck Surg 2005;132(2):334–335

31. Ducatman BS, Scheithauer BW, Piepgras DG, Reiman HM, Ilstrup DM. Malignant peripheral nerve sheath tumors. A clinicopathologic study of 120 cases. Cancer 1986;57(10):2006–2021

32. Vege DS, Chinoy RF, Ganesh B, Parikh DM. Malignant peripheral nerve sheath tumors of the head and neck: a clinico-pathological study. J Surg Oncol 1994;55(2):100–103

33. Shugar MA, Montgomery WW, Reardon EJ. Management of paranasal sinus schwannomas. Ann Otol Rhinol Laryngol 1982;91(1 Pt 1):65–69

34. Howard DJ, Lund VJ. The role of midfacial degloving in modern rhinological practice. J Laryngol Otol 1999;113(10):885–887

35. Howard DJ, Lund VJ, Wei WI. Craniofacial resection for tumors of the nasal cavity and paranasal sinuses: a 25-year experience. Head Neck 2006;28(10):867–873

36. Ramina R, Mattei TA, Sória MG, et al. Surgical management of trigeminal schwannomas. Neurosurg Focus 2008;25(6):E6, discussion E6

37. Gupta SK. Trans-sylvian transtentorial approach for skull base lesions extending from the middle fossa to the upper petro-clival region. Br J Neurosurg 2009;23(3):287–292

38. Klossek JM, Ferrie JC, Goujon JM, Fontanel JP. Endoscopic approach of the pterygopalatine fossa: report of one case. Rhinology 1994;32(4):208–210

39. Pasquini E, Sciarretta V, Farneti G, Ippolito A, Mazzatenta D, Frank G. Endoscopic endonasal approach for the treatment of benign schwannoma of the sinonasal tract and pterygopalatine fossa. Am J Rhinol 2002;16(2):113–118

40. Esposito F, Cappabianca P, Del Basso De Caro M, Cavallo LM, Rinaldi C, De Divitiis E. Endoscopic endonasal transsphenoidal removal of an intra-suprasellar schwannoma mimicking a pituitary adenoma. Minim Invasive Neurosurg 2004;47(4):230–234

41. Kanaan HA, Gardner PA, Yeaney G, et al. Expanded endoscopic endonasal resection of an olfactory schwannoma. J Neurosurg Pediatr 2008;2(4):261–265

42. Kassam AB, Prevedello DM, Carrau RL, et al. The front door to Meckel's cave: an anteromedial corridor via expanded endoscopic endonasal approach—technical considerations and clinical series. Neurosurgery 2009;64(3 Suppl):ons71–82; discussion ons82–83

43. Kurschel S, Gellner V, Clarici G, Braun H, Stammberger H, Mokry M. Endoscopic rhino-neurosurgical approach for non-adenomatous sellar and skull base lesions. Rhinology 2011;49(1):64–73

44. Sanchez-Mejia RO, Pham DN, Prados M, et al. Management of a sporadic malignant subfrontal peripheral nerve sheath tumor. J Neurooncol 2006;76(2):165–169

Malignant Triton Tumor

Definition and Etiology

Malignant triton tumor (MTT) is an exceptionally rare tumor originally described in 1932 by Masson as a malignant schwannoma with rhabdomyoblastic differentiation.[1] It acquired the name "malignant triton tumor" some 40 years later,[2] the term being coined to indicate its ability for pluridirectional differentiation, based on the ability of the Triton salamander to generate supernumerary limbs.

The most likely explanation for the tumor composition is that neoplastic Schwann cells transform into striated muscle in keeping with the capacity of neural crest tissue to undergo mesenchymal differentiation.

Site

There is a small number of sinonasal case reports in the literature, the largest number of cases being gathered by Heffner and Gnepp in 1992.[3] Of the eight cases discussed by Nicolai et al, all affected the nasal cavity and in three cases extended into adjacent sinuses.[4] Since then there have been a few case reports of lesions in the sinonasal region.[5–7] Four of seven cases reported by Terzic et al[6] affected the sinonasal region, the others affecting the mandible, petrous bone, and occiput. They also reviewed 46 other patients in the literature, in 24 of whom the tumor affected the sinonasal tract.

Diagnostic Features

Over half the cases are associated with NF1 (57%) and radiation may be a factor in their development.[6] Generally the tumor affects younger patients of either sex. Terzic et al found an age range of 3 to 83 years (mean 40 years) in the literature, with 29 male and 24 female patients in the entire head and neck cohort, although the age was lower (mean 26 years) if the tumor was associated with NF1.[6]

Sinonasal lesions mainly produce nasal obstruction or epistaxis. Rarely, metastatic spread occurs to the lungs, brain, liver, breast, and bones, but this is exceptional from the nasal lesions.

Histopathological criteria for diagnosis require the MTT to involve a peripheral nerve or, in a patient with NF1, to show growth characteristics of a Schwann cell tumor and to contain true neoplastic rhabdomyoblasts.[8]

Imaging is nonspecific but should include both CT and MRI to best define the mass.

Treatment and Outcome

Treatment has largely relied on surgery, to which radiotherapy has been added when surgery has been incomplete. Radical surgery produces significantly better outcomes than one might expect ($p = 0.036$) and endoscopic resection has been proposed in the more recent cases, as was undertaken in our single case. However, the small number of cases precludes discussion of the advantage of additional radiotherapy or chemotherapy. Overall, for triton tumors affecting the head and neck, survival at 5 years was 49%, and was 37% at 10 years with no deaths reported after 6.5 years' survival.[6] The overall prognosis for the sinonasal lesions appears much better than elsewhere in the body, with over 80% surviving 5 years and beyond,[6] in contrast to the outcome for MTT elsewhere in the body, where crude and specific survival figures of 11% and 26%, respectively, have been reported.[8,9]

References

1. Mason P. Recklinghausen's neurofibromatosis, sensory neuromas and motor neuromas. In: Libman Anniversary. Vol 2. New York: International Press; 1932:793–802
2. Woodruff JM, Chernik NL, Smith MC, Millett WB, Foote FW Jr. Peripheral nerve tumors with rhabdomyosarcomatous differentiation (malignant "Triton" tumors). Cancer 1973;32(2):426–439
3. Heffner DK, Gnepp DR. Sinonasal fibrosarcomas, malignant schwannomas, and "Triton" tumors. A clinicopathologic study of 67 cases. Cancer 1992;70(5):1089–1101
4. Nicolai P, Tomenzoli D, Berlucchi M, Facchetti F, Morassi L, Maroldi R. Malignant triton tumor of the ethmoid sinus and nasal cavity. Ann Otol Rhinol Laryngol 2000; 109(9):880–886
5. López Alvarez F, Llorente Pendás JL, Coca Pelaz A, Fernández García MS, Cuello Bueno G, Suárez Nieto C. Malignant triton tumor of the infratemporal fossa. J Craniofac Surg 2009;20(4):1282–1286
6. Terzic A, Bode B, Gratz KW, Stoeckli SJ. Prognostic factors for the malignant triton tumor of the head and neck. Head Neck 2009;31(5):679–688
7. Xue T, Wei L, Qiao L, Zha DJ, Chen XD, Qiu JH. Malignant triton tumour of right paranasal sinuses: case report. J Laryngol Otol 2009;123(5):e16
8. Woodruff JM, Perino G. Non-germ-cell or teratomatous malignant tumors showing additional rhabdomyoblastic differentiation, with emphasis on the malignant Triton tumor. Semin Diagn Pathol 1994;11(1):69–81
9. Yakulis R, Manack L, Murphy AI Jr. Postradiation malignant triton tumor. A case report and review of the literature. Arch Pathol Lab Med 1996;120(6):541–548

Neurofibroma and Neurofibromatosis

Definition

(ICD-O code 9540/0)

A nonencapsulated tumor of Schwann cells differing from a schwannoma in its structure and clinical behavior.

Etiology

These tumors may occur spontaneously as solitary lesions or in association with neurofibromatosis type 1 (NF1). This is a relatively common inherited disorder; the inheritance is autosomal dominant with variable penetrance. The gene responsible for NF1 has been localized to chromosome 17. NF2, by contrast, is classically associated with acoustic neuromas (actually schwannomas) and is due to a lesion on chromosome 22q. Specific criteria for diagnosis of NF1 and NF2 have been developed by the national health institutions.[1,2]

For NF1 two or more of the following criteria have to be present to make the diagnosis:

1. Six or more café au lait spots
2. More than two neurofibromas of any type or one plexiform neurofibroma
3. Hyperpigmentation of the axilla or intertriginous areas
4. More than two iris hamartomas
5. Distinctive bony abnormality, such as sphenoid dysplasia
6. A first-degree relative with NF1

Synonyms

Von Recklinghausen described NF1 in the late nineteenth century.[3]

Incidence

If associated with NF1, this condition is found in 1 in 4,000 live births. NF1 accounts for 90% of neurofibromas generally[4–6] and is also associated with other neurogenic tumors such as optic gliomas.[7]

In our own series of 5 sinonasal cases, none were associated with NF1.

Site

Solitary or multiple neurofibromas can occur throughout the upper aerodigestive tract. They remain rare in the sinonasal tract and it can be difficult to determine the precise peripheral nerve sheath of origin. Plexiform lesions, as part of NF1, may be seen more often in the orbit. Isolated lesions have been reported in the nasal cavity, for example, on the inferior turbinate[8,9] or septum[10,11] or paranasal sinuses.[12]

Diagnostic Features

Clinical Features

Although neurofibromas often occur as single lesions, other signs of neurofibromatosis should be sought. The age at presentation appears younger than for schwannomas, particularly when associated with NF1, usually 20 to 40 years or younger. The sex incidence is equal and there does not appear to be any ethnic predisposition.

Solitary tumors grow slowly though in NF1 they may be painful. The symptoms, as might be anticipated, are initially nasal obstruction, then possible displacement of the eye, and sinus obstruction.

In our 5 cases, there were 2 men and 3 women, aged 37 to 53 years (mean 47.8 years). Four presented via the ophthamologists with slowly progressive proptosis, the fifth with unilateral nasal obstruction, reflecting their sites of origin (Table 15.7).

Imaging

The lesions may appear well circumscribed (though not encapsulated) or plexiform. Both CT and MRI may be required, particularly if intracranial abnormalities are also suspected and to distinguish inflammation and sinus secretion from tumor (Fig. 15.9). MRI is preferentially used for monitoring or post therapy.

Table 15.7 Neurofibromas: personal series

No.	Sex	Age (y)	Site	Treatment	Outcome
1	M	53	Orbit	Lateral orbitotomy and lateral skull base resection	AWR 10 y
2	F	42	Orbit	Lateral orbitotomy and midfacial degloving	A&W 9 y
3	F	48	Orbit	Midfacial degloving	AWR 8 y
4	M	59	Lateral skull base	Lateral skull base resection	A&W 8 y
5	F	37	Lateral nasal wall	Endoscopic resection	A&W 5 y

Abbreviations: A&W, alive and well; AWR, alive with recurrence; F, female; M, male; y, year(s).

Histological Features and Differential Diagnosis

(See **Table 15.8**.)

Macroscopically the lesion may be obviously and intimately related to the nerve of origin. Microscopically they are composed of a rather uniform mix of spindle cells with serpentine or wavy nuclei, collagenous fibers, and a myxoid matrix. The spindle cells may be fibroblasts, neurites, and Schwann cells, so there may be some positivity to S100 on immunohistochemistry as well as to CD34.

Plexiform neurofibromas look like a thickened and distorted nerve trunk.

The distinction that should be made is from a schwannoma, which may be difficult on small biopsies. Neurofibromas may also be confused with myxomas, fibromas, hemangiomas, and MPNSTs.

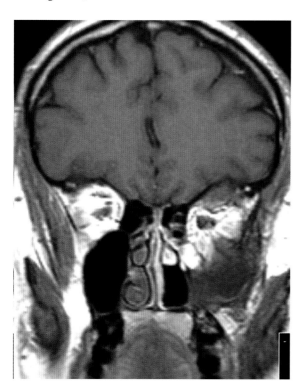

Fig. 15.9 Coronal MRI (T1W post gadolinium enhancement) showing a neurofibroma affecting the left orbit and maxillary sinus.

Five different variants of solitary neurofibromas have been described in the past[13]:

1. Myxoid—abundant mucin is present in the matrix; S100 positivity distinguishes this from myxoma.
2. Collagenous—thick collagen bundles are present in the matrix.
3. Epithelioid—tumor cells are rounded with eosinophilic cytoplasm.
4. Granular—cells contain granular periodic acid-Schiff–positive, diastase-resistant cytoplasm.
5. Pigmented—scattered cells contain melanin; positive to S100 and HMB45 (monoclonal mouse antihuman melanosome) and to melanin A.

Malignant transformation is rare, particularly in solitary tumors but may occur with multiple lesions as in NF1. This is evidenced by increased cellularity, mitoses, atypia, and invasive growth (see MPNSTs, p. 343). These lesions must be differentiated from fibrosarcomas.

Natural History

Neurofibromas are slow-growing tumors producing symptoms by pressure as much as local infiltration. Bone erosion per se does not indicate malignant transformation. However, rapid growth in an existing lesion, especially in NF1, is highly suspicious.

Treatment and Outcome

As with virtually all benign tumors, complete excision results in cure but may be difficult to achieve. Depending on the site and extent, excision may be effected by an endoscopic approach or any one of several external approaches.[14] In our series, four required lateral orbitotomies/lateral skull base resections, facilitated in two by midfacial degloving. Only one was amenable to an endonasal endoscopic resection. The infiltrative nature in relation to the orbital apex and cavernous sinus in patients with residual vision means that total excision was not achieved in two individuals and they remain under regular review with MRI and orbital assessment.

Plexiform lesions are particularly difficult to extirpate and tumors that have undergone malignant

Table 15.8 Pathological differences between fibroblastic and Schwann cell tumors

	Fibrosarcoma	Neurilemmoma	Neurofibroma	Neurogenic sarcoma
Border	Infiltrative	Encapsulated	Infiltrative	Infiltrative
Low-power appearance	Moderate cellularity	Highly cellular (Antoni A)	Moderate cellularity	Highly cellular
Fibrous tissue	Decreasing with increased cellularity	Variable	Small amounts	Small amounts
Myxoid tissue	Unusual	Focally (Antoni B)	Prominent	?
Nuclear appearance	Spindle-shaped	Tapered	Tapered	Spindle-shaped
Nuclear pleomorphism	Minimal	Bizarre	Bizarre	Minimal
Mitotic activity	Moderate	Few	Few	Numerous

Source: After reference 7.

transformation are especially resistant to cure (see MPNSTs), with most patients succumbing to their disease despite many operations and adjunctive therapies.

References

1. National Institutes of Health Consensus Development Conference. Neurofibromatosis. Conference statement. Arch Neurol 1988;45(5):575–578
2. Gutmann DH, Aylsworth A, Carey JC, et al. The diagnostic evaluation and multidisciplinary management of neurofibromatosis 1 and neurofibromatosis 2. JAMA 1997; 278(1):51–57
3. Von Recklinghausen J. Die fibrose oder deformiende osteite. Festschrift R Virchow zei Seinem. Berlin: Geburtage; 1881
4. Riccardi VM. Neurofibromatosis: past, present, and future. N Engl J Med 1991;324(18):1283–1285
5. Friedman JM. Epidemiology of neurofibromatosis type 1. Am J Med Genet 1999;89(1):1–6
6. Greenberg M. Handbook of Neurosurgery. 6th ed. New York: Thieme; 2006
7. Perzin KH, Panyu H, Wechter S. Nonepithelial tumors of the nasal cavity, paranasal sinuses and nasopharynx. A clinicopathologic study. XII: Schwann cell tumors (neurilemoma, neurofibroma, malignant schwannoma). Cancer 1982;50(10):2193–2202
8. Moreno PM, Meseguer DH. Solitary neurofibroma of the inferior nasal turbinate. Auris Nasus Larynx 1998; 25(3):329–331
9. Manganaris A, Tsompanidou C, Manganaris T. A peripheral nerve sheath tumour as a cause of nasal obstruction. J Laryngol Otol 2006;120(12):e44
10. Annino DJ Jr, Domanowski GF, Vaughan CW. A rare cause of nasal obstruction: a solitary neurofibroma. Otolaryngol Head Neck Surg 1991;104(4):484–488
11. Kim YD, Bai CH, Suh JS, Song KW. Transnasal endoscopic excision of an isolated neurofibroma of the nasal septum. Rhinology 1997;35(2):89–91
12. Stevens DJ, Kirkham N. Neurofibromas of the paranasal sinuses. J Laryngol Otol 1988;102(3):256–259
13. Batsakis J. Pathology of the nasal cavity and paranasal sinuses. In: Thawley S, Panje W, Batsakis J, Lindberg R, eds. Comprehensive Manual of Head and Neck Cancer. Philadelphia: WB Saunders; 1999:144–148
14. Hirao M, Gushiken T, Imokawa H, Kawai S, Inaba H, Tsukuda M. Solitary neurofibroma of the nasal cavity. J Laryngol Otol 2001;115:1012–1014

Meningioma

Definition

(ICD-O code 9530/0)

A benign tumor of the central nervous system that is believed to originate in arachnoid cap cells of the meninges.

Etiology

Involvement of the upper aerodigestive tract can occur in several ways:

- An intracranial neoplasm directly extends extracranially.
- Extracranial growth from arachnoid cells accompanies cranial nerves (e.g., the optic nerve), as they exit the skull foramina.
- There may be extracranial growth without overt intracranial connection arising from ectopic arachnoid cells.
- An intracranial tumor metastasizes.[1]

Intracranial meningiomas can occur in association with neurofibromatosis 2 (NF2)[2] and are increased by exposure to radiation.

Incidence

Meningioma is generally an intracranial tumor (90%), in which site it accounts for 15% of primary tumors. True extracranial meningiomas, by contrast, are relatively rare as arachnoid cells are not normally found in the sinonasal region.

Site

Meningiomas may occur wherever arachnoid cells are located and therefore can also occur in the spine (9%), but other extracranial lesions in the head and neck have been described (1%). Anterior skull base meningiomas account for 40% of intracranial lesions, involving the olfactory groove, tuberculum sellae and sphenoidal ridge, from where they may affect the orbit on one or both sides.[3-5] About 20% have an extracranial component. In descending order, the sites of these extensions are: orbit, outer table of the cranium and soft tissue of the scalp, sinonasal, and pterygoid regions.[6] Those in the olfactory groove may spread inferiorly through the cribriform plate into the ethmoids. This has been estimated to occur in 15% of cases.[7]

Extracranial meningiomas may affect the sinuses, or less commonly the nasal cavity, according to the case reports as large series are not found in the literature. One of the largest is that of Perzin et al who reported 12 cases in 1984.[8] A subsequent review of the literature by Thompson in 2000 found 98 cases to which a few case reports have been subsequently been published.[9] An intracranial source should be assumed until proven otherwise by appropriate imaging and some early reported cases that lacked adequate investigation may have simply been

extracranial extensions. In our series of 11 meningiomas that presented extracranially, the frontal region and orbit were most often affected (Tables 15.9 and 15.10).

Diagnostic Features

Clinical

Intracranial lesions peak age at presentation is 40 to 60 years and they are more common in females. The specific neurological deficit obviously depends on site and size. In the olfactory groove loss of smell can be anticipated, even though this may not be a source of immediate concern to the patient. Visual loss and headache are associated with meningiomas of the tuberculum sellae.[10,11]

Extracranial sinonasal lesions occur over a wide age range (9–76 years, mean 43 years) and are said to affect men and women equally, although they appeared to be slightly commoner in men in an analysis of nearly 100 cases.[9] In our small cohort, 8 were men, 3 women, their

Table 15.9 Extracranial meningiomas: personal series

Male	Female	Age (y)	Site	Treatment	Outcome
1		38	Frontal bone	Frontal craniotomy (×2)	DOD 14 y
				Radiotherapy	
				Craniofacial resection	
1		73	Frontal bone	Craniofacial resection	A&W 6 y
				Titanium plate	
1		39	Frontal bone	Craniofacial resection	DOD 2 y
				Craniotomy	
1		14	Orbit	Orbital explorations (×6)	9-y FU
				Bifrontal craniotomy	AWR then lost
				Craniofacial resection and orbital clearance	
1		61	Orbit	Orbital clearance	A&W 11 y
1		25	Orbit	Lateral orbitotomy (×2)	A&W 16 y
				Craniotomy	
				Orbital clearance	
	1	40	Ethmoid, skull base	Craniofacial (×2)	DOD 10 y
	1	75	Frontoethmoid region	Lateral rhinotomy	DICD 10 y
1		64	Nasal septum	Lateral rhinotomy ×1	A&W 26 y
				Craniofacial resection	
	1	40	Olfactory groove, skull base	Craniofacial resection	A&W 2 y then lost to FU

Abbreviations: A&W: alive and well; AWR: alive with recurrence; DOD: dead of disease; DICD: dead of intercurrent disease; FU: follow-up; y, year(s).

Table 15.10 Extracranial meningioma: cases published in literature and personal cohort

All cases[a]	n = 121
Sex	
Female	60
Male	45
Age at presentation	
Range	9–76 y
Average	46.1 y
Females (average)	50.5 y
Males (average)	39.0 y
Length of symptoms	
Range	0.1–40 y
Average	5.1 y
Tumor location	
Ethmoid sinus alone	5
Frontal sinus alone	11
Nasal cavity alone	4
Nasopharynx alone	6
Maxillary sinus alone	5
Sphenoid sinus alone	17
Paranasal sinuses alone	19
Nasal cavity and sinuses (NOS)	51
Orbit	3
CNS connection	
Yes	38
No	65
Unknown	18
Evidence of recurrence/residual disease	47

Abbreviations: NOS, not otherwise specified; y, year(s).

[a] Parameter was not always stated in the report and therefore the numbers do not necessarily equal the total values in the columns.

ages ranged from 14 to 75 years (mean 49 years). Most patients present with the effects of a mass, that is, nasal obstruction, hyposmia, cosmetic deformity such as a frontal mass,[12–14] and sometimes produce epistaxis. Lesions affecting the orbit will produce proptosis, visual field changes, and loss of color vision.[15] Regrettably meningioma is one of the few tumors that can lead to bilateral blindness due to chiasmal involvement and it did so in 3 of our patients.

A firm polyp may be found on nasal examination. Even bilateral "polyps" have been described.[16]

Imaging

CT with contrast and MRI are the mainstay of diagnosis and follow-up,[3] though they may be corroborated by endoscopic biopsy in some cases (**Figs. 15.10, 15.11, 15.12, 15.13, 15.14**).[17] Meningiomas are isodense to slightly hyperdense on CT, homogeneous, and demarcated by contrast. There is often marked adjacent hyperostosis, which indeed may alert the ENT surgeon to the presence of a meningioma. Intracranial lesions may have surrounding edema and calcification.

On T1W MRI the lesion is isodense to hypodense; on T2W images the appearances are variable and can be hyperdense. The tumor enhances with gadolinium contrast medium and a dural "tail" may be seen. Other techniques may be used to further delineate neurovascular relationships.

Imaging of extracranial lesions in this area may be diagnosed by a combination of the hyperostosis in adjacent bone and soft tissue mass ± calcification seen on CT, further elucidated by MRI. It is important to confirm that there is no intracranial connection or component. The cause of the hyperostosis is unknown as it can occur some distance from the lesion, suggesting some additional growth factor. However, sometimes a soft tissue mass alone may fill and expand a sinus, giving the appearance of a mucocele.[18]

Pneumosinus dilatans, an abnormal dilatation of the paranasal sinuses, can be associated with meningioma (as well as benign fibro-osseous disease). First described by Benjamins in 1918[19] it can affect any of the sinuses except the maxillary. Between 20% and 38% of skull base meningiomas are reported as associated with this condition.

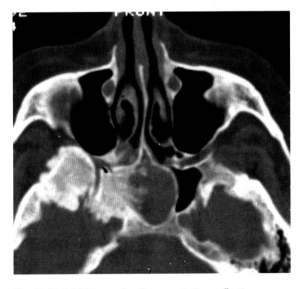

Fig. 15.10 Axial CT scan showing a meningioma affecting the sphenoid sinus and bone with soft tissue and calcified components.

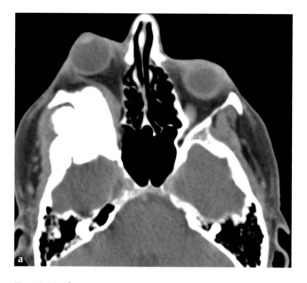

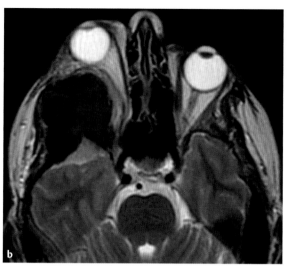

Fig. 15.11a, b

a Axial CT scan showing hyperostosis in the greater wing of the sphenoid due to meningioma compressing the left orbit.

b Axial MRI (T2W) in the same patient showing signal void from a calcified mass.

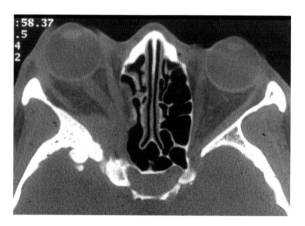

Fig. 15.12 Axial CT scan showing the postoperative situation after removal of the medial wall of the orbit to decompress the apex compressed by soft tissue and a hyperostotic mass of sphenoid meningioma.

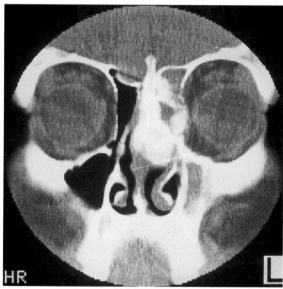

Fig. 15.13 Coronal CT showing a meningioma in the left nasal cavity and ethmoid with areas of hyperdensity.

Histological Features and Differential Diagnosis

These lesions are classically circumscribed and rubbery in consistency. Some grow en plaque as opposed to forming masses. Several grades have been defined.[3,5,20]

- Grade I: fibroblastic, transitional, psammomatous meningotheliomatous (angiomatous)
- Grade II: atypical showing hypercellularity, frequent mitoses, and necrosis
- Grade III: malignant or anaplastic, which are invasive, recur but rarely metastasize

The majority of lesions (90%) are grade I. Psammoma bodies are laminated calcified lesions associated with meningiomas but are not pathognomonic as they can be found in thyroid carcinoma and certain ovarian tumors.[21]

Extracranial meningiomas have the same histological features and are usually grade I meningotheliomatous composed of whorled nodules of plump spindle cells. Rarely, grades II and III are encountered. Psammoma bodies are found in about one-third of cases.

Immunohistochemistry may be helpful to confirm the diagnosis, specifically positivity to epithelial membrane

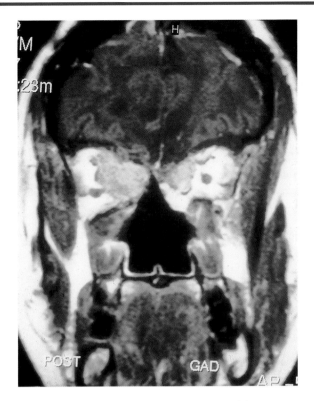

Fig. 15.14 Meningioma. Coronal MRI (T1W post gadolinium enhancement) in a patient showing bilateral orbital disease despite previous craniotomy and craniofacial resection.

antigen (EMA) and vimentin.[9] About 50% of meningiomas have immunoreactivity with antibodies to progesterone receptors, whereas a small number react to cytokeratin and estrogen receptor antibodies. However, it should be noted that the differential diagnosis includes other neuroectodermal tumors such as schwannoma, neurofibroma, and even malignant melanoma or olfactory neuroblastoma as well as paraganglioma and aggressive psammomatoid ossifying fibroma.

Natural History

These tumors generally grow slowly and may never present clinically. The rate of growth seems to relate to some extent to the age of the individual, being an indolent lesion in the elderly. However, it has been our and others' experience that in the young males growth is rapid and locally destructive, often with fatal consequences despite radical surgery.

Treatment

Extracranial sinonasal lesions can reasonably be expected to be excised completely in many cases using external, endoscopic, or combined techniques. Lateral rhinotomy and external frontoethmoidectomy have been used in the past, and craniofacial resection for the more

extensive lesions.[22] Endoscopic techniques are also being employed[23] but in our cohort, all underwent radical open procedures (**Table 15.9**). However, whatever technique is used, because meningiomas more often infiltrate the surrounding normal structures, wide radical excision is necessary. In particular, any adjacent thickened bone must be assumed to be infiltrated microscopically with disease and should be removed.

For intracranial lesions four possible management strategies are adopted:

- Observation ± regular imaging for incidental asymptomatic lesions and small tumors or in patients where major surgery is not appropriate
- Surgical resection for symptomatic lesions[24]
- Stereotactic radiosurgery for residual, recurrent, or surgically inaccessible lesions
- Conventional radiotherapy or stereotactic techniques possibly for malignant lesions

The neurosurgical techniques for intracranial lesions are beyond the scope of this book, but those involving the skull base and orbit increasingly come within the ambit of the rhinological surgeon.[25-34] Suffice to say that a range of combined external (e.g., subfrontal, supraorbital, or midfacial) approaches and endoscopic techniques are being applied to lesions involving the tuberculum sellae.[35-39]

Approaching these intracranial tumors endoscopically from below facilitates early devascularization of the meningeal blood supply without brain retraction and minimizes morbidity as there is less manipulation of adjacent structures, in particular of the optic nerve and chiasm. Kassam and colleagues have developed a modular approach to the skull base, dividing them broadly into midline sagittal (rostrocaudal axis) and paramedian (coronal plane).[34] In general lesions extending between the plane of the superior rectus muscles bilaterally may be approached endoscopically. These resections initially posed significant difficulties in reconstruction but these have to a large extent been remedied by the development of vascularized flaps such as the Haddad nasoseptal flap,[40] reducing postoperative CSF leaks from 40% to 5%.

Decompression of the orbital apex, optic canals, and chiasm can also be undertaken by external and endoscopic approaches.[15,41] While not curing the problem, this can achieve useful improvement in vision for prolonged periods of time in patients who are often elderly. Endoscopic removal of the medial bony wall from 0 to 180° is undertaken from anterior to posterior, including the medial wall of the sphenoid. This is usually combined with incision of the periosteal sheath if there is intraperiosteal involvement. The incisions should be performed in the upper medial quadrant to avoid damage to the ophthalmic artery, which can lie in the inferior medial quadrant of the optic nerve sheath (estimated at 15% by Lang[42]).

Outcome

Generally meningiomas have a good long-term prognosis with 5-year survival figures of 90% quoted in the neurosurgical literature.[43] However, this should not necessarily be equated with disease-free survival and late "recurrence" can occur even with ostensible complete excision. Those arising in the skull base may be technically challenging and associated with potentially a higher morbidity.[44–46] In our group of patients, 4 died of disease (2–14 years), 4 are alive and well (6–26 years), one died of intercurrent disease 10 years after treatment, and 2 have been lost to follow-up. These numbers are too small for any meaningful analysis but 55% required more than one major procedure.

Up to 2010, 82 patients have been reported[34] (Table 15.10[17,47–55]) as undergoing an extended endoscopic endonasal approach for meningioma involving the skull base, with follow-up ranging from 1 month to 51 months. These mainly arose in the tuberculum sellae. These patients are a heterogeneous group, making comparisons difficult, but complications included transient visual deterioration (6.5%), diabetes insipidus (transient 4.9%, permanent 3.7%), meningitis (1.2%), significant hemorrhage (1.2%), pneumocephalus (1.2%), and death (1.2%). These figures compare well with the recent literature for transcranial approaches to meningiomas of the tuberculum sellae. Similar resection rates are quoted for the different approaches (86.4% total resection by transcranial route vs. 86.9% total or near total by endoscopic techniques), but there is a quantum difference in numbers (487 vs. 41) and patient selection may vary significantly. CSF leakage is higher after endoscopic surgery but visual function appears to be better in terms of both post-operative deterioration and overall improvement.[34]

A similar comparison may also be made between olfactory groove meningiomas treated conventionally and endoscopically[34] (Table 15.11). There are obviously many cases that cannot be tackled endoscopically, in particular any lesion lateral to cranial nerves where conventional approaches must be used. Experience with all possible neurosurgical techniques and an understanding of the natural history of this tumor are prerequisites of deciding on the best approach. As always the surgical approach is determined by the disease not the other way around.

Endoscopic orbital apex decompression in 12 female patients, all with significant visual impairment, resulted in both subjective and objective improvement in visual functions, including acuity, density of RAPD (relative afferent papillary defect), visual fields, ocular balance, motility, reduced proptosis, and lack of complications.[15] Follow-up was a mean of 45 months (range 5–96 months) with further deterioration noted in two patients but not until 4 to 5 years later.

Whatever the management, patients generally require long-term follow-up.

References

1. Friedman CD, Costantino PD, Teitelbaum B, Berktold RE, Sisson GA Sr. Primary extracranial meningiomas of the head and neck. Laryngoscope 1990;100(1):41–48
2. Barnholtz-Sloan JS, Kruchko C. Meningiomas: causes and risk factors. Neurosurg Focus 2007;23(4):E2
3. Drummond KJ, Zhu JJ, Black PM. Meningiomas: updating basic science, management, and outcome. Neurologist 2004;10(3):113–130
4. Greenberg M. Meningiomas. Handbook of Neurosurgery. 5th ed. New York: Thieme; 2001:407–410
5. Whittle IR, Smith C, Navoo P, Collie D. Meningiomas. Lancet 2004;363(9420):1535–1543
6. Batsakis JG. Pathology consultation. Extracranial meningiomas. Ann Otol Rhinol Laryngol 1984;93(3 Pt 1):282–283
7. Hentschel SJ, DeMonte F. Olfactory groove meningiomas. Neurosurg Focus 2003;14(6):e4
8. Perzin KH, Pushparaj N. Nonepithelial tumors of the nasal cavity, paranasal sinuses, and nasopharynx. A clinicopathologic study. XIII: Meningiomas. Cancer 1984;54(9):1860–1869
9. Thompson LD, Gyure KA. Extracranial sinonasal tract meningiomas: a clinicopathologic study of 30 cases with a review of the literature. Am J Surg Pathol 2000;24(5):640–650
10. Swain RE Jr, Kingdom TT, DelGaudio JM, Muller S, Grist WJ. Meningiomas of the paranasal sinuses. Am J Rhinol 2001;15(1):27–30

Table 15.11 Comparison of transcranial and endoscopic approaches for olfactory groove meningiomas

	Transcranial	Endonasal endoscopic
N	234	20
Total removal (mean)	90.7%	75%
Mortality (mean)	1%	0%
Overall complication rate		
Mean	25.5%	
Range	0–46.6%	
CSF leaks		
Mean	9.4%	25%
Range	0–20%	
Source: After reference 34.		

11. Chi JH, McDermott MW. Tuberculum sellae meningiomas. Neurosurg Focus 2003;14(6):e6

12. Sadar ES, Conomy JP, Benjamin SP, Levine HL. Meningioma of the paranasal sinuses, benign and malignant. Neurosurgery 1979;4(3):227–232

13. Papavasiliou A, Sawyer R, Lund V. Effects of meningiomas on the facial skeleton. Arch Otolaryngol 1982;108(4):255–257

14. Min JH, Kang SH, Lee JB, Chung YG, Lee HK. Hyperostotic meningioma with minimal tumor invasion into the skull. Neurol Med Chir (Tokyo) 2005;45(9):480–483

15. Lund VJ, Rose GE. Endoscopic transnasal orbital decompression for visual failure due to sphenoid wing meningioma. Eye (Lond) 2006;20(10):1213–1219

16. Ismail H, Burnley H, Harries PG. Recurrent extracranial sinonasal meningioma presenting 27 years after complete surgical eradication of right frontal meningioma. Acta Otolaryngol 2004;124(6):751–753

17. Liu HS, Di X. Endoscopic endonasal surgery for biopsy of cavernous sinus lesions. Minim Invasive Neurosurg 2009;52(2):69–73

18. Daneshi A, Asghari A, Bahramy E. Primary meningioma of the ethmoid sinus: a case report. Ear Nose Throat J 2003;82(4):310–311

19. Benjamins C Pneumosinus frontalis dilatans. Acta Otolaryngol 1918;1:412–422

20. Commins DL, Atkinson RD, Burnett ME. Review of meningioma histopathology. Neurosurg Focus 2007;23(4):E3

21. Granich MS, Pilch BZ, Goodman ML. Meningiomas presenting in the paranasal sinuses and temporal bone. Head Neck Surg 1983;5(4):319–328

22. Howard DJ, Lund VJ, Wei WI. Craniofacial resection for tumors of the nasal cavity and paranasal sinuses: a 25-year experience. Head Neck 2006;28(10):867–873

23. Kainuma K, Takumi Y, Uehara T, Usami S. Meningioma of the paranasal sinus: a case report. Auris Nasus Larynx 2007;34(3):397–400

24. Rockhill J, Mrugala M, Chamberlain MC. Intracranial meningiomas: an overview of diagnosis and treatment. Neurosurg Focus 2007;23(4):E1

25. Jho HD, Carrau RL. Endoscopic endonasal transsphenoidal surgery: experience with 50 patients. J Neurosurg 1997;87(1):44–51

26. Cappabianca P, Cavallo LM, Colao A, et al. Endoscopic endonasal transsphenoidal approach: outcome analysis of 100 consecutive procedures. Minim Invasive Neurosurg 2002;45(4):193–200

27. Cavallo LM, Messina A, Cappabianca P, et al. Endoscopic endonasal surgery of the midline skull base: anatomical study and clinical considerations. Neurosurg Focus 2005;19(1):E2

28. Kassam A, Snyderman CH, Mintz A, Gardner P, Carrau RL. Expanded endonasal approach: the rostrocaudal axis. Part I. Crista galli to the sella turcica. Neurosurg Focus 2005;19(1):E3

29. de Divitiis E, Cavallo LM, Cappabianca P, Esposito F. Extended endoscopic endonasal transsphenoidal approach for the removal of suprasellar tumors: Part 2. Neurosurgery 2007;60(1):46–58, discussion 58–59

30. Kassam A, Thomas AJ, Snyderman C, et al. Fully endoscopic expanded endonasal approach treating skull base lesions in pediatric patients. J Neurosurg 2007; 106(2, Suppl)75–86

31. de Divitiis E, Esposito F, Cappabianca P, Cavallo LM, de Divitiis O. Tuberculum sellae meningiomas: high route or low route? A series of 51 consecutive cases. Neurosurgery 2008;62(3):556–563, discussion 556–563

32. Schwartz TH, Fraser JF, Brown S, Tabaee A, Kacker A, Anand VK. Endoscopic cranial base surgery: classification of operative approaches. Neurosurgery 2008;62(5):991–1002, discussion 1002–1005

33. Dehdashti AR, Ganna A, Witterick I, Gentili F. Expanded endoscopic endonasal approach for anterior cranial base and suprasellar lesions: indications and limitations. Neurosurgery 2009;64(4):677–687, discussion 687–689

34. Lund VJ, Stammberger H, Nicolai P, et al. European position paper on endoscopic management of tumours of the nose, paranasal sinuses and skull base. Rhinol Suppl 2010;(22):1–143

35. Arai H, Sato K, Okuda, et al. Transcranial transsphenoidal approach for tuberculum sellae meningiomas. Acta Neurochir (Wien) 2000;142(7):751–756, discussion 756–757

36. Jane J, Dumont A, Vance M, Laws E. The transsphenoidal transtuberculum sellae approach for suprasellar meningiomas. Semin Neurosurg 2003;14:211–218

37. Cook SW, Smith Z, Kelly DF. Endonasal transsphenoidal removal of tuberculum sellae meningiomas: technical note. Neurosurgery 2004;55(1):239–244, discussion 244–246

38. Dusick JR, Esposito F, Kelly DF, et al. The extended direct endonasal transsphenoidal approach for nonadenomatous suprasellar tumors. J Neurosurg 2005;102(5):832–841

39. Jane JA Jr, Han J, Prevedello DM, Jagannathan J, Dumont AS, Laws ER Jr. Perspectives on endoscopic transsphenoidal surgery. Neurosurg Focus 2005;19(6):E2

40. Ganna A, Dehdashti AR, Karabatsou K, Gentili F. Frontobasal interhemispheric approach for tuberculum sellae meningiomas; long-term visual outcome. Br J Neurosurg 2009;23(4):422–430

41. Hadad G, Bassagasteguy L, Carrau RL, et al. A novel reconstructive technique after endoscopic expanded endonasal approaches: vascular pedicle nasoseptal flap. Laryngoscope 2006;116(10):1882–1886

42. Kennerdell JS, Maroon JC. Intracanalicular meningioma with chronic optic disc edema. Ann Ophthalmol 1982;14:80–83

43. Lang J. Clinical Anatomy of the Nose, Nasal Cavity and Paranasal Sinuses. Stuttgart: Georg Thieme Verlag; 1989:128

44. Nakasu S, Fukami T, Jito J, Nozaki K. Recurrence and regrowth of benign meningiomas. Brain Tumor Pathol 2009;26(2):69–72

45. DeMonte F. Surgical treatment of anterior basal meningiomas. J Neurooncol 1996;29(3):239–248

46. Little KM, Friedman AH, Sampson JH, Wanibuchi M, Fukushima T. Surgical management of petroclival meningiomas: defining resection goals based on risk of neurological morbidity and tumor recurrence rates in 137 patients. Neurosurgery 2005;56(3):546–559, discussion 546–559

47. Samii M, Gerganov VM. Surgery of extra-axial tumors of the cerebral base. Neurosurgery 2008; 62(6, Suppl 3)1153–1166, discussion 1166–1168

48. Laufer I, Anand VK, Schwartz TH. Endoscopic, endonasal extended transsphenoidal, transplanum transtuberculum approach for resection of suprasellar lesions. J Neurosurg 2007;106(3):400–406

49. de Divitiis E, Esposito F, Cappabianca P, Cavallo LM, de Divitiis O, Esposito I. Endoscopic transnasal resection of anterior cranial fossa meningiomas. Neurosurg Focus 2008;25(6):E8

50. Gardner PA, Kassam AB, Thomas A, et al. Endoscopic endonasal resection of anterior cranial base meningiomas. Neurosurgery 2008;63(1):36–52, discussion 52–54

51. Kassam AB, Prevedello DM, Thomas A, et al. Endoscopic endonasal pituitary transposition for a transdorsum sellae approach to the interpeduncular cistern. Neurosurgery 2008; 62(3, Suppl 1)57–72, discussion 72–74

52. Ceylan S, Koc K, Anik I. Extended endoscopic approaches for midline skull-base lesions. Neurosurg Rev 2009; 32(3):309–319, discussion 318–319

53. Kassam AB, Prevedello DM, Carrau RL, et al. The front door to Meckel's cave: an anteromedial corridor via expanded

endoscopic endonasal approach—technical considerations and clinical series. Neurosurgery 2009;64(3 Suppl):ons71–82; discussion ons82–83

54. Wang Q, Lu XJ, Li B, Ji WY, Chen KL. Extended endoscopic endonasal transsphenoidal removal of tuberculum sellae meningiomas: a preliminary report. J Clin Neurosci 2009;16(7):889–893

55. Kurschel S, Gellner V, Clarici G, Braun H, Stammberger H, Mokry M. Endoscopic rhino-neurosurgical approach for non-adenomatous sellar and skull base lesions. Rhinology 2011;49(1):64–73

Neuroendocrine Carcinoma

- Carcinoid (well-differentiated neuroendocrine carcinoma) (ICD-O code 8240/3)
- Atypical carcinoid (moderately differentiated neuroendocrine carcinoma) (ICD-O code 8249/3)
- Small cell carcinoma (poorly or undifferentiated neuroendocrine carcinoma) (ICD-O code 8041/3)

Neuroendocrine carcinomas of a wide range of differentiation can be found in the upper aerodigestive tract, mainly in the larynx.[1] However, the term has caused some confusion; it is important that they should be distinguished from olfactory neuroblastoma[2] and their relationship with sinonasal undifferentiated tumors has been much debated.[3] As they also represent a wide range of behavior, accurate diagnosis is important.

Definition

Tumors of neuroendocrine origin of varying differentiation and aggressiveness.

Etiology

No predisposing factors are known.

Synonyms

In addition to the degree of differentiation, they may be referred to by grade (1 to 3, with carcinoid being grade 1 and small cell being grade 3). The generic acronym "SNEC" (sinonasal neuroendocrine carcinoma) is often used. Atypical or moderately differentiated lesions are sometimes called large cell whereas the small cell type has been called "oat cell." Small cell carcinoma has also been called small cell undifferentiated (neuroendocrine) carcinoma or poorly differentiated neuroendocrine carcinoma.[4]

Incidence

These lesions are rare but they may have been underdiagnosed in the past. They are more often encountered in the submucosa of the supraglottis. The first case at this site was described by Goldman in 1969.[5] The atypical or moderately differentiated neuroendocrine carcinoma and small cell variants are commoner than the well-differentiated carcinoid tumors and, of the three, the small cell variant is the one that is also found in the sinonasal tract.[6] Only a handful of cases of sinonasal carcinoid carcinoma have been described. Up to 2000, only around 30 small cell carcinomas had been described in the sinonasal region, but on review a number were probably sinonasal undifferentiated carcinomas (SNUCs) so the true number would have been somewhat less.[7–10] By 2004 Georgiou and colleagues reported that the number of documented cases had risen to 61,[11] but no series have more than 10 cases.[12]

Site

From the very small number of validated cases, it is impossible to generalize about the site of origin except to say that lesions have occurred in the nasal cavity, ethmoid, maxillary and, in one case, sphenoid sinuses.[13–16] Specifically, they can arise on the nasal septum[17] but in many other cases no site of origin can be accurately determined.[2]

Diagnostic Features

Clinical

(See Table 15.12.)

In the larynx these rare tumors are generally much commoner in men, occurring in the fifth to sixth decades, whereas in the nose this male predilection is not so evident and the age range is wider (26 to 77 years, median 48 years). Nasal obstruction and epistaxis are the main symptoms and a smooth polypoid mass or area of granular thickening have been observed.[9,10] One of the largest cohorts was reported by Babin et al in 2006,[18] who considered 21 patients with neuroendocrine carcinoma presenting between 1989 and 2003 to several French hospitals. There were 12 men and 9 women, with a mean age of 55 years (range 27–79 years). The majority were T4 and three had bilateral neck nodes, the rest being N0. One patient had distant metastases at presentation. Our 7 cases comprised 5 men and 2 women, aged 32 to 70 years (mean 47.2 years). All presented with advanced disease affecting the skull base and including skin and bone metastases in 2 cases. Three presented with disease in the antroethmoid, 2 in the sphenoid, and 2 in the nasal cavity.

Some case reports describe presentation with inappropriate secretion of antidiuretic hormone associated with a neuroendocrine carcinoma in the sinonasal region.[19,20]

In keeping with the degrees of differentiation, cervical metastases are more common in atypical and small cell tumors, occurring in 22 to 30% at presentation with atypical tumors and 50% with small cell tumors.[21,22]

Table 15.12 Clinical and pathological features of neuroendocrine carcinomas of the upper aerodigestive tract

	Carcinoid tumor	Atypical carcinoid tumor	Small cell carcinoma	Poorly differentiated, large cell neuroendocrine carcinoma (including SNUC)
Age (y)	50–60	50–60	50–60	50–60
Sex	M > F	M > F	M > F	M > F
Site	Supraglottic larynx	Supraglottic larynx	Supraglottic larynx and other sites including sinonasal tract	All sites, especially sinonasal tract
Survival, 5 y	>90%	~50%	<10%	<10%[a]
Atypia	None	Mild to moderate	Marked	Marked
Mitoses	None	Few, scattered	Numerous	Numerous
Necrosis	None	None to little	Abundant	Abundant

Abbreviations: F, female; M, male; SNUC, sinonasal undifferentiated carcinoma; y, year(s)

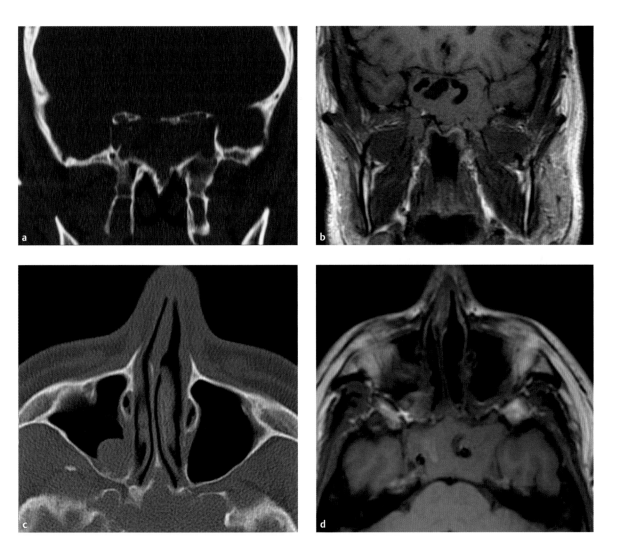

Fig. 15.15a–d Extensive neuroendocrine carcinoma filling the sphenoid region and encasing the carotid arteries.

a Coronal CT scan.
b Coronal MRI (T1W unenhanced).

c Axial CT scan.
d Axial MRI (T1W unenhanced).

Imaging

Apart from a markedly enhancing soft tissue mass, there are no specific features to distinguish these tumors. Flow voids are seen on MRI, indicating the vascularity of these lesions.[23] Small cell tumors show areas of necrosis (**Fig. 15.15**).

Histological Features and Differential Diagnosis

The histological appearances of these tumors are the same as elsewhere in the body, in particular in the lung, and their immunoreactivity to neuroendocrine markers helps distinguish SNECs from SNUCs.[15]

Well-differentiated neuroendocrine carcinomas are comprised of nests, ribbons, and trabeculae of small homogeneous epithelioid cells. Both the nuclei and cytoplasm of these cells may be granular. Mitoses and necrosis are rare.

Carcinoid tumors are usually immunoreactive to keratins, NSE (neuron specific enolase), chromogranin, synaptophysin, and specific endocrine antigens such as serotonin.[1]

In the larynx, the principal differentiation is from paragangliomas, which are also very rare but are not immunoreactive to cytokeratins and have a typical sustentacular pattern of staining with S100. In the sinonasal region, neuroendocrine carcinomas are often confused with olfactory neuroblastoma.

Atypical or moderately differentiated neuroendocrine carcinomas have similar microscopic appearances as their well-differentiated counterparts but with more nuclear and cellular pleomorphism. The nucleoli may be offset to the periphery of the cell. Their immunohistochemistry is also the same, although curiously ~ 75% react with antibodies to calcitonin[24] so they must be distinguished from medullary thyroid cancer by their lack of staining with thyroid transcription factor-1.

Amyloid may be seen in both well- and moderately differentiated tumors. The term "atypical" should be subject to caution as it belies an aggressive tumor with a rather poor prognosis.

Small cell carcinomas have a sheetlike growth pattern of cells with a high nuclear/cytoplasmic ratio and many mitoses and also show marked necrosis and vascular invasion. The immunoreactivity can be less specific, and even with a wide battery of agents there can be considerable overlap with SNUCs and olfactory neuroblastoma (**Table 15.1**).[3] The other differentials include basaloid squamous cell carcinoma and lymphoma.

Natural History

The behavior of these tumors is predicted by their histological differentiation. Increasing locoregional and systemic metastases are associated with moderate and poorly differentiated tumors.[25] Bone, lung, liver, and skin deposits have been reported.[8,10]

Treatment and Outcome

Surgery is the treatment of choice for well- and moderately differentiated tumors and some have advocated an elective neck dissection for moderately differentiated tumors occurring in the larynx. Their rarity in the nose and sinuses and paucity of lymphatic drainage make this strategy less relevant at this site, so neck dissection is confined to proven positive lymphadenopathy.

The choice of surgical approach, as ever, would be determined by the site and extent of the lesion, although it should be noted that these tumors can be quite vascular. Thus, anything from craniofacial to endoscopic resection has been described, through lateral rhinotomy and midfacial degloving.[23,26]

The outcome for the few cases of well-differentiated sinonasal carcinoid is reasonable if the tumor is completely excised, but no robust statistics are available. One of the largest series comprises 18 patients from the MD Anderson Cancer Center, 14 of whom had surgery and 12 chemotherapy resulting in 5-year survival of 64%.[27] Five-year local failure was 21.4%, regional failure was 13%, and distant metastases occurred in 14%. However, the situation with atypical/moderately differentiated neoplasms is worse, certainly in the larynx, where 5-year survival is <50%, with two-thirds dead by 10 years.

With small cell carcinoma the outlook is even worse, with <5% alive at 5 years irrespective of treatment. The MD Anderson series included 7 patients, all with advanced disease, 5 of whom were treated with chemoradiotherapy and with only one long-term survivor. Consequently, chemotherapy and radiation employing protocols developed for pulmonary disease have been advocated rather than radical surgery.[28]

Cisplatin and etoposide seem to be the drugs of choice for all neuroendocrine tumors, be it induction,[28] combined with radiotherapy,[29] or for small cell carcinoma.[30]

In a series of 21 patients with SNECs reported by Babin et al, 52% had surgery, 66% radiotherapy, and 57% chemotherapy (usually cisplatin and etoposide).[18] Forty-seven percent developed local recurrence, 23% had regional or systemic metastases, and 10 out of 21 (48%) died of disease within 4 years of diagnosis, with only one long-term survivor. Reviews by Their and Silva et al[2,18] of SNEC patients show that in addition to intracranial extent of tumor, the presence of ectopic hormone syndrome increased mortality, whereas, interestingly, intrinsic size of tumor and number of mitoses did not correlate with recurrence, metastases, or survival.

In our small group of 7 SNEC cases, all patients received chemoradiotherapy and 5 subsequently underwent radical surgery including craniofacial resection and removal of the eye (1 case). Unfortunately, we have no long-term survivors, with death occurring between 3 and 48 months after treatment.

References

1. Ferlito A, Barnes L, Rinaldo A, Gnepp DR, Milroy CM. A review of neuroendocrine neoplasms of the larynx: update on diagnosis and treatment. J Laryngol Otol 1998; 112(9):827–834

2. Silva EG, Butler JJ, Mackay B, Goepfert H. Neuroblastomas and neuroendocrine carcinomas of the nasal cavity: a proposed new classification. Cancer 1982;50(11):2388–2405

3. Mills SE. Neuroectodermal neoplasms of the head and neck with emphasis on neuroendocrine carcinomas. Mod Pathol 2002;15(3):264–278

4. Iezzoni JC, Mills SE. "Undifferentiated" small round cell tumors of the sinonasal tract: differential diagnosis update. Am J Clin Pathol 2005;124(Suppl):S110–S121

5. Goldman NC, Hood CI, Singleton GT. Carcinoid of the larynx. Arch Otolaryngol 1969;90(1):64–67

6. Perez-Ordonez B, Caruana SM, Huvos AG, Shah JP. Small cell neuroendocrine carcinoma of the nasal cavity and paranasal sinuses. Hum Pathol 1998;29(8):826–832

7. Raychowdhuri RN. Oat-cell carcinoma and paranasal sinuses. J Laryngol Otol 1965;79:253–255

8. Koss LG, Spiro RH, Hajdu S. Small cell (oat cell) carcinoma of minor salivary gland origin. Cancer 1972;30(3):737–741

9. Rejowski JE, Campanella RS, Block LJ. Small cell carcinoma of the nose and paranasal sinuses. Otolaryngol Head Neck Surg 1982;90(4):516–517

10. Weiss MD, deFries HO, Taxy JB, Braine H. Primary small cell carcinoma of the paranasal sinuses. Arch Otolaryngol 1983;109(5):341–343

11. Georgiou AF, Walker DM, Collins AP, Morgan GJ, Shannon JA, Veness MJ. Primary small cell undifferentiated (neuroendocrine) carcinoma of the maxillary sinus. Oral Surg Oral Med Oral Pathol Oral Radiol Endod 2004;98(5):572–578

12. Renner G. Small cell carcinoma of the head and neck: a review. Semin Oncol 2007;34(1):3–14

13. Soussi AC, Benghiat A, Holgate CS, Majumdar B. Neuroendocrine tumours of the head and neck. J Laryngol Otol 1990;104(6):504–507

14. Chaudhry MR, Akhtar S, Kim DS. Neuroendocrine carcinoma of the ethmoid sinus. Eur Arch Otorhinolaryngol 1994;251(8):461–463

15. Smith SR, Som P, Fahmy A, Lawson W, Sacks S, Brandwein M. A clinicopathological study of sinonasal neuroendocrine carcinoma and sinonasal undifferentiated carcinoma. Laryngoscope 2000;110(10 Pt 1):1617–1622

16. Westerveld GJ, van Diest PJ, van Nieuwkerk EB. Neuroendocrine carcinoma of the sphenoid sinus: a case report. Rhinology 2001;39(1):52–54

17. Galm T, Turner N. Primary carcinoid tumour of nasal septum. J Laryngol Otol 2009;123(7):789–792

18. Babin E, Rouleau V, Vedrine PO, et al. Small cell neuroendocrine carcinoma of the nasal cavity and paranasal sinuses. J Laryngol Otol 2006;120(4):289–297

19. Vasan NR, Medina JE, Canfield VA, Gillies EM. Sinonasal neuroendocrine carcinoma in association with SIADH. Head Neck 2004;26(1):89–93

20. Rossi P, Suissa J, Bagneres D, et al. [Syndrome of inappropriate antidiuretic hormone secretion disclosing a sinonasal neuroendocrine carcinoma: case report]. Rev Med Interne 2007;28(6):426–428

21. Wenig BM, Gnepp DR. The spectrum of neuroendocrine carcinomas of the larynx. Semin Diagn Pathol 1989; 6(4):329–350

22. Woodruff JM, Senie RT. Atypical carcinoid tumor of the larynx. A critical review of the literature. ORL J Otorhinolaryngol Relat Spec 1991;53(4):194–209

23. Furuta A, Kudo M, Kanai K, Ohki S, Suzaki H. Typical carcinoid tumor arising in the nose and paranasal sinuses—case report. Auris Nasus Larynx 2010;37(3):381–385

24. Woodruff JM, Huvos AG, Erlandson RA, Shah JP, Gerold FP. Neuroendocrine carcinomas of the larynx. A study of two types, one of which mimics thyroid medullary carcinoma. Am J Surg Pathol 1985;9(11):771–790

25. Lund V. Distant metastases from sinonasal cancer. ORL 2001;63:212–213

26. Lee DH, Cho HH, Cho YB. Typical carcinoid tumor of the nasal cavity. Auris Nasus Larynx 2007;34(4):537–539

27. Rosenthal DI, Barker JL Jr, El-Naggar AK, et al. Sinonasal malignancies with neuroendocrine differentiation: patterns of failure according to histologic phenotype. Cancer 2004;101(11):2567–2573

28. Rischin D, Coleman A. Sinonasal malignancies of neuroendocrine origin. Hematol Oncol Clin North Am 2008; 22(6):1297–1316, xi

29. Fitzek MM, Thornton AF, Varvares M, et al. Neuroendocrine tumors of the sinonasal tract. Results of a prospective study incorporating chemotherapy, surgery, and combined proton-photon radiotherapy. Cancer 2002; 94(10):2623–2634

30. González-García R, Fernández-Rodríguez T, Naval-Gías L, Rodríguez-Campo FJ, Nam-Cha SH, Díaz-González FJ. Small cell neuroendocrine carcinoma of the sinonasal region. A propose of a case. Br J Oral Maxillofac Surg 2007;45(8):676–678

Sinonasal Undifferentiated Carcinoma

Definition

(ICD-O code 8020/3)

Sinonasal undifferentiated carcinoma (SNUC) is a rare aggressive malignancy of the sinonasal region that is generally regarded as being of neuroendocrine origin.[1-4] The World Health Organization subsequently defined SNUC as a highly aggressive and clinicopathologically distinct carcinoma of uncertain histiogenesis.[5]

Etiology

Sinonasal undifferentiated carcinoma was originally described by Frierson in 1986, but its precise etiology is unknown.[6]

Synonyms

Anaplastic carcinoma.

Incidence

This tumor is increasingly diagnosed and was undoubtedly overlooked in the past. Between 1986 and 2009, 28 papers with 152 patients were published, so close to 200 cases have been reported since the condition was recognized in 1986, with numbers increasing every year.[7]

Site

The rapid growth of this tumor can make determination of the exact site of origin difficult as more than one area

Table 15.13 SNUCs: personal series

	n	Age		Sex	Surgery				Medical oncology	
		Range (y)	Mean (y)	M:F	CFR	MFD	LR	ESS	CRT	RT
Outcome	24	21–79	53	7:5	5	2	1	2	10	13
Follow-up										
A&W	8	6 mo–12 y								
AWR	3	6 mo–6 y								
DOD	7	5 mo–4 y								
Lost	5									

Abbreviations: A&W, alive and well; AWR, alive with recurrence; CFR, craniofacial resection; CRT, chemoradiotherapy; DOD, dead of disease; ESS, endoscopic sinus surgery; F, female; LR, lateral rhinotomy; M, male; MFD, midfacial degloving; mo, month(s); RT, radiotherapy; SNUC, sinonasal undifferentiated carcinoma; y, year(s).

of the nose and sinuses is usually involved, often with intracranial and orbital extension at presentation. Generally the nasal cavity, ethmoid, and maxilla are affected (Table 15.13).[6]

Diagnostic Features

Clinical Features

The mean age at diagnosis is the sixth decade[8] but a range of third to ninth decades is reported and the condition can occur at any age from childhood onward.[1,9]

In the literature SNUCs are reported to be slightly commoner in males (2:1 to 3:1).[1] In our cohort of 24 patients, there are 14 men and 10 women, and their ages at presentation ranged from 21 to 79 years (mean 53 years) (Table 15.13).

Patients usually present with advanced disease as the tumor is associated with rapid growth into adjacent structures such as the orbit and cranial cavity. Patients initially have the usual symptoms of nasal obstruction and epistaxis or serosanguinous discharge, followed by signs of orbital involvement such as proptosis, diplopia, epiphora, and ultimately chemosis and visual loss. Cranial nerve deficits may also occur though intracranial extension is often silent.

Up to one-third may present with cervical lymphadenopathy, although systemic metastases are less common initially.[2,10–13] Only 8% of our cohort (2/24) had cervical lymphadenopathy.

Imaging and Staging

CT and MRI appearances have been described by Philips et al in a series of 11 cases.[14] On CT a homogeneous opacification was evident with significant bone destruction and without calcification. MRI differentiated tumor from obstructed sinuses and presented generally an isodense mass on T1W images and a range of density on

T2 weighting, tending to the hyperdense. Use of contrast medium produced heterogeneous enhancement (Figs. 15.16 and 15.17).

The TNM, AJCC, and Kadish staging systems originally designed for olfactory neuroblastoma have been applied to SNUCs. The majority of reported cases fall into T4, Stage IV or Stage C, respectively,[7,10,15,16] as was the finding in our own cohort.

Screening of the neck by ultrasonography and imaging of the neck, thorax, and abdomen should be considered in this particular tumor due to the propensity for early spread, and PET-CT is increasingly used to stage disease.

Histological Features and Differential Diagnosis

Diagnosis is often one of exclusion as the tumor is undifferentiated by definition and falls into a large group of potential tumors (Table 15.14). SNUCs are composed of medium-sized cells that grow in nests, ribbons, sheets, and wide trabeculae, with many mitoses and apoptosis. There is a high nuclear-to-cytoplasmic ratio with prominent nucleoli. Necrosis and vascular invasion are prominent features and there is both mucosal surface growth and extension into surface mucosal glands.[7,17]

Table 15.14 Tumors that may be microscopically undifferentiated

- Sinonasal undifferentiated carcinoma
- Olfactory neuroblastoma
- Small cell neuroendocrine carcinoma
- Malignant melanoma
- Rhabdomyosarcoma
- Lymphomas, e.g., T/NK lymphoma
- Primitive neuroectodermal tumor
- Ewing's sarcoma
- Nasopharyngeal carcinoma
- NK—natural killer

Source: After reference 3.

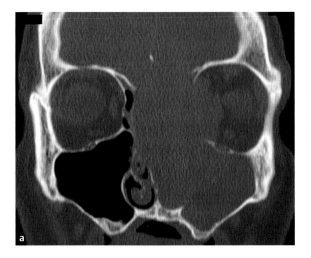

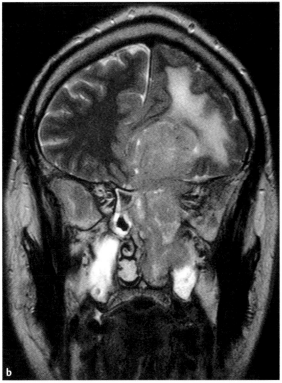

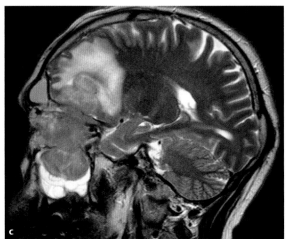

Fig. 15.16a–c

a Coronal CT showing extensive SNUC eroding and infiltrating into the orbit and anterior cranial fossa with complete opacification of the left nasal cavity, ethmoids, and maxillary sinus.

b Coronal MRI (T2W) in the same patient showing the degree of extension into the orbit and anterior cranial fossa with associated cerebral edema.

c Sagittal MRI (T2W) in the same patient.

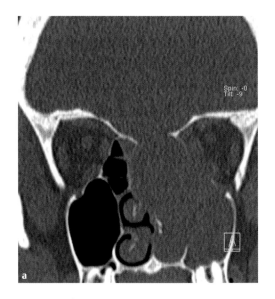

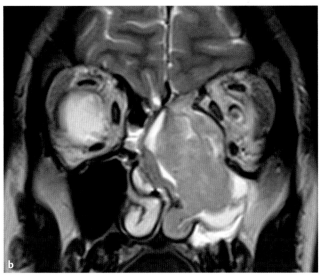

Fig. 15.17a, b

a Coronal CT showing less extensive SNUC occupying the left nasal cavity and maxillary and ethmoid sinuses.

b Coronal MRI (T2W) in the same patient showing tumor expanding but not infiltrating into adjacent structures.

Adjunctive analyses such as immunohistochemistry, molecular biology, and electron microscopy are usually required to confirm the diagnosis. Indeed, immunohistochemistry is regarded as mandatory to confirm the diagnosis (Table 15.1)[18] and specifically shows positivity to parakeratins, cytokeratin 7 and 8,[19] and neuroendocrine markers such as NSE and synaptophysin but not as intensely as olfactory neuroblastoma (which is negative to cytokeratin). It is for this reason that it is now classified with other neuroendocrine tumors. Epstein-Barr virus status and melanocytic and lymphoid antigens should not be present to differentiate the tumor from NPC, melanoma, and lymphomas.[1,9,20] The other important differentiation is from basaloid squamous carcinoma and adenoid cystic carcinoma (solid variant). In our entire cohort of nearly 1,000 malignant sinonasal tumors, apart from the 24 proven SNUCs, there is an additional group of 20 patients who, prior to the immunohistochemistry available from the early 1980s, were diagnosed as having anaplastic forms. It is quite possible that these were also SNUCs but we have excluded them from this discussion and they demonstrate the difficulties of estimating accurate incidence.

It has also been suggested recently that some SNUCs may be part of an unusual group of aggressive midline carcinomas characterized by genetic translocations that involve the gene nuclear protein in testis (*NUT*), a novel gene on chromosome 15.[21] These tumors often involve the upper aerodigestive tract in younger people and appear undifferentiated, although may have some focal squamous differentiation. This may explain some of the debate whether SNUCs are of epidermoid or neuroendocrine origin.

Natural History

In addition to the usually large tumor mass at presentation, cervical lymphadenopathy is reported at between 10% and 30%.[2,10–13,22] While distant metastases are uncommon at diagnosis, subsequent spread can occur and the cerebrospinal fluid may be seeded, leading to "drop metastases."[23] Time to metastasis ranges from 2 to 30 months.[24]

Treatment and Outcome

All permutations of surgery, radiotherapy, and chemotherapy have been used for this aggressive tumor. However, two broad strategies have been adopted. If the tumor is resectable, a craniofacial resection followed by radiotherapy has been employed with some success[16,25,26] and has been our approach in the past 20 years. Endoscopic excision has also been described, either alone or combined with craniotomy plus chemoradiotherapy[27] in a small number of patients[7] with at least comparable results. Overall and disease-free survival of 57% with a

mean follow-up of 32.3 months was reported. This would be in keeping with our own experience but our numbers are too small to undergo robust statistical analysis. However, the majority of patients who present with advanced disease are now managed by chemoradiotherapy after biopsy, usually using cisplatin-based regimes, with surgery reserved for residual or recurrent disease.[12,16] It could be argued that this is one tumor for which endoscopic debulking as opposed to oncological resection is an acceptable approach.

A case can also be made for irradiation of the N0 neck.[26] Intensity-modulated radiotherapy and/or proton beam therapy may offer some benefit in the future but this is essentially speculative. High-dose chemotherapy combined with autologous marrow transplantation has also been advocated but lack of numbers precludes comment.[28]

In a meta-analysis of the literature up to 2009, results are often compromised by relatively short follow-up which has ranged from 1 to 195 months (mean 23.2 months, median 14 months).[29] However, overall the tumor has a poor prognosis with 5-year disease-free survival less than 25% despite dramatic initial responses. Twenty-two percent were reported as alive with disease and 52.6% dead of disease. Lin et al[13] reviewed 19 patients treated over 13 years in a single institution who at 2 years had local and regional control rates of 83% and regional control of 50%. However, at 5 years, overall survival was 22%. Indeed, one study suggested a median survival of 4 months, others less than a year.[1,22] Death occurs from extensive local disease and distant metastases to liver, bone, brain, and elsewhere. However, in our own series there are several long-term survivors (Table 15.13) and Rosenthal and colleagues, who reviewed 72 individuals with neuroendocrine tumors of which 16 were SNUCs, suggested that survival may be improving, either due to better histological differentiation from small cell carcinoma or/and the addition of chemotherapy.[15] The difficulty remains that with small numbers treated with a range of therapeutic options it has been difficult to prove that one strategy was superior to another. However, the meta-analysis by Reiersen in 2009[29] comparing similarly staged disease (irrespective of the system of staging) demonstrated that the best patient survival was obtained with combined surgery, radiotherapy, and chemotherapy.

References

1. Jeng YM, Sung MT, Fang CL, et al. Sinonasal undifferentiated carcinoma and nasopharyngeal-type undifferentiated carcinoma: two clinically, biologically, and histopathologically distinct entities. Am J Surg Pathol 2002; 26(3):371–376
2. Musy PY, Reibel JF, Levine PA. Sinonasal undifferentiated carcinoma: the search for a better outcome. Laryngoscope 2002;112(8 Pt 1):1450–1455

3. Ejaz A, Wenig BM. Sinonasal undifferentiated carcinoma: clinical and pathologic features and a discussion on classification, cellular differentiation, and differential diagnosis. Adv Anat Pathol 2005;12(3):134–143
4. Enepekides DJ. Sinonasal undifferentiated carcinoma: an update. Curr Opin Otolaryngol Head Neck Surg 2005; 13(4):222–225
5. Iezzoni J, Mills S. 'Undifferentiated' small round cell tumors of the sinonasal tract. Differential diagnosis update. Am J Clin Path 2005;124:S110–121
6. Frierson HF Jr, Mills SE, Fechner RE, Taxy JB, Levine PA. Sinonasal undifferentiated carcinoma. An aggressive neoplasm derived from schneiderian epithelium and distinct from olfactory neuroblastoma. Am J Surg Pathol 1986;10(11):771–779
7. Schmidt ER, Berry RL. Diagnosis and treatment of sinonasal undifferentiated carcinoma: report of a case and review of the literature. J Oral Maxillofac Surg 2008; 66(7):1505–1510
8. Frierson HF Jr, Bellafiore FJ, Gaffey MJ, McCary WS, Innes DJ Jr, Williams ME. Cytokeratin in anaplastic large cell lymphoma. Mod Pathol 1994;7(3):317–321
9. Cerilli LA, Holst VA, Brandwein MS, Stoler MH, Mills SE. Sinonasal undifferentiated carcinoma: immunohistochemical profile and lack of EBV association. Am J Surg Pathol 2001;25(2):156–163
10. Miyamoto RC, Gleich LL, Biddinger PW, Gluckman JL. Esthesioneuroblastoma and sinonasal undifferentiated carcinoma: impact of histological grading and clinical staging on survival and prognosis. Laryngoscope 2000;110(8):1262–1265
11. Smith SR, Som P, Fahmy A, Lawson W, Sacks S, Brandwein M. A clinicopathological study of sinonasal neuroendocrine carcinoma and sinonasal undifferentiated carcinoma. Laryngoscope 2000;110(10 Pt 1):1617–1622
12. Rischin D, Porceddu S, Peters L, Martin J, Corry J, Weih L. Promising results with chemoradiation in patients with sinonasal undifferentiated carcinoma. Head Neck 2004;26(5):435–441
13. Lin EM, Sparano A, Spalding A, et al. Sinonasal undifferentiated carcinoma: a 13-year experience at a single institution. Skull Base 2010;20(2):61–67
14. Phillips CD, Futterer SF, Lipper MH, Levine PA. Sinonasal undifferentiated carcinoma: CT and MR imaging of an uncommon neoplasm of the nasal cavity. Radiology 1997; 202(2):477–480
15. Rosenthal DI, Barker JL Jr, El-Naggar AK, et al. Sinonasal malignancies with neuroendocrine differentiation: patterns of failure according to histologic phenotype. Cancer 2004;101(11):2567–2573
16. Mendenhall WM, Mendenhall CM, Riggs CE Jr, Villaret DB, Mendenhall NP. Sinonasal undifferentiated carcinoma. Am J Clin Oncol 2006;29(1):27–31
17. Bellizzi AM, Bourne TD, Mills SE, Stelow EB. The cytologic features of sinonasal undifferentiated carcinoma and olfactory neuroblastoma. Am J Clin Pathol 2008;129(3):367–376
18. Stelow E, Mills SE. Biopsy Interpretation of the Upper Aerodigestive Tract and Ear. Philadelphia: Wolters Kluwer/ Lippincott Williams and Wilkins; 2008:150
19. Iezzoni JC, Mills SE. "Undifferentiated" small round cell tumors of the sinonasal tract: differential diagnosis update. Am J Clin Pathol 2005;124(Suppl):S110–S121
20. Lopategui JR, Gaffey MJ, Frierson HF Jr, et al. Detection of Epstein-Barr viral RNA in sinonasal undifferentiated carcinoma from Western and Asian patients. Am J Surg Pathol 1994;18(4):391–398
21. Stelow EB, Bellizzi AM, Taneja K, et al. NUT rearrangement in undifferentiated carcinomas of the upper aerodigestive tract. Am J Surg Pathol 2008;32(6):828–834
22. Righi PD, Francis F, Aron BS, Weitzner S, Wilson KM, Gluckman J. Sinonasal undifferentiated carcinoma: a 10-year experience. Am J Otolaryngol 1996;17(3):167–171
23. Ghosh S, Weiss M, Streeter O, Sinha U, Commins D, Chen TC. Drop metastasis from sinonasal undifferentiated carcinoma: clinical implications. Spine 2001;26(13):1486–1491
24. Kim BS, Vongtama R, Juillard G. Sinonasal undifferentiated carcinoma: case series and literature review. Am J Otolaryngol 2004;25(3):162–166
25. Howard DJ, Lund VJ, Wei WI. Craniofacial resection for tumors of the nasal cavity and paranasal sinuses: a 25-year experience. Head Neck 2006;28(10):867–873
26. Tanzler ED, Morris CG, Orlando CA, Werning JW, Mendenhall WM. Management of sinonasal undifferentiated carcinoma. Head Neck 2008;30(5):595–599
27. Revenaugh PC, Seth R, Pavlovich JB, Knott PD, Batra PS. Minimally invasive endoscopic resection of sinonasal undifferentiated carcinoma. Am J Otolaryngol 2011;32(6):464–469
28. Stewart FM, Lazarus HM, Levine PA, Stewart KA, Tabbara IA, Spaulding CA. High-dose chemotherapy and autologous marrow transplantation for esthesioneuroblastoma and sinonasal undifferentiated carcinoma. Am J Clin Oncol 1989;12(3):217–221
29. Reiersen D. Sinonasal undifferentiated carcinoma. A 24 year meta-analysis. Otolaryngol Head Neck Surg 2010;143(2 Suppl):P202

Primitive Peripheral Neuroectodermal Tumor and Extraosseous Ewing's Sarcoma

Definition

(ICD-O codes 9364/3 PNET; 9260/3 Ewing's sarcoma)

A primitive neuroectodermal round cell tumor with variable evidence of neural differentiation, genetically characterized with a translocation t(11;22)(q24;q12).

Synonyms

Ewing's sarcoma (ES) and peripheral or primitive neuroectodermal tumor (pPNET) are now known to represent a single entity over a spectrum. ES represents the undifferentiated most primitive end of the spectrum and PNET the more neurally defined opposite end. It was described by James Ewing in 1921[1] in the ulna of a 14-year-old girl; she initially responded to radiotherapy but died a year later due to metastases. Hart and Earle introduced the term "PNET" in 1973.[2] The additional terms of peripheral neuroepithelioma and peripheral neuroblastoma have also been used.

Incidence

A rare family of tumors only occasionally reported in the head and neck, these account for 4% of childhood and adolescent malignancies and are slightly more common in males.[3]

Site

These tumors can occur anywhere in the body; in children ~20% of ES/PNET affect the head and neck. Of 130 cases of Ewing's sarcoma reported by Raney et al, 23 occurred in the head and neck.[3] Approximately 20% of head and neck cases occur in the sinonasal tract, usually in the nasal cavity and maxillary sinus. Nothwithstanding this, ~20 cases of pPNETs in the maxilla have been reported up to 2010.[4-6]

Diagnostic Features

Clinical

ES/PNETs may develop at any age but tend to occur in the first three decades of life, which has been our experience.[7] The peak incidence is said to be 18 years[8] with a slight male preponderance. Although expressing evidence of neural differentiation, most tumors are anatomically not associated with neurologic structures. We have treated 3 patients with ES (2 male of 14 and 38 years, and 1 female of 8 years) and 3 patients with PNETs (2 male of 40 and 58 years, 1 female of 17 years). The Ewing's sarcoma occurred in the chest and spread to the frontoethmoid region, and in the maxilla (2 cases), whereas the PNETs affected the ethmoid sinuses in all three cases.

Symptoms are nonspecific though rapid (mean 3.6 months)[9] and relate to the mass or metastatic spread, in particular to the bone and lungs. The tumor may present as a polypoid mass when arising in the nasal cavity, or as a soft tissue mass deforming the nasal dorsum.[10,11]

Imaging

There are no specific features other than a soft tissue destructive mass with evidence of bone and soft tissue infiltration.

A staging protocol imaging the neck, thorax, and abdomen and a skeletal survey should be undertaken.

Histological Features and Differential Diagnosis

Macroscopically the tumors are circumscribed but not encapsulated. Histologically these tumors are composed of small blue cells in common with several other tumors from which they must be distinguished[12] such as embryonal rhabdomyosarcoma, olfactory neuroblastoma, and lymphomas. Cells are arranged in sheets and nests with intervening fibrous bands. Homer Wright–like rosettes with centrally located fibrillary material have been described. The cells have a high nuclear-to-cytoplasmic ratio and mitoses are frequent.

Consequently there is considerable reliance on immunoreactivity (**Tables 15.1 and 15.15**) and if possible, cytogenetic analysis, which characteristically reveals

Table 15.15 Histological hallmarks of EW/PNETs

- Small blue tumors
- Immunostaining with 2 or more neural markers
- Ultrastructure
- Evidence of abnormal t(11,22)(q24;q12) translocation

t(11;22)(q24;q12).[13] Immunohistochemistry shows reactivity with antibodies to synaptophysin, NSE, S100, and CD99. Antibodies to FLl1 may also prove helpful as PNETs express this antigen secondarily to their classic translocation that unites the Ewing's sarcoma gene on chromosome 22 with the FLl1 gene on chromosome 11.[14]

Virtually all neuroblastomas are nonreactive for vimentin, while MIC-2 is expressed in 90% of PNET/extraosseous Ewing's sarcoma (EOE) compared with 0% of neuroblastomas.[15]

Natural History

These tumors are locally aggressive and can spread at an early stage. Pulmonary metastases are estimated to occur in 15 to 30% of cases within 6 months of diagnosis and are a common cause of death. Even when patients survive, they may go on to develop a second sarcoma. This occurred in 6.5% of those with Ewing's sarcoma who received >60 Gy.[16]

Treatment and Outcome

Originally outcome was extremely poor with most individuals dead within 2 years, but this situation has improved considerably with triple therapy[17,18]—that is, radical surgical excision combined with chemoradiotherapy. However, bearing in mind that there is a spectrum of disease, overall 5-year survival for PNET was 30% compared with 70% for extraosseous Ewing's sarcoma, which seems to do better in the sinonasal tract than elsewhere.[4,19-21] Surgery has ranged from craniofacial resection (in our own series[22]) to endoscopic resection[23,24] but its role has more recently become secondary to chemoradiotherapy, reserved for residual disease.[25]

There is no standard protocol to treat these tumors but most have favored multiagent chemotherapy including vincristine, cyclophosphamide, doxorubicin alternating with ifosfamide, and etoposide.[3] All our patients underwent radical chemoradiotherapy and two of the PNETs had craniofacial resections in addition. Unfortunately, we have only one long-term survivor, the patient with secondary disease from the chest to the frontoethmoidal region, who is still alive 7 years later.

Those tumors demonstrating EWS/FLI1 gene fusion appear to have an improved prognosis independent of tumor site, size, or stage.[26]

References

1. Ewing J. Diffuse endothelioma of the bone. Proc New York Path Soc 1921;21:17–24

2. Hart MN, Earle KM. Primitive neuroectodermal tumors of the brain in children. Cancer 1973;32(4):890–897

3. Raney RB, Asmar L, Newton WA Jr, et al. Ewing's sarcoma of soft tissues in childhood: a report from the Intergroup Rhabdomyosarcoma Study, 1972 to 1991. J Clin Oncol 1997;15(2):574–582

4. Hafezi S, Seethala RR, Stelow EB, et al. Ewing's family of tumors of the sinonasal tract and maxillary bone. Head Neck Pathol 2011;5:8–16

5. Mohindra P, Zade B, Basu A, et al. Primary PNET of maxilla: an unusual presentation. J Pediatr Hematol Oncol 2008;30(6):474–477

6. Hormozi AK, Ghazisaidi MR, Hosseini SN. Unusual presentation of peripheral primitive neuroectodermal tumor of the maxilla. J Craniofac Surg 2010;21(6):1761–1763

7. Howard DJ, Lund VJ. Primary Ewing's sarcoma of the ethmoid bone. J Laryngol Otol 1985;99(10):1019–1023

8. Dehner LP. Primitive neuroectodermal tumor and Ewing's sarcoma. Am J Surg Pathol 1993;17(1):1–13

9. Windfuhr JP. Primitive neuroectodermal tumor of the head and neck: incidence, diagnosis, and management. Ann Otol Rhinol Laryngol 2004;113(7):533–543

10. Pontius KI, Sebek BA. Extraskeletal Ewing's sarcoma arising in the nasal fossa. Light- and electron-microscopic observations. Am J Clin Pathol 1981;75(3):410–415

11. Howard DJ, Daniels HA. Ewing's sarcoma of the nose. Ear Nose Throat J 1993;72(4):277–279

12. Folpe AL, Goldblum JR, Rubin BP, et al. Morphologic and immunophenotypic diversity in Ewing family tumors: a study of 66 genetically confirmed cases. Am J Surg Pathol 2005;29(8):1025–1033

13. Turc-Carel C, Aurias A, Mugneret F, et al. Chromosomes in Ewing's sarcoma. I. An evaluation of 85 cases of remarkable consistency of t(11;22)(q24;q12). Cancer Genet Cytogenet 1988;32(2):229–238

14. Folpe AL, Hill CE, Parham DM, O'Shea PA, Weiss SW. Immunohistochemical detection of FLI-1 protein expression: a study of 132 round cell tumors with emphasis on CD99-positive mimics of Ewing's sarcoma/primitive neuroectodermal tumor. Am J Surg Pathol 2000;24(12):1657–1662

15. Weidner N, Tjoe J. Immunohistochemical profile of monoclonal antibody O13: antibody that recognizes glycoprotein p30/32MIC2 and is useful in diagnosing Ewing's sarcoma and peripheral neuroepithelioma. Am J Surg Pathol 1994;18(5):486–494

16. Kuttesch JF Jr, Wexler LH, Marcus RB, et al. Second malignancies after Ewing's sarcoma: radiation dose-dependency of secondary sarcomas. J Clin Oncol 1996;14(10):2818–2825

17. Ahmad R, Mayol BR, Davis M, Rougraff BT. Extraskeletal Ewing's sarcoma. Cancer 1999;85(3):725–731

18. Ludwig JA. Ewing sarcoma: historical perspectives, current state-of-the-art, and opportunities for targeted therapy in the future. Curr Opin Oncol 2008;20(4):412–418

19. Shimada H, Newton WA Jr, Soule EH, Qualman SJ, Aoyama C, Maurer HM. Pathologic features of extraosseous Ewing's sarcoma: a report from the Intergroup Rhabdomyosarcoma Study. Hum Pathol 1988;19(4):442–453

20. Marina NM, Etcubanas E, Parham DM, Bowman LC, Green A. Peripheral primitive neuroectodermal tumor (peripheral neuroepithelioma) in children. A review of the St. Jude experience and controversies in diagnosis and management. Cancer 1989;64(9):1952–1960

21. Schmidt D, Herrmann C, Jürgens H, Harms D. Malignant peripheral neuroectodermal tumor and its necessary distinction from Ewing's sarcoma. A report from the Kiel Pediatric Tumor Registry. Cancer 1991;68(10):2251–2259

22. Howard DJ, Lund VJ, Wei WI. Craniofacial resection for tumors of the nasal cavity and paranasal sinuses: a 25-year experience. Head Neck 2006;28(10):867–873

23. Iseri M, Ozturk M, Filinte D, Corapcioglu F. A peripheral primitive neuroectodermal tumour arising from the middle turbinate and transnasal endoscopic approach for its surgical treatment. Int J Pediatr Otorhinolaryngol 2007;2:180–184

24. Hayes SM, Jani TN, Rahman SM, Jogai S, Harries PG, Salib RJ. Solitary extra-skeletal sinonasal metastasis from a primary skeletal Ewing's sarcoma. J Laryngol Otol 2011;125(8):861–864

25. Gradoni P, Giordano D, Oretti G, Fantoni M, Ferri T. The role of surgery in children with head and neck rhabdomyosarcoma and Ewing's sarcoma. Surg Oncol 2010;19(4):e103–e109

26. de Alava E, Kawai A, Healey JH, et al. EWS-FLI1 fusion transcript structure is an independent determinant of prognosis in Ewing's sarcoma. J Clin Oncol 1998;16(4):1248–1255

Olfactory Neuroblastoma

Definition

(ICD-O 9522/3)

Olfactory neuroblastoma is a malignant neuroendocrine neoplasm that generally arises from the olfactory mucosa.

Synonyms

After it was first described by Berger and colleagues in 1924, the name "esthesioblastoma" was frequently used.[1] However, a wide range of other terms have been used including esthesioneurocytoma, esthesioneuroma, intranasal neuroblastoma, and olfactory neuroepithelial tumor; in the English literature it is most commonly referred to as "olfactory neuroblastoma" (ONB) in recognition of its likely origin.

Incidence

While ONB is relatively rare, as with all tumors of the anterior skull base, it is now recognized as one of the more common histologies encountered. In 1966, Skolnik et al[2] found only 97 cases reported in 42 papers in the English literature with most authors only treating two or three cases, and by 1989 O'Connor estimated that fewer than 300 cases had been published, which represented 1 to 5% of all malignant tumors of the nasal cavity.[3] However, this number had risen to 945 by 1997,[4] in a report which did not include a large series from the Armed Forces Institute of Pathology[5] nor one from the Institut Gustave-Roussy.[6] In 2000, the National Cancer Database included 664 cases from over 500 US hospitals over a 10-year period (1985 to 1995). In recent years increasing numbers of this tumor are being described, almost certainly due to increasing awareness and improved histological techniques for diagnosis. Working in a tertiary referral center, we have had the opportunity of managing 80 cases since 1970 (Table 15.16).

Etiology and Epidemiology

Hitherto, unlike some other sinonasal tumors, occupational factors in the development of olfactory neuroblastoma have not been identified in humans apart from the occasional anecdotal case,[7] whereas in rodents the administration of N-nitroso compounds has been reported to produce esthesioneuroepitheliomas[8-10] when administered parenterally, orally, or topically. Bischloromethyl ether has been shown to have a similar effect.[11] In a recent series of 54 patients with olfactory neuroblastoma, questionnaires and/or structured interviews were administered to evaluate possible etiological factors. This revealed 4 individuals (8%) who were dental practitioners[2] or dental nurses,[2] whereas only one other member of the dental profession (a case of adenocarcinoma) has previously been found in a cohort of over 700 other sinonasal malignancies. Further enquiry has not determined which chemical, if any, could be associated with this, but is worthy of continued observation.

Site

Olfactory neuroblastoma generally arises in the upper nasal cavity, corresponding to the anatomical distribution of the olfactory epithelium that extends from the olfactory niche onto the upper nasal septum and superior turbinates on the lateral wall. The presence of neurofilaments supports the proposition that olfactory neuroblastoma arises from the neural crest, but evidence for its origin from specialized olfactory epithelium is somewhat circumstantial[4,5] and tumors that occasionally arise outside this distribution have been ascribed to ectopic olfactory epithelium.

The olfactory stem cell or basal reserve cell is thought to be the precise cell of origin, but possible sources include the vomeronasal organ, sphenopalatine ganglion, ectodermal olfactory placode, autonomic ganglia in the nasal mucosa as well as the olfactory epithelium. Tumors arising in the cribriform niche can easily spread superiorly along olfactory fibers into the anterior cranial fossa to affect the olfactory bulb and tracts.[12] The superior septum is often involved and from there the tumor may spread to the contralateral side and into the ethmoids and adjacent orbit.

As tumors sometimes recur intracranially many years later with distant dural deposits, it must be presumed that microscopic embolic spread can occur early but remains inactive until some time later.

Diagnostic Features

Clinical Features

In the literature there appears to be a slight male preponderance and the tumor can occur over a wide age range

Table 15.16 Olfactory neuroblastoma: personal series 1976–2010

	n	Age		M:F	CFR	ESS	MFD	LR	No surgery
		Range (y)	Mean (y)						
	80	12–88	48	45:35	47	26	3	2	2
Radiotherapy	58				28	25	2	1	2
Chemotherapy	23				9	14	–	–	–
Local recurrence					11 (23%)	2 (7.6%)	1 (33%)	1 (50%)	2 (100%)
Survival									
5 y					75%	89%			
10 y					52%				
15 y					40%				
Staging[a]									
T1					2	4			
T2					11	16			
T3					24	6			
T4					10	0			

Abbreviations: CFR, craniofacial resection; ESS, endoscopic sinus surgery; F, female; LR, lateral rhinotomy; M, male; MFD, midfacial degloving; y, year(s).
[a] Staging according to Dulgerov.[13]

(3–90 years) and some authors have reported a bimodal peak in the second/third decades and sixth/seventh decades.[3,13-17] No racial predilection has been reported. In our own series of 80 cases, the gender ratio is 1.3:1 male to female and the age range is 12 to 88 years (mean 48 years). No bimodal distribution was observed, the majority of cases presenting between 40 and 69 years (**Table 15.16**).

Unilateral nasal obstruction, serosanguinous discharge, or frank epistaxis and reduced smell accompany the tumor but may be quite insidious and as a consequence there is often considerable delay in diagnosis, with some patients waiting for more than a year (24% of 40 cases reported by Schwabb et al[6]). In a series of 42 of our own patients, unilateral obstruction occurred in 93%, epistaxis in 55%, and rhinorrhea in 30%.[16] On endoscopic examination the tumor is usually a purplish red and bleeds easily (**Fig. 15.18**). Although characteristically early invasion of the anterior cranial fossa occurs, it is generally silent. Patients may experience epiphora, displacement of the eye, diplopia, and eventually visual loss as the tumor spreads laterally. Ocular symptoms occurred in 11% of our patients.[16] Surprisingly, in this series the left side was more often affected (62%) than the right (29%), with both sides affected at presentation in 9%.

Occasionally the tumor spreads into the nasopharynx and basisphenoid and en route may produce eustachian dysfunction.

As there are few large series in the literature, the true incidence of cervical metastases is difficult to estimate accurately.[15] A retrospective review[18] suggested an incidence of 27% based on 10 series that included 207 cases. In our original series,[19] only one case out of 20 developed

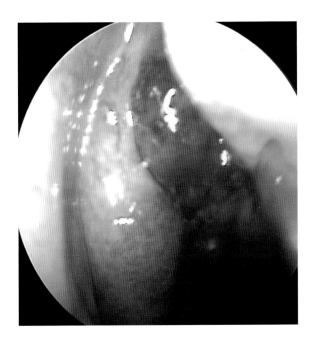

Fig. 15.18 Endoscopic view of ONB in the upper left nasal cavity.

neck disease, in contrast to the experience of Morita et al[20] who reported 20.4% (10/49) in a series from the Mayo Clinic. In a recent review of 320 cases in 15 series, Rinaldo et al[15] reported a lymph node metastatic frequency of 23.4% (range 5–100%), although only 8 studies validated the diagnosis of ONB with immunohistochemistry.

Distant metastases can occur with and without locoregional disease and may be widespread, including skin and eye as well as lungs, liver, bone, and other parts of the central nervous system.

As ONB is a neuroendocrine tumor, it can be associated with syndromes caused by inappropriate hormone production such as Cushing's syndrome or antidiuretic (ADH) secretion.[6,21-24]

Imaging

All patients should undergo a sinonasal tumor preoperative imaging protocol that combines high-resolution contrast-enhanced CT (coronal and axial planes) with three-plane MRI enhanced with gadolinium DTPA,[25-27] including the neck. There are no pathognomonic features of ONB but the position of a mass in the olfactory cleft at the top of the nasal cavity ± extension into the anterior cranial fossa is highly suspicious. Coronal CT remains the most accurate method of demonstrating early anterior skull base erosion, while contrast enhancement and MRI show extent of intracranial and orbital spread (**Figs. 15.19a, b, 15.20a, b**). The vascular nature of the tumor produces hyperdensity on precontrast T2W spin echo sequences and strong enhancement with gadolinium on T1W sequences.[28] Enhancement may be homogeneous or heterogeneous on both CT and MRI. Peripheral areas of cystic degeneration, though not particularly common, when present are highly suspicious of ONB (**Fig. 15.21**).[29] Areas of calcification may also be observed, but less than with chondrosarcoma. However, even the most modern imaging still cannot demonstrate unequivocal involvement of the dura and orbital periosteum, which can only be determined by surgery with histological confirmation.

After treatment all patients should be followed regularly for life using MRI (combined with formal examination and biopsy when indicated under general anesthesia), every 3 to 4 months for the first 2 years and then 6-monthly thereafter, in addition to regular endoscopy as an outpatient (**Figs. 15.19c, 15.20c**).[30,31] PET/CT may have value in the future for follow-up[32] and increased uptake by technetium Tc 99m ethylcysteinate dimer (^{99m}Tc-EDC) has been used to demonstrate tumors of neural crest origin.[33]

Ultrasound of the neck combined with fine needle aspiration cytology is an important screening technique with a high degree of accuracy[34] and is routinely employed as part of our initial work-up. Retropharyngeal metastases have also been reported in addition to the more usual cervical sites.[35] Although metastatic spread can occur outside the head and neck, it is rare at presentation and

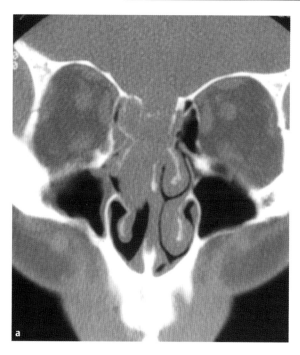

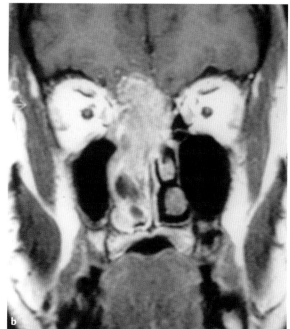

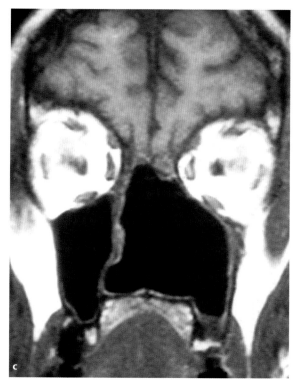

Fig. 15.19a–c

a Coronal CT showing ONB in the upper right nasal cavity with suggestion of skull base erosion.

b Coronal MRI (T1W post gadolinium enhancement) in the same patient showing obvious intracranial extension of ONB into the anterior cranial fossa.

c Coronal MRI (T1W unenhanced) following craniofacial resection and radiotherapy at 5 years in the same patient.

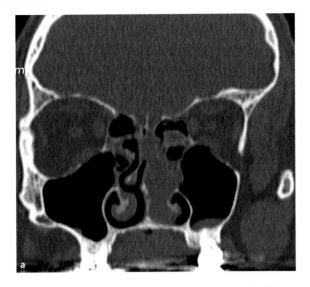

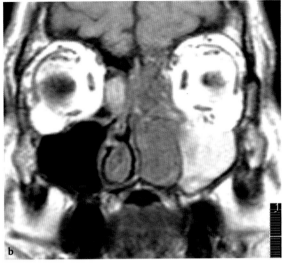

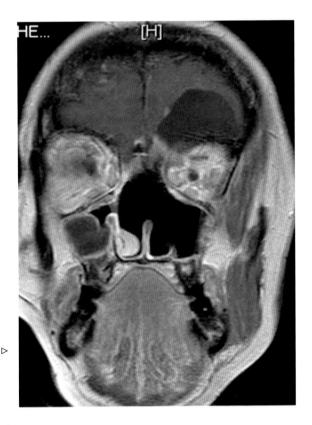

Fig. 15.20a–c

a Coronal CT showing a mass of ONB filling the left nasal cavity without obvious erosion of the skull base.

b Coronal MRI (T1W unenhanced) in the same patient showing tumor confined to the nasal cavity.

c Coronal MRI (T1W unenhanced) showing follow-up appearances at 1 year after endoscopic resection and postoperative radiotherapy.

Fig. 15.21 Coronal MRI (T1W post gadolinium enhancement) showing a cystic lesion in the anterior cranial fossa in a patient following craniofacial resection of extensive ONB together with high signal from the buccal lymph node, 6 years after initial surgery and radiotherapy. ▷

therefore it is not the authors' practice to undertake more extensive body imaging at this stage. Collection of urine for estimation of vanillylmandelic acid, a breakdown product of norepinephrine is no longer used as a marker of disease.

Histological Features and Differential Diagnosis

Macroscopically, the tumor is characteristically a polypoid reddish gray mass that bleeds readily. Microscopically, the tumor often grows in nests or classically in rosettes around eosinophilic fibrillary material, but the appearances are variable. The rosettes have been further divided into "true rosettes" and "pseudorosettes."

It was originally thought that ONB was part of the Ewing group of tumors but the typical t(11;22) found on cytogenetic analysis and associated with these tumors has not been demonstrated in ONB.[36,37] Other genetic markers have been suggested to distinguish ONB from other poorly differentiated tumors[38] and cytogenetic characterization continues to be an area of interest[39,40] that could assist diagnosis. This has also included examination of *p53* which in a small study on 18 cases did not seem to be relevant to initial development of ONB but might be important in a more aggressive subset.[41]

ONB falls into that group of small cell tumors that can pose diagnostic difficulties to the general pathologist, which prompted Ogura and Schenck to describe ONB as the "great imposter" (**Table 15.17**).[42] As a consequence, immunohistochemistry using a broad panel of antibodies is usually used to confirm the diagnosis, including general neuroendocrine markers such as neuron-specific enolase (NSE), synaptophysin, chromogranin, and protein gene product 9.5 (PGP-9.5), which are usually positive.[43,44] S100 positivity can be demonstrated at the periphery of the tumor nests and some tumors are also positive using MNF 116 and CAM 5.2, both stains for certain cytokeratins. Conversely, LP 34 (a high–molecular weight cytokeratin stain), EMA, carcinoembryonic antigen (CEA), and glial fibrillary acidic protein (GFAP) are generally negative (**Table 15.1**).

Various grading systems have been proposed based on the histological features (for example, Hyams from grade 1 [most differentiated] to grade 4 [undifferentiated]) but these have been largely superseded by immunohistochemistry.[5,43]

Staging

Several staging systems have been proposed, of which that of Kadish et al[45] has been most used, crudely dividing the tumors into three stages:

- Stage A: lesions confined to the nasal cavity
- Stage B: involvement of nasal cavity + one or more of the paranasal sinuses
- Stage C: involvement beyond the nasal cavity including the orbit, skull base, intracranial cavity, cervical lymph nodes, or systemic metastases

A modified Kadish system that proposes a stage D for metastases has been adopted by some authors (**Table 15.18**).[20,24]

Using the TNM classification, Dulguerov, Allal and Calcaterra[13] proposed a further staging system (**Table 15.19**).

Natural History

ONB arises from the olfactory epithelium in many cases and thus lies in immediate proximity to the cribriform plate and anterior cranial fossa. Histological studies based on early craniofacial specimens showed microscopic spread into the olfactory bulbs and tracts even

Table 15.17 Differential diagnoses for olfactory neuroblastoma

- Adenoid cystic carcinoma
- Small cell (high-grade neuroendocrine) carcinoma
- Sinonasal undifferentiated carcinoma
- Peripheral neuroectodermal tumor (PNET)/Ewing's sarcoma
- Lymphoma (diffuse large B cell)
- Basaloid squamous cell carcinoma
- Malignant melanoma

Table 15.18 Olfactory neuroblastoma: staging according to Kadish et al[45] and modified by Morita et al[20]

Type	Extension
A	Tumor limited to the nasal cavity
B	Tumor involving the nasal and paranasal sinuses
C	Tumor extending beyond the nasal and paranasal sinuses, including involvement of the cribriform plate, base of the skull, orbit or intracranial cavity
D	Tumor with metastasis to cervical nodes or distant sites

Table 15.19 Olfactory neuroblastoma: staging system after Dulguerov et al[13]

Stage	Characteristics
T1	Tumor involving the nasal cavity and/or paranasal sinuses (excluding the sphenoid sinus), sparing the most superior ethmoidal cells
T2	Tumor involving the nasal cavity and/or paranasal sinuses (including the sphenoid sinus), with extension to or erosion of the cribriform plate
T3	Tumor extending into the orbit or protruding into the anterior cranial fossa, without dural invasion
T4	Tumor involving the brain
N0	No cervical lymph node metastases
N1	Any form of cervical lymph node metastases
M0	No metastases
M1	Any distant metastases

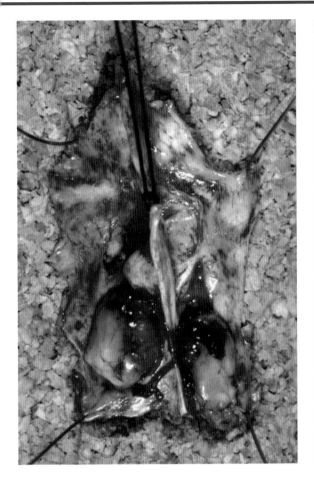

Fig. 15.22 ONB. Operative specimen taken at craniofacial resection showing dura and olfactory bulbs and tracts, with macroscopic swelling of both bulbs due to tumor infiltration.

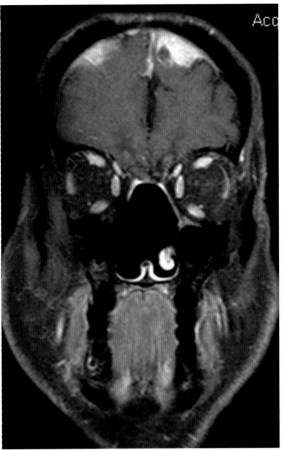

Fig. 15.23 Coronal MRI (T1W with gadolinium) showing multiple dural deposits of olfactory neuroblastoma.

when not macroscopically obvious (**Fig. 15.22**),[12] which supported the routine resection of the dura and adjacent olfactory system. There is also an increasing recognition that cervical involvement occurs relatively early and more frequently than is seen with many other sinonasal malignancies.[15] ONB is one of the few sinonasal tumors to spread to nodes in the cheek and parotid region or the contralateral neck. Systemic spread is estimated to occur in 10 to 15%; it is rarely evident at presentation and is generally found in the presence of residual or recurrent local disease.

Intriguingly, ONB can pop up anywhere in the midface. We have had several cases where a second deposit has occurred in the contralateral eye and a common late feature of locoregional disease is the appearance of dural plaques, which may develop *en cuirasse* to encase the brain; these are often slow-growing but generally resistant to all forms of treatment (**Fig. 15.23**). This can occur without evidence of local recurrence, which is difficult to explain in terms of routes of spread or reasons for activation but may be due to spread through the venous channels or CSF.

Treatment

The advent of craniofacial resection has revolutionized the treatment of ONB, doubling survival figures, and is now regarded as the "gold standard." In a meta-analysis, Dulguerov et al confirmed that this procedure combined with radiotherapy was the treatment of choice[13] and others have confirmed that neither surgery nor radiotherapy alone is sufficient for optimum results.[16,46]

Surgery

Craniofacial resection was introduced in the 1970s by Ketcham and others, providing the combination of an en bloc oncologic resection with low morbidity and excellent cosmesis.[47–49] By approaching the tumor from the nose and anterior cranial fossa, the operation directly addresses the origin and local spread of this tumor, allowing resection of dura and the olfactory system including the olfactory epithelium, cribriform plate, olfactory bulb, and tracts. This directly deals with macro- and microscopic spread of disease, reducing local recurrence.[50,51]

There are many variations on the technique but essentially all involve some form of craniotomy together with a nasal approach using various incisions and forms of repair. Using a coronal incision in the scalp and a sublabial incision for midfacial degloving, these scars can be hidden. However, an extended lateral rhinotomy or a supraorbital spectacle incision are difficult to discern once healed. The skull base repair may be effected with a pericranial flap or fascia lata and split skin. In our series, which extends over 27 years, using this technique of craniofacial resection in 308 patients, postoperative hospital stay has been on average 14 days and major complications have been low (**Table 15.16**).[51]

Prior to craniofacial resection, conventional wisdom dictated that the orbit should be sacrificed if tumor was either adjacent to or had transgressed the periosteum. However, it is clear that it is possible to salvage a proportion of these eyes without compromising survival. If the tumor has not penetrated through the full thickness of orbital periosteum on frozen section, it is possible to resect it widely and skin graft the area. Nonetheless, the orbit should be cleared if there is full-thickness periosteal penetration or frank infiltration of orbital contents.

More recently endoscopic resection has been used for selected cases, usually those without significant skull base erosion, or for patients who are a poor anesthetic risk. The endoscopic approach should not be regarded as a limited procedure but rather as a craniofacial resection performed via an endonasal approach that includes a similar wide-field resection of tissue under excellent direct visualization.[52] The ability to perform skull base resection and repair via an endoscopic approach has facilitated this[31,53] and indeed some surgeons have advocated undertaking extensive intracranial resection from below in teams that involve neurosurgical input.[54] Alternatively, the endoscopic approach can be combined with an external craniotomy.[55–57] Patients should be appraised that both might be required or that an endoscopic approach may need to be extended to include a formal craniotomy.

In a recent series of 49 patients with malignant sinonasal tumors undergoing endoscopic resection with curative intent, 11 were olfactory neuroblastomas, one of which was converted to craniofacial resection at one year.[52] Other published cohorts of malignant tumors have also included olfactory neuroblastoma[58–62] and, as in this series, complications, if any, have been at very low rates. In our own series, hospital stay has been on average 4 days and postoperative radiotherapy has been started very promptly. It should also be noted that endoscopic surgery can have a role following conventional craniofacial resection in the management of localized recurrence.

The neck is not traditionally treated prophylactically, although a selective neck dissection is undertaken in the presence of disease.[63]

Radiotherapy

Radiation in this area must be carefully administered to deliver the maximum dose while preserving the adjacent brain and optic nerves. An external megavoltage beam and three-field technique has generally been used. An anterior port combined with wedged lateral fields delivers a dose of 55 to 65 Gy. Because of the proximity of the optic chiasm, the dose given must remain below normal tissue tolerance and the advent of intensity-modulated radiotherapy may be of some advantage in this respect. Generally, radiotherapy has been used as an adjunct to surgery, both open and endoscopic,[16,64,65] and postoperative delivery is preferred.

Other authors have combined stereotactically guided radiotherapy with surgery, which may offer improved local control with minimal collateral damage,[66,67] but again numbers and follow-up preclude definitive evidence.

The role of elective neck irradiation remains unproven in the small numbers thus far considered.[68,69]

Chemotherapy

The use of concomitant chemotherapy has not been fully evaluated, although chemosensitivity has been found in retrospective series. ONB has been shown to respond to platinum-based regimens[70,71] and chemotherapy has been used as an adjunct to radiotherapy in combination with craniofacial resection with comparable results in several centers.[72] University of Virginia researchers have used cyclophosphamide, doxorubicin, cisplatin, and etoposide for stage 3 disease in combination with radiotherapy and surgery with reasonable results.[73,74] Eight of 18 patients between 1999 and 2005 who received radiotherapy also received cisplatin, which suggested a reduced recurrence rate, although the number of patients precludes any reliable statistical conclusions.[75] Notwithstanding this, all our ONB patients are offered two courses of this adjunctive chemotherapy at the beginning and half-way through their postoperative course of radiotherapy. Similar regimes have been employed in Korea and Japan[71,76] in combination with radiotherapy and/or surgery, but the side effects, albeit temporary, were considerable and the numbers were small (11 and 12, respectively).

Palliative chemotherapy using cisplatin-based regimes or docetaxel plus irinotecan have also been reported, but the benefits of short-term response should again be weighed against the potential morbidity of the treatment.[77]

Outcome and Prognosis

ONB characteristically has a long natural history punctuated by locoregional recurrence. Thus in common with most sinonasal tumors, a lifetime's follow-up is required and 5-year survival does not equate to cure. We have observed de novo recurrence after 12 years of regular follow-up including MRI.

Prior to craniofacial resection, the use of lateral rhinotomy and radiotherapy provided poor results[78-80] of <40%, largely due to the inability to deal with intracranial spread. Craniofacial resection specifically addresses this area and allows removal of the olfactory bulbs and tracts where microscopic disease may be residing undetected. Thus, when large series with long-term follow-up after craniofacial resection are considered, the 5-year survival is seen to have improved significantly[51,81-86] or even doubled as in our own series to 77%[16] or 89% in that of Diaz et al and Gabory et al.[85,86] However, there is continued loss over time and local recurrence can occur up to 12 years after treatment (range 12–144 months, mean 37 months). In our series of 42 cases, disease-free survival drops from 77% at 5 years to 53% at 10 years. In a further study of this cohort enlarged to 56 individuals, 15-year survival fell to 40%, which emphasizes the importance of long-term follow-up (**Fig. 15.24**).[30,51]

The most frequent recurrence is local and occurred in 17% of our series, in keeping with other published series using craniofacial resection and radiotherapy. Local recurrence has been shown to be decreased by the addition of radiotherapy, but it does not seem to matter whether this is given before or after surgery. In our series radiotherapy was originally reserved for those patients who had disease above the skull base, but on analysis the recurrence rate was higher in those with more limited disease (28%) than in those with more advanced cases (4%). This resulted in our offering postoperative radiotherapy to all patients with ONB thereafter. Interestingly, previous treatment did not seem to affect 5-year actuarial survival either, and in patients who developed local recurrence 5-year survival after further salvage treatment was 54%.

In a retrospective population-based cohort study in the United States of 311 patients, with a modified Kadish staging, presence of lymph nodes, type of treatment, and age proved to be significant predictors of disease-specific survival.[87] Similar findings have been reported by Loy et al[74] and, with the exception of age, by Ozsahin et al.[88]

Kane et al[89] analyzed 205 published studies that included 956 patients with a median follow-up of 3 years. In contrast to our series, they were not able to demonstrate benefit from the addition of radiotherapy to surgical management, but this may have related to the relatively short length of follow-up. Relevant prognostic factors on univariate analysis included histological grade, staging, and being >65 years of age at presentation. However, multivariate analysis showed that tumors with Hyam grades 3 and 4 carried the worst prognosis (proportional hazard = 4.83, $p < 0.001$) with 5- and 10-year survivals of 47% and 31%.

Multivariate analysis of the craniofacial series shows that involvement of the brain and orbit are independent factors affecting outcome.[16] When survival was considered according to orbital involvement, 5-year actuarial survival was 97% when the eye was not affected and 49% when the periosteum was affected, but when the eye was frankly infiltrated even when the eye was sacrificed, there were no 5-year survivors ($p = 0.0067$) (**Fig. 15.25**). This supports the philosophy of sacrificing the eye only when there is frank infiltration or full-thickness penetration of the periosteum.

When skull base and intracranial involvement were considered, there was a difference between those whose tumor was confined to the nasal cavity and those in whom the skull base was affected, those in whom the olfactory tracts were involved, those in whom the dura was additionally infiltrated, and those in whom the brain was affected ($p = 0.035$). When patients with tumor in the nasal cavity and/or skull base were compared with the other groups, there was as might be expected a statistical difference between these patients and those with dura and/or olfactory tract involvement ($p = 0.006$) and those with brain involvement ($p = 0.039$) (**Fig. 15.26**).

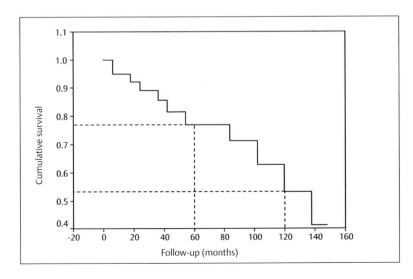

Fig. 15.24 Kaplan–Meier graph showing disease-free survival of ONB patients following craniofacial resection.

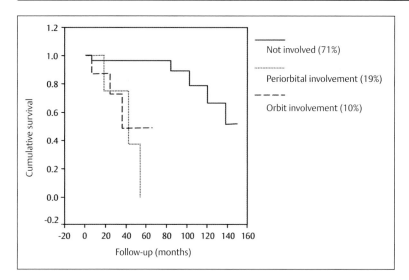

Fig. 15.25 Kaplan–Meier graph showing survival in ONB patients with orbital involvement following craniofacial resection.

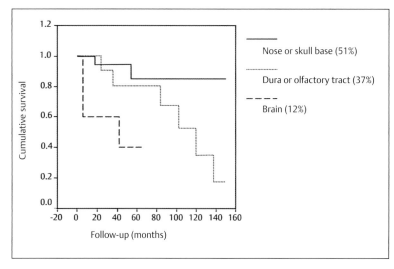

Fig. 15.26 Kaplan–Meier graph showing survival in ONB patients with intracranial involvement following craniofacial resection.

Until recently those patients treated by endoscopic approaches were too limited in number and follow-up for any meaningful comparison to be made, but it is clear that in carefully selected individuals early results are at least as good as those of craniofacial resection.[52,58–62,67,90] The meta-analysis by Devaiah and Andreoli[91] compared open and endoscopic approaches reported in 23 articles, considering 361 cases that met their inclusion criteria, and showed comparable results for the two methods, taking into account that larger tumors were more often treated with the open techniques as in our own cohort. The advantage of the endoscopic approaches is obviously that the complication rate and morbidity are commensurately less than with craniofacial resection while the resection can be comparable in extent.[92,93]

As previously indicated, cervical lymphadenopathy constitutes an important prognostic factor.[87] Koka et al[24] showed 29% survival with nodes versus 64% without and

this was supported by several subsequent meta-analyses.[13,15,17] Distant metastases with locoregional control are relatively rare (<10%[16,73]) and inevitably carry a poor prognosis.

Key Points

- Olfactory neuroblastoma requires surgery and radiotherapy.
- The role of adjunctive chemotherapy remains to be determined.
- Combined craniofacial resection and radiotherapy is the "gold standard" of treatment and has more than doubled overall survival.
- Endoscopic resection can encompass comparable surgery in selected cases.
- Follow-up must be life-long as recurrence can occur over 10 years later.

References

1. Berger L, Luc R, Richard D. L'estheioneuroepitheliome olfactif. Bull Assoc Fr Etud Cancer 1924;13:410–421

2. Skolnik EM, Massari FS, Tenta LT. Olfactory neuroepithelioma. Review of the world literature and presentation of two cases. Arch Otolaryngol 1966;84(6):644–653

3. O'Connor TA, McLean P, Juillard GJ, Parker RG. Olfactory neuroblastoma. Cancer 1989;63(12):2426–2428

4. Broich G. Pagliaria, Ottaviani F. Esthesioneuroblastoma: a general review of the cases published since the discovery of the tumour in 1924. Anticancer Res 1927;17:2683–2706

5. Hyams VJ. Olfactory neuroblastoma. In: Hyams VJ, Baksakis JG, Michaels L, eds. Tumours of the Upper Respiratory Tract and Ear. Washington, DC: Armed Forces Institute of Pathology; 1998:240–248

6. Schwaab G, Micheau C, Le Guillou C, et al. Olfactory esthesioneuroma: a report of 40 cases. Laryngoscope 1988;98(8 Pt 1):872–876

7. Magnavita N, Sacco A, Bevilacqua L, D'Alessandris T, Bosman C. Aesthesioneuroblastoma in a woodworker. Occup Med (Lond) 2003;53(3):231–234

8. Magee PN, Montesano R, Preussmann R. *N*-nitroso compounds and related carcinogens. In: Searle CE, ed. Chemical Carcinogens. Washington DC: American Chemical Society; 1976:491–625

9. Herrold KM. Induction of olfactory neuroepithelial tumors in Syrian hamsters by diethlynitrosamine. Cancer 1964;17:114–121

10. Vollrath M, Altmannsberger M, Weber K, Osborn M. Chemically induced tumors of rat olfactory epithelium: a model for human esthesioneuroepithelioma. J Natl Cancer Inst 1986;76(6):1205–1216

11. Leong BK, Kociba RJ, Jersey GC. A lifetime study of rats and mice exposed to vapors of bis(chloromethyl)ether. Toxicol Appl Pharmacol 1981;58(2):269–281

12. Harrison D. Surgical pathology of olfactory neuroblastoma. Head Neck Surg 1984;7(1):60–64

13. Dulguerov P, Allal AS, Calcaterra TC. Esthesioneuroblastoma: a meta-analysis and review. Lancet Oncol 2001;2(11):683–690

14. Kumar M, Fallon RJ, Hill JS, Davis MM. Esthesioneuroblastoma in children. J Pediatr Hematol Oncol 2002;24(6):482–487

15. Rinaldo A, Ferlito A, Shaha AR, Wei WI, Lund VJ. Esthesioneuroblastoma and cervical lymph node metastases: clinical and therapeutic implications. Acta Otolaryngol 2002;122(2):215–221

16. Lund VJ, Howard D, Wei W, Spittle M. Olfactory neuroblastoma: past, present, and future? Laryngoscope 2003;113(3):502–507

17. Gore MR, Zanation AM. Salvage treatment of late neck metastasis in esthesioneuroblastoma: a meta-analysis. Arch Otolaryngol Head Neck Surg 2009;135(10):1030–1034

18. Davis RE, Weissler MC. Esthesioneuroblastoma and neck metastasis. Head Neck 1992;14(6):477–482

19. Harrison DFN, Lund VJ. Neuroectodermal lesions. Tumours of the Upper Jaw. London: Churchill Livingstone; 1993:295–328

20. Morita A, Ebersold MJ, Olsen KD, Foote RL, Lewis JE, Quast LM. Esthesioneuroblastoma: prognosis and management. Neurosurgery 1993;32(5):706–714, discussion 714–715

21. Singh W, Ramage C, Best P, Angus B. Nasal neuroblastoma secreting vasopressin. A case report. Cancer 1980;45(5):961–966

22. Srigley JR, Dayal VS, Gregor RT, Love R, van Nostrand AW. Hyponatremia secondary to olfactory neuroblastoma. Arch Otolaryngol 1983;109(8):559–562

23. Myers SL, Hardy DA, Wiebe CB, Shiffman J. Olfactory neuroblastoma invading the oral cavity in a patient with inappropriate antidiuretic hormone secretion. Oral Surg Oral Med Oral Pathol 1994;77(6):645–650

24. Koka VN, Julieron M, Bourhis J, et al. Aesthesioneuroblastoma. J Laryngol Otol 1998;112(7):628–633

25. Kairemo KJ, Jekunen AP, Kestilä MS, Ramsay HA. Imaging of olfactory neuroblastoma—an analysis of 17 cases. Auris Nasus Larynx 1998;25(2):173–179

26. Lloyd GAS, Lund VJ, Howard DJ, Savy L. Optimum imaging for sinonasal malignancy. J Laryngol Otol 2000;114(7):557–562

27. Madani G, Beale TJ, Lund VJ. Imaging of sinonasal tumors. Semin Ultrasound CT MR 2009;30(1):25–38

28. Pickuth D, Heywang-Köbrunner SH, Spielmann RP. Computed tomography and magnetic resonance imaging features of olfactory neuroblastoma: an analysis of 22 cases. Clin Otolaryngol Allied Sci 1999;24(5):457–461

29. Som P, Brandwein M. Tumors and tumor-like conditions. In: Som P, Curtin D, eds. Head and Neck Imaging. 4th ed. St Louis, MO: Mosby; 2003:261–373

30. Lund VJ, Howard DJ, Wei WI, Cheesman AD. Craniofacial resection for tumors of the nasal cavity and paranasal sinuses—a 17-year experience. Head Neck 1998;20(2):97–105

31. Lund VJ, Stammberger H, Nicolai P, et al. European position paper on endoscopic management of tumours of the nose, paranasal sinuses and skull base. Rhinol Suppl 2010;(22):1–143

32. Nguyen BD, Roarke MC, Nelson KD, Chong BW. F-18 FDG PET/CT staging and posttherapeutic assessment of esthesioneuroblastoma. Clin Nucl Med 2006;31(3):172–174

33. Prado GL, Itabashi Y, Noda H, Miura H, Mariya Y, Abe Y. Olfactory neuroblastoma visualized by technetium-99m-ECD SPECT. Radiat Med 2001;19(5):267–270

34. Collins BT, Cramer HM, Hearn SA. Fine needle aspiration cytology of metastatic olfactory neuroblastoma. Acta Cytol 1997;41(3):802–810

35. Zollinger LV, Wiggins RH III, Cornelius RS, Phillips CD. Retropharyngeal lymph node metastasis from esthesioneuroblastoma: a review of the therapeutic and prognostic implications. AJNR Am J Neuroradiol 2008;29(8):1561–1563

36. Argani P, Perez-Ordoñez B, Xiao H, Caruana SM, Huvos AG, Ladanyi M. Olfactory neuroblastoma is not related to the Ewing family of tumors: absence of EWS/FLI1 gene fusion and MIC2 expression. Am J Surg Pathol 1998;22(4):391–398

37. Kumar S, Perlman E, Pack S, et al. Absence of EWS/FLI1 fusion in olfactory neuroblastomas indicates these tumors do not belong to the Ewing's sarcoma family. Hum Pathol 1999;30(11):1356–1360

38. Mhawech P, Berczy M, Assaly M, et al. Human achaete-scute homologue (hASH1) mRNA level as a diagnostic marker to distinguish esthesioneuroblastoma from poorly differentiated tumors arising in the sinonasal tract. Am J Clin Pathol 2004;122(1):100–105

39. Bockmühl U, You X, Pacyna-Gengelbach M, Arps H, Draf W, Petersen I. CGH pattern of esthesioneuroblastoma and their metastases. Brain Pathol 2004;14(2):158–163

40. Holland H, Koschny R, Krupp W, et al. Comprehensive cytogenetic characterization of an esthesioneuroblastoma. Cancer Genet Cytogenet 2007;173(2):89–96

41. Papadaki H, Kounelis S, Kapadia SB, Bakker A, Swalsky PA, Finkelstein SD. Relationship of p53 gene alterations with tumor progression and recurrence in olfactory neuroblastoma. Am J Surg Pathol 1996;20(6):715–721

42. Ogura JH, Schenck NL. Unusual nasal tumors. Problems in diagnosis and treatment. Otolaryngol Clin North Am 1973;6(3):813–837

43. Lund VJ, Milroy C. Olfactory neuroblastoma: clinical and pathological aspects. Rhinology 1993;31(1):1–6

44. Hirose T, Scheithauer BW, Lopes MB, et al. Olfactory neuroblastoma. An immunohistochemical, ultrastructural, and flow cytometric study. Cancer 1995;76(1):4–19

45. Kadish S, Goodman M, Wang CC. Olfactory neuroblastoma. A clinical analysis of 17 cases. Cancer 1976; 37(3):1571–1576

46. Gruber G, Laedrach K, Baumert B, Caversaccio M, Raveh J, Greiner R. Esthesioneuroblastoma: irradiation alone and surgery alone are not enough. Int J Radiat Oncol Biol Phys 2002;54(2):486–491

47. Clifford P. Transcranial approach for cancer of the antroethmoidal area. Clin Otolaryngol Allied Sci 1977;2(2):115–130

48. Terz JJ, Young HF, Lawrence W Jr. Combined craniofacial resection for locally advanced carcinoma of the head and neck I. Tumors of the skin and soft tissues. Am J Surg 1980;140(5):613–617

49. Ketcham AS, Van Buren JM. Tumors of the paranasal sinuses: a therapeutic challenge. Am J Surg 1985;150(4):406–413

50. Shah JP, Kraus DH, Bilsky MH, Gutin PH, Harrison LH, Strong EW. Craniofacial resection for malignant tumors involving the anterior skull base. Arch Otolaryngol Head Neck Surg 1997;123(12):1312–1317

51. Howard DJ, Lund VJ, Wei WI. Craniofacial resection for tumors of the nasal cavity and paranasal sinuses: a 25-year experience. Head Neck 2006;28(10):867–873

52. Lund V, Howard DJ, Wei WI. Endoscopic resection of malignant tumours of the nose and sinuses. Am J Rhinol 2007;21(1):89–94

53. Lund VJ. Endoscopic management of cerebrospinal fluid leaks. Am J Rhinol 2002;16(1):17–23

54. Kassam A, Horowitz M, Welch W, et al. The role of endoscopic assisted microneurosurgery (image fusion technology) in the performance of neurosurgical procedures. Minim Invasive Neurosurg 2005;48(4):191–196

55. Thaler ER, Kotapka M, Lanza DC, Kennedy DW. Endoscopically assisted anterior cranial skull base resection of sinonasal tumors. Am J Rhinol 1999;13(4):303–310

56. Devaiah AK, Larsen C, Tawfik O, O'Boynick P, Hoover LA. Esthesioneuroblastoma: endoscopic nasal and anterior craniotomy resection. Laryngoscope 2003; 113(12):2086–2090

57. Yuen AP, Fan YW, Fung CF, Hung KN. Endoscopic-assisted cranionasal resection of olfactory neuroblastoma. Head Neck 2005;27(6):488–493

58. Draf W, Schick B, Weber R, et al. Endoscopic micro-endoscopic surgery of nasal and paranasal sinus tumours. In: Stamm AC, Draf W, eds. Micro-Endoscopic Surgery of the Paranasal Sinuses and the Skull Base. Berlin: Springer; 2000:481–488

59. Goffart Y, Jorissen M, Daele J, et al. Minimally invasive endoscopic management of malignant sinonasal tumours. Acta Otorhinolaryngol Belg 2000;54(2):221–232

60. Walch C, Stammberger H, Anderhuber W, Unger F, Köle W, Feichtinger K. The minimally invasive approach to olfactory neuroblastoma: combined endoscopic and stereotactic treatment. Laryngoscope 2000;110(4):635–640

61. Casiano RR, Numa WA, Falquez AM. Endoscopic resection of esthesioneuroblastoma. Am J Rhinol 2001;15(4):271–279

62. Batra PS, Citardi MJ, Worley S, Lee J, Lanza DC. Resection of anterior skull base tumors: comparison of combined traditional and endoscopic techniques. Am J Rhinol 2005;19(5):521–528

63. Zanation AM, Ferlito A, Rinaldo A, et al. When, how and why to treat the neck in patients with esthesioneuroblastoma: a review. Eur Arch Otorhinolaryngol 2010; 267(11):1667–1671

64. Foote RL, Morita A, Ebersold MJ, et al. Esthesioneuroblastoma: the role of adjuvant radiation therapy. Int J Radiat Oncol Biol Phys 1993;27(4):835–842

65. Castelnuovo P, Bignami M, Delù G, Battaglia P, Bignardi M, Dallan I. Endonasal endoscopic resection and radiotherapy in olfactory neuroblastoma: our experience. Head Neck 2007;29(9):845–850

66. Zabel A, Thilmann C, Milker-Zabel S, et al. The role of stereotactically guided conformal radiotherapy for local tumor control of esthesioneuroblastoma. Strahlenther Onkol 2002;178(4):187–191

67. Unger F, Haselsberger K, Walch C, Stammberger H, Papaefthymiou G. Combined endoscopic surgery and radiosurgery as treatment modality for olfactory neuroblastoma (esthesioneuroblastoma). Acta Neurochir (Wien) 2005;147(6):595–601, discussion 601–602

68. Monroe AT, Hinerman RW, Amdur RJ, Morris CG, Mendenhall WM. Radiation therapy for esthesioneuroblastoma: rationale for elective neck irradiation. Head Neck 2003;25(7):529–534

69. Noh OK, Lee SW, Yoon SM, et al. Radiotherapy for esthesioneuroblastoma: is elective nodal irradiation warranted in the multimodality treatment approach? Int J Radiat Oncol Biol Phys 2011;79(2):443–449

70. McElroy EA Jr, Buckner JC, Lewis JE. Chemotherapy for advanced esthesioneuroblastoma: the Mayo Clinic experience. Neurosurgery 1998;42(5):1023–1027, discussion 1027–1028

71. Kim DW, Jo YH, Kim JH, et al. Neoadjuvant etoposide, ifosfamide, and cisplatin for the treatment of olfactory neuroblastoma. Cancer 2004;101(10):2257–2260

72. Dulguerov P, Calcaterra T. Esthesioneuroblastoma: the UCLA experience 1970–1990. Laryngoscope 1992; 102(8):843–849

73. Levine PA, Gallagher R, Cantrell RW. Esthesioneuroblastoma: reflections of a 21-year experience. Laryngoscope 1999;109(10):1539–1543

74. Loy AH, Reibel JF, Read PW, et al. Esthesioneuroblastoma: continued follow-up of a single institution's experience. Arch Otolaryngol Head Neck Surg 2006;132(2):134–138

75. Nikapota A, Sevitt T, Lund VJ, et al. Outcomes of radical conformal radiotherapy and concomitant cisplatin chemotherapy for olfactory neuroblastoma—review of a single centre experience. J Clin Oncol 2006;24(18 Suppl):5555 [ASCO Annual Meeting Proceedings (Post-Meeting Edition)]

76. Mishima Y, Nagasaki E, Terui Y, Irie T, Takahashi S, Ito Y, et al. Combination chemotherapy (cyclophosphamide, doxorubicin, and vincristine with continuous-infusion cisplatin and etoposide) and radiotherapy with stem cell support can be beneficial for adolescents and adults with esthesioneuroblastoma. Cancer 2004;101(6):1437–1444

77. Yoh K, Tahara M, Kawada K, et al. Chemotherapy in the treatment of advanced or recurrent olfactory neuroblastoma. Asia Pac J Clin Oncol 2006;2:180–184

78. Bailey BJ, Barton S. Olfactory neuroblastoma. Management and prognosis. Arch Otolaryngol 1975;101(1):1–5

79. Shah JP, Feghali J. Esthesioneuroblastoma. Am J Surg 1981;142(4):456–458

80. Appelblatt NH, McClatchey KD. Olfactory neuroblastoma: a retrospective clinicopathologic study. Head Neck Surg 1982;5(2):108–113

81. Eriksen JG, Bastholt L, Krogdahl AS, Hansen O, Joergensen KE. Esthesioneuroblastoma—what is the optimal treatment? Acta Oncol 2000;39(2):231–235

82. Resto VA, Eisele DW, Forastiere A, Zahurak M, Lee DJ, Westra WH. Esthesioneuroblastoma: the Johns Hopkins experience. Head Neck 2000;22(6):550–558

83. Patel SG, Singh B, Polluri A, et al. Craniofacial surgery for malignant skull base tumors: report of an international collaborative study. Cancer 2003;98(6):1179–1187
84. Constantinidis J, Steinhart H, Koch M, et al. Olfactory neuroblastoma: the University of Erlangen-Nuremberg experience 1975-2000. Otolaryngol Head Neck Surg 2004;130(5):567–574
85. Diaz EM Jr, Johnigan RH III, Pero C, et al. Olfactory neuroblastoma: the 22-year experience at one comprehensive cancer center. Head Neck 2005;27(2):138–149
86. de Gabory L, Abdulkhaleq HM, Darrouzet V, Bébéar J-P, Stoll D. Long-term results of 28 esthesioneuroblastomas managed over 35 years. Head Neck 2011;33(1):82–86
87. Jethanamest D, Morris LG, Sikora AG, Kutler DI. Esthesioneuroblastoma: a population-based analysis of survival and prognostic factors. Arch Otolaryngol Head Neck Surg 2007;133(3):276–280
88. Ozashin M, Gruber G, Olszyk O, et al. Outcome and prognostic factors in olfactory neuroblastoma: a rare cancer network study. Int J Radiat Oncol Biol Phys 2010;78(4):992–997
89. Kane AJ, Sughrue ME, Rutkowski MJ, et al. Posttreatment prognosis of patients with esthesioneuroblastoma. J Neurosurg 2010;113(2):340–351
90. Folbe A, Herzallah I, Duvvuri U, et al. Endoscopic endonasal resection of esthesioneuroblastoma: a multicenter study. Am J Rhinol Allergy 2009;23(1):91–94
91. Devaiah AK, Andreoli MT. Treatment of esthesioneuroblastoma: a 16-year meta-analysis of 361 patients. Laryngoscope 2009;119(7):1412–1416
92. Snyderman CH, Carrau RL, Kassam AB, et al. Endoscopic skull base surgery: principles of endonasal oncological surgery. J Surg Oncol 2008;97(8):658–664
93. Ganly I, Patel SG, Singh B, et al. Complications of craniofacial resection for malignant tumors of the skull base: report of an International Collaborative Study. Head Neck 2005;27(6):445–451

Mucosal Malignant Melanoma

Definition

(ICD-O code 8720/3)

Mucosal malignant melanomas (MMMs) are aggressive tumors arising from melanin producing cells (melanocytes), derived from neural crest tissue.

Etiology

While exposure to sun is well established in the development of skin melanoma, no such association could be considered relevant in the clefts and cavities of the nose and sinuses. However, there has been some interest in occupational exposure to formaldehyde.[1,2] Further enquiry among British ENT surgeons revealed 181 cases, 26% of which had occurred in the Midlands (Leicestershire, Nottinghamshire, and Birmingham) but unfortunately the rarity of the tumor has precluded any robust epidemiological studies and the concern remains anecdotal. Formaldehyde has been shown to be a respiratory carcinogen in animal models such as the rat[3] but nasal MMM has not been reported in embalmers, who might

reasonably be expected to be most at risk. However, they do have a higher incidence of skin melanoma and carcinoma of the colon.[4]

Comparative genomic hybridization has identified chromosomal abnormalities such as 1q and 6p gains not usually seen with cutaneous melanomas.[5,6]

Incidence

Cutaneous melanomas are the most common type of which 15 to 33% occur in the skin of the head and neck region.[1] Melanocytes are also found in mucosa, secretory glands, nasal stroma, and supporting cells of the olfactory epithelium,[7] where they can undergo malignant transformation. MMMs are rare, however, accounting for 1.3% of all malignant melanomas, 55% of which occur in the head and neck region.[8] Of these, two-thirds originate in the sinonasal region and a quarter in the oral cavity.[1,9–13] Overall, less than 1% of malignant melanomas are sinonasal.[1,10,14,15] Of the diverse range of sinonasal malignancies, melanoma accounts for ~4%.[15]

Site

The most common subsite for sinonasal malignant melanomas is the lateral nasal wall followed by, in order of frequency, septum, maxillary sinus, and ethmoids.[15] They rarely originate in the sphenoid sinus, nasopharynx, or nasal vestibule.

In our series of 115 cases, 90 cases (78.3%) originated in the nasal cavity, 12 (10.5%) in the ethmoids with/without nasal cavity involvement, and 7 (6.1%) involved the maxilla (in 6 cases disease was too extensive for site of origin to be determined).

Although rarer still, the possibility of the sinonasal lesion representing a metastasis should be considered. This has occurred on two occasions in our series of cases.

Diagnostic Features

Clinical Features

Sinonasal melanomas are equally common in men and women. In previously reported series the mean age (64.3 years) has been older than for those with cutaneous melanomas.[1] The incidence is much higher in Japan, where mucosal melanomas make up a one-quarter to one-third of all melanomas, and they may be more common in black populations.[10,16] In our own series of 115 cases, which is the largest series of sinonasal mucosal malignant melanomas from a single institution and was collected prospectively for 47 years (1963–2010), 64 patients were female (55.7%) and 51 male (44.3%). The mean age at the time of initial treatment was 65.9 years (range 15 to 91 years).

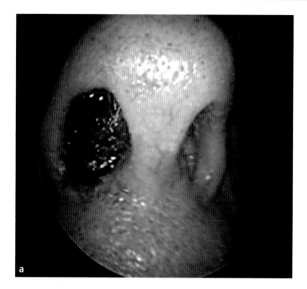

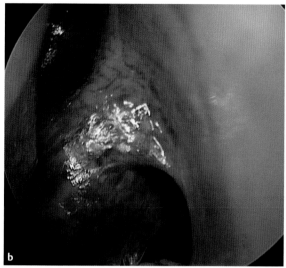

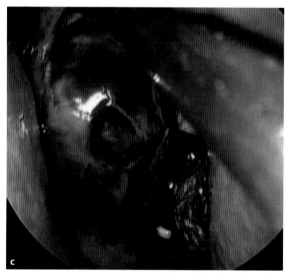

Fig. 15.27a–c Endoscopic views of MMM.
a MMM presenting in the right vestibule.
b MMM presenting as a vascular lesion filling the middle meatus.
c A pigmented lesion, bleeding to the touch and filling the nasal cavity.

Imaging

There are no specific features of MMM other than a uniform soft tissue mass on CT with erosion of adjacent bone, and even this may not be marked (**Fig. 15.28**). Similarly, MRI shows the mass with surrounding inflammation and retained secretions, so it must be distinguished from SCC, adenocarcinoma, and lymphoma.

Imaging of the neck (or ultrasound), chest, and liver may be considered for staging. It has been suggested that PET may be more sensitive in the detection of metastatic disease.[13,17]

Histological Features and Differential Diagnosis

Melanoma by definition arises from melanocytes, embryological derivatives of neural crest. These are widely distributed in skin and mucosa, including that of the nose, and are found in the glands, in superficial and deep stroma of the septum and turbinates, and in association with the supporting cells of the olfactory epithelium. Early studies[7] suggested that they were absent in fetal and neonatal nasal mucosa.

Obvious melanosis is seen quite commonly in the oral cavity and it has been estimated that a proportion proceed to malignancy (though the range is wide, 0.5 to 30%[18]).

The tumor can pose some difficulties in diagnosis, composed as it is of many polygonal or spindle-shaped cells with many mitoses and must, therefore, be distinguished from sinonasal undifferentiated carcinoma (SNUC), lymphoma, and nasopharyngeal carcinoma

Presentation, as with other sinonasal malignancies, may mimic inflammatory conditions, leading to a delayed diagnosis. Unilateral nasal obstruction, a visible mass, and in particular frank epistaxis, are the most common features (**Fig. 15.27**). On endoscopic examination the lesion may appear pigmented but may be amelanotic in at least 10%. It is often vascular and may be necrotic as it outgrows its blood supply. While there may be a polypoid friable mass, the lesion can also be spreading and more sessile. Furthermore, there may be satellite lesions anywhere on the mucosa of one or both sides of the nose and in addition patches of melanosis may be observed that histologically are made up of melanin within macrophages. Thus, determination of the true extent of the tumor can often be difficult. Diplopia, epiphora, and proptosis are late features and only 1 in 10 present with cervical lymphadenopathy, although both this and systemic metastases can develop at any point.

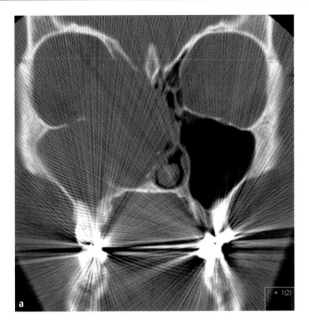

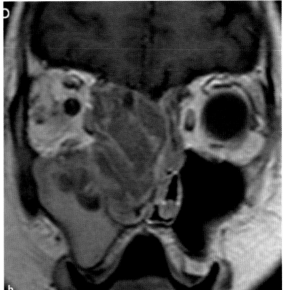

Fig. 15.28a, b

a Coronal CT scan showing opacification of the right nasal cavity, ethmoid and maxillary sinuses with displacement of the septum and erosion and infiltration into the orbit.

b Coronal MRI (T1W post gadolinium enhancement) defining the tumor mass in the upper nasal cavity involving the eye and invaginating into the maxillary sinus, which also contains obstructed secretion.

(NPC). Immunohistochemistry is required to confirm the diagnosis by demonstrating protein S100 (expressed by virtually all), VIM, HMB-45, melan-A, tyrosinase, and MIFT (microphthalmia transcription factor) in addition to the presence of intracellular melanin itself (**Table 15.1**).

Staging

Cutaneous melanomas are staged according to thickness,[19] according to thickness and ulceration (TNM), or in relation to dermal levels (Clarke's levels).[12,14,19,20] These staging systems are backed up by large numbers of cases and closely relate to prognosis. Sinonasal mucosal melanomas do not lend themselves to these staging systems because there are no dermal landmarks, lack of orientation makes measuring depth of penetration difficult, and thickness does not strongly relate to outcome. Many staging systems have been proposed for sinonasal melanomas, including a new section for mucosal melanomas in the 7th edition of the American Joint Committee on Cancer (AJCC) staging manual.[12] The AJCC omit T1 and T2, making the lowest tumor categorization of mucosal melanoma T3, due to its aggressive behavior. This leaves a choice of only stage III or IV disease. Most series have failed to show any relationship between the nasal cavity or sinus TNM staging system for carcinomas and malignant sinonasal melanoma outcomes, the exception being from the MD Anderson Center in Texas, USA.[15] A simple and frequently used system was proposed by Ballantyne:

stage I for localized lesions, stage II for cervical lymph node metastasis, and stage III for distant metastasis.[21] This has been criticized as most patients present with an array of local diseases (stage I) that are not differentiated in this system.[22] Prasad et al proposed a staging system based upon depth of mucosal invasion, with level I defined as melanoma in situ or with "microinvasion," level II as melanoma invading up to the lamina propria, and level III as melanoma with deep tissue invasion.[23] They showed this to be an independent predictor of survival. Thompson et al reviewed 115 cases and proposed a TNM-like system for sinonasal and nasopharyngeal mucosal malignant melanomas in which T1 = 1 subsite and T2 = 2 or more subsites; nodal status was N0 or N1 and the presence of metastatic deposits M1.[1] However, this has not been widely adopted and it is recognized by many that there is a lack of correlation between tumor size and outcome in this most capricious of malignant tumors.[13]

Natural History

The majority of patients present with local disease alone and ultimately succumb to local recurrence, which may occur on multiple occasions during the course of the disease. However, a number will present with cervical lymphadenopathy (10 and 18%) and occasionally distant metastasis (4%). Distant spread becomes a major feature of advancing disease; it can occur anywhere but has a predilection for lung, liver, brain, and bone.

In our series at the time of diagnosis 101 patients (91%) had no identifiable lymph node involvement (N−), 10 (9%) had involved lymph nodes (N+), and the status was unknown in 4 of the early cases.

Treatment

In the literature the mainstay of treatment for sinonasal malignant melanomas has been surgical resection, sometimes in combination with postoperative radiotherapy.[8,10,15,22,24–27] Traditionally, radical surgery via an open approach was utilized but, as results were unpredictable and generally poor, there has been a growing trend toward endoscopic techniques. Ideally, clear margins should be obtained[28] but the proximity or spread of sinonasal tumors to the skull base, orbit, and other vital structures makes this a challenge.

Open approaches have included lateral rhinotomy, midfacial degloving, maxillectomy, rhinectomy, or craniofacial resection with or without orbital clearance with varying degrees of associated morbidity.[29–33] Endoscopic resection can often facilitate a similar resection which, although piecemeal, should not be regarded as a less extensive operation.[34] The endoscope provides a more detailed (magnified) view of the anatomy and assessment of tumor margins than open techniques, which is particularly important when dealing with a disease that may have satellite lesions, amelanotic areas, and submucosal spread that can be better assessed and meticulously removed. Morbidity is reduced with decreased surgical time, decreased hospital stay, less discomfort, and improved cosmetic outcome.[8,35,36] As always, endoscopic techniques can also be combined with open approaches.

Melanoma is traditionally considered a radioresistant tumor but may respond to high doses of radiation.[37] Protocols differ from unit to unit but radiotherapy is generally given as adjuvant treatment rather than as a single modality. New radiotherapy techniques such as IMRT and neutron beams are being employed, as is the gamma knife for smaller recurrences.[38,39] Despite the lack of statistical proof, the use of postoperative radiotherapy may be justified in patients who are well enough and in the presence of positive margins after resection or of unresectable or recurrent disease.

Future developments are likely to include improved staging techniques such as sentinel node assessment and the use of molecular markers such as S100 and tyrosinase to identify high-risk patients.[40–43]

Outcome

(See Tables 15.20 and 15.21.)

The prognosis for sinonasal melanomas is poor—worse than for its cutaneous counterpart—and the rarity of the tumor will continue to pose the same difficulties in performing randomized prospective trials. Five-year survival is typically less than 25%, with reports varying between 8% and 48% with a median overall survival of 12.5 to 19.3 months.[1,10,11,13,15,22,24,25,46–55] Death is usually a consequence of both local recurrence and metastatic disease.

In our series, virtually all cases were treated with a curative intent. Patients underwent surgery, with selected cases receiving postoperative radiotherapy and/or chemotherapy. Follow-up ranged from 2 to 360 months, mean 37.5 months, in the 109 patients whose follow-up was recorded, 6 being lost to follow-up. The primary management in all cases was surgery, the majority undergoing lateral rhinotomy (n = 71) but this has largely been superseded by endoscopic resection (ESS) (n = 31) in the last 20 years. In addition, 4 patients had a craniofacial resection and 4 a midfacial degloving approach, and all procedures were performed by the same surgeon. Sixty-four (55.7%) had surgery alone, 51 (44.3%) had radiotherapy, 10 received chemotherapy in addition to the adjuvant radiotherapy, and 5 were given adjuvant chemotherapy alone. As can be seen from Table 15.20, the overall median survival was 24 months (standard error [SE] = 5.127; 95% confidence interval [CI] = 13.952–34.048) (Fig. 15.29), 5-year overall survival was 28% and 10-year survival 19.4%. Median disease-free survival as expected was less at 21 months (SE 2.943; 95% CI = 15.232–26.768) with a 5-year disease-free survival of 23.7% and 10-year figure of 9.7%.

If lymph nodes were involved at diagnosis (N+) the overall survival, local control rate, and disease-free survival were significantly worse (Mantel-Cox p < 0.001) with no survivors at 5 years in the N+ group (Fig. 15.30). Postoperative radiotherapy did not confer a survival advantage, either overall or disease-free, nor did it improve local control, but this may reflect a selection bias in addition to the small numbers involved (Fig. 15.31). Consequently, the decision to offer patients postoperative radiotherapy must be on an individual basis and after informed discussion.

Interestingly, when endoscopic resection was compared with open approaches, there was a significant improved overall survival with endoscopic surgery up to 5 years (Mantel-Cox p = 0.013). There was a similar trend, albeit not reaching statistical significance, favoring the endoscopic technique for local control (p = 0.225) and disease-free survival. This cannot be explained simply in terms of extent of disease as the endoscopic technique has been applied to all comers irrespective of stage, and this group is directly comparable to those who underwent lateral rhinotomy and midfacial degloving, which it has replaced in the hands of the same surgeon.

Thus it appears that endoscopic surgery carries a better prognosis than the lateral rhinotomy, midfacial degloving, or rhinectomy group (median 19 months, SE = 4.297; CI = 10.578–27.422), which in turn had a better prognosis than the craniofacial resection or maxillectomy group (median 7 month overall survival, SE = 7.115; CI = 0–20.946) (Figs. 15.32 and 15.33). Several series have now

Table 15.20 Malignant mucosal melanoma: personal series (survival statistics, 5-year, 10-year, and median for overall survival, disease-free survival, and local control)

		5-year survival (%)	10-year survival (%)	Median (months)
Overall		**28**	**19.4**	**24**
Lymph node				
	N0	31.5	21.8	32
	N1	0	0	11
Radiotherapy				
	None	31.7	20.3	28
	Given	24.1	19.3	24
Surgical approach				
	Endoscopic	45.6	N/A	59
	Open minor	24	16.9	19
	Open major	10	10	7
Disease-free survival		23.7	9.7	21
Lymph node				
	N0	27.1	11.1	24
	N1	0	0	11
Radiotherapy				
	None	28.2	12.9	18
	Given	18.8	6.5	21
Surgical approach				
	Endoscopic	31.3	N/A	36
	Open minor	27.7	11.6	18
	Open major	9.1	0	7
Local control		27.7	11.3	21
Lymph node				
	N0	31.8	13.0	28
	N1	0	0	11
Radiotherapy				
	None	31.9	14.6	23
	Given	23.7	8.1	21
Surgical approach				
	Endoscopic	40.2	N/A	50
	Open minor	25.3	12.9	18
	Open major	10.6	0	15

Table 15.21 Results of treatment of sinonasal malignant melanoma in the literature

Authors	Number of patients (n)	Primary treatment to local recurrence	Primary treatment to regional recurrence	Primary treatment to distant metastases	Survival and disease-free interval
Brandwein et al[44]	25	N/A	N/A	N/A	60% survival at a mean of 21 mo 44% disease-free at 5 y
Lund et al[30] (open radical surgery ± radiotherapy)	58	8 mo (mean)	N/A	N/A	28% A&W at 5 y 20% at 10 y
Thompson et al[1] (wide local excision + some radiotherapy/ chemotherapy)	115	N/A	N/A	N/A	45% alive at a mean of 2.3 y 22% alive at 5 y
Bridger et al[45] (radical surgery and radiotherapy)	27	14.7 mo (mean)	N/A	23.2 mo (mean)	46% alive at 5 y mean survival 52 mo
Huang et al[46] (surgery + some with radiotherapy/ chemotherapy)	15	5 mo (mean)	7.45 mo (mean)	10.3 mo (mean)	49.5% alive at 2 y 33% at 5 y
Lund et al[35] (all endoscopic resection, ITC, prospective)	11	N/A	N/A	N/A	36% disease-free at 2 y
Dauer et al[33] (wide local excision + some radiotherapy)	61	9 mo (mean)	N/A	13 mo (mean)	48.9% alive at 3 y 22.1% at 5 y Median survival 19 mo
Nicolai et al[36] (endoscopic resection, probable radiotherapy but not detailed)	14	N/A	N/A	N/A	18% disease-free mean follow-up of 34.1 mo
Roth et al[13] (13 endoscopic, 6 open surgery, 7 radiotherapy, 6 palliative: ITC in 19)	25	Median disease-free interval 22 mo	N/A	N/A	33% alive at 5 y Median survival 47 mo in ITC group
Lund et al: present series (31 endoscopic, 78 open, ± radiotherapy)	109	21 mo (median)	N/A	N/A	ESS: 45.6% alive at 5 y Open:10–24% alive at 5 y Median survival 59 vs. 18 mo ESS vs. open

Abbreviations: A&W, alive and well; ESS, endoscopic sinus surgery; ITC, intention to cure; mo, month(s); N/A, not available or applicable; y, year(s).
Source: Modified from reference 8 with permission of *Rhinology*.

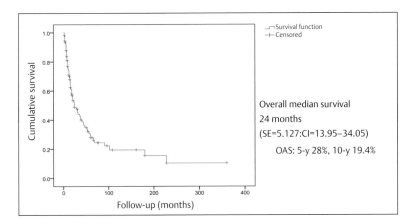

Fig. 15.29 Kaplan–Meier graph of overall survival of 109 sinonasal malignant melanoma patients.

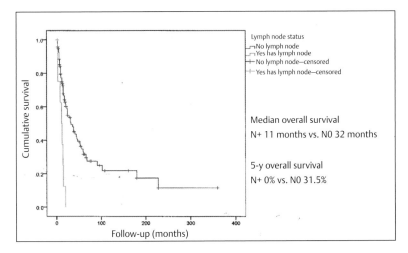

Fig. 15.30 Kaplan–Meier graph of overall survival comparing cases of sinonasal melanoma with lymph node involvement (N+) at diagnosis to those without (N0).

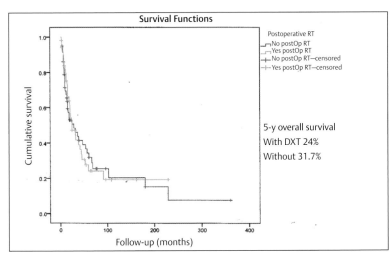

Fig. 15.31 Kaplan–Meier graph of overall survival comparing postoperative radiotherapy with no postoperative radiotherapy.

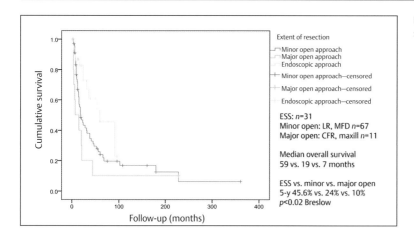

Fig. 15.32 Kaplan–Meier graph of overall survival comparing surgical approaches.

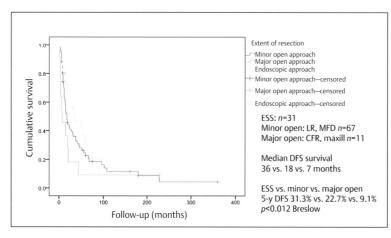

Fig. 15.33 Kaplan–Meier graph of disease-free survival comparing surgical approaches.

shown comparable, if not improved, outcomes with endoscopic techniques for MMM when compared with open approaches.[13,22,35,36] Even allowing for selection and surgical bias, which may be of less relevance in this disease, it appears that endoscopic resection does not adversely affect the outcome in selected cases with appropriately skilled surgeons and may even improve survival. A possible explanation may relate to the low morbidity associated with endoscopic procedures in a disease that exhibits an exquisite immunological balance with its host, often an elderly patient. Why this benefit should persist for some years and then disappear is unknown and requires further investigation.

In common with some other series, we have shown no correlation between prognosis and tumor site of origin.[11] Some have suggested that septal lesions fare better, perhaps because they present earlier, while tumors originating in the maxillary or ethmoid sinuses have a worse prognosis than those in the nasal cavity.[13,33,54] This could be a consequence of later presentation or because tumors in these sites are less amenable to resection with clear margins due to orbital or skull base involvement, both likely to be negative predictive factors.[13,35]

In the literature, the most relevant outcome predictors would seem to be the presence of lymph node involvement (as demonstrated in this series) or distant metastasis.[15] Locoregional recurrence frequently precedes the occurrence of metastases and may be an independent predictor of survival in sinonasal melanomas.[55,56]

In our series, radiotherapy was originally administered to patients in whom complete resection with clear margins had not been achieved or for more advanced disease. Our first analysis,[30] although it did not demonstrate a statistical advantage, indicated a trend to benefit that might have been compromised by the numbers of patients available for analysis at that time. Subsequently, from 1996, all patients were given the choice of radiotherapy irrespective of extent of disease and this was accepted by 30 of the 50 patients (60%). Again in this larger cohort, if radiotherapy does have some limited benefit, it fails to show statistical significance. The few series examining the effects of radiation on mucosal melanoma typically used pooled series from all head and neck sites. These are summarized by Krengli et al in a literature analysis.[38] They conclude that postoperative radiotherapy improves local control and recommend its use for unresectable disease, but there is no evidence to show that it alters survival.[38] The series of Moreno et al from the MD Anderson Center retrospectively looked at 58 cases, 33 of which had received postoperative radiotherapy. Although there was no survival benefit, those receiving 54 Gy or more had a statistically lower rate of locoregional recurrence than those receiving 30 to 50 Gy.[15] This further highlights the need for high doses of radiotherapy to achieve any response. This is often limited in sinonasal disease by the close proximity of vital structures such as the optic nerve. Other series that claim benefit with adjuvant radiotherapy are based on small numbers and/or lack statistical proof,[13,32,33,38] and conversely there are several large series, including our own, that do confirm this benefit in local control.[29–31]

The only study to report on radiotherapy as a primary treatment modality resulted in an 18% 5-year survival, lower than in most surgical series.[37]

Insufficient patients have been treated with chemotherapy or vaccines thus far to comment on the likely success in MMM. Various protocols using chemotherapy such as cisplatin and hyperfractionated radiotherapy or iodine 125 have been reported in individual cases.[57,58] In contrast, Eigentler et al were able to perform a meta-analysis on 41 RCTs on palliative treatment in cutaneous melanoma.[59] However, Hocker et al have reviewed some novel techniques based on an increased understanding of the genetics of melanoma, including agents that target the Bcl-2 signaling network.[60] Lotem et al considered the use of interleukin-2 in combination with DNP-modified autologous vaccine in metastatic melanoma[61] and there is also interest in targeting anti-cytotoxic T-lymphocyte antigen (CTLA-4) monoclonal antibodies, either as monotherapy or combined with chemotherapy or vaccines.[62,63] Whether any benefits in skin melanoma can be translated into mucosal disease remains to be seen. Finally, although malignant melanoma is regarded as a molecularly heterogeneous disease, it has been shown that the mucosal tumors show a variable frequency of KIT mutations[64,65] and this may have therapeutic implications for the future with the introduction of new biological agents such as imatinib, sorafinib, and dasatinib.[66,67]

Key Points

- Malignant melanoma is the most capricious and unpredictable of sinonasal tumors.
- Endoscopic resection offers outcomes similar to if not better than those from radical open procedures.
- The role of radiotherapy is unproven.

References

1. Thompson LD, Wieneke JA, Miettinen M. Sinonasal tract and nasopharyngeal melanomas: a clinicopathologic study of 115 cases with a proposed staging system. Am J Surg Pathol 2003;27(5):594–611

2. Holmstrom M, Lund VJ. Malignant melanomas of the nasal cavity after occupational exposure to formaldehyde. Br J Ind Med 1991;48(1):9–11

3. Monticello TM, Morgan KT. Cell proliferation and formaldehyde-induced respiratory carcinogenesis. Risk Anal 1994;14(3):313–319

4. Walrath J, Fraumeni JF Jr. Mortality patterns among embalmers. Int J Cancer 1983;31(4):407–411

5. Cohen Y, Rosenbaum E, Begum S, et al. Exon 15 BRAF mutations are uncommon in melanomas arising in nonsun-exposed sites. Clin Cancer Res 2004;10(10):3444–3447

6. van Dijk M, Sprenger S, Rombout P, et al. Distinct chromosomal aberrations in sinonasal mucosal melanoma as detected by comparative genomic hybridization. Genes Chromosomes Cancer 2003;36(2):151–158

7. Zak FG, Lawson W. The presence of melanocytes in the nasal cavity. Ann Otol Rhinol Laryngol 1974;83(4):515–519

8. Lund VJ, Stammberger H, Nicolai P, et al. European position paper on endoscopic management of tumours of the nose, paranasal sinuses and skull base. Rhinol Suppl 2010;(22):1–143

9. Andersen LJ, Berthelsen A, Hansen HS. Malignant melanoma of the upper respiratory tract and the oral cavity. J Otolaryngol 1992;21(3):180–185

10. Mendenhall WM, Amdur RJ, Hinerman RW, Werning JW, Villaret DB, Mendenhall NP. Head and neck mucosal melanoma. Am J Clin Oncol 2005;28(6):626–630

11. Bachar G, Loh KS, O'Sullivan B, et al. Mucosal melanomas of the head and neck: experience of the Princess Margaret Hospital. Head Neck 2008;30(10):1325–1331

12. Edge SBBD, Compton CC, Fritz AG, Greene FL, Trotti A. AJCC Cancer Staging Manual. 7th ed. New York: Springer; 2010

13. Roth TN, Gengler C, Huber GF, Holzmann D. Outcome of sinonasal melanoma: clinical experience and review of the literature. Head Neck 2010;32(10):1385–1392

14. Chang AE, Karnell LH, Menck HR; The American College of Surgeons Commission on Cancer and the American Cancer Society. The National Cancer Data Base report on cutaneous and noncutaneous melanoma: a summary of 84,836 cases from the past decade. Cancer 1998;83(8):1664–1678

15. Moreno MA, Roberts DB, Kupferman ME, et al. Mucosal melanoma of the nose and paranasal sinuses, a contemporary experience from the M. D. Anderson Cancer Center. Cancer 2010;116(9):2215–2223

16. Thompson AC, Morgan DA, Bradley PJ. Malignant melanoma of the nasal cavity and paranasal sinuses. Clin Otolaryngol Allied Sci 1993;18(1):34–36

17. Goerres GW, Stoeckli SJ, von Schulthess GK, Steinert HC. FDG PET for mucosal malignant melanoma of the head and neck. Laryngoscope 2002;112(2):381–385

18. Shah JP, Huvos AG, Strong EW. Mucosal melanomas of the head and neck. Am J Surg 1977;134(4):531–535

19. Breslow A. Thickness, cross-sectional areas and depth of invasion in the prognosis of cutaneous melanoma. Ann Surg 1970;172(5):902–908

20. Clark WH Jr, From L, Bernardino EA, Mihm MC. The histogenesis and biologic behavior of primary human malignant melanomas of the skin. Cancer Res 1969;29(3):705–727

21. Ballantyne AJ. Malignant melanoma of the skin of the head and neck. An analysis of 405 cases. Am J Surg 1970;120(4):425–431

22. Moreno MA, Hanna EY. Management of mucosal melanomas of the head and neck: did we make any progress? Curr Opin Otolaryngol Head Neck Surg 2010;18(2):101–106

23. Prasad ML, Patel SG, Huvos AG, Shah JP, Busam KJ. Primary mucosal melanoma of the head and neck: a proposal for microstaging localized, Stage I (lymph node-negative) tumors. Cancer 2004;100(8):1657–1664

24. Owens JM, Roberts DB, Myers JN. The role of postoperative adjuvant radiation therapy in the treatment of mucosal

melanomas of the head and neck region. Arch Otolaryngol Head Neck Surg 2003;129(8):864–868

25. Temam S, Mamelle G, Marandas P, et al. Postoperative radiotherapy for primary mucosal melanoma of the head and neck. Cancer 2005;103(2):313–319

26. Howard DJ, Lund VJ, Wei WI. Craniofacial resection for tumors of the nasal cavity and paranasal sinuses: a 25-year experience. Head Neck 2006;28(10):867–873

27. Wagner M, Morris CG, Werning JW, Mendenhall WM. Mucosal melanoma of the head and neck. Am J Clin Oncol 2008;31(1):43–48

28. Penel N, Mallet Y, Mirabel X, Van JT, Lefebvre JL. Primary mucosal melanoma of head and neck: prognostic value of clear margins. Laryngoscope 2006;116(6):993–995

29. Nandapalan V, Roland NJ, Helliwell TR, Williams EM, Hamilton JW, Jones AS. Mucosal melanoma of the head and neck. Clin Otolaryngol Allied Sci 1998;23(2):107–116

30. Lund VJ, Howard DJ, Harding L, Wei WI. Management options and survival in malignant melanoma of the sinonasal mucosa. Laryngoscope 1999;109(2 Pt 1):208–211

31. Patel SG, Prasad ML, Escrig M, et al. Primary mucosal malignant melanoma of the head and neck. Head Neck 2002;24(3):247–257

32. Kingdom TT, Kaplan MJ. Mucosal melanoma of the nasal cavity and paranasal sinuses. Head Neck 1995;17(3):184–189

33. Dauer EH, Lewis JE, Rohlinger AL, Weaver AL, Olsen KD. Sinonasal melanoma: a clinicopathologic review of 61 cases. Otolaryngol Head Neck Surg 2008;138(3):347–352

34. Zada G, Kelly DF, Cohan P, Wang C, Swerdloff R. Endonasal transsphenoidal approach for pituitary adenomas and other sellar lesions: an assessment of efficacy, safety, and patient impressions. J Neurosurg 2003;98(2):350–358

35. Lund V, Howard DJ, Wei WI. Endoscopic resection of malignant tumors of the nose and sinuses. Am J Rhinol 2007;21(1):89–94

36. Nicolai P, Battaglia P, Bignami M, et al. Endoscopic surgery for malignant tumors of the sinonasal tract and adjacent skull base: a 10-year experience. Am J Rhinol 2008;22(3):308–316

37. Gilligan D, Slevin NJ. Radical radiotherapy for 28 cases of mucosal melanoma in the nasal cavity and sinuses. Br J Radiol 1991;64(768):1147–1150

38. Krengli M, Jereczek-Fossa BA, Kaanders JH, Masini L, Beldì D, Orecchia R. What is the role of radiotherapy in the treatment of mucosal melanoma of the head and neck? Crit Rev Oncol Hematol 2008;65(2):121–128

39. Combs SE, Konkel S, Thilmann C, Debus J, Schulz-Ertner D. Local high-dose radiotherapy and sparing of normal tissue using intensity-modulated radiotherapy (IMRT) for mucosal melanoma of the nasal cavity and paranasal sinuses. Strahlenther Onkol 2007;183(2):63–68

40. Fernández JM, Santaolalla F, Del Rey AS, Martínez-Ibargüen A, González A, Iriarte MR. Preliminary study of the lymphatic drainage system of the nose and paranasal sinuses and its role in detection of sentinel metastatic nodes. Acta Otolaryngol 2005;125(5):566–570

41. Stárek I, Koranda P, Benes P. Sentinel lymph node biopsy: A new perspective in head and neck mucosal melanoma? Melanoma Res 2006;16(5):423–427

42. Vermeeren L, Valdés Olmos RA, Klop WM, et al. SPECT/CT for sentinel lymph node mapping in head and neck melanoma. Head Neck 2011;33(1):1–6

43. Andrés R, Mayordomo JI, Visus C, et al. Prognostic significance and diagnostic value of protein S-100 and tyrosinase in patients with malignant melanoma. Am J Clin Oncol 2008;31(4):335–339

44. Brandwein MS, Rothstein A, Lawson W, Bodian C, Urken ML. Sinonasal melanoma. A clinicopathologic study of 25 cases and literature meta-analysis. Arch Otolaryngol Head Neck Surg 1997;123(3):290–296

45. Bridger AG, Smee D, Baldwin MA, Kwok B, Bridger GP. Experience with mucosal melanoma of the nose and paranasal sinuses. ANZ J Surg 2005;75(4):192–197

46. Huang SF, Liao CT, Kan CR, Chen IH. Primary mucosal melanoma of the nasal cavity and paranasal sinuses: 12 years of experience. J Otolaryngol 2007;36(2):124–129

47. Trapp TK, Fu YS, Calcaterra TC. Melanoma of the nasal and paranasal sinus mucosa. Arch Otolaryngol Head Neck Surg 1987;113(10):1086–1089

48. Stern SJ, Guillamondegui OM. Mucosal melanoma of the head and neck. Head Neck 1991;13(1):22–27

49. Guzzo M, Grandi C, Licitra L, Podrecca S, Cascinelli N, Molinari R. Mucosal malignant melanoma of head and neck: forty-eight cases treated at Istituto Nazionale Tumori of Milan. Eur J Surg Oncol 1993;19(4):316–319

50. Loree TR, Mullins AP, Spellman J, North JH Jr, Hicks WL Jr. Head and neck mucosal melanoma: a 32-year review. Ear Nose Throat J 1999;78(5):372–375

51. Pandey M, Abraham EK, Mathew A, Ahamed IM. Primary malignant melanoma of the upper aero-digestive tract. Int J Oral Maxillofac Surg 1999;28(1):45–49

52. Prasad ML, Busam KJ, Patel SG, Hoshaw-Woodard S, Shah JP, Huvos AG. Clinicopathologic differences in malignant melanoma arising in oral squamous and sinonasal respiratory mucosa of the upper aerodigestive tract. Arch Pathol Lab Med 2003;127(8):997–1002

53. Narasimhan K, Kucuk O, Lin HS, et al. Sinonasal mucosal melanoma: a 13-year experience at a single institution. Skull Base 2009;19(4):255–262

54. McLean N, Tighiouart M, Muller S. Primary mucosal melanoma of the head and neck. Comparison of clinical presentation and histopathologic features of oral and sinonasal melanoma. Oral Oncol 2008;44(11):1039–1046

55. Clifton N, Harrison L, Bradley PJ, Jones NS. Malignant melanoma of nasal cavity and paranasal sinuses: report of 24 patients and literature review. J Laryngol Otol 2011;125(5):479–485

56. Lee SP, Shimizu KT, Tran LM, Juillard G, Calcaterra TC. Mucosal melanoma of the head and neck: the impact of local control on survival. Laryngoscope 1994;104(2):121–126

57. Albertsson M, Tennvall J, Andersson T, Biörklund A, Elner A, Johansson L. Malignant melanoma of the nasal cavity and nasopharynx treated with cisplatin and accelerated hyperfractionated radiation. Melanoma Res 1992;2(2):101–104

58. De Meerleer GO, Vermeersch H, van Eijkeren M, et al. Primary sinonasal mucosal melanoma: three different therapeutic approaches to inoperable local disease or recurrence and a review of the literature. Melanoma Res 1998;8(5):449–457

59. Eigentler TK, Caroli UM, Radny P, Garbe C. Palliative therapy of disseminated malignant melanoma: a systematic review of 41 randomised clinical trials. Lancet Oncol 2003;4(12):748–759

60. Hocker TL, Singh MK, Tsao H. Melanoma genetics and therapeutic approaches in the 21st century: moving from the benchside to the bedside. J Invest Dermatol 2008;128(11):2575–2595

61. Lotem M, Shiloni E, Pappo I, et al. Interleukin-2 improves tumour response to DNP-modified autologous vaccine for the treatment of metastatic malignant melanoma. Br J Cancer 2004;90(4):773–780

62. Weber J. Overcoming immunologic tolerance to melanoma: targeting CTLA-4 with ipilimumab (MDX-010). Oncologist 2008;13(Suppl 4):16–25

63. Nisticò P, Capone I, Palermo B, et al. Chemotherapy enhances vaccine-induced antitumor immunity in melanoma patients. Int J Cancer 2009;124(1):130–139

64. Curtin JA, Fridlyand J, Kageshita T, et al. Distinct sets of genetic alterations in melanoma. N Engl J Med 2005; 353(20):2135–2147
65. Curtin JA, Busam K, Pinkel D, Bastian BC. Somatic activation of KIT in distinct subtypes of melanoma. J Clin Oncol 2006;24(26):4340–4346
66. Woodman SE, Trent JC, Stemke-Hale K, et al. Activity of dasatinib against L576P KIT mutant melanoma: molecular, cellular, and clinical correlates. Mol Cancer Ther 2009;8(8):2079–2085
67. Handolias D, Hamilton AL, Salemi R, et al. Clinical responses observed with imatinib or sorafenib in melanoma patients expressing mutations in KIT. Br J Cancer 2010;102(8):1219–1223

Melanocytic Neuroectodermal Tumor of Infancy

Definition

(ICD-O code 9363/0)

A benign neuroectodermally-derived melanocytic tumor with a predilection for the anterior maxilla of children <1 year old.

Etiology

There is some debate concerning the origin of this tumor but it is now generally agreed to derive from the neural crest. The finding of high levels of urinary vanillylmandelic acid originally supported this,[1] subsequently confirmed by ultrastructural studies.[2,3]

Synonyms

Pigmented ameloblastoma, melanotic ameloblastic odontoma, melanotic prognoma, pigmented epulis, congenital melanocarcinoma.

Incidence

Since melanotic neuroectodermal tumor of infancy (MNTI) was first described by Krompecker in 1918 (congenital melanocarcinoma), around 400 cases have been reported in the literature.[4]

Site

This lesion is found predominantly in the maxilla. Indeed, 80% of all reported cases have affected the premaxilla[5–7] although lesions elsewhere in the skull (15.7%), mandible (6.4%), and oropharynx have been reported.[6,8,9] Other sites include brain, epididymis, thigh, femur, and mediastinum.[10,11]

Diagnostic Features

Clinical Features

The majority of cases reported by Johnson et al and Hupp et al presented within the first year of life and affected boys and girls equally.[5,6] The child presents with a firm painless mass often appearing blue-black through normal mucosa. The lesion grows rapidly to involve the alveolar-buccal sulcus, which may affect suckling, and ultimately the dentition can be displaced. Judging by the literature, these patients more often present to maxillofacial surgeons but may be encountered by ENT, pediatric, and plastic surgeons.[12]

Imaging

CT shows a cystic, lytic mass in the premaxilla that is poorly demarcated and shows varying degrees of bone destruction and dental displacement. Contrast helps to delineate the margins and MRI demonstrates a soft tissue tumor with nonenhancing heterogeneous tissue density.[13,14]

Histological Features and Differential Diagnosis

The tumor has a pigmented surface and may appear to be encapsulated. Microscopically it is composed of two cell populations within a fibrous stroma. One group are large cuboidal epithelioid cells containing melanin granules that line numerous alveolar spaces and the other group are small dark neuroblastlike cells arranged in an alveolar pattern.

Immunohistochemistry is positive for cytokeratin, synaptophysin, HMB45, NSE, epithelial membrane antigen, glial fibrillary acidic protein, and Leu-7.[3,15] De Souza reported diffuse immunoreactivity of melanin-containing epithelioid cells for MDM-2 and a complete absence of p53 expression.[16]

Ultrastructural examination by Cutler et al[8] has revealed three types of melanin granule formation; many cells had a single cilium, and cell junctions of the "close" or "modified-light" type were seen but no desmosomes were found. This supports the concept that MNTI arises from neural crest cells.

In the study of Barrett et al[3] on 8 cases, the most mitotically active tumor also showed the most aggressive behavior and was the only one to show membrane expression of CD99 and have a detectable Ki-67-positive fraction.

The differential diagnosis includes metastatic neuroblastoma, primitive neuroectodermal tumor, and rhabdomyosarcoma, but MNTI may be distinguished from these by its biphasic cell population together with the presence of pigmentation.[17]

Natural History

These lesions are generally considered benign but are capable of rapid expansion and a high local recurrence of up to 36% despite surgical excision,[8,13,18] possibly due to a multifocal origin. Malignant transformation may occur (estimated at between 2% and 7%)[8,13] so the possibility of locoregional and systemic metastases should be considered and can lead to death, as in a case in a 4-month-old boy described by Dehner et al.[2] The frequency of cervical metastases was found to be 6.6% in a review of 195 cases by Pettinato et al.[19]

Treatment and Outcome

In the past simple curettage was undertaken, which almost certainly accounted for the local "recurrence." Wide excision with clear margins should be curative but may have a deleterious effect on the dentition. Thus, partial maxillectomy and midfacial degloving approaches have been utilized with later reconstruction if required.

Radiotherapy and combination chemotherapy (vincristine, ifosfamide, etoposide, cyclophosphamide, doxorubicin, and dactinomycin) have been used for recurrence, after margin-positive resection,[20,21] or when the lesion is not amenable to resection.[4]

Although many authors report local recurrences, some long-term disease-free cases are described up to 10 years.[21] A 20% recurrence rate has been reported, mainly in the maxilla, usually within the first 4 months of life and mostly within 4 weeks of surgery.[4] Recurrence after 6 months of age is exceptional but has been reported.[22] Chaudhary and colleagues reported a mean survival time of 189.7 months (95% confidence interval, 103.7–157.8 months) in a group of 18 patients.[23]

References

1. Borello ED, Gorlin RJ. Melanotic neuroectodermal tumor of infancy—a neoplasm of neural crese origin. Report of a case associated with high urinary excretion of vanilmandelic acid. Cancer 1966;19(2):196–206
2. Dehner LP, Sibley RK, Sauk JJ Jr, et al. Malignant melanotic neuroectodermal tumor of infancy: a clinical, pathologic, ultrastructural and tissue culture study. Cancer 1979;43(4):1389–1410
3. Barrett AW, Morgan M, Ramsay AD, Farthing PM, Newman L, Speight PM. A clinicopathologic and immunohistochemical analysis of melanotic neuroectodermal tumor of infancy. Oral Surg Oral Med Oral Pathol Oral Radiol Endod 2002;93(6):688–698
4. Kruse-Lösler B, Gaertner C, Bürger H, Seper L, Joos U, Kleinheinz J. Melanotic neuroectodermal tumor of infancy: systematic review of the literature and presentation of a case. Oral Surg Oral Med Oral Pathol Oral Radiol Endod 2006;102(2):204–216
5. Hupp JR, Topazian RG, Krutchkoff DJ. The melanotic neuroectodermal tumor of infancy. Report of two cases and review of the literature. Int J Oral Surg 1981;10(6):432–446
6. Johnson RE, Scheithauer BW, Dahlin DC. Melanotic neuroectodermal tumor of infancy. A review of seven cases. Cancer 1983;52(4):661–666
7. Tan O, Atik B, Ugras S. Melanotic neuroectodermal tumor in a newborn. Int J Pediatr Otorhinolaryngol 2005; 69(10):1441–1444
8. Cutler LS, Chaudhry AP, Topazian R. Melanotic neuroectodermal tumor of infancy: an ultrastructural study, literature review, and reevaluation. Cancer 1981;48(2):257–270
9. Matsumoto M, Sakuma J, Suzuki K, Kawakami M, Sasaki T, Kodama N. Melanotic neuroectodermal tumor of infancy in the skull: case report and review of the literature. Surg Neurol 2005;63(3):275–280
10. Misugi K, Okajima H, Newton W. Mediastinal origin of a melanotic prognoma or retinal anlage tumour. Ultrastructural evidence for neural crest origin. Cancer 1965;18:477–484
11. Elli M, Aydin O, Pinarli FG, et al. Melanotic neuroectodermal tumor of infancy of the femur. Pediatr Hematol Oncol 2006;23(7):579–586
12. el-Saggan A, Bang G, Olofsson J. Melanotic neuroectodermal tumour of infancy arising in the maxilla. J Laryngol Otol 1998;112(1):61–64
13. Fowler DJ, Chisholm J, Roebuck D, Newman L, Malone M, Sebire NJ. Melanotic neuroectodermal tumor of infancy: clinical, radiological, and pathological features. Fetal Pediatr Pathol 2006;25(2):59–72
14. Nazira B, Gupta H, Chaturvedi AK, Rao SA, Jena A. Melanotic neuroectodermal tumor of infancy: discussion of a case and a review of the imaging findings. Cancer Imaging 2009;9:121–125
15. Nelson ZL, Newman L, Loukota RA, Williams DM. Melanotic neuroectodermal tumour of infancy: an immunohistochemical and ultrastructural study. Br J Oral Maxillofac Surg 1995;33(6):375–380
16. de Souza PE, Merly F, Maia DM, Castro WH, Gomez RS. Cell cycle-associated proteins in melanotic neuroectodermal tumor of infancy. Oral Surg Oral Med Oral Pathol Oral Radiol Endod 1999;88(4):466–468
17. Mills S, Gaffey M, Frierson H. Tumors of the Upper Aerodigestive Tract and Ear. Atlas of Tumor Pathology. Third Series. Fascicle 26. Washington: Armed Forces Institute of Pathology; 2000:138
18. Brekke JH, Gorlin RJ. Melanotic neuroectodermal tumor of infancy. J Oral Surg 1975;33(11):858–865
19. Pettinato G, Manivel JC, d'Amore ES, Jaszcz W, Gorlin RJ. Melanotic neuroectodermal tumor of infancy. A reexamination of a histogenetic problem based on immunohistochemical, flow cytometric, and ultrastructural study of 10 cases. Am J Surg Pathol 1991;15(3):233–245
20. Woessmann W, Neugebauer M, Gossen R, Blütters-Sawatzki R, Reiter A. Successful chemotherapy for melanotic neuroectodermal tumor of infancy in a baby. Med Pediatr Oncol 2003;40(3):198–199
21. Neven J, Hulsbergen-van der Kaa C, Groot-Loonen J, de Wilde PC, Merkx MA. Recurrent melanotic neuroectodermal tumor of infancy: a proposal for treatment protocol with surgery and adjuvant chemotherapy. Oral Surg Oral Med Oral Pathol Oral Radiol Endod 2008;106(4):493–496
22. Omodaka S, Saito R, Kumabe T, et al. Melanotic neuroectodermal tumor of the brain recurring 12 years after complete remission: case report. Brain Tumor Pathol 2010;27(1):51–57
23. Chaudhary A, Wakhlu A, Mittal N, Misra S, Mehrotra D, Wakhlu AK. Melanotic neuroectodermal tumor of infancy: 2 decades of clinical experience with 18 patients. J Oral Maxillofac Surg 2009;67(1):47–51

16 Germ Cell Tumors

Germ cell tumors are rare in the head and neck, and histologically are almost identical to those that arise in the gonads (Table 16.1).

Immature Teratoma

(ICD-O code 9080/3)

Incidence and Site

Teratomas are not uncommon tumors in children, but the vast majority arise in the sacrococcygeal area and Tapper and Lack[1] reviewing a 54-year experience from a children's hospital in Boston, Massachusetts, found only 5% of the tumors arising in the head and neck from a total of 254 patients. None arose from the sinonasal region and only a single case from the nasopharynx. Further cases of nasopharyngeal teratoma have been described[2,3] and additionally two in the maxillary sinus[4] and in the ethmoid sinus[5] and sphenoid sinus.[6]

The subsequent appearance of both embryonal carcinoma[7] and squamous cell carcinoma[8] arising in inadequately resected immature teratomas has been reported. Lack's review of 16 cases in the head and neck details four large tumors that involve both oropharynx and nasopharynx and adjacent tissues. One of these cases was attached by a narrow stalk to the posterior nasal septum and presented as a polypoidal mass passing through the nasopharynx and into the oropharynx as far inferiorly as the laryngeal inlet.

Diagnostic Features

Clinical Features

Teratoma is most commonly seen in newborn children as, by the time of birth, they have often attained a significant size to produce either a visible mass or symptoms related to the site of origin, such as respiratory distress, feeding difficulties, and dysphagia. An emergency tracheostomy is frequently necessary in the neonates with the larger cervical tumors and those affecting the oropharynx and nasopharynx.

Histological Features

Teratomas of the head and neck have been reported in a large range of sizes ranging from 3 to 11 cm in diameter and may be solid or cystic. Those involving the sinonasal tract and nasopharynx have been described as containing mature and immature tissues from the three embryonic germ layers, and the variable immature element is mostly neuroepithelial. In addition to the primitive neuroepithelial tissue, the cystic spaces may be lined with ciliated pseudostratified epithelium. Cellular atypia are not common, although mitotic figures are usually seen in the immature areas. Immature teratomas are rarely malignant but, as mentioned above, malignant transformation has to be excluded, particularly following inadequate treatment.

Treatment and Prognosis

The general recommendation for treatment of germ cell malignancies in all sites of the body is for complete surgical resection when possible. Both the treatment and prognosis ultimately depend on the age of the patient, the site of involvement, and the tumor histology. Examples of immature and mature teratoma tissue in cervical lymph nodes have been described, but it does not seem to alter the favorable prognosis if complete surgical resection is achieved. The pathologist has an important role in germ cell tumors of accurate determination of histological grade, adequate resection, and the presence or absence of unfavorable histological elements such as embryonal carcinoma. However, in neonates and infants, the histological grade of immature teratomas arising in the head and neck region does not seem to be a reliable predictor of biological behavior.

Teratoma with Malignant Transformation

(ICD-O code 9084/3)

In the sinonasal tract and nasopharynx, teratomas with malignant transformation are extremely rare. This neoplasm has a somatic malignancy in addition to benign tissue elements of all three germinal layers and, as described above, both embryonal carcinoma[5] and squamous carcinoma[6] have been reported. These cases require adjuvant treatment with radiotherapy and chemotherapy on an individual basis in relation to the site, extent, and type of malignancy.

Table 16.1 Germ cell neoplasms

Immature teratomas	ICD-O 9080/3
Teratoma with malignant transformation	ICD-O 9084/3
Sinonasal yolk sac tumor	ICD-O 9071/3
Sinonasal teratocarcinoma	No ICD-O code
Mature teratoma	ICD-O 9080/0
Dermoid cyst	ICD-O 9084/0

Sinonasal Yolk Sac Tumor (Endodermal Sinus Tumor)

(ICD-O code 9071/3)

These extremely rare tumors in the sinonasal tract have identical histology to the yolk sac tumor (endodermal sinus tumor) of the gonads. The two reported cases have occurred in adults aged 34 and 43 years. In one of these adult cases, there was an accompanying area of sinonasal nonkeratinizing carcinoma.

Sinonasal Teratocarcinosarcoma

Definition

(No ICD-O code)

As the name implies, this is a malignant sinonasal lesion with features of both teratoma and carcinosarcoma. Most commonly, it has both epithelial elements which are benign as well as malignant. There are mesenchymal and neural elements including blastomatous immature tissues. Seminoma, embryonal carcinoma, and choriocarcinoma features are absent.

Etiology

There are no known etiological factors and, contrary to the tumor currently being classified under germ cell tumors, recent work would suggest that it is unlikely to be of germ cell origin. In a detailed analysis of the ultrastructural and immunohistochemical evidence, Shimazaki et al[9] feel that sinonasal teratocarcinoma is essentially a neuroectodermal tumor with a capacity to differentiate into divergent types of somatic cells.

Incidence and Site

There are ~60 cases to date in the literature, with the vast majority arising in the nasal cavity with the ethmoid and maxillary sinuses subsequently involved. The tumor has a marked male predominance and is exclusive to adults, being described up to an age of 79 years.[10–16]

Diagnostic Features

Clinical Features

The commonest symptoms at presentation are nasal obstruction and epistaxis; in contrast to many other tumors within the sinonasal area, **the duration of symptoms in these patients is often short**. In the study by Heffner et al[10] of 20 cases, the duration of symptoms ranged from 2 to 10 weeks. Only two of their patients complained of pain or headache, and only one was associated with proptosis. On examination, the nasal masses have been described as being moderately firm, red to red-purple, with friable and necrotic areas in some cases. Bleeding in association with examination was common.

Imaging

CT and MRI reveal a soft tissue mass with surrounding bony destruction, but no particular imaging features of note.

Histological Features

These tumors show a complex histological pattern with mature and immature glands, benign squamous and malignant poorly differentiated epithelium, and neuroepithelial elements, often with rosettes and neuroblastomalike areas. The mesenchymal areas may range from immature tissues such as cartilage to sarcomas, notably with rhabdomyoblastic differentiation and elements akin to fibrosarcoma. There may be additional small round cells that are difficult to classify.

Immunohistochemical Features

As might be expected in a tumor containing so many different elements, the reported immunohistochemical findings vary considerably, but in general the primitive cells are often positive for cytokeratin, epithelial membrane antigen, vimentin, and neurospecific enolase. The rhabdomyoblast components are positive for desmin, muscle actin (HHF35), α smooth muscle actin, myoglobin, and cytokeratin. Components of squamous cell differentiation may be positive for cytokeratin, epithelial membrane antigen, and neuron-specific enolase. MyoD1 and myogenin may be expressed in the primitive cells, glandular cells, and rhabdomyoblasts. The stroma may contain a small number of S100-positive cells.

Differential Diagnosis

As with so many rare tumors, inadequate biopsy may lead to incorrect diagnosis and the possibilities with this tumor are wide-ranging, varying from olfactory neuroblastoma, undifferentiated carcinoma, adenocarcinoma, malignant salivary gland–type tumors, and adenosquamous carcinoma. Adequate biopsy material is absolutely essential and may require a general anesthetic to allow sufficient material to be obtained.

Treatment and Prognosis

These lesions are highly malignant, presenting with short histories, and are quickly locally aggressive, invading bone, soft tissue, the orbit, the skull base, and the intracranial compartment.[16] The oft-quoted figures of survival from Heffner's clinicopathological study of 20 cases reported in 1984[10] are that the average survival is <2 years, with 60% of patients not surviving beyond 3 years. Spread to regional lymph nodes and distant sites, particularly the lungs, is described in publications from the 1980s and 1990s. However, what is significant in evaluating papers from this period is that these patients have not been treated with complete resection by modern craniofacial surgery followed by appropriate radical radiotherapy plus or minus chemotherapy. It is possible that earlier and accurate diagnosis of the tumor combined with complete resection and postoperative radiotherapy might improve the treatment outcome in these patients. The clinical effectiveness of chemotherapy in the reported cases cannot be evaluated because of the small numbers of patients and inadequate detail.[17]

Mature Teratoma

Definition

(ICD-O code 9080/0)

Mature teratomas of the sinonasal area and skull base are similar to the same lesion within the gonads or other gonadal locations. They are composed of varying amounts of mature tissues that are foreign to the sinonasal site and typically contain tissues derived from three germ layers, but occasionally only two.

Etiology

As with other germ cell tumors, the main discussion is whether they are derived from primordial germ cells or primitive somatic cells that have escaped the control of the normal influence of cell organizers and growth factors.[1]

Synonyms

Benign teratoma and teratoid tumor are the most commonly used synonyms. Hairy polyp and hamartomata have also been used.

Incidence and Site

Teratomas in the head and neck account for ~6% of all teratomas, but mature teratomas in the sinonasal tract are rare. Most of these cases have been described in neonates and older infants with an approximately equal sex distribution.[18] These lesions have been associated with maternal polyhydramnios, fetal malpresentation, prematurity, and stillbirth. They may be diagnosed in the antenatal period by routine ultrasonography. The maxillary sinuses are the most frequently affected areas, but cases originating from the sphenoid sinus and nasopharynx have also been reported.[6,7,19,20]

Diagnostic Features

Clinical Features

Antenatal diagnosis of nasopharyngeal teratomas is uncommon, but the use of antenatal ultrasonography in the diagnosis of various congenital anomalies, especially when the mother presents with polyhydramnios, is well documented. The hydramnios is associated with congenital malformation in ~20% of patients. Eighteen percent of cervical teratomatous lesions are associated with polyhydramnios, but this finding is much rarer in sinonasal and nasopharyngeal teratomas.[21–23] Elevated alpha-fetoprotein (AFP) has been associated with nasopharyngeal teratomas.[24] If the antenatal ultrasonography does show a substantial head and neck mass, the likelihood of perinatal airway obstruction is high and appropriate management is required.

Teratomas have been associated with other congenital deformities of the head and neck, including cleft palate, hemicrania, and anencephaly.[25]

There is some confusion in the older literature with regard to nasopharyngeal dermoids and nasopharyngeal teratomas. Chaudhry et al in 1978 reviewed 113 cases and reported that nasopharyngeal dermoids are frequently pedunculated and attached to the lateral nasopharyngeal wall, or onto the nasopharyngeal aspect of the soft palate, whereas true teratomas were more often larger sessile lesions.[26] More recently, Coppit et al 2000[23] reviewed the literature and presented a case series clarifying the differences between nasopharyngeal teratomas and dermoids.

We have only one case of mature teratoma that impinged on the nasal cavity via the infratemporal and pterygopalatine fossae. This was in a young man who had previously had a teratoma of the parotid treated as a young child and then re-presented with nasal obstruction 12 years later.

Imaging

In addition to antenatal ultrasonography, CT and MRI scanning of neonates and infants confirms the soft tissue mass filling the nasopharynx and often extending inferiorly to involve the oropharynx, hypopharynx, or larynx to varying degrees, in addition to the parapharyngeal space. CT demonstrates bony dehiscence, and cystic formation and calcification are not uncommon.[27]

Histological Features

Even within the nasopharynx and sinonasal area, teratomas may achieve a considerable size but remain **encapsulated** masses with varying degrees of solid cystic and multiloculated areas. They are composed of widely varying mixtures of tissues such as skin and skin appendages, fat, smooth muscle, bone, cartilage, glial tissue, salivary glands, and so on. Neural tissues are most commonly seen in sinonasal and nasopharyngeal teratomas; prior to the advent of modern imaging, aspiration of the mass to test for CSF and glucose content was advocated.

Differential Diagnosis

Although the features of a mature teratoma are not usually particularly difficult, the differential diagnoses include intranasal glioma, meningoencephalocele, encephalocele, congenital rhabdomyosarcoma, hemangioma, neurofibromatosis, and lymphatic malformations. High-quality scanning should discern the important differences between these lesions.

Treatment and Prognosis

With the possibility of prenatal diagnosis, there are multiple reports of planned deliveries, mainly by cesarean section, that indicate the importance of careful planning to improve the outcome for the affected neonate. The size of the lesion and the compromise of the airway, along with any other congenital anomalies, determine whether the maternal fetal circulation has to be maintained while a tracheostomy is undertaken, or whether endotracheal intubation or simple observation are the most appropriate forms of management. Coppit et al[23] noted that all nasopharyngeal cases associated with polyhydramnios required either intubation or tracheostomy.

Once an adequate airway is established, treatment of these lesions is by complete surgical excision. The majority of smaller lesions can be resected transorally and transpalatally, but meticulous dissection external to the capsule of the lesion is required as those cases reported with recurrence in the literature are felt to be a consequence of inadequate resection of the original tumor. Larger nasopharyngeal lesions involving the oropharynx, hypopharynx, and parapharyngeal space may require combined exposure through the neck, in addition to transorally. One of the authors, D.J.H., has personal experience of three patients presenting as infants with similar large, immature teratomas occupying the parapharyngeal space and involving both oropharynx and nasopharynx as far as the skull base. The patients presented at the ages of 1 week, 6 weeks, and 2 months, and all were treated by complete excision via an upper cervical approach. All three patients were alive and well at follow-up at 10 years with no significant functional or aesthetic deficit.

The extremely rare sinonasal lesions can be removed by midfacial degloving, which avoids any subsequent facial scars in the child. This was the surgical approach utilized in our single case in 2003 without evidence of recurrence to date.

The prognosis is related directly to obtaining clear surgical margins and there have been no subsequent reported malignancies in sinonasal and nasopharyngeal teratomas.[24] Reported deaths are usually attributable to associated congenital anomalies,[23] although a single death from a nasopharyngeal teratoma is reported.[28]

Dermoid Cyst

Definition

(ICD-O code 9084/0)

Dermoid cysts are benign developmental lesions derived from both ectoderm and mesoderm, but with no endodermal component. Keratinizing squamous epithelium is usually present along with dermal derivatives such as sweat and sebaceous glands, hair follicles, smooth muscle, and adipose tissue.

Etiology

Dermoid cysts of the head and neck are considered to be of the congenital inclusion type, forming along the lines of embryological fusion and containing both dermal and epidermal derivatives. Many embryogenetic theories have been proposed concerning the etiology of dermoid cysts, but none of these have been absolutely verified. Similar theories have been proposed for other anatomical lesions in the area, including gliomas and encephaloceles.

Several examples of familial cases have been reported, initially by New and Erich in 1937 and by Khan and Gibb, who described four members of the same family who were affected.[29,30]

Synonyms

The terms dermoid, cystic dermoid, nasal dermoid sinus cyst, and pediatric dermoid cyst are all used in the literature.

Incidence and Site

Approximately 10% of all dermoids arise in the head and neck region and have a male predominance in most significant series. Approximately one-third are present at birth and around one-half are detected in children before the age of 6 years.[31] Dermoid cysts involving the nose comprise ~3% of all dermoids.[32] The most commonly reported sites in the head and neck area are periorbital, nasal, submental, and suprasternal.[33–36] While they present most commonly in the subcutaneous tissue of the supraorbital ridge, in the nose the prenasal space present during development extends from the skull base to the nasal tip, and hence while the dermoids occur most commonly over the bridge of the nose in the midline, the glabella, nasal septum, nasal tip, and columella may also present with these lesions. A few cases have been reported originating from the paranasal sinuses.[36]

We have a small cohort of 7 cases, 3 originating in the orbit, 3 in the nose, and 1 affecting the sphenoid.

Essentially, ectodermal tissue is retained along the lines of closure at the junctions of bone, soft tissues, and embryonic membranes.[37] The cartilaginous nasal capsule is present at the second month of intrauterine life and delineates the prenasal space extending from the skull base to the nasal tip. The prenasal space is also between the membranous ossification centers of the nasal bones. Diverticula of dura project anteriorly through the fonticulus frontalis and may extend inferiorly in these prenasal space with or without accompanying neural tissues. These diverticula may come into contact with the skin and normally regress with time. It is postulated that incomplete regression leaves ectodermal residue in either the prenasal or nasofrontal region at any point from the foramen cecum to the tip of the nose. The inherent problems with dermoid cysts in these areas lie in their possible intracranial extension. The frequency of intracranial extension varies considerably in the literature of those substantially reported series, probably as a result of varying imaging capabilities in the older series and whether or not there was contact with an intact skull base, the dura mater, or extension into the falx cerebri. Denoyelle et al[31] noted a variation between 4% and 45% in 8 reported series of nasal dermoid cysts in children. The cyst developing in the periorbital region appears along the naso-optic groove between the maxillary and mandibular processes during embryonal closure.

The most widely accepted theory of dermoid formation was first presented by Grunvald in 1910 and later expanded on by Bradley,[38] who termed it the cranial theory in 1983.

Diagnostic Features

Clinical Features

By far the commonest presentation of a nasal dermoid is a palpable mass overlying the nasal bridge, glabella, or nasal tip. Approximately half will have an accompanying obvious midline fistula opening onto dorsal skin, and Denoyell et al[31] reported 36% of their patients as being diagnosed following local infections producing fistulization on the lateral aspect of the nose. This has been our own experience (**Fig. 16.1**). In a small percentage of cases, infection of the cyst has followed nasal injury. Although diagnosis has followed intracranial complications, including meningitis, cerebral abscess, and cavernous sinus thrombosis, these events are rare and are not described in most series.[39,40] Additionally, the frequency of these patients presenting with associated multiple congenital anomalies also varies greatly in the literature, with 5% in Denoyelle's series of 49 patients and 41% reported by Wardinsky et al.[31,39] The only specific syndrome associated with nasal dermoid cysts has been the case of Gorlin's syndrome. This autosomal dominant multisystem disorder is characterized by multiple basal cell nevi, cysts of the jaw, skeletal anomalies, and a variety of other defects. The author has postulated that the common tissue of origin between basal cell nevi, cysts of the jaw, and dermoid cysts bodes an association of the two rare conditions is probably not a chance occurrence. Bradley

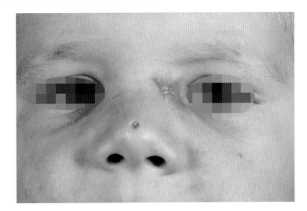

Fig. 16.1 Clinical photograph of a 4-year-old child with a fistula in the left medial canthus where dacrocystorhinostomy had been performed, and a fistula on the nasal tip.

in 1983[38] concluded that the appearance of a sinus or fistula on the nasal dorsal skin gave no indication of the potential superior extension, but Paller et al[41] suggested that patients with a visible ostium had a higher risk of cranial involvement (44%) than those with an isolated cystic mass (10%). Denoyelle et al[31] found that only 5 out of 26 patients with a sinus or fistula ostium had superior extensions (19%) **so this simple clinical sign is not a reliable indication on intracranial extension.**

In addition to a palpable mass, nasal sinus, or fistula, there may be actual broadening of the nasal bridge and notable widening of the nasal septum on intranasal examination. In addition to purulent discharge from any ostia, there may be surrounding cellulitis. Keratin debris and sebum may fill the lumen of any ostia and the underlying cyst may be palpable varying from soft and fluctuant to firm.

Of our 7 cases, there were 4 males and 3 females, aged 3–68 years, of whom 4 were children (**Table 16.2**). Four presented with a nasal mass, three of whom had fistulas, two on the tip of the nose and one iatrogenically created by a misguided dacrocystorhinostomy (**Fig. 16.1**). The others presented to ophthalmologists with displacement of the globe (**Fig. 16.2**).

Imaging

Bearing in mind the variability of clinical features, the detection of any intracranial extension relies heavily on imaging. Prior to the 1980s, reports detailed mainly facial tomographic studies coupled at times with fistulography. In the last three decades, CT scanning, including axial and coronal planes, has been increasingly used, but is now generally supplemented by MRI in all three planes. **A combination of CT, particularly using bony windows, and MRI now allows accurate assessment in the majority of patients in deciding whether extension reaches the skull base or dura, or whether there is any rare intradural component. This remains an important**

Table 16.2 Dermoid cysts: personal series

Age (y)/Sex	Presenting lesion	Site	Surgical approach	Long-term follow-up
3/M	Nasal mass affecting bridge and septum. Fistula on nasal tip	Nasal bridge from tip to crista galli	MFD, revision 8 mo later via external rhinoplasty	A&W 20 y
4/F	Nasal obstruction	Nasal bridge and septum	MFD	A&W 5 y
8/M	Nasal obstruction and fistula	Nasal bridge and septum	MFD	A&W 7 y
29/M	Nasal obstruction	Sphenoid	Craniotomy	A&W 17 y
10/F	Mass in medial canthus with fistula after 3 DCRs	Orbit	External frontoethmoidectomy	A&W 19 y
27/M	Orbital mass	Orbit	Lateral craniotomy	A&W 14 y
68/F	Orbital mass displacing eye	Orbit	Lateral craniotomy	A&W 4 y

Abbreviations: A&W, alive and well; DCR, dacrocystorhinostomy; F, female; M, male; MFD, midfacial degloving; mo, month(s); y, year(s).

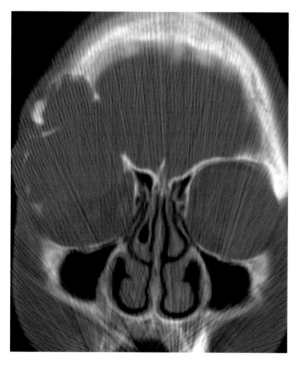

Fig. 16.2 Coronal CT showing a large dermoid cyst in the right upper lateral orbit displacing the eye.

point in what is often a neonatal or infant diagnosis as the interpretation of the skull base here is not always easy. The ossification process of the perpendicular plate of the ethmoid initially appears in its central section as tissue that extends upward and forward toward the crista galli process. These changes occur in children up to the age of 5 years and can be interpreted as an intracranial extension.[42]

The accepted criteria for evidence of intracranial extension include bifidity of the crista galli and enlargement of the foramen cecum according to Pensler et al who felt that **these criteria are particularly conclusive if they are absent**.[43] The variability of imaging studies may in itself explain the marked variation among reported series detailing intracranial extension rates. It may also explain why several series report negative findings for extension on intracranial exploration. Irrespective of the results from historical series, **a combination of MRI and CT with bony windows is now the standard of care** to confirm any suspected intracranial extension so as to avoid any unnecessary intracranial procedures with their attendant risks. Bradley et al reported a 5% incidence of postsurgical epilepsy.[44]

Histological Features

On average, the cystic lesion extends between 1 and 2 cm, although cysts have been reported as large as 12 cm. The lumen generally contains white/yellowish cheeselike material surrounded by mature keratinizing squamous epithelium. Additional cutaneous appendages are usually found in the cyst wall but, unlike with teratoma, there are no endodermal components. This is also in contrast to epidermal inclusion cysts, which macroscopically may resemble dermoid cysts but do not contain any adnexa and occur almost exclusively in adults rather than neonates, infants, and children.

Treatment and Prognosis

All publications agree that complete excision of these lesions is necessary, regardless of the site and extension. Some authors have suggested that, provided there is no intracranial extension, the operation can be deferred until the neonate or infant is older.[30] However, we, in common with others, recommend that cases discovered in neonates or early infancy should be operated on within the first few months of life as the possibility of an infective complication is unpredictable and when they result in severe infection and spontaneous fistulization, this can make subsequent surgery more difficult and give rise to significant scarring at the site of any spontaneous discharge. Intracranial complications from any intracranial extension are extremely rare, but are another reason for considering early operation.

In the earlier literature, the midline and vertical incision on the nasal dorsum was the most frequently used, but its unsatisfactory aesthetic consequences were noted by Bradley, evaluating a series of 32 patients reported in 1982.[45] **A variety of horizontal and H-shaped incisions over the glabella and superior nasal dorsum have also been described, and while they generally give more satisfactory results than vertical midline incisions, these scars may widen significantly with growth of the child and are rarely, if ever, necessary as an excellent exposure can be obtained by an external rhinoplasty approach with medial crura section or an even greater exposure obtained by midfacial degloving, without the need for any facial skin incisions**.

Both the external rhinoplasty approach using a midcolumella and anterior vestibular incision, and the midfacial degloving using a bilateral sublabial incision allow for wide exposure, improved control of any osteotomies, and excision of the tract all the way to the skull base. Occasionally, a combined paracanthal approach may be necessary for cysts located in the nasofrontal angle, but both of these approaches allow for excision of the tract all the way to the skull base and, combined with endoscopic surgery or concomitant use of the operating microscope, dura may be resected and repaired without the need for a craniotomy. A further modification has been advocated by Bartlett et al[46] and Pensler et al[43] whereby the superior aspect of the tract is excised and submitted to histopathology. If the most superior portion is composed of fibrous tissue without any dermoid tissue, an intracranial procedure is not performed. This does not seem to have been associated with higher recurrence rates and regular postoperative MRI surveillance is necessary should there be any doubt. If an intracranial mass is detected, an appropriate intracranial exploration and excision can then be undertaken.

With the use of magnification and these modern surgical approaches, recurrence rates should be <5%,[37] in contrast to recurrence rates of up to 50% reported in the literature from the 1950s and 1960s.[47,48]

We managed to achieve an apparent cure in all of our seven cases though two had had several operations done elsewhere and two required revision surgery by ourselves. The details are shown in Table 16.2.

Key Points

- Dermoid cysts are developmental lesions containing both dermal and epidermal derivatives.
- They most often present in childhood but can occur in later life.
- They commonly affect the orbit and nose where midline structures are affected from the crista galli to the nasal tip.
- Classically they present with a mass, sometimes associated with a fistula.
- CT and MRI are required to assess extent.
- Complete surgical excision of the entire tract must be undertaken to avoid "recurrence" and often requires an external rhinoplasty or midfacial degloving approach.

References

1. Tapper D, Lack EE. Teratomas in infancy and childhood. A 54-year experience at the Children's Hospital Medical Center. Ann Surg 1983;198(3):398–410
2. Rowe LD. Neonatal airway obstruction secondary to nasopharyngeal teratoma. Otolaryngol Head Neck Surg (1979) 1980;88(3):221–226
3. Igarashi Y, Suzuki JI. Nasopharyngeal teratoma. Report of a case. Auris Nasus Larynx 1980;7(2):73–79
4. Guarisco JL, Butcher RB II. Congenital cystic teratoma of the maxillary sinus. Otolaryngol Head Neck Surg 1990;103(6):1035–1038
5. Patchefsky A, Sundmaker W, Marden PA. Malignant teratoma of the ethmoid sinus. Report of a case. Cancer 1968;21(4):714–721
6. Morita T, Fujiki N, Sudo M, Miyata K, Kurata K. Neonatal mature teratoma of the sphenoidal sinus: a case report. Am J Otolaryngol 2000;21(6):398–401
7. Lack EE. Extragonadal germ cell tumors of the head and neck region: review of 16 cases. Hum Pathol 1985;16(1):56–64
8. Kuhn JJ, Schoem SR, Warnock GR. Squamous cell carcinoma arising in a benign teratoma of the maxilla. Otolaryngol Head Neck Surg 1996;114(3):447–452
9. Shimazaki H, Aida S, Tamai S, Miyazawa T, Nakanobou M. Sinonasal teratocarcinosarcoma: ultrastructural and immunohistochemical evidence of neuroectodermal origin. Ultrastruct Pathol 2000;24(2):115–122
10. Heffner DK, Hyams VJ. Teratocarcinosarcoma (malignant teratoma?) of the nasal cavity and paranasal sinuses A clinicopathologic study of 20 cases. Cancer 1984;53(10):2140–2154
11. Fernández PL, Cardesa A, Alós L, Pinto J, Traserra J. Sinonasal teratocarcinosarcoma: an unusual neoplasm. Pathol Res Pract 1995;191(2):166–171, discussion 172–173
12. Pai SA, Naresh KN, Masih K, Ramarao C, Borges AM. Teratocarcinosarcoma of the paranasal sinuses: a clinicopathologic and immunohistochemical study. Hum Pathol 1998;29(7):718–722
13. Terasaka S, Medary MB, Whiting DM, Fukushima T, Espejo EJ, Nathan G. Prolonged survival in a patient with sinonasal teratocarcinosarcoma with cranial extension. Case report. J Neurosurg 1998;88(4):753–756
14. Rotenberg B, El-Hakim H, Lodha A, MacCormick A, Ngan BY, Forte V. Nasopharyngeal teratocarcinosarcoma. Int J Pediatr Otorhinolaryngol 2002;62(2):159–164
15. Wellman M, Kerr PD, Battistuzzi S, Cristante L. Paranasal sinus teratocarcinosarcoma with intradural extension. J Otolaryngol 2002;31(3):173–176
16. Smith SL, Hessel AC, Luna MA, Malpica A, Rosenthal DI, El-Naggar AK. Sinonasal teratocarcinosarcoma of the head and neck: a report of 10 patients treated at a single institution and comparison with reported series. Arch Otolaryngol Head Neck Surg 2008;134(6):592–595

17. Takasaki K, Sakihama N, Takahashi H. A case with sinonasal teratocarcinosarcoma in the nasal cavity and ethmoid sinus. Eur Arch Otorhinolaryngol 2006;263(6):586–591
18. Guarisco JL, Butcher RB II. Congenital cystic teratoma of the maxillary sinus. Otolaryngol Head Neck Surg 1990;103(6):1035–1038
19. Shaheen KW, Cohen SR, Muraszko K, Newman MH. Massive teratoma of the sphenoid sinus in a premature infant. J Craniofac Surg 1991;2(3):140–145
20. Mwang'ombe NJ, Kirongo G, Byakika W. Fronto-ethmoidal teratoma: case report. East Afr Med J 2002;79(2):106–107
21. Mills RP, Hussain SS. Teratomas of the head and neck in infancy and childhood. Int J Pediatr Otorhinolaryngol 1984;8(2):177–180
22. Stocks RM, Egerman RS, Woodson GE, Bower CM, Thompson JW, Wiet GJ. Airway management of neonates with antenatally detected head and neck anomalies. Arch Otolaryngol Head Neck Surg 1997;123(6):641–645
23. Coppit GL III, Perkins JA, Manning SC. Nasopharyngeal teratomas and dermoids: a review of the literature and case series. Int J Pediatr Otorhinolaryngol 2000;52(3):219–227
24. Marras T, Poenaru D, Kamal I. Perinatal management of nasopharyngeal teratoma. J Otolaryngol 1995; 24(5):310–312
25. Abemayor E, Newman A, Bergstrom L, Dudley J, Magidson JG, Ljung BM. Teratomas of the head and neck in childhood. Laryngoscope 1984;94(11 Pt 1):1489–1492
26. Chaudhry AP, Loré JM Jr, Fisher JE, Gambrino AG. So-called hairy polyps or teratoid tumors of the nasopharynx. Arch Otolaryngol 1978;104(9):517–525
27. Carpenter LM, Merten DF. Radiographic manifestations of congenital anomalies affecting the airway. Radiol Clin North Am 1991;29(2):219–240
28. Moriarty AJ, McEwan IP. Pharyngeal teratoma. Anaesthesia 1993;48(9):792–794
29. New G, Erich J. Dermoid cysts of the head and neck. Surg Gynecol Obstet 1937;65:48–55
30. Khan MA, Gibb AG. Median dermoid cysts of the nose familial occurrence. J Laryngol Otol 1970;84(7):709–718
31. Denoyelle F, Ducroz V, Roger G, Garabedian EN. Nasal dermoid sinus cysts in children. Laryngoscope 1997; 107(6):795–800
32. Zerris VA, Annino D, Heilman CB. Nasofrontal dermoid sinus cyst: report of two cases. Neurosurgery 2002; 51(3):811–814, discussion 814
33. Taylor BW, Erich JB, Dockerty MB. Dermoids of the head and neck. Minn Med 1966;49(10):1535–1540
34. McAvoy JM, Zuckerbraun L. Dermoid cysts of the head and neck in children. Arch Otolaryngol 1976;102(9):529–531
35. Torske KR, Benson GS, Warnock G. Dermoid cyst of the maxillary sinus. Ann Diagn Pathol 2001;5(3):172–176
36. Pryor SG, Lewis JE, Weaver AL, Orvidas LJ. Pediatric dermoid cysts of the head and neck. Otolaryngol Head Neck Surg 2005;132(6):938–942
37. Pratt L. Midline cyst of the nasal dorsum: embryological origin and treatment. Laryngoscope 1965;75:968–975
38. Bradley PJ. The complex nasal dermoid. Head Neck Surg 1983;5(6):469–473
39. Maniglia AJ, Goodwin WJ, Arnold JE, Ganz E. Intracranial abscesses secondary to nasal, sinus, and orbital infections in adults and children. Arch Otolaryngol Head Neck Surg 1989;115(12):1424–1429
40. Wardinsky TD, Pagon RA, Kropp RJ, Hayden PW, Clarren SK. Nasal dermoid sinus cysts: association with intracranial extension and multiple malformations. Cleft Palate Craniofac J 1991;28(1):87–95
41. Paller AS, Pensler JM, Tomita T. Nasal midline masses in infants and children. Dermoids, encephaloceles, and gliomas. Arch Dermatol 1991;127(3):362–366
42. Barkovich AJ, Vandermarck P, Edwards MS, Cogen PH. Congenital nasal masses: CT and MR imaging features in 16 cases. AJNR Am J Neuroradiol 1991;12(1):105–116
43. Pensler JM, Bauer BS, Naidich TP. Craniofacial dermoids. Plast Reconstr Surg 1988;82(6):953–958
44. Bradley PJ, Singh SD. Congenital nasal masses: diagnosis and management. Clin Otolaryngol Allied Sci 1982;7(2):87–97
45. Bradley PJ. Results of surgery for nasal dermoids in children. J Laryngol Otol 1982;96(7):627–633
46. Bartlett SP, Lin KY, Grossman R, Katowitz J. The surgical management of orbitofacial dermoids in the pediatric patient. Plast Reconstr Surg 1993;91(7):1208–1215
47. Nydell CC Jr, Masson JK. Dermoid cysts of the nose: a review of 39 cases. Ann Surg 1959;150:1007–1016
48. Taylor P, Erich J. Dermoid cysts of the nose. Mayo Clin Proc 1967;42:488–494

17 Metastases to the Nasal Cavity and Paranasal Sinuses

Definition

A malignant deposit emanating from a site outside the nose and paranasal sinuses. The majority derive from below the clavicle.

Etiology

Distant metastasis from sinonasal cancer is a relatively rare occurrence except in the terminal stages of the disease,[1] but primaries from elsewhere in the body occasionally spread via the bloodstream into the sinonasal region and may be the first indication of the problem.

Incidence

Perls in 1872 first described such a lesion, which involved the sphenoid and arose from the bronchus.[2] A thyroid secondary was reported by Von Eiselberg in 1893, and the first secondary from a renal tumor was reported by Albrecht in 1905.[3,4] The frequency with which they occur is difficult to estimate with any accuracy but they appear to be exceptionally rare. This has been attributed to the paucity of bone marrow or lymph nodes in this area, which are thought to be prerequisites for metastases to occur.[5] The mandible is a much commoner site than the maxilla (93:20 in Batsakis and McBurney's study[5]). Hematogenous spread is thought to occur via the vertebral venous plexus or via (occult) lung metastases.[6]

In our series of 1,635 malignant sinonasal tumors, we have seen 10 cases (**Table 17.1**).

Site

The most frequent source of sinonasal metastases is renal cell carcinoma to the maxilla and ethmoid sinuses.[7] It is estimated that 8% of renal carcinomas present with secondaries in the head and neck, of which half affect the sinonasal region. They made up 80% in Friedmann and Osborn's series of sinonasal metastases, although they were around 42% of those reported in the past 140 years.[8] Tumors from many other sites can also do this—lung, breast, thyroid, gastrointestinal tract, prostate, pancreas, adrenal gland, liver, and skin malignant melanoma (**Table 17.2**).

The most frequent site for metastases is the maxilla, followed by ethmoid, nasal cavity, and frontal with the sphenoid sinuses least affected. Occasionally the alveolar ridge and palate can be affected. Very rarely they can be bilateral.[6,59,89]

Diagnostic Features

Clinical Features

There are no particular features other than epistaxis (especially with renal tumors[19]), nasal obstruction, and pain, followed by a mass or facial swelling and various orbital and neurologic symptoms. These symptoms predate those from the primary in 50% of cases by up to 6 years[90] but can also occur some time after the primary has been treated,[20,91,92] between 10 months and 17 years later. In our group, half presented with the secondary and an unsuspected primary that manifested itself up to 8 months later, and in the other 5 the secondary appeared up to 9 years after the originating primary was diagnosed (**Table 17.1**). The deposit may be associated with cervical lymphadenopathy.[89,93] In the literature a wide age range is reported of 17 months to 80 years and the metastatic deposit can be solitary in the sinonasal region or part of more systemic spread.

Imaging

Imaging shows a generally destructive process with bone erosion and spread into the orbit and anterior cranial fossa (**Fig. 17.1a**). For some, such as intestinal adenocarcinoma, areas of calcification may be seen. In the case of prostatic carcinoma (and sometimes breast), an osteosclerotic process may be seen as well as osteolytic lesions, and the deposit may be in the frontal bone adjacent to the sinus (**Fig. 17.1b**).

Once a metastasis is suspected, full-body screening is needed using CT of the thorax and abdomen and/or PET-CT if available.

Histological Features and Differential Diagnosis

A low threshold for the possibility of a metastasis on the part of the histopathologist is the most important thing. In the case of renal carcinoma, the appearances are quite characteristic, with clusters of large clear vacuolated cells with a high glycogen content. The stroma is vascular, hence the epistaxis. Immunohistochemical confirmation of lipid and glycogen is useful. Cytoplasmic inclusions and microvilli can be seen on electron microscopy.

Resto et al[94] looked for an immunohistochemical distinction between intestinal-type sinonasal adenocarcinoma and metastatic adenocarcinoma of intestinal origin. In a small number of cases they showed that tumors with CK7[+], CK20[+], MUC2[+] immunophenotype are more

Table 17.1 Metastases to the upper jaw: personal cases

No.	Site of origin	Age (y)	Sex	Site	Histology	Relation of primary to secondary	Treatment of secondaries	Outcome
1	Kidney	49	M	Ethmoid	Clear cell adenocarcinoma	Secondary appeared first	External fronto-ethmoidectomy, radiotherapy	Died after 8 y
2	Pancreas	56	M	Ethmoid	Adenocarcinoma	Primary appeared 4 mo later	Craniofacial, radiotherapy	Died after 4 mo
3	Pancreas	61	M	Ethmoid	Anaplastic	Primary appeared 8 mo later	Craniofacial, radiotherapy, chemotherapy	Lost to follow-up, presumed dead
4	Malignant melanoma on skin of back	34	M	Nasal cavity	Malignant melanoma	Secondary appeared 2 y later	Craniofacial, radiotherapy, chemotherapy	Died after 27 mo
5	Malignant melanoma on leg	55	F	Nasal cavity	Malignant melanoma	Secondary appeared 9 y later	Lateral rhinotomy	Alive and well at 6 y
6	Prostate	72	M	Frontal	Poorly dif-ferentiated adenocarcinoma	Secondary appeared first	Chemotherapy	Died after 4 mo
7	Pancreas	55	M	Antroethmoid	Adenocarcinoma	Secondary appeared first	Chemoradio-therapy	Died after 2 mo
8	Skin	24	M	Posterior ethmoid + sphenoid	Malignant melanoma	Secondary appeared 4 y after primary	Lateral rhinotomy + radiotherapy	Died after 4 mo
9	Prostate	59	M	Ethmoid	Adenocarcinoma	Secondary appeared after primary	ESS, radiotherapy	Lost to follow-up
10	Ovary	68	F	Sphenoid	Adenocarcinoma	Secondary appeared after primary	ESS, chemoradio-therapy	Died after 6 mo

Abbreviations: ESS, endoscopic sinus surgery; F, female; M, male; mo, month(s); y, year(s).

likely to be primary sinonasal tumors, whereas tumors with the CK7[-], CK20[+], MUC2[+] profile may be metastases and require further investigation for another primary.

Clear cell tumors may mimic acinic cell carcinoma.

Natural History

In unsuspected cases, the sinonasal lesion may be treated, only for the actual primary to declare itself later. We have had this experience on two occasions with pancreatic adenocarcinomas that declared themselves respectively 4 and 8 months after craniofacial resection in the early part of our series. This raises the question whether it is cost-effective to do full-body screening for all cases of adenocarcinoma not arising in a woodworker.

Treatment and Outcome

Treatment of a metastasis is usually palliative, but with modern surgical and medical oncology, surgical resection, be it endoscopic and even craniofacial resection, together with targeted chemoradiotherapy in addition to the treatment of the primary, may provide a useful period of survival as long as it is without significant morbidity.[95] Having said this, in the past average survival with secondaries affecting the maxillary sinus was reported as 20 months[90] and in most of the case reports no follow-up is given. Survival as short as 1 or 2 months is given after diagnosis of metastases from breast, stomach, and bladder, whereas longer periods of 24 months or more can be seen with kidney, bronchus, and adrenal gland. In our

Table 17.2 Metastases to the upper jaw in the literature

Site	No.	Age		M:F	Histology	Site of metastasis					
		Range (y)	Mean (y)			M	E	F	S	NC	Other
Kidney[7,9-27]	112	34–85	61	2:1	Hypernephroma (clear cell)	38	34	14	5	16	5
Breast[6,9,24,25,28-38]	28	34–83	62	1:27	Adenocarcinoma	15	5	2	3	2	1
Bronchus[9,39-43]	20	38–81	60	6:1	SCC, anaplastic adenoid cystic, adenocarcinoma	6	1	3	2	3	5
Thyroid[9,24,44-49]	18	28–81	–	1:2	Follicular carcinoma papillary	4	2	4	7	1	–
Colon/rectum[9,24,25,50-55]	16	33–78	–	1:1	Adenocarcinoma	7	–	3	3	–	3
Prostate[9,56-65]	16	57–87	68	16:0	Adenocarcinoma	3	2	6	2	3	–
Hepatic[9,66-73]	12	49–71	59	5:1	Hepatocellular	6	–	–	2	4	–
Testicle[9,74-77]	12	24–69	50	12:0	Seminoma, lymphoma, choriocarcinoma	7	1	1	–	1	2
Uterus, cervix, fallopian tube[9,78-81]	11	3/12–77	–	0:11	Leiomyosarcoma, choriocarcinoma	5	–	2	1	–	3
Stomach/esophagus[9,82]	6	45–70	58	1:1	Adenocarcinoma, SCC	4	2	–	–	–	–
Skin[9,83,84]	5	21–47	33	2:1	Malignant melanoma	3	–	–	–	2	–
Bladder[9,85-87]	5	67–80	74	3:2	SCC, transitional cell carcinoma	3	2	–	–	–	–
Adrenal[9,88]	3	17/12, 5, 8	–	1:1	Neuroblastoma	2	–	–	–	–	1
Pancreas[9,27]	2	33,65	–	1:1	Anaplastic	1	1	–	–	1	–
Total	266					104	50	35	25	33	20

Abbreviations: E, ethmoid; F, frontal; M, maxillary; NC, nasal cavity; S, sphenoid; SCC, squamous cell carcinoma.

Notes: Multiple sites are affected in some reports. Harrison and Lund[9] covers the majority of references pre-1990.

10 cases, the outcome was uniformly poor with all dying of disease within a few months of diagnosis (**Table 17.1**).

References

1. Lund VJ. Distant metastases from sinonasal cancer. ORL J Otorhinolaryngol Relat Spec 2001;63(4):212–213
2. Beitrage zur Geschwulstlehre M. Virchow Arch Pathol Anat Histol (Berlin) 1872;56:437–444
3. Von Eiselberg A. Uber Knochen-Metastasen des Schilddrusen Krebses. Verhandlungen der Deutschen Gesellschaft fur Chirurgie 1893;22:255–259
4. Albrecht P. Hypernephrom in Siebeingebeit. Archiv fur Klinische Chirurgie 1905;77:1073
5. Batsakis JG, McBurney TA. Metastatic neoplasms to the head and neck. Surg Gynecol Obstet 1971;133(4):673–677
6. Monserez D, Vlaminck S, Kuhweide R, Casselman J. Symmetrical ethmoidal metastases from ductal carcinoma of the breast, suggesting transcribrosal spread. Acta Otorhinolaryngol Belg 2001;55(3):251–257
7. Miyamoto R, Helmus C. Hypernephroma metastatic to the head and neck. Laryngoscope 1973;83(6):898–905
8. Friedmann I, Osborn D. Pathology of Granulomas and Neoplasms of the Nose and Paranasal Sinuses. Edinburgh: Churchill Livingstone; 1983:300
9. Harrison D, Lund V. Tumours of the Upper Jaw. London: Churchill Livingstone; 1993:125–126
10. Sgouras ND, Gamatsi IE, Porfyris EA, et al. An unusual presentation of a metastatic hypernephroma to the frontonasal region. Ann Plast Surg 1995;34(6):653–656
11. Gottlieb MD, Roland JT Jr. Paradoxical spread of renal cell carcinoma to the head and neck. Laryngoscope 1998;108(9):1301–1305

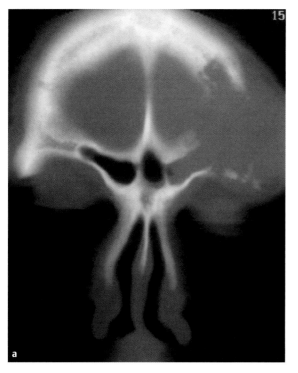
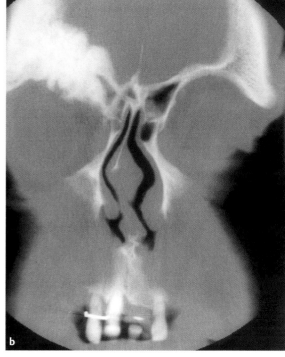

Fig. 17.1a, b

a Metastasis. Coronal CT scan showing a highly destructive lesion of the left frontal and temporal region from adenocarcinoma of the prostate.

b Metastasis. Coronal CT scan showing a metastasis from adenocarcinoma of the prostate in the right frontal region producing massive hyperostosis.

12. Terada N, Hiruma K, Suzuki M, Numata T, Konno A. Metastasis of renal cell cancer to the ethmoid sinus. Acta Otolaryngol Suppl 1998;537(Suppl):82–86
13. Simo R, Sykes AJ, Hargreaves SP, et al. Metastatic renal cell carcinoma to the nose and paranasal sinuses. Head Neck 2000;22(7):722–727
14. Yee LL, Keng CG. A rare case of renal cell carcinoma metastatic to the sinonasal area. Ear Nose Throat J 2001;80(7):462–467
15. Lang EE, Patil N, Walsh RM, Leader M, Walsh MA. A case of renal cell carcinoma metastatic to the nose and tongue. Ear Nose Throat J 2003;82(5):382–383
16. Maheshwari GK, Baboo HA, Patel MH, Usha G. Metastatic renal cell carcinoma involving ethmoid sinus at presentation. J Postgrad Med 2003;49(1):96–97
17. Nason R, Carrau RL. Metastatic renal cell carcinoma to the nasal cavity. Am J Otolaryngol 2004;25(1):54–57
18. Singh I, Khaitan A. Diplopia - an unusual primary manifestation of metastatic renal cell carcinoma. Urol Int 2004;73(3):285–286
19. Lee HM, Kang HJ, Lee SH. Metastatic renal cell carcinoma presenting as epistaxis. Eur Arch Otorhinolaryngol 2005; 262(1):69–71
20. Ziari M, Shen S, Amato RJ, Teh BS. Metastatic renal cell carcinoma to the nose and ethmoid sinus. Urology 2006; 67(1):199
21. Cobo-Dols M, Alés-Díaz I, Villar-Chamorro E, et al. Solitary metastasis in a nasal fossa as the first manifestation of a renal carcinoma. Clin Transl Oncol 2006;8(4):298–300
22. Brener ZZ, Zhuravenko I, Jacob CE, Bergman M. An unusual presentation of renal cell carcinoma with late metastases to the small intestine, thyroid gland, nose and skull base. Nephrol Dial Transplant 2007;22(3):930–932
23. Sawazaki H, Segawa T, Yoshida K, et al. Bilateral maxillary sinus metastasis of renal cell carcinoma: a case report. [Article in Japanese] Hinyokika Kiyo 2007;53(4):231–234
24. Huang HH, Fang TJ, Chang PH, Lee TJ. Sinonasal metastatic tumors in Taiwan. Chang Gung Med J 2008;31(5):457–462
25. Kaminski B, Kobiorska-Nowak J, Bień S. Distant metastases to nasal cavities and paranasal sinuses, from the organs outside the head and neck. [Article in Polish] Otolaryngol Pol 2008;62(4):422–425
26. Doğan S, Can IH, Sayın M, et al. The nasal septum: an unusual presentation of metastatic renal cell carcinoma. J Craniofac Surg 2009;20(4):1204–1206
27. Duque-Fisher CS, Casiano R, Vélez-Hoyos A, Londoño-Bustamante AF. Metastasis to the sinonasal region. [Article in Spanish] Acta Otorrinolaringol Esp 2009;60(6):428–431
28. Wanamaker JR, Kraus DH, Eliachar I, Lavertu P. Manifestations of metastatic breast carcinoma to the head and neck. Head Neck 1993;15(3):257–262
29. Austin JR, Kershiznek MM, McGill D, Austin SG. Breast carcinoma metastatic to paranasal sinuses. Head Neck 1995;17(2):161–165
30. Pitkäranta A, Markkola A, Malmberg H. Breast cancer metastasis presenting as ethmoiditis. Rhinology 2001; 39(2):107–108
31. Monserez D, Vlaminck S, Kuhweide R, Casselman J. Symmetrical ethmoidal metastases from ductal carcinoma of the breast, suggesting transcribrosal spread. Acta Otorhinolaryngol Belg 2001;55(3):251–257
32. Pignataro L, Peri A, Ottaviani F. Breast carcinoma metastatic to the ethmoid sinus: a case report. Tumori 2001; 87(6):455–457

33. Hiromura Y, Dejima K, Imamura Y, Wada Y. Breast carcinoma metastatic to the sphenoid sinus: a case report. Otolaryngol Head Neck Surg 2003;129(6):756–758

34. Asproudis I, Gorezis S, Charalabopoulos K, Stefaniotou M, Peschos D, Psilas K. Breast carcinoma metastasis to the orbit and paranasal sinuses: a case report. Exp Oncol 2004;26(3):246–248

35. Marchioni D, Monzani D, Rossi G, Rivasi F, Presutti L. Breast carcinoma metastases in paranasal sinuses, a rare occurrence mimicking a primary nasal malignancy. case report. Acta Otorhinolaryngol Ital 2004;24(2):87–91

36. Fyrmpas G, Televantou D, Papageorgiou V, Nofal F, Constantinidis J. Unsuspected breast carcinoma presenting as orbital complication of rhinosinusitis. Eur Arch Otorhinolaryngol 2008;265(8):979–982

37. Darouassi Y, Fetohi M, Touiheme N, Ichou M, Abrouq A, Azendour B. Nasosinusal metastasis of a breast cancer in a man. [Article in French] Presse Med 2010; 39(12):1340–1342

38. Liao HS, Hsueh C, Chen SC, Chen IH, Liao CT, Huang SF. Solitary nasal cavity metastasis of breast cancer. Breast J 2010;16(3):321–322

39. Ii T, Doutsu Y, Ashitani J, et al. A case of pulmonary adenocarcinoma in a young man with multiple metastasis to the nasopharynx and paranasal sinuses. [Article in Japanese] Nihon Kyobu Shikkan Gakkai Zasshi 1992;30(10):1884–1888

40. Clarkson JH, Kirkland PM, Mady S. Bronchogenic metastasis involving the frontal sinus and masquerading as a Pott's puffy tumour: a diagnostic pitfall. Br J Oral Maxillofac Surg 2002;40(5):440–441

41. Rombaux P, Hamoir M, Liistro G, Bertrand B. Frontal sinus tumor as the first sign of adenocarcinoma of the lung. Otolaryngol Head Neck Surg 2005;132(5):816–817

42. Huang CT, Hong RL. Nasion swelling as the presenting symptom of lung adenocarcinoma. J Thorac Oncol 2009;4(4):555–558

43. Khorsandi AS, Silberzweig JE, Wenig BM, Urken ML, Holliday RA. Adenoid cystic carcinoma of the trachea metastatic to the nasal cavity: a case report. Ear Nose Throat J 2009;88(12):E9–E11

44. Cumberworth VL, Ohri A, Morrissey G, Stirling R. Late sino-nasal metastasis from follicular thyroid carcinoma. J Laryngol Otol 1994;108(11):1010–1011

45. Yamasoba T, Kikuchi S, Sugasawa M, Higo R, Sasaki T. Occult follicular carcinoma metastasizing to the sinonasal tract. ORL J Otorhinolaryngol Relat Spec 1994;56(4):239–243

46. Freeman JL, Gershon A, Liavaag PG, Walfish PG. Papillary thyroid carcinoma metastasizing to the sphenoid-ethmoid sinuses and skull base. Thyroid 1996;6(1):59–61

47. Altman KW, Mirza N, Philippe L. Metastatic follicular thyroid carcinoma to the paranasal sinuses: a case report and review. J Laryngol Otol 1997;111(7):647–651

48. Coca Pelaz A, Llorente JL, Suárez C. Infratemporal metastasis from occult follicular thyroid carcinoma. J Craniofac Surg 2009;20(1):165–167

49. Nishijima H, Kitahara N, Murata M, Egami N. A case of papillary thyroid carcinoma metastatic to the sphenoid sinus presenting with epistaxis. [Article in Japanese] Nippon Jibiinkoka Gakkai Kaiho 2010;113(2):62–66

50. Robiony M, Polini F, Costa F, Politi M. Disfiguring nasal metastasis from colorectal adenocarcinoma: a case report. Otolaryngol Head Neck Surg 2001;125(1):103–104

51. Cama E, Agostino S, Ricci R, Scarano E. A rare case of metastases to the maxillary sinus from sigmoid colon adenocarcinoma. ORL J Otorhinolaryngol Relat Spec 2002;64(5):364–367

52. Somali I, Yersal O, Kilçiksiz S. Infratemporal fossa and maxillary sinus metastases from colorectal cancer: a case report. J BUON 2006;11(3):363–365

53. Tanaka K. A case of metastases to the paranasal sinus from rectal mucinous adenocarcinoma. Int J Clin Oncol 2006;11(1):64–65

54. bin Sabir Husin Athar PP, bte Ahmad Norhan N, bin Saim L, bin Md Rose I, bte Ramli R. Metastasis to the sinonasal tract from sigmoid colon adenocarcinoma. Ann Acad Med Singapore 2008;37(9):788-3

55. Conill C, Vargas M, Valduvieco I, Fernández PL, Cardesa A, Capurro S. Metastasis to the nasal cavity from primary rectal adenocarcinoma. Clin Transl Oncol 2009;11(2):117–119

56. McClatchey KD, Lloyd RV, Schaldenbrand JD. Metastatic carcinoma to the sphenoid sinus. Case report and review of the literature. Arch Otorhinolaryngol 1985;241(3):219–224

57. Matsumoto I, Furusato M, Inomata I, Wada T, Aizawa S. Prostatic cancer presenting as metastatic adenocarcinoma of sphenoid sinus. Acta Pathol Jpn 1986;36(11):1753–1756

58. Gil Sánz MJ, González Enguita C, Roncales Badal A, Tello Royloa C, Rioja Sánz LA. Metastasis in maxillary sinus as presentation form of adenocarcinoma of the prostate. [Article in Spanish] Actas Urol Esp 1992;16(3):272–274

59. Fortson JK, Bezmalinovic ZL, Moseley DL. Bilateral ethmoid sinusitis with unilateral proptosis as an initial manifestation of metastatic prostate carcinoma. J Natl Med Assoc 1994;86(12):945–948

60. Saleh HA. A case of prostatic cancer metastatic to the orbit and ethmoid sinus. Ann Otol Rhinol Laryngol 1996;105(7):584

61. Jiménez Oliver V, Lazarich Valdés A, Dávila Morillo A, et al. Frontal ethmoid metastases of prostatic carcinoma. Report of one case and review of the literature. [Article in Spanish] Acta Otorrinolaringol Esp 2001;52(2):151–154

62. Prescher A, Brors D. Metastases to the paranasal sinuses: case report and review of the literature. [Article in German] Laryngorhinootologie 2001;80(10):583–594

63. Lavasani L, Zapanta PE, Tanna N, Sadeghi N. Metastasis of prostatic adenocarcinoma to the sphenoid sinus. Ann Otol Rhinol Laryngol 2006;115(9):690–693

64. Llarena Ibarguren R, García-Olaverri Rodríguez J, Villafruela Mateos A, Azurmendi Arin I, Olano Grasa I, Pertusa Peña C. Metastases in the paranasal sinuses secondary to prostatic adenocarcinoma. [Article in Spanish] Arch Esp Urol 2007;60(9):137–140

65. Viswanatha B. Prostatic carcinoma metastatic to the paranasal sinuses: a case report. Ear Nose Throat J 2008; 87(9):519–520

66. Sim RS, Tan HK. A case of metastatic hepatocellular carcinoma of the sphenoid sinus. J Laryngol Otol 1994;108(6):503–504

67. Kleinjung T, Held P. Metastasis in the frontal skull base from hepatocellular carcinoma. [Article in German] HNO 2001;49(2):126–129

68. Okada H, Kamino Y, Shimo M, et al. Metastatic hepatocellular carcinoma of the maxillary sinus: a rare autopsy case without lung metastasis and a review. Int J Oral Maxillofac Surg 2003;32(1):97–100

69. Yoo SJ, Cheon JH, Lee SW, et al. Extrahepatic metastasis of hepatocellular carcinoma to the nasal cavity manifested as massive epistaxis: a case report. [Article in Korean] Korean J Hepatol 2004;10(3):228–232

70. Satake N, Yoshida S, Jinnouchi O, Sekita T. Adenoid cystic carcinoma of maxillary sinus with metastatic hepatocellular carcinoma. Case report. APMIS 2005;113(6):450–455

71. Matsuda H, Tanigaki Y, Yoshida T, Matsuda R, Tsukuda M. A case of metastatic hepatocellular carcinoma in the nasal cavity. Eur Arch Otorhinolaryngol 2006;263(4):305–307

72. Chang CW, Wang TE, Chen LT, et al. Unusual presentation of metastatic hepatocellular carcinoma in the nasal

septum: a case report and review of the literature. Med Oncol 2008;25(3):264–268

73. Kurisu Y, Tsuji M, Takeshita A, Hirata K, Shibayama Y. Cytologic findings of metastatic hepatocellular carcinoma of the nasal cavity: a report of 2 cases. Acta Cytol 2010; 54(5, Suppl)989–992

74. Andaz C, Alsanjari N, Garth RJ, Dearnaley DP. Metastatic seminoma of the sphenoid sinus. J Laryngol Otol 1991;105(12):1075–1078

75. Weiss JN, Ziegelbaum M, Hirschfield L. An unusual manifestation of testicular lymphoma. N Y State J Med 1992;92(6):270–272

76. Tariq M, Gluckman P, Thebe P. Metastatic testicular teratoma of the nasal cavity: a rare cause of severe intractable epistaxis. J Laryngol Otol 1998;112(11):1078–1081

77. Xanthopoulos J, Assimakopoulos D, Noussios G, Mouratidou D. Testicular tumor metastatic to the nose. A case report. Acta Otorhinolaryngol Belg 2000;54(4):479–482

78. Merimsky O, Inbar M, Groswasser-Reider I, Neudorfer M, Chaitchik S. Sphenoid and cavernous sinuses involvement as first site of metastasis from a fallopian tube carcinoma. Case report. Tumori 1993;79(6):444–446

79. Scott A, Raine M, Stansbie JM. Ethmoid metastasis of endometrial carcinoma causing mucocoele of maxillary antrum. J Laryngol Otol 1998;112(3):283–285

80. Sandruck J, Escobar P, Lurain J, Fishman D. Uterine leiomyosarcoma metastatic to the sphenoid sinus: a case report and review of the literature. Gynecol Oncol 2004;92(2):701–704

81. Ilvan S, Akyildiz EU, Calay Z, Celikoyar M, Sahinler I. Endometrial clear cell carcinoma metastatic to the paranasal sinuses: a case report and review of the literature. Gynecol Oncol 2004;94(1):232–234

82. Owa AO, Gallimore AP, Ajulo SO, Cheesman AD. Metastatic adenocarcinoma of the ethmoids in a patient with previous gastric adenocarcinoma: a case report. J Laryngol Otol 1995;109(8):759–761

83. Hassard AD, Boudreau SF. Malignant melanoma of the maxillary sinus. Ear Nose Throat J 1989;68(6):469–471

84. Nicolai P, Peretti G, Cappiello J, Renaldini G, Cavaliere S, Morassi ML. Melanoma metastatic to the trachea and nasal cavity: description of a case and review of the literature. [Article in Italian] Acta Otorhinolaryngol Ital 1991;11(1):85–92

85. Nanbu A, Tsukamoto T, Kumamoto Y, et al. Squamous cell carcinoma of bladder diverticulum with initial symptoms produced by metastasis to maxillary sinus. Eur Urol 1988;15(3-4):285–286

86. Kawai N, Asakura K, Sambe S, Kataura A, Enomoto K. Metastatic squamous cell carcinoma of the paranasal sinuses from a primary squamous cell carcinoma of the urinary bladder. J Laryngol Otol 1989;103(6):602–604

87. Torrico Román P, Mogollón Cano-Cortés T, López-Ríos Velasco J, Fernández de Mera JJ, Blasco Huelva A. Bladder transitional cell carcinoma with metastasis to the maxillary sinus as first symptom. [Article in Spanish] Acta Otorrinolaringol Esp 2001;52(7):622–624

88. Ogawa T, Hara K, Kawarai Y, et al. A case of infantile neuroblastoma with intramucosal metastasis in a paranasal sinus. Int J Pediatr Otorhinolaryngol 2000;55(1):61–64

89. Matsumoto Y, Yanagihara N. Renal clear cell carcinoma metastatic to the nose and paranasal sinuses. Laryngoscope 1982;92(10 Pt 1):1190–1193

90. Kent SE, Majumdar B. Metastatic tumours in the maxillary sinus. A report of two cases and a review of the literature. J Laryngol Otol 1985;99(5):459–462

91. Achar MV. Metastatic hypernephroma occurring in nasal septum. AMA Arch Otolaryngol 1955;62(6):644–648

92. Edwards WG. Epistaxis from metastatic renal carcinoma. J Laryngol Otol 1964;78:96–102

93. Robinson D. Antral metastases from carcinoma. J Laryngol Otol 1973;87(6):603–609

94. Resto VA, Krane JF, Faquin WC, Lin DT. Immunohistochemical distinction of intestinal-type sinonasal adenocarcinoma from metastatic adenocarcinoma of intestinal origin. Ann Otol Rhinol Laryngol 2006;115(1):59–64

95. Bernstein JM, Montgomery WW, Balogh K Jr. Metastatic tumors to the maxilla, nose, and paranasal sinuses. Laryngoscope 1966;76(4):621–650

18 Conditions Simulating Neoplasia and Granulomatous Disorders

There is a range of conditions, inflammatory or infective, that may affect the sinonasal region and produce clinical features and in some cases imaging appearances that may resemble those of a neoplastic process. Some can also coexist with a neoplasm, so it seems appropriate to consider them for completeness. For this reason we have included them to assist with differential diagnosis (Table 18.1).

These conditions include:

- Mucoceles
- Fungal disease
- Maxillary hematoma
- Rhinosporidiosis/rhinoscleroma
- Tuberculosis
- Wegener's granulomatosis
- Sarcoidosis
- Churg-Strauss syndrome
- Relapsing polychondritis
- Cholesterol granuloma

Mucoceles

Definition

A mucocele is an epithelium-lined sac completely filling the paranasal sinus and capable of expansion,[1] as opposed to an obstructed sinus which simply contains mucus.

Etiology

Prevailing theories of mucocele formation include obstruction and inflammation, but these states occur in many more patients than those who develop a mucocele. The normal metabolic process of bone resorption and regeneration alters in favor of resorption, leading to expansion;[2,3] others have suggested that it is pressure erosion that results in the bone erosion,[4] but the histological appearances are against this (see below). In either case it is an active process that can be accelerated by additional infection, or exacerbation of preexisting infection, when a "pyocele" forms. Cystic degeneration of glandular tissue has also been proposed, but if this occurs one would expect to see early stages before the cyst completely fills the sinus and a double wall to the mucocele. The only circumstance when this might occur is in the "mucoceles" described quite frequently 16 to 19 years after Caldwell-Luc procedures in the Japanese.[5] In the Western literature, cysts are found as incidental and asymptomatic phenomena in the maxillary sinus, the rarest site of all for a mucocele,[6] in over 30% of normal individuals, so this proposition seems highly unlikely.

Table 18.1 Granulomatous disorders of the nose

Infectious	
Bacterial	
• Tuberculosis	*Mycobacterium tuberculosis*
• Leprosy	*Mycobacterium leprae*
• Rhinoscleroma	*Klebsiella rhinoscleromatis*
• Syphilis	*Treponema pallidum*
• Actinomycosis	*Actinomyces israeli*
Fungal	
• Aspergillus	*A. fumigatus, A. flavus, A. niger*
• Zygomycosis	*Conidiobolus coronatus* *Rhizopus oryzae*
• Dematiacetes	*Curvularia* *Alternaria* *Bipolaris*
• Rhinosporidiosis	*Rhinosporidiosis seeberi*
• Blastomycosis	*Blastomyces dermatitidis* *Cryptococcus neoformans*
• Histoplasmosis	*Histoplasma capsulatum*
• Sporotrichosis	*Sporotrichum schenkii*
• Coccidioidomycosis	*Coccidiodes immitis*
Protozoal	
• Leishmaniasis	*Leishmania* spp.
Inflammatory	
Wegener's granulomatosis	
Sarcoidosis	
Churg-Strauss syndrome	
Cholesterol granuloma	
Neoplastic	
NK/T-cell lymphoma (midline lethal granuloma)	
Eosinophilic granuloma	

Some bone-resorbing factors have been shown in mucocele mucosa, including PGE2, leukotrienes, and a range of cytokines.[2] Compared with normal controls, chronic rhinosinusitis, and mucosa from obstructed sinuses, IL-1α, IL-1β, and tumor necrosis factor-α (TNF-α) are increased and there is upregulation of the vascular adhesion molecules e-selectin, and I-CAM.[3] This suggests that more than just obstruction of sinus outflow is needed for a mucocele to form. It is therefore proposed that following obstruction, superadded infection leads to chronic inflammation mediated by bacterial antigens, which in turn leads to an acceleration of bone resorption outstripping bone formation; but it is still unclear what predisposes an individual to this process.

Thus, while it is not clear why mucoceles form when sinus inflammation in general is so common, in ~2/3 of patients a possible initiating factor can be determined (Table 18.2).[7] This includes various forms of trauma to the sinus outflow, often related to road traffic accidents and other pathology such as osteomas and Paget's disease.[8,9] However, the largest group comprises chronic rhinosinusitis, nasal polyps, and allergic/eosinophilic fungal disease, and the contents can be composed of a variety of secretions including the "peanut-butter" of fungal material and polypoid tissue itself. Many of these patients have also undergone previous sinus surgery, often multiple, and one-quarter have had external frontoethmoidectomy. There are also patients who have undergone surgery for nonsinus conditions such as orbital decompression and oncological surgery. There is often a significant time lag between the event and presentation with the mucocele. In the case of surgery or trauma, a mean time of 23 years elapses as compared with 22 months after an acute infection.[7]

Table 18.2 Possible etiological factors in mucocele formation: personal series

Factor	Number	Details of factors
None	99	
Trauma	20	
Polyps/chronic rhinosinusitis	85	
Previous sinus surgery	52	External frontoethmoidectomy (12) Osteoplastic flap (2) Polypectomy (45) Multiple in some cases
Acute infection	21	
Other pathology	14	Paget's disease, osteoma
Other surgery	12	Orbital exenteration (1)
		Dacryocystorhinostomy (1)
		Orbital decompression (6)
		Lateral rhinotomy (1)
		Craniofacial resection (1)
		Repair blow-out (1)
		Pituitary surgery (1)
Total	303	
Please note, factors are multiple in some patients.		

Synonyms

The first description of a pyocele possibly relates to the case of Francis I, king of France (1494–1547).[10] Lagenbeck[11] described a "hydatid" in the sinuses in 1819 and in 1896 Rollet used the term "mucocele."[12]

Incidence

Mucoceles are relatively rare given the proposed etiology and there is no predisposing factor in at least one-third. Around 10% are bilateral and 8% are multiloculated, usually associated with nasal polyps. Our personal cohort comprises 266 cases which is largely the result of referrals from the United Kingdom's postgraduate ophthalmic hospital, Moorfields, with which we have had a longstanding relationship. Other large series are shown in Table 18.3.

Site

(See Table 18.3.)

Mucoceles most often affect the frontal sinus and frontoethmoidal region, but individual ethmoidal cells (mainly anterior), the sphenoid, and occasionally the maxillary sinus can be affected. A concha bullosa can also house a mucocele.

In our series the majority occur in the frontal and frontoethmoidal region (86%), followed by the ethmoid (8.6%). As in other series, the maxilla is the rarest site (2%), but the sphenoid may be commoner than our 3.4% as they may also present to neurology. This distribution may relate to the complexity of drainage from the respective sinuses but is not otherwise easy to explain. The right and left sides are affected equally.

Diagnostic Features

Clinical Features

Nasal symptoms are usually quite minor or absent and the majority of patients present to ophthalmologists with orbital displacement with axial proptosis (91%), although over half also have lateral (55%) or inferior displacement (59%). As a consequence, many have some degree of diplopia (95%) usually in the extremes of the visual fields and the mass effect of the mucocele limits ocular mobility in 55%. Unless a pyocele occurs, vision is rarely at risk, with acuity reduced in only 9%. Epiphora can result from compression of the lacrimal system. However, patients in another, smaller, group do present to neurologists and neurosurgeons with sudden visual compromise, ophthalmoplegia, or vertex headache due to a sphenoid mucocele. Meningitis and raised intracranial pressure have also been reported.[21]

Mucoceles have been reported from 23 months to 79 years. The age range of patients in our series of 266 cases

Table 18.3 Endoscopic management of mucoceles in the literature

	No. of mucoceles	Site				Age		Female: Male	Previous surgery	Follow-up		Recurrence
		F	E	S	M	Range (y)	Mean (y)			Range	Mean	
Kennedy et al 1989[13]	16	9	5	2	–	10–76	44.7	8:10	5 (31%)	2–42 mo	17.6mo	0%
Moriyama et al 1992[14]	49 (47 pts)	–	41	8	–	20–69	46.2	14:33	37 (78%)	2–10 y	?	?
Beasley and Jones 1995[15]	34 (25 pts)	21	10	1	2	23–76	51	7:18	18 (72%)	6 mo–3 y	2 y	6% (both had previous external surgery)
Benninger et al 1995[16]	15	–	7	8	–	?	?	10:5	5 (33%)	5–40 mo	20 mo	13%
Lund 1998[17]	20 (ESS)	12	6	2	–	4–89	42.6	10:10	0	7–61 mo	34 mo	0%
	28 (Combined ESS and external)	28				25–83	59	11:17	9 (42%)	10–76 mo	44 mo	11%
Conboy and Jones 2003[18]	68 (59 pts) 44 ESS 14 EFE 9 Comb	42	16	4	6	14–90	56	?	21 (31%)	3 mo–10.2 y	6.2 y	13% (9% post-ESS) (26% post-external ops)
Khong et al 2004[19]	41 (28 pts)	32	3	1	5	15–83	52	11:17	At least 18 (64%)	1–42 mo	18 mo	0%
Bockmuhl et al 2006[20]	290 (255 pts) 185 ESS	148	41	29	72	10–80	52	85:170	168 (66%)	4–21 y	?	2%
Lund et al (unpublished)	266	228	23	9	6	4–89	53	1:1.5		3 mo–25 y	65% >5 y	
ESS	103											2%
Combined ESS/external	43											12%
External only	120											14%

Abbreviations: Comb, combined endoscopic and external approaches; E, ethmoid; EFE, external frontoethmoidectomy; ESS, endoscopic sinus surgery; F, frontal; M, maxillary; mo, month(s); pt, patient; S, sphenoid; y, year.

is 4 to 89 years (mean 53 years) and the male-to-female ratio is 1.5:1.

Mucoceles are rare in children, our cohort of 7 being one of the larger reported,[22] and all followed an infection.

Endoscopic examination may show a smooth expansion of the mucosa over the mass but often there is little obvious to see. In addition to the displacement of the eye, a firm swelling may be palpable in the superior medial quadrant of the orbit or extending into the forehead or cheek, which may or may not have a bony shell but which can be very thin producing an egg-shell cracking sensation on palpation. A fistula in the upper lid has been observed in 18 of our cases, either occurring spontaneously or produced iatrogenically.[23]

Imaging

(See **Figs. 18.1, 18.2, 18.3, 18.4, 18.5.**)

CT is the primary imaging modality, and coronal, axial, and sagittal (for frontal lesions) views are ideally required. The bony outline of the sinus becomes rounded as the bone remodels and scalloping and septations disappear.[24] There is expansion of the sinus walls, particularly where the bone is thinnest, together with smooth erosion. The appearances are those of a balloon being gradually blown up rather than the craggy, irregular bone destruction of a malignant tumor. Thus the bony interface between sinuses and the orbit disappears first, and in the frontal, expansion occurs into the contralateral sinus. The posterosuperior wall of the frontal frequently erodes and sometimes mucoceles of spectacular dimensions can be found extending into the anterior cranial fossa with frontal lobe displacement and compression with few clinical symptoms.[25,26] In the sphenoid, erosion of the medial wall of the optic canal and elevation of the planum sphenoidale occurs. In the maxilla, the rarest site, there is expansion of all walls leading to upward displacement of the eye, bowing into the nasal cavity, and swelling of the cheek.

The attenuation of the content may increase with time as the protein content increases (from 10–18 HU [Hounsfield units] to 20–40 HU in older lesions). Contrast is rarely used but will show enhancement of the lining mucosa.[24] Other pathologies such as osteoma, Paget's disease, and polyps will be shown.

MRI is not routinely undertaken but can be helpful if there is doubt about the diagnosis. The usual signal characteristics are low T1 and high T2 but degree of hydration or a recent bleed will alter these and any signal intensity can be observed from the contents. Generally the older the mucocele, the shorter the T1 relaxation time. Post gadolinium imaging usually shows signal absent from the contents.

Histological Features and Differential Diagnosis

The mucosal lining is generally a pseudostratified columnar epithelium with some squamous metaplasia, goblet cell hyperplasia, and a cellular infiltration dependent on the degree of chronic or acute-on-chronic inflammation. This includes neutrophils, eosinophils, macrophages, monocytes, and plasma cells. Fibroblastic activity is increased, as is vascularity of the submucosa.[27] With time, the epithelium becomes more flattened or cuboidal but not atrophic as might be expected with high

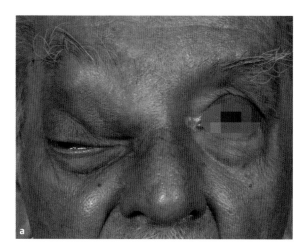

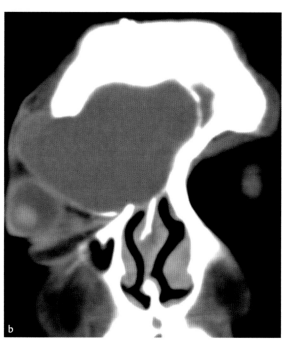

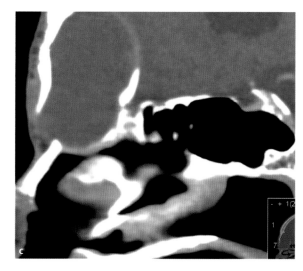

Fig. 18.1a–c

a Clinical photograph of a patient with a large frontal mucocele.
b Coronal CT scan showing a large frontal mucocele.
c Sagittal CT scan showing a large frontal mucocele.

intramucocele pressure or keratinization, which if present in the maxilla would suggest an odontogenic keratocyst. The underlying bone shows woven and lamellar bone, with frequent osteoclasts and osteoblasts, indicative of the active bone turnover and remodeling.

The differential diagnosis includes fungal disease, cholesterol granuloma, benign and malignant neoplasms (schwannoma, inverted papilloma, mucinous adenocarcinoma), and, in the maxilla, dental or odontogenic cysts.

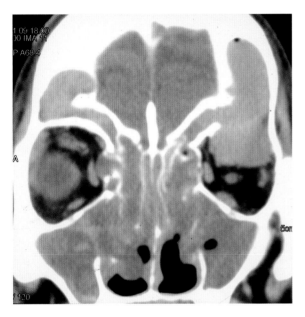

Fig. 18.2 Coronal CT scan showing severe polyposis associated with bilateral "polypoceles" in lateral compartments of the frontal sinuses.

Sphenoidal mucoceles must be distinguished from nasopharyngeal and pituitary lesions.

Natural History

The natural progression of the mucocele is slow expansion over many years, often unrecognized by the patient but brought to light by someone who has not seen them for some time and who notes the cosmetic change. An acute infection can result in rapid change, which can precipitate presentation. Up to 17 mm of axial proptosis has been observed in some elderly individuals, with minimal visual symptoms.

Treatment

In the vast majority of cases mucoceles in all the sinuses can be adequately marsupialized using an endoscopic approach, providing the contents are liquid enough to drain, as it is not necessary to strip away the mucosal lining.[28] Exceptions to this can therefore be a frontal sinus where there may be other pathologies such as a large osteoma or a "fungocele" compartmentalized in the most lateral part of the frontal sinus or severe polyposis, although both of these latter conditions may be managed by surgery combined with aggressive medical management. Furthermore, the mucocele itself may be in a compartment of the frontal sinus that lies lateral to the midpoint of the orbit. In these cases, a small external incision may assist drainage in the rare circumstances when a binasal Draf III approach is not adequate. Occasionally, in the case of multiloculated "mucopolypoceles" often associated with aspirin-sensitive asthma (Samter's triad), an osteoplastic flap may be required (**Fig. 18.2**).

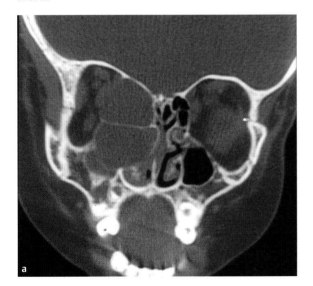

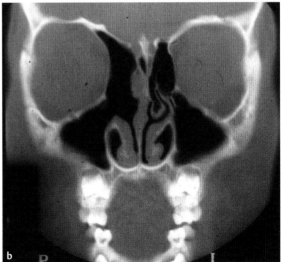

Fig. 18.3a, b

a Coronal CT showing a biloculated ethmoidal mucocele in a 6-year-old child.

b Coronal CT following endoscopic drainage performed 4 years later at another hospital as the child was complaining of headaches.

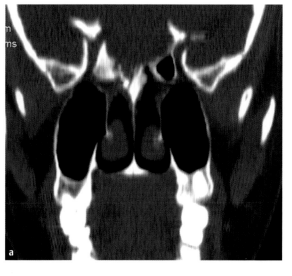

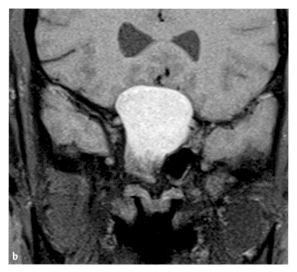

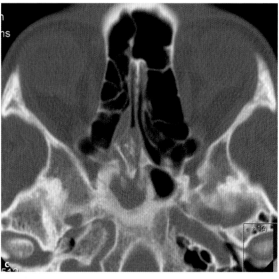

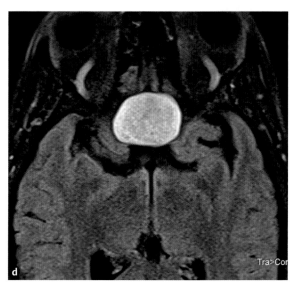

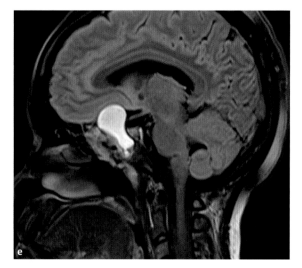

Fig. 18.4a–e Sphenoidal mucocele secondary to fungal material in the sphenoethmoidal recess with visual loss in the left eye that recovered post surgery.

a Coronal CT showing an expanded sphenoid sinus with bone loss superiorly and sclerosis inferiorly.

b Coronal MRI (T1W post gadolinium enhancement with fat saturation) showing high-signal material filling the sphenoidal mucocele.

c Axial CT scan showing sclerosis of the left sphenoid sinus together with hyperdensity in the sphenoethmoidal recess due to fungal material.

d Axial MRI (FLAIR) showing high-signal material filling the sphenoidal mucocele.

e Sagittal MRI (T1W post gadolinium enhancement) showing high-signal material in the sphenoidal mucocele.

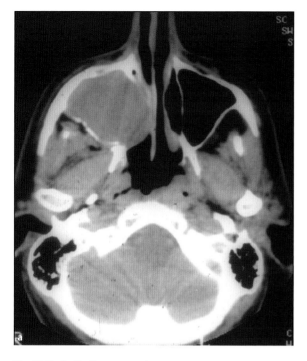
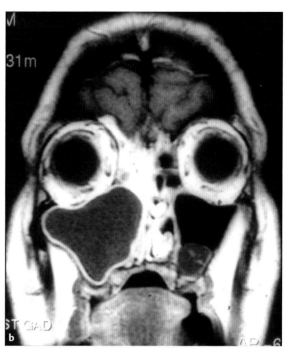

Fig. 18.5a, b Maxillary mucocele.

a Axial CT scan showing an expanded maxillary mucocele.

b Coronal MRI (T1W post gadolinium enhancement) showing low-signal contents in the expanded maxillary sinus.

Previous surgery and sclerotic bone may also make an endoscopic approach technically impossible (**Table 18.4**). If an external approach is used, the lateral support of the frontonasal recess must not be undermined by removal of bone as this will result in medialization of the orbital contents and is the main reason why the Lynch-Howarth type procedures fell into disrepute.

The standard endoscopic approach under general anesthesia is utilized with wide marsupialization of the mucocele.[17] Image-guidance may assist for some frontal mucoceles but is rarely necessary. Once the mucocele is opened a large quantity of mucus can be aspirated; this may comprise various components depending on the precipitation of the contents into clear or proteinaceous fluid. In frontal mucoceles, this, combined with transmitted pulsation from the dura if bone is missing posterosuperiorly, can be quite alarming when first encountered as it immediately suggests a CSF leak. However, the situation rapidly becomes clear as the flocculating, colored, and thicker contents appear!

Once the mucocele sac has been opened, usually with a sickle knife or cutting instrument, the opening should be made as large as the anatomy will allow. This can be done with circumferential cutting mushroom punches, through-biting instruments, or powered instrumentation. Specimens for microbiology should be taken but this is positive in only <30% and, if fungus is suspected, histopathology of the secretion should also be requested.

In most cases there will be areas where erosion of bone exposes orbital periosteum or dura covered only by mucosa. Gentle pressure on the eye will readily demonstrate this. There is absolutely no necessity to repair these areas as there is no risk of CSF leak or meningitis unless mucosa is stripped away. In younger patients, evidence of recalcification has been observed at these areas of interface.

As the mucocele is drained, the position of the eye will normalize. The degree to which this happens will depend on how much bone is missing. Usually there is significant improvement immediately, but there will be continued improvement as the bone remodels over subsequent months. The degree of diplopia following endoscopic surgery is much less than that after external procedures, due in part to the more progressive nature of improvement but also to the lack of disturbance of the trochlea region, which frequently occurs with conventional external fronto-ethmoidectomy. Lund and Rolfe[29] reported diplopia in 7/22 (32%) of a prospective study of mucocele patients undergoing Lynch-Howarth procedures. Consequently, patients should be warned that diplopia may occur, or may worsen if preexisting. This can be improved by wearing a prism on spectacles postoperatively and occasionally strabismus surgery is required. This has never been needed after endoscopic drainage but was undertaken in one of our patients having external operations in a prospective study of 22 patients.

Table 18.4 Advantages and contraindications of surgical approaches

Advantages	Contraindications
Endoscopic approach	
• Quick • Short stay • Low morbidity and excellent cosmesis • Good visualization • Diplopia absent or minor • Can be used for recurrence	• When contents cannot be accessed or the mucocele is adequately marsupialized • Secretion too solid, e.g., fungal material • Bone too thick, e.g., sclerosis secondary to chronic infection, Paget's disease • Pathology inappropriate, e.g., large osteoma, extensive malignancy • Mucocele too lateral, e.g., beyond midpoint of orbit • Previous external surgery, e.g., fibrosis, medialization of orbital contents
External approaches (i.e. modified Lynch-Howarth, osteoplastic flap)	

• Can be combined with endoscopic approach when
  – Mucocele lateral to midpoint of orbit
  – Multiloculated mucocele
  – For copathology that cannot be encompassed by endoscopic surgery alone, e.g., large osteoma
	• None specifically but associated with potential additional complications of paresthesia, visible incision, and diplopia due to superior oblique underaction

No packing is required and virtually all patients treated endoscopically are day cases.

Routine postoperative medications such as saline douching and intranasal steroids can be given, but it is important to see the patient within the first few weeks to check that the opening into the mucocele remains widely patent.

Outcome

The results of endoscopic drainage of mucoceles, both in our own hands and in the literature, are excellent. A success rate of 98% can be anticipated with long-term follow-up (**Table 18.3**). In our series the follow-up ranges from 3 months to 25 years and is >5 years in 65%. There was only one recurrence in the endoscopic group of 103 cases, which was revised endoscopically. In the combined group of endoscopic and external approaches the recurrence rate was 12%, one-third of which were revised endoscopically. The rest, a mainly historical group that predates 1990, had a recurrence rate of 14%, some having re-presented many years later. Endoscopic drainage of sphenoid mucoceles is especially successful and may reverse visual loss if undertaken within 24 hours of it occurring.[16,30,31] Although rarest, maxillary sinus mucoceles are also highly amenable to endoscopic drainage.[32]

The advantages of this approach are the short duration of the procedure, short stay in hospital, minimal morbidity, and excellent visualization. Endoscopic techniques can also be used for recurrent disease.

In those requiring additional approaches, the recurrence rate is inevitably higher (11%) due to the complexity of the cases. These cofactors include multiple previous operations, nasal polyposis, and eyelid fistula.

Resolution or improvement in displacement of the globe and diplopia can be anticipated in most patients and the complications of the surgery itself are minimal. In contrast, external procedures potentially carry the cosmetic disadvantages of the external incision,[33] problems with bone flaps (frontal bossing or loss of bone), and even skin necrosis.[34] The cosmetic advantages of endoscopic drainage are particularly important in the younger patients.[35]

Key Points

- The pathogenesis of mucoceles is unknown but includes obstruction and inflammation.
- Mucoceles are characterized by bone erosion and sinus expansion.
- Most patients present with orbital symptoms and signs.
- CT scanning is the primary mode of imaging.
- Most mucoceles can be managed endoscopically.

References

1. Natvig K, Larsen TE. Mucocele of the paranasal sinuses. A retrospective clinical and histological study. J Laryngol Otol 1978;92(12):1075–108
2. Lund VJ, Harvey W, Meghji S, Harris M. Prostaglandin synthesis in the pathogenesis of fronto-ethmoidal mucoceles. Acta Otolaryngol 1988;106(1–2):145–151
3. Lund VJ, Henderson B, Song Y. Involvement of cytokines and vascular adhesion receptors in the pathology of fronto-ethmoidal mucocoeles. Acta Otolaryngol 1993;113(4):540–546
4. Kass ES, Fabian RL, Montgomery WW. Manometric study of paranasal sinus mucoceles. Ann Otol Rhinol Laryngol 1999;108(1):63–66

5.   Hasegawa M, Saito Y, Watanabe I, Kern E. Post-operative mucoceles of the maxillary sinus. Rhinology 1979;17:253–256
6.   Kanagalingam J, Bhatia K, Georgalas C, Fokkens W, Miszkiel K, Lund VJ. Maxillary mucosal cyst is not a manifestation of rhinosinusitis: results of a prospective three-dimensional CT study of ophthalmic patients. Laryngoscope 2009;119(1):8–12
7.   Lund VJ. Anatomical considerations in the aetiology of fronto-ethmoidal mucoceles. Rhinology 1987;25(2):83–88
8.   Shady JA, Bland LI, Kazee AM, Pilcher WH. Osteoma of the frontoethmoidal sinus with secondary brain abscess and intracranial mucocele: case report. Neurosurgery 1994;34(5):920–923, discussion 923
9.   Brunori A, Bruni P, Delitala A, Greco R, Chiappetta F. Frontoethmoidal osteoma complicated by intracranial mucocele and hypertensive pneumocephalus: case report. Neurosurgery 1995;36(6):1237–1238
10. Hackett F. Francis I. New York: Doubleday Doran and Co.; 1934:313–316
11. Lagenbeck C. Neue Bibliothek fur die Chirurgie und Ophthalmologie. Hahn Hanover 1896;2:365
12. Rollet M. Mucocele de l'angle supero-interne des orbites. Lyon Med 1896;81:573–575
13. Kennedy DW, Josephson JS, Zinreich SJ, Mattox DE, Goldsmith MM. Endoscopic sinus surgery for mucoceles: a viable alternative. Laryngoscope 1989;99(9):885–895
14. Moriyama H, Nakajima T, Honda Y. Studies on mucocoeles of the ethmoid and sphenoid sinuses: analysis of 47 cases. J Laryngol Otol 1992;106(1):23–27
15. Beasley N, Jones N. Paranasal sinus mucoceles: modern management. Am J Rhinol 1995;9:251–256
16. Benninger MS, Marks S. The endoscopic management of sphenoid and ethmoid mucoceles with orbital and intranasal extension. Rhinology 1995;33(3):157–161
17. Lund VJ. Endoscopic management of paranasal sinus mucocoeles. J Laryngol Otol 1998;112(1):36–40
18. Conboy PJ, Jones NS. The place of endoscopic sinus surgery in the treatment of paranasal sinus mucocoeles. Clin Otolaryngol Allied Sci 2003;28(3):207–210
19. Khong JJ, Malhotra R, Selva D, Wormald PJ. Efficacy of endoscopic sinus surgery for paranasal sinus mucocele including modified endoscopic Lothrop procedure for frontal sinus mucocele. J Laryngol Otol 2004;118(5):352–356
20. Bockmühl U, Kratzsch B, Benda K, Draf W. Surgery for paranasal sinus mucocoeles: efficacy of endonasal micro-endoscopic management and long-term results of 185 patients. Rhinology 2006;44(1):62–67
21. Davis CH, Small M, Lund V. An 'empty' sphenoid mucocele. Br J Neurosurg 1992;6(4):381–383
22. Hartley BE, Lund VJ. Endoscopic drainage of pediatric paranasal sinus mucoceles. Int J Pediatr Otorhinolaryngol 1999;50(2):109–111
23. Rossman D, Verity DH, Lund VJ, Rose GE. Eyelid fistula: a feature of occult sinus disease. Orbit 2007;26(3):159–163
24. Lloyd G, Lund VJ, Savy L, Howard D. Optimum imaging for mucoceles. J Laryngol Otol 2000;114(3):233–236
25. Delfini R, Missori P, Iannetti G, Ciappetta P, Cantore G. Mucoceles of the paranasal sinuses with intracranial and intraorbital extension: report of 28 cases. Neurosurgery 1993;32(6):901–906, discussion 906
26. Voegels RL, Balbani AP, Santos Júnior RC, Butugan O. Frontoethmoidal mucocele with intracranial extension: a case report. Ear Nose Throat J 1998;77(2):117–120
27. Lund VJ, Milroy CM. Fronto-ethmoidal mucocoeles: a histopathological analysis. J Laryngol Otol 1991;105(11):921–923
28. Lund V. Endoscopic surgery for fronto-ethmoidal mucoceles. Oper Tech Otolaryngol Head Neck Surg 1995; 6:221–224
29. Lund VJ, Rolfe ME. Ophthalmic considerations in fronto-ethmoidal mucocoeles. J Laryngol Otol 1989; 103(7):667–669
30. Li J, Stankiewicz J. The endoscopic approach to the lateral accessory sphenoid sinus. Otolaryngol Head Neck Surg 1991;105(4):608–612
31. Yumoto E, Hyodo M, Kawakita S, Aibara R. Effect of sinus surgery on visual disturbance caused by spheno-ethmoid mucoceles. Am J Rhinol 1997;11(5):337–343
32. Makeieff M, Gardiner Q, Mondain M, Crampette L. Maxillary sinus mucocoeles—10 cases—8 treated endoscopically. Rhinology 1998;36(4):192–195
33. Rubin J, Lund VJ, Salmon B. Fronto-ethmoidectomy in the treatment of mucoceles: a neglected operation. Arch Otolaryngol Head Neck Surg 1985;112:434–436
34. Hardy JM, Montgomery WW. Osteoplastic frontal sinusotomy: an analysis of 250 operations. Ann Otol Rhinol Laryngol 1976;85(4 Pt 1):523–532
35. Zrada SE, Isaacson GC. Endoscopic treatment of pediatric ethmoid mucoceles. Am J Otolaryngol 1996;17(3):197–201

Fungal Rhinosinusitis

Definition

Sinonasal inflammation resulting from fungi.

This can be broadly divided into noninvasive and invasive which is defined by the absence or presence of fungal hyphae within the sinus mucosa.[1] It is not defined by the presence of bone erosion which may be found in both invasive and non-invasive forms. The classification can be seen in **Table 18.5**.[2]

Etiology

The range of associated organisms is large (**Table 18.6**). Of these the *Aspergillus* species was previously regarded as one of the principal agents, but in recent years the importance of the dematiaceous fungal genera *Alternaria*, *Bipolaris* and *Curvularia* has been recognized. This relates to many factors including geographical predilection. Noninvasive forms have been reported in high numbers from Poitiers (France), Graz (Austria), and the southern states of the United States,[3] whereas chronic invasive disease seems commoner in India, the Middle East, and Sudan.[4] In addition, the zygomycetes *Rhizopus* and *Conidiobolus* can be the cause of invasive fungal disease. The former classically produces a rhinocerebral zygomycosis (mucomycosis) and the latter a rhinofacial zygomycosis.

The host response to environmental exposure is also key to the development of the various conditions. Acute fulminant forms of the condition are most often found in individuals with immune compromise, whereas this is not necessarily the case for chronic invasive and rarely a feature of noninvasive forms.

Interest has focused on the noninvasive forms as it was increasingly recognized that fungi might be a more common cause of inflammation than had previously been realized. This followed the description of "allergic fungal

Table 18.5 Classification of fungal rhinosinusitis[a]

Noninvasive	Invasive
Fungal ball	Acute fulminant
Allergic or eosinophilic fungal rhinosinusitis	Chronic • Immunocompetent • Immunocompromised
	Sclerosing
	Granulomatous (mycetoma)

[a]After De Shazo[2].

rhinosinusitis" in patients with "allergic bronchopulmonary aspergillosis," first by Millar and then Katzenstein et al in the 1980s.[5,6] The term "allergic" reflected the large number of eosinophils found in the mucosa and secretions and the dramatic response to corticosteroids. It appears now that the reaction is more likely to be an antiparasitic one to fungal material. The frequent finding of eosinophilic inflammation led to the suggestion that all chronic rhinosinusitis with and without nasal polyps was provoked by fungi and a considerable debate ensued that is still not completely resolved.[7–9] However, it is generally acknowledged that fungi are only one of several entities responsible for the generation and perpetuation of chronic sinonasal inflammation; it is beyond the scope of this book to go into further detail and the topic is widely discussed in the literature.[10–12]

Synonyms

The term "fungal ball" has sometimes been replaced by "mycetoma," but it is now agreed that the latter term should be reserved for a specific granulomatous reaction involving fungi.

Table 18.6 Range of fungi responsible for sinonasal disease

Aspergillus spp.	*A. fumigatus*
	A. flavus
	A. niger
Dematiaceous	*Alternaria*
	Bipolaris
	Curvularia
Zygomycetes	*Conidiobolus coronatus*
	Rhizopus oryzae (*Mucor*)
Rhinosporidium seeberi	
Cryptococcus neoformans	
Histoplasma capsulatum	
Sporothrix schenckii	
Candida	

Similarly "allergic fungal rhinosinusitis" is also more appropriately referred to as "eosinophilic fungal rhinosinusitis."

Incidence

Given the difficulty with the recognition of fungal diseases and wide geographical variation, the true incidence is almost impossible to calculate. Perhaps "commoner than originally thought, but not the sole cause of sinonasal inflammation" would best encapsulate the situation. In most practices the noninvasive forms are much commoner and/or more frequently recognized than the invasive ones, which are fortunately rare.[13] In our own cohort of 91 histologically confirmed cases, the vast majority are noninvasive, eosinophilic fungal rhinosinusitis being 3 times commoner than fungal balls (**Table 18.7**).

Site

All sinuses can be affected as single sites or as a more diffuse process in both noninvasive and invasive forms. In the majority of our eosinophilic fungal cases both right and left sides were affected and most sinuses (>80%) were involved on both sides, though one side might predominate. Of the 22 cases of fungal balls, 2 affected the ethmoid, 8 the sphenoid, and 12 the maxillary sinus. The invasive forms affected multiple sinuses, the orbit, and the intracranial compartment in most cases.

Diagnostic Features

Clinical Features

The fungal ball is often an incidental finding and occurs in normal, nonatopic individuals, although two of our patients had had previous road traffic accidents and facial fractures. Secondary bacterial infection, particularly with *Staphylococcus aureus* or anaerobes, may bring the condition to light and there may be a history of dental work, as it has been suggested that zinc oxide–eugenol paste used in root canal filling in the past promoted the growth of *Aspergillus*.[14] Thus there may be purulent secretion, cacosmia, nasal obstruction, and pain. The fungal mass may have sporangia on the surface or simply present a mass of dark solid "peanut butter" or "axle grease" material (**Fig. 18.6**).

Eosinophilic fungal rhinosinusitis presents as a diffuse polyposis with nasal obstruction, reduced olfaction, and rhinorrhea but rarely pain unless there is significant secondary bacterial infection. There may be expansion of the ethmoids leading to pseudohypertelorism, orbital displacement with proptosis, and sometimes diplopia due to "fungocele" formation. These collections can reach impressive proportions in the anterior cranial fossa without significant symptoms. It is not uncommon for patients to have significant pain in the distribution of the

Table 18.7 Sinonasal fungal disease: personal series

	Eosinophilic fungal rhinosinusitis	Fungal ball	Acute invasive	Chronic invasive	Sclerosing	Total group
n	60	22	2	6	1	91
Male:female	25:35	8:14	1:1	5:1	0:1	42:49
Age						
Range (y)	7–79	7–79	45, 49	32–70	22	7–79
Mean (y)	44.3	45		39		44
Surgery	ESS (45) External ± ESS (15) EFE (8) LR (2) MFD (2) CFR (2) OPF (1)	ESS 22	Radical surgery: CFR+OC (1) ESS (1)	Radical surgery: LR (3) MFD (1) CFR (2)	CFR	

Abbreviations: CFR, craniofacial resection; EFE, external frontoethmoidectomy; LR, lateral rhinotomy; MFD, midfacial degloving; OC, orbital clearance; OPF, osteoplastic flap.

trigeminal nerve that can persist even after treatment and several patients have presented with an orbital apex syndrome from sphenoid involvement.[15] The patients are often young adults, men and women being equally affected and most, if not all, have asthma. They often have allergic rhinitis and some do have positive skin prick reactions to *Aspergillus* and *Cladosporium*, but it is not certain how relevant this is and the lack of standardized extracts make testing for other fungi difficult. As before, the secretion ranges from a tenacious lemon-colored jelly to more solid dark green-brown material.

Chronic invasive fungal disease presents with the mass effect (nasal obstruction, swelling of the cheek), involvement of adjacent structures such as the eye (proptosis, diplopia, visual loss), and sometimes neurologic problems such as headache or cranial nerve palsies. There may be polypoid or granulomatous tissue in the nasal cavity and biopsy is required to distinguish it from the noninvasive forms. These patients may be immunocompetent or compromised by conditions such as diabetes mellitus or high-dose corticosteroids.

Acute fulminant fungal rhinosinusitis is a highly aggressive disease that can kill the often immunocompromised patient in a matter of hours. Thus, patients with poorly controlled diabetes, immunosuppressed oncology patients, and those with acquired immune deficiency syndrome (AIDS) or tuberculosis are particularly at risk. The patient may feel unwell and have minor nasal symptoms that progress with crusting, discharge, pain, and progressive destruction of soft tissues and bone. This results in fistulas in the septum, palate, and skin, loss of structure in the face, and destruction of the eye with visual loss. Neuropathies develop as the cranial nerves are progressively involved, affecting swallowing and other functions.

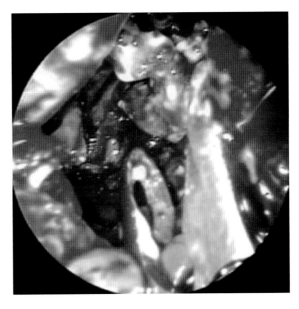

Fig. 18.6 Endoscopic photograph of fungal material within the right maxillary sinus.

Endoscopic examination reveals large amounts of adherent crust on necrotic tissue or eschar which appears atrophic or black. There is little bleeding with débridement.

Sclerosing invasive fungal disease is very rare and only a few cases have been reported, mainly from the Middle East and Africa. Here the fungal hyphae provoke a fibrotic reaction, producing a space-occupying mass that gradually enlarges to give a mass effect in the nose, face, and orbit with associated symptoms. It is a slowly progressive disease and in some cases spreads to the subcutaneous tissues of the nose and orbit.

Finally, the granulomatous invasive fungal disease (or true mycetoma) is a rare condition mainly confined to the Sudan usually secondary to *Aspergillus flavus*, and often presenting with proptosis.

Imaging

CT is the primary imaging modality, although MRI can add important information.[16] Three planar scans are needed (coronal, axial, and sagittal for frontal sinus involvement) using both bone and soft tissue protocol (**Table 18.8**). This will optimally show the extent of the disease as well as the high-density areas that are characteristic though not absolutely pathognomonic of noninvasive fungal disease. This high density is due to dystrophic calcification and/ or high–atomic number elements such as manganese, calcium, zinc, and iron.[17] It is difficult to distinguish non-invasive from chronic invasive forms radiologically.

MRI with and without gadolinium enhancement is necessary to show intracranial extension but the signal will depend on the amount of proteinaceous secretion and paramagnetic material. Thus a very low signal may be given from the sinus contents on T1W sequences and a signal void on T2W sequences. If MRI alone is used this may mislead the clinician into thinking the sinus is "empty," but closer inspection shows that the lining mucosa has an irregular inflammation or "fuzzy felt" appearance that should raise suspicion.

A **fungal ball** affects one sinus, the maxillary most commonly, the ethmoids including a concha bullosa, or the sphenoid. The opacification may be partial, or complete when there is often expansion of the sinus with thinning and erosion of the bony walls (**Fig. 18.7**). Conversely, sclerosis can also be seen.[18] Most show hyperdensity (80%) and consequently can present a "signal void" on MRI that may fool the unwary.

In **eosinophilic fungal rhinosinusitis** the process is more widespread. It was previously described as mainly unilateral, but this has not been our experience, where 88% of cases had problems on both sides. The process is

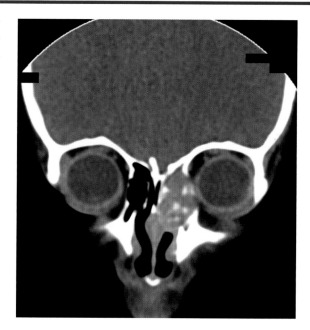

Fig. 18.7 Noninvasive fungal ball on coronal CT scan showing opacification with areas of hyperdensity in an anterior ethmoidal cell expanding into the orbit.

one of polyposis mixed with thick secretion, so a mixed density is seen in 83%. Again significant expansion can be seen and bone erosion is found in 70 to 80%.[16,19,20] The multiple areas affected produce a characteristic appearance on MRI (**Fig. 18.8**).

Chronic invasive disease produces a similar appearance to the noninvasive form but with greater extension into surrounding structures. There is often invasion of the orbit, cavernous sinus, and anterior and posterior cranial fossae. Bone erosion and heterogeneous density are also features. MRI will assist in determining orbital and intra-cranial extension (**Fig. 18.9**).

Acute fulminant invasive forms are much feared due to their extremely rapid progression associated with massive tissue necrosis and skull base destruction, resembling a malignant process. Mixed high density is not a feature and MRI may also suggest a malignant process but will define spreading inflammation and necrosis (**Fig. 18.10**).

Sclerosing invasive forms are rare and produce a fibrotic space-occupying lesion in the midline, usually involving both orbits and the anterior cranial fossa. MRI demonstrates low signal from the fibrotic mass. Some forms spread to involve the subcutaneous tissues (**Fig. 18.11**).

Histological Features and Differential Diagnosis

The fungal ball is composed of masses or nodules of entwined fungal mycelia and is easy to diagnose.

In eosinophilic fungal rhinosinusitis, the diagnosis can be surprisingly difficult to confirm even when there is a strong clinical suspicion, often due to the paucity of fungal material in the secretion and soft tissues.[21,22]

Table 18.8 Imaging protocol for fungal rhinosinusitis

CT	3-planar (coronal, axial, sagittal)
	Bone protocol • Window widths ~2000 HU[a] • Centered −250/−200
	Soft tissue protocol • Window widths 300–350 HU[a] • Centered +30
Add contrast enhancement or proceed to MRI when intracranial or intraorbital extension is suspected	
MRI	3-planar (coronal, axial, sagittal)
	T1 ± gadolinium contrast enhancement
	T2 sequences
[a]Depending on scanner.	

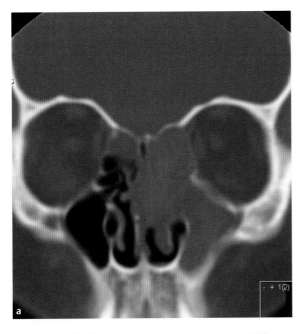

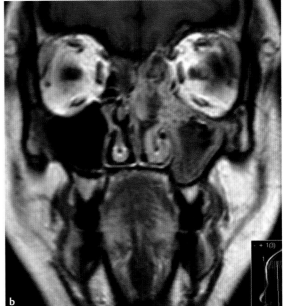

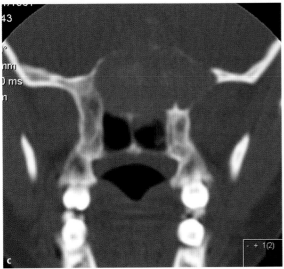

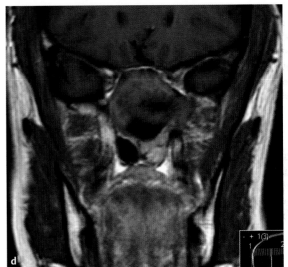

Fig. 18.8a–d Noninvasive eosinophilic (allergic) fungal rhinosinusitis.

a Coronal CT showing unilateral opacification with mild heterogeneous signal in the maxillary and ethmoid sinuses.

b Coronal MRI (T1W post gadolinium enhancement) of the same patient showing mixed signal from fungal material within the maxillary and ethmoid sinuses.

c Coronal CT of the same patient showing opacification of the sphenoid with expansion, bone erosion, and mildly heterogeneous signal.

d Coronal MRI (T1W post gadolinium enhancement) of same patient showing mixed signal from fungal material within sphenoid sinus with areas of signal void.

Specimens should be sent for both microbiology (mycology) and histopathology as fungal stains (Gomori methenamine silver/Grocott or periodic acid-Schiff) may be more successful, or even chitin stains may be used. The fungal mucin typically shows large numbers of eosinophils, Charcot-Leyden crystals (resulting from the dead eosinophils), and hopefully fungal hyphae. The fungal fragments, if found, often branch at 45-degree angles and may have conidia.[23] More often a report will describe the specimen as "consistent with" rather than diagnostic as the fungal elements have not been found. It should be noted, however, that with careful harvesting fungal elements can be found in most cases of sinus inflammation as well as in normal controls.[7,8] Kuhn and colleagues devised strict criteria for diagnosis of this condition that included the demonstration of fungi,[20] but others recognized the inherent problems in fulfilling these in every case.[21]

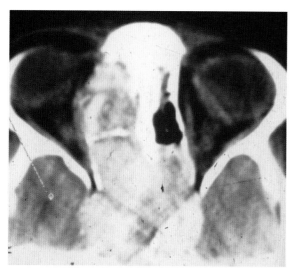

◁ **Fig. 18.9** Axial CT scan showing chronic invasive fungal rhinosinusitis with infiltration of both cavernous sinuses.

▽ **Fig. 18.10a–d** Acute fulminant fungal rhinosinusitis.

a Coronal CT at presentation showing an inflammatory process affecting both sides and infiltrating the left orbit.

b Sagittal CT at presentation showing an inflammatory process infiltrating the lower left orbit as far as the apex together with involvement of the maxilla, posterior ethmoid, and sphenoid.

c Axial MRI (T1W post gadolinium enhancement with fat saturation) at presentation showing a high-signal inflammatory process also affecting the infratemporal and temporal lobe dura.

d Coronal MRI 2 weeks later, after radical débridement of midfacial structures including orbital exenteration.

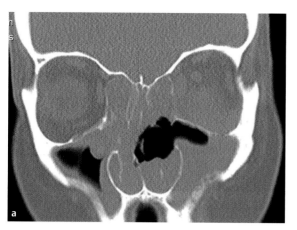

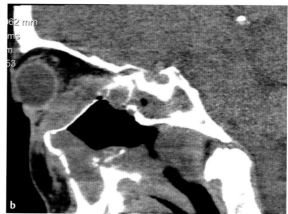

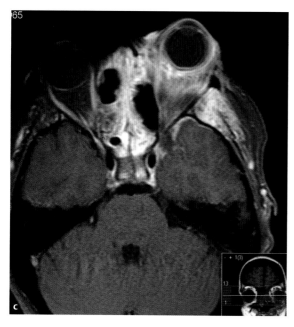

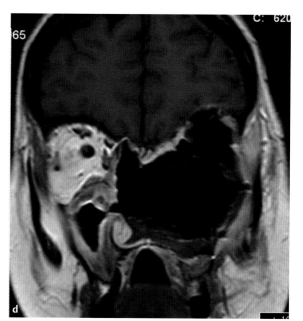

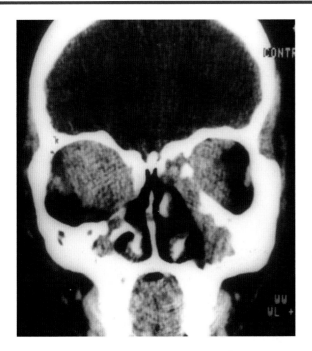

Fig. 18.11 Coronal CT of the sinuses showing a soft tissue mass infiltrating both orbits with a central surgical defect in sclerosing fungal rhinosinusitis.

Aspergillus and the dematiaceous fungi are implicated in noninvasive, chronic invasive, and sometimes acute fulminant forms, but one of the phycomycetes, *Rhizopus oryzae* or *Mucor*, is frequently responsible for the acute fulminant forms. The fungi invade the tissue and in particular vascular structures, leading to thrombosis and infarction.[24] Surrounding inflammation is often minimal but necrosis is common. *Mucor/Rhizopus* hyphae are nonseptate and have nonparallel walls, whereas *Aspergillus* has branching septate hyphae. These may be obvious on hematoxylin and eosin (H&E) staining, *Rhizopus* staining deeply with hematoxylin, but special fungal stains should also be used if available.

In any case, mucosa adjacent to the secretion must always be examined histologically for fungal invasion as well as being sent for culture. In all cases, but especially in the acute situation, representative tissue must be taken as the superficial material may only be composed of slough and necrotic debris.

In the rare sclerosing form, hyphae are very difficult to find among the fibrous tissue and must be meticulously sought histologically. This can be associated with *Conidiobolus coronatus*. These present irregular branching and very occasional septae, often embedded in eosinophilic material. Staining with H&E shows the eosinophilic material surrounding the clear empty hyphae.

In the invasive granulomatous form, a nonnecrotizing granulomatous inflammation is seen as well as tissue invasion with *Aspergillus flavus*.

On imaging, the areas of hyperdensity on CT suggest inverted papilloma, chondrosarcoma, and even adenocarcinoma, all of which may show areas of hyperdensity/calcification. The differential diagnosis on CT also includes mucoceles and cholesterol granuloma, although MRI will clarify the situation. The acute fulminant form must be distinguished from other midline destructive pathologies such as NK/T-cell lymphoma, Wegener's granulomatosis, and necrotizing fasciitis.

Natural History

The fungal ball and eosinophilic fungal rhinosinusitis cases grumble on over long periods, gradually enlarging the sinus cavity until treated. Thus, impressive collections of material can accrue in the anterior cranial cavity with few symptoms, even though the disease is extradural and noninvasive, but necessitating major surgery (**Fig. 18.12**). Recurrence after treatment is high with eosinophilic disease and it can appear on the contralateral side some time later.

Chronic invasive fungal disease also follows a rather indolent course unless the immune status of the patient changes. However, progressive involvement of adjacent orbit and cranial fossa can lead to the demise of the patient if not tackled aggressively.

Acute fulminant disease, by contrast, is a rapidly progressive condition capable of overwhelming the patient in a few hours or days as the progressive shutdown of vascular supply leads to an advancing wave of necrosis across the skull base, affecting any structure in its path including cranial nerves, bone, and soft tissue.

Treatment

As a general principle the fungal material needs to be removed.[25] This can almost always be accomplished by an endoscopic approach, although the secretion is often difficult to clean out as it blocks the suckers and has an impressive tensile strength that resists pulling or irrigation. However, with perseverance, time, and powered instrumentation, it can and should be removed in its entirety.[26]

In two-thirds of our patients, an entirely endoscopic approach was sufficient to extirpate disease but in one-third this was combined with external approaches (**Table 18.7**). This was mainly to deal with disease in the lateral compartment of a well-pneumatized frontal sinus or lateral "fungocele" or with major intracranial extension. In some cases a "second look" is undertaken a few months later after initial clearance and medical therapy.

In the case of fungal balls and in many areas of "eosinophilic" disease, the underlying mucosa looks remarkably normal. The combination of removing the material and ventilation will deal with the fungal ball and in all of our cases this was accomplished by an endoscopic approach.

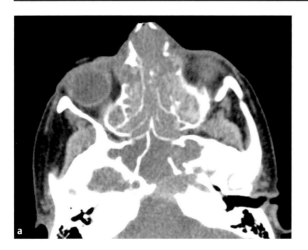

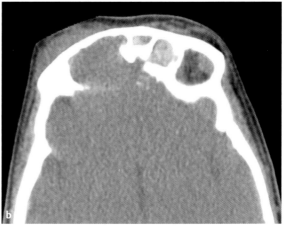

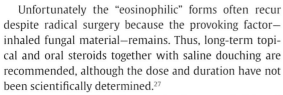

Fig. 18.12a, b

a Axial CT showing bilateral opacification of sinuses with expansion and bone loss of the posterior sphenoid wall.

b Axial CT showing bilateral heterogenous opacification of frontal sinuses with expansion and bone erosion of posterior wall into anterior cranial fossa.

Unfortunately the "eosinophilic" forms often recur despite radical surgery because the provoking factor—inhaled fungal material—remains. Thus, long-term topical and oral steroids together with saline douching are recommended, although the dose and duration have not been scientifically determined.[27]

The use of antifungal agents has been much debated in recent years. Amphotericin has been used as a douche but has mainly been investigated in chronic rhinosinusitis rather than overt fungal disease where it has not been shown in randomized controlled trials to be superior to douching alone.[28–31] Furthermore the antifungal agents have been developed for invasive disease so their efficacy in noninvasive disease is unknown and they carry potential adverse effects on renal and hepatic function, which must be monitored. Nonetheless, high-dose postoperative oral itraconazole combined with oral and topical steroids in a cohort of 139 patients with eosinophilic fungal rhinosinusitis was shown to reduce the need for revision surgery to a rate of 20.5%.[32]

In chronic invasion, surgical ventilation and débridement, ideally to remove all infected tissue, is advisable, although extension into the cavernous sinus and intracranial cavity poses technical difficulties. It may be possible to employ an endoscopic approach, but more radical surgery can necessitate craniofacial resection, maxillectomy, and orbital exenteration in some advanced cases even in the apparently immunocompetent. In addition here, the use of an antifungal agent is mandatory for 8 to 12 weeks. The choice will depend on the organism, but oral itraconazole is often used. In more severe cases intravenous liposomal amphotericin or newer antifungal agents such as voriconazole and posaconazole are used. A lifetime dose should not be exceeded and renal and liver function must be closely monitored.

In the acute fulminant form, rapid diagnosis and prompt action are paramount if the patient is to survive. The characteristic imaging and presence of necrotic tissue should prompt urgent débridement even before a formal identification of the pathogen in some cases, and similarly intravenous antifungal therapy should be initiated.[33] Frozen section can help confirm the presence of fungal fragments. Necrotic material must be removed back to "normal" bleeding tissue, even if this means removal of the eye and skull base. Thus, while endoscopic surgery can be of assistance, more major external surgery is usually needed. In our most recent case, a 45-year-old woman who was not overtly immunocompromised, radical débridement was required before the process was arrested. This included the eye, the entire nasal cavity, all sinuses, an extended maxillectomy, and resection of the pterygopalatine region and skull base. She has survived and is now undergoing reconstruction.

The sclerosing form is primarily treated with surgery as the penetration of antifungals is poor in the fibrous tissue. Our only case, a 23-year-old woman, underwent a formal craniofacial resection as well as receiving amphotericin.

Outcome

Complete removal of the fungal ball can be anticipated to cure the patient. None of our patients has developed recurrence in the original sinus, but one individual had a second fungal ball in the contralateral maxilla. However, with eosinophilic fungal rhinosinusitis, whatever strategy is employed, recurrence rates are high, varying from 32 to 100%.[25,34] This in part relates to the postoperative medication and consciousness of follow-up. In our own cohort, with a follow-up that ranges from 6 months to 19 years, the recurrence rate has been around 30% if all patients with further polypoid change are counted, although many of these are controlled with further oral and topical steroids. Follow-up MRI is recommended for those with initial intracranial extension if the area cannot be adequately visualized endoscopically.

Chronic invasive forms can usually be controlled but often with significant morbidity depending on the extent of disease at presentation. Acute invasive forms carry high morbidity and potential mortality between 25 and 75% in the literature.[35]

Key Points

- Fungal rhinosinusitis may be divided into invasive and noninvasive forms according to the presence of fungal hyphae within the tissue but not depending on the presence of bone erosion, which can occur in any form.
- The diagnosis can be difficult and often requires histological confirmation rather than positive culture.
- The secretion and imaging show characteristic features, although these are not pathognomonic. MRI alone is not recommended as the diagnosis may be missed due to signal void from the sinus contents.
- Surgical removal of the fungal material is required in all forms.
- Corticosteroids are used in eosinophilic fungal rhinosinusitis; antifungals have a limited role in this condition but are necessary in most invasive forms, which carry high morbidity and mortality.

References

1. Schubert MS. Fungal rhinosinusitis: diagnosis and therapy. Curr Allergy Asthma Rep 2001;1(3):268–276
2. deShazo RD, Chapin K, Swain RE. Fungal sinusitis. N Engl J Med 1997;337(4):254–259
3. Ferguson BJ, Barnes L, Bernstein JM, et al. Geographic variation in allergic fungal rhinosinusitis. Otolaryngol Clin North Am 2000;33(2):441–449
4. Schwietz LA, Gourley DS. Allergic fungal sinusitis. Allergy Proc 1992;13(1):3–6
5. Millar J, Johnston A, Lamb D. Allergic aspergillosis of the maxillary sinuses. Thorax 1981;36:710
6. Katzenstein AL, Sale SR, Greenberger PA. Allergic Aspergillus sinusitis: a newly recognized form of sinusitis. J Allergy Clin Immunol 1983;72(1):89–93
7. Ponikau JU, Sherris DA, Kern EB, et al. The diagnosis and incidence of allergic fungal sinusitis. Mayo Clin Proc 1999;74(9):877–884
8. Braun H, Buzina W, Freudenschuss K, Beham A, Stammberger H. 'Eosinophilic fungal rhinosinusitis': a common disorder in Europe? Laryngoscope 2003;113(2):264–269
9. Hamilos DL, Lund VJ. Etiology of chronic rhinosinusitis: the role of fungus. Ann Otol Rhinol Laryngol Suppl 2004;193:27–31
10. Fokkens WJ, Lund VJ, Mullol J, et al. EPOS 2012: European position paper on rhinosinusitis and nasal polyps 2012. A summary for otorhinolaryngologists. Rhinology 2012;50(1, Suppl 23)1–12
11. Kern RC, Conley DB, Walsh W, et al. Perspectives on the etiology of chronic rhinosinusitis: an immune barrier hypothesis. Am J Rhinol 2008;22(6):549–559
12. Fokkens WJ, Ebbens F, van Drunen CM. Fungus: a role in pathophysiology of chronic rhinosinusitis, disease modifier, a treatment target, or no role at all? Immunol Allergy Clin North Am 2009;29(4):677–688
13. Lund V. The mushroom explosion. ENT News 2000;9:55
14. Willinger B, Beck-Mannagetta J, Hirschl AM, Makristathis A, Rotter ML. Influence of zinc oxide on Aspergillus species: a possible cause of local, non-invasive aspergillosis of the maxillary sinus. Mycoses 1996;39(9-10):361–366
15. Jonathan D, Lund V, Milroy C. Allergic aspergillus sinusitis—an overlooked diagnosis? J Laryngol Otol 1989;103(12):1181–1183
16. Lund VJ, Lloyd G, Savy L, Howard D. Fungal rhinosinusitis. J Laryngol Otol 2000;114(1):76–80
17. Zinreich SJ, Kennedy DW, Malat J, et al. Fungal sinusitis: diagnosis with CT and MR imaging. Radiology 1988;169(2):439–444
18. Som PM, Dillon WP, Fullerton GD, Zimmerman RA, Rajagopalan B, Marom Z. Chronically obstructed sinonasal secretions: observations on T1 and T2 shortening. Radiology 1989;172(2):515–520
19. Bent JP III, Kuhn FA. Diagnosis of allergic fungal sinusitis. Otolaryngol Head Neck Surg 1994;111(5):580–588
20. Mukherji SK, Figueroa RE, Ginsberg LE, et al. Allergic fungal sinusitis: CT findings. Radiology 1998;207(2):417–422
21. Ferguson BJ. Eosinophilic mucin rhinosinusitis: a distinct clinicopathological entity. Laryngoscope 2000;110(5 Pt 1):799–813
22. Karpovich-Tate N, Dewey FM, Smith EJ, Lund VJ, Gurr PA, Gurr SJ. Detection of fungi in sinus fluid of patients with allergic fungal rhinosinusitis. Acta Otolaryngol 2000;120(2):296–302
23. Torres C, Ro JY, el-Naggar AK, Sim SJ, Weber RS, Ayala AG. Allergic fungal sinusitis: a clinicopathologic study of 16 cases. Hum Pathol 1996;27(8):793–799
24. McGill TJ, Simpson G, Healy GB. Fulminant aspergillosis of the nose and paranasal sinuses: a new clinical entity. Laryngoscope 1980;90(5 Pt 1):748–754
25. Lund V. What is the place of endonasal surgery in fungal sinusitis? In: Stamm A, Draf W, eds. Microscopic and Endoscopic Surgery of the Nose and Sinuses. Berlin: Springer; 2000:309–314
26. Kuhn FA, Javer AR. Allergic fungal rhinosinusitis: perioperative management, prevention of recurrence, and role of steroids and antifungal agents. Otolaryngol Clin North Am 2000;33(2):419–433
27. Schubert MS. Medical treatment of allergic fungal sinusitis. Ann Allergy Asthma Immunol 2000;85(2):90–97, quiz 97–101
28. Ebbens FA, Scadding GK, Badia L, et al. Amphotericin B nasal lavages: not a solution for patients with chronic rhinosinusitis. J Allergy Clin Immunol 2006;118(5):1149–1156
29. Weschta M, Rimek D, Formanek M, Podbielski A, Riechelmann H. Effect of nasal antifungal therapy on nasal cell activation markers in chronic rhinosinusitis. Arch Otolaryngol Head Neck Surg 2006;132(7):743–747
30. Ebbens FA, Georgalas C, Luiten S, et al. The effect of topical amphotericin B on inflammatory markers in patients with chronic rhinosinusitis: a multicenter randomized controlled study. Laryngoscope 2009;119(2):401–408
31. Liang KL, Su MC, Shiao JY, et al. Amphotericin B irrigation for the treatment of chronic rhinosinusitis without nasal polyps: a randomized, placebo-controlled, double-blind study. Am J Rhinol 2008;22(1):52–58
32. Rains BM III, Mineck CW. Treatment of allergic fungal sinusitis with high-dose itraconazole. Am J Rhinol 2003;17(1):1–8
33. Rizk SS, Kraus DH, Gerresheim G. Mudan S. Aggressive combination treatment for invasive fungal sinusitis in immunocompromised patients. Ear Nose Throat J 2000;79(4):278–280, 282, 284–285

34. Manning SC, Schaefer SD, Close LG, Vuitch F. Culture-positive allergic fungal sinusitis. Arch Otolaryngol Head Neck Surg 1991;117(2):174–178
35. Blitzer A, Lawson W. Fungal infections of the nose and paranasal sinuses. Part I. Otolaryngol Clin North Am 1993;26(6):1007–1035

Maxillary Sinus Hematoma

Definition

The formation of a hematoma within the maxillary sinus is a very rare cause of a mass that may be mistaken for a tumor.

Etiology

There is sometimes a history of trauma, but not in all cases, and it has been described in bleeding diatheses such as von Willebrand's disease.[1,2] It is postulated that there is leakage of blood at a rate that exceeds mucociliary clearance so that it can accumulate.[3,4]

Synonym

Maxillary sinus hematoma is sometimes referred to as organized hematoma or hemorrhagic pseudotumor.

Diagnostic Features

Maxillary sinus hematoma presents with a range of symptoms, the commonest of which is epistaxis or blood-stained nasal mucus, that also includes nasal obstruction, swelling of the face, and orbital displacement. Endoscopic examination shows only smooth medialization of the lateral nasal wall.

Imaging

Imaging reveals a nonenhancing opaque expanded mass on CT that may be mistaken for an antral mucocele or a benign tumor such as a schwannoma (**Fig. 18.13**). The mass may be homogeneous or show some heterogeneity due to calcification. Local expansion is sometimes accompanied by compression of adjacent structures and erosion of bone, although the exact mechanism is unknown.[4,5] MRI will assist in the diagnosis as it is nonenhancing on both T1W and T2W sequences, but blood of different ages can produce a heterogeneous signal.

Histological Features

Histology shows a mass composed of fibrin and red blood cells. Focal areas of dystrophic calcification can be seen in mature lesions and there is a fibrous capsule. However, there are sometimes areas of irregular blood vessels with

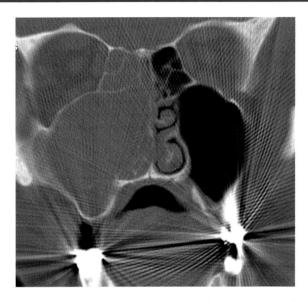

Fig. 18.13 Maxillary hematoma. Coronal CT showing an expanded maxillary sinus with homogeneous mass.

bizarre endothelial cells and granulation tissue, leading to a misdiagnosis of a malignant vascular tumor.

Treatment and Outcome

Twelve cases have been reported in the literature, whose ages range from 18 to 78 years and in whom external approaches were used including lateral rhinotomy and Caldwell-Luc. However, surgical removal of all the material, which is essentially organized clot, can be undertaken endoscopically through a large middle meatal antrostomy. This was done successfully in our only case of this condition, in a 56-year-old woman who on endoscopic examination had no evidence of recurrence at 1 year.[6]

References

1. Ozhan S, Araç M, Isik S, Oznur II, Atilla S, Kemaloglu Y. Pseudotumor of the maxillary sinus in a patient with von Willebrand's disease. AJR Am J Roentgenol 1996;166(4):950–951
2. Lee PK, Wu JK, Ludemann JP. Hemorrhagic pseudotumour of the maxillary sinus. J Otolaryngol 2004;33(3):206–208
3. Unlu HH, Mutlu C, Ayhan S, Tarhan S. Organized hematoma of the maxillary sinus mimicking tumor. Auris Nasus Larynx 2001;28(3):253–255
4. Tabaee A, Kacker A. Hematoma of the maxillary sinus presenting as a mass—a case report and review of literature. Int J Pediatr Otorhinolaryngol 2002;65(2):153–157
5. Lee BJ, Park HJ, Heo SC. Organized hematoma of the maxillary sinus. Acta Otolaryngol 2003;123(7):869–872
6. Lim M, Lew-Gor S, Beale T, Ramsay A, Lund VJ. Maxillary sinus haematoma. J Laryngol Otol 2008;122(2):210–212

Rhinosporidiosis/Rhinoscleroma

Rhinosporidiosis

Definition and Etiology

Rhinosporidiosis is a chronic disease of the nose and eye characterized by polypoid change in the nose and said to be caused by *Rhinosporidium seeberi*, which has yet to be cultured in vitro. Transmission is thought to occur from animal hosts such as horses and cattle via stagnant water. The actual organism may be a cyanobacterium, *Microcystis aeruginosa*, which is associated with the fungus.[1]

Incidence

It can occur anywhere but is most commonly found in southern India and Sri Lanka. We have treated one case, a 47-year-old man of Indian origin who was referred with residual disease unresponsive to medical therapies.

Diagnostic Features

Clinical Features

The polyps can be single or multiple, pedunculated or sessile, and are fleshy with an irregular surface. If they are unilateral, they may be mistaken for a tumor. Symptoms are of a mass effect and imaging is nonspecific (**Figs. 18.14 and 18.15**).

Natural History

The organism replicates in the tissues and forms a sporangium that releases thousands of spores. This process produces a chronic inflammatory response with eosinophils and giant cells. Histology is required to identify the sporangia.[2,3]

Treatment and Outcome

The condition has proved difficult to treat and a range of medications including dapsone, griseofulvin, amphotericin, and diaminodiphenylsulfone have all been tried without much success. Surgical debulking is also sometimes offered and in our patient, a radical endoscopic resection of affected tissue combined with KTP laser was undertaken of both sides of the nose and lateral postnasal space. This appears to have proved successful with a follow-up of 2 years.

Rhinoscleroma

Diagnosis and Etiology

Rhinoscleroma is a chronic granulomatous condition caused by *Klebsiella rhinoscleromatis*. It was first described by Von Hebra in 1870 but the causative organism was isolated by Von Frisch in 1882.[4]

Incidence

It is found worldwide but is endemic to Africa, Central and South America, eastern Europe, the Middle East, and

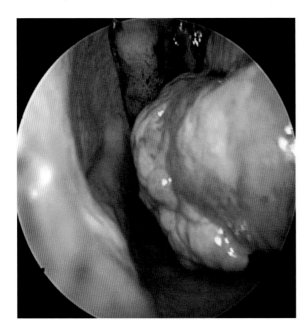

Fig. 18.14 Rhinosporidiosis. Endoscopic view of the left side of the nose showing a bulky granulomatous inferior turbinate.

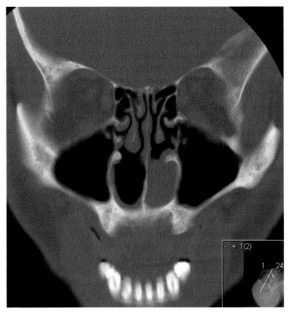

Fig. 18.15 Coronal CT scan showing rhinosporidiosis affecting the left side of the nose; previous surgical treatment is shown in the inset at right.

China. It is occasionally seen in Europe and the United States. We have treated only one case.

Diagnostic Features

Clinical Features

The infection affects the nasal cavity but it can extend into the nasopharynx, pharynx, and larynx and can produce crusting, purulent discharge and nasal blockage followed by nasal deformity with time. A study of 80 patients by Gamea[5] showed that all had involvement of the nasal vault, 22% of the maxillary sinus, 27% of the eustachian tube, and 26% of the larynx. The patients are usually young, in their teens or early twenties, as was the case in our patient, a girl of 15 years of Mediterranean origin. She had developed nasal blockage secondary to a smooth expansion of the nasal septum, confirmed on CT and MRI, so her presentation is not entirely typical.[6]

Although transmissible, the infection requires long-term contact, usually within a family setting.[7]

Diagnosis

The condition goes through several stages, exudative, proliferative, and cicatricial or fibrotic. The exudative or atrophic phase is characterized by inflammation, suppurative necrosis, and microabscesses. The proliferative or granulomatous phase shows chronic inflammation with characteristic foamy macrophages that have ingested the bacillus (Mikulicz cells), plasma cells, and Russell bodies. Nonulcerative nodules develop that are initially bluish red. Special silver staining reveals gram-negative coccobacilli consistent with *Klebsiella rhinoscleromatis*, but diagnosis is confirmed by culture on blood agar or MacConkey agar.[3] Immunohistochemistry with capsular antigen O2K3 is available and is the basis for immunoperoxidase testing.[8] The fibrotic phase is characterized by dense scar tissue.

Treatment and Outcome

The disease is often self-limiting but can leave significant scarring. The causative organism is resistant to many antibiotics as it resides intracellularly. Originally streptomycin, tetracycline, and trimethoprim-sulfamethoxazole have been given for prolonged periods, but better results have been achieved with long-term ciprofloxacin (500 mg orally twice a day for 8 weeks).[9–11] This may be because quinolones are concentrated within macrophages.[12] Our patient remained well with negative biopsies for 1 year and then developed further problems. She had a further 3-month course of ciprofloxacin and has subsequently remained disease-free for 2 years but will need long-term follow-up.

Surgery, except for diagnosis and late reconstruction, is not required.

References

1. Ahluwalia KB, Maheshwari N, Deka RC. Rhinosporidiosis: a study that resolves etiologic controversies. Am J Rhinol 1997;11(6):479–483
2. Arseculeratne SN. Recent advances in rhinosporidiosis and Rhinosporidium seeberi. Indian J Med Microbiol 2002;20(3):119–131
3. Batsakis JG, el-Naggar AK. Rhinoscleroma and rhinosporidiosis. Ann Otol Rhinol Laryngol 1992;101(10):879–882
4. Winstead W, Connely TV, Raff MJ. Rhinoscleroma: a case report and clinical update. Am J Rhinol 1993;7:282–285
5. Gamea AM. Role of endoscopy in diagnosing scleroma in its uncommon sites. J Laryngol Otol 1990;104(8):619–621
6. Badia L, Lund VJ. A case of rhinoscleroma treated with ciprofloxacin. J Laryngol Otol 2001;115(3):220–222
7. Shaw HJ, Martin H. Rhinoscleroma—a clinical perspective. J Laryngol Otol 1961;75:1011–1039
8. Andraca R, Edson RS, Kern EB. Rhinoscleroma: a growing concern in the United States? Mayo Clinic experience. Mayo Clin Proc 1993;68(12):1151–1157
9. Trautmann M, Held T, Ruhnke M, Schnoy N. A case of rhinoscleroma cured with ciprofloxacin. Infection 1993;21(6):403–406
10. Avery RK, Salman SD, Baker AS. Rhinoscleroma treated with ciprofloxacin: a case report. Laryngoscope 1995;105(8 Pt 1):854–856
11. Valor García C, Castillo Serrano E, Martín del Guayo G, et al. Rhinoscleroma. A case report. [Article in Spanish] Acta Otorrinolaringol Esp 1999;50(4):321–323
12. Hooper DC, Wolfson JS. Fluoroquinolone antimicrobial agents. N Engl J Med 1991;324(6):384–394

Sinonasal Tuberculosis

Definition and Etiology

Infection of the nose and sinuses by *Mycobacterium tuberculosis*.

Incidence

Apart from lupus vulgaris, tuberculosis (TB) within the nose and sinuses is rather uncommon. We have seen two cases in the past 30 years. However, there is a resurgence in association with HIV and social deprivation. Thirty-five cases have been reported in the English-language literature over the past 95 years.[1]

Site

The nose and sinuses can be the primary site or secondary to more widespread infection. The nasal cavity is more common than the sinuses, but cases have been described in the frontal and sphenoid.[2–4]

Diagnostic Features

Clinical

The symptoms are chronic nasal obstruction, rhinorrhea, and epistaxis together with crusting and ulceration. Any part of the nasal cavity and nasopharynx is affected and the ulceration can lead to palatal and septal fenestration.[5-7] There is generalized ulceration and sloughing, which may suggest other chronic granulomatous conditions such as Wegener's granulomatosis and sarcoid. Cervical lymphadenopathy may be present, due either to TB or a secondary inflammation.

Our patients, both women (42 and 65 years old), were otherwise fit and well and no other site of infection was determined. In both there was extensive involvement of the nasal vestibule, cavity, and nasopharynx and both had palatal ulceration. A predominance in middle-aged women is typical.

Imaging

Nonspecific inflammatory changes with some degree of cartilage and bone destruction are seen on CT scanning. Imaging of the chest should obviously be undertaken.

Histological Features and Differential Diagnosis

Representative biopsy will reveal caseating granulomas with Langerhans giant cells, and staining and culture for acid-fast bacilli will be positive.

Other granulomatous conditions must be excluded and the pseudoepitheliomatous reaction that can occur must be differentiated from squamous cell carcinoma.[8]

Treatment and Outcome

Once the condition is diagnosed, the assistance of infectious disease physicians will be invaluable in the evaluation of the patient and the choice and duration of antibiotic regime.

References

1. Butt AA. Nasal tuberculosis in the 20th century. Am J Med Sci 1997;313(6):332–335
2. Mohasseb G, Nasr B, Lahoud S, Halaby G. Hypophyseal tuberculosis. A case report. [Article in French] Neurochirurgie 1983;29(2):167–170
3. Shah GV, Desai SB, Malde HM, Naik G. Tuberculosis of sphenoidal sinus: CT findings. AJR Am J Roentgenol 1993;161(3):681–682
4. Sierra C, Fortún J, Barros C, et al. Extra-laryngeal head and neck tuberculosis. Clin Microbiol Infect 2000;6(12):644–648
5. Waldman SR, Levine HL, Sebek BA, Parker W, Tucker HM. Nasal tuberculosis: a forgotten entity. Laryngoscope 1981;91(1):11–16
6. Waldron J, Van Hasselt CA, Skinner DW, Arnold M. Tuberculosis of the nasopharynx: clinicopathological features. Clin Otolaryngol Allied Sci 1992;17(1):57–59
7. Kim YM, Kim AY, Park YH, Kim DH, Rha KS. Eight cases of nasal tuberculosis. Otolaryngol Head Neck Surg 2007;137(3):500–504
8. Sim DW, Crowther JA. Primary nasal tuberculosis masquerading as a malignant tumour. J Laryngol Otol 1988;102(12):1150–1152

Wegener's Granulomatosis or Granulomatosis with Polyangiitis

Definition

An idiopathic chronic inflammatory disease characterized by necrotizing granulomatous lesions and systemic vasculitis strongly associated with antineutrophil cytoplasmic antibodies (C-ANCA).

Etiology

The cause is unknown but this is probably an autoimmune disease. Several recent studies, both in vitro and in vivo, are now indicating that ANCA induce the systemic vasculitis[1] by binding to and activating neutrophils, which causes the release of oxygen radicals, lytic enzymes, and inflammatory cytokines. ANCA may also induce immune complex formation and may directly adhere to and kill endothelial cells, thereby causing vasculitis.[2] While PR3-ANCA (proteinase-3) is highly specific for Wegener's granulomatosis, the initial trigger may be infection or other environmental factors, possibly combined with a genetic susceptibility. Exposure to silica is one possibility. However, *Staphylococcus aureus* colonization of the nose, which is found more frequently in Wegener's granulomatosis, has been strongly implicated as a causative agent, especially in relapses.[3,4] A strong association with HLA-DPB1*0401 has also been described.[5]

Synonyms

First described by Klinger in 1932, this condition was ascribed to Wegener after his publication in 1936.[6,7] In recent times it has been referred to as C-ANCA positive granulomatosis and **most recently the nomenclature has been changed to granulomatosis with polyangiitis (GPA)**.[8]

Incidence

The true incidence of Wegener's granulomatosis (WG) has been underestimated in the past. Even with the advent of the ANCA test, many localized forms of the disease may go unrecognized. In Europe a prevalence of 23.7 per million has been reported; in the United States, 30 per million.[9]

The overall incidence ranges from 2.9 to 12 per million per year depending on the geographic region.

Site

Classically WG affected the nose, lungs, and kidneys. However, it can present in any system and limited forms of the disease are now well recognized, having been first described by Carrington and Liebow in 1966.[10] In addition to the nose, the audiovestibular system, larynx, and cranial nerves may be affected. Any organ can be affected, including the eye, skin, heart, gastrointestinal tract, and nervous systems.

Diagnostic Features

Clinical Features

The peak incidence is in the fourth to fifth decades but the condition can occur at any age (range 13 to 78 years). The average age at diagnosis was 50 years in a study we performed on a cohort of 199 patients.[11] It seems to be more aggressive in younger people. Men and women appear equally affected and the vast majority are white (93%).[12–15] However, there is some evidence that males are more likely to have "severe" disease and females the more "limited" phenotype.[13]

Two-thirds of patients initially present with an ENT-related symptom, of which 41% were rhinological, 16% otological, and 6% laryngopharyngeal in our study (**Fig. 18.16**).[11] Nasal symptoms were commoner in those diagnosed at <40 years (55%) than in those >60 years (27%). Typically the patient presents with nasal symptoms of

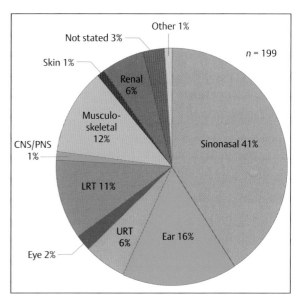

Fig. 18.16 Pie diagram showing the distribution of WG patients by initial presenting system. (CNS, central nervous system; LRT, lower respiratory tract; PNS, peripheral nervous system; URT, upper respiratory tract.) (Modified from Srouji et al.[11])

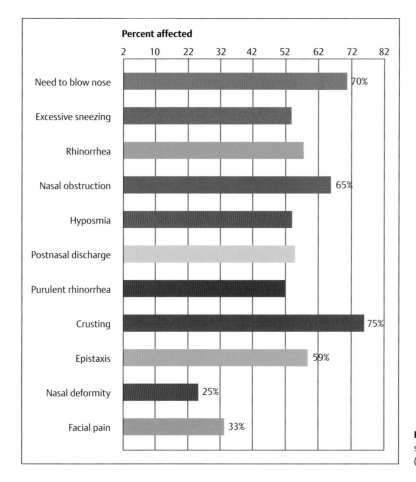

Fig. 18.17 Histogram showing the sinonasal symptom pattern in WG patients (n = 199). (Modified from Srouji et al.[11])

crusting (75%), discharge (70%), nasal stuffiness (65%), bleeding (59%), reduced sense of smell (52%), and facial pain (33%). The hyposmia may be simply a result of mechanical obstruction of the olfactory region or specific cranial nerve involvement. Deep-seated facial pain is quite a distressing symptom and may be secondary to sinus changes, but may also be due to an osteitis of midfacial bone, indicative of disease activity (**Fig. 18.17**). When all sinonasal symptoms are ranked, crusting and epistaxis are first and second in importance.[14]

The external appearances of the nose may change in ~25% of patients, with a characteristic supratip collapse that is somewhat different from that seen after nasal septal trauma and only seen in WG and relapsing polychondritis (**Fig. 18.18**). The nose folds inwards and looks as though it could be pulled out. This may or may not be associated with septal perforation. Sometimes the entire internal structure of the nose disappears, creating a large featureless cavity. On endoscopic examination the nasal mucosa is often very friable, granular, and covered with old blood and crust (**Fig. 18.19**). Adhesions may be present and the condition should be suspected in patients who develop significant adhesions after minor nasal surgery. As the condition progresses, there can be bone erosion of the skull base and patients may occasionally develop meningitis.

The ears can also be involved in a variety of ways. Patients may develop a chronic serous otitis media, and if grommets are inserted a persistent discharge that should be a clue to the presence of WG. Hearing loss can be conductive due to this, sensorineural due to cranial nerve involvement, or mixed. Scarring in the nose and eustachian region will often lead to persistent middle ear problems. Patients may also present with balance problems or a facial nerve palsy. In our study on 199 patients, 50% had aural fullness and 42% experienced dizziness. Otalgia was also complained of by one-third.[11]

In the mouth there may be gingivitis, ulceration, and oroantral fistulas, although midline palatal necrosis is rare in contrast to the situation with cocaine abuse (see below) (**Fig. 18.20**).

An area that is frequently overlooked is the larynx, and in particular the subglottis where stenosis may occur.[16] This can be a presenting problem but may be overshadowed or confused with lower respiratory tract symptoms. This condition should be considered in any patients with dyspnea, hoarseness, or inspiratory stridor and is estimated to occur in ~16% of WG patients.[17] It is commoner when WG starts in childhood.[18] In addition, the vocal fold mobility may be affected by cranial neuropathy.

Although WG can present in a myriad of ways, in many patients relatively minor upper respiratory symptoms are associated with disproportionate unwellness, fatigue, weight loss, and night sweats, heralding generalized WG, the systemic symptoms and signs of which are legion (**Table 18.9**). In the lungs, the necrotizing vasculitis leads

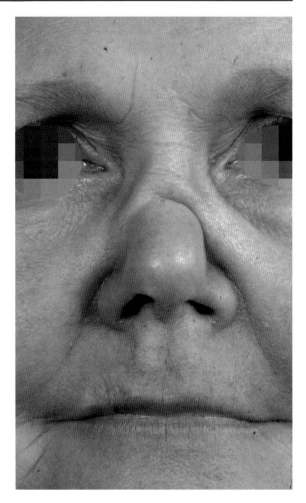

Fig. 18.18 Clinical photograph showing the typical collapse of the external nose in WG.

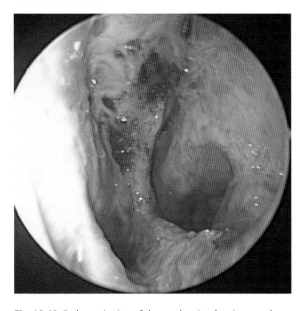

Fig. 18.19 Endoscopic view of the nasal cavity showing septal perforation and widespread granular change with some old blood.

to hemoptysis and cough, and pleuritic pain with gradual dyspnea as lung function is lost. The necrotic cavities may heal by fibrosis or form encapsulated abscesses. It is important to distinguish this from the effects of subglottic stenosis, which may be overlooked.

Renal involvement can occur in 75% of patients and eventually leads to renal failure.

In the orbit, granulomatous infiltration and vasculitis can result in proptosis (~2%) and corneal exposure, pain, and visual loss (~8%).[17] Patients may also have epiphora and dacrocystoadenitis. They may present with a "red eye" due to episcleritis or keratitis, which is seen in 15% of early-stage WG.[18] About half of patients have some ocular problems during the course of their disease.[19]

There can be arthralgia; skin lesions such as purpura, subcutaneous nodules, ulcers, vesicles, and papules; pericardial effusions; and neuropathies; as a result patients may be seen by a wide range of specialists (**Table 18.9**).

Not surprisingly the quality of life in these patients is significantly affected. In our study of 199 patients with WG using two validated quality of life (QoL) instruments— general (SF-36) and rhinosinusitis-specific quality of life (Sinonasal Outcome Test-SNOT-22)—a significant effect of sinonasal involvement on the general QoL was demonstrated.[14] This also showed that Wegener's-related sinonasal morbidity is at least as significant as that in the general rhinosinusitis population, which may in part explain the delay in diagnosis of this disease.

Diagnosis

Prior to the advent of the ANCA test, diagnosis relied on clinical signs and symptoms supported by raised ESR (erythrocyte sedimentation rate), CRP (C-reactive protein), altered renal function on blood and urine testing, and chest radiography, which might show evidence of granulations, infiltration, necrotic cavitation, and fibrosis. Urine testing can still be helpful if it shows proteinuria, microscopic hematuria, and red cell casts.

However, the ANCA test was first described in 1985 by Van Der Woude and colleagues and has significantly helped in the diagnosis of WG and other vasculitides.[20] It is 99% specific with a sensitivity of 73% using combined

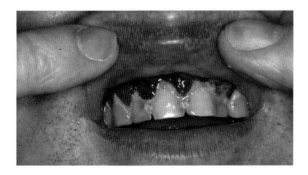

Fig. 18.20 Clinical photograph showing marked gingivitis.

Table 18.9 Symptoms associated with different system involvement in Wegener's granulomatosis/PGA

Bodily system	Manifestation
Ear, nose, throat	Nasal obstruction, crusting, bleeding, sinusitis
	Otalgia, otorrhea, deafness
	Oral lesions, laryngitis
Upper respiratory tract	Stridor, cord palsy/fixation
	Tracheal stenosis
Lower respiratory tract	Pulmonary infiltrates, nodules or hemorrhage
Ophthalmic	Scleritis, episcleritis, retinitis, retro-orbital granuloma
Cardiac	Arrhythmias, effusion, infarction, myocarditis
Renal	Nephritis, renal impairment, renal failure
Gastrointestinal	Diarrhea, bleeding
Peripheral nervous system	Sensory or motor polyneuropathy, mononeuritis
Central nervous system	CNS lesions, meningeal vasculitis
Skin	Purpura, nonhealing ulceration
Musculoskeletal	Arthralgia, myalgia

immunofluorescence and enzyme-linked immunosorbent assay (ELISA) techniques.

Up to 95% of patients with active systemic disease are ANCA positive and in most patients the ANC antibodies are directed against proteinase 3 (PR3). In vitro and animal models suggest that the interaction of ANCA with cytokine-primed neutrophils results in premature activation, respiratory burst, and degranulation of neutrophil granulocytes, with subsequent endothelial cell damage and necrotizing vasculitis. Altered T cell responses with predominant T_H1-type cytokine release might facilitate autoantigen recognition in WG.[1]

Sequential monitoring of the c-ANCA is a very useful tool in management and as early as 1989 a 4-fold increase in titer was shown to indicate a relapse,[21] but it is recognized that not all patients show the classical pattern of fluctuation with disease activity.[22] The c-ANCA was only positive in 68% of relapses.[15] In addition, unfortunately, the c-ANCA lacks sensitivity in the limited forms of the disease (dropping to 50%) and/or following therapy with corticosteroids, so a negative ANCA does not exclude WG. Interestingly, a few patients (~5%) have a positive MPO-ANCA.

The American College of Rheumatology proposed a clinical classification in 1990 to distinguish WG from other vasculitides (**Table 18.10**) and a range of validated indices have been developed to semiquantify disease activity (e.g., Birmingham vasculitis activity score), extent, and damage.

Cocaine Abuse

It is now well-recognized that cocaine abuse in the form of "snorting" can induce midline destruction of the nose and palate.[23] This may be preceded by progressive nasal obstruction, epistaxis, and crusting, which closely resemble the sinonasal symptoms of WG. Ulceration of the mucosa is followed by septal perforation and serious destruction of the midface can ensue (**Fig. 18.21**). Furthermore, the c-ANCA and PR-3 can be positive, making differentiation between the conditions extremely difficult.[23,24] However, on further investigation, there are some subtle differences in the ANCA between the two groups[25] and it seems that massive apoptosis with abundant caspase-3 and -9 expression is found in the cocaine users but not in WG patients.[26] ANCA react with human neutrophil elastase in the cocaine group but not in autoimmune vasculitis,[27] so this may help with the differential diagnosis.

Table 18.10 Definitions and criteria for Wegener's granulomatosis (WG)[1]

The American College of Rheumatology proposed clinical classification criteria (vasculitis must be present) for Wegener's granulomatosis (1990)[a]
• Nasal or oral inflammation (painful or painless oral ulcers or purulent or bloody nasal discharge)
• Abnormal chest radiograph showing nodules, fixed infiltrates, or cavities
• Abnormal urinary sediment (microscopic hematuria with or without red cell casts)
• Granulomatous inflammation on biopsy of an artery or perivascular area
Definition and classification of Wegener's granulomatosis according to the Chapel Hill Consensus (1994)
• Granulomatous inflammation involving the respiratory tract, and necrotizing vasculitis affecting small to medium-sized vessels (i.e., capillaries, venules, arterioles, and arteries)
• Necrotizing glomerulonephritis is common
• Cytoplasmic pattern ANCA (c-ANCA) with antigen specificity for proteinase 3 (PR3) is a very sensitive marker for Wegener's granulomatosis
[a] For classification purposes, a patient shall be said to have WG if he/she has satisfied any two or more of these four criteria. This rule is associated with a sensitivity of 88.2% and a specificity of 92.0%.

Imaging

Imaging of the sinuses can be helpful as there are characteristic features on CT and MRI. In a patient without a history of previous sinonasal surgery, a combination of bone destruction and new bone formation on CT is virtually diagnostic of WG, especially when accompanied on MRI by a fat signal from the sclerotic sinus wall ("tramlines") giving a high signal on T1W sequences. In a series of 28 patients, 86% showed nonspecific mucosal thickening in the nose or paranasal sinuses, 75% showed evidence of bone destruction, and 50% evidence of new bone formation in the walls of the sinuses.[28] These changes were present in both localized and systemic forms of WG. Progressive midfacial loss can be observed and can mimic that seen in NK/T-cell lymphoma. Concomitant bone destruction in the skull base can also be seen in some individuals (**Figs. 18.22, 18.23, 18.24, 18.25**).

When scans are done in this area it is always worth asking for an additional series with bone widths, which optimally show the orbits as these are involved in at least a third of cases where sinus changes are present and may occur independently. Appearances on CT are of an ill-defined soft tissue mass completely obscuring the optic nerve and extraocular muscles, often starting in the retro-orbit, with associated local bony destruction. The process can advance so that the entire orbital is overwhelmed by the process. On MRI, low to intermediate signal granulomas on T1W and T2W imaging may be distinguished from surrounding fat and ocular muscles.[29] With time, the granulomatous tissue may be replaced by fibrosis, altering the tissue signals.

Furthermore, any patients with dyspnea, hoarseness, stridor, or other airway problems should be considered for imaging of the larynx to show subglottic stenosis.

Imaging of the lungs can reveal diffuse infiltration, multiple pulmonary nodules (2–4 cm in diameter) or large necrotic cavitating granulomatous masses (10 cm diameter or larger), some with fluid levels, which may compress or discharge into adjacent bronchi. On CT there may be ground-glass shadowing around the nodules, probably due to hemorrhage.[29] Progressive consolidation and scarring occur with time. Pleural effusions and hilar lymphadenopathy are less common than in other granulomatoses.

Histological Features and Differential Diagnosis

WG is characterized by three key findings:
• Granulomatous inflammation
• Necrosis
• Vasculitis

The granulomas are composed of CD4[+] and CD8[+] T cells, CD28[−] T cells, histiocytes, CD20[+] B lymphocytes, neutrophil granulocytes, macrophages, and multinucleated

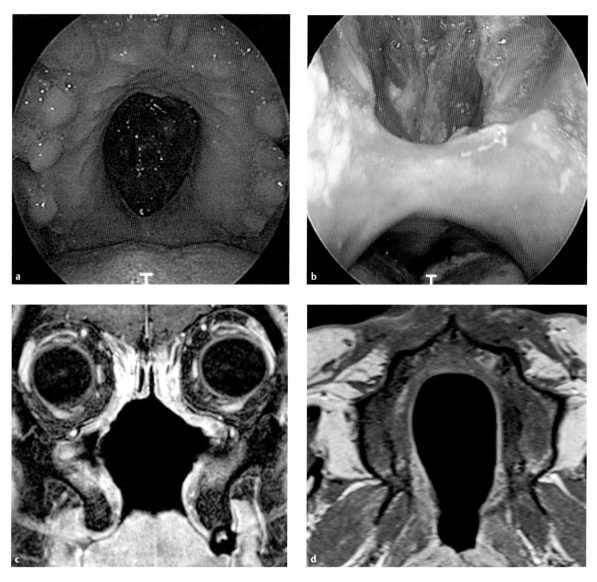

Fig. 18.21a–d Effects of cocaine abuse. (Courtesy of Dr. Matteo Trimarchi.)

a Clinical photograph of the oral cavity showing a midpalatal fistula.

b Endoscopic view of the nasal cavity showing the loss of central structures and palatal fistula.

c Coronal MRI showing the loss of midline structures.

d Axial MRI showing the loss of midline structures.

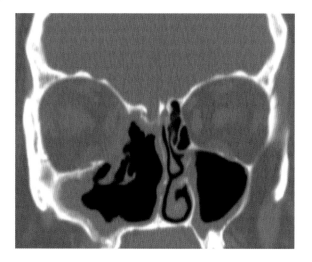

Fig. 18.22 Coronal CT scan showing loss of structure in the right nasal cavity, with inflammatory change particularly in the right maxillary sinus and ethmoids and bone erosion and early orbital infiltration. Tram lines are seen on the lateral wall of the maxillary sinus, which are pathognomonic for WG.

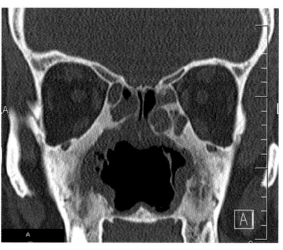

Fig. 18.23 Coronal CT scan showing loss of the nasal septum and new bone formation, and obliterative change in the lateral walls of the sinuses.

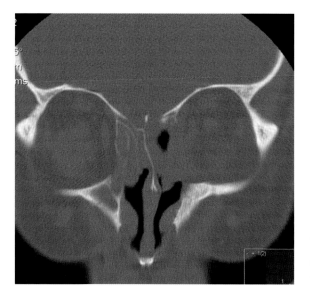

Fig. 18.24 Coronal CT scan showing inflammatory change in the upper nasal cavities with early bone erosion of the left skull base and lamina papyracea.

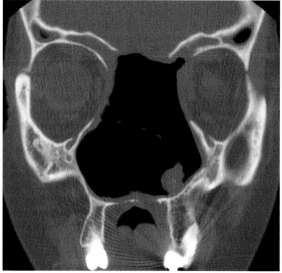

Fig. 18.25 Coronal CT scan showing marked loss of midline structures with significant erosion of the skull base in a patient who developed meningitis.

giant cells surrounding an area of central necrosis. Occasional eosinophils may confuse the diagnosis with Churg-Strauss syndrome.

The vasculitis predominantly affects small to medium-sized vessels (capillaries, venules, arterioles, and arteries) and again is associated with necrosis. In the kidneys a rapidly progressive glomerulonephritis can occur and diagnosis can be confirmed by renal or lung biopsy. However, it can be very difficult for the diagnosis to be made on the histological findings alone, which are usually reported as "consistent with" rather than definitive. Many nasal biopsies are taken, particularly from the edge of incidental septal perforations, more in hope than expectation as they are rarely diagnostic of WG even when the condition is present.[30,31] Abnormal tissue from the sinuses is likely to provide a better yield.[32]

The differential diagnosis is from any of the other granulomatous conditions (Table 18.1) including sarcoid, T-cell lymphoma, and a range of infectious conditions such as tuberculosis, and fungal conditions, particularly rhinosporidiosis and rhinoscleroma.

Natural History

Prior to the advent of systemic cytotoxic therapy, WG was a serious disease that generally had a fatal outcome within 2 years, usually due to renal failure. Before 1970, only 50% of patients survived 5 months from diagnosis and 82% were dead within 1 year.[33] Even the advent of corticosteroids only improved mean survival to 12.5 months.[34] Fortunately, that situation improved enormously with the combination of corticosteroids and cyclophosphamide, a regimen introduced by Fauci and colleagues, but remission was often followed by relapses and treatment-related toxicity was substantial.[35] Modern regimens aim to rapidly induce remission to limit organ damage and maintain this while minimizing side effects of the medications.

However, WG should still be regarded as potentially life-threatening, particularly as there is often delay in diagnosis. Some patients are overwhelmingly ill within a couple of days; in others the condition takes months to be recognized by the patient and their doctor. A survey conducted on over 700 patients in the United States[36] revealed that a third of patients waited 6 months or longer before their diagnosis was made. In a study of 199 British patients, the delay was even longer with 43% waiting over 6 months and 23% undiagnosed after 12 months from their initial presentation.[11] Furthermore, there did not seem to be any improvement over the years in this delay to diagnosis. The delay was greatest when patients presented with eye symptoms (>14 months) but ENT symptoms were associated with the second longest delay (of >8 months). This is particularly disappointing as over half the patients (56%) saw an ENT surgeon prior to their diagnosis.

As ENT surgeons we see manifestations of either limited or systemic forms of the disease. The European Vasculitis Study Group (EUVAS) distinguishes "localized" (i.e., WG restricted to the respiratory tract) and "early systemic" WG (i.e., nonimminent WG without renal organ involvement) from "generalized" WG (Table 18.11).[37] The majority of patients ultimately develop systemic disease within a few months or several years, but whether all localized forms go on to systemic disease, and if so what determines progression and the speed with which it happens, is unknown. This clearly has important implications for treatment as the medications are not without their potential side effects nor is it known whether treatment of limited disease prevents dissemination.

The condition also has a fluctuating course that is different from individual to individual and the disease is a classic example of "snakes and ladders" in which, as medication is reduced to minimize adverse effects or other events such as infection occur, patients may experience recrudescences of disease activity. These can also be triggered by many events from an episode of influenza to pregnancy.

If the patient survives these relapses (and their treatment), in many individuals the disease does eventually burn out.

Table 18.11 Clinical subgroups of Wegener's granulomatosis (WG) according to the definitions of the European Vasculitis Study Group (EUVAS)

Subgroup	Organ involvement	Constitutional symptoms	Presence of ANCA
Localized WG	Upper and/or lower respiratory tract	No	Yes/no
Early systemic WG	Any except renal involvement or imminent organ failure	Yes	Usually yes
Generalized WG	Renal with serum creatinine ≤500 µmol/L and/or other imminent organ failure	Yes	Yes
Severe renal WG	Renal with serum creatinine >500 µmol/L	Yes	Yes
Refractory WG	Progressive disease despite therapy with glucocorticoids and cyclophosphamide	Yes	Yes/No

Source: After reference 36.

Treatment

To obtain rapid remission, steroids are usually used in combination with cyclophosphamide in the severe systemic forms. Both may be used parenterally or orally. Cyclophosphamide is often given in pulsed form together with bolus doses of methylprednisolone in the acute situation and then orally for maintenance (EUVAS).[37] The typical daily dose of cyclophosphamide is 2 mg/kg and generally should not exceed 200 mg/day, with lower doses in the elderly or those with renal problems. However, the long-term side effects of both drugs are an issue and not all patients are steroid responsive. Cyclophosphamide can cause significant leukopenia, alopecia, and hemorrhagic cystitis and is associated with a significantly increased risk of certain malignancies. There is an 11-fold increase in the chances of lymphoma or leukemia in the longer term[17] and a 33-fold increase in the chances of bladder cancer. In addition, fertility is affected, with 60% of women of child-bearing age developing ovarian failure.

Methylprednisolone is used up to 1 g/day intravenously in severe cases, tapering down to oral prednisolone from a maximum of ~ 80 mg/day. The aim is to reduce the prednisolone within the first 6 to 9 months if patients do well in order to minimize the side effects, either to stopping the drug altogether or to a low maintenance dose of 5 to 7.5 mg/day.[38] The long-term multisystem side effects of corticosteroids include osteoporosis, diabetes, hypertension, changes in skin and muscle, and classic "steroid facies" to name but a few.

For longer-term maintenance, in addition to prednisolone, azathioprine and more recently mycophenolate mofetil, an inhibitor of purine synthesis, are being used. These may be "steroid-sparing," thus reducing the requisite dose of prednisolone or be monotherapy for longer-term maintenance, and are less often associated with significant side effects.[37,39] In the United Kingdom, among 199 patients, 71% were on oral steroids and 41% on azathioprine for maintenance.[11] A prospective randomized study by Jayne et al showed that substituting azathioprine for cyclophosphamide once a patient was in remission did not increase the rate of relapse.[38]

Plasmapheresis is used in those with severe renal involvement. Immunoglobulin replacement and other cytotoxic agents such as methotrexate are sometimes used. Methotrexate is given once a week (typically 15–20 mg/week), usually in combination with oral steroids, and patients should receive supplemental folic acid. Again this drug must be given with caution if there is renal damage. It is probably best used for longer-term maintenance rather than for the initial induction of remission.[40]

Most recently monoclonal antibodies, in particular the anti-CD20 antibody rituximab, have been used with some success,[32] and the RAVE (Rituximab for ANCA-associated Vasculitis) study[41] on 197 patients showed intermittent infusion of rituximab to be equivalent to daily cyclophosphamide for induction of remission and possibly superior in relapsing disease. TNF-α inhibitors such as infliximab and etanercept have been less convincing versus placebo.[42]

Patients require frequent monitoring so that the treatments can be titrated against the activity of the condition and also for the side effects of the drugs. Thus, regular ANCA tests as well as full blood counts, ESR, CRP, and renal function tests are needed.

Bone densitometry and prophylaxis against osteoporosis should be considered, although the routine use of bisphosphonate treatment has been questioned as an association with osteonecrosis of the jaws has been reported, albeit mainly in patients taking the drug for malignancy.[43] Calcium and vitamin D supplements, and hormone replacement therapy in postmenopausal women, can all be considered.

Once the disease has burnt out, some individuals will continue to require a small dose of prednisolone (e.g., 5 mg/day) to provide baseline replacement of their corticosteroid requirement.

The possible role of an infectious agent such as *Staphylococcus aureus* led to the use of long-term oral co-trimoxazole (trimethoprim-sulfamethoxazole) and topical antistaphylococcal creams in the nose. There is some evidence that co-trimoxazole reduces relapses in the respiratory tract,[44] and can also reduce the chance of *Pneumocystis* pneumonia infection.

ENT Treatment

Nose

Topical medications such as some form of douching, a topical intranasal corticosteroid, and/or nasal lubricant such as glucose and glycerin drops or an aqueous gel can be helpful. Surgery has a limited role, but it is sometimes worthwhile endoscopically exploring the sinuses if only to confirm that the opacification is granulation/fibrosis rather than infection. The skull base may need reinforcement in selected patients who develop meningitis secondary to bone erosion, which again can be effected endoscopically using established on-lay techniques.

Repair of the septal perforation is unlikely to be successful, but many younger patients now request "cosmetic" improvement of the external nasal deformity. As long as the disease has been quiescent for a reasonable period of time (e.g., 1 year), this can be undertaken with success.

Larynx

There is no consensus as to the management of subglottic and tracheobronchial stenosis in WG, but good results were obtained in a cohort of 18 patients treated with intralesional steroids, conservative laser surgery, and endoluminal dilation.[45] Using this strategy, mean intervention-free intervals of around 2 years were obtained and no patients required tracheostomy or stenting.

In the ear, grommets are probably best avoided but patients may benefit from a hearing aid.

Outcome

The best outcomes are derived from a multidisciplinary approach, combining specialists covering the many systems that may be affected, but usually under the leadership of a physician with a special interest in the condition. This allows regular monitoring of renal and pulmonary function and ANCA titers. Sequential ESR or CRP are cheap and quick but nonspecific as they will be affected by other events such as infection. However, they can still be a helpful indicator.

The primary goal of treatment is to achieve remission, but it is not known how long therapy must be given and this is the subject of several ongoing trials (Table 18.12).

Although overall the outcome for most patients has improved significantly in recent years, ~10% never achieve remission, relapses occur in up to 50% of individuals, and mortality rates of 5% or higher are still reported.[15]

Key Points

- Suspect WG when:
  - ENT symptoms do not improve with conventional treatment
  - There is nasal crusting and bleeding + feeling unwell
  - Adhesions, septal perforation, nasal collapse occur after minor nasal surgery
  - Persistent discharge occurs after grommet insertion in an adult
  - Subglottic stenosis occurs "spontaneously."
- c-ANCA is useful if positive but a negative test does not rule out WG.
- If in doubt, refer to a colleague with an interest in vasculitis/granulomatoses.

References

1. Gross W, Aries P, Lamprecht P. Granulomatosis: Wegener's disease. Encyclopedia of Respiratory Medicine. Elsevier; 2006:255–261
2. Jennette JC, Xiao H, Falk RJ. Pathogenesis of vascular inflammation by anti-neutrophil cytoplasmic antibodies. J Am Soc Nephrol 2006;17(5):1235–1242
3. Stegeman CA, Tervaert JW, Sluiter WJ, Manson WL, de Jong PE, Kallenberg CG. Association of chronic nasal carriage of Staphylococcus aureus and higher relapse rates in Wegener granulomatosis. Ann Intern Med 1994;120(1):12–17
4. Popa ER, Tervaert JW. The relation between Staphylococcus aureus and Wegener's granulomatosis: current knowledge and future directions. Intern Med 2003;42(9):771–780
5. Jagiello P, Gross WL, Epplen JT. Complex genetics of Wegener granulomatosis. Autoimmun Rev 2005;4(1):42–47
6. Klinger H. Grenzformen der periarteritis nodosa. Frankfurt J Pathol 1931;42:455–480
7. Wegener F. Uber generaliserle, septische geffasserkrankugen. Verhandlungen Deutschen Gesselschaft Pathol 1936; 29:202–210
8. Jennette J, Falk R, Bacon P, et al. 2012 Revised International Chapel Hill Consensus Conference Nomenclature of Vasculitides. Arthritis Rheum 2013;65(1):1–11.

Table 18.12 Criteria for relapse in Wegener's granulomatosis according to the European Vasculitis Study Group (EUVAS)

Major relapse
Recurrence or new appearance of major organ involvement, if attributable to active vasculitis. Such as:
1. An increase in serum creatinine of >30% or reduction in creatinine clearance of >25%, within a period of 3 months or histological evidence of active, focal, necrotizing glomerulonephritis
2. Clinical, radiological, or bronchoscopic evidence of pulmonary hemorrhage or granulomas
3. Threatened vision, e.g., increasing orbital granuloma or retinal vasculitis
4. Significant subglottic or bronchial stenosis
5. New multifocal lesions on brain MRI suggestive of cerebral vasculitis
6. Motor mononeuritis multiplex
7. Gastrointestinal hemorrhage or perforation
Minor relapse
Recurrence of disease activity of less severity, if attributable to active vasculitis. Such as:
1. ENT: epistaxis, crusting, pain, new deafness, active nasal ulceration, or proliferative mass at nasal endoscopy
2. Mouth ulcers
3. Rash
4. Myalgia, arthralgia, or arthritis
5. Episcleritis or scleritis
6. Pulmonary symptoms with or without minor radiological changes, e.g., cough, wheeze, dyspnea
Source: After reference 36.

9. Cotch MF, Hoffman GS, Yerg DE, Kaufman GI, Targonski P, Kaslow RA. The epidemiology of Wegener's granulomatosis. Estimates of the five-year period prevalence, annual mortality, and geographic disease distribution from population-based data sources. Arthritis Rheum 1996;39(1):87–92

10. Carrington CB, Liebow A. Limited forms of angiitis and granulomatosis of Wegener's type. Am J Med 1966; 41(4):497–527

11. Srouji IA, Andrews P, Edwards C, Lund VJ. Patterns of presentation and diagnosis of patients with Wegener's granulomatosis: ENT aspects. J Laryngol Otol 2007; 121(7):653–658

12. O'Devaney K, Ferlito A, Hunter BC, Devaney SL, Rinaldo A. Wegener's granulomatosis of the head and neck. Ann Otol Rhinol Laryngol 1998;107(5 Pt 1):439–445

13. Stone JH; Wegener's Granulomatosis Etanercept Trial Research Group. Limited versus severe Wegener's granulomatosis: baseline data on patients in the Wegener's granulomatosis etanercept trial. Arthritis Rheum 2003; 48(8):2299–2309

14. Srouji IA, Andrews P, Edwards C, Lund VJ. General and rhinosinusitis-related quality of life in patients with Wegener's granulomatosis. Laryngoscope 2006;116(9):1621–1625

15. Sproson EL, Jones NS, Al-Deiri M, Lanyon P. Lessons learnt in the management of Wegener's granulomatosis: long-term follow-up of 60 patients. Rhinology 2007;45(1):63–67

16. Hoare TJ, Jayne D, Rhys Evans P, Croft CB, Howard DJ. Wegener's granulomatosis, subglottic stenosis and antineutrophil cytoplasm antibodies. J Laryngol Otol 1989; 103(12):1187–1191

17. Hoffman GS, Kerr GS, Leavitt RY, et al. Wegener granulomatosis: an analysis of 158 patients. Ann Intern Med 1992;116(6):488–498

18. Rasmussen N. Management of the ear, nose, and throat manifestations of Wegener granulomatosis: an otorhinolaryngologist's perspective. Curr Opin Rheumatol 2001; 13(1):3–11

19. Taylor S, Simon R, Salama A, Pusey CD, Lightman SL. Ocular manifestations of Wegener's granulomatosis. Expert Rev Ophthalmol 2007;2:91–103

20. van der Woude FJ, Rasmussen N, Lobatto S, et al. Autoantibodies against neutrophils and monocytes: tool for diagnosis and marker of disease activity in Wegener's granulomatosis. Lancet 1985;1(8426):425–429

21. Tervaert JW, van der Woude FJ, Fauci AS, et al. Association between active Wegener's granulomatosis and anticytoplasmic antibodies. Arch Intern Med 1989; 149(11):2461–2465

22. Lund VJ, Cambridge G. Immunologic aspects of Wegener's granulomatosis. In: Passali D, Veldman J, Lim D, eds. New Frontiers in Immunobiology. The Hague: Kugler Publications; 2000:195–207

23. Trimarchi M, Gregorini G, Facchetti F, et al. Cocaine-induced midline destructive lesions: clinical, radiographic, histopathologic, and serologic features and their differentiation from Wegener granulomatosis. Medicine (Baltimore) 2001;80(6):391–404

24. Trimarchi M, Nicolai P, Lombardi D, et al. Sinonasal osteocartilaginous necrosis in cocaine abusers: experience in 25 patients. Am J Rhinol 2003;17(1):33–43

25. Peikert T, Finkielman JD, Hummel AM, et al. Functional characterization of antineutrophil cytoplasmic antibodies in patients with cocaine-induced midline destructive lesions. Arthritis Rheum 2008;58(5):1546–1551

26. Trimarchi M, Miluzio A, Nicolai P, Morassi ML, Bussi M, Marchisio PC. Massive apoptosis erodes nasal mucosa of cocaine abusers. Am J Rhinol 2006;20(2):160–164

27. Wiesner O, Russell KA, Lee AS, et al. Antineutrophil cytoplasmic antibodies reacting with human neutrophil elastase as a diagnostic marker for cocaine-induced midline destructive lesions but not autoimmune vasculitis. Arthritis Rheum 2004;50(9):2954–2965

28. Lloyd G, Lund VJ, Beale T, Howard D. Rhinologic changes in Wegener's granulomatosis. J Laryngol Otol 2002;116(7):565–569

29. Allen SD, Harvey CJ. Imaging of Wegener's granulomatosis. Br J Radiol 2007;80(957):757–765

30. Devaney KO, Travis WD, Hoffman G, Leavitt R, Lebovics R, Fauci AS. Interpretation of head and neck biopsies in Wegener's granulomatosis. A pathologic study of 126 biopsies in 70 patients. Am J Surg Pathol 1990;14(6):555–564

31. Raynaud P, Garrel R, Rigau V, et al. How can the diagnostic value of head and neck biopsies be increased in Wegener's granulomatosis: a clinicopathologic study of 49 biopsies in 21 patients. [Article in French] Ann Pathol 2005;25(2):87–93

32. Erickson VR, Hwang PH. Wegener's granulomatosis: current trends in diagnosis and management. Curr Opin Otolaryngol Head Neck Surg 2007;15(3):170–176

33. Walton EW. Giant-cell granuloma of the respiratory tract (Wegener's granulomatosis). BMJ 1958;2(5091):265–270

34. Hollander D, Manning RT. The use of alkylating agents in the treatment of Wegener's granulomatosis. Ann Intern Med 1967;67(2):393–398

35. Fauci AS, Wolff SM, Johnson JS. Effect of cyclophosphamide upon the immune response in Wegener's granulomatosis. N Engl J Med 1971;285(27):1493–1496

36. Abdou NI, Kullman GJ, Hoffman GS, et al. Wegener's granulomatosis: survey of 701 patients in North America. Changes in outcome in the 1990s. J Rheumatol 2002;29(2):309–316

37. EUVAS – European Vasculitis Study Group. Trial protocol for randomized trial of daily oral versus pulse cyclophosphamide as therapy for ANCA associated systemic vasculitis. Biomed-2 2005:BMH4-CT97-2328

38. Jayne D, Rasmussen N, Andrassy K, et al; European Vasculitis Study Group. A randomized trial of maintenance therapy for vasculitis associated with antineutrophil cytoplasmic autoantibodies. N Engl J Med 2003;349(1):36–44

39. Langford CA, Talar-Williams C, Sneller MC. Mycophenolate mofetil for remission maintenance in the treatment of Wegener's granulomatosis. Arthritis Rheum 2004;51(2):278–283

40. De Groot K, Rasmussen N, Bacon PA, et al. Randomized trial of cyclophosphamide versus methotrexate for induction of remission in early systemic antineutrophil cytoplasmic antibody-associated vasculitis. Arthritis Rheum 2005;52(8):2461–2469

41. Stone JH, Merkel PA, Spiera R, et al; RAVE-ITN Research Group. Rituximab versus cyclophosphamide for ANCA-associated vasculitis. N Engl J Med 2010;363(3):221–232

42. Wung PK, Stone JH. Therapeutics of Wegener's granulomatosis. Nat Clin Pract Rheumatol 2006;2(4):192–200

43. Marx RE, Sawatari Y, Fortin M, Broumand V. Bisphosphonate-induced exposed bone (osteonecrosis/osteopetrosis) of the jaws: risk factors, recognition, prevention, and treatment. J Oral Maxillofac Surg 2005;63(11):1567–1575

44. Stegeman CA, Tervaert JW, de Jong PE, Kallenberg CG; Dutch Co-Trimoxazole Wegener Study Group. Trimethoprim-sulfamethoxazole (co-trimoxazole) for the prevention of relapses of Wegener's granulomatosis. N Engl J Med 1996;335(1):16–20

45. Nouraei SA, Obholzer R, Ind PW, et al. Results of endoscopic surgery and intralesional steroid therapy for airway compromise due to tracheobronchial Wegener's granulomatosis. Thorax 2008;63(1):49–52

Sarcoidosis

Definition

Sarcoidosis is a chronic granulomatous disease, the first description of which is sometimes ascribed to Besnier in 1889, who coined the term "lupus pernio" for the cutaneous lesions.[1] Boeck and Hutchinson both recognized the more generalized nature of the condition in the late1890s.[2,3]

Etiology and Pathophysiology

The etiology of sarcoidosis remains unknown, although a wide range of agents have been suggested. This includes infective agents such as mycobacteria or propionibacteria, chemicals (beryllium and zirconium), pine pollen, and peanut dust. It is one of the few pulmonary diseases commoner in nonsmokers.

It is known to be associated with cell-mediated and humoral immune abnormalities.

The pathology is characterized by an accumulation of $CD4^+$ T cells followed by a noncaseating granuloma.

Incidence

Sarcoidosis has an interesting distribution, being commoner in northern Europe (Sweden, Iceland), affecting an estimated 64/100,000 of the population, but is also found in the southern United States and Australia. It is 10 to 20 times more prevalent in blacks than in whites. It is commoner in women than in men, with an onset in the third to fourth decades, although any age can be affected.

Site

Sarcoidosis is classically a multisystem disease and can therefore present in protean ways, the distribution of which reflects the origin of the individual series. However, it has a propensity for the lower respiratory tract (Table 18.13). The upper respiratory tract is affected in ~4% of patients with generalized disease,[4,5] notably the nose with blockage, crusting, and bleeding (Table 18.14). However, the ears, mouth, and larynx may also be affected as shown.[6–8]

Diagnostic Features

Clinical Features

In a series of 148 patients with proven sarcoid and referred to a specialist rhinological practice, nearly 90% suffer nasal congestion or blockage and two-thirds have crusting. Bleeding or spotting of blood affects 40%, and nearly one-quarter have facial pain. Anosmia can result from mechanical obstruction of the olfactory region and/or be sensorineural.[4] This means that many of these

Table 18.13 Systemic symptoms of sarcoidosis

Chest	Dyspnea, cough
Lymphatic	Hilar and peripheral lymphadenopathy
Skin	Rash, erythema nodosum, lupus pernio
Parotid	Parotitis (Heerfordt's syndrome)
Eye	Epiphora, uveitis, iridocyclitis, keratoconjunctivitis
	Lacrimal enlargement
Other organs	Hepatosplenomegaly
	Cardiac failure and ventricular arrhythmia
	Myalgia, arthralgia
	Polyneuritis, peripheral mononeuritis, myelopathy
	Dactylitis

Table 18.14 ENT manifestations of sarcoidosis

Ears	Sensorineural deafness
	Conductive deafness (granulomas in middle ear, eustachian involvement)
	Vestibular dysfunction
	Facial; nerve paralysis
Nose	Nasal obstruction, crusting, blood-stained discharge
	Facial pain
	Anosmia
	Nasal bones—rarefaction and soft tissue infiltration
Mouth	Cranial nerve palsies
Larynx	Supraglottic granulomas
	Vocal fold palsies

patients may present to the ENT community, but—as with other granulomatous diseases[9]—it may be anticipated that they can go unrecognized. To put this in context, the diagnosis of nasal sarcoid was made in 23 patients who presented with "chronic rhinosinusitis" in a cohort of 5,000 patients presenting to the aforementioned rhinology clinic and this has been the experience of others.[6,8,10]

On endoscopic examination, the mucosa has been described as a "strawberry skin" with small pale granulomas dotted over an erythematous and granular mucosa (Fig. 18.26). These appearances may be obscured by extensive crusting and eventually may become atrophic. Within the nasal cavity, the inferior turbinate and adjacent nasal septum are particularly affected. However, any of the paranasal sinuses, nasopharynx, soft palate, hypopharynx, and supraglottis can be involved.

Imaging

CT scanning of the nose and sinuses, when the patient is symptomatic, shows a nonspecific generalized opacification similar to that seen in chronic rhinosinusitis (**Fig. 18.27**). This may be due to an active granulomatous process, fibrosis after the condition has regressed, and/or nonspecific inflammation or infection.

The nasal bones may show rarefaction or punctuate osteolysis similar to that seen in the metacarpals or metatarsals (**Fig. 18.28**).

It is worth noting the lacrimal glands, which may be enlarged bilaterally.

CT of the lungs may show multiple nodules or nodular infiltration but occasionally these may be solitary or unilateral, between 1 and 5 cm in diameter (**Fig. 18.29**).

Histological Features and Differential Diagnosis

(See **Table 18.15**.)

The classic appearance is of a noncaseating granuloma composed of a central area of tightly packed epithelioid giant cells, CD4[+] T cells surrounded by CD8[+] T and B lymphocytes, and fibroblasts at the periphery. Unfortunately, biopsying the nose if the mucosa appears macroscopically normal is generally unrewarding, where 92% will be negative. Conversely, biopsy of macroscopically abnormal mucosa is 91% positive.[4]

Unfortunately, there are no specific pathognomonic tests for sarcoidosis since the withdrawal of the Kveim test due to untested health and safety concerns. Diagnosis is one of exclusion and relies on a combination of clinical manifestations, imaging of the chest, and immunological, biochemical, and histological investigations.

An elevated serum angiotensin-converting enzyme is suggestive, although this can be raised in other conditions such as TB, lymphoma, leprosy, and Gaucher disease. Serum calcium may be raised in 11% of patients with systemic disease.

Gallium 67 (^{67}Ga) perfusion scanning can demonstrate increased uptake in the sarcoid granuloma, and MRI of the brain may show granulomatous involvement of the basal meninges.

Pulmonary investigations include a CT scan, respiratory function tests, perfusion studies, and bronchoalveolar lavage.

The differential diagnosis must be between other granulomatous diseases such as syphilis, tuberculosis, rhinoscleroma, Wegener's granulomatosis, and Churg-Strauss syndrome as well as berylliosis, leprosy, and fungal disease.

Natural History and Outcome

In many cases, particularly stage 1 disease (bilateral hilar lymphadenopathy, normal lung fields), the disease undergoes spontaneous remission within 2 years without specific treatment. Of those with stage 2 (hilar

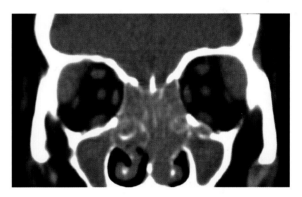

Fig. 18.27 Coronal CT scan of the sinuses showing nonspecific opacification of all the sinuses in nasal sarcoidosis.

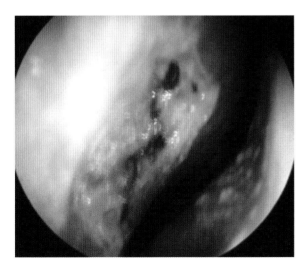

Fig. 18.26 Endoscopic view of the nasal mucosa showing a "strawberry skin" appearance ± crusting on the septum seen in nasal sarcoidosis.

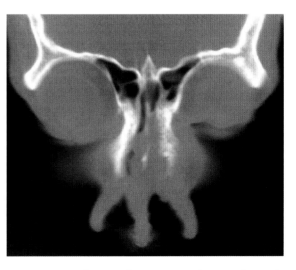

Fig. 18.28 Coronal CT scan showing osteitic changes in the nasal bones with overlying soft tissue swelling in nasal sarcoidosis.

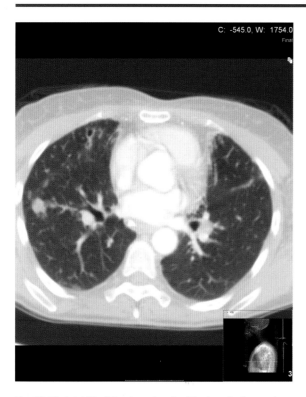

Fig. 18.29 Axial CT of the chest showing hilar lymphadenopathy and pulmonary fibrosis.

Table 18.15 Diagnostic tests for sarcoidosis[a]

ESR, FBC, globulin, Ca^{2+} (raised in 11%)
ACE (angiotensin-converting enzyme) (raised in 76%)
Pulmonary – Imaging (CT) – RFTs – Perfusion studies – Bronchoalveolar lavage
Gallium 67 scan
MRI of brain
CT of sinuses
Biopsy
Abbreviations: ACE, angiotensin-converting enzyme; ESR, erythrocyte sedimentation rate; FBC, full blood count; RFT, respiratory function tests. [a] Kveim test (93%+) no longer available

lymphadenopathy and lung disease), 65% spontaneously regress; those with stage 3 with just lung disease have a 30% chance of remission. By contrast 85% of those with erythema nodosum and acute arthritis remit spontaneously. Those with more advanced disease as evidenced by raised SACE or extrapulmonary involvement will usually require treatment and ~50% may experience a relapse, with 1 in 10 developing serious disability. Severe cardiac

Table 18.16 Medical and surgical treatment of sarcoidosis

Medical—Systemic	Corticosteroids—oral or inhaled
	Methotrexate
	Hydroxychloroquine
	Cyclophosphamide
	Ciclosporin
	Azathioprine
	Tumor necrosis factor antagonists, e.g., infliximab
Medical—Local	Alkaline douche
	Glucose and glycerin drops
	Betamethasone sodium phosphate 0.1% drops
Surgical	Debulking of inferior turbinate or polypoid masses ONLY
	Endoscopic sinus surgery for sinus involvement

or pulmonary involvement may lead to death in some cases and lung transplantation has been undertaken, although up to two-thirds develop recurrence in the allograft.[11] FDG-PET is being used to monitor response in severe cases.

Treatment

(See **Table 18.16.**)

The mainstay of treatment remains oral corticosteroids to which hydroxychloroquine and steroid-sparing cytotoxic agents such as methotrexate (weekly) may be added. The chloroquines are especially helpful for cutaneous manifestations but can cause retinal toxicity. Most recently there has been some interest in TNF-α antagonists such as infliximab.[12]

Nasal symptoms may be ameliorated by standard topical treatments with douching, corticosteroids, and lubricants.

Surgery has a very limited role, confined to biopsy, rarely debulking of granulomatous masses, and occasional endoscopic sinus surgery to elucidate CT changes.[13] Nasal reconstruction and resurfacing have also been anecdotally described, mainly for persistent lupus pernio.[14,15]

In the larynx, minimally invasive endoscopic surgery with intralesional corticosteroid injection and laser reduction has proved successful in controlling the disease and maintaining an airway.[16]

References

1. Besnier E. Lupus pernio de la face. Ann Dermatol Syphiligr (Paris) 1889;10:333–336
2. Boeck C. Multiple benign sarcoid of the skin. J Cutaneous Genito-Urinary Dis 1899;17:543–550
3. Hutchinson J. Cases of Mortimer's malady. Arch Surg 1898; 9:307–314

4. Wilson R, Lund VJ, Sweatman M, Mackay IS, Mitchell DN. Upper respiratory tract involvement in sarcoidosis and its management. Eur Respir J 1988;1(3):269–272
5. Lund VJ. Granulomatous diseases and tumours of the nose and sinuses. In: Kennedy DW, Bolger WE, Zinreich SJ, eds. Diseases of the Sinuses. Diagnosis and Management. Philadelphia: BC Dekker; 2001:85–106
6. Schwartbauer HR, Tami TA. Ear, nose, and throat manifestations of sarcoidosis. Otolaryngol Clin North Am 2003;36(4):673–684
7. Aubart FC, Ouayoun M, Brauner M, et al. Sinonasal involvement in sarcoidosis: a case–control study of 20 patients. Medicine (Baltimore) 2006;85(6):365–371
8. Braun JJ, Gentine A, Pauli G. Sinonasal sarcoidosis: review and report of fifteen cases. Laryngoscope 2004; 114(11):1960–1963
9. Srouji IA, Andrews P, Edwards C, Lund VJ. General and rhinosinusitis-related quality of life in patients with Wegener's granulomatosis. Laryngoscope 2006;116(9):1621–1625
10. Zeitlin JF, Tami TA, Baughman R, Winget D. Nasal and sinus manifestations of sarcoidosis. Am J Rhinol 2000;14(3):157–161
11. Ma Y, Gal A, Koss MN. The pathology of pulmonary sarcoidosis: update. Semin Diagn Pathol 2007;24(3):150–161
12. Paramothayan S, Lasserson TJ, Walters EH. Immunosuppressive and cytotoxic therapy for pulmonary sarcoidosis. Cochrane Database Syst Rev 2006;3(3):CD003536
13. Kay DJ, Har-El G. The role of endoscopic sinus surgery in chronic sinonasal sarcoidosis. Am J Rhinol 2001; 15(4):249–254
14. Gürkov R, Berghaus A. Nasal reconstruction in advanced sinunasal sarcoidosis. Rhinology 2009;47(3):327–329
15. Smith R, Haeney J, Gulraiz Rauf Kh. Improving cosmesis of lupus pernio by excision and forehead flap reconstruction. Clin Exp Dermatol 2009;34(5):e25–e27
16. Butler CR, Nouraei SA, Mace AD, Khalil S, Sandhu SK, Sandhu GS. Endoscopic airway management of laryngeal sarcoidosis. Arch Otolaryngol Head Neck Surg 2010; 136(3):251–255

Churg-Strauss Syndrome Vasculitis

Definition

Churg-Strauss syndrome (CSS) is a rare form of vasculitis characterized by adult-onset asthma, severe rhinitis, nasal polyps, and other systemic manifestations as a result of widespread eosinophilic granulomatous infiltration of tissues. The Chapel Hill consensus defined it as "eosinophil-rich granulomatous inflammation of the respiratory tract and necrotizing vasculitis of small to medium-sized vessels, associated with eosinophilia."[1]

Etiology

The etiology is unknown but this is probably an autoimmune disorder affecting eosinophils, endothelial cells, and lymphocytes. It has been suggested that exposure to certain drugs, corticosteroid withdrawal, vaccination, and pulmonary infection may initiate the inflammatory cascade.[2] An interesting phenomenon has been described in relation to the use of antileukotriene antagonists such as zafirlukast.[3] When these have been used in the treatment of asthma in some patients, it may unmask CSS if oral glucocorticosteroids are withdrawn (as opposed to actually precipitating the condition per se). Several other drugs have also been implicated including antibiotics, estrogen replacement therapy, and carbamazepine, suggesting a hypersensitivity reaction.

There is also some evidence for a genetic predisposition in respect of the HLA-DRB1 and 4 loci.[4]

Synonyms

Churg and Strauss described the syndrome that bears their names in 1951.[5] It has sometimes been called "allergic granulomatosis and angiitis."

Incidence

The UK incidence of the condition has most recently been reported at 4.2 per million per year, less than half as common as Wegener's granulomatosis, but 4 to 8 times higher than figures from other European countries.[6]

Among asthma patients the incidence is as high as 67 per million.[7]

Site

Both the nasal cavity and any or all of the paranasal sinuses can be affected.

Diagnostic Features

Clinical Features

Patients with CSS classically have allergic rhinitis, nasal polyps, and asthma, but these symptoms may predate the vasculitis by many years (mean 8 years).[3] As a consequence they are frequently seen by the ENT community, who may not appreciate the potential for a more serious systemic disease. In 25 patients with CSS[8] whom we examined, 80% had active sinonasal symptoms at the time of the study. Overall, 28% of CSS patients reported worsening of their nasal symptoms as the main event leading to their diagnosis, but interestingly 48% of CSS patients had undergone nasal surgery. Nasal symptoms of particular relevance to this patient group were nasal obstruction (95%), rhinorrhea (95%), anosmia (90%), and excessive sneezing (80%). Other symptoms included nasal crusting (75%), purulent nasal discharge (65%), and epistaxis (60%). These symptoms are rather higher than those described in two other studies.[9,10] Patients may also develop comorbidities such as serous otitis media and mucoceles secondary to sinus obstruction and inflammation (**Fig. 18.30**). Septal perforation may occur due to the condition or to ill-judged surgery.

There may be a slight preponderance of women—in our series there were 10 men (40%) and 15 women (60%),

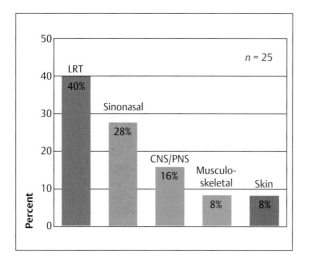

Fig. 18.30 The main presenting system in CSS patients that led to their diagnosis. (LRT, lower respiratory tract; CNS, central nervous system; PNS, peripheral nervous system.)

whereas others report equality or slight male predilection. The majority were white (92%) and the average age at diagnosis with CSS was 55.4 years (range 31.7 to 79.3, SD 14.5 years). The breakdown for predominant presenting symptoms leading to the diagnosis of CSS with respect to the different bodily systems is demonstrated in **Fig. 18.30** and a comparison with patients with Wegener's granulomatosis is shown in **Fig. 18.31**.[11]

Another characteristic manifestation is peripheral nervous system involvement (50 to 78%), which may include the cranial nerves and again present to ENT surgeons.[12] However, this is a multisystem disease that affects the lungs, producing asthma, the skin, the musculoskeletal system, and the heart (**Table 18.17**). Patients may complain of malaise and fever and one should suspect an underlying vasculitis in any patient who does not improve with conventional therapy of the nose and feels unwell disproportionately to the clinical findings.

Together with Wegener's granulomatosis (WG) and microscopic polyangiitis (MPA), CSS is one of the anti-neutrophil cytoplasmic antibody (ANCA)-associated vasculitides. However, with only around 50% (35–77%) of CSS patients displaying raised myeloperoxidase (MPO)-specific p-ANCA titers, diagnosis is often quite challenging. This is particularly so in the ENT setting, where it presents with the all too common findings of allergic rhinitis and nasal polyps. Thus, pinpointing the diagnosis with certainty remains difficult, not least due to the modest sensitivity of laboratory tests and low predictive values of the continuously evolving clinical criteria for CSS diagnosis.[1,13,14]

Imaging

A simple investigation such as chest radiography and/or a CT of the chest may demonstrate atypical "fluffy" or nodular pulmonary infiltrates.

Sinus CT does not show anything other than what would be expected in diffuse polypoid rhinosinusitis, that is, pan-opacification. Expansion and bone erosion may be seen in the ethmoid complex, with widening of the intercanthal distance. In addition, there may be evidence of mucocele formation, notably in the frontoethmoidal region (**Fig. 18.32**).

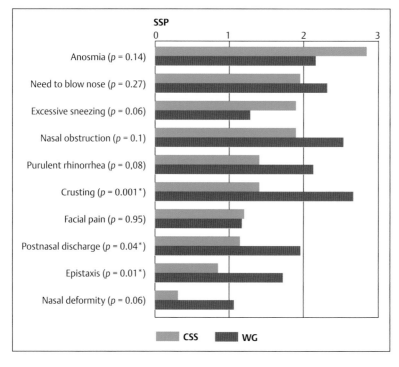

Fig. 18.31 Rhinological symptom severity product (SSP) values for CSS (n = 20) and WG patients (n = 127) with nasally active vasculitis (p values and statistical significance are indicated by *, two-tailed t-test, Statistica Version 6). (Modified from Srouji et al[9] with permission of *Laryngoscope*.)

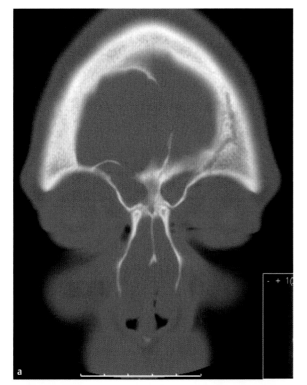

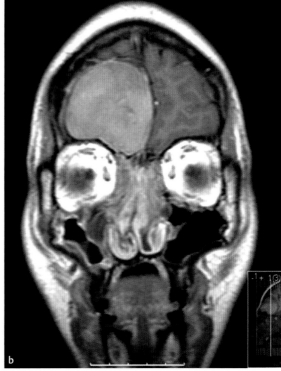

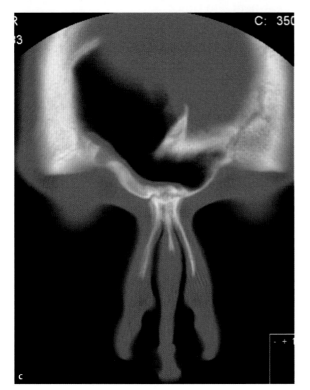

Fig. 18.32a–c A male patient with Churg-Strauss syndrome, asthma, nasal polyps, eosinophilia, and a large clinically silent "polypocele" expanding from the right frontal sinus into the anterior cranial fossa.

a Coronal CT scan showing an expanded frontal sinus with significant bone erosion.

b Coronal MRI (T1W post gadolinium enhancement) showing heterogeneous signal from the sinus contents, consisting of inspissated eosinophilic mucus suggestive of an eosinophilic fungal rhinosinusitis although no fungus could be demonstrated.

c Coronal CT scan showing aeration and contracture of the cavity 6 months after a combined osteoplastic flap and endoscopic approach. This scan was performed because the patient had complained of headache.

Table 18.17 Disease manifestations in Churg-Strauss syndrome in the literature[a]

Disease manifestations		Percentage
Asthma		96–100
Peripheral eosinophilia		91–100
Granulomatous inflammation		
	Paranasal sinus	52–74
	Lung	27–72
Vasculitis		100
	Peripheral nerve	66–76
	Skin	51–70
	Kidney	25–58
	Joint	19–57
Gastrointestinal		13–59
Endomyocardial		13–47
Pericardial		8–32

[a]Modified from reference [7].

Changes in pulmonary and sinus imaging are two of the six diagnostic criteria for the American College of Rheumatology definition of CSS.[13]

Histological Features and Differential Diagnosis

The condition is characterized by eosinophilic inflammation, extravascular granulomas, and necrotizing vasculitis in the presence of asthma. However, the granulomas themselves show necrosis and peripheral palisading of histiocytes. The granulomas are surrounded by a marked abundance of eosinophils, more so than that seen in WG. The polyps are histologically of the benign eosinophilic type seen in a "normal" group of patients.

The differential diagnosis is from other eosinophilic pneumonias, idiopathic hypereosinophilic syndrome, c-ANCA-positive (Wegener's) granulomatosis, and microscopic polyangiitis. In addition, sarcoid, allergic bronchopulmonary aspergillosis, and parasitic infection need to be considered.

Although the histology is important, it must be combined with clinical criteria to make the diagnosis.[1,13,14]

Natural History

Patients often present with sinonasal symptoms, which can be quite severe. A QoL assessment using a self-administered SNOT-22[15] revealed significantly increased scores compared with the normal population, but still only reaching average values similar to those of patients from the general rhinosinusitis population. This may explain the delay in diagnosis that many patients experience. The average reported delay in diagnosis was 18.5 months (range 1–71 months, SD 21.6 months) from presenting to the physician with worsening of symptoms that eventually led to a diagnosis of CSS. Ten patients (40%) reported worsening of their asthma or new pulmonary findings as the most prominent event leading to their diagnosis. A significant proportion of patients (28%) reported that their initial diagnosis was mostly related to worsening of their nasal symptoms.

Once the diagnosis is made, referral to physicians with a special interest in vasculitis provides other therapeutic possibilities, leading to significant improvements in patients' quality of life. Furthermore, early diagnosis and treatment may improve overall outcome by minimizing irreversible vasculitic tissue damage, although this assumption has yet to be confirmed by clinical studies. However, in this multisystem disease mortality is most commonly related to cardiac or severe gastrointestinal involvement.

It has been suggested that various subtypes of CSS exist, dependent on p-ANCA positivity. Those with ANCA positivity more frequently suffer from renal disease, peripheral nervous system involvement, and/or alveolar hemorrhage, whereas ANCA-negative patients have more frequent infiltrations in the heart and lungs and/or systemic manifestations.[16]

Treatment and Outcome

In most patients, disease control is achieved with immunosuppressant therapy, usually oral prednisolone ± cytotoxic drugs such as cyclophosphamide, azathioprine, mycophenolate, and methotrexate depending on the severity of the disease at presentation. Pulsed cyclophosphamide had less toxic side effects than regular oral dosage.[17] Monoclonal antibodies such as rituximab are also being used[18] and other new biological therapies may be valuable, for example, anti-interleukin 5 or anti-immunoglobulin E monoclonal antibodies.[19]

Long-term studies have shown that overall remission rates are good, ranging from 81 to 92%, but over a quarter do relapse either within the first year of treatment or much later. Overall mortality in treated patients who relapsed was only 3.1%. Factors predicting poor outcome are creatininemia >140 µmol/L, proteinuria >1 g/day, and central nervous system, gastrointestinal, or myocardial involvement. If one of these factors is present at onset, the 5-year mortality is 25.9%; when two or more are present, this increases to 46% at 5 years.[20]

Long-term survival means it is the chronic symptoms that produce significant morbidity and require symptomatic treatment. In the case of the nose and sinuses, this includes local therapies with alkaline douches, topical intranasal corticosteroids, and surgery for the nasal symptoms and comorbidities, for example, insertion of grommets or marsupialization of paranasal sinus mucoceles. In our series of 25 patients, 48% had undergone nasal surgery, usually polypectomy and often multiple times.

Key Points

- Churg-Strauss syndrome is a systemic vasculitis affecting small-to-moderate vessels that is characterized by nasal polyps and asthma with tissue and blood eosinophilia.

- Diagnosis can be difficult to confirm but may be suspected in the presence of a raised ESR, and positive p-ANCA.

- Other systems may also be involved; if this is suspected, refer to a physician with a particular interest in vasculitis.

References

1. Jennette JC, Falk RJ, Andrassy K, et al. Nomenclature of systemic vasculitides. Proposal of an international consensus conference. Arthritis Rheum 1994;37(2):187–192
2. Noth I, Strek ME, Leff AR. Churg-Strauss syndrome. Lancet 2003;361(9357):587–594
3. Wechsler ME, Garpestad E, Flier SR, et al. Pulmonary infiltrates, eosinophilia, and cardiomyopathy following corticosteroid withdrawal in patients with asthma receiving zafirlukast. JAMA 1998;279(6):455–457
4. Vaglio A, Martorana D, Maggiore U, et al; Secondary and Primary Vasculitis Study Group. HLA-DRB4 as a genetic risk factor for Churg-Strauss syndrome. Arthritis Rheum 2007;56(9):3159–3166
5. Churg J, Strauss L. Allergic granulomatosis, allergic angiitis, and periarteritis nodosa. Am J Pathol 1951;27(2):277–301
6. Lane SE, Watts R, Scott DG. Epidemiology of systemic vasculitis. Curr Rheumatol Rep 2005;7(4):270–275
7. Keogh KA, Specks U. Churg-Strauss syndrome. Semin Respir Crit Care Med 2006;27(2):148–157
8. Srouji I, Lund V, Andrews P, Edwards C. Rhinologic symptoms and quality-of-life in patients with Churg-Strauss syndrome vasculitis. Am J Rhinol 2008;22(4):406–409
9. Lane SE, Watts RA, Shepstone L, Scott DGI. Primary systemic vasculitis: clinical features and mortality. QJM 2005;98(2):97–111
10. Bacciu A, Bacciu S, Mercante G, et al. Ear, nose and throat manifestations of Churg-Strauss syndrome. Acta Otolaryngol 2006;126(5):503–509
11. Srouji IA, Andrews P, Edwards C, Lund VJ. General and rhinosinusitis-related quality of life in patients with Wegener's granulomatosis. Laryngoscope 2006;116(9):1621–1625
12. Hattori N, Ichimura M, Nagamatsu M, et al. Clinicopathological features of Churg-Strauss syndrome-associated neuropathy. Brain 1999;122(Pt 3):427–439
13. Lanham JG, Elkon KB, Pusey CD, Hughes GR. Systemic vasculitis with asthma and eosinophilia: a clinical approach to the Churg-Strauss syndrome. Medicine (Baltimore) 1984;63(2):65–81
14. Masi AT, Hunder GG, Lie JT, et al. The American College of Rheumatology 1990 criteria for the classification of Churg-Strauss syndrome (allergic granulomatosis and angiitis). Arthritis Rheum 1990;33(8):1094–1100
15. Piccirillo JF, Merritt MG Jr, Richards ML. Psychometric and clinimetric validity of the 20-Item Sino-Nasal Outcome Test (SNOT-20). Otolaryngol Head Neck Surg 2002;126(1):41–47
16. Pagnoux C, Guillevin L. Churg-Strauss syndrome: evidence for disease subtypes? Curr Opin Rheumatol 2010; 22(1):21–28
17. Gayraud M, Guillevin L, Cohen P, et al; French Cooperative Study Group for Vasculitides. Treatment of good-prognosis polyarteritis nodosa and Churg-Strauss syndrome: comparison of steroids and oral or pulse cyclophosphamide in 25 patients. Br J Rheumatol 1997;36(12):1290–1297
18. Koukoulaki M, Smith KG, Jayne DR. Rituximab in Churg-Strauss syndrome. Ann Rheum Dis 2006;65(4):557–559
19. Pagnoux C, Guilpain P, Guillevin L. Churg-Strauss syndrome. Curr Opin Rheumatol 2007;19(1):25–32
20. Guillevin L, Lhote F, Amouroux J, Gherardi R, Callard P, Casassus P. Antineutrophil cytoplasmic antibodies, abnormal angiograms and pathological findings in polyarteritis nodosa and Churg-Strauss syndrome: indications for the classification of vasculitides of the polyarteritis Nodosa Group. Br J Rheumatol 1996;35(10):958–964

Relapsing Polychondritis

Definition

Relapsing polychondritis (RP) is an autoimmune disease characterized by episodic and progressive inflammation of cartilage throughout the body.[1-3]

Etiology

The cause is unknown but this is thought to be an autoimmune disease. The allele HLA DR4 is found in 56% of affected individuals.[4]

Synonyms

The disorder was first described by Jaksch-Wartenhorst in 1923 who called it "polychondropathia."[5] The term "relapsing polychondritis" was introduced by Pearson et al when they described 12 cases in 1960.[6]

Site

RP can affect multiple structures throughout the body but in the head and neck can affect the pinna cartilage, the larynx, and the nose. The eustachian tubes may be affected as may the trachea, ribs, and joints. The condition can also extend to the heart, kidneys, and skin.

Diagnostic Features

Clinical Features

In 29 cases described from the Mayo Clinic, the ages ranged from 16 to 77 years (mean 49 years), with men outnumbering women 1.6:1.[7] RP is rare in children (<5%).[8] In 76% the external pinna cartilage was involved, in 62% the nose was affected, and in 52% the larynx. Involvement of the laryngeal cartilages, epiglottis, and subglottis leads to progressive collapse and loss of airway. Initially, patients may have hoarseness or a breathy voice, inspiratory stridor and increasing dyspnea that may lead to collapse of the airway, necessitating tracheostomy.

In addition, patients may present with hearing loss (conductive, sensorineural, or mixed) (46%) and vestibular problems (6%).

The external nose collapses in a rather characteristic way that is only seen in this condition and Wegener's

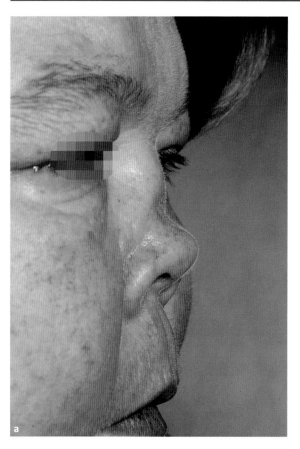

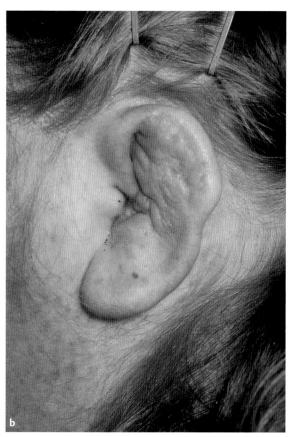

Fig. 18.33a, b

a Clinical photograph showing collapse of the external nose.

b Clinical photograph showing loss of the cartilaginous structure of the pinna.

granulomatosis (**Fig. 18.33a**). Endoscopically there may be diffuse crusting and a friable mucosa.

The pinnae, often bilaterally, become swollen and lose their contour, mimicking the changes that may occur following hematoma resolution (cauliflower ear),[9] and this is the most frequent presenting feature for most patients (**Fig. 18.33b**).

Other systemic manifestations include arthritis, heart valve disease, and neurologic, ocular, and renal disease.

Apart from a raised ESR, there are few specific laboratory investigations, although antinuclear antibodies (5–20%), rheumatoid factor, and antineutrophil cytoplasmic antibody titers[10] may be abnormal as the condition can be associated with other autoimmune diseases such as systemic lupus erythematosus, rheumatoid arthritis, and myelodysplasia in ~30% of affected adults.

Histological Features and Differential Diagnosis

Diagnosis is generally based on clinical appearances but is corroborated by histology. Two phases can be observed—an active phase followed by a quiescent phase. In the active phase there is chondrolysis and chondritis. Microscopically the cartilage shows loss of basophilia

or metachromasia with perichondrial acute and chronic inflammation. Cartilage destruction and its replacement by fibrous tissue are also seen in the second, quiescent phase. These changes are, however, not specific to RP.

The main differential diagnosis is from Wegener's granulomatosis, which can be difficult.

Natural History

The course of the condition is repeated acute attacks of cartilage inflammation punctuated by months or years of quiescence. Eventually severe deformity of the affected areas results and deaths can occur from involvement of the heart, kidneys, and airway.

Treatment and Outcome

The rarity of the condition has not permitted clinical trials, so treatment has mirrored that in other autoimmune diseases such as Wegener's granulomatosis or sarcoidosis, relying on corticosteroids and immunosuppressants such as azathioprine, cyclophosphamide, methotrexate, mycophenolate mofetil, hydroxychloroquine, and ciclosporin. Newer drugs such as tumor necrosis factor α-antagonists such as infliximab have also been tried. As a consequence of prompt medical treatment, the mortality rate has fallen from 30% to 6%.[11,12]

Surgical correction of the deformity, be it nasal or pinna, should be postponed until the condition has been quiescent for at least 2 years.

In a systematic review by Belot et al, one-third of all reported cases of pediatric RP underwent tracheotomy versus 6% of adults.[8] Pulsed high-dose corticosteroids have also been used.

References

1. Batsakis JG, Manning JT. Relapsing polychondritis. Ann Otol Rhinol Laryngol 1989;98(1 Pt 1):83–84
2. Damiani JM, Levine HL. Relapsing polychondritis—report of ten cases. Laryngoscope 1979;89(6 Pt 1):929–946
3. Trentham DE, Le CH. Relapsing polychondritis. Ann Intern Med 1998;129(2):114–122
4. Lang B, Rothenfusser A, Lanchbury JS, et al. Susceptibility to relapsing polychondritis is associated with HLA-DR4. Arthritis Rheum 1993;36(5):660–664
5. Jaksch-Wartehorst R. Polychondropathia. Wiener Archiv für innere Medizin 1923;6:93–100
6. Pearson CM, Kline HM, Newcomer VD. Relapsing polychondritis. N Engl J Med 1960;263:51–58
7. McCaffrey T, McDonald T, McCaffrey L. Head and neck manifestations of relapsing polychondritis: review of 29 cases. Otolaryngol 1978;86(3 Pt 1):ORL473–478
8. Belot A, Duquesne A, Job-Deslandre C, et al. Pediatric-onset relapsing polychondritis: case series and systematic review. J Pediatr 2010;156(3):484–489
9. Bachor E, Blevins NH, Karmody C, Kühnel T. Otologic manifestations of relapsing polychondritis. Review of literature and report of nine cases. Auris Nasus Larynx 2006;33(2):135–141
10. Geffriaud-Ricouard C, Noël LH, Chauveau D, Houhou S, Grünfeld JP, Lesavre P. Clinical spectrum associated with ANCA of defined antigen specificities in 98 selected patients. Clin Nephrol 1993;39(3):125–136
11. McAdam LP, O'Hanlan MA, Bluestone R, Pearson CM. Relapsing polychondritis: prospective study of 23 patients and a review of the literature. Medicine (Baltimore) 1976;55(3):193–215
12. Michet CJ Jr, McKenna CH, Luthra HS, O'Fallon WM. Relapsing polychondritis. Survival and predictive role of early disease manifestations. Ann Intern Med 1986;104(1):74–78

Cholesterol Granuloma

Definition

A condition characterized by a foreign body reaction to the presence of cholesterol.

Etiology

It is usually suggested that the area has been traumatized, resulting in hemorrhage into the mucosa. However, in addition, disturbed ventilation and impaired drainage are also required.[1] In the petrous apex, another theory has been proposed by Jackler and Cho[2] who suggested that exposed marrow is also a major contributory factor. Only 2 of our 6 sinonasal cases had undergone some form of trauma.

Synonyms

Confusingly, this condition has been referred to as orbital cholesteatoma, chocolate cyst, or even intraorbital hematoma.

Incidence

A small number of cases have been described, around 50 in the literature, 37 of which were reviewed by Chao and colleagues who included 2 of their own in 2006.[1,3–9] We have seen 6 cases in 20 years in contrast to 177 mucoceles in the same period.

Site

These lesions are more often encountered in the ear but are described in the paranasal sinuses, particularly in the maxilla and occasionally in the frontal region. This is the opposite distribution to that of mucoceles. In our 6 sinonasal cases, 3 affected the orbit, 2 involved the frontal region, and 1 arose in the sphenoid; all were referred by ophthalmologists (Table 18.18).

Table 18.18 Cholesterol granuloma: personal series

No.	Age (y)	Sex	Site	Treatment	Outcome	Possible etiology
1	56	F	Orbit	EFE	A&W 11 y	Trauma
2	89	M	Orbit	EFE	A&W 9 y	
3	31	M	Greater wing of sphenoid	LC	A&W 16 y	
4	63	M	Orbit	EFE × 2	Recurrence at 5 y, A&W 8 y	
5	46	M	Frontal	EFE	A&W 8 y	Previous surgery
6	70	M	Frontal	ESS	A&W 6 mo	Anticoagulation

Abbreviations: A&W, alive and well; EFE, external frontoethmoidectomy; F, female; LC, lateral craniotomy; M, male; mo, month(s); y, year(s).

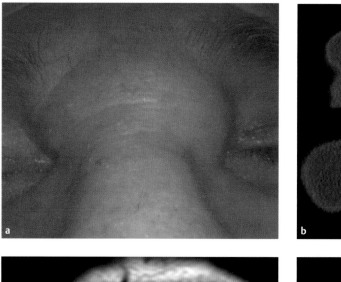

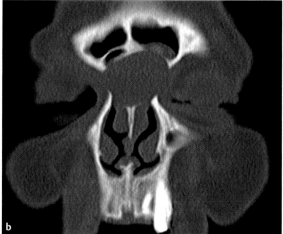

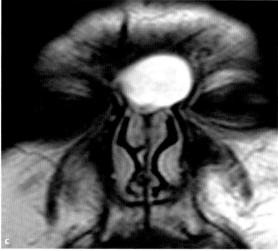

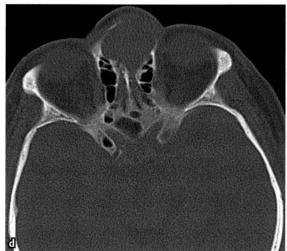

Fig. 18.34a–e Sinonasal cholesterol granuloma presenting in the glabellar region.

a Clinical appearance.
b Coronal CT scan showing a fluctuant mass in the glabellar region.
c Coronal MRI (T2W) showing a high-signal mass in the glabellar region.
d Axial CT scan showing a fluctuant mass in the glabellar region.
e Axial MRI (T2W) showing a fluctuant mass in the glabellar region.

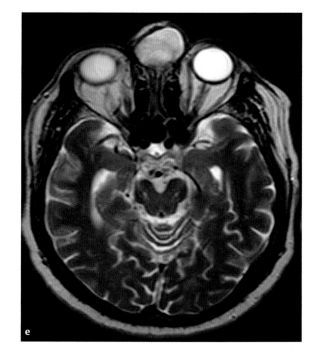

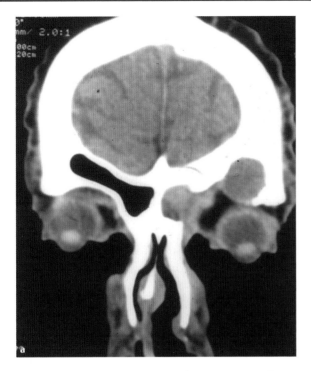
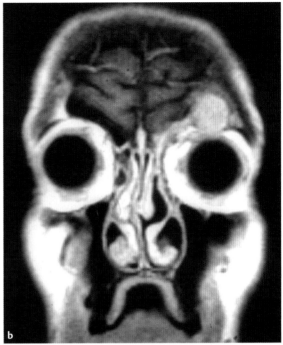

Fig. 18.35a, b Orbital cholesterol granuloma presenting with proptosis.

a Coronal CT showing a lesion excavating the left superolateral orbit.

b Coronal MRI (T1W post gadolinium enhancement) showing a lesion excavating the left superolateral orbit.

Diagnostic Features

Clinical

The lesion expands the sinus and so nasal obstruction, postnasal discharge, and facial pain may mimic chronic rhinosinusitis. The lesion may erode into the adjacent structures such as the cheek or orbit, displacing the eye.

In our series of 6 cases, the ages range from 31 to 89 years (mean 59 years), with a male preponderance of 5:1. In the orbital literature it is even more common in men (8:1).[10] The mean duration of symptoms was 3 years, range 3 months to 10 years.

Imaging

The typical appearances are of a cystlike expansion of the sinus cavity with thinning and/or erosion of the walls on CT. The opacification is of the same density as brain and does not enhance. However, on MRI the lesion gives a very high signal on all sequences, which distinguishes it from a dermoid, which is hypointense on T1W sequences (**Fig. 18.34**).[11,12] The signal may be heterogeneous on T2W sequences due to layering of the contents. Those lesions affecting the orbit may be located lateral to the frontal sinus cavity itself, presenting in the lateral superior quadrant of the orbit (**Fig. 18.35**).

Histological Features and Differential Diagnosis

The lesion has a bluish color and may be mistaken as a cyst. When opened, it contains golden glistening liquid due to the copious cholesterol crystals and more solid tissue also rich in hemosiderin in the histiocytes and extensive cholesterol clefts with a foreign body reaction.[3,4] When dissolved by the alcohol during histological processing, the crystals leave characteristic large needle-shaped spaces against an inflammatory cell background.[8]

The differential diagnosis includes mucoceles, dermoid and epidermoid cysts, and leukemic deposits or chloroma. Histology will resolve the situation if imaging does not.

Natural History

Once initiated, the process continues slowly to enlarge.

Treatment

Complete surgical drainage and marsupialization is required to prevent recurrence, which is usually possible when a sinus cavity is affected and can often be accomplished endoscopically.[13–15] The lesions in the lateral orbit are more problematic. First, they require some form of external incision, as by definition they lie lateral to the midpoint of the orbit and are therefore not amenable to an endoscopic approach. This incision can be a small incision under the brow, taking care not to damage the adjacent neurovascular bundles if possible, or a lateral orbitotomy or osteoplastic flap may be needed for the larger lesions. Second, if they cannot be connected to the adjacent frontal sinus, the contents including the lining mucosa must be completely exenterated and the underlying bone drilled. Particular care is needed if dura is exposed. It is not recommended to obliterate the cavity with fat as this will simply add to confusion when follow-up imaging is undertaken.

Outcome

As the lesion can recur, long-term follow-up is recommended, including orbital assessment if there was proptosis preoperatively. Whether it is necessary to perform regular MRI and for how long is open to debate.

In our series, one lesion recurred in the lateral orbit after 5 years and required further surgery.

References

1. Graham J, Michaels L. Cholesterol granuloma of the maxillary antrum. Clin Otolaryngol Allied Sci 1978;3(2):155–160
2. Jackler RK, Cho M. A new theory to explain the genesis of petrous apex cholesterol granuloma. Otol Neurotol 2003;24(1):96–106, discussion 106
3. Friedmann I, Osborn D. Pathology of Granulomas and Neoplasms of the Nose and Paranasal Sinuses. Edinburgh: Churchill Livingstone; 1982:26
4. Hellquist H, Lundgren J, Olofsson J. Cholesterol granuloma of the maxillary and frontal sinuses. ORL J Otorhinolaryngol Relat Spec 1984;46(3):153–158
5. Milton CM, Bickerton RC. A review of maxillary sinus cholesterol granuloma. Br J Oral Maxillofac Surg 1986; 24(4):293–299
6. Niho M. Cholesterol crystals in the temporal bone and the paranasal sinuses. Int J Pediatr Otorhinolaryngol 1986; 11(1):79–95
7. Gunes HA, Almac A, Canbay E. Cholesterol granuloma of the maxillary antrum. J Laryngol Otol 1988;102(7):630–632
8. Bütler S, Grossenbacher R. Cholesterol granuloma of the paranasal sinuses. J Laryngol Otol 1989;103(8):776–779
9. Chao T-K. Cholesterol granuloma of the maxillary sinus. Eur Arch Otorhinolaryngol 2006;263(6):592–597
10. McNabb A, Wright J. Orbitofrontal cholesterol granuloma. Ophthalmology 1990;97:28–32
11. Lloyd G, Lund VJ, Savy L, Howard D. Optimum imaging for mucoceles. J Laryngol Otol 2000;114(3):233–236
12. Shykhon ME, Trotter MI, Morgan DW, Reuser TT, Henderson MJ. Cholesterol granuloma of the frontal sinus. J Laryngol Otol 2002;116(12):1041–1043
13. Marks SC, Smith DM. Endoscopic treatment of maxillary sinus cholesterol granuloma. Laryngoscope 1995;105(5 Pt 1):551–552
14. Kikuchi T, So E, Ishimaru K, Miyabe Y, Abe K, Kobayashi T. Endoscopic sinus surgery in cases of cholesterol granuloma of the maxillary sinus. Tohoku J Exp Med 2002;197(4):233–237
15. London SD, Schlosser RJ, Gross CW. Endoscopic management of benign sinonasal tumors: a decade of experience. Am J Rhinol 2002;16(4):221–227

Section I C Treatment Options

19 Surgery

Informed Consent

As emphasized throughout this book, sinonasal tumors are rare, present late, and are often difficult to cure. Patients and their families must understand this from the outset so that a strong relationship of trust is developed. It is important that they understand the rationale for all the treatment options, the chances of success, and the potential complications that accompany them so that a genuinely informed consent may be taken. The increased availability of information means that patients can choose to be involved in the decisions about their treatment to a much greater extent than in the past; but with that power comes responsibility, so it is important that the consequences of a particular choice are fully discussed. This of course can be difficult and the extent of patient involvement will differ from person to person. However, doctors should always be prepared to discuss their expertise in dealing with the specific condition and be prepared to involve other colleagues if appropriate.

In discussing a particular operation such as the choice between an open craniofacial resection and an endonasal endoscopic technique, it may be appropriate to obtain consent for both procedures in case the tumor is found to be more extensive than indicated by preoperative imaging. As Wolfgang Draf has so wisely remarked, "the operation must fit the tumor, not the tumor made to fit a particular operation."

Endonasal Endoscopic Surgical Approaches

The introduction of endoscopic endonasal surgery in the 1980s, underpinned by access to CT and then MRI, revolutionized our approach to the diagnosis and management of virtually all rhinological conditions. Beginning with inflammatory and infective conditions, it was rapidly extended to the interfaces with the orbit and skull base, encouraging cross-specialty interaction and leading to the development of new techniques particularly for repair of dura and orbital periosteum. It was thus a natural progression to the resection of benign sinonasal tumors and then, albeit with some trepidation, to malignant tumors. Similarly, it became clear that disease arising outside the sinuses might be accessed via endonasal routes, beginning with the pituitary and extending to cranial and orbital lesions. The collaboration of rhinological surgeons with neurosurgeons and ophthalmologists has proved beneficial for all concerned, not least the patients, who may avoid some of the morbidity of conventional external approaches and, as a consequence, often enjoy shorter hospital stays. This in turn has led to a new genre of surgery—neuroendoscopic or minimal access skull base surgery that is based on detailed anatomical studies of the skull base anatomy from an endoscopic perspective, the use of new instrumentation and intraoperative image guidance, and often two senior surgeons or more working together, depending on the complexity of the case.

As a consequence, the anterior, middle, and posterior cranial fossae can now be reached using extended endonasal approaches (EEAs).[1,2] These techniques have been developed in several centers around the world, which to some extent has led to the concentration of some of these rare pathologies. The feasibility and the safety of these approaches is now well established and has been published widely (**Table 19.1**).[3–13] However, not all tumors can be resected by endoscopic endonasal approaches and it is important that the full range of surgical procedures and other therapies is available in managing these difficult and generally rare conditions.

One of the major criticisms of EEAs is the often piecemeal nature of the resection. However, anyone undertaking any form of major sinonasal surgery will know that after removal of the main specimen, further surrounding tissue is almost always removed. As long as all the tumor is excised and clear margins are obtained, which can be confirmed with frozen section, there is no hard evidence that piecemeal resection is detrimental to cure.[14] Indeed it has been argued that the visualization afforded by the endoscope significantly improves complete resection and is a reason for combining endoscopic techniques with an open approach if the latter is undertaken. The concept of an "en bloc" resection, originally conceived in relation to

Table 19.1 Advantages and disadvantages of extended endoscopic approaches

Advantages	Disadvantages

• Reduced morbidity
• Reduced surgical time
• Reduced hospital stay
• Direct approach with minimal disturbance of normal tissues
  – Soft tissue planes
  – Brain parenchyma
  – Neurovascular structures
• Early tumor devascularization
• Direct decompression of orbit
• No external incision
• Comparable oncological results to those obtained with traditional open approaches for similar staged disease
	• Piecemeal resection of malignant tumors?
	• Not all tumors amenable due to size, vascularity, locoregional invasion, etc.

colon cancer, may not be justifiably applied to the sino-nasal area. The term "debulking" should also be regarded with some circumspection as it implies that there will be residual tumor at the end of this process. This should definitively **not** be the aim in most instances, unless the situation is palliative or some degree of decompression is sought—for example, of the orbit—while obtaining tissue for diagnosis. Resection with intent to cure should be the guiding principle via whatever approach is appropriate. A much more appropriate term, coined by Piero Nicolai, Paolo Castelnuovo, and colleagues, is "tumor disassembly."

The limits of EEA are constantly changing, although factors such as the histology, the extent of disease, and its relationship to major neurovascular structures and invasion of dura, brain, and eye are important determining factors as well as the experience of the surgeon and the facilities of the institution and not forgetting factors related to the patients themselves.[13] Access to the lesion with minimal manipulation of normal neurovascular structures while maintaining good visualization and hemostasis[15] is critical, and the ability to manage vascular complications and to perform the necessary reconstruction[16-18] after resection is essential for optimal surgical results (**Fig. 19.1**). Ultimately the same oncological principles must be applied, irrespective of the surgical approach.

Technique

The details of the various EEAs are widely available in the literature but it is helpful to consider them in the three broad categories described by Nicolai, Castelnuovo, and colleagues[19]:

- Endonasal endoscopic resection (EER)
- EER with transnasal craniectomy (ERTC)
- Cranioendoscopic resection (CER)

EER may be used for all tumors involving the nasal cavity and paranasal sinuses that reach the skull base but do not require extensive skull base removal or dural resection. ERTC encompasses those tumors that have involved and/or transgressed the skull base with contact or focal infiltration of the dura. It should also be considered for tumors such as olfactory neuroblastoma, where the olfactory tract is likely to be involved. Finally, there are those tumors that have extensively involved the skull base or dura, particularly with lateral extension over the orbital roof and/or brain involvement, where the endoscope may assist a conventional craniofacial resection with or without a facial incision (CER).

Adequate Access

A common mistake is to think of resection via an EEA as somehow smaller. It is true that there may be less collateral damage of normal tissue, but the actual resection of tumor and its margin will be comparable to that achieved via an open approach. However, adequate access and visualization of the operative field is mandatory. Thus, for tumors involving the maxillary sinus, an endoscopic medial maxillectomy should be undertaken to allow complete subperiosteal dissection of tumor and removal of mucosa and any involved bone. For sellar and skull base lesions, a binarial approach is frequently utilized to allow for a two-surgeon, three- or four-hand technique.[20] Bimanual dissection is facilitated by bilateral nasal access, often combined with some form of postero-superior nasal septectomy as it provides the necessary space for instrument manipulation and movement of the scope and improves the angle for dissection. Out-fracture or removal of some of the structures on the lateral wall, for example, inferior and middle turbinates, may be needed to provide a wider access to the posterior and superior nasal cavity and skull base as well as to confirm complete excision and absence of field-change in the case of certain malignant tumors.

Many surgeons advocate extending the septectomy into the frontal sinuses (Draf III) so that this area may

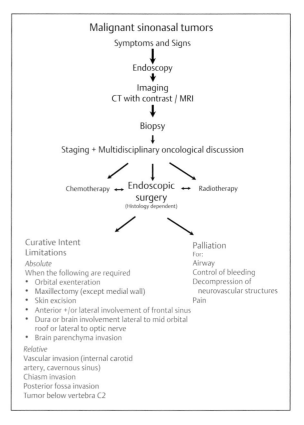

Fig. 19.1 An algorithm for management of sinonasal malignancy with endoscopic sinus surgery. (Modified and with permission from Figs. 14.7 to 14.9, Lund et al. European position paper on endoscopic management of tumours of the nose, paranasal sinuses and skull base. Rhinology Suppl 2010; (22):105.)

be readily visualized postoperatively and similarly wide bilateral sphenoidotomies are usually performed.[21] These may be extended laterally to the level of the pterygoid plates and lateral wall of the sphenoid sinus, superiorly to the planum sphenoidale and inferiorly to the floor of the sphenoid sinus. Even if the lateral wall is not involved, a middle meatal antrostomy is often recommended either as part of staging or to optimize postoperative visualization and to avoid secondary inflammation/infection particularly if radiotherapy will be given.

Resection

The extent of the tumor resection should be the same whether undertaken endoscopically, using a microscope, or with the naked eye. The main difference is the necessity in many cases to endoscopically debulk the lesion, although it may still be possible to circumnavigate it, taking a cuff of normal mucosa and mucoperiosteum and removing the tumor as one piece. This will be determined by the position, size, and consistency of the lesion. A small osteoma can be removed in its entirety; a large one will need to be drilled out from within and "imploded." Tumor removal may involve suction, powered instrumentation (debriders), drills, through-cutting forceps, and ultrasonic aspiration. Intracranial lesions in particular will require sequential capsular mobilization, extracapsular dissection of neurovascular structures, coagulation, and then removal of the capsule.

The stages of EER/ERTC have been divided into six main steps (**Figs. 19.2** and **19.3**)[19,22]:

1. Tumor debulking or disassembly
2. Septal resection
3. Opening of adjacent sinuses (usually including Draf III, total ethmoidectomy, medial maxillectomy, and median sphenoidotomy) and wide field removal of nasal and sinus mucosa and periosteum
4. Removal of bone adjacent to tumor—lamina papyracea, skull base
5. Removal of the orbital periosteum, dura, olfactory bulbs, and tracts if tumor is adjacent, adherent, or infiltrating
6. Repair and reconstruction of the skull base and orbit

When CER is undertaken, four phases have been defined:
1. Endoscopic
2. Transcranial
3. Simultaneous removal of the "ethmoid box" from above and below
4. Skull base reconstruction

The concept of endoscopic endonasal modules based on anatomical corridors has been widely popularized by Kassam, Carrau, and colleagues using the sphenoid sinus as the pivot point for the sagittal and coronal planes (**Table 19.2**).[1,2,14,23] The sagittal plane modules extend from the frontal sinus to the second cervical vertebra, enabling

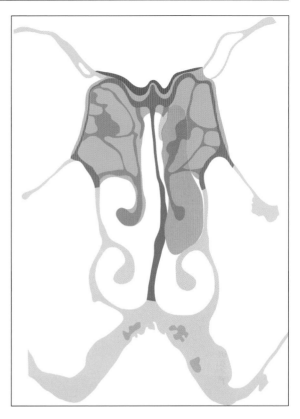

Fig. 19.2 Coronal section through a midfacial block showing stages of endoscopic surgical resection. (Modified from references 19, 22, 82.)

1. Tumor debulking or disassembly (orange).
2. Septal resection (blue).
3. Opening of adjacent sinuses (usually including Draf III, total ethmoidectomy, medial maxillectomy, and median sphenoidotomy) and wide-field removal of nasal and sinus mucosa and periosteum (green).
4. Removal of bone adjacent to tumor—i.e., lamina papyracea, skull base (red).
5. Removal of the orbital periosteum, dura, olfactory bulbs and tracts if tumor is adjacent, adherent, or infiltrating (light blue).
6. Repair and reconstruction of skull base (purple).

access through the crista galli, planum, tuberculum, dorsum sella, and clivus. The EEA approaches in the coronal plane are divided into anterior, middle, and posterior, corresponding to the relevant cranial fossae.

Transcribriform Approach

The transcribriform approach[1] is the approach most often utilized for sinonasal neoplasia affecting the anterior skull base, although it may also be used to repair CSF leaks, remove meningoencephaloceles, and access benign intracranial tumors such as olfactory groove meningiomas. This approach can be performed unilaterally or bilaterally. Its anterior limits are the crista galli and the frontal sinuses (i.e., transfrontal approach), the posterior limit is the planum sphenoidale. Laterally, it is bounded

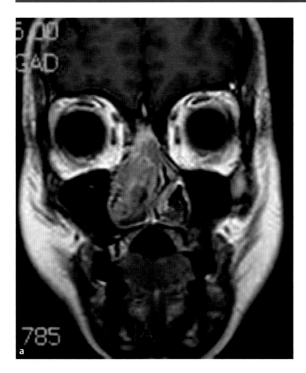

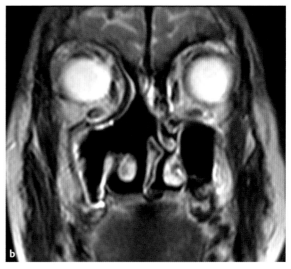

Fig. 19.3a–c

a Preoperative coronal MRI (T1W post gadolinium enhancement) showing malignant melanoma in the right nasal cavity.

b Postoperative coronal MRI (T2W) 6 months after endoscopic surgical removal.

c Endoscopic view of the surgical cavity 6 months after surgery.

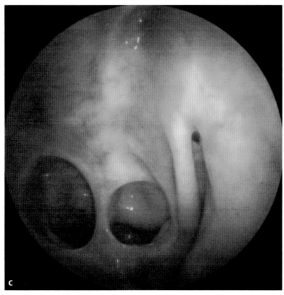

by the roof of the ethmoid sinus (fovea ethmoidalis) and medial orbital wall (lamina papyracea).

A complete fronto-ethmo-sphenoidectomy may be performed together with resection of the anterior nasal septum from the skull base. This allows complete staging of the disease in cases of malignancy and allows excellent visualization of the postoperative cavity. If not already performed, large middle meatal antrostomies will avoid subsequent maxillary sinusitis, particularly if radiotherapy will be given.

The lamina papyracea can be removed together with orbital periosteum if required (see Management of the Orbit, below). The ethmoidal arteries (AEA and PEA) can be identified, coagulated and transected medial to the lamina papyracea, aiding devascularization of the tumor (as may the sphenopalatine vessels). A frontal sinusotomy may be undertaken depending on the extent of disease and the exposure required. This is often a Draf III (or endoscopic Lothrop), which includes the bilateral removal of the sinus floors and intersinus septum, or just an ipsilateral resection may suffice (Draf II).[21]

The skull base may then be removed using osteotomies around the cribriform plate, or by drilling away the bone after removal of the nasal mucosa, or by thinning the bone to facilitate piecemeal resection together with coagulation of ethmoidal vessels and olfactory filaments. Once the cribriform plate has been removed, the crista galli is drilled/dissected out. Dural prolongations on either side of the crista need to be coagulated as they carry CSF and/or venous channels.

The exposed dura is coagulated and incised on each side of the falx and the tumor is removed by approaching from each side, exposing the free edges of the falx. After coagulation of the falx and any feeding vessels arising from the associated arteries, the dura is incised and the rest of the tumor is removed. Ideally, dura anterior to the tumor–brain junction is not opened, to prevent frontal lobe herniation. Considerable care is now required using gentle countertraction and sharp dissection, especially if dissection of the upper extent of the tumor involves the interhemispheric fissure, as the A2 and frontopolar arteries will be draped over the tumor surface. Similarly the dissection inferoposteriorly may bring one into close

Table 19.2 Classification of endonasal approaches to the ventral skull base

Sagittal plane
Transcribriform
Transfrontal
Transtuberculum/Transplanum
Transsellar

Transclival
• Superior third
   – Transsellar (intradural)
   – Subsellar (extradural)
• Middle third
• Panclival

Transodontoid and foramen magnum/craniovertebral approach
Coronal plane
Anterior coronal plane • Supraorbital • Transorbital
Middle coronal plane • Medial petrous apex • Petroclival approaches • Inferior cavernous sinus/quadrangular space • Superior cavernous sinus • Infratemporal approach

Posterior coronal plane
• Infrapetrous
• Transcondylar
• Transhypoglossal
• Parapharyngeal space
   – Medial (jugular foramen)
   – Lateral

Source: Lund et al. European position paper on endoscopic management of tumours of the nose, paranasal sinuses and skull base. Rhinology Suppl 2010; (22):19. With permission.

contact with the optic nerves and the anterior communicating artery. If there is any concern that safe excision from below cannot be accomplished, the decision should be made to proceed to an open craniofacial approach, ideally at that time, and patients should provide consent for both procedures if there is any doubt.

Transsellar Approach

The transsellar approach[1] is primarily used for pituitary pathology such as pituitary adenomas and Rathke cleft cysts. The endoscope affords a panoramic view, ensuring complete tumor removal. In the event of cavernous sinus extension, the medial cavernous wall can be examined from within the sella. Since the carotid siphon is usually displaced anteriorly, the space between the posterior

clinoid and the siphon offers an ideal corridor to enter the cavernous sinus. A considerable literature may be found on this approach, which is beyond the scope of this book.[13]

Transtuberculum/Transplanum Approach

Extrasellar pituitary adenomas with suprasellar extension, meningiomas and select craniopharyngiomas require a combined transsellar/transplanum approach[1] with removal of the tuberculum. This allows one-stage removal of the entire tumor with direct visualization.

Transclival Approach

The clivus can be divided into three portions along the rostral-caudal direction.[23] The upper third includes the dorsum sella and posterior clinoids down to the level of Dorello's canal. The middle third extends from Dorello's canal down to the jugular foramen. The lower third extends from jugular foramen through the cervicomedullary junction and foramen magnum. Indications include the surgical treatment of meningiomas, chordomas, and chondrosarcomas, which are the most common tumors in this region.

Transodontoid and Foramen Magnum/ Craniovertebral Approach

Exposure of the foramen magnum and odontoid requires additional soft tissue removal following the panclival module and may be utilized for surgery on the odontoid itself, for recurrent nasopharyngeal carcinoma, and for access to structures within the foramen magnum and cervical spinal cord down to the level C1-C2. Caudal exposure is limited by the inability to move the instruments beyond the nasal bones anterosuperiorly and the hard palate posteroinferiorly. The line connecting these two points is defined as the nasopalatine line (NPL). The NPL accurately predicts the most inferior extent of an endoscopic endonasal approach.[23-25]

Anterior Coronal Plane: Supraorbital and Transorbital Approaches

In the supraorbital approach, the medial wall of the orbit is removed and the orbital soft tissues are displaced to visualize the orbital roof. The transorbital approach is used for intraconal lesions that are inferior and medial to the optic nerve. Access is gained between the inferior and medial rectus muscle with preservation of extraocular muscle function.

Middle Coronal Plane

These approaches are defined by their relationship to the petrous carotid artery.[2] Infrapetrous approaches give access to the medial petrous apex and the petroclival junction, whereas the suprapetrous approaches give access to the inferior and superior cavernous sinus as well as the infratemporal/middle fossa.

Medial Petrous Apex Approach

Large bilateral sphenoidotomies are undertaken followed by removal of the basipharyngeal fascia from the face of the sphenoid down to the clivus. The sphenoid floor is then drilled down to the clival recess and the clivus itself may also be partially removed if needed. The posterior wall of the maxillary sinus is accessed via a large middle meatal antrostomy and the posterior wall is removed to expose the pterygopalatine fossa. The sphenopalatine arteries are identified and coagulated at the foramen, remembering that there may be up to 11 branches.[26] The base of the pterygoid plate is exposed by elevation of the soft tissues of the pterygopalatine fossa and the vidian canal (pterygoid canal), identified just lateral to the junction of the sphenoid floor with the medial pterygoid plate (MPP). The canal is important as lesions such as angiofibroma often involve it and from there infiltrate the basisphenoid. The canal also leads directly to the anterior genu of the internal carotid artery (ICA) as its petrous portion turns up to form the vertical paraclival ICA.

The medial pterygoid plate may be drilled medial and inferior to the vidian canal while following it posteriorly, toward the foramen lacerum. After identifying the anterior genu of the ICA, the lateral and superior part of the MPP can be removed. To access the petrous apex, drilling of the bone covering the paraclival carotid may be required if the ICA needs to be mobilized laterally.[27] Greater access can also be provided by drilling a portion of the lateral clivus at its junction with the petrous apex.

Petroclival Approaches

Kassam and colleagues have described extending the medial petrous apex approach, by drilling the vidian canal circumferentially and following it back to the anterior genu of the ICA.[28,29] The anterior genu of the ICA represents the lateral margin of this approach and is the most important landmark. The bone overlying the genu, the horizontal petrous, and the vertical paraclival segments of the ICA can be removed to uncover the carotid, allowing its lateral displacement. The medial portion of the clivus may then be safely drilled after identification of the anterior genu of the ICA. The lateral portion of the clivus at the petroclival junction is drilled up to the clival recess of the sphenoid. The cavernous sinus represents the superior boundary of this exposure, and the middle fossa the lateral boundary.

Inferior Cavernous Sinus/Quadrangular Space Approach

This is an extension of the petroclival approach. Removal of the posterior wall of the maxillary antrum is extended laterally until the maxillary branch (V2) of the trigeminal nerve is identified traveling superiorly toward the foramen rotundum. The MPP is drilled inferiorly and medially to the vidian canal. Next, the bone between the vidian canal and V2 is drilled away, accepting that this bony corridor narrows progressively as it deepens. Removal of this bone gives access to the quadrangular space that is defined by the parasellar ICA medially, V2 and dura of middle cranial fossa laterally, the horizontal petrous ICA inferiorly, and the sixth cranial nerve superiorly. Bone covering the horizontal petrous ICA, the anterior genu, and parasellar ICA may need to be removed if mobilization of the carotid is required. Access to the inferior cavernous sinus is gained by opening the dura from the genu of the ICA (medial) toward the V2 (lateral).

Superior Cavernous Sinus Approach

This module requires a similar amount of bone removal and ICA exposure as for the inferior cavernous sinus module. However, before incising the dura, the medial margin of the ICA in the sella should be identified so that it can be protected during this maneuver. The dural incision is begun directly over the superolateral portion of the cavernous sinus and performed in a medial-to-lateral direction. If, as is often the case, the cavernous sinus has thrombosed, little venous bleeding occurs during initial opening but this can dramatically change once the tumor is removed. This approach has been used for tumors unresponsive to medical treatment or radiosurgery and for patients with established cranial nerve deficits.[30]

Infratemporal Approach

Once the medial pterygoid plate has been dissected, the vidian canal has been identified, and the maxillary antrostomy completed, the plate is removed flush with the middle cranial fossa and foramen rotundum. The internal maxillary artery and its branches must be identified and ligated and the anterior genu of the ICA and horizontal petrous segment of the ICA identified before tumor removal commences. Dissection may be extended laterally until the lateral pterygoid plate is identified, and this may also be drilled rostrally until flush with the middle cranial fossa and foramen ovale. Bleeding from the pterygopalatine venous complex can be profuse and it may be necessary to pack the area and perform further resection at a later date, after the venous complex has thrombosed.

Posterior Coronal Plane

The posterior coronal plane extends from the foramen magnum across the occipital condyle and hypoglossal canal to the jugular foramen; it is rarely needed for sinonasal tumors but is included for completeness.

Infrapetrous Approach

After identifying the maxillary nerve (V2), the vidian canal, and the anterior genu of the ICA, the medial pterygoid plate is drilled flush with the middle cranial fossa and foramen rotundum.[2] As the lateral pterygoid plate is resected, the mandibular branch of the trigeminal nerve (V3) is identified along its posterior edge and guides drilling, also flush with the middle fossa and the foramen ovale. The cartilaginous segment of the eustachian tube is resected for ~1 cm. The inferior surface of the petrous apex is reached by drilling the bone between the horizontal petrous segment of the ICA and the eustachian tube, medial to V3. The horizontal petrous and vertical paraclival segments of the ICA are identified and skeletonized. Further drilling and tumor dissection may be undertaken inferiorly to the petrous ICA into the petrous apex.

Other endoscopic approaches along the posterior coronal plane, such as the transcondylar, transhypoglossal, and parapharyngeal space approaches, have been described to address other skull base lesions, but not sinonasal pathologies.

Reconstruction

The advent of extended applications of EEAs was accompanied by the recognition that reconstruction would be required in many cases. While bony skull base defects resulting from certain pathologies (e.g., mucoceles) require no reinforcement after drainage, congenital or acquired dehiscences are usually associated with the risk of prolapse of intracranial contents, meningitis, and/or cerebrospinal fluid (CSF) leakage and thus require repair. When iatrogenic injury to the skull base was found to accompany the spread of EEAs around the world in a small but significant number of patients (<0.2%), it also fortunately became clear that a wide range of methods and materials could be employed to repair the damage, either immediately or as a secondary procedure. It was quickly established that an endoscopic repair was highly successful and as a consequence these techniques were rapidly adopted for the repair of skull base defects in general, with overall success rates of >90% quoted for most series of nonneoplastic cases.[13] The main exception to this is a well-established "spontaneous" leak in the obese patient, which is associated with an aberrant CSF metabolism.[31]

There are, however, several specific considerations in an oncological case.
1. It must be ensured that the graft does not contain tumor and has not undergone a field change.
2. The repair may need to be robust enough to withstand radiotherapy.
3. The surgical defect may be large and complex.

A wide range of techniques and a long list of materials have been used, ranging from free grafts to local mucoperiosteal vascularized flaps (Table 19.3). Autologous free grafts are generally preferred as these avoid the potential dangers of transmissible diseases such as HIV, hepatitis, and bovine spongiform encephalopathy.[16,17,32–38]

If a free homograft is used, it should come from the contralateral side of the nose in the presence of a benign tumor but may not be appropriate at all in malignant tumors such as adenocarcinoma or olfactory neuroblastoma, which can be associated with field change or dysplasia and/or may recur anywhere in the nose.

In general the repair techniques may be divided into underlay, overlay, and the fat plug technique, the last being mainly applicable to smaller defects.[39] For oncology cases, several layers of free graft material in combinations of overlay and underlay are usually used, for which fascia lata has provided the most reliable large source of material. However, as resections got larger, particularly in the middle cranial fossa, it became clear that conventional free grafts, even of fascia lata, would not be sufficient. Persistent CSF leaks were a major problem despite refinements in the grafting techniques[16,40–43] and led to the development of a vascular pedicled nasoseptal flap that utilizes the mucoperichondrium/mucoperiosteum of the septum on one side, pedicled posteriorly on the sphenopalatine artery.[44]

The Hadad-Bassagasteguy flap (HBF) is posteriorly based on the nasoseptal arteries, which are branches of the posterior nasal artery, one of the terminal branches of the internal maxillary artery. Two parallel incisions are made along the axis of the nasal septum, the lower one over the maxillary crest and the upper incision 1 to 2 cm below the most superior aspect of the septum to preserve

Table 19.3 Materials used to repair skull base defects in EEAs

Free grafts
Homograft • Mucoperiosteum—septum, inferior or middle turbinate • Fascia—temporalis, lata • Bone—septum, turbinate • Cartilage—septum, pinna • Fat—pinna, abdomen
Allograft • Lyophilized dura
Local flap
Nasoseptal
Inferior turbinate
Middle turbinate
Regional flap
Transpterygoid
Temporoparietal
Transfrontal pericranial
Oliver palatal

the olfactory epithelium. A vertical incision at the muco-cutaneous junction joins these two horizontal incisions anteriorly. Posteriorly, the superior incision extends laterally over the rostrum of the sphenoid sinus at the level of the inferior aspect of the sphenoid ostium, while the inferior incision extends along the posterior free border of the nasal septum and then laterally along the arch of the posterior choana. The strip of mucosa between the sphenoid rostrum incisions contains the posterior septal arteries and forms a relatively long and narrow pedicle that has a long reach and wide arc of rotation. A wider flap can be harvested by placing the horizontal incisions along the lateral nasal floor or closer to the nasal bones superiorly. The flap is raised in the subperichondrial plane and is then stored in the nasopharynx or inside the antrum, while the resection proceeds, to avoid damage.[45–48]

The HBF provides an area of vascularized tissue of ~25 cm^2,[49] which is adequate to cover most anterior skull base/cribriform, planar/sellar, or clival defects when addressed independently. This surface area is usually sufficient to cover two adjacent areas such as cribriform and planum or sella and clivus. However, in children the dimensions of the nasal septum are not adequate to cover a large skull base defect until around 12 years of age.[50] Preoperative imaging can be used to estimate both the dimensions of the defect and the flap if there is concern of a potential shortfall,[49,50] and postoperative imaging provides a way to examine the adequacy of the reconstruction by establishing the position of the flap in relation to the defect.[51] If the flap falls away from the defect, reexploration should be considered. Similarly, lack of contrast enhancement may indicate ischemia of the flap and reexploration or removal of the nasal packing to relieve the pressure should be considered.

The HBF has become the mainstay for reconstructing large skull base defects. It can be applied to free nonmucosal grafts and its use has led to a significant decrease in postoperative CSF leaks to <5%,[44–48,50] which in turn has led to an increasing acceptance of EEA techniques.

Other vascular pedicled flaps have been developed, providing alternatives for skull base defects of various sizes and locations when the Hadad-Bassagasteguy flap is not suitable or not available due to the site and extent of the tumor or previous treatment. This might include tumors that involve the septum, pterygopalatine fossa, or sphenoid rostrum and those where there has been disruption of the blood supply to the septal flap due to previous posterior septectomy or large sphenoidotomies. In these cases, other options such as posterior pedicled inferior or middle turbinate flaps, the temporoparietal fascia flap, the transfrontal pericranial flap, and the Oliver pedicled palatal flap may be considered.

The posterior pedicle inferior turbinate flap (PPITF) is based on the inferior turbinate artery, which is a terminal branch of the posterolateral nasal artery (PLNA), a branch of the sphenopalatine artery (SPA).[52] Two parallel incisions are made along the axis of the inferior turbinate, one above on the lateral nasal wall and one below along its caudal margin. These are joined anteriorly with a vertical cut made on the head of the turbinate. The medial mucoperiosteum is elevated, providing around 5 cm^2 of surface area, which, due to the posterolateral position of its pedicle, makes it fit better into caudal defects, such as those in the sella or clivus. However, its use is limited by its being narrow and significantly smaller than the HBF even if the inferior incision is made on the medial side of the turbinate or the nasal floor. Occasionally, bilateral flaps or a combination with another pedicled flap can be used.

The posterior pedicle middle turbinate flap (PPMTF) is based on a branch of the sphenopalatine artery through its posterior attachment. It can be used for defects at the cribriform plate, fovea ethmoidalis, planum sphenoidale, or sella turcica.[53] A vertical incision is made at the most anterior aspect of the middle turbinate and a horizontal incision is made on its medial surface just below the skull base and parallel to its vertical attachment. The mucoperiosteum is elevated in a superior-to-inferior direction, exposing the turbinate bone medially and laterally and the turbinate bone is nibbled away to expose the lateral mucosal attachment, which is then released using another horizontal incision. Further elevation of the flap posteriorly exposes the pedicle, which can be mobilized and released from all surrounding attachments.

However, it is a difficult flap to raise, and this may be hindered further by anatomical variations such as concha bullosa, paradoxical turbinate, or hypoplasia.[53] On average the surface area of the PPMTF is around 5.6 cm^2 but it can vary significantly. An advantage is that it can reach defects of the planum sphenoidale, sella, and fovea ethmoidalis area better than the PPITF but needs to be longer than 4 cm to reach the sella.

The temporoparietal fascia flap (TPFF) is a pedicled flap based on the anterior branch of the superficial temporal artery (STA), one of the terminal branches of the external carotid artery.[54] In addition to the repair of skull base defects after traditional craniofacial resections, it has been used elsewhere in the head and neck: for example, for oronasal and nasocutaneous fistulas. After making a large maxillary antrostomy, the sphenopalatine and posterior nasal arteries are dissected into the pterygopalatine fossa with removal of the posterior wall of the maxillary sinus. The lateral wall of the maxillary sinus is then removed, creating a wide communication into the infratemporal fossa. The soft tissues of the pterygopalatine fossa are mobilized to expose the anterior aspect of the pterygoid plates and these are drilled away to produce the tunnel for transposition of the flap.[54]

Through a hemicoronal incision, the superficial layer of the deep temporal fascia is incised vertically and elevated away from the underlying temporalis muscle. A tunnel is created by separating the temporalis muscle from the lateral orbital wall and from the pterygomaxillary fissure that connects the temporal fossa, the infratemporal fossa, and the transpterygoid approach. Further enlargement of this tunnel can be achieved using dilators such as those used for a percutaneous tracheotomy with a guide wire. The TPFF can be tied to the guide wire and pulled into the nasal cavity. A stitch and artery clip could also be used. The flap has a long vascular pedicle and a large surface area that can be used for the reconstruction of large defects of planum, sella, clivus, and craniovertebral junction.

The pericranial and galeopericranial pedicled axial flaps are most commonly used to reconstruct the skull base after conventional craniofacial resections. They are based on the supraorbital and supratrochlear arteries and provide a large surface area.[55] The flap is harvested via a standard coronal incision or using an endoscopically assisted technique,[56] utilizing several 2-cm incisions along the coronal plane of the scalp. The supraorbital and supratrochlear arteries can be located by Doppler ultrasound if necessary and are included in a 3 cm wide pedicle. If using an endoscopic technique, a 1-cm glabellar incision is made and a subperiosteal tunnel is developed to communicate with the subperiosteal plane of the flap dissection. A bony window through the nasion allows the transposition of the flap through the nasofrontal recesses into the endonasal surgical field. A Draf III frontal procedure is necessary to facilitate passage of the flap and to secure the drainage of the frontal sinuses. Due to the position of the pedicle, the endoscopically assisted pericranial flap is suitable for the reconstruction of cribriform and planar defects but it can be extended to cover defects of the sella and clivus.

The Oliver modification of the palatal flap (OPPF) transposes the vascularized mucoperiosteal tissue of the hard palate into the nasal cavity through the greater palatine foramen.[57,58] A mucosal incision is made around the hard palate extending to within 2 to 5 mm of alveolar ridge laterally and at the limit of the hard palate posteriorly. The mucoperiosteum of the hard palate is raised subperiosteally, preserving one of the greater palatine neurovascular bundles. Using a drill or bone forceps, the greater palatine foramen is enlarged to allow the passage of the flap. Through a wide middle meatal antrostomy, the posterior wall of the maxillary sinus is removed to expose the junction between the sphenopalatine and descending palatine arteries within the pterygopalatine fossa. A horizontal incision placed 2.5 to 3 cm posterior to the pyriform aperture allows the elevation of nasal floor mucosa. The bony canal of the pterygopalatine canal is opened and the descending palatine artery is released from the canal. Then, the flap is passed into the nasal cavity and mobilized to cover the defect. This flap provides a large surface area of between 12 and 18.5 cm^2 and its long pedicle allows a wide arc of rotation so that a large part of the skull base can be reached, in particular the

planum, sella, and clivus.[57,58] It is particularly helpful if other reconstructive options are not available due to previous surgery or the disease itself but it may be marred by the persistence of an oronasal fistula unless mucosa from the nasal floor is preserved to cover the defect.

However, maintaining the position of the grafts and flaps can also be problematic. Biological glues, dissolvable packing, and traditional packs soaked in solutions such as Whitehead's varnish have all been used. (Whitehead's varnish is a compound iodoform paint: iodoform, benzoin, prepared storax, tolu balsam, and the solvent ether.) Inflatable balloons and U clips have also been employed to secure the grafts against gravity[13,59,60] and other methods are being explored. There is no consensus on how long packs should be left in place. In our own practice, the Whitehead's gauze is usually left for ~7 to 10 days and then removed under a short general anesthetic.

Similarly, the use of lumbar drains, the duration of bed-rest, the use of diuretics, antibiotics, or DVT prophylaxis, and the postoperative advice on physical activity are all up for debate as no trials have been conducted on any of these aspects. Suffice to say that a commonsense approach is probably the best policy, with a few days' bed rest depending on the extent of repair and avoidance of major physical exertion that raises intracranial pressure, such as lifting heavy weights, for some weeks or months. Lumbar drains are generally not recommended routinely by most surgeons, particularly where there is a risk of entraining air (for example, with underlay techniques) as this may produce a pneumoencephalocele.

Training

For optimum results with minimal complications, a comprehensive training in all aspects of endoscopic techniques is required as well as experience of open approaches, alternative therapies, and a full understanding of the diagnostic options and natural history of the relevant pathology. This cannot be acquired easily or quickly, but a staged surgical progression is fundamental in acquiring the necessary skills and judgment. This may take the form of courses, mentoring, and fellowships. Much has been written about the "learning curve" for endoscopic surgery, both in the nose and sinuses and elsewhere,[61,62] but it is difficult to be didactic about the number of cases needed as it will vary from surgeon to surgeon. A training format that is incremental and modular has been proposed for all endonasal surgeons, irrespective of their specialty, and this is highly recommended (see **Table 19.4**).[14] It should be recognized that not everyone will ever reach Level V, nor is there a need for everyone to do so because the number of cases requiring these techniques is limited. However, it is important that competence at each level is achieved before progression to the next stage, which represents greater difficulty and risk. Even in the most expert hands, serious

Table 19.4 Suggested training program for endonasal cranial base surgery[13]

Level	Procedures
Level I	Endoscopic sinonasal surgery
	Endoscopic sphenoethmoidectomy
	Sphenopalatine artery ligation
	Endoscopic frontal sinusotomy
Level II	Advanced sinus surgery
	Cerebrospinal fluid leaks
	Lateral recess sphenoid
	Sella/pituitary (intrasellar)
Level III (extradural)	Medial orbital decompression
	Optic nerve decompression
	Sella/pituitary (extrasellar)
	Petrous apex (medial expansion)
	Transclival approaches (extradural)
	Transodontoid approach (extradural)
Level IV (intradural)	A. Presence of a cortical cuff • Transplanum approach • Transcribriform approach • Preinfundibular lesions
	B. Absence of cortical cuff (direct vascular contact) • Transplanum approach • Transcribriform approach • Infundibular lesions • Retroinfundibular lesions • Transclival approach • Foramen magnum approach
	C. ICA dissection
Level V	A. Middle coronal plane (paramedian) • Suprapetrous carotid approaches • Infrapetrous carotid approaches • Transpterygoid approach • Infratemporal approach
	B. Posterior coronal plane (paramedian)
	C. Vascular surgery

Source: Lund et al. European position paper on endoscopic management of tumours of the nose, paranasal sinuses and skull base. Rhinology Suppl 2010;(22):23. With permission.

complications and mortality can occur, although given a comparable case mix of intracranial pathology, these are of no greater order than with craniofacial resection or open neurosurgery. Indeed, for sinonasal tumors affecting the skull base, the morbidity is considerably less (see below).[13]

Complications

(See **Table 19.5**.)

As mentioned above, certain complications may occur with any surgical (or nonsurgical) therapies but have generally been less frequent after EEAs. However, as these techniques are extended further intracranially, they may inevitably result in catastrophic events. Surgeons undertaking this surgery should be well versed in the management of these problems and be able to deal with them. Thus, the combination of multidisciplinary teams, with access to neurosurgical and ophthalmological expertise as well as interventional radiology, is mandatory for the more extended surgical approaches.

Minor problems such as postoperative crusting and postnasal discharge barely count as complications but are generally less than with conventional craniofacial resection. In a study of 63 patients undergoing endoscopic skull base surgery, the median time to absence of crusting was 101 days, and that for the remucosalization of the nasoseptal flap, if used, was 89 days. However, this was longer in more complex cases and few in this cohort received radiotherapy.[63]

Significant hemorrhage is the most difficult intraoperative complication and, if anticipated, may be mitigated by embolization, availability of blood, and preparation for major vessel injury with appropriate equipment and personnel.

The issue of persistent CSF leakage has been largely overcome by the various repair techniques now available (see above).[64]

Table 19.5 Complications of endonasal endoscopic sinus surgery (not including systemic—pulmonary embolism, chest infection, etc.)

Immediate or early	Late
Loss of olfaction and perception of flavor	CSF leak
Visual loss	Prolapse of intracranial contents through skull base defect
Diplopia	Epilepsy
Epiphora	Frontal osteomyelitis
Enophthalmos	Mucocele formation
CSF leak	
Meningitis	
Intra- or extradural abscess	
Pneumoencephalocele	
Hemorrhage	
Cerebrovascular accident or neurologic deficit	
Confusion	
Death	

Orbital complications may occur with open or endoscopic techniques and, apart from visual loss, are largely treatable either at the time of surgery or subsequently. Loss of olfaction has a significant effect on quality of life[65] but was an inevitable consequence of conventional craniofacial resection. As a result, attempts have been made to preserve the olfactory system on one side in some endoscopic resections. However, any subsequent radiotherapy is likely to adversely affect residual function.

Overall significant complications range from 0 to 28% but usually range around 14 to 15% in the larger published series, and the majority of these were CSF leaks. In the series of Villaret et al, the prevalence of CSF leakage correlated with advanced tumor stage, dural involvement, and the earlier period of treatment: that is, 2004 to 2006 versus 2007 to 2008,[19] suggesting a learning curve related to the type of repair.

Outcomes

The results for individual tumors managed endoscopically are covered in the respective sections, but it is helpful to consider the literature on EEAs as a whole. The application of endoscopic resection for benign sinonasal tumors began during the late 1980s and has continued ever since, with increasingly larger lesions and extension into the orbit and through the skull base being undertaken in many centers worldwide. The earliest tentative reports of entirely endoscopic resection of malignant sinonasal tumor with curative intent began appearing in the late 1990s and early 2000s,[66–68] but there was understandable caution and the majority of series to this day are generally composed of relatively small numbers, mixed histologies, and short follow-up. A few authors described using an endoscope during conventional craniofacial resection to aid visualization or preferred to combine a conventional craniotomy with an endoscopic endonasal resection (endoscopically assisted craniofacial resection), but making a comparison between the results of these series and conventional craniofacial procedure is especially difficult for the same reasons.[69,70] An initiative of the European Rhinologic Society to review the entire topic resulted in the "European position paper on endoscopic management of tumours of the nose, paranasal sinuses and skull base."[13] This considered all aspects of the subject, including the evidence thus far for diagnosis and endoscopic techniques in the context of existing treatments; it proposed algorithms for management of the different tumors and offered guidance for outcome measures for future research. Perhaps most importantly, it stimulated the development of an international database that will allow the prospective collection of detailed (and anonymized) data.

Table 19.6[19,22,67,71–87] shows some of the main series published in this area, from which it will be seen that cumulatively quite large numbers of malignant tumors are being accrued but that we still lack numbers with long-term follow-up to make direct statistical comparison with the established "gold standard" of craniofacial resection. However, there are some authors who have followed their patients now for prolonged periods (median 100 months) and are showing that recurrence and patient loss continue to occur for as long as surveillance continues.[67,87] Furthermore, though staging is not always mentioned, generally the lesions chosen for EEAs are likely to be less extensive in their involvement of prognostically important areas such as the orbit and skull base. Notwithstanding this caveat, one can say that EEAs provide at least comparable results in the shorter term, and emerging evidence suggests in the longer term as well with significantly reduced complications and morbidity.[83,84,88,89] It is therefore reasonable to assume that as long as the oncological principles are observed and the natural history of the individual tumors is understood, EEAs provide a viable alternative to open approaches for most T1, T2 and some T3 sinonasal malignancies. In addition, they may also play a role in the palliative management of T4+ tumors when genuine "debulking" may be undertaken.

What are the limitations of endoscopic tumor resection for malignant tumors? Depending on the histological type and extent, these will also differ from unit to unit, surgeon to surgeon, and day to day. It is likely, as these techniques are increasingly accepted, that more and more cases will be undertaken by these approaches, but we should be conscious of the fact that (a) they require considerable technological support that is not available worldwide; (b) open techniques will still be required in some instances; and (c) their application to inappropriate cases by teams with inadequate experience of these pathologies will lead to poor results for patients, which will be a disservice to all concerned.

As a general principle, the following areas are difficult to assess and adequately resect and may be considered as exclusion criteria for an entirely endoscopic approach:

1. Nasolacrimal system
2. Orbit—extension beyond the orbital periosteum and infiltration of orbital fat
3. Frontal sinus—significant mucosal involvement or any involvement of the bone itself
4. Maxillary sinus—involvement of bony walls (except medial)
5. Significant extension into the pterygopalatine and infratemporal fossae
6. Inferior erosion through the floor of the nasal cavity and maxilla to involve the hard palate, upper alveolus, and dentition
7. Erosion into nasal bones
8. Intracranial—significant dural involvement
   - Infiltration of the superior sagittal sinus
   - Infiltration of brain parenchyma
9. Nasopharyngeal—significant extension

Table 19.6 Malignant tumors resected by an entirely endoscopic approach—main published series

Author	Histology	n	Mean follow-up (mo)	Survival	RT (± Chemo)
Walch et al 2000[71]	ON	6	57	100% 1 CFR	100%
Goffart et al 2000[67]	Mixed	66	26	66% (2 y)	90%
Casiano et al 2001[72]	ON	5 (3 primary)	31	80% DFS	100%
Roh et al 2004[73]	Mixed	13 (8[a])	26	68% (86%[a]) DFS	79%
Bockmuhl et al 2005[74]	Adeno, ON, SCC	29	65	78% 5-y survival	?
Poetker 2005[75]	Mixed	16 (14[a])	51	87% overall	69%
Shipchandler et al 2005[76]	SCC	7	31	91% at 31.5 mo (OS & DFS)	73%
Carrau et al 2006[77]	Mixed	20	11–46	95% OS	5%
Castelnuovo et al 2006[22]	Mixed	49 (33[a])	25	61% at 19.8	51%
Dave et al 2007[78]	Mixed	17 (14[a])	34	94% local control	82%
Lund et al 2007[79]	Mixed	49	36	88% OS 68% DFS	76% (28%)
Nicolai et al 2007[80]	Adeno (12) SCC (4)	16	47	87% DFS 93% DSS	50%
Podboj and Smid 2007[81]	Mixed	15	67	87% overall	63%
Bogaerts et al 2008[82]	Adeno	44	36	81% OS 91% DSS 73% local control	100%
Nicolai et al 2008[83]	Mixed	134	34	91% DSS	43%
Eloy et al 2009[84]	Mixed	18	26	94% OS	78% (11%)
Folbe et al 2009[85]	ON	19	45	89% local control	70%
Jardeleza et al 2009[86]	Adeno	12	30	92% OS & DFS	92% (8%)
Villaret et al 2010[19]	Mixed	62	17.5	80% 5-y OS 81% 5-y DSS 85% 5-y DFS	56%
Van Gerven et al 2011[87]	Adeno	44	61	63% 5-y OS 82% 5-y DSS 60% 5-y DFS 53% 100-mo OS 72% 100-mo DSS 54% 100-mo DFS	100%

Abbreviations: Adeno, adenocarcinoma; Chemo, chemotherapy; DFS, disease-free survival; DSS, disease-specific survival; mo, month(s); ON, olfactory neuroblastoma; OS, overall survival; SCC, squamous cell carcinoma; y, year(s).
[a] Curative and entirely endoscopic.

References

1. Kassam A, Snyderman CH, Mintz A, Gardner P, Carrau RL. Expanded endonasal approach: the rostrocaudal axis. Part I. Crista galli to the sella turcica. Neurosurg Focus 2005;19(1):E3
2. Kassam AB, Gardner P, Snyderman C, Mintz A, Carrau R. Expanded endonasal approach: fully endoscopic, completely transnasal approach to the middle third of the clivus, petrous bone, middle cranial fossa, and infratemporal fossa. Neurosurg Focus 2005;19(1):E6
3. Laufer I, Anand VK, Schwartz TH. Endoscopic, endonasal extended transsphenoidal, transplanum transtuberculum approach for resection of suprasellar lesions. J Neurosurg 2007;106(3):400–406
4. Frank G, Pasquini E, Doglietto F, et al. The endoscopic extended transsphenoidal approach for craniopharyngiomas. Neurosurgery 2006; 59(1, Suppl 1)ONS75–ONS83, discussion ONS75–ONS83
5. de Divitiis E, Cappabianca P, Cavallo LM, Esposito F, de Divitiis O, Messina A. Extended endoscopic transsphenoidal approach for extrasellar craniopharyngiomas. Neurosurgery 2007; 61(5, Suppl 2)219–227, discussion 228
6. de Divitiis E, Cavallo LM, Cappabianca P, Esposito F. Extended endoscopic endonasal transsphenoidal approach for the removal of suprasellar tumors: Part 2. Neurosurgery 2007;60(1):46–58, discussion 58–59
7. Carrabba G, Dehdashti AR, Gentili F. Surgery for clival lesions: open resection versus the expanded endoscopic endonasal approach. Neurosurg Focus 2008;25(6):E7
8. de Divitiis E, Esposito F, Cappabianca P, Cavallo LM, de Divitiis O, Esposito I. Endoscopic transnasal resection of anterior cranial fossa meningiomas. Neurosurg Focus 2008;25(6):E8
9. Gardner PA, Kassam AB, Snyderman CH, et al. Outcomes following endoscopic, expanded endonasal resection of suprasellar craniopharyngiomas: a case series. J Neurosurg 2008;109(1):6–16
10. Dehdashti AR, Ganna A, Witterick I, Gentili F. Expanded endoscopic endonasal approach for anterior cranial base and suprasellar lesions: indications and limitations. Neurosurgery 2009;64(4):677–687, discussion 687–689
11. Fatemi N, Dusick JR, de Paiva Neto MA, Malkasian D, Kelly DF. Endonasal versus supraorbital keyhole removal of craniopharyngiomas and tuberculum sellae meningiomas. Neurosurgery 2009; 64(5, Suppl 2)269–284, discussion 284–286
12. Fraser JF, Nyquist GG, Moore N, Anand VK, Schwartz TH. Endoscopic endonasal transclival resection of chordomas: operative technique, clinical outcome, and review of the literature. J Neurosurg 2010;112(5):1061–1069
13. Lund VJ Stammberger H, Nicolai P, et al. European position paper on endoscopic management of tumours of the nose, paranasal sinuses and skull base. Rhinol Suppl 2010;(22):1–143
14. Snyderman CH, Carrau RL, Kassam AB, et al. Endoscopic skull base surgery: principles of endonasal oncological surgery. J Surg Oncol 2008;97(8):658–664
15. Kassam A, Snyderman CH, Carrau RL, Gardner P, Mintz A. Endoneurosurgical hemostasis techniques: lessons learned from 400 cases. Neurosurg Focus 2005;19(1):E7
16. Kassam A, Carrau RL, Snyderman CH, Gardner P, Mintz A. Evolution of reconstructive techniques following endoscopic expanded endonasal approaches. Neurosurg Focus 2005;19(1):E8
17. Kassam AB, Thomas A, Carrau RL et al. Endoscopic reconstruction of the cranial base using a pedicled nasoseptal flap. Neurosurgery 2008;63(1 Suppl 1): ONS44–52; discussion ONS52–53
18. Zanation AM, Snyderman CH, Carrau RL, Kassam AB, Gardner PA, Prevedello DM. Minimally invasive endoscopic pericranial flap: a new method for endonasal skull base reconstruction. Laryngoscope 2009;119(1):13–18
19. Villaret AB, Yakirevitch A, Bizzoni A, et al. Endoscopic transnasal craniectomy in the management of selected sinonasal malignancies. Am J Rhinol Allergy 2010;24(1):60–65
20. Castelnuovo P, Pistochini A, Locatelli D. Different surgical approaches to the sellar region: focusing on the "two nostrils four hands technique". Rhinology 2006;44(1):2–7
21. Draf W. Endonasal micro-endoscopic frontal sinus surgery; the Fulda concept. Oper Tech Otolaryngol Head Neck Surg 1991;2:234–240
22. Castelnuovo P, Battaglia P, Locatelli D, Delu G, Sberze F, Bignami M. Endonasal micro-endoscopic treatment of malignant tumors of the paranasal sinuses and anterior skull base. Oper Tech Otolaryngol Head Neck Surg 2006;17:152–167
23. Kassam A, Snyderman CH, Mintz A, Gardner P, Carrau RL. Expanded endonasal approach: the rostrocaudal axis. Part II. Posterior clinoids to the foramen magnum. Neurosurg Focus 2005;19(1):E4
24. Kassam AB, Snyderman C, Gardner P, Carrau R, Spiro R. The expanded endonasal approach: a fully endoscopic transnasal approach and resection of the odontoid process: technical case report. Neurosurgery 2005; 57(1, Suppl) E213, discussion E213
25. Messina A, Bruno MC, Decq P, et al. Pure endoscopic endonasal odontoidectomy: anatomical study. Neurosurg Rev 2007;30(3):189–194, discussion 194
26. Simmen DB, Raghavan U, Briner HR, Manestar M, Groscurth P, Jones NS. The anatomy of the sphenopalatine artery for the endoscopic sinus surgeon. Am J Rhinol 2006;20(5):502–505
27. Zanation AM, Snyderman CH, Carrau RL, Gardner PA, Prevedello DM, Kassam AB. Endoscopic endonasal surgery for petrous apex lesions. Laryngoscope 2009;119(1):19–25
28. Kassam AB, Vescan AD, Carrau RL, et al. Expanded endonasal approach: vidian canal as a landmark to the petrous internal carotid artery. J Neurosurg 2008;108(1):177–183
29. Osawa S, Rhoton AL Jr, Seker A, Shimizu S, Fujii K, Kassam AB. Microsurgical and endoscopic anatomy of the vidian canal. Neurosurgery 2009; 64(5, Suppl 2)385–411, discussion 411–412
30. Kassam A, Snyderman C, Carrau R. Expanded endonasal approach: Transplanum approach. Skull Base Interdiscip Approach 2004;14(Suppl 1):10
31. Badia L, Loughran S, Lund VJ. Primary spontaneous cerebrospinal fluid rhinorrhea and obesity. Am J Rhinol 2001;15(2):117–119
32. Anand VK, Murali RK, Glasgold MJ. Surgical decisions in the management of cerebrospinal fluid rhinorrhoea. Rhinology 1995;33(4):212–218
33. Hughes RG, Jones NS, Robertson IJ. The endoscopic treatment of cerebrospinal fluid rhinorrhoea: the Nottingham experience. J Laryngol Otol 1997;111(2):125–128
34. Marshall AH, Jones NS, Robertson IJ. CSF rhinorrhoea: the place of endoscopic sinus surgery. Br J Neurosurg 2001;15(1):8–12
35. Lopatin AS, Kapitanov DN, Potapov AA. Endonasal endoscopic repair of spontaneous cerebrospinal fluid leaks. Arch Otolaryngol Head Neck Surg 2003;129(8):859–863
36. Al-Sebeih K, Karagiozov K, Elbeltagi A, Al-Qattan F. Nontraumatic cerebrospinal fluid rhinorrhea: diagnosis and management. Ann Saudi Med 2004;24(6):453–458
37. Tabaee A, Kassenoff TL, Kacker A, Anand VK. The efficacy of computer assisted surgery in the endoscopic management of cerebrospinal fluid rhinorrhea. Otolaryngol Head Neck Surg 2005;133(6):936–943

38. Alameda YA, Busquets JM, Portela JC. Anterior skull base cerebrospinal fluid fistulas in Puerto Rico: treatment and outcome. Bol Asoc Med P R 2009;101(2):29–33

39. Wormald PJ, McDonogh M. 'Bath-plug' technique for the endoscopic management of cerebrospinal fluid leaks. J Laryngol Otol 1997;111(11):1042–1046

40. Castelnuovo PG, Delú G, Locatelli D, et al. Endonasal endoscopic duraplasty: our experience. Skull Base 2006;16(1):19–24

41. Leong JL, Citardi MJ, Batra PS. Reconstruction of skull base defects after minimally invasive endoscopic resection of anterior skull base neoplasms. Am J Rhinol 2006;20(5):476–482

42. Locatelli D, Rampa F, Acchiardi I, Bignami M, De Bernardi F, Castelnuovo P. Endoscopic endonasal approaches for repair of cerebrospinal fluid leaks: nine-year experience. Neurosurgery 2006;58(4 Suppl 2):ONS-246–256; discussiom ONS-256–257

43. Castelnuovo P, Dallan I, Bignami M, Pistochini A, Battaglia P, Tschabitscher M. Endoscopic endonasal management of petroclival cerebrospinal fluid leaks: anatomical study and preliminary clinical experience. Minim Invasive Neurosurg 2008;51(6):336–339

44. Hadad G, Bassagasteguy L, Carrau RL, et al. A novel reconstructive technique after endoscopic expanded endonasal approaches: vascular pedicle nasoseptal flap. Laryngoscope 2006;116(10):1882–1886

45. El-Sayed IH, Roediger FC, Goldberg AN, Parsa AT, McDermott MW. Endoscopic reconstruction of skull base defects with the nasal septal flap. Skull Base 2008;18(6):385–394

46. Kassam AB, Thomas A, Carrau RL, et al. Endoscopic reconstruction of the cranial base using a pedicled nasoseptal flap. Neurosurgery 2008; 63(1, Suppl 1)ONS44–ONS52, discussion ONS52–ONS53

47. Zanation AM, Carrau RL, Snyderman CH, et al. Nasoseptal flap reconstruction of high flow intraoperative cerebral spinal fluid leaks during endoscopic skull base surgery. Am J Rhinol Allergy 2009;23(5):518–521

48. Harvey RJ, Nogueira JF, Schlosser RJ, Patel SJ, Vellutini E, Stamm AC. Closure of large skull base defects after endoscopic transnasal craniotomy. Clinical article. J Neurosurg 2009;111(2):371–379

49. Pinheiro-Neto CD, Prevedello DM, Carrau RL, et al. Improving the design of the pedicled nasoseptal flap for skull base reconstruction: a radioanatomic study. Laryngoscope 2007;117(9):1560–1569

50. Shah RN, Surowitz JB, Patel MR, et al. Endoscopic pedicled nasoseptal flap reconstruction for pediatric skull base defects. Laryngoscope 2009;119(6):1067–1075

51. Kang MD, Escott E, Thomas AJ, et al. The MR imaging appearance of the vascular pedicle nasoseptal flap. AJNR Am J Neuroradiol 2009;30(4):781–786

52. Fortes FS, Carrau RL, Snyderman CH, et al. The posterior pedicle inferior turbinate flap: a new vascularized flap for skull base reconstruction. Laryngoscope 2007;117(8):1329–1332

53. Prevedello DM, Barges-Coll J, Fernandez-Miranda JC, et al. Middle turbinate flap for skull base reconstruction: cadaveric feasibility study. Laryngoscope 2009;119(11):2094–2098

54. Fortes FS, Carrau RL, Snyderman CH, et al. Transpterygoid transposition of a temporoparietal fascia flap: a new method for skull base reconstruction after endoscopic expanded endonasal approaches. Laryngoscope 2007;117(6):970–976

55. Yoshioka N, Rhoton AL Jr. Vascular anatomy of the anteriorly based pericranial flap. Neurosurgery 2005; 57(1, Suppl)11–16, discussion 11–16

56. Zanation AM, Snyderman CH, Carrau RL, Kassam AB, Gardner PA, Prevedello DM. Minimally invasive endoscopic pericranial flap: a new method for endonasal skull base reconstruction. Laryngoscope 2009;119(1):13–18

57. Oliver CL, Hackman TG, Carrau RL, et al. Palatal flap modifications allow pedicled reconstruction of the skull base. Laryngoscope 2008;118(12):2102–2106

58. Hackman T, Chicoine MR, Uppaluri R. Novel application of the palatal island flap for endoscopic skull base reconstruction. Laryngoscope 2009;119(8):1463–1466

59. Lim M, Lew-Gor S, Sandhu G, Howard D, Lund VJ. Whitehead's varnish nasal pack. J Laryngol Otol 2007;121(6):592–594

60. Gardner P, Kassam A, Snyderman C, Mintz A, Carrau R, Moossy JJ. Endoscopic endonasal suturing of dural reconstruction grafts: a novel application of the U-Clip technology. Technical note. J Neurosurg 2008;108(2):395–400

61. Dagash H, Chowdhury M, Pierro A. When can I be proficient in laparoscopic surgery? A systematic review of the evidence. J Pediatr Surg 2003;38(5):720–724

62. Stankiewicz JA. Complications in endoscopic intranasal ethmoidectomy: an update. Laryngoscope 1989;99(7 Pt 1):686–690

63. de Almeida JR, Snyderman CH, Gardner PA, Carrau RL, Vescan AD. Nasal morbidity following endoscopic skull base surgery: a prospective cohort study. Head Neck 2011;33(4):547–551

64. Harvey RJ, Smith JE, Wise SK, Patel SJ, Frankel BM, Schlosser RJ. Intracranial complications before and after endoscopic skull base reconstruction. Am J Rhinol 2008;22(5):516–521

65. Jones E, Lund VJ, Howard DJ, Greenberg MP, McCarthy M. Quality of life of patients treated surgically for head and neck cancer. J Laryngol Otol 1992;106(3):238–242

66. Yuen AP, Fung CF, Hung KN. Endoscopic cranionasal resection of anterior skull base tumor. Am J Otolaryngol 1997;18(6):431–433

67. Goffart Y, Jorissen M, Daele J, et al. Minimally invasive endoscopic management of malignant sinonasal tumours. Acta Otorhinolaryngol Belg 2000;54(2):221–232

68. Stammberger H, Anderhuber W, Walch C, Papaefthymiou G. Possibilities and limitations of endoscopic management of nasal and paranasal sinus malignancies. Acta Otorhinolaryngol Belg 1999;53(3):199–205

69. Thaler ER, Kotapka M, Lanza DC, Kennedy DW. Endoscopically assisted anterior cranial skull base resection of sinonasal tumors. Am J Rhinol 1999;13(4):303–310

70. Har-El G. Anterior craniofacial resection without facial skin incisions—a review. Otolaryngol Head Neck Surg 2004;130(6):780–787

71. Walch C, Stammberger H, Anderhuber W, Unger F, Köle W, Feichtinger K. The minimally invasive approach to olfactory neuroblastoma: combined endoscopic and stereotactic treatment. Laryngoscope 2000;110(4):635–640

72. Casiano RR, Numa WA, Falquez AM. Endoscopic resection of esthesioneuroblastoma. Am J Rhinol 2001;15(4):271–279

73. Roh H-J, Batra PS, Citardi MJ, Lee J, Bolger WE, Lanza DC. Endoscopic resection of sinonasal malignancies: a preliminary report. Am J Rhinol 2004;18(4):239–246

74. Bockmühl U, Minovi A, Kratzsch B, Hendus J, Draf W. Endonasal micro-endoscopic tumor surgery: state of the art. [Article in German] Laryngorhinootologie 2005;84(12):884–891

75. Poetker DM, Toohill RJ, Loehrl TA, Smith TL. Endoscopic management of sinonasal tumors: a preliminary report. Am J Rhinol 2005;19(3):307–315

76. Shipchandler TZ, Batra PS, Citardi MJ, Bolger WE, Lanza DC. Outcomes for endoscopic resection of sinonasal squamous cell carcinoma. Laryngoscope 2005;115(11):1983–1987

77. Carrau R, Kassam A, Snyderman C, Duvvuri U, Mintz A, Gardner P. Endoscopic transnasal anterior skull base

resection for the treatment of sinonasal malignancies. Oper Tech Otolaryngol Head Neck Surg 2006;17:102–110

78. Dave SP, Bared A, Casiano RR. Surgical outcomes and safety of transnasal endoscopic resection for anterior skull tumors. Otolaryngol Head Neck Surg 2007;136(6):920–927

79. Lund V, Howard DJ, Wei WI. Endoscopic resection of malignant tumors of the nose and sinuses. Am J Rhinol 2007;21(1):89–94

80. Nicolai P, Castelnuovo P, Lombardi D, et al. Role of endoscopic surgery in the management of selected malignant epithelial neoplasms of the naso-ethmoidal complex. Head Neck 2007;29(12):1075–1082

81. Podboj J, Smid L. Endoscopic surgery with curative intent for malignant tumors of the nose and paranasal sinuses. Eur J Surg Oncol 2007;33(9):1081–1086

82. Bogaerts S, Vander Poorten V, Nuyts S, Van den Bogaert W, Jorissen M. Results of endoscopic resection followed by radiotherapy for primarily diagnosed adenocarcinomas of the paranasal sinuses. Head Neck 2008;30(6):728–736

83. Nicolai P, Battaglia P, Bignami M, et al. Endoscopic surgery for malignant tumors of the sinonasal tract and adjacent skull base: a 10-year experience. Am J Rhinol 2008;22(3):308–316

84. Eloy JA, Vivero RJ, Hoang K, et al. Comparison of transnasal endoscopic and open craniofacial resection for malignant tumors of the anterior skull base. Laryngoscope 2009;119(5):834–840

85. Folbe A, Herzallah I, Duvvuri U, et al. Endoscopic endonasal resection of esthesioneuroblastoma: a multicenter study. Am J Rhinol Allergy 2009;23(1):91–94

86. Jardeleza C, Seiberling K, Floreani S, Wormald PJ. Surgical outcomes of endoscopic management of adenocarcinoma of the sinonasal cavity. Rhinology 2009;47(4):354–361

87. Van Gerven L, Jorissen M, Nuyts S, Hermans R, Vander Poorten V. Long-term follow-up of 44 patients with adenocarcinoma of the nasal cavity and sinuses primarily treated with endoscopic resection followed by radiotherapy. Head Neck 2011;33(6):898–904

88. Devaiah AK, Larsen C, Tawfik O, O'Boynick P, Hoover LA. Esthesioneuroblastoma: endoscopic nasal and anterior craniotomy resection. Laryngoscope 2003;113(12):2086–2090

89. Batra PS, Citardi MJ, Worley S, Lee J, Lanza DC. Resection of anterior skull base tumors: comparison of combined traditional and endoscopic techniques. Am J Rhinol 2005;19(5):521–528

External Surgery

The **late presentation**, extensive nature and aggressive biology of a wide variety of sinonasal tumors necessitates surgery in the management of the majority of cases. The significant improvements in imaging with CT and MRI have allowed us ever-increasing preoperative accuracy with regard to the extent of the lesions. This improved imaging, combined with improved pathology-diagnostic techniques, has allowed us to more appropriately use the wide variety of surgical techniques available, which vary from endoscopic to major open skull base resection. Larger procedures may involve removal of intracranial structures, the bone of the skull base itself, and extensive components of the subcranial area when disease involves the orbit, nose, sinuses, and adjacent tissues. The surgeon, preferably part of a multidisciplinary team, attempts to combine a definitive cure with preservation of function, cosmesis, and quality of life.

The surgery in these areas is often complex and may require the careful coordination of several members of the multidisciplinary team to safely carry out the resection and reconstruction (should the latter be necessary). Much has been written about these evolving surgical techniques, but most of the variants of approaches to the anterior and anterolateral areas of the skull base by open surgery have now been with us for a sufficient time for us to have substantial long-term figures with regard to morbidity, mortality, and cure rates. Endoscopic surgery continues to be increasingly utilized but, as yet, the long-term outcomes of a substantial number of patients, particularly those treated for malignant disease, remain limited.

Despite our ever-increasing experience with these operative procedures, cure is still not possible in a significant proportion of these patients and is nearly always at a price of some morbidity. While the last three decades of craniofacial surgery have revealed low mortality and morbidity figures, it is to be hoped that endoscopic procedures, newer forms of radiotherapy, new chemotherapy and novel molecular biological agents will have an increasing amount to offer.

This book is not intended to replace the many excellent manuals published in recent years of operative surgery techniques for nose, sinus, and skull base tumors, but the following represents an assessment of the respective roles and limitations of the different surgical options.

When *Tumors of the Upper Jaw* was published in 1993, we stated that the immensely improved optics afforded by rigid and flexible endoscopes had greatly facilitated our examination technique and the hope was that this might ultimately lead to earlier diagnosis of disease. Sadly, while this may have occurred in some fortunate individual cases, **the rarity of these diseases continues to be associated with a late clinical presentation** as a consequence of both patients and doctors ignoring the early innocuous symptoms of sinonasal malignancy. **The simple and extremely common symptoms** of nasal block, discharge, and facial pain are often present for periods of between 6 months and 1 year, and it is only with advent of bleeding, facial swelling, orbital symptoms, and oral problems, or the appearance of a mass that prompts presentation of the patient. Endoscopes have allowed us to carry out far more accurate, specific, and multiple biopsies of many lesions, but there are still many patients in whom only imaging reveals the extensive nature of the disease and in whom obtaining appropriate biopsies can still be difficult. A high index of suspicion has to be maintained both in primary practice and in ENT outpatient clinics to detect these rare cases. **Unilateral nasal and sinus symptoms**, particularly in association with unpleasant nasal discharge or bleeding and inappropriate facial pain and paresthesia, should always be carefully assessed. Two further groups of patients are worthy of note in that, with the increase in modern scanning available around the world, asymptomatic patients may have lesions detected during investigation for other, unrelated problems. For those undertaking tertiary referral care, it is unfortunately the case that a substantial number of patients have had prior failed primary treatment and are referred with persisting/recurrent disease.

Clinical Features

Unilateral nasal symptoms of recent onset require as a minimum a good quality nasal examination and evaluation of any orbital, oral, or neurologic symptoms. If a short course of appropriate medical therapy does not produce a prompt resolution, patients should be referred for specialist assessment.

Following further examination in an appropriate ENT clinic, preferably with rigid and/or fiberoptic telescopes, further imaging studies may be indicated.

Imaging

This evaluation plays a key role in the pretreatment planning of both benign and malignant lesions involving the nose, paranasal sinuses, nasopharynx, and adjacent skull base. **Both CT and MRI are frequently required** as they are complementary when assessing lesions in this area and both are required to gain maximum accuracy in assessing the local regional extent of the involved tissues (**Fig. 19.4**).[1]

The individual imaging for each of the pathologies is outlined in the respective chapters and in Chapter 5. Since 1986, our own protocol has been to employ preoperative imaging by a combination of high-resolution contrast-enhanced CT (in coronal and axial planes) with 3 planar MRI enhanced with gadolinium diethylenetriamine pentaacetic acid (Gd-DTPA). **This combination of imaging gives the best overall assessment of the tumors**. It is important to understand that pain management may be required to allow a person to undergo this type of scanning and occasionally sedation is indicated as some patients confined in a magnetic resonance or CT scanner can find the experience very upsetting if they suffer from claustrophobia and the extent and nature of the procedure has not been explained to them.

Additional evaluation by modalities such as ultrasound or PET-CT scanning may be indicated depending on the tumor type and extent. It is important to discuss the outcome of the scans and any additional testing with the patient as well as at the multidisciplinary meeting with all colleagues. This is best done in association with the results of pathology from any biopsies.

Imaging may be of further importance as an added parameter to **intraoperative** guidance and is essential for long-term follow-up. However, **posttreatment imaging** undertaken with a different modality from the preoperative imaging, on a different machine with different settings, and then reported on by a different radiologist (often without access to the original imaging and no multidisciplinary discussion with the treating team) can be a complete disaster. Inappropriately early posttreatment imaging before treatment changes have resolved (less than 12 weeks and often longer) can also be seriously misleading. The patient's and the team's desire for early confirmation of "cure" can be disastrous. Additionally,

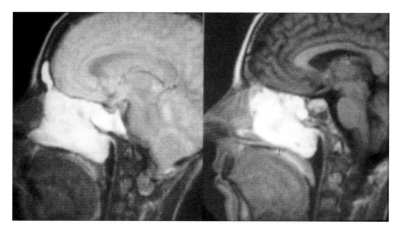

Fig. 19.4 MRI (T1W pre and post gadolinium enhancement) clearly distinguishing between the tumor mass, adjacent inflamed nasal and sinus mucosa, and retained secretions in the frontal and sphenoid sinus.

too-early "repeat" posttreatment biopsy, again before a minimum of 12 weeks post treatment, can cause considerable confusion and distress if the pathologist reports what seems to be "residual" disease, when in fact this is nonviable.

All scanning techniques—CT, MRI, PET—become far more reliable at predicting " cure" after 4 months and preferably 6 months post treatment.

Histopathology

The diversity of pathology found within tumors of the nose, paranasal sinuses, nasopharynx, and adjacent skull base, is as great as any area of the human body. This is clearly documented in the WHO classification of tumors, *Pathology and Genetics of Head and Neck Tumors* edited by Leon Barnes et al in 2005—outlined in **Table 4.2** on pages 42–44.

This list of tumors has been added to in this book with a variety of further conditions with potential for high morbidity and, in some cases, mortality.

Perioperative Patient Care— The Multidisciplinary Team

The **multidisciplinary head and neck surgical team** has existed for more than 30 years in our institution and combined clinics with our radiation oncology colleagues date back to 1952. However, in many institutions around the world, the multidisciplinary team is a relatively recent thing and, in some countries, is still not the accepted way of working. Within the United Kingdom, the head and neck surgical multidisciplinary team meets on a weekly basis, but in the last 10 years, there has been an increasing emphasis on an additional skull base team comprising those surgeons from ENT, neurosurgery, plastics, and maxillofacial with a particular interest in this group of patients. For more than 30 years our multidisciplinary teams have included colleagues from pathology, radiology, and radiation oncology and, at times, varying levels and numbers of specialist surgeons. Senior nurses, including over the past 15 years clinical nurse specialists, head and neck trained nurses, dieticians, social workers, nutritionists, speech therapists, physiotherapists, and ward clerks, have all been involved within the team. The **key worker** in the team has changed in emphasis from the senior ward sister to the clinical nurse specialist, but this situation varies in different hospitals and different countries. It remains extremely important that a particular individual can be in constant contact with the patient, whether at home or within the hospital. In many instances, a busy multidisciplinary group requires a coordinator to carry out administration, improve communications, mobilize test results, and collate/produce detailed

documentation for multidisciplinary team meetings. The coordinator should ensure that data collection, both locally and nationally, are completed and logged. In addition, some coordinators are involved in clinic scheduling and research organization, although there are, unfortunately, multidisciplinary teams in the United Kingdom without coordinators and various members of the team undertake many of these functions.

For a young trainee surgeon, the emphasis is often on acquiring the surgical expertise but an understanding of the natural history of the disease and the use of all aspects of the multidisciplinary team can involve considerably more work and study to obtain a full understanding. It is vital for the trainee to understand this requirement and in particular to study the varying natural history of these diseases.

Preoperative Counseling and Patient/ Relation Education

The benign and malignant diseases outlined in this book often require frank and detailed discussion with the patients and other family members. The topics covered are many and varied but may include:

- Pain control
- The effects of any environmental exposure at work
- Smoking, alcohol use, obesity, and lifestyle in general
- Poor nutrition, weight loss
- The individual fears of cancer of both the patient and family
- The issues related to the upcoming surgery, radiotherapy, and/or chemotherapy
- The early and long-term postoperative treatment in relation to breathing, speech, swallowing, cosmesis, eyesight, smell, taste, hearing, and restoration of normal or limited activities

Lack of information with regard to the potential changes, morbidity, and indeed mortality, often leads to inadequate ability of the patients and their families to cope, not only with the possibilities of even moderate or major surgery but with the issues of radiotherapy and chemotherapy. Obtaining informed consent from this group of patients requires care and time, and while this is not always easily available in a busy therapeutic, tertiary referral practice, it is extremely important to put aside this time and for all the members of the multidisciplinary team to be well informed with regard to the patient's preoperative situation. A high proportion of these patients present with advanced disease with a far from certain outcome as to whether or not they can be cured; it is important to establish a real and definite area of cooperation and trust within the multidisciplinary team, the patient, and their family. With specific surgical procedures often being done by one or more surgeons, it is important that one, and preferably more, of the surgeons take a specific interest in each patient along with their key worker, who is usually the clinical nurse specialist. While multidisciplinary team efforts have been advocated for many years, it is still essential that a main operating surgeon and the patient have appropriate time together to discuss the overall situation, both pre- and postoperatively.

The Head and Neck Clinical Nurse Specialist

In the United Kingdom, the clinical nurse specialists are frequently former senior nurses and many of them have been ward sisters on head and neck and neurosurgical wards. As such, they are **advocates for the patients** and have considerable clinical nursing expertise, but added to this, many of them understand the roles of all the staff involved in the multidisciplinary team and can act as advisers, counselors, teachers, and researchers and generally liaise throughout the team. They are specifically able to provide continuity of care for the patients and must be involved from a point of early initial contact right through to discharge to home and subsequent communications with the family practitioner, visits to home, and the patient's return to the clinic. This is a demanding but incredibly satisfying role for the right individual and another keystone for improved care for the patient. They are however, **not a substitute for full and careful communication between the treating physician/surgeon and the patient**.

Initial Assessment and Symptom Management

Patients with relatively early tumors of the nose, paranasal sinuses, and skull base may have little in the way of symptoms as alluded to above, but any that present late or having had previous failed treatment do have important problems with regard to pain control and symptoms such as epistaxis, epiphora or double vision, trismus, dental problems, and so on. While immediate consideration is given to establishing an accurate diagnosis if this has not already been undertaken, it is important before considering investigations, or certainly at the same time, for the consulting doctor and the team to address the patient's pain control and other needs. Diseases of this area rarely result in major nutritional issues as most patients are still able to take food orally, unless the disease is so extensive as to involve the oral cavity or to produce severe trismus. However, **weight loss**, as with cancer in general, may already be significant and early assessment by the dietician, irrespective of the subsequent form of treatment, is essential.

Pain management is increasingly undertaken by specialist members of the team and morphine and its derivatives may be required immediately and, on occasion, immediate patient admission may be necessary to address the issues of pain and epistaxis. Only when these problems have been brought under control, should the team proceed with imaging, biopsies, and so forth.

Hospice Care

Unfortunately, **advanced disease in these areas may be unresectable** and inappropriate to be treated with either chemotherapy or radiotherapy; it is important that the multidisciplinary team agree on these issues and that the patient and the family receive immediate supportive care, and that any primary physicians receive adequate and early information with referral of the patient and family to an appropriate local hospice, if this exists in the country in which they present. When patients are transferred from hospital to hospice, or are returning to their home with appropriate primary care, pain control and nursing must be clearly communicated and documented to the ongoing carers.

Nutrition

The importance of nutrition in all forms of major head and neck tumor treatment cannot be overemphasized. As in other areas of cancer, there has been an increasing international literature over the last three decades that shows that it is important to establish nutritional parameters:
1. Prior to treatment
2. Throughout the treatment
3. During the posttreatment phase, particularly when combined therapy has been instituted

Patients with malignant disease of the nose, sinuses, and skull base are, unfortunately, no different from any others within the general population in that obesity, diabetes, respiratory, cardiovascular, and gastrointestinal disease and arthritis are all common accompanying factors. The overall weight of the patient and any loss or gain in recent times should be clearly established along with the present state of nutrition, which may require intervention and careful planning with correction prior to any major treatment considerations, either surgical, radiotherapeutic or chemotherapeutic. A nutritional plan is individualized for each patient and reassessed at regular intervals throughout any subsequent treatment. There is a wide variation in patients' tolerance with regard to oral feeding or nasogastric or parental feeding with a wide variety of nutritional support and hence the need for a continuous and expert input if this is available. **In those countries where dietetic/nutritionist expertise is not available** these considerations must be taken on by the surgical team. Irrespective of the expertise of any surgeon, good postoperative results with low morbidity and mortality will not be obtained if operating on nutritionally compromised, dehydrated, and poorly prepared patients.

A proportion of patients with advanced disease of the skull base have significant cranial nerve deficits preoperatively, but these may be markedly increased following surgery and/or radiotherapy and may be accompanied by problems such as silent aspiration. In these patients, early assessment of these problems and their long-term care may be absolutely crucial to a successful outcome. They may require a full swallowing rehabilitation program and close cooperation between the nutritionists and speech therapists (speech pathologist).

Social Services

A proportion of the elderly patients who may present with diseases in this area will live on their own and may not have significant family support. For other patients, even ones who have significant family help, **social service issues may need to be addressed from the outset** and considered prior to any significant surgery. The important issues of coping on return to home may require adaptation. For instance, if it is necessary to remove the patient's eye or maxilla or to carry out substantial facial reconstruction, then additional support may be necessary to help the patient cope with their **subsequent return to home and, if possible, work. A patient's comorbidity, dependence on alcohol, and drug history** may also be part of the important mix of their requirements; social assessment and nursing evaluation needs, again, may be channeled through the clinical nurse specialist, depending on the circumstances within each given team or the country in which the patient is being treated. The patient may require a variety of aids both in and out of the home and help to deal with issues of disfigurement, mobility, ability to drive, and so on.

As in all forms of cancer surgery, occasionally, pretreatment assessment may require expert psychiatric opinion and certainly this is necessary in a small number of patients who survive the more arduous forms of combined treatment and find it difficult to reestablish a reasonable quality of life.[2] These issues cannot be ignored as the cure of many of these unfortunate patients is only the beginning of a **long period of rehabilitation**.

Dental Assessment; Osseointegration Prosthetics

The history of **prosthetic rehabilitation** after maxillectomy extends back to Syme in 1835. By the early part of the 20th century, prosthetic and dental restoration after maxillectomy were well developed, with Woodman's seminal description of the technique of an initial plaster cast, a temporary denture, and subsequently a permanent denture, being described in 1923 (**Fig. 19.5**). These techniques have been continuously improved with the use of an ever-increasing range of modern materials so that in our own hospital, preoperative assessment and fashioning of an upper jaw prosthesis, which was subsequently placed at the time of the ablative surgery, dates back for more than 60 years (**Fig. 19.6**). In contrast, **thorough pretreatment oral and dental evaluation by an oncologically orientated dentist** documenting oral and dental pathology prior to any cancer treatment is far from universal. Many treating surgeons and physicians still fail to remember how important it is before treatment to **reduce or remove any sources of potential infection** and to consider **osseointegrated implantation** at the time of the ablative surgery to aid subsequent rehabilitation even if there is to be postoperative radiotherapy and chemotherapy. The surgeon, radiation oncologist, and

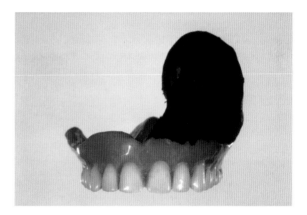

Fig. 19.5 Clinical photograph of the initial temporary obturator fashioned using gutta percha applied to the plate made preoperatively. This obturator is fitted immediately following removal of the maxilla under the same anesthetic following wound closure.

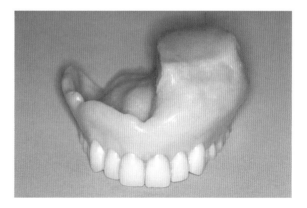

Fig. 19.6 Subsequent lightweight permanent obturator made after full healing and stabilization of the maxillectomy cavity.

medical oncologist should be able to assess oral pathology secondary to poor dental status, notably advanced periodontal disease, gross dental caries, poorly fitting existing dentures, and poor oral hygiene. As part of the initial assessment, the patient should be referred to a dental colleague to undertake thorough oral and dental assessment with appropriate radiographs, which may include occlusal, panoramic, periapical, and bitewing views. **These are relatively easy and inexpensive investigations in comparison with CT and MRI and may be extremely important in the long-term care of the patient**. This is particularly the case if an extensive nasal, paranasal, sinus, or skull base lesion involves the interior aspect of the upper jaw and **prosthetic rehabilitation depends on stable anchorage of any prosthesis to remaining teeth on the opposite side** (Fig. 19.7).

Teeth with potentially poor prognosis require extraction before postoperative chemotherapy or irradiation. With forward planning, this may be done under the same general anesthetic as the ablative surgery. Performing these removals at the time of the primary surgery may decrease the workload for the team and the waiting time for the patient. There is considerable potential room for improvement with regard to this aspect of patient care as subsequent **osteoradionecrosis remains a serious and debilitating problem** with a generally poor outcome. Dental assessment is frequently required in the postoperative and posttreatment period, particularly with

patients who undergo additional irradiation because—even with the more modern techniques of IMRT—they may still experience some dry mouth (xerostomia) and an increased incidence of dental disease, particularly of the upper jaw in this group of patients. Patients may require continual encouragement to use simple measures such as a fluoride rinse and to attend their general dentist for routine care in the long term after their treatment.

There have been steady improvements in the extraoral application of osseointegrated techniques to allow improved retention of intraoral/maxillectomy/orbital/nasal/hemifacial prostheses in the last 20 years (see Chapter 21). While reconstruction of maxillectomy defects with free flaps is becoming increasingly popular in those countries able to undertake the technique, it does not always provide the best alternative to a well-constructed obturator prosthesis, particularly if the latter can be secured in an excellent manner on any remaining teeth and with additional osseointegrated implants. There are cases, particularly those patients who are edentulous, where the free flap reconstruction may offer an acceptable aesthetic and functional result, but in older patients the prolonged operating time may be a contraindication. In contrast, for some of the older edentulous patients and less capable individuals who are unable to maintain and accurately place a prosthesis, a free flap reconstruction may be beneficial. Careful consideration must be given to each individual patient.

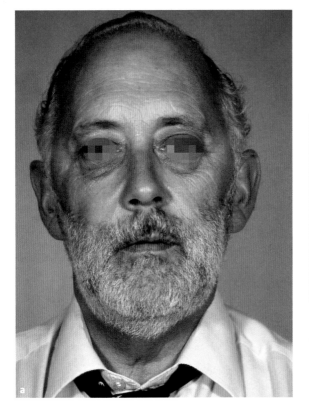

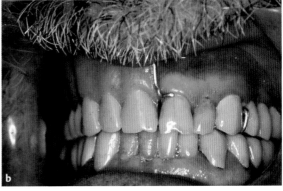

Fig. 19.7a, b

a Clinical photograph of a patient 6 months after right total maxillectomy for extensive adenoid cystic carcinoma.

b The same patient with a right maxillary obturator firmly anchored with clips to the remaining left upper dentition, giving excellent swallowing and speech.

Overview

Insufficient attention has frequently been paid in the past to understanding patients' concerns with regard to proposed treatment of their nose, paranasal sinus, and skull base tumors. The multidisciplinary team needs to be sensitive to these issues and to understand that a patient's ability to take in information under the stress of this situation is, to say the least, suboptimal. The use of medical terms rather than understandable everyday language is inappropriate, and the whole patient journey requires patients to be cared for and supported in a positive manner. The unique aspects of surgery in this region and the possibility of additional radiotherapy and chemotherapy require frank discussion with the patient and their family members; and the patient's individual fears about why they have presented with these cancers and the issues around complications, morbidity, disfigurement, and overall changes from their normal activities require thorough discussion. Informed consent should be obtained by senior members of the team, preferably the consultant surgeon undertaking the procedure and with the clinical nurse specialist present. The patient, the relatives, and the team members will all benefit from the establishment of an atmosphere of mutual trust, particularly where the situation is likely to change over the passage of time, and there is always the possibility of failure of therapy or recurrence of disease in addition to the morbidity and occasional mortality.

Key Points

- Surgery in these areas is often complex and requires the careful coordination of several members of a multidisciplinary team.
- The rarity of these diseases, in contrast to their often common presenting symptoms, means that the majority of patients still present with advanced disease.
- A high index of suspicion for **unilateral** nasal and sinus symptoms is needed in primary practice and with ENT outpatients to detect these rare diseases.
- Both CT and MRI are usually required for imaging as they are complementary and provide maximum accuracy in assessing locoregional tumor extent.
- The diversity of pathology found within tumors of the nose, paranasal sinuses, nasopharynx, and skull base is greater than in any other area of the human body.
- Multidisciplinary team-working improves the care and outcomes for these patients.
- Young surgeons need to acquire a thorough knowledge of the pathology and natural history of these diseases.
- Preoperative counseling of these patients and their relatives is essential.
- A dedicated head and neck clinical nurse specialist is an invaluable member of the team.

- Pain control management and nutritional assessment are essential in advanced disease.
- **Pre**treatment dental assessment and prosthetic rehabilitation are important considerations in selected patients.
- Thorough pretreatment of oral and dental disease to remove or reduce infection and to consider osseointegrated implantation is essential in many patients, but particularly those undergoing radiotherapy ± chemotherapy and maxillary sinus surgery.
- Appropriate pre- and postoperative information, care, and support are essential for these patients.

Surgical Treatment

This component of the book is not designed to replace the many excellent major surgical manuals that are available on these subjects and clearly such issues as operative equipment and the positioning, prepping, draping, and overall planning of any operative procedure will depend on the individual operation. What is important in all cases is close **cooperation and clear exchange of information with anesthesiology colleagues**, particularly in the circumstances of patients with notable trismus or other possible airway difficulties. The positioning of any endotracheal tube or the establishment of a tracheostomy needs careful consideration depending on the approach to be used to the tumor.

Experienced circulating and scrub nurse personnel are an important requirement, as too is the recovery and postoperative nursing care. While many postoperative wards and intensive care units may contain highly qualified nursing staff, various problems can arise if they are not familiar with the specific requirements of patients undergoing surgery for tumors in these areas. Postoperative neurological monitoring, care of the airway, care and use of any prosthesis and any reconstruction by means of flaps and grafts all require appropriate understanding along with the general principles of wound care and postoperative patient management.

Key Points

- Cooperation and clear exchange of information with anesthetic colleagues is essential.
- Perioperative and specialist postoperative nursing care are essential.

Selection of a Particular Operative Procedure

In selecting a particular procedure for an individual patient, the site, size, histology, and natural history of the patient's disease and any additional comorbidities are extremely important. Surgeons are influenced by their personal philosophy, past experience, and technical capability. A professional approach is required if patients who are curable are to be cured and **the aim of any surgery is total removal of the tumor**. Combined approaches to any cancer require the availability of a wide range of expertise and often individuals of compatible experience may not be available in most multidisciplinary clinics and democratic discussion may be weighted toward one particular discipline. In many countries, unfortunately, financial issues take part in the decision-making process and an undesirable, competitive element between different departments may further complicate the issues. However, if we are to improve the overall poor long-term control rates for many of these diseases, and the persistence of the crippling and mutilating effects of many surgical resections, then these procedures require careful consideration. **Mere acquisition of multiple surgical technical skills does not necessarily produce appropriate selection for patients and this whole area is fraught with philosophical considerations**. In particular, the advantages of successful surgery must outweigh the risks and subsequent morbidity and the surgeons must ask themselves whether they are able to perform the procedure to an accepted level of competence, bearing in mind **what is the best treatment for any particular patient** with any specific disease. If this is not the case, they should consider referring the case to a more experienced colleague or an alternative multidisciplinary team dealing specifically with these rare tumors.

Much of the surgery in this area aimed at cure or long-term palliation is associated with a degree of mutilation, and certainly notable interference with function. In some countries, such disabilities preclude social acceptance and facial disfigurement is still an important problem in most communities. Even excellent external prostheses only act as camouflage and considerable damage to the patient's self-image may present a serious problem, with them requiring considerable support to return to work or other aspects of daily life (**Figs. 19.8 and 19.9**).

In contrast, however, electing a conservative procedure with little hope of cure may only allow the disease to progress and cause the patient far more in the way of symptoms prior to an unpleasant death. While the patient may pay a price for a "cure at any cost" philosophy, inadequate "debulking" and reliance on "chemotherapy" can produce devastating sequelae.

Key Points

- The aim of any surgery is **total** resection of the tumor.
- Appropriate selection of patients for surgery is extremely important.

Anterior External Approaches to the Nose, Sinuses, and Skull Base

A wide variety of anterior and anterolateral approaches to tumors of the nose, sinuses, and skull base have been advocated for over a hundred years and there are multiple variations described of every approach. The following descriptions are certainly not exhaustive but are those that we have found useful in our own practice in dealing with more than 1,600 benign and malignant tumors described within this book.

Lateral Rhinotomy

Up until the description of this operation in 1902 by E. J. Moure (Professor of Otolaryngology in Bordeaux, France), most tumors arising within the nasal passages were generally removed by intranasal resection and electrocauterization.[3] Moure's external approach to the ethmoid labyrinth introduced a new concept to nasal and sinus surgery; with the passage of time, his original procedure has undergone minor modifications but essentially, it gives excellent access and good cosmetic results when approaching tumors within the nasal passages and adjacent sinuses. While in our own practice it has often been replaced by midfacial degloving, it is still a useful and rapid procedure, particularly in an older age group of patients.

Incision

Moure described a skin incision that extended from the inferior part of the frontal bone above the inner margin of the eyebrow and down to the corresponding nostril. While this incision or slight variations of it might be appropriate when undertaking a limited craniofacial approach for tumors extending up to and through the

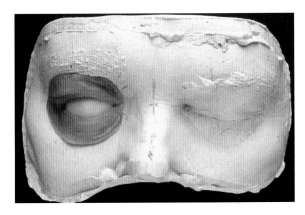

Fig. 19.8 A facial mold has been taken to allow the initial stages of an orbital implant to be fashioned.

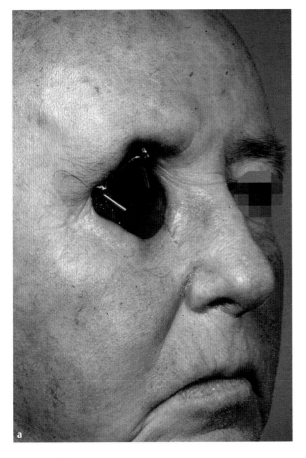 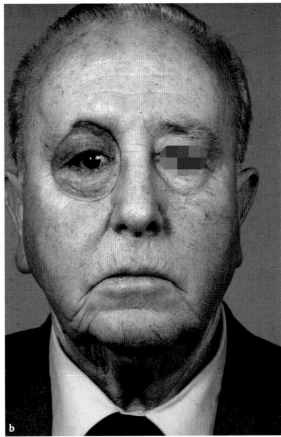

Fig. 19.9a, b

a Clinical photograph of a patient following right lateral rhinotomy and orbital exenteration for malignant melanoma with osseointegrated implants and gold bar onto which the retaining clips of the orbital prosthesis attach.

b The osseointegrated orbital prosthesis in place. Unfortunately, over time (2 years) the color match of the prosthesis to surrounding facial skin has changed. A revision of the prosthesis was indicated but the patient was satisfied and had returned to full-time work.

cribriform plate, for most lesions within the nasal cavity, ethmoids, and medial maxilla **the upper limit of the incision may need to go no higher than to a point just below the medial canthal ligament** (Fig. 19.10a). This avoids detachment of this important structure and markedly improves the subsequent cosmetic result. The incision may remain entirely in the nasomaxillary groove, curving round the alar margin to enter the nose, although modifications of this incision on to the lateral aspect of the nasal dorsum have also been proposed but there is no substantiating evidence to show that these give a better cosmetic appearance in a large series of patients. The dorsal framework of the nose may then be detached from the pyramidal opening and swung round medially, exposing the underlying bone (**Fig. 19.10b, c**).

The superior labial branches running to the vestibule in the alar portion of the incision usually require diathermy or ligation. Depending on the degree of access required, the skin and periosteum over the nasal bone and frontonasal process are mobilized accordingly. Likewise, lateral access is gained across the face of the maxilla and to the orbital rim.

If necessary the medial canthal ligament can be detached from the lacrimal crests (though this is often not necessary) and the lacrimal sac displaced laterally to allow the orbital periosteum to be mobilized widely from the lamina papyracea. Additionally the ethmoidal vessels can be cauterized/clipped and divided to improve access.

Key Points

- In many patients the incision need not go above the medial canthal ligament.

473

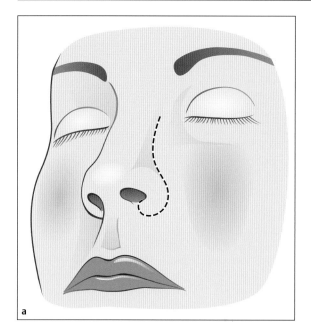

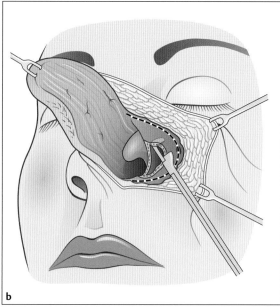

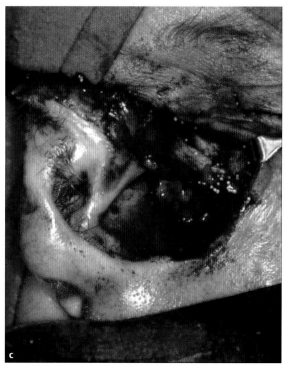

Fig. 19.10a–c

a Drawing showing the lateral rhinotomy incision, running from just below the level of the medial canthal ligament, equidistant from the dorsum of the nose and the medial canthus, down the nasomaxillary groove and accurately following the ala into the nasal cavity.

b All layers are divided and the lateral wall tissue can be retracted with a stay suture. Underlying bone removal is variable, depending on the pathology.

c Intraoperative view of right lateral rhinotomy for extensive recurrent inverted papilloma in the early 1980s, which nowadays would have been managed by an endonasal endoscopic approach.

Removal of Bone (Medial Maxillectomy)

How much bone requires removal will obviously vary depending on the underlying pathology but can include both the nasal and frontonasal process, lacrimal fossa, and lamina papyracea (preserving the infraorbital rim), the complete lateral wall of the nose and nasal septum, and the bone of the anterior wall of the maxilla, as far laterally as dissection of the soft tissues of the cheek will allow. This is frequently to a point beyond a vertical plane from the infraorbital foramen and in older patients it may be possible to access the lateral wall of the maxilla. This open procedure can, of course, be combined with endoscopic or microscopic techniques. Importantly, irrespective of the degree of removal of underlying bone, primary closure is always obtained and usually cosmetically acceptable in adults, although children are frequently unhappy about it in the long term (**Fig. 19.11**). Postoperative crusting is the only significant long-term morbidity and is significantly reduced and controlled by regular nasal douching with saline.

Key Point

- The site and quantity of the bone removal depends on the position, extent and type of pathology.

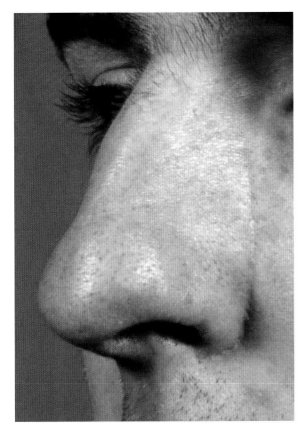

Fig. 19.11 This young man would be judged by many to have a good cosmetic result following the excision of his angiofibroma in 1984 via a left lateral rhinotomy, but he was unhappy with the slight alar retraction.

Indication

A wide variety of benign and malignant pathologies may be removed by this approach.[4]

If required, the medial canthal tendon can be elevated by sharp dissection of the tendon (with care to reattach it to precisely the same point and tension subsequently) and the medial orbital periosteum raised to allow a complete external ethmoidectomy depending on the extent of the tumor. Should the tumor be involving the orbital periosteum, the periosteum may be removed in this medial aspect and submitted for histological frozen section evaluation to see whether the tumor has invaded through the periosteum. If this is evident with substantial involvement of the medial aspect of the orbital muscle and fat, then the eye should be removed. Likewise, if the lacrimal sac and ducts are invaded by aggressive malignancies with additional involvement of the eye, then orbital clearance (or rarely exenteration) is necessary. If involved orbital periosteum can be resected with clear margins, we have utilized an underlay fascia lata graft and onlay split-thickness skin graft to fill the defect and preserve the eye.

Key Points

- Children may be unhappy with the facial scar from a lateral rhinotomy in the long term.
- A wide variety of benign and malignant pathologies may be removed by this approach.

Extended Lateral Rhinotomy Approaches

The lateral rhinotomy incision may be turned laterally at the level of the medial canthal ligament running around the edges of both the upper and lower aspects of the palpebral fissure to the lateral canthal area. Following this dissection of both upper and lower eyelids, orbital clearance can be undertaken in many patients with preservation of both eyelids to close the subsequent defect (**Fig. 19.12**). The policy for orbital clearance or exenteration (which includes excision of the eyelids) in addition to lateral rhinotomy or a craniofacial procedure will be discussed in the separate section on orbital management (p. 505).

Midfacial Degloving

Introduction

We described the application of the midfacial degloving approach in 36 cases of sinonasal pathology in 1992.[5] The continued experience of this technique was reported for 86 patients in 1999.[6] The series now has more than 200 patients treated with a wide variety of sinonasal and skull base pathology (**Table 19.7**). Unilateral exposure of the midfacial skeleton via an intraoral incision with subperiosteal elevation was originally described by Converse in 1950.[7] This technique was subsequently extended to combine a bilateral sublabial incision with elevation of the external nasal tissues via intercartilaginous and transfixion incisions to mobilize the soft tissues of the entire middle third of the face.[8]

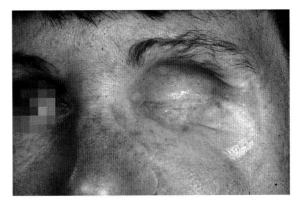

Fig. 19.12 Left lateral rhinotomy and orbital clearance with preservation of both eyelids, providing an excellent skin-lined orbital socket for rehabilitation.

Table 19.7 Midfacial degloving: personal series by histopathology

Benign histopathologies	
Angiofibroma	89
Inverted papilloma	12
Fibro-osseous disease	11
Dermoid cyst	5
Odontogenic cyst	4
Fungal infection	3
HHT	2
Neurolemmoma	3
Ameloblastoma	2
Hemangioma	3
Hemangiolymphoma	1
Facial	1
Cherubism	1
Lipoma	1
Meningoencephaloceles	2
Mucocele	1
n	141
Malignant histopathologies	
Nasopharyngeal carcinoma	13
Adenoid cystic carcinoma	6
Chondrosarcoma	7
Olfactory neuroblastoma	4
Other sarcomas	5
Malignant schwannoma	2
Rhabdomyosarcoma	3
Squamous cell carcinoma	7
Transitional cell carcinoma	3
Adenocarcinoma	2
Plasmacytoma	1
Malignant melanoma	2
Lymphoma	1
Basal cell carcinoma	1
Fibrosarcoma	1
Teratoma	1
n	59

Note: Some of these pathologies have changed their nomen-clature since the WHO classification in 2005 which is used elsewhere in this book.

Casson and colleagues originally described this procedure for cases of fibrous dysplasia but it has subsequently been a useful approach for midfacial fractures, craniofacial dysostosis, and a wide range of nasal, sinus, and skull base neoplasia. Maniglia and Phillips in 1995 published a

further review of the procedure in 30 cases of their own, treated between 1986 and 1994.[9]

Surgical Technique

The procedure is performed under general anesthesia with the endotracheal tube positioned centrally in the mouth. The patient is supine in the reversed Trendelenberg position with ~15° of head-up tilt and the head placed in a head ring. Constriction of the soft tissues is assisted by instilling Moffat's solution into the nose[10] and injecting 2% lidocaine, 1/80,000 epinephrine into the sites of incision: intercartilaginous, columella, and buccogingival sulcus (**Fig. 19.13a**). The cornea must be protected by temporary tarsorrhaphies (**Fig. 19.13b**) or appropriate shields and taping.

A bilateral, sublabial incision is made straight down to bone, running **from the maxillary tuberosity to the opposite maxillary tuberosity to gain maximal access** (**Fig. 19.13c**). An inadequate length to this incision makes subsequent mobilization of the soft tissues more difficult and decreases the use and value of this approach. (The old surgical maxim that incisions heal from side to side and not end to end is very appropriate here. A short incision seriously compromises the operation and does not "improve" healing.) The frenulum in the buccogingival sulcus is carefully marked so that it can be accurately reconstituted at the time of closure.

The periosteum and soft tissues of the cheek are raised as for a Caldwell-Luc approach, taking care with the exposure of the infraorbital nerves and allowing the infraorbital margin to be clearly identified.

Intercartilaginous incisions, made as in a routine rhinoplasty, give access to the soft tissues on the dorsum of the nose, which are elevated with the dissection extending laterally onto the anterior face of the maxilla to meet the subperiosteal approach. The intercartilaginous incisions are continued into a transfixion incision along the dorsal and caudal borders of the cartilaginous septum, separating it from the medial crura of the lower lateral cartilages (**Fig. 19.13d**). This incision is continued across the floor of the nose to join the intercartilaginous incision laterally. **It is often helpful to enter the nasal cavity inferiorly from the sublabial incision to allow better placement of the inferior cuts** (**Fig. 19.13e**). At the lateral end of the intercartilaginous incision, if the incision is turned downward and posteriorly to the piriform aperture rather than continuing in a circular manner to meet the inferior incision, this stepped incision acts to lessen the possibility of vestibular stenosis postoperatively. Further careful dissection of the skin and soft tissues of the dorsum of the nose now allows the middle third of the face to be degloved completely and gives excellent access to both nasal cavities, maxillary sinus, ethmoids, sphenoid, pterygopalatine and infratemporal fossae, and nasopharynx (**Fig. 19.13f**).

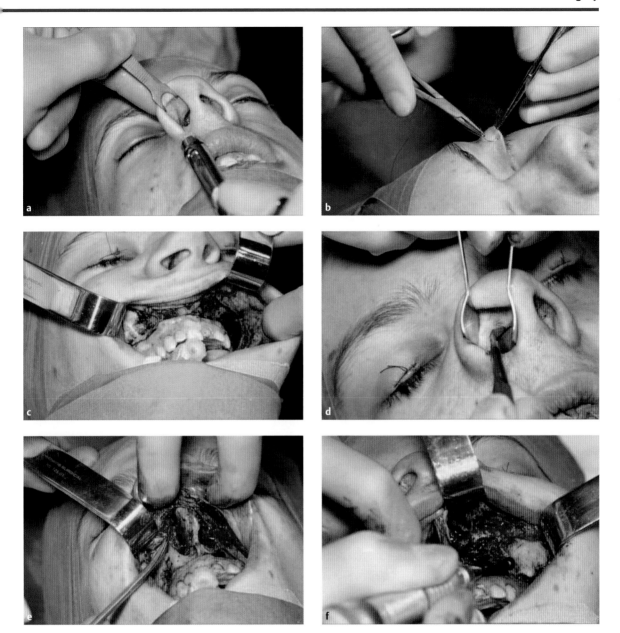

Fig. 19.13a–k Steps in the midfacial degloving operation.

a Injection of 2% lidocaine with 1:80,000 epinephrine into incision sites and nasal dorsal soft tissue.

b Bilateral temporary tarsorrhaphies with horizontal mattress sutures.

c Bilateral sublabial incision from maxillary tuberosity to the opposite maxillary tuberosity. The periosteum and soft tissues have been initially elevated from the right maxillary face.

d Right intercartilaginous incision. Note the bilateral tarsorrhaphies.

e Elevation of soft tissues of the midface after joining sublabial intercartilaginous and transfixion incisions to expose the septum.

f Opening the face of the left maxillary sinus with a drill, preserving the orbital rim superiorly and the alveolar bone inferiorly.

Fig. 19.13g–k ▷

◁ continued

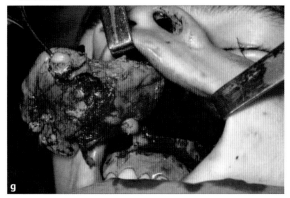

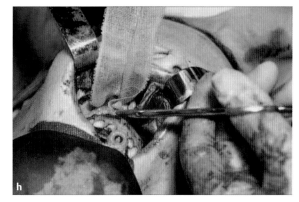

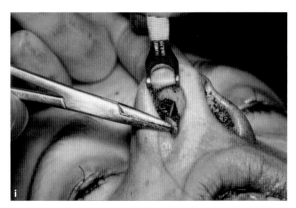

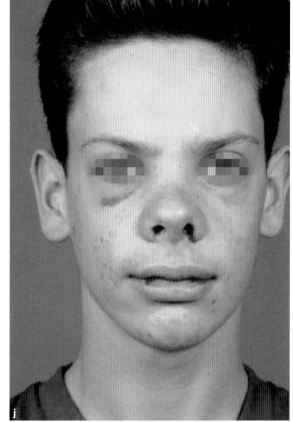

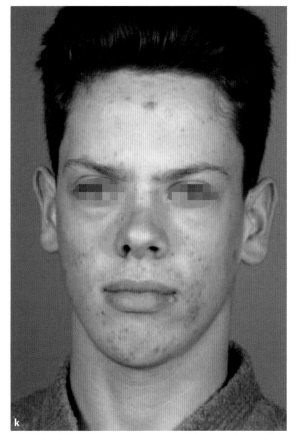

g Mobilization of stage IIIb (Radowski staging) angiofibroma through midfacial degloving with a superb view by operating microscope of the basisphenoid and surrounding skull base. This allows careful drilling out of the basisphenoid to remove any remnant of angiofibroma that has invaded the bone and vidian canal. This part of the procedure is the most important factor in preventing recurrence.

h Packing of the surgical cavity with Whitehead's varnish–soaked gauze.

i Suturing of the intercartilaginous incisions with resorbable interrupted sutures.

j Clinical photograph of the patient on the fourth postoperative day (day of discharge from hospital).

k Clinical photograph of the same patient 3 months after surgery.

The posterior wall of the sphenoid sinus, pterygoid plates, and attached muscles and posterior wall of the nasophyarynx are generally the posterior limits of the resection. The superior limit is formed by the cribriform plate and roof of the ethmoids and, laterally, the exploration can continue to the coronoid process of the mandible. The extent of resection will obviously be determined by the pathology, but a bilateral radical maxillectomy can readily be undertaken and may be combined with orbital clearance if required. The approach is particularly appropriate when combined with a coronal incision, allowing extensive craniofacial surgery without any subsequent facial scars.

The approach is also particularly appropriate for excision of an angiofibroma, allowing excellent exposure of the lesion and direct control of the internal maxillary artery and its branches prior to any attempted removal of the angiofibroma (**Fig. 19.13g**).

Postoperative hemostasis is greatly facilitated by packing of the cavity with Whitehead's varnish gauze (**Fig. 19.13h**) or similar antiseptic material. Considerable care must be exercised when suturing the incisions to minimize complications (**Fig. 19.13i**); failure to do so may result in vestibular stenosis or oroantral fistula. A simple resorbable suture may be used and routine rhinoplasty taping of the nose will reduce facial edema and bruising. It is important to warn patients and their relatives about the immediate postoperative bruising. The duration of packing will vary and may require a short general anesthetic for its removal if a substantial amount is used. Use of modern packing materials such as Nasopore may obviate the need for removing Whitehead's varnish packing.

Immediate postoperative complications include hemorrhage and paresthesia of the overlying skin of the cheek, but the latter is temporary if care is taken with the infraorbital nerves, particularly during retraction. Crusting of the cavity is the inevitable long-term consequence but this resolves gradually as regrowth of mucosa occurs. It may last for periods of up to 18 months and regular saline douching is required to lessen and control the degree of crusting. The initial facial swelling usually settles over a period of ~2 weeks (**Fig. 19.13j**) and **some excess tearing** may occur if the nasolacrimal duct is disturbed (**Fig. 19.13k**). Vestibular stenosis is the most common significant problem needing to be rectified and is therefore best avoided by careful repair of the stepped circumferential intranasal incisions.

Indications

A wide range of benign pathology including angiofibroma, schwannoma, odontogenic lesions, and fibrous dysplasia can be treated by this approach, as well as selected malignant conditions depending on their size and site. The approach is obviously contraindicated if the anterior soft tissues of the cheek are involved by malignant disease. It has always been somewhat surprising to us that the midfacial technique has not received more attention and has achieved only limited popularity when it has the attraction of combining the facial plastic skills of the rhinoplasty surgeon with an oncological approach. It offers excellent bilateral exposure of the nasal cavities, the mid third of the face, and the central skull base and can readily be modified and extended. Comparison is clearly to be made with the lateral rhinotomy and Weber–Fergusson incisions, which are quicker to perform but have the significant disadvantage of a facial scar for the remainder of the patient's life (**Fig. 19.14**). They are both associated with epiphora, and while the lateral rhinotomy incision can be associated with upward contracture of the alar margin, the Weber–Fergusson approach may give rise to upper lip and nasomaxillary groove asymmetry and medial canthal deformity and may prolong lower eyelid edema (**Fig. 19.15**). The midfacial degloving can also be used in combination with an endoscopic approach to give an excellent view when dealing with pathologies such as extensive inverted papilloma, larger angiofibromas, and fibro-osseous disease.

The application of the technique for sinonasal malignancy should only be attempted in those selected cases that can be successfully encompassed by the exposure (**Fig. 19.16**). The midfacial degloving may be combined with a coronal incision to undertake a craniofacial resection with an anterior craniotomy. Excellent subsequent cosmesis is obtained (**Fig. 19.17**).

As there is no compromise of the midfacial soft tissue blood supply, the approach may be combined with a wide variety of other facial incisions and neither previous or postoperative radiotherapy nor chemotherapy offers any contraindication to the approach. Additionally, the use of modern prosthetic techniques, such as osseointegrated implants, ensures excellent functional rehabilitation for those patients undergoing unilateral or bilateral maxillectomy through this approach.

Despite the cosmetic advantages, notably in young

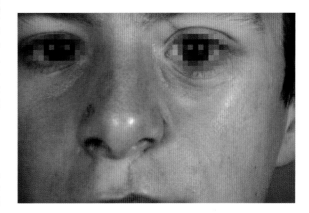

Fig. 19.14 Clinical photograph of a patient who underwent a Weber–Fergusson approach to remove an angiofibroma elsewhere, showing the cosmetic problems associated with the incision.

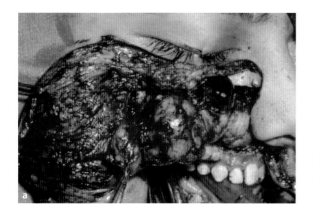

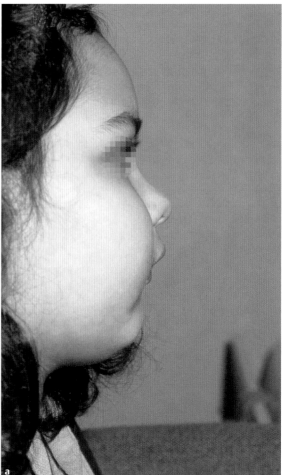

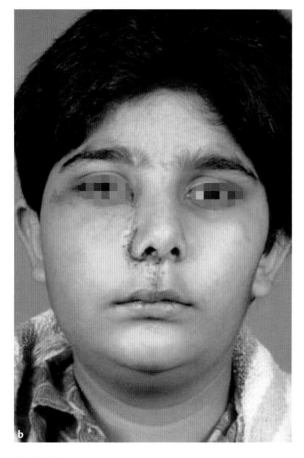

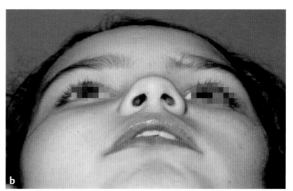

Fig. 19.15a, b

a Intraoperative photograph showing a Weber–Fergusson approach in another patient in 1984 to remove a stage IIIa angiofibroma.

b Clinical photograph of the same patient 10 days after operation showing the external incision. There are many aspects of this early postoperative result that a surgeon would consider as "good," but the patient was very unhappy with his facial scar in later life, despite no recurrence of his disease.

Fig. 19.16a–f

a, b Clinical photographs of a 10-year-old girl with a large malignant schwannoma of the right maxilla and nasal cavity in 1988. She had been advised to have it removed via a Weber–Fergusson incision. Note the displacement of the anterior maxillary sinus wall and distortion of the cheek.

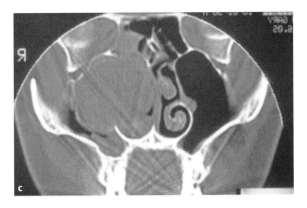

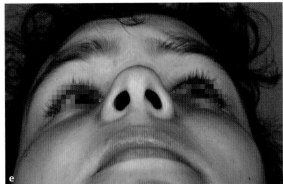

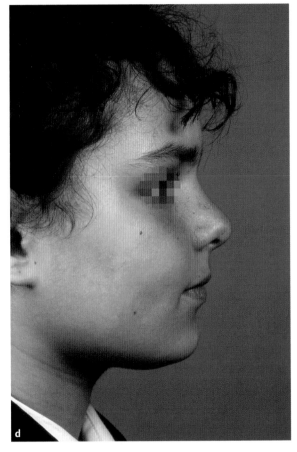

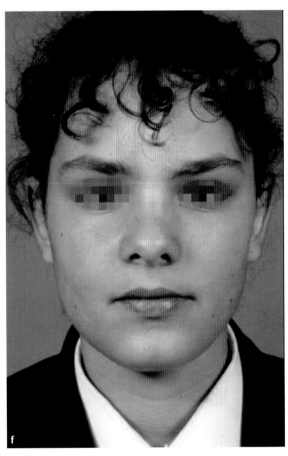

c Coronal CT scan showing tumor in the nasal cavity and maxillary sinus.

d Clinical photograph showing the same patient 2 years after midfacial degloving to remove the tumor. The result is in contrast to the patient in **Fig.19.15b**.

e Another clinical postoperative view of the same patient.

f Clinical photograph of same patient 3 years later. She has an excellent stable right maxillary prosthesis and normal facial development.

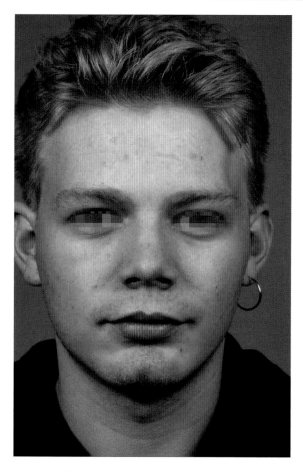

Fig. 19.17 Clinical photograph of 18-year-old man, 4 years after anterior craniofacial resection using a combination of coronal scalp incision and midfacial degloving to remove an extensive cholesterol granuloma of the anterior skull base.

patients, an initial concern was that radical surgery might affect midfacial development, but our long-term study using standardized sequential photography and lateral cephalometry on all children showed that there is no significant cosmetic sequelae resulting from this type of surgery as long as the integrity of the cartilaginous septum is preserved.[11]

Key Points

- The bilateral sublabial incision runs from the maxillary tuberosity to the opposite maxillary tuberosity to gain maximal access.
- The "stepped" lateral component of the circumvestibular incision acts to lessen the postoperative complication of vestibular stenosis.
- The midfacial degloving approach may be combined with a coronal incision and anterior craniotomy or transfacial subcranial approach allowing extensive craniofacial surgery without facial scars.

- A wide variety of benign tumors and selected malignant lesions can be treated with this approach.

Extended Transmaxillary Procedure

If it is necessary to obtain additional access into the temporal fossa, the infratemporal fossa, the floor of the middle cranial fossa, the cavernous sinus, and the paralateral pharyngeal space, then the posterolateral bone of the maxilla, the lateral wall, and the anterolateral pillar can be removed. This allows an excellent extended view that can be augmented by the use of the operating microscope. If necessary, Le Fort I osteotomies, performed bilaterally, will further increase exposure, although this is rarely necessary.

Extended Unilateral Maxillotomy Approach

This technique has been advocated for removal of rare extracranial skull base craniocervical lesions that extend from the roof of the sphenoid to the fourth cervical vertebra, essentially between the carotid canals.[12] The midfacial degloving is used to give a full bilateral exposure of the anterior maxilla, nose, masseter muscle, coronoid process of the mandible, medial and lateral pterygoid plates, and zygoma. The mucoperiosteum of the hard palate is divided vertically in an AP direction on the contralateral side of the lesion. A transnasal flap comprising the mucoperichondrium of the lateral inferior meatal wall, the floor of nose, and the adjacent posterior septum is elevated first and preserved. To achieve the maxillotomy exposure of the skull base, osteotomies are performed through the superior maxilla, preserving the infraorbital nerve but allowing the lower maxilla and the lower half of the zygoma to be mobilized, pedicled on the intact ipsilateral soft palate. This portion of the maxilla can then be rotated and retracted to the contralateral side and the posterior, medial, and lateral walls of the maxillary sinus with the superior and middle turbinates can be removed and a total ethmoidectomy and sphenoidectomy performed if necessary. Additionally, the posterior half of the nasal septum may be removed and this then allows the middle and lateral skull base compartments, as well as the infratemporal fossa, to be fully exposed. Further retropharyngeal and cervical spine exposure can additionally be undertaken.

In contrast to the standard Le Fort I operation, this procedure divides the maxilla through the middle meatus rather than through the inferior meatus. This permits the inferior turbinate to remain attached to the retracted maxilla but still gives a substantial exposure of the skull base and upper cervical region. This more extensive procedure is not recommended as a bilateral procedure as fragmentation of the maxilla into more than one segment on both sides carries a high risk of maxillary necrosis.[13] While this extended procedure gives a low morbidity when excising the larger nose and paranasal sinus tumors, the morbidity notably increases for management of major disease, particularly malignancies at the skull base and cervical spine. The wide view does allow excellent use of the operating microscope and manipulation of surgical instruments at a comfortable working distance within the operative field.

Total Maxillectomy

Introduction

The maxilla is essentially a bony box with four processes—zygomatic, frontal, alveolar, and palatine—which must be divided for its removal. Additionally, the bony box has four surfaces—nasal, anterior, orbital, and infratemporal, any of which may have been breached by disease depending on the type and extent of disease process. Maxillectomy has a long history and the first total maxillectomy is usually assigned to Gensoul in 1827.[14] Lizars described a maxillectomy in the United Kingdom in 1829[15] and Syme undertook a similar procedure in the same year.[16] (See Chapter 2 for more information.)

Operative Procedure

The operation is performed under general anesthesia with the patient supine in the reverse Trendelenberg position. A cuffed endotracheal tube is usually passed through the nasal cavity on the opposite side to the disease, which allows postmaxillectomy prosthesis or free flap reconstruction to be assessed for satisfactory dental occlusion while the patient remains under anesthesia. Corneal protection is necessary and is usually achieved by a temporary tarsorrhaphy on both sides.

Incision

The classic Weber–Fergusson incision runs ~3 to 5 mm below the lower lash margin on the affected side and allows skin to be detached from the underlying orbicularis oculi. If the incision is placed too low, disfiguring edema can result. If it is placed too close to the lid margin, ectropion may occur. The incision may be extended below and lateral to the lateral canthus but medially is continued from the level of the medial canthus down the nasomaxillary groove along the side of the nose, as for a lateral rhinotomy, cutting straight through to the underlying bone and nasal mucosa. The incision curves around the ala to the midpoint of the columella and then divides the lip in the midline. Multiple variations of the medial and lower part of the incision have been described, including darts in the nasal sill and at the skin vermilion junction and extension down the philtral crest rather than through the midline. All have their advocates but none gives consistently perfect results. Accurate closure of the skin vermilion line is certainly an important consideration. It

is important to make the angle at the medial canthus as obtuse as possible as the blood supply to this corner may be jeopardized, particularly if the patient has had previous radiotherapy. Subsequent breakdown at this point can be a major problem (**Fig. 19.18a**).

The upper lip can be held back with a retractor while the rest of the incision is completed. The cut continues in the alveolar buccal sulcus, passing round the maxillary tuberosity, and crosses the palate at the junction of the soft and hard palates. A cutting diathermy may be used to minimize bleeding. The incision is then continued from posterior to anterior through the mucous membrane of the hard palate at a point which, if possible, can be lateral to the midline, thus providing some retained mucosal covering to the medial aspect of the bone cut. However, the exact siting of this part of the incision will depend on the extent of the disease within the maxilla, the nasal cavity, and the adjacent nasal septum. The incision usually joins the alveolar buccal margin in the region of the first incisor, which, if present, must be removed (**Fig. 19.18b**). Again, exactly which tooth is removed will depend on the degree of radicality of the procedure and good teeth must be preserved as far as possible laterally on the side of the disease without compromise of the oncological resection. This allows the best possible anchorage and function for any prosthesis.

The entire facial skin flap, including buccinator, can now be raised, revealing the maxillary bone and piriform aperture and laterally the zygomatic arch and malar bone. The orbital rim is defined and the orbital periosteum is carefully dissected to reveal the orbital floor. Careful inspection of this region, particularly along the infraorbital canal, is important to ensure that no tumor invasion has occurred, which would require additional orbital clearance. Similarly, the lamina papyracea and its adjacent periosteum on the medial wall must be examined along its length as far as the orbital apex if necessary.

High-speed drills may be used to undertake the osteotomies but the malar bone may be divided by a Gigli saw passed into the lateral part of the infraorbital fissure with curved forceps. The osteotomies through the floor of the orbit and through the frontal process join the piriform aperture (**Fig. 19.18c**). A drill, a Gigli saw, or a curved osteotome may be used to divide the hard palate starting from the incisor socket and passing posteriorly lateral to the attachment of the nasal septum. Following division of the hard palate only the pterygoid plates need to be separated posteriorly; this is best done with a large curved osteotome inserted behind the tuberosity in the groove between it and the pterygoid plates (**Fig. 19.18d**). A variable amount of carefully controlled force and leverage will detach the bone, but the pterygoid muscle fibers must be cut with curved strong scissors before the specimen is free. After removal of the maxilla, it is useful to place a hot pack (60–70°C) in the cavity immediately to diminish bleeding from the internal maxillary artery.

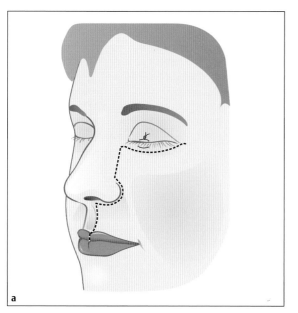

a

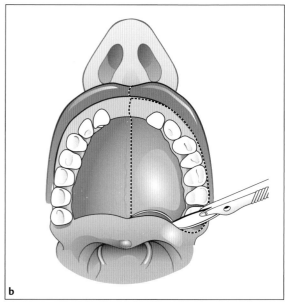

b

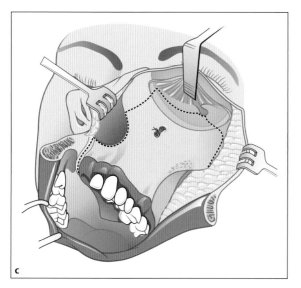

c

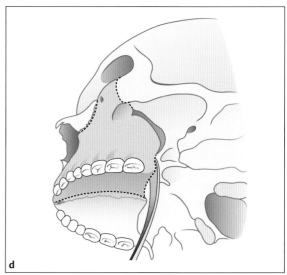

d

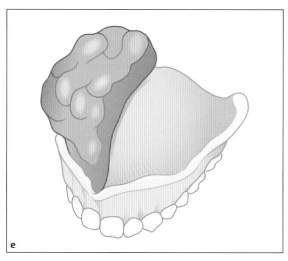

e

Fig. 19.18a–e

a Drawing showing classical Weber–Fergusson incision. (See Chapter 2 for more information.)

b Drawing showing the palatal incision just lateral to the midline, if possible to preserve a medial portion of mucosa to cover the medial aspect of the underlying bone cut.

c Drawing showing the osteotomies for a left total maxillectomy, including the orbital floor.

d Drawing showing the curved osteotome used to separate the hard palate from the pterygoid plates posteriorly.

e Drawing of a temporary obturator using gutta percha on a preformed denture.

After several minutes, the cavity can be inspected and, if necessary, the artery ligated.

Further removal of pterygoid muscle, vessels, nerves, and pterygoid plates may be necessary to encompass all the disease. The anterior wall of the sphenoid may be opened and the ethmoid labyrinth exenterated. Additional orbital clearance or exenteration may be required. If this is not the case, the maxillectomy cavity is checked for hemostasis and a 5 cm wide ribbon gauze soaked in Whitehead's varnish is inserted, sufficient to line the cavity without obstructing the fitting of any prosthesis.

The prosthodontist can now fashion a temporary obturator using gutta percha or other similar malleable material on the preformed denture that attaches to the existing dentition and fills the palatal defect, restoring the contour of the roof of the oral cavity and face (**Fig. 19.18e**). The combined use of Whitehead's varnish and obturator prevents contracture of the maxillectomy cavity and obviates the need for skin grafting of the cavity. Indeed, the cavity will mucosalize with normal mucosa given time, which is preferable to that of a skin graft. Normal speech and diet can thus be achieved in the immediate postoperative period. Some prosthodontists prefer that the skin flap be laid back and closed with subcutaneous and skin sutures prior to the fashioning of the obturator. This makes the fitting a little more difficult but makes evaluation of the facial contour more accurate. Particular care with the skin sutures must be taken in the medial canthal region and at the vermilion border.

Having removed the tarsorrhaphy sutures, the eye is carefully rinsed of blood, chloramphenicol ointment is introduced, and an eye pad is applied followed by a light pressure dressing for 24 hours. Preservation of the suspensory ligament of Lockwood, the medial palpebral and lateral palpebral ligaments, and often the posterior portion of the orbital floor provides adequate support for the eye, giving excellent function in most patients.

Indications

This procedure is most commonly indicated for removal of malignancy arising within the maxilla, either within the sinus or the bone itself or from the odontogenic tissues. To satisfy oncological criteria, disease should be confined to within the sinus cavity, but due to late presentation, this is actually rarely the case. Additional orbital clearance is often required with exenteration of the adjacent ethmoid labyrinth. **With extensive ethmoidal involvement where there is any possibility of compromise of the cribriform plate, the disease is generally better managed by craniofacial resection, which can be combined with maxillectomy and orbital clearance.** Occasionally, removal of extensive benign pathology affecting the maxilla is required and usually these lesions occur after years of neglect with significant disfigurement such as with gross fibro-osseous conditions. Usually total maxillectomy is employed as a last resort.

In the past, the Weber–Fergusson incision has been overused and employed for many procedures that can now be undertaken by midfacial degloving or by endoscopic procedures, avoiding the necessity for this large facial incision. In the past, many patients with extensive anteroethmoidal disease underwent total maxillectomy and orbital clearance; nowadays this would be treated by craniofacial resection following an accurate radiological reappraisal showing the intracranial spread.

Key Points

- Care is required with the correct placement of the incision.
- Preserve the maximal number of teeth without compromising the oncological resection.
- The immediate fitting of a prosthesis at the end of the excision is extremely beneficial to patients, allowing them to speak and eat immediately after surgery.
- Consideration needs to be given to endoscopic procedures or midfacial degloving techniques, which may obviate the need for total maxillectomy.

Orbital Clearance

Many large nasal cavity, antroethmoid, and maxillary sinus malignancies may have invaded the orbit at presentation. Indeed, it may be impossible to know exactly where large-scale malignancies initially arose. There is an important point here that is of particular concern and of advantage to the patient in that, while orbital clearance may be necessary in many cases, orbital exenteration where the eyelids are also removed is rarely necessary and is of no oncological advantage. If the eyelid is not involved, as is frequently the case with nose and paranasal sinus tumors (in contrast to facial skin tumors), the eyelid skin and orbicularis oculi provide a composite flap that is excellent for closure of the orbit and allows the use of any subsequent osseointegrated implants or other orbital prosthetic techniques.

The other important point about orbital clearance that has stood the test of time is our approach to disease involving the orbit. Our philosophy has been one of **periosteal resection and grafting if the disease from the nose and sinuses has involved the orbital periosteum but has not breached it to extensively invade the contents of the orbit**. This situation can be assessed intraoperatively by frozen section and allows the "halfway house" of resecting orbital periosteum and grafting it with fascia lata and split-thickness skin graft in those patients where only the periosteum is involved; this is in contrast to orbital clearance when malignant disease involves the orbital fat, musculature, and globe. This philosophy has been vindicated by our results with over 25 years of experience of the craniofacial operation, which confirms that there is no prognostic disadvantage with this approach, even if a small number of eyes require to be sacrificed at a later date.[17] From the perspective of the patient, there are clear functional and cosmetic advantages to this approach.[18] (See Management of the Orbit below.)

If orbital clearance is required, a modified Weber–Dieffenbach incision is used that skirts both lash margins of the upper and lower lids (**Fig. 19.19a**). Attention again has to be given to the acuity of the angle of the nasofacial incision extending inferiorly and this incision may simply be an extension of a lateral rhinotomy as well as the full Weber–Fergusson type incision which is used for total maxillectomy. Using stay sutures, the eyelid skin can be retracted and elevated from the underlying tarsal plates. It is preferable to keep the orbicularis in both the upper and lower eyelid flaps.

The clearance of the orbit is completed after elevation of these flaps. There is no advantage in performing the orbital clearance in continuity with the maxillectomy, which is actually facilitated by the initial clearance of orbital contents. Thus, in the case of obvious gross orbital disease, the orbital clearance is undertaken prior to the maxillectomy (**Fig. 19.19b**). The orbital periosteum is elevated and freed around the entire bony socket, bearing in mind its adherence to the suture lines and the trochlea. The medial and lateral suspensory ligaments are detached and a finger can be swept around the socket to complete the dissection. Other authors have advocated the use of a right-angled clamp to clip the orbital apex, but the tissue of the orbital apex may be divided with curved Mayo scissors, which are introduced from laterally and follow the natural curve of the orbital wall, allowing the tissues of the orbital apex to be removed more completely than if a clamp is already placed there. Care is taken not to unduly traumatize the globe, which we subsequently send for use in corneal grafting.

Rather than a clamp, a 10 cm × 10 cm gauze immersed in hot sterile water (~60–70°C) is available at this point of the operation to be inserted into the orbit while the excised orbital tissues are inspected to define tumor invasion at their most posterior extent. The hot gauze is removed after ~5 minutes and may have achieved complete hemostasis or at least clearly defined the ophthalmic artery, which then may be ligated as necessary.

An important point here is that tumor penetration at the orbital apex is an extremely important margin. Depending on the tumor extent seen, and if necessary evaluated by frozen section, on the posterior aspect of the orbital clearance, a greater amount of orbital apical tissue may need to be resected. The fibrous ring of the annulus of Zinn is firmly attached to the bone around the optic nerve and further definitive resection may be required to free this origin of the ocular muscles. Meticulous removal of all tissue around the optic nerve may be required and division of the optic nerve stump and ophthalmic artery as they exit the optic canal. Further frozen section may be taken at this point. If necessary, a margin of healthy tissue may be obtained by drilling away the optic canal. If necessary, this dissection can be continued to the optic chiasm, but if there is gross tumor involvement at this point, **conversion to a craniofacial procedure is required** to

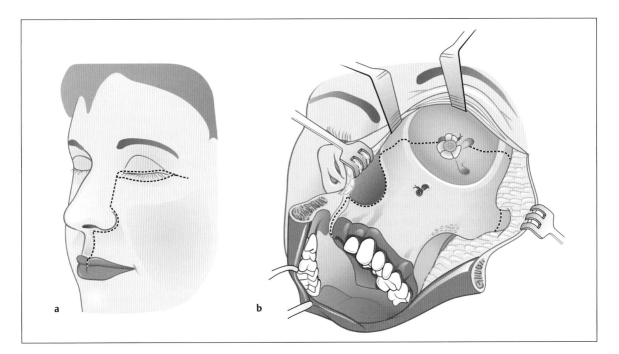

Fig. 19.19a, b

a Drawing showing a modified Weber–Dieffenbach incision allowing preservation of both eyelids when orbital clearance is being undertaken.

b Drawing showing extended osteotomies that are possible following removal of the orbital contents.

give the necessary additional intracranial exposure. If the superior orbital fissure is involved by tumor, a craniotomy may be required to access the middle fossa. Finally, if operative-microscope evaluation or frozen section analysis confirms obvious infraorbital nerve involvement then this may require additional removal of skull base bone around the foramen rotundum and assessment of the nerve up to the dura. Depending on the type of tumor, the patient's characteristics, and the results of frozen section, additional intracranial exploration of Meckel's cave may be required.

Once the excisional portion of the procedure is complete, the orbit is lightly packed with Gelfoam at the apex, followed by Whitehead's varnish ribbon gauze above the maxillectomy cavity, which may contain further Whitehead's plus the temporary obturator. The edges of the eyelids are carefully approximated with two layers of fine, absorbable suture, the first through the orbicularis muscle and the second in the skin itself. No attempt should be made to remove this suture material at a later date. With this careful approximation and elasticity of the normal eyelid, skin will eventually fall back to line the socket under the influence of respiration; in the first few weeks, this will be seen to draw the skin into the socket. The packing is removed 7 to 10 days after surgery under general anesthesia and this additionally allows reevaluation and any needed alteration of the obturator that was fitted and positioned at the end of the initial operation.

If facilities are available, the first stage of placing osseointegrated implants around the superior circumference of the orbital socket may be undertaken before the eyelids are sutured together. The second stage of implant placement may be undertaken between 3 months and 1 year later depending on circumstances such as postoperative radiotherapy and the preferences of the treating team. Once the skin of the orbital socket is well seated, an orbital prosthesis can be fashioned based on preoperative photographs and this may be attached to spectacles or self-retained in the cavity using biological glues and osseointegrated implants. (See section Management of the Orbit for further information.)

Key Points

- Orbital clearance rather than orbital exenteration is often possible in the management of nose and paranasal sinus tumors. The retained eyelids provide excellent reconstruction of the socket.
- Orbital periosteum may be excised and grafted to preserve the function and position of the eye.
- Orbital clearance may be undertaken **prior** to the maxillectomy part of the procedure.
- Clearance of the tumor at the orbital apex is essential.
- Conversion to a craniofacial procedure may be required with extensive unsuspected disease at the orbital apex.

Extended Total Maxillectomy

Involvement of the anterior cheek skin will necessitate resection and reconstruction, occasionally with local flaps or pedicle flaps, but if there is extensive involvement a free myocutaneous flap procedure may be indicated. Extension through the posterior wall of the maxilla into the pterygoid musculature will naturally require further clearance of this region and, if necessary, the infratemporal fossa may be cleared. Radioactive seeding of areas of the skull base has been advocated and, as detailed above, further additional craniofacial surgery may be indicated.

Extended Transfacial Subcranial Approach

With the increasing confidence that many surgeons have acquired as a result of performing standard anterior craniofacial procedures with an associated anterior craniotomy, an anterior subcranial technique is now commonly used through a **lateral rhinotomy type approach** (Fig. 19.20a). This obviates the necessity for a craniotomy and any associated brain mobilization and retraction that may accompany it. However, the relatively narrow exposure of the roof of the ethmoid and cribriform plate area makes it essential that this procedure is only used for limited anterior dural and intracranial disease (Fig. 19.20b). Intracranial exposure is small and the subcranial exposure of the dura and adjacent structures is limited even when augmented by visualization with an endoscope or microscope. Indeed, it was for exactly this reason that the pioneers in this area of surgery began the standard craniofacial procedure with its anterior craniotomy component. Prior to the introduction of craniofacial surgery, surgeons removed the tumor from the nasal cavity and ethmoids but residual tumor on the roof of the ethmoid and level of the cribriform plate was left for fear of complications and the patient was referred for radiation therapy in the hope of curing the disease. In the precraniofacial era, 5-year results of 23 to 38% were usual for malignant lesions even if treated by additional maxillectomy and orbital clearance as well as radiotherapy.[19–24]

In contrast today, for appropriate tumors with minimal invasion of the skull base, the majority of the tumor is first removed from within the nasal cavities and ethmoid sinus, leaving only the small portion penetrating the skull base. This area of tumor must be outlined by osteotomies, using small cutting burs or blades giving a margin of at least 5 mm. Using endoscopes or the operating microscope, care is taken not to penetrate the dura, but if the dura is invaded then the area is resected, again with a minimum margin of 5 mm for most types of pathology. If, at this point, significant brain invasion becomes obvious then the subcranial approach should be abandoned and a formal craniotomy procedure continued. **Frozen section margins** are often necessary to assist in checking complete tumor excision but are, of course, not available in all centers and in themselves are not totally reliable,

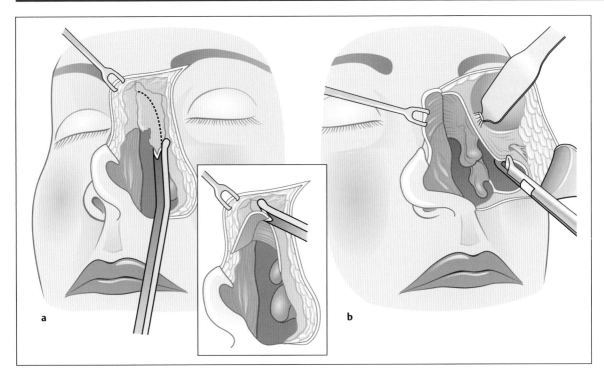

Fig. 19.20a, b

a Drawing showing the extended lateral rhinotomy approach. The upper part of the incision may be turned laterally into the eyebrow or medially into the glabellar region. The nasal bones are hinged medially to allow an operating microscopic (or endoscopic) view of the superior ethmoids, nasal cavity, and skull base.

b Drawing showing the removal of bone and soft tissue of the lateral nasal wall, maxilla, and orbit depending on the extent of disease.

depending much on the quantity and quality of the specimen and the experience of the laboratory technician and the reporting pathologist. Once again an understanding of the natural history of the disease is of paramount importance; for example, it would be inappropriate to rely on frozen sections in this limited approach with a patient suffering from an adenoid cystic carcinoma, particularly of the dural margins and the olfactory bulbs. In the case of an olfactory neuroblastoma involving the cribriform niche, a portion of olfactory tract will require removal.

The dural defect is closed by a graft that may be stitched in place in addition to using tissue glue and/or other additional grafting material as favored by a variety of authors. If the disease does not involve the nasal septum then a vascularized septal flap may augment the graft closure. If the nasal bone and frontonasal process have been removed as a unit free of disease, they may be replaced with microplating, but all too often the deeper aspect of the bone is involved by tumor. This transfacial subcranial approach is now often termed a type IA approach; if it includes orbital exenteration, this is labeled as a type IB approach. If an additional maxillectomy is incorporated into the excision, then this is termed a type II operative

procedure,[25] although other authors reserve this term for the standard anterior craniotomy craniofacial procedure.

Key Point

* This approach gives a relatively confined exposure of the roof of the ethmoid and cribriform plate areas.

Subcranial Extended Anterior Craniofacial Approach

The extended anterior subcranial approach was initially used in the 1970s for craniofacial congenital anomalies and high-velocity skull base trauma. It was further developed by Raveh et al in the 1980s for excision of benign and malignant tumors of the nose, sinuses, and skull base.[26,27] In this approach, the osteotomies of the frontonasal orbital external skeleton provide excellent access to the anterior skull base, and orbital and sphenoethmoidal planes, and hence to the nasal and paranasal cavities. This approach avoids significant frontal lobe retraction and external facial incisions as the approach is undertaken by a coronal scalp incision. The optic canal, optic nerve, and posteriorly the anterior and medial aspect of the cavernous sinus can also be evaluated. Because of the lack of intradural frontal lobe manipulation and external facial incisions, postoperative complications and cosmetic problems related to these factors are generally avoided.

Surgical Technique

A coronal scalp flap is raised in a subperiosteal plane and the pericranium is preserved for possible use in any subsequent reconstruction. The coronal flap is raised down to the frontozygomatic suture lines bilaterally and to the piriform aperture in the midline. The periorbital periosteum is dissected to a varying degree from the superior, medial, and lateral walls of the orbit back to the apex on either side and the anterior ethmoid arteries are ligated. Care is required raising the scalp and face flaps as they produce some traction on the orbital contents (**Fig. 19.21a**).

Depending on the size of the nose, paranasal sinus, or skull base lesion, the extent of the nasofrontal osteotomies is variable. Titanium miniplates are applied prior to completion of the osteotomy lines. Raveh has advocated a technique for these osteotomies using preliminary bur-holes and then insertion of a dissector to protect the frontal lobe dura while the osteotomies proceed. We have used an alternative technique using a 2 mm rose-head bur to blue-line the dura in the same manner as when we approach the semicircular canals during temporal bone surgery. The osteotomies can be made to carefully outline the known degree of underlying disease and designed to remove a frontonasal segment of a size no larger than required to offset complications or subsequent deformity. Once the blue-lining procedure is complete across the frontal bone, supraorbital ridge, medial orbital wall, and nasal bones, a small osteotome is used to crack the

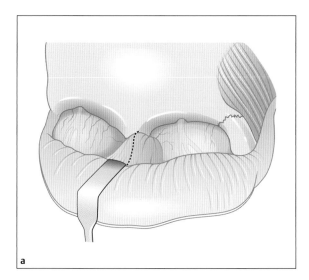

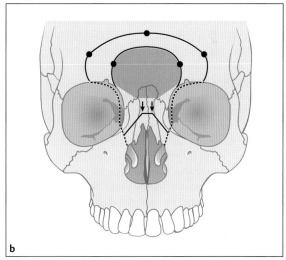

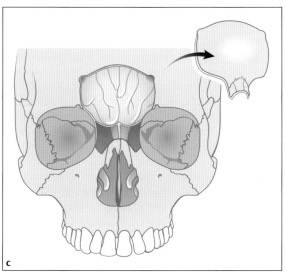

Fig. 19.21a–c

a A coronal scalp flap raised in the subperiosteal plane beyond the frontozygomatic suture lines bilaterally. A midline releasing incision in the periosteum may be required to assist the dissection over the nasal bones. The degree of periosteal dissection along the superior, medial, and lateral walls of the orbit will vary according to the extent of the disease.

b, c The overall size of the frontal osteotomies can be varied according to the underlying tumor. Our preference has been to leave the inferior aspect of the nasal bones in place and not to disrupt the attachment of the upper lateral cartilages to the nasal bones as this additional component of exposure is rarely required. If there is extensive disease in the inferior aspect of the nasal cavity or maxilla, our combined coronal and midfacial degloving procedure is preferred.

extremely thin layer of residual bone and the segment can then be removed whether small or large. The pre-removal application of 1.7-mm titanium miniplates means that extremely precise replacement is possible.

As described by Raveh, there are essentially two types of osteotomy:

- Type 1, which removes the anterior wall of the frontal sinus because of the known possibility of the posterior wall being involved with tumor
- Type 2, in which the anterior and posterior walls of the frontal sinus are removed when there is no indication that the tumor is involving the posterior wall

The overall size of these osteotomies can be varied according to the underlying tumor and occasionally, for unilateral tumors, the contralateral olfactory filaments may be preserved, particularly if there is no significant intracranial extension (**Fig. 19.21b, c**). Additional bone from the orbital and sphenoidal roofs may be removed to enable satisfactory resection of the tumor and, passing posteriorly, the medial aspect of the optic nerve canal and the optic chiasm can be exposed. Special retractors have been advocated to avoid pressure on the orbital contents or damage to the periorbital periosteum during the procedure, but we have found that careful use of soft, malleable copper retractors will also suffice and additionally the retraction is provided gently and intermittently in contrast to prolonged retraction.

Reconstruction of the area will depend on the extent of tumor resection and while, as in all craniofacial surgery, small dural defects can be sutured, larger areas of dural involvement that have been excised may be patched with fascia lata and covered by a split-thickness skin graft or a pericranial flap. The medial orbital periosteal defects may be reconstructed using a variety of materials such as fascia lata and skin grafts. Using this technique we have not found it necessary to replace the medial orbital wall with cartilage or bone grafts. The combination of a fascia lata graft with a second layer of onlay split thickness skin provides a strong alternative to the resected lamina bone and orbital periosteum. The subsequent slight contraction of the skin graft also aids support of the orbital contents. Only rarely are free osseomyocutaneous flaps necessary if a very extensive resection of the skeletal skull base frame has been necessary.

Exact repositioning of the nasofrontal segment is required and, most importantly, medial canthal ligament refixation is necessary. Raveh describes achieving this by a nonabsorbable suture through the ligament and then passage of this suture under the nasofrontal segment to the contralateral anterior frontal sinus wall at the supraorbital rim. Bilateral tightening of this suture results in a downward, inward, and medial traction on the canthal ligament to achieve correct positioning along the vertical, horizontal, and sagittal planes. This is an extremely important point in the reconstruction as asymmetry of

the medial canthal ligament and palpebral fissure gives a notable long-term cosmetic anomaly. We have used a similar technique with a prolene suture double passed through the medial canthal tendon and through two drill holes in the frontal process of the maxilla just superior and posterior to the anterior lacrimal crest. This suture is further passed through two 1.5-mm holes drilled through the contraglabellar area in the frontonasal bone segment before it is replaced (this makes the drilling and placing of the suture an easy matter). Once the nasofrontal segment is replaced, these sutures are tightened until the canthus is firmly secured. Unfortunately, both these techniques may be complicated by canthal drift.

Postoperative Complications

This excellent procedure provides an overall low rate of complications. While frontal lobe contusion with associated edema is generally low in reported series, CSF leakage does occur in a small proportion of patients and the incidence of orbital cranial nerve dysfunction (i.e., optic nerve, trochlear, abducent, and oculomotor nerves), enophthalmos, and medial canthal problems are more common than with other transfacial or coronal anterior craniotomy craniofacial procedures.

Key Points

- Intradural frontal lobe manipulation and external facial incisions are avoided by this approach.
- The frontonasal osteotomies can be varied according to the site, extent, and type of underlying disease.
- Medial canthal refixation is necessary and is an extremely important point in the reconstruction.
- Exact repositioning of the nasofrontal segment is required.

Craniofacial Resection

Introduction

It became increasingly recognized in the latter part of the last century that the poor prognosis associated with malignant tumors of the nose and paranasal sinuses was engendered by local recurrence as a consequence of inadequate resection. The realization that every tumor affecting the inferior surface of the cribriform plate and the roof of the ethmoid theoretically had spread intracranially, led to the development of the craniofacial approach, which offered access to the area and a more rational resection depending on anatomical considerations. Additionally, disease involving the orbit intraperiosteally or extending through the roof of the orbit into the anterior cranial fossa would also be better assessed and resected. As a consequence, the combined anterior craniofacial procedure has become well established. The operation was originally described in 1954[28] and was subsequently developed most notably by Ketcham, Smith, Van Buren, and colleagues.[29]

There has been considerable evolution of the technique used in our unit since 1978 but it has resulted in an operation that satisfies oncological criteria while being associated with a low morbidity and excellent cosmesis. A variety of neurosurgical techniques are used and the procedure is most commonly undertaken nowadays by a combined team of surgeons, but in our unit the procedure has been primarily otolaryngological and undertaken by only three ENT/head and neck surgeons over a thirty-year period.

Anatomy and Spread

The anatomical relationship of the roof of the nasal cavity and ethmoid complex is well seen in the coronal section shown in **Fig. 19.22**. The figure shows the narrow cribriform plate compared with the adjacent ethmoid roof. Tumors arising in the nose and sinuses can spread quickly through the thin, bony boundaries and preexisting holes of the olfactory plate into the anterior cranial fossa and orbit, and while dura and orbital periosteum resist disease for a remarkably long time, brain and orbital contents are eventually involved.

Disease can escape through the posteromedial orbital wall into the optic canal or posterolaterally into the sphenoid pterygoid palatine fossa and middle cranial fossa, or bilaterally from one side of the ethmoid to the other via the septum. The ability to excise the whole ethmoid block with an osteotomy that encompasses the roofs of both ethmoid and cribriform plate regions, passing through the frontal sinus anteriorly and the sphenoid posteriorly, was an obvious and significant oncological advance (**Figs. 19.23 and 19.24**).

Key Points

- Tumors arising in the nose and sinuses can potentially spread quickly through their thin bony boundaries and preexisting holes in the skull base.

Surgical Technique

Two techniques have predominantly been used in our unit. In younger patients for the last two decades, we have

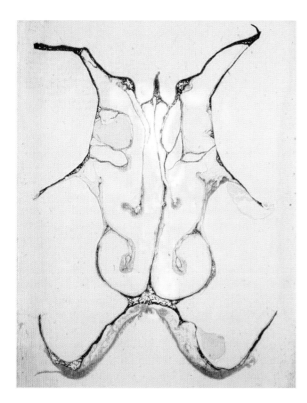

Fig. 19.22 Coronal midfacial section showing the thin orbital walls, ethmoid roofs, and cribriform plate that separate nose and sinus tumors from these important prognostic areas.

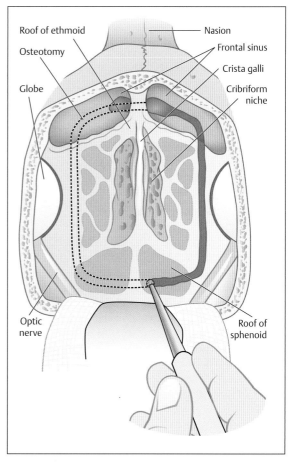

Fig. 19.23 Drawing demonstrating the view through our shield-shaped anterior window craniotomy, the osteotomies encompassing the entire ethmoid block, cribriform plate, additional medial orbital roof, and planum sphenoidale as necessary depending on the extent of the disease.

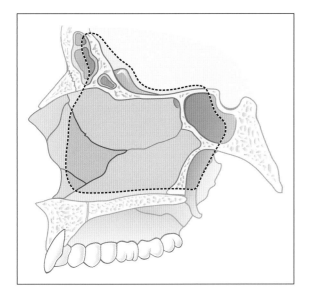

Fig. 19.24 Drawing showing the sagittal view of the lines of resection in a standard craniofacial procedure. Further bone and soft tissue removal may obviously be required for more extensive disease.

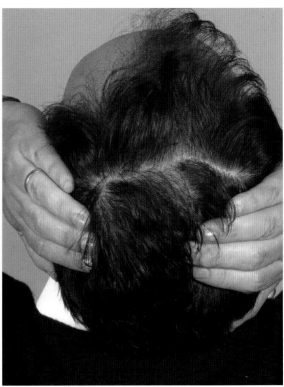

Fig. 19.25 Postoperative photograph showing the healed coronal scalp incision. It is important to angle the incision through the scalp in line with the hair follicles to minimize subsequent alopecia along the line of the incision and to place it sufficiently posteriorly to the existing hairline, bearing in mind subsequent male-pattern baldness.

favored a midfacial degloving procedure combined with a coronal scalp incision (**Fig. 19.25**). In older patients we have used an extension of the Moure lateral rhinotomy incision, which allows rapid access and gives an excellent cosmetic result. This is used on the side of the lesion, being extended vertically onto the forehead along the line of the vertical skin crease just lateral to the midline as far as the hairline (**Fig. 19.26a, b**).

Extended Lateral Rhinotomy Incision

After bilateral temporary tarsorrhaphies and skin infiltration with epinephrine (1 in 200,000), an extended lateral rhinotomy incision is made. The soft tissues are dissected off the underlying facial bones with careful preservation of the periosteum (**Fig. 19.26c**). Full access to the anterior cranial fossa is effected via a "shield-shaped" window craniotomy that has miniplates placed initially to allow exact replacement following its removal and completion of the excisional part of the operative procedure. This small craniotomy bone flap is ~2.5 cm × 2.5 cm with the inferior point based over the frontal sinuses but not involving the supraorbital ridge (**Fig. 19.26d**). The bone flap is defined using a high-speed 2 mm rosehead drill. The bone, including the posterior wall of the frontal sinus, is drilled almost to dura and when sufficiently thin it can be fractured outward using a small curved elevator resulting in minimal trauma to the dura (**Fig. 19.26e**).

The dura is elevated over a wide front bilaterally and falls back posteriorly, obviating the need for any significant retraction on the frontal lobes even when progressing posteriorly onto the planum sphenoidale. Releasing

the dura laterally from the frontal bone is key to this part of the procedure. The initial dissection toward the cribriform plate and ethmoidal roof proceeds extradurally to allow assessment of the degree of dural invasion by tumor (**Fig. 19.26f**), but an incision through the dura anterosuperiorly often becomes necessary to assess the extent of invasion through the dura and involvement of the olfactory bulbs, tracts, and adjacent frontal lobe (**Fig. 19.26g**). This allows assessment and decision making with regard to safe margins, excision of tumor, and placement of the osteotomies in the anterior cranial fossa floor (**Fig. 19.26h**).

The dissection is performed under the operating microscope, which gives excellent illumination and magnification of the entire orbital roofs, ethmoidal block, and cribriform plate area extending posteriorly to the posterior extent of the planum sphenoidale. Frontal lobe tissue is protected by 10 cm × 2 cm moistened neurosurgical patties and the anterior and posterior ethmoidal vessels are clearly defined and bipolar coagulated or clipped as appropriate (**Fig. 19.26i**).

Shrinkage of the brain is facilitated by deliberate hyperventilation to produce a pCO_2 of 2.7 to 3.3 kPa (20

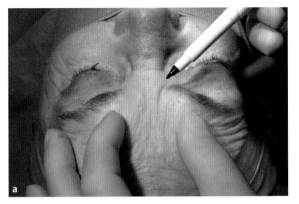

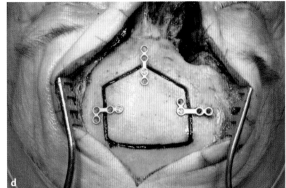

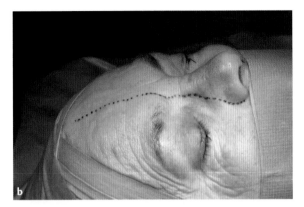

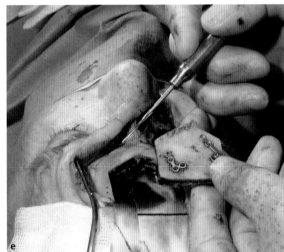

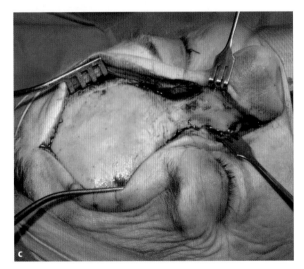

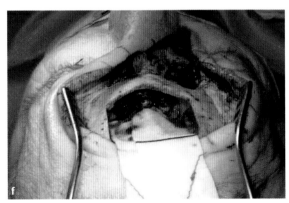

Fig. 19.26a–t

a, b Operative photographs showing placement of the extended lateral rhinotomy incision. Note that the vertical portion on the forehead is along the line of the natural skin crease, which is lateral to the exact midline, and the use of bilateral horizontal mattress tarsorrhaphies. Also note that in this patient it was not necessary to completely detach the right alar margin. Both these points improve the ultimate cosmetic result.

c Through the opened incision, an initial intranasal evaluation of this high-grade adenocarcinoma showed involvement of the right nasal bone, requiring resection, which was confirmed by subsequent histological analysis. Skin and periosteum are held back by four-pronged self-retaining retractor. Note the small horizontal scratch marks in the skin creases to assist accurate skin closure at the end of the procedure.

d A view of the same patient looking from superior to inferior. Note the initial resection of right nasal bone, right lamina papyracea, and the medial part of the supraorbital ridge adjacent to the trochlea. The anterior shield-shaped window has been outlined and 1.7-mm miniplates have been fitted and drilled prior to removal of the window.

e Anterior craniotomy removed. Note the moistened neurosurgical patties overlying the dura.

f Evaluation showed tumor in the right frontal sinus and extensive involvement of the right orbital periosteum. The posterior wall of the frontal sinus has been resected and the orbital periosteum over a wide area will be sent for histological analysis.

Fig. 19.26g–t ▷

◁ continued

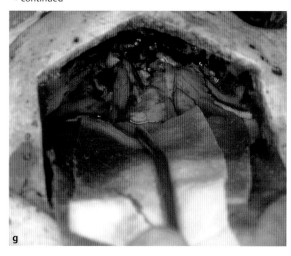

g

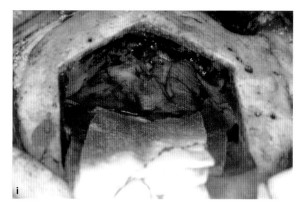

i

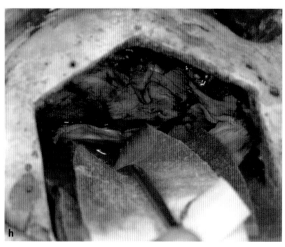

h

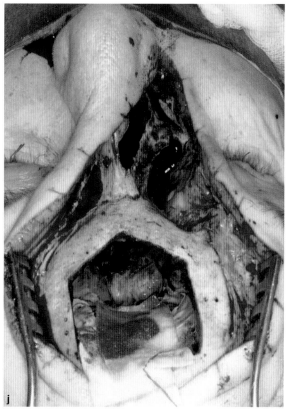

j

g An anterosuperior incision in the dura allows intradural inspection confirming disease involving the dura over the right medial orbital roof, ethmoid roof, right cribriform niche, and olfactory bulb. The photograph shows the wide exposure possible through the shield-shaped craniotomy and the beginning of the dural division along the lateral border of the left ethmoidal roof.

h The involved area of dura has now been outlined around its whole extent with adequate margins, checked by frozen section. Both olfactory tracts have been divided.

i A further view just prior to commencement of anterior cranial floor osteotomies. Note that other than three neurosurgical patties overlying the dura and frontal lobes, no form of permanent retraction has been used at any time during the procedure.

j The view following completion of the anterior cranial fossa floor osteotomies and removal of the entire central specimen and tumor. Note the extensive removal of orbital periosteum.

k On this view, the edges of the dural excision are being inspected and the adjacent frontal lobe had not been involved by disease but the entire roof of the sphenoid sinus on both sides has been removed and the entire mucosa has been stripped. There was invasive disease in the right sphenoid sinus.

l A further view showing clearance of the sphenoid sinus and clearance of the posterior nasal cavity onto the basisphenoid with particular attention being paid to the pterygomaxillary fissure on the right side to be sure that disease had not entered at this point. Note also clearance of the medial orbital wall almost to its apex. Access to the superomedial canal could have been obtained if necessary.

m A view of the right medial aspect of the orbit to show the extensive removal of orbital periosteum. A frozen section confirmed extensive invasion of the external aspect of the periosteum but not invasion through the full thickness into the intraorbital contents. Thus the decision was made to graft this area and preserve the orbit.

n Dural defect closed with fascia lata underlay technique and fibrin glue.

o Split-thickness skin graft overlying dura.

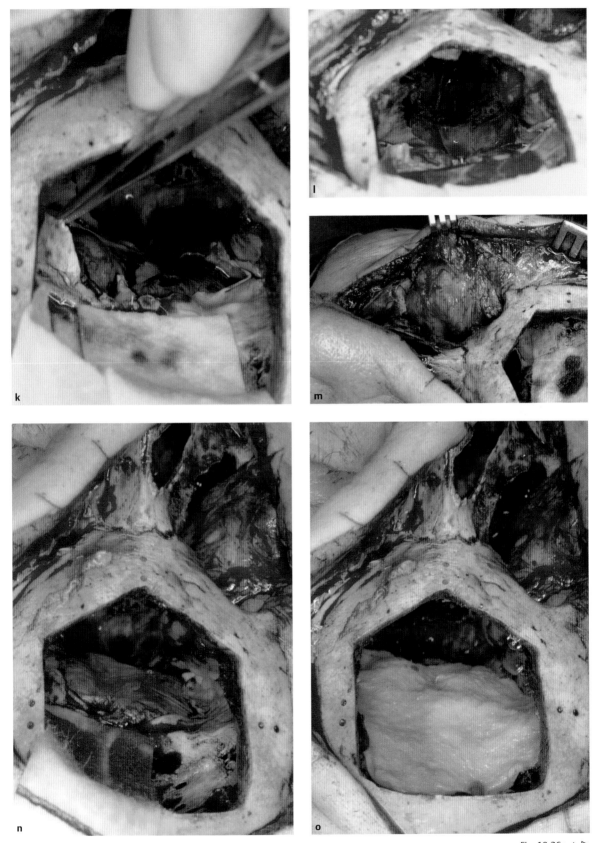

Fig. 19.26p–t ▷

◁ continued

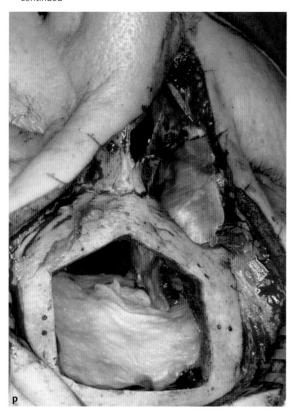

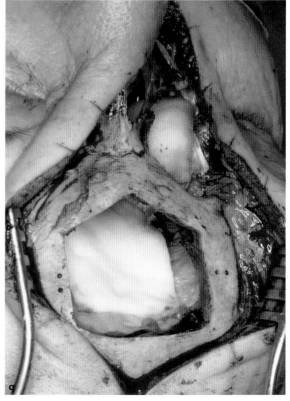

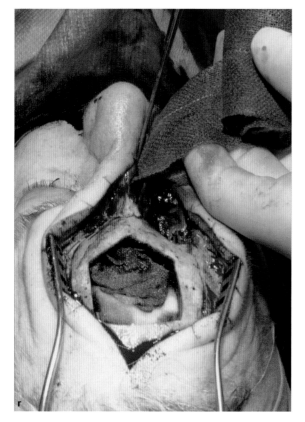

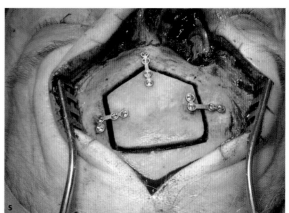

p Fascia lata repair to the right medial orbit.

q Additional split-thickness skin graft to the right medial orbital repair. Grafts are covered with gelatin sponge soaked in Sofradex antibiotic drops (framycetin sulfate, gramicidin, dexamethasone).

r The craniofacial cavity lightly packed with 5-cm ribbon gauze soaked with Whitehead's varnish (compound iodoform varnish).

s The anterior window osteotomy replaced.

◁ continued

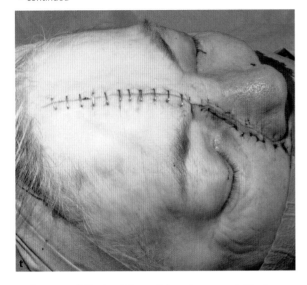

t The patient following right medial canthopexy and skin closure.

to 25 mm Hg). A head up tilt of 15 to 20° and hypertension of 70 to 90 mm Hg systolic pressure is also used and, if insufficient, intravenous mannitol may be added (rarely required). The wide lateral freeing of the dura over the orbital plates facilitates the dura moving posteriorly and often placement of two or three 10 cm × 2 cm moistened neurosurgical patties is all that is required to allow excellent visualization of the floor of the anterior cranial fossa without any form of additional brain retraction.

En bloc removal of both ethmoidal complexes, cribriform plate, and the superior aspect of the nasal septum can now be performed via the osteotomies. The cranial osteotomy is outlined with a 2 mm rosehead burr to encompass both ethmoids and the anterior wall of the sphenoid sinus. Anteriorly, they are completed with a fissure burr through the frontonasal ducts into the orbit thus uniting intra- and extracranial cuts (**Fig. 19.26j**).

The specimen is freed by dividing the perpendicular plate of the ethmoid from the rest of the septum and delivered via the facial approach. Depending on the extent of disease, additional resection of overlying skin, nasal bones, frontal sinuses, orbital walls and contents, maxilla, pterygopalatine fossa, infratemporal fossa, dura, and brain may be undertaken, under frozen-section control where appropriate (**Fig. 19.26k**).

Accurate evaluation of orbital involvement is possible as the procedure gives excellent visualization of the posterior extent of the medial orbital wall (**Fig. 19.26l**). In cases in which the medial bony wall of the orbit has been breached but the periosteum is intact, the compromised area of the periosteum can be resected (**Fig. 19.26m**).

The dural defect is repaired with fascia lata in an underlay manner, placed between brain and remaining dura and carefully sutured or glued to give a cerebrospinal fluid–proof repair (**Fig. 19.26n**). A thin split-thickness skin graft is applied to this inferiorly and held in place with tissue glue (**Fig. 19.26o**). The resected area of periosteum is grafted with a fascia lata and split-thickness skin graft, preserving the globe and its musculature. Contraction of the graft results in remarkably little disturbance of ocular function (**Fig. 19.26p**).

A layer of absorbable gelatin sponge soaked in Sofradex (framycetin sulfate, gramicidin, and dexamethasone) ear drops is placed over any skin-grafted areas (**Fig. 19.26q**) and the whole cavity packed with 5-cm ribbon gauze soaked in Whitehead's varnish (**Fig. 19.26r**). The shield of frontal bone is microplated back into position (**Fig. 19.26s**) and the periosteum and skin are closed in three layers (**Fig. 19.26t**).

Patients with very advanced disease may require additional modifications at closure, including median forehead and glabellar skin flaps to cover defects due to resection of involved skin over the nasal bones, or additional temporalis muscle flaps after removal of superolateral aspect of the orbit for extensive neoplasms. Occasional free flaps with microvascular anastomosis are necessary if there is an extensive area of the skull base necrosed by a tumor or previous radical radiotherapy. Iliac bone grafts may be used to replace significant quantities of bone resected frontonasally for extensive frontal sinus involvement. A

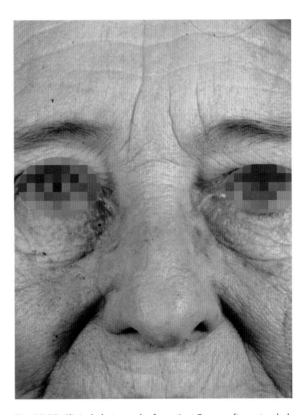

Fig. 19.27 Clinical photograph of a patient 5 years after extended right lateral rhinotomy incision for craniofacial resection.

moderate pressure scalp bandage is applied for 24 hours and the patients are kept lying at 30° for 3 to 4 days postoperatively. The Whitehead's varnish packing is removed under general anesthesia 10 days after operation, at which time the cavity may be inspected. In older patients the cosmetic result of the procedure is satisfactory (**Fig. 19.27**).

Key Points

- The craniofacial operation was a significant oncological advance.
- Dura is elevated from the bone on a wide front, particularly laterally.
- Involved orbital periosteum may be resected and grafted if significant intraorbital invasion is absent.
- Frozen section control with an experienced pathologist is beneficial.
- Moistened neurosurgical patties and controlled hyperventilation and hypertension obviate the need for brain retraction.
- Excellent light and magnification are provided by the operating microscope.

Complications and Morbidity

In 2006, we published a 25-year experience of craniofacial resection for tumors of the nasal cavity, paranasal sinuses, and skull base, presenting the analysis of 308 patients.[30] **Table 19.8** shows the complications in our series associated with craniofacial resection. Overall, the complications of this surgery remain low, with most of the more serious ones occurring in the early part of the series in older patients. Many of the long-term complications such as epiphora, diplopia, and serous otitis media have been managed with relative ease. Patients are commenced on phenytoin 100 mg twice daily, 48 hours prior to surgery, which they continue postoperatively for 2 months. Prophylactic antibiotics (cefuroxime axetil 750 mg 8-hourly and metronidazole 500 mg 8-hourly) are given intravenously with the premedication and for 48 hours perioperatively. They are then continued orally until removal of the nasal pack 10 days later.

Results of Craniofacial Surgery

Table 19.9 shows the malignant and benign histology of the craniofacial patients. Malignant conditions predominate in this series but virtually every histological type occurring in this area has been encountered by us. The most common was adenocarcinoma (62 cases) followed by olfactory neuroblastoma (56 cases), squamous cell carcinoma (34 cases), and chondrosarcoma (24 cases). Malignant conditions predominated (84%) but included in the benign group were a small number of extensive nonneoplastic conditions that necessitated radical treatment by craniofacial surgery.

Table 19.8 Craniofacial resection: complications in personal series

	No.	Results
Immediate		
Convulsions	1	No sequelae
Hemorrhage	2	1 controlled by embolization, 1 death
Air embolism	1	Recovery
Decreased vision	4	3 recovery, 1 permanent
Intermediate/late		
CVA	2	1 partial recovery, 1 death
Confusion	6	Recovery
Pulmonary embolism	2	1 death, 1 recovery
Meningitis	2	Recovery
CSF leak	8	4 repaired, 4 spontaneous recovery
Aerocele (pneumoencephalocele)	2	Recovery
Frontal abscess/ encephalitis	4	2 death, 2 recovery
Bone necrosis/fistula	6/8	Recovery after repair
Epilepsy	7	Anticonvulsant control
Epiphora	11	7 DCR, 2 Jones tube
Diplopia	6	Repair or spontaneous recovery
Serous otitis media	15	Grommets
Sinusitis/mucocele	3/2	Surgery
Pituitary deficiency	1	Replacement therapy

Abbreviations: CSF, cerebrospinal fluid; CVA, cerebrovascular accident; DCR, dacryocystorhinostomy.

Although it is difficult to assess the exact site of origin of the larger tumors, most tumors in our series arose in the ethmoid or nasal cavity or were determined as antroethmoid when the disease was extensive in these areas.

Only half of the patients (49%) had received no previous treatment at the point of referral for craniofacial resection and the rest had received surgery, radiotherapy, chemotherapy, or a combination thereof. However, there was no statistical difference in survival between those who had undergone previous treatment, more notably some form of surgery, before the craniofacial resection and those who had not (*p* = 0.20). Forty percent of our patients were given additional treatment following craniofacial surgery and revision craniofacial resection was performed in 6.5% of cases between a total of one and six times for recurrent disease. Five percent of our patients underwent subsequent neck dissection, in two cases bilateral.

Table 19.9 Craniofacial resection: personal series by histopathology

Benign histopathologies		Malignant histopathologies	
Meningioma	9	Adenocarcinoma	62
Fibro-osseous disease	6	Olfactory neuroblastoma	54
Phycomycetes granuloma	6	Squamous cell carcinoma	34
Osteoma	5	Chondrosarcoma	24
Reparative granuloma	2	Adenoid cystic carcinoma	19
Osteoblastoma	2	SNUC	15
Leiomyoblastoma	2	Malignant melanoma	8
Meningoencephalocele	2	Cylindrical cell carcinoma	9
Hemangioma	2	Primitive neuroblastoma	6
Osteomyelitis	2	Rhabdomyosarcoma	5
Neurofibroma	2	Osteogenic sarcoma	5
Angiofibroma	2	Metastases	4
Dermoid	2	Carcinosarcoma	4
Cholesterol granuloma	1	Malignant fibrous histiocytoma	2
Pseudotumor	1	Angiosarcoma	1
Angioma	1	Spindle cell carcinoma	1
Pleomorphic adenoma	1	Hemangiopericytoma	1
Craniopharyngioma	1	Alveolar soft part sarcoma	1
n	49	Malignant schwannoma	1
		Mucoepidermoid carcinoma	1
		Ewing's sarcoma	1
		Plasmacytoma	1
		n	259

Note: Some of these pathologies have changed their nomenclature since the WHO classification in 2005 that is used elsewhere in this book.

The Orbit

All tissue removed in our craniofacial resection series was submitted for detailed histopathology and patients were stratified according to orbital and intracranial involvement as these were felt, early on, to be important factors affecting survival. No orbital involvement was found in 187 of the 308 patients (56%). Fifty-three patients (17%) underwent orbital clearance at the time of craniofacial resection and 50 (16%) underwent resection of orbital periosteum with preservation of the eye. Five of these individuals subsequently underwent secondary orbital clearance 5 months to 4 years later. Thus, the overall number of patients in our series requiring orbital clearance was 63 (20.5%).

Seventy-three patients (24%) had dural involvement and 17% had frontal lobe infiltration. A mean hospital stay was 14 days and the average operating time for the entire procedure was 3.3 hours.

Long-Term Follow-Up

The mean follow-up period of our 25-year study was 63 months and the actuarial disease-free survival for malignant tumors was 59% at 5 years, 40% at 10 years, and 33% at 15 years. For benign tumors, the actuarial disease-free survival was 92% at 5 years, falling to 82% at 10 years and 76% at 15 years. A disease-free survival for the larger cohorts of individual histologies is shown in **Table 19.10**. Multivariate analysis employing the Cox regression method identified brain involvement, type of malignancy, and orbital involvement as the three significant prognostic factors in our group as a whole. As in an earlier evaluation of this cohort, our strategy of resection of orbital periosteum with preservation of the eye in selected cases was supported by a statistically improved prognosis as compared with those undergoing orbital clearance. The 50 patients undergoing resection of orbital periosteum would initially have undergone an orbital clearance at the

Table 19.10 Craniofacial resection: survival in whole group and individual histologies in personal series

Histology	Survival			No of patients
	5 years (%)	10 years (%)	15 years (%)	
Overall	65	47	41	308
Benign	92	82	76	49
Malignant	59	40	33	259
Adenocarcinoma	58	40	33	62
Olfactory neuroblastoma	74	50	40	56
Squamous cell carcinoma	53	35	35	34
Chondrosarcoma	94	56	37	24
Adenoid cystic carcinoma	61	31	31	19

time of the craniofacial resection but only five of these patients subsequently lost the eye and without an apparent effect on prognosis (**Fig. 19.28**).

Preoperative or Postoperative Radiotherapy

For those patients receiving combined therapy, there was no statistical significance on the outcome, whether the radiotherapy was given before or after craniofacial resection ($p = 0.87$) (**Fig. 19.29**).

Survival Figures

The actuarial disease-free survival in our craniofacial series for malignant tumors was 59% at 5 years, 40% at 10 years, and 33% at 15 years. For benign conditions, actuarial disease-free survival was 92% at 5 years, falling to 82% at 10 years and 76% at 15 years. These figures emphasize the fact that "benign" is a relative term for

tumors affecting the anterior skull base. Meningioma is the prominent cause of these deaths and, together with chondrosarcoma from the malignant group, may render patients blind in both eyes before their demise as a result of bilateral involvement of the chiasm and orbital apices. As seen in **Table 19.10**, local recurrences occurred at up to 12 years with some histologies such as olfactory neuroblastoma and adenoid cystic carcinoma and this has continued in the long term. In 2009 a patient who had undergone a craniofacial resection at the age of 29 years for an adenoid cystic carcinoma developed bilateral lung metastases 20 years postoperatively despite there being no evidence of local recurrence at the primary site. She remains well and disease-free after bilateral segmental lung resections for the metastases.

Multivariate analysis employing the Cox regression method had identified brain involvement, type of malignancy, and orbital involvement as the three significant

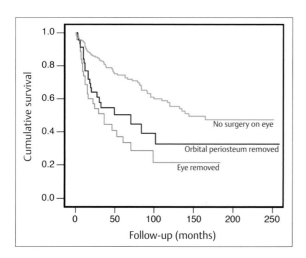

Fig. 19.28 Kaplan–Meier curve showing the effects on survival of orbital management. (Modified from reference 11.)

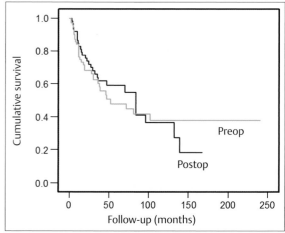

Fig. 19.29 Kaplan–Meier curve showing the effects on survival of pre- and postoperative radiotherapy.

prognostic factors in our group of patients as a whole. Since the development of craniofacial resection during the 1970s and 1980s, this procedure has become the standard of care in many countries for tumors involving the anterior skull base. The ability to perform a radical resection combined with other forms of medical oncology has led to significant improvements in the survival of patients with these rare tumors, which by virtue of their site are prone to late presentation. While the diverse histopathology that can occur in the region has made it difficult to accrue large cohorts of sufficient size to provide robust statistical analysis, this has led by necessity to multicenter and multisurgeon cohort analyses with their intrinsic disadvantages.[31] This, coupled with the ability of most of these tumors to recur beyond 5 years, has meant that we have only recently been in a position to genuinely assess the impact of this procedure. This is particularly appropriate at the moment when increasing numbers of surgeons are advocating surgery by completely endoscopic approaches in this region.

Our cohort of 308 patients presents a substantial single-institution cohort accrued over 25 years by three surgeons and treated, when required, predominantly by one radiotherapist/medical oncologist. Continuous analysis of our group of patients has shown improvement in overall survival (possibly related to earlier presentation as the series became known nationally), and improvement in surgical techniques and postoperative support and in adjuvant management and patient selection. In particular, we have paid meticulous attention under microscopic and/or endoscopic control to wide-field dural and periosteal resection, to the sphenopalatine area and pterygomaxillary fissure, the infratemporal fossa, the roof of the nasopharynx, and the apex of the orbit.

Individual, larger histological groups from our series, including adenocarcinoma, olfactory neuroblastoma, and chondrosarcoma have shown sustained improvement as compared with previous figures, notably olfactory neuroblastoma at 74% 5-year survival and chondrosarcoma at 94%. However, in all cases, there is still a continuous loss with time as evidenced by 10-year and 15-year figures, and these are in keeping with those published by other investigators and with our own previous intermediate analysis (**Fig. 19.30**).[32–35]

Our analysis, along with others', has demonstrated the importance of craniofacial resection for accurate staging and for oncologically encompassing the extension of disease up to and including the olfactory tracts and bulbs, which is particularly relevant for tumors such as olfactory neuroblastoma and is reflected in survival rates more than double that produced in the previous era of lateral rhinotomy plus radiotherapy.[32] However, irrespective of histology, involvement of the brain gives a particularly poor prognosis with few survivors in the long term.

Key Points

- Half of our craniofacial patients had received previous unsuccessful treatment.
- Forty percent required additional treatment post craniofacial resection.
- Multivariate analysis identified type of malignancy, brain, and orbital involvement as the most important prognostic factors.
- The outcome is identical in combined treatment whether the radiotherapy is given pre- or postoperatively.
- Meningioma is the principal cause of death in the benign group of tumors.
- Survival has been more than doubled for many of the malignant tumors by craniofacial resection.
- The long-term study of craniofacial surgery acts as a baseline for future treatments in this group of tumors.

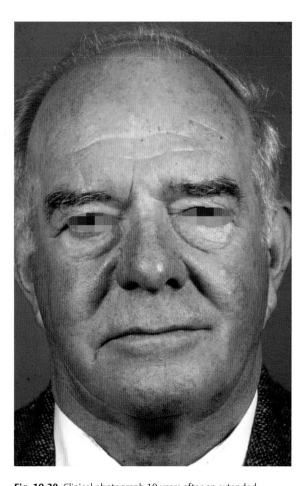

Fig. 19.30 Clinical photograph 10 years after an extended right lateral rhinotomy incision for craniofacial resection of an extensive olfactory neuroblastoma. The patient developed a dural recurrence after 11 years.

Recurrent Disease

In common with other authors' experience,[36-38] our most frequent form of recurrent disease was local and amenable to treatment with intention to cure in 44 patients (14% of our series). Most of these (91%) underwent surgery, most commonly revision craniofacial resection, which in one individual was undertaken six times to successfully treat a chondrosarcoma long term, emphasizing both the importance of the low morbidity and the palliative role of the procedure.

Regional recurrence occurred in 17 of our 308 patients, 16 of whom underwent neck dissection. This low instance of cervical node metastases has generally been the finding of other investigators.[37,39] Distant metastases with locoregional control are rare but carry a poor prognosis with rapid demise of the patient.

Key Point

- Recurrence beyond 5 years is not uncommon in this tumor group and long-term follow-up is required and worthwhile.

Comparison with Endoscopic Surgery

The increasing interest in extended radical endoscopic sinus surgery and/or intensity of modulated radiotherapy for malignant tumors of the anterior skull base[40-42] makes it appropriate to continue to provide statistical analysis of long-term cohorts of patients who have undergone craniofacial resection. Clearly, it will be some time before meaningful comparisons can be made with the newer, alternative treatments but, until then, the craniofacial resection remains the gold standard for sinonasal tumors affecting the skull base.[42]

Total Rhinectomy

The nose and eyes are arguably the most prominent and important features of facial appearance and rhinectomy is not an operation to undertake lightly, but as already discussed in the sections on vestibular and nasal septal malignancy, late presentation or recurrent disease, particularly of squamous carcinoma and malignant melanoma, may on occasions necessitate the operation to palliate serious symptoms, most notably epistaxis and fungation (**Fig. 19.31**). On occasion, total cure is possible with this procedure combined with other adjuvant treatment, but this is certainly not the case in malignant melanoma, although long-term palliation may be possible.[43]

Surgical Technique

The external nose is composed of bone and hyaline cartilage and the cartilaginous component may be removed to leave an intact piriform bony aperture. The nasal cartilage and overlying soft tissues are easily freed by an incision beginning at the lateral edge of one naris and following the edge of the pyramidal opening, which is easy to discern. After both lateral components have been sectioned, excision of the columella and anterior septum can be performed under direct vision. This then allows excellent inspection of the remaining nasal cavity, preferably under the operating microscope, and allows further removal of bony septum, nasal bones, and lateral wall of the nose if there is any doubt regarding clear tumor margins.

Extension inferiorly to involve the premaxilla is important as this is a common area for squamous carcinoma and adenoid cystic carcinoma to spread and this requires in-continuity resection with sufficient palatal removal, at times creating an additional intraoral defect. Modern prostheticists may easily design a nasal prosthesis that can lock into an intraoral prosthetic device and give excellent stability and adequate sealing.

The nasal bones should be preserved if possible to provide good seating for the nasal prosthesis, but undercutting of the bony edge of the pyramidal opening does assist in promoting nasal coverage and rapid epithelialization of the margins (**Fig. 19.32**). Skin grafting is rarely necessary as coverage may be obtained from surrounding skin and any substantial loss of the upper lip tissues may be augmented by nasolabial flaps, either unilateral or bilateral.

Bleeding from the alar and septal branches of the facial artery is easily controlled but, if necessary, the intranasal component of the operation can be packed with Whitehead's varnish gauze or the surgeon's alternative choice. Initial long-term crusting requires saline nasal douching whether the patient has a prosthetic or facial plastic reconstruction.

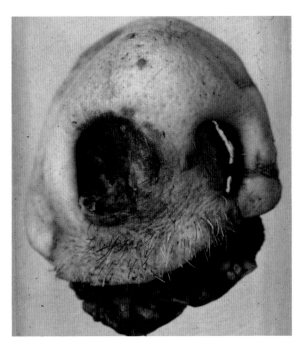

Fig. 19.31 Total rhinectomy for extensive malignant mucosal melanoma that presented with severe epistaxis.

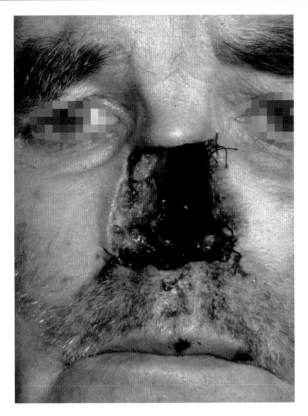

Fig. 19.32 Clinical photograph of a patient 4 days postoperatively showing skin and mucosal apposition possible on the left side, but the inferior aspect of the nasal bones and the entire septum were sacrificed. Long-term saline douches are necessary.

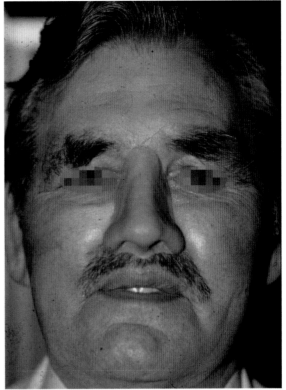

Fig. 19.33 Clinical photograph of the same patient as in Fig. 19.32 with a nasal prosthesis that was an excellent compromise for someone with a short life span. The patient died in 11 months.

Reconstruction after Rhinectomy

It remains doubtful whether even the most ingenious and technically able reconstructive surgeon can match the abilities of modern prosthetics, and since most patients have a total rhinectomy for neoplasia, which may be associated with failure of previous treatment such as radiotherapy, custom-made prostheses are often the most appropriate choice (**Fig. 19.33**). Prostheses have the advantage of allowing frequent inspection of the remaining nasal passages as well as easy replacement to match changing skin coloration. While they may be attached with recent osseointegrated techniques, where these are not available simple attachment to spectacle frames will ensure sufficient stability (**Fig. 19.34**).

Summary

Irrespective of the pathology necessitating total rhinectomy, it is considered to be an aesthetically disturbing procedure for both patient and surgeon, but the disfigurement produced by uncontrolled neoplasia involving the nasal framework is extremely unpleasant and the operation provides effective access for long-term palliation in many patients and can be curative for vestibular and septal carcinoma. In a similar manner to orbital clearance and/or exenteration, it is rare to regret carrying out the operation, but unless the patient receives careful counseling, there can be considerable delay in undertaking the procedure, which means an increased level of resection and a greater degree of prosthetic or facial plastic reconstruction.

References

1. Lloyd G, Lund VJ, Howard D, Savy L. Optimum imaging for sinonasal malignancy. J Laryngol Otol 2000; 114(7):557–562
2. Jones E, Lund VJ, Howard DJ, Greenberg MP, McCarthy M. Quality of life of patients treated surgically for head and neck cancer. J Laryngol Otol 1992;106(3):238–242
3. Moure E. Traitement des tumeurs malignes primitives de l'ethmoid. Rev Laryngol Otol Rhinol (Bord) 1902; 23:401–412
4. Harrison DF. Lateral rhinotomy: a neglected operation. Ann Otol Rhinol Laryngol 1977;86(6 Pt 1):756–759
5. Howard DJ, Lund VJ. The midfacial degloving approach to sinonasal disease. J Laryngol Otol 1992;106(12):1059–1062
6. Howard DJ, Lund VJ. The role of midfacial degloving in modern rhinological practice. J Laryngol Otol 1999;113(10):885–887

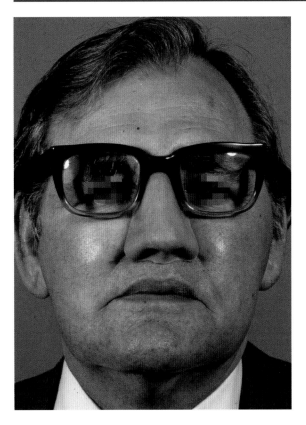

Fig. 19.34 A prosthesis attached to eyeglasses provides greater stability and partially disguises the edge for the patient (same patient as in Fig. 19.32 and Fig. 19.33).

7. Converse JM. Restoration of facial contour by bone grafts introduced through the oral cavity. Plast Reconstr Surg (1946) 1950;6(4):295–300
8. Casson PR, Bonanno PC, Converse JM. The midface degloving procedure. Plast Reconstr Surg 1974;53(1):102–103
9. Maniglia AJ, Phillips DA. Midfacial degloving for the management of nasal, sinus, and skull-base neoplasms. Otolaryngol Clin North Am 1995;28(6):1127–1143
10. Moffatt A. Postural instillation. A method of inducing local anaesthesia in the nose. J Laryngol Otol 1941;56:429–436
11. Lund V, Howard D, Gardner A. Sinonasal surgery on the developing face. In: Tos M, Thomsen J, Balle V, eds. Rhinology: State of the Art. Amsterdam: Kugler; 1995:211–216
12. Cocke EW Jr, Robertson JH, Robertson JT, Crook JP Jr. The extended maxillotomy and subtotal maxillectomy for excision of skull base tumors. Arch Otolaryngol Head Neck Surg 1990;116(1):92–104
13. Lanigan DT, Hey JH, West RA. Aseptic necrosis following maxillary osteotomies: report of 36 cases. J Oral Maxillofac Surg 1990;48(2):142–156
14. Gensoul P. Lettre Chirurgicale sur Quelques Maladies Graves du Sinus Maxillaire avec Atlas de Huit Planches en Couleur. Paris: Baillière; 1833
15. Lizars J. Removal of the superior maxillary bone. London Med Gaz 1829;30(V):92–93
16. Syme J. Excision of the upper jaw. Edinburgh Med Surg J 1829;XXXII:238–239
17. Howard DJ, Lund VJ, Wei WI. Craniofacial resection for tumors of the nasal cavity and paranasal sinuses: a 25-year experience. Head Neck 2006;28(10):867–873
18. Lloyd S, Devesa-Martinez P, Howard DJ, Lund VJ. Quality of life of patients undergoing surgical treatment of head and neck malignancy. Clin Otolaryngol Allied Sci 2003;28(6):524–532
19. Harrison D. The management of malignant tumours affecting the maxillary and ethmoidal sinuses. J Laryngol Otol 1973;87:749–772
20. Weymuller EA Jr, Reardon EJ, Nash D. A comparison of treatment modalities in carcinoma of the maxillary antrum. Arch Otolaryngol 1980;106(10):625–629
21. Lee F, Ogura JH. Maxillary sinus carcinoma. Laryngoscope 1981;91(1):133–139
22. St-Pierre S, Baker SR. Squamous cell carcinoma of the maxillary sinus: analysis of 66 cases. Head Neck Surg 1983;5(6):508–513
23. McNicoll W, Hopkin N, Dalley VM, Shaw HJ. Cancer of the paranasal sinuses and nasal cavities. Part II. Results of treatment. J Laryngol Otol 1984;98(7):707–718
24. Lindeman P, Eklund U, Petruson B. Survival after surgical treatment in maxillary neoplasms of epithelial origin. J Laryngol Otol 1987;101(6):564–568
25. Donald P. Surgery of the Skull Base. Philadelphia: Lippincott-Raven; 1998: 292–298
26. Raveh J, Vuillemin T. Subcranial-supraorbital and temporal approach for tumor resection. J Craniofac Surg 1990;1(1):53–59
27. Raveh J, Turk JB, Lädrach K, et al. Extended anterior subcranial approach for skull base tumors: long-term results. J Neurosurg 1995;82(6):1002–1010
28. Smith RR, Klopp CT, Williams JM. Surgical treatment of cancer of the frontal sinus and adjacent areas. Cancer 1954;7(5):991–994
29. Ketcham AS, Wilkins RH, Vanburen JM, Smith RR. A combined intracranial facial approach to the paranasal sinuses. Am J Surg 1963;106:698–703
30. Howard DJ, Lund VJ, Wei WI. Craniofacial resection for tumors of the nasal cavity and paranasal sinuses: a 25-year experience. Head Neck 2006;28(10):867–87
31. Ganly I, Patel SG, Singh B, et al. Craniofacial resection for malignant paranasal sinus tumors: Report of an International Collaborative Study. Head Neck 2005;27(7):575–584
32. Lund VJ, Howard D, Wei W, Spittle M. Olfactory neuroblastoma: past, present, and future? Laryngoscope 2003;113(3):502–507
33. Catalano PJ, Hecht CS, Biller HF, et al. Craniofacial resection. An analysis of 73 cases. Arch Otolaryngol Head Neck Surg 1994;120(11):1203–1208
34. Levine PA, Scher RL, Jane JA, et al. The craniofacial resection—eleven-year experience at the University of Virginia: problems and solutions. Otolaryngol Head Neck Surg 1989;101(6):665–669
35. Shah JP, Kraus DH, Bilsky MH, Gutin PH, Harrison LH, Strong EW. Craniofacial resection for malignant tumors involving the anterior skull base. Arch Otolaryngol Head Neck Surg 1997;123(12):1312–1317
36. Patel SG, Singh B, Polluri A, et al. Craniofacial surgery for malignant skull base tumors: report of an international collaborative study. Cancer 2003;98(6):1179–1187
37. Bhattacharyya N. Cancer of the nasal cavity: survival and factors influencing prognosis. Arch Otolaryngol Head Neck Surg 2002;128(9):1079–1083
38. Porceddu S, Martin J, Shanker G, et al. Paranasal sinus tumors: Peter MacCallum Cancer Institute experience. Head Neck 2004;26(4):322–330
39. Gullane PJ, Conley J. Carcinoma of the maxillary sinus. A correlation of the clinical course with orbital involvement, pterygoid erosion or pterygopalatine invasion and cervical metastases. J Otolaryngol 1983;12(3):141–145

40. Kühn UM, Mann WJ, Amedee RG. Endonasal approach for nasal and paranasal sinus tumor removal. ORL J Otorhinolaryngol Relat Spec 2001;63(6):366–371
41. Goffart Y, Jorissen M, Daele J, et al. Minimally invasive endoscopic management of malignant sinonasal tumours. Acta Otorhinolaryngol Belg 2000;54(2):221–232
42. Lund VJ Stammberger H, Nicolai P, et al. European position paper on endoscopic management of tumours of the nose, paranasal sinuses and skull base. Rhinol Suppl 2010;(22):1–143
43. Harrison DF. Total rhinectomy—a worthwhile operation? J Laryngol Otol 1982;96(12):1113–1123

Management of the Orbit

The proximity of the orbit to all the paranasal sinuses and the nasal cavity makes it vulnerable to involvement and invasion by any neoplastic or expansile process occurring in these sites. Involvement of the orbit is an important predictor of survival and this is reflected in the staging classifications, where any malignant tumor becomes T3 or T4 once the orbit is affected.[1,2] Involvement of the orbital apex constitutes T4b, indicating the worst outcome. Even benign tumors may have a profound effect on the eye by displacement and compression of the orbital contents if neglected. Extreme examples may be seen with benign fibro-osseous lesions and even benign inverted papilloma can occasionally breach the periosteum. Visual symptoms accompany at least 50% of malignant sinonasal tumors and may be the reason patients present to their doctors (see Table 4.1, p. 40),[3] unilateral proptosis, diplopia, and epiphora being the commonest problems.

Iannetti et al[4] have classified orbital invasion into three stages (**Fig. 19.35**):
1. Erosion or destruction of the medial orbital wall
2. Extraconal invasion of the periorbital fat
3. Invasion of the medial rectus muscle, optic nerve, ocular bulb, or the skin overlying the eyelid

Whether the tumor is extra- or intraperiosteal, it may track posteriorly into the apex and thence reach the cavernous sinus and middle cranial fossa.

It should also be remembered that the nasolacrimal system may be directly or indirectly involved by compression or infiltration.[5]

Fifty years ago conventional wisdom dictated the removal of the eye if a malignant tumor was even abutting the orbital periosteum.[6] However, with time a more conservative approach has prevailed without any evidence that this compromises cure (**Fig. 19.36**).[7,8] The lamina papyracea is eroded with relative ease, but it is often the case—even with quite large tumors—that a plane exists between the tumor and the orbital periosteum, for example in adenocarcinoma (**Fig. 19.37**). In these circumstances, the periosteum can be widely resected

and repaired with split skin or fascia, assuming that frozen section confirms that the tumor has not penetrated microscopically through the full thickness of periosteum. An anterior incision through the periosteum allows dissection between this and the orbital fat and a generous portion can be resected without major problems. Care is required posteriorly where the medial rectus muscle is most readily encountered.

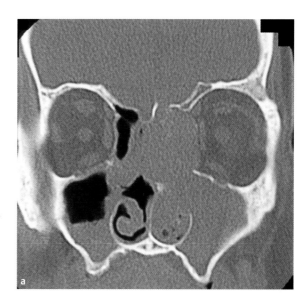

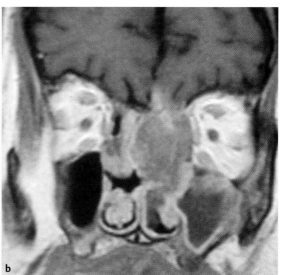

Fig. 19.35a–e
a Coronal CT showing adenocarcinoma eroding the lamina papyracea and pushing against the orbital periosteum.
b Coronal MRI (T1W post gadolinium enhancement) suggesting tumor adjacent to but not adherent to periosteum, subsequently confirmed at surgery and histologically.

Fig. 19.35c–e ▷

◁ continued

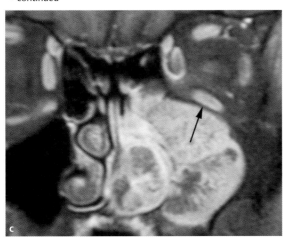

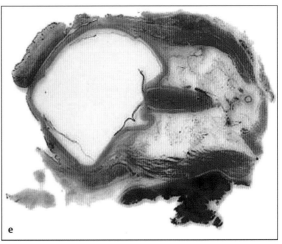

c Coronal MRI (T1W post gadolinium enhancement with fat
saturation) showing squamous cell carcinoma in the maxillary
sinus having eroded the bone of the roof and probably
adherent to the orbital periosteum but not through into orbital
fat, confirmed at surgery and histologically. (Courtesy of Dr. T.
Beale.)

d Coronal MRI (T1W post gadolinium enhancement) showing
squamous cell carcinoma in the maxillary sinus having
penetrated through bone and periosteum and appearing to
be involving the inferior rectus muscle. This was confirmed at
operation and orbital clearance was undertaken. (Courtesy of
Dr. T. Beale.)

e Histological section through the orbital contents showing
tumor infiltrating the inferior rectus muscle. (Courtesy of Dr. A.
Gallimore.)

To offset enophthalmos due to medial prolapse of
orbital fat into the nasal cavity, various grafts have been
utilized including skin, fascia, and mucosa. Of these, split
skin has the advantage of shrinkage with time, which
counteracts the enophthalmos to some extent. The graft
is held in place with a few drops of biological glue, gelatin
sponge soaked in an antibiotic solution, and insertion of
a pack (e.g., Whitehead's[9])which is left in place for 7 to
10 days and then removed, usually under a short general
anesthetic. Even if periosteum of the entire medial wall
is resected, the function of the eye is surprisingly good
after grafting, although patients should always be warned
about diplopia and enophthalmos, which may require
subsequent corrective surgery.

Previously the orbit was approached through an external incision that facilitated assessment of the situation
and subsequent resection of periosteum. However, with

the increasing application of endoscopic techniques, it
is possible in many cases to also manage the orbit endoscopically, as resection of the periosteum may be undertaken and repaired through this approach. However, it is
technically difficult to deal with the most anterior medial
wall by this approach and in these circumstances an
external incision should be considered.

Nonetheless, there are still circumstances when
the eye has to be removed, when the tumor has spread
through the periosteum in individuals who, but for the
eye involvement, are curable. As preseptal spread is rare
and there is no anterior lymphatic drainage, the eyelids
can usually be spared. This constitutes an orbital clearance as opposed to orbital exenteration, where the lids
are sacrificed. The latter is most often required with
extensive squamous or basal cell carcinomas in the
medial canthal region.

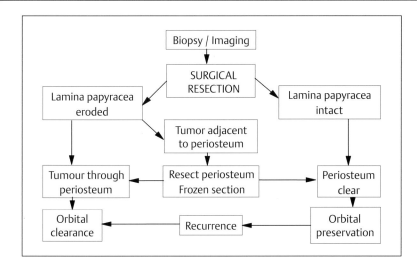

Fig. 19.36 Algorithm for management of the orbit. (Modified from reference 11.)

Orbital Clearance

In orbital clearance the globe, muscles, fat, and periorbita are removed, while the lids and palpebral conjunctiva remain. When preserving the lids, cuts are made leaving the lash margin on the specimen and the skin and subcutaneous tissues are dissected off the tarsal plates. A circumferential incision is made around the socket, down to bone, and the canthal ligaments are divided. The periosteum is then elevated from the walls of the socket using a Freer elevator and ribbon gauze soaked in 1:1000 epinephrine, taking care not to extend out through the inferior or superior orbital fissures. Once the orbital contents are mobilized, the anesthetist should be warned that the apex is about to be divided as patients often develop a marked bradycardia as the optic nerve is cut. The apex is divided using large curved Mayo scissors introduced into the orbital socket from lateral to medial and thus following the curve of the lateral wall and removing the maximal tissue at the orbital apex with the first cut. This maneuver should be done with reasonable speed as significant bleeding is usually encountered from the ophthalmic artery. However, this quickly vasoconstricts and can be encouraged to do so with a gauze that has been soaked in boiling water and then wrung out. The water must be hot because anything less will actually encourage vasodilation. Care must also be taken that the delicate skin of the lids is not in contact with the gauze. The bleeding may also be controlled with a curved artery clip and further clearance of the apex can be undertaken, but this must be done with care. It is advisable to put a stay suture through the optic neurovascular bundle not only for hemostasis but also to close the cerebrospinal fluid space around the nerve.

Reconstruction

The lids are closed without tension using dissolvable 5/0 sutures in two layers. The first layer of interrupted sutures is in the preserved orbicularis muscle. The second fine continuous layer is in the skin itself. No attempt is subsequently made to remove these sutures and with time the skin will sink back to line the socket (**Fig. 19.37**). This provides an excellent socket with additional stability for an orbital prosthesis irrespective of whether or not osseointegrated implants are subsequently used. However, the skin is fragile and will sometimes break down, especially after radiotherapy, or may be intentionally sacrificed in an exenteration, so a decision may be made to fill the socket from the outset with a free microvascular flap or a temporalis muscle flap to which a split skin graft can be applied. The entire temporalis muscle, pedicled on its insertion on the coronoid process, may be transferred into the socket through a 3 cm × 2 cm window in the lateral orbital wall with preservation of the lateral orbital rim.[10]

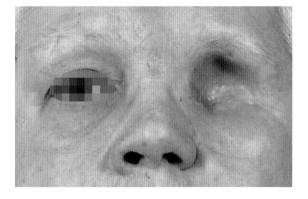

Fig. 19.37 Clinical photograph showing the socket lined with eyelid skin.

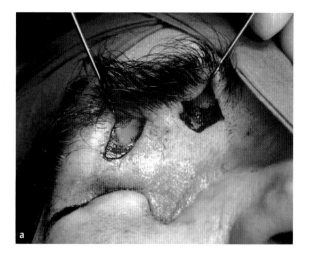

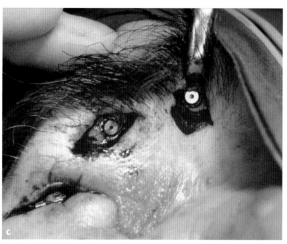

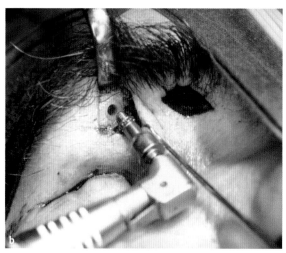

Fig. 19.38a–c

a Peroperative photograph of the first stage of insertion of the osseointegrated implants at the time of orbital clearance and prior to the two-layer closure of the preserved eyelid skin. Small incisions are being made.

b Slow-speed insertion of the first implant following drilling and tapping of the orbital rim. This insertion is done under continuous cooling saline irrigation (not shown).

c First stage of implantation complete. The titanium implants have covering caps.

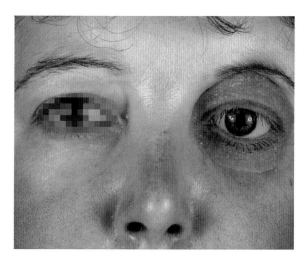

Osseointegrated implants may be placed in the orbital rim at the time of the resection or any time thereafter, but integration can take up to a year in this area especially if radiotherapy is given (**Fig. 19.38**).[11] An orbital prosthesis held with adhesives or on a spectacle frame can be fitted while integration takes place (**Figs. 19.39 and 19.40**).

If the orbital contents are preserved, consideration should be given to repair of any significant defect of the floor to minimize functional loss, particularly if the orbital periosteum has been resected (see below). A variety of techniques have been described including fascial or muscle slings, bone grafts, or synthetic meshes (propylene or titanium) together with a variety of free or pedicled muscle or osseomusculocutaneous flaps. These may involve the rectus abdominis, latissimus dorsi, scapula, rib, or fibula.[11] These tissues can also be used to reconstruct larger defects after total maxillectomy and orbital clearance.[12,13]

Conventional prosthetic obturators still have a role and have the advantage of allowing inspection of the surgical cavity.

Fig. 19.39 Clinical photograph of a left orbital prosthesis held in place with adhesive prior to the second stage of osseointegrated implantation. The skin color match required further adjustments.

Outcome

As previously noted, orbital involvement has an adverse effect on survival and, together with involvement of the brain and histology, is one of the most important prognostic factors on multivariate analysis of our and other craniofacial patients (see **Fig. 19.28**).[8,14] A similar finding was reported by Suarez et al,[15] who also showed that involvement of the orbital periosteum alone did not

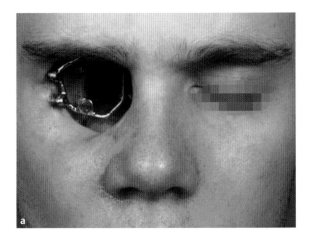

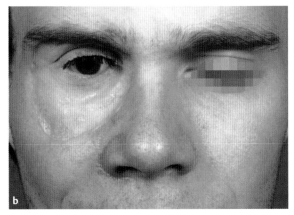

Fig. 19.40a, b

a Clinical photograph showing an open orbital defect but with excellent titanium osseointegrated implants and gold bar fitting.

b An osseointegrated prosthesis clipped firmly onto the underlying gold bar. This form of fixation allows a fine feathered edge on the orbital prosthesis.

affect survival. By contrast, involvement of the orbital apex adversely affects outcome[14,16,17] and is not improved by orbital clearance. Orbital involvement is also a significant prognostic factor in maxillary sinus malignancy[18,19]; it was associated with a 5-year survival of 17% as compared with 49% without orbital invasion, and again was not improved by orbital clearance.[18]

Some authors have sought to differentiate the effects of orbital involvement based on histological type, although the results are somewhat unclear. Nishino et al[20] showed patients with squamous cell carcinoma who had orbital involvement did better than those with other histologies (74% versus 40% 5-year survival) but this was not the conclusion of Imola and Schramm.[21] This may in part be due to the numbers of patients and definition of orbital involvement. Of note, however, are histological studies that have shown that in 25 maxillectomy and orbital clearance specimens for squamous cell carcinoma, the invasion of the orbit was limited to the periorbita[22]

probably due to a thin fascial layer surrounding the periocular fat.

While the strategy of orbital conservation adopted since the 1980s by ourselves and others, if the periosteum has not been penetrated, has not been shown to adversely affect outcome, either in terms of local control or actuarial survival,[7,8,18,21,23,24] patients must be prepared to undergo orbital clearance at a later date if disease recurs. Interestingly this was only necessary in 5/50 of our patients who initially had had orbital periosteal resection and was undertaken between 5 months and 4 years later. However, not everyone has agreed with this approach[25] and the studies may suffer from selection bias due to patients with more extensive disease undergoing orbital clearance.

Others have gone further and undertaken piecemeal debulking combined with high-dose radiotherapy ± chemotherapy.[20,26,27] Overall survival rates at 5 years of 59%, 60%, and 68% were reported respectively in these publications and in the Jansen study overall survival was significantly better than those treated with radiotherapy alone (9%) (n = 18 radiotherapy alone vs. 50 radiotherapy + debulking), though the groups differed in disease extent.

Orbital Function

Conservation of the orbital contents can come at a price. Imola and Schramm[21] reported on 54 patients and divided them into functional without impairment (54%), functional with impairment (37%), and nonfunctional (9%). The commonest result was malposition of the globe in 63% but this was often asymptomatic and only 9% had persistent diplopia. This was generally due to orbital floor resection and argues in favor of reconstruction of the defect. By contrast, removal of the medial orbital wall has little effect on orbital function, whatever the approach.[8,10,28]

The addition of radiotherapy increases the chances of orbital problems such as cataract formation, optic atrophy, excessive dryness, and ectropion.

Key Points

- The orbit is frequently affected by sinonasal tumors but can be asymptomatic.
- Orbital symptoms include unilateral proptosis, diplopia, epiphora, and ultimately visual loss.
- If the orbital periosteum has not been completely transgressed, the periosteum can be resected and the eye preserved, without adversely affecting survival.
- Orbital clearance is indicated for involvement of the orbital apex, full-thickness invasion through the periorbita into retrobulbar fat, extension into the extraocular muscles, and invasion of the bulbar conjunctiva or sclera.
- Orbital exenteration is indicated when the eyelids are involved.

References

1. Sorbin L, Gospodarowicz M, Wittekind C. TNM Classification of Malignant Tumours. 7th ed. Chichester: Wiley-Blackwell; 2009:50
2. Greene F, Compton C, Fritz A, Shah J, Winchester D. American Joint Committee on Cancer Staging Manuel. New York: Springer; 2010:69–78
3. Lund VJ. Malignant tumours of the nasal cavity and paranasal sinuses. ORL J Otorhinolaryngol Relat Spec 1983; 45(1):1–12
4. Iannetti G, Valentini V, Rinna C, Ventucci E, Marianetti TM. Ethmoido-orbital tumors: our experience. J Craniofac Surg 2005;16(6):1085–1091
5. Lloyd GAS, Lund VJ, Howard DJ, Savy L. Optimum imaging for sinonasal malignancy. J Laryngol Otol 2000; 114(7):557–562
6. Ketcham AS, Van Buren JM. Tumors of the paranasal sinuses: a therapeutic challenge. Am J Surg 1985;150(4):406–413
7. McCary WS, Levine PA, Cantrell RW. Preservation of the eye in the treatment of sinonasal malignant neoplasms with orbital involvement. A confirmation of the original treatise. Arch Otolaryngol Head Neck Surg 1996;122(6):657–659
8. Howard DJ, Lund VJ, Wei WI. Craniofacial resection for tumors of the nasal cavity and paranasal sinuses: a 25-year experience. Head Neck 2006;28(10):867–873
9. Lim M, Lew-Gor S, Sandhu G, Howard D, Lund VJ. Whitehead's varnish nasal pack. J Laryngol Otol 2007; 121(6):592–594
10. Suárez C, Ferlito A, Lund VJ, et al. Management of the orbit in malignant sinonasal tumors. Head Neck 2008; 30(2):242–250
11. Lund VJ, Howard DJ, Wei WI, Cheesman AD. Craniofacial resection for tumors of the nasal cavity and paranasal sinuses—a 17-year experience. Head Neck 1998; 20(2):97–105
12. Cordeiro PG, Santamaria E. A classification system and algorithm for reconstruction of maxillectomy and midfacial defects. Plast Reconstr Surg 2000;105(7):2331–2346, discussion 2347–2348
13. Pryor SG, Moore EJ, Kasperbauer JL. Orbital exenteration reconstruction with rectus abdominis microvascular free flap. Laryngoscope 2005;115(11):1912–1916
14. Ganly I, Patel SG, Singh B, et al. Craniofacial resection for malignant paranasal sinus tumors: Report of an International Collaborative Study. Head Neck 2005;27(7):575–584
15. Suarez C, Llorente JL, Fernandez De Leon R, Maseda E, Lopez A. Prognostic factors in sinonasal tumors involving the anterior skull base. Head Neck 2004;26(2):136–144
16. Cantù G, Solero CL, Mariani L, et al. Anterior craniofacial resection for malignant ethmoid tumors—a series of 91 patients. Head Neck 1999;21(3):185–191
17. Patel SG, Singh B, Polluri A, et al. Craniofacial surgery for malignant skull base tumors: report of an international collaborative study. Cancer 2003;98(6):1179–1187
18. Nazar G, Rodrigo JP, Llorente JL, Baragaño L, Suárez C. Prognostic factors of maxillary sinus malignancies. Am J Rhinol 2004;18(4):233–238
19. Carrillo JF, Güemes A, Ramírez-Ortega MC, Oñate-Ocaña LF. Prognostic factors in maxillary sinus and nasal cavity carcinoma. Eur J Surg Oncol 2005;31(10):1206–1212
20. Nishino H, Ichimura K, Tanaka H, et al. Results of orbital preservation for advanced malignant maxillary sinus tumors. Laryngoscope 2003;113(6):1064–1069
21. Imola MJ, Schramm VL Jr. Orbital preservation in surgical management of sinonasal malignancy. Laryngoscope 2002;112(8 Pt 1):1357–1365
22. Tiwari R, van der Wal J, van der Waal I, Snow G. Studies of the anatomy and pathology of the orbit in carcinoma of the maxillary sinus and their impact on preservation of the eye in maxillectomy. Head Neck 1998;20(3):193–196
23. Stern SJ, Goepfert H, Clayman G, Byers R, Wolf P. Orbital preservation in maxillectomy. Otolaryngol Head Neck Surg 1993;109(1):111–115
24. Carrau RL, Segas J, Nuss DW, et al. Squamous cell carcinoma of the sinonasal tract invading the orbit. Laryngoscope 1999;109(2 Pt 1):230–235
25. Dulguerov P, Jacobsen MS, Allal AS, Lehmann W, Calcaterra T. Nasal and paranasal sinus carcinoma: are we making progress? A series of 220 patients and a systematic review. Cancer 2001;92(12):3012–3029
26. Itami J, Uno T, Aruga M, Ode S. Squamous cell carcinoma of the maxillary sinus treated with radiation therapy and conservative surgery. Cancer 1998;82(1):104–107
27. Jansen EP, Keus RB, Hilgers FJ, Haas RL, Tan IB, Bartelink H. Does the combination of radiotherapy and debulking surgery favor survival in paranasal sinus carcinoma? Int J Radiat Oncol Biol Phys 2000;48(1):27–35
28. Lund VJ, Howard DJ, Wei WI. Endoscopic resection of malignant tumors of the nose and sinuses. Am J Rhinol 2007;21(1):89–94

Post-Therapy Follow-Up

As has been emphasized throughout this book, tumors arising in the sinonasal tract behave in idiosyncratic ways that make them different from neoplasia elsewhere in the body. The traditional use of 5-year survival as the breakpoint for "cure" can rarely be applied to sinonasal malignancy, which requires a lifetime's surveillance to confidently assert that the patient no longer has anything to fear. As a consequence, we have developed protocols for follow-up that include regular outpatient visits with endoscopic examination, regular imaging (generally with MRI), and formal admission for examination under anesthesia and biopsy when appropriate. The exact intervals are open to debate and the cost-effectiveness of such an intensive strategy remains to be determined in the present financial climate. However, only by carefully assessing our patients over many years will we be able to determine optimal treatment for these rare conditions. These assessments may be combined with sequential measures of quality of life such as the Short Form 36 (SF-36), Sino-Nasal Outcome Test (SNOT) 22, or European Organization for Research and Treatment of Cancer Quality of Life Core Questionnaire (EORTC-QLQ-C30),[1–6] although a wide range of rhinological instruments is available (**Tables 19.11, 19.12, 19.13**).[7–26] These may be broadly divided into general health questionnaires, which may focus on cancer and to which a small number of rhinology questions have been added (**Table 19.11**); those designed for allergic rhinitis and chronic rhinosinusitis (**Table 19.12**); and those directed at skull base surgery (**Table 19.13**). None is completely "fit for purpose" but they will doubtless be modified and merged with time.

Some have considered the effects of anterior skull base surgery using craniofacial resection, showing generally good results,[23] but interestingly, loss of smell was

Table 19.11 Shortlist of general QoL instruments

Instrument	Special features	Reference
Short Form 36 Health Survey (SF-36)	36 items (8 scales)	Ware[2] www.sf-36.org
Short Form 12 Health Survey (SF-12)	12 items	Ware et al[3] www.sf-36.org/tools/sf12.shtml
Glasgow Benefit Inventory (GBI)	18 items	Robinson et al[4]
European Quality of life 5 dimensions (EQ-5D)	5 dimensions	Rabin and de Charro[5] www.euroquol.org
Child Health Questionnaire (CHQ) CHQ-50PF (parent form) CHQ-87CF (child form)	50 items (CH-50PF) 87 items (CH-87CF)	Solans et al[6]
European Organization for Research and Treatment of Cancer Quality of Life Core Questionnaire (EORTC-QLQ-C30)	30 items	King[7] http://groups.eortc.be/qol/question-naires_qlqc30.htm
Functional Assessment of Cancer Therapy–General (FACT-G); Head and Neck (FACT-HandN)	27 items (FACT-G) 11 items (FACT-HandN)	List et al[8]
University of Washington Quality of Life Scale (UWQLS)	9 items	Hassan and Weymuller[9]
Hospital Anxiety and Depression Scale (HADS)	14 items	Bjelland et al[10]

Source: Modified and with permission from Table 11.1, Lund et al. European position paper on endoscopic management of tumours of the nose, paranasal sinuses and skull base. Rhinology Suppl 2010(22):1–143.

Table 19.12 QOL instruments addressing sinonasal diseases

Instrument	Special features	Reference
Nasal Symptom Questionnaire	12 items	Fairley et al[11]
Chronic Sinusitis Survey–Severity Based (CSS-S)	4 items (CSS-S)	Gliklich and Metson[12]
Chronic Sinusitis Survey–Duration Based (CSS-D)	6 items (CSS-D)	
Rhinosinusitis Disability Index (RSDI)	30 items	Benninger and Senior[13]
Rhinosinusitis Outcome Measure (RSOM-31)	31 items	Piccirillo et al[14]
General Nasal Patient Inventory (GNPI)	45 items	Douglas et al[15]
Sino-Nasal Outcome Test (SNOT-16)	16 items (modification of the RSOM-31)	Anderson et al[16]
Sino-Nasal Outcome Test (SNOT-20)	20 items (modification of the RSOM-31)	Piccirillo et al[17]
Sino-Nasal Outcome Test (SNOT-22)	22 items (modification of the RSOM-31)	Hopkins et al[18]
Sino-Nasal Assessment Questionnaire 11 (SNAQ-11)	3 items	Fahmy et al[19]
Sinonasal-5 Quality of Life Survey (SN-5)	5 domains (children)	Kay and Rosenfeld[20]
Rhinosinusitis Quality of Life Survey (RhinoQol)	17 items	Atlas et al[21]

Table 19.13 Disease-specific QOL instruments addressing skull base diseases

Instrument	Special features	Reference
Questionnaire "craniofacial tissue-integrated prosthesis"	Assessment of appearance and functional deficits related to implant-supported prostheses (20 items)	Sloan et al[22]
Midface Dysfunction Scale (MDS)	Assessment of midface function (4 items: vision, smell, taste, crusting)	Palme et al[23]
Youth Quality of Life Instrument –Facial Differences; Youth Quality of Life Instrument–Craniofacial Surgery module	Assessment of QOL in adolescents with congenital and acquired craniofacial differences	Edwards et al[24]
Skull Base Quality of Life Questionnaire	General assessment of QOL in patients undergoing anterior skull base surgery (35 items)	Gil et al[25,26]
Source: Modified and with permission from Tables 11.2 and 11.3 Lund et al. European position paper on endoscopic management of tumours of the nose, paranasal sinuses and skull base. Rhinology Suppl 2010;(22):1–143.		

regarded as more of a problem than the presence of a simple facial scar[27] while not surprisingly survival is the most important consideration of patients.[8] This is in contradistinction to the effect of more disfiguring resections necessitating major reconstruction.[29] It is also not surprising that persistent local problems such as crusting, nasal obstruction, epiphora, diplopia, and facial paresthesia adversely affect quality of life.[25,28–31]

For benign tumors such as inverted papilloma, follow-up is recommended for a minimum of 3 years or longer if the patient has already had a "recurrence" after surgery. Imaging is not routinely required unless the surgical cavity cannot be adequately assessed endoscopically in the outpatient setting, when MRI might be performed (**Fig. 19.41**). Benign fibro-osseous lesions generally require little follow-up if the surgeon is confident of complete removal. It is our practice to undertake a baseline CT scan after surgery in selected cases and to rescan only if there are any subsequent concerns, although generally patients are discharged after a couple of visits.

The situation with angiofibroma is similar to that in inverted papilloma, with a minimum follow-up of 3 years including regular MRI. The interpretation of all of these follow-up scans requires considerable skill and the ability to make direct comparison with previous images to pick up subtle interval change (**Fig. 19.42**).

Our present protocol for malignant tumors includes regular outpatient visits 4- to 6-weekly, increasing to 3-monthly over the first 2 years, then 4- to 6-monthly up to 5 years, and thereafter 9- to 12-monthly depending on the pathology, with direct access if the patient has any causes for concern in the meantime. MRI is undertaken ~3 months after treatment, which allows post-therapy changes to settle; and then 3- to 4-monthly for the first year and 6-monthly up to 5 years. In most cases we then offer to scan every 6 to 9 months for as long as the patient is willing and able (**Fig. 19.43**).

However, in chondrosarcoma the initial postsurgical scan is best done with CT, although MRI may be used thereafter until such time as a specific abnormality is detected when again CT may be considered. The MRI should be extended inferiorly to include the neck in certain tumors such as olfactory neuroblastoma. Additional follow-up imaging of the chest may be considered in adenoid cystic carcinoma.

Finally, it is very important that accurate data are collected prospectively and to this end an electronic database has been devised which allows anonymized data entry and analysis. This will be vital if we are to collect sufficient information on the wide range of sinonasal tumors to allow comparison between the different forms of management.

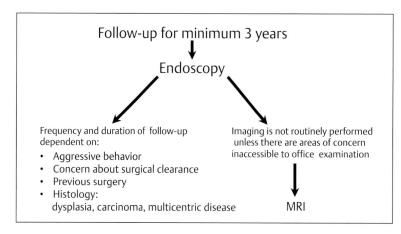

Fig. 19.41 Follow-up algorithm for inverted papilloma. (Modified and with permission from Figures 14.7 to 14.9, Lund et al. European position paper on endoscopic management of tumours of the nose, paranasal sinuses and skull base. Rhinology Suppl 2010; (22):107.)

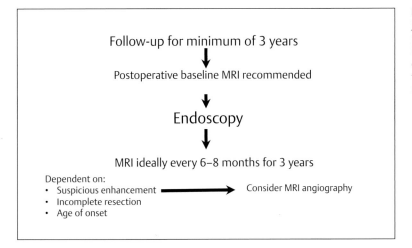

Fig. 19.42 Follow-up algorithm for juvenile angiofibroma. (Modified and with permission from Figures 14.7 to 14.9, Lund et al. European position paper on endoscopic management of tumours of the nose, paranasal sinuses and skull base. Rhinology Suppl 2010; (22):107.)

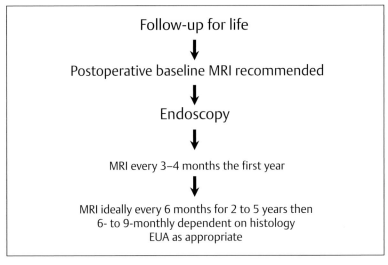

Fig. 19.43 Follow-up algorithm for malignant sinonasal tumors. (Modified and with permission from Figures 14.7 to 14.9, Lund et al. European position paper on endoscopic management of tumours of the nose, paranasal sinuses and skull base. Rhinology Suppl 2010;(22):107.)

References

1. Lund VJ Stammberger H, Nicolai P, et al. European position paper on endoscopic management of tumours of the nose, paranasal sinuses and skull base. Rhinol Suppl 2010;(22):1–143
2. Ware J. SF-36 Health Survey: Manual and Interpretation Guide. Boston: New England Medical Center, Health Institute; 1993
3. Ware JE Jr, Kosinski M, Keller SD. A 12-Item Short-Form Health Survey: construction of scales and preliminary tests of reliability and validity. Med Care 1996;34(3):220–233
4. Robinson K, Gatehouse S, Browning GG. Measuring patient benefit from otorhinolaryngological surgery and therapy. Ann Otol Rhinol Laryngol 1996;105(6):415–422
5. Rabin R, de Charro F. EQ-5D: a measure of health status from the EuroQol Group. Ann Med 2001;33(5):337–343
6. Solans M, Pane S, Estrada MD, et al. Health-related quality of life measurement in children and adolescents: a systematic review of generic and disease-specific instruments. Value Health 2008;11(4):742–764
7. King MT. The interpretation of scores from the EORTC quality of life questionnaire QLQ-C30. Qual Life Res 1996;5(6):555–567
8. List MA, D'Antonio LL, Cella DF, et al. The Performance Status Scale for Head and Neck Cancer Patients and the Functional Assessment of Cancer Therapy-Head and Neck Scale. A study of utility and validity. Cancer 1996;77(11):2294–2301
9. Hassan SJ, Weymuller EA Jr. Assessment of quality of life in head and neck cancer patients. Head Neck 1993;15(6):485–496
10. Bjelland I, Dahl AA, Haug TT, Neckelmann D. The validity of the Hospital Anxiety and Depression Scale. An updated literature review. J Psychosom Res 2002;52(2):69–77
11. Fairley JW, Yardley MPJ, Durham LH, Parker AJ. Reliability and validity of a nasal symptom questionnaire for use as an outcome measure in clinical research and audit of functional endoscopic sinus surgery. Clin Otolaryngol 1993;18:436–437
12. Gliklich RE, Metson R. Techniques for outcomes research in chronic sinusitis. Laryngoscope 1995;105(4 Pt 1):387–390
13. Benninger MS, Senior BA. The development of the Rhinosinusitis Disability Index. Arch Otolaryngol Head Neck Surg 1997;123(11):1175–1179
14. Piccirillo JF, Edwards D, Haiduk A, Yonan C, Thawley SE. Psychometric and clinimetric validity of the 31-item rhinosinusitis outcome measure (RSOM-31). Am J Rhinol 1995;9:297–306
15. Douglas SA, Marshall AH, Walshaw D, Robson AK, Wilson JA. The development of a General Nasal Patient Inventory. Clin Otolaryngol Allied Sci 2001;26(5):425–429
16. Anderson ER, Murphy MP, Weymuller EA Jr. Clinimetric evaluation of the Sinonasal Outcome Test-16. Student

Research Award 1998. Otolaryngol Head Neck Surg 1999;121(6):702–707

17. Piccirillo JF, Merritt MG Jr, Richards ML. Psychometric and clinimetric validity of the 20-item Sino-Nasal Outcome Test (SNOT-20). Otolaryngol Head Neck Surg 2002;126(1):41–47

18. Hopkins C, Gillett S, Slack R, Lund VJ, Browne JP. Psychometric validity of the 22-item Sinonasal Outcome Test. Clin Otolaryngol 2009;34(5):447–454

19. Fahmy FF, McCombe A, Mckiernan DC. Sino nasal assessment questionnaire, a patient focused, rhinosinusitis specific outcome measure. Rhinology 2002;40(4):195–197

20. Kay DJ, Rosenfeld RM. Quality of life for children with persistent sinonasal symptoms. Otolaryngol Head Neck Surg 2003;128(1):17–26

21. Atlas SJ, Metson RB, Singer DE, Wu YA, Gliklich RE. Validity of a new health-related quality of life instrument for patients with chronic sinusitis. Laryngoscope 2005;115(5):846–854

22. Sloan JA, Tolman DE, Anderson JD, Sugar AW, Wolfaardt JF, Novotny P. Patients with reconstruction of craniofacial or intraoral defects: development of instruments to measure quality of life. Int J Oral Maxillofac Implants 2001;16(2):225–245

23. Palme CE, Irish JC, Gullane PJ, Katz MR, Devins GM, Bachar G. Quality of life analysis in patients with anterior skull base neoplasms. Head Neck 2009;31(10):1326–1334

24. Edwards TC, Patrick DL, Topolski TD, Aspinall CL, Mouradian WE, Speltz ML. Approaches to craniofacial-specific quality of life assessment in adolescents. Cleft Palate Craniofac J 2005;42(1):19–24

25. Gil Z, Abergel A, Spektor S, et al. Quality of life following surgery for anterior skull base tumors. Arch Otolaryngol Head Neck Surg 2003;129(12):1303–1309

26. Gil Z, Abergel A, Spektor S, Shabtai E, Khafif A, Fliss DM. Development of a cancer-specific anterior skull base quality-of-life questionnaire. J Neurosurg 2004;100(5):813–819

27. Jones E, Lund VJ, Howard DJ, Greenberg MP, McCarthy M. Quality of life of patients treated surgically for head and neck cancer. J Laryngol Otol 1992;106(3):238–242

28. Alberty J, Hermann W, Mueller C, Rudack C, Stoll W. Aesthetic outcome of transfacial sinus surgery: the patient's view. Arch Otolaryngol Head Neck Surg 2006;132(11):1190–1195

29. Fukuda K, Saeki N, Mine S, et al. Evaluation of outcome and QOL in patients with craniofacial resection for malignant tumors involving the anterior skull base. Neurol Res 2000;22(6):545–550

30. Klimek T, Atai E, Schubert M, Glanz H. Inverted papilloma of the nasal cavity and paranasal sinuses: clinical data, surgical strategy and recurrence rates. Acta Otolaryngol 2000;120(2):267–272

31. Lindemann J, Leiacker R, Sikora T, Rettinger G, Keck T. Impact of unilateral sinus surgery with resection of the turbinates by means of midfacial degloving on nasal air conditioning. Laryngoscope 2002;112(11):2062–2066

20 Principles and Techniques of Radiotherapy and Chemotherapy for Nasal Cavity and Paranasal Sinus Tumors

S. J. Frank, A. S. Garden, and K. K. Ang

Sinonasal malignancies are relatively rare tumors of the head and neck accounting for less than 1% of all malignancies and ~3% of upper respiratory tract tumors.[1]

Tumors originating within the nasal vestibule, nasal fossa, and paranasal sinuses each have a unique natural history and biological behavior. The therapeutic principles and techniques also vary for each type of tumor, although for any tumor type special consideration is always given to organ preservation, organ function, and overall cosmesis. A multidisciplinary team approach involving experts in head and neck cancer surgery, radiotherapy, chemotherapy, imaging, and pathology is best suited for managing cases of disease in this region to provide patients with the best chance of cure and optimal quality of life. Primary and adjuvant radiotherapy have essential roles in the overall treatment strategy for tumors in this complex anatomical location. This chapter focuses primarily on the principles and techniques of radiotherapy and chemotherapy for carcinomas of the nasal cavity and paranasal sinuses.

Tumors of the Nasal Cavity

Treatment Principles

Nasal Vestibule Tumors

The definitive treatment for nasal vestibule tumors is either surgery, primary radiotherapy, or—when indicated because of tumor size or positive surgical findings—surgery followed by adjuvant radiation therapy. The role of systemic chemotherapy has not been established for tumors of this type. For small superficial tumors, standard treatment approaches are surgery or primary radiotherapy, delivered as external beam radiotherapy, brachytherapy, or a combination of the two. Either approach (surgery or primary radiotherapy) can yield high control rates with excellent cosmesis. Small invasive tumors are treated with either surgery or primary radiotherapy. Adjuvant radiation is indicated in cases involving positive surgical margins, positive lymph nodes, or perineural invasion. For large invasive tumors, the combination of surgery and radiotherapy—with radiotherapy given either before or after surgery—is the mainstay of treatment. Older patients and patients with poor performance status may be treated with radiotherapy alone.

The presence of cartilage invasion should not be considered a contraindication for radiotherapy because the risk of necrosis is low after fractionated radiotherapy.[2]

Patients with large defects after surgery and adjuvant radiation for large invasive tumors can be fitted with custom-made nasal prostheses by experienced prosthodontists.

Several retrospective studies of the use of radiotherapy for nasal vestibule tumors[3-11] suggest that either brachytherapy or external beam radiotherapy can produce cure rates approximating 90% for patients with small lesions (<2 cm in diameter) (Table 20.1). For lesions 2 to 4 cm in diameter, external beam radiotherapy can control 70 to 80% of tumors. Although nodal spread of disease is relatively rare for lesions smaller than 2 cm, up to 40% of patients with larger primary tumors have metastases to the cervical nodes at presentation. With the use of appropriate radiation techniques and fractionation schedules (described further below), severe and late complications after radiation therapy are uncommon (Table 20.1).

Nasal Fossa Tumors

Either primary radiotherapy or surgery for early-stage nasal fossa lesions can produce similarly high control rates. The size and location of the tumor as well as the anticipated cosmetic outcome generally guides the choice of treatment. Surgery is the mainstay of treatment for posterior septum lesions or locally advanced lesions. Primary radiotherapy, given as brachytherapy, is appropriate for small anterior-inferior septal lesions; external beam radiotherapy may produce the best cosmetic result for lateral wall lesions extending to the nasal ala.

Documentation of treatment outcomes for nasal fossa tumors comes mostly from retrospective studies.[12-15] Locoregional control rates range from 60 to 85%, and the rate of isolated regional recurrence in patients who did not receive elective nodal irradiation is ~5%. The most common complications after radiotherapy were soft tissue necrosis, visual impairment, and nasal stenosis (Table 20.2). Ang et al reported better primary disease control and survival rates for patients with tumors located in the septum (86%) versus patients with tumors on the lateral

Table 20.1 Studies of treatment outcomes for nasal vestibule tumors

Study institution and reference	Local control rates	Regional control rates	Late complications
MD Anderson Cancer Center, USA[4]	BT: 11/11 (100%) EBRT: 20/21 (95%) Total: 31/32 (97%)	Small lesions: 11/11 Large lesions: ELI:12/12 (100%) No ELI: 5/9 (56%) Total: 28/32 (88%)	Osteonecrosis: 1 Epistaxis: 1
Princess Margaret Hospital, Canada[3]	<2 cm (n = 34): 97% ≥2 cm (n = 16) + size not recorded (n = 6): 57%	No ELI: 51/54 (94%)	Osteonecrosis: 2 Nasal stenosis: 2 Epistaxis: 1
Dr. Daniel den Hood Cancer Center, Netherlands[6]	BT alone: 35/36 (97%) EBRT alone: 13/15 (87%) EBRT + BT: 5/8 (62%)	N0: 93%	Not reported
VU University Medical Center, Netherlands[7]	Overall at 2 years: 79% (ultimate at 5 years [after salvage]: 95%) <1.5 cm (n = 32): 83% (Ultimate: 94%) ≥1.5 cm (n = 24): 74% (Ultimate: 96%)	Routine ELI to the moustache region Overall at 2 years: 87% Ultimate at 5 years: 97%	Rhinorrhea: 45% Nasal dryness: 39% Epistaxis: 15% Adhesions: 4% Skin necrosis: 3 Nasal-vestibule sarcoma: 1
University of Florida College of Medicine, USA[5,8]	Overall at 5 years: 87% RT: 60/71 (86%) Surgery → RT: 8/8 (100%) Ultimate local control: 94%	T1–T2: 39/43 (91%) T4: 30/36 (83%) N0 control: 87% (ultimate: 97%) N0/no ENI: 47/54 (87%) Ultimate neck control: 97%	Soft tissue necrosis: 15 Severe complications: 3
Queens Medical Centre, UK	RT only: 8/13 Surgery only: 8/10	Not reported	Radionecrosis: 1
DAHANCA, Denmark[10]	5-year locoregional control: 67% T1: 79% T2: 54% T3: 35%	No ENI: 89%	Not reported
Queensland Radium Institute, Australia[11]	Surgery → RT: 4/6 (66%) RT: 13/22 (59%)	Surgery → RT: 57% RT: 86%	Septal necrosis: 2 Nasobuccoalveolar fistula: 1 Fistula: 1

Abbreviations: BT, brachytherapy; EBRT, external beam radiotherapy; ELI, elective lymph node irradiation; ENI, elective neck irradiation; RT, radiotherapy; .

wall or floor of the nasal fossa (68%).[12] In that study, patients with nasal septum carcinomas who underwent elective nodal irradiation had no nodal relapses, whereas 2 of 8 patients who did not undergo nodal irradiation experienced recurrence in the ipsilateral subdigastric nodes. Distant metastasis was more common among patients with lateral wall and floor disease, and ultimately survival rates were best among patients with nasal septum tumors. However, Badid et al[13] and Hawkins et al[15] found no differences in results for tumors at various sites within the nasal cavity. Results of treatment for early-stage tumors are equally good after radiotherapy or surgery; Bosch et al. found that the T1 lesions were well controlled with either surgery or radiotherapy and were associated with a 5-year overall survival rate of 91%.[14]

Esthesioneuroblastoma (Olfactory Neuroblastoma)

Single-modality therapy with either primary radiotherapy or surgery can produce locoregional control rates exceeding 90% when esthesioneuroblastoma lesions are confined to the nasal cavity (i.e., stage A).[16] Single-modality therapy has also been used for lesions involving the nasal cavity and one or more paranasal sinuses (stage B), as has surgery followed by adjuvant radiation therapy. However, the optimal therapy for stage B lesions is not clear because of the heterogeneity of these tumors. Disease that extends beyond the nasal cavity and paranasal sinuses (stage C) seems to be best treated with a combination of surgery and radiotherapy. Chemotherapy may

Table 20.2 Studies of treatment outcomes for nasal fossa tumors

Study institution and reference	No. of patients treated	Survival rates at 5 years	Late complications: number of patients
MD Anderson Cancer Center[12]	RT only: 18 RT → Surgery: 2 Surgery → RT: 25	Overall: 75% Disease-specific: 83%	Radiation-induced blindness: 2 Surgical blindness: 2 Maxillary necrosis: 3 Nasal stenosis: 2 Septal perforation: 1 Severe dental decay: 1
Roswell Park Memorial Institute[13]	RT only: 30 Surgery only: 13 Surgery → RT: 14	Crude overall 56% Disease-free 67%	Not reported
University of Puerto Rico[14]	RT only: 34 Surgery only: 6	Overall: 56%	Not reported
Mallinckrodt Institute of Radiology[15]	RT only: 28 RT → surgery: 18 Surgery → RT: 10	Overall: 52%	Soft tissue necrosis: 2 Cataract: 1 Nasal synechiae: 1 Severe otitis media: 2 Hemorrhage (fatal): 2 Optic neuropathy: 1 Brain necrosis: 1

Abbreviation: RT, radiotherapy.

have a role in the management of stage C disease. Elective nodal irradiation is not generally recommended because the incidence of nodal relapse is less than 15%. Distant metastasis is uncommon (10%) even among patients presenting with locally advanced disease. At this time, the role of systemic therapy for esthesioneuroblastoma is considered investigational; moreover, prospective studies to identify the optimal therapy are unlikely because of the rarity of this disease.

Radiotherapy Techniques[17]

Nasal Vestibule Tumors

External Beam Radiotherapy

Thin superficial nasal vestibule lesions can be treated with either orthovoltage X-rays or electrons with skin bolus; thicker lesions are generally treated with electrons. For definitive therapy, well-differentiated tumors that are circumscribed and up to 1.5 cm in diameter are generally treated to a dose of 66 to 70 Gy with a 1- to 2-cm margin, with a small treatment-field reduction after 50 Gy to boost the dose to the gross disease. Tumors larger than 1.5 cm and poorly differentiated are treated with a wider 2- to 3-cm margin, with irradiation of the bilateral facial nodes, submandibular nodes, and subdigastric nodes. For patients presenting with palpable neck adenopathy, the entire neck is treated with at least a subclinical dose of 50 Gy, and the gross disease plus a 1- to 2-cm margin is then treated with an additional 16 to 20 Gy.

For the larger nasal vestibule lesions, the lower half of the nose and the upper lip are treated with an anterior appositional field using 20-MeV electrons and 6-MV photons weighted 4 to 1. The right and left facial lymphatics are irradiated with anterior appositional fields using ~15-degree gantry rotation to the respective side with 6-MeV electron fields. The medial border is matched to the lateral border of the anterior primary field. The anterior border extends down from the oral commissure to the middle of the horizontal ramus of the mandible, whereas the posterior border extends from the upper edge of the anterior field to just above the angle of the mandible. The inferior border splits the horizontal ramus of the mandible and is matched to the upper neck field. The upper neck nodes are treated with parallel-opposed lateral photon fields. The primary tumor is treated to 60 Gy (at 90%) in 30 fractions, and the electively treated facial and upper neck nodes are treated to 50 Gy in 25 fractions.

When postoperative radiotherapy is indicated for close or positive surgical margins, perineural invasion, or tumors larger than 5 cm in diameter, the operative bed plus a 1- to 1.5-cm margin is treated to a dose of 60 to 66 Gy. Postoperative radiation doses to the neck depend on whether the neck was dissected and the presence of nodal disease: if dissection reveals positive lymph nodes, the dose is 60 Gy; if dissection reveals no evidence of nodal disease, the dose is 56 Gy; and if dissection was not done and nodal disease is not evident, the dose is 50 Gy, all delivered in 2-Gy fractions.

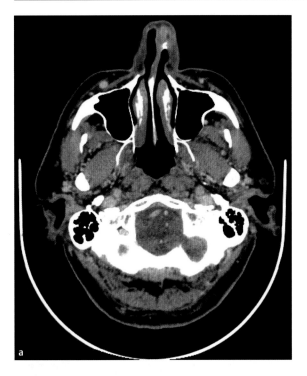

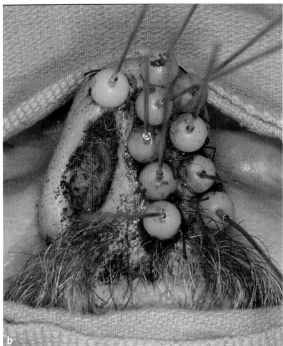

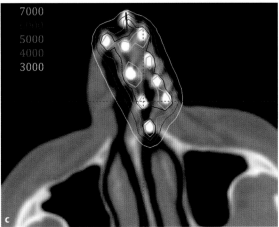

Fig. 20.1a–d An 87-year-old man presented with epistaxis. A biopsy of a 1-cm lesion at the anterior left nasal septum was positive for well-differentiated squamous cell carcinoma. CT of the head and neck reveals the lesion (**a**). He was treated with brachytherapy. Ten stainless-steel needles were placed in the left nasal ala, nasal tip, and left nasal septum (**b**) and were afterloaded with ^{192}Ir wires. A total dose of 60 Gy was delivered over 3.5 days. CT dosimetry was obtained and isodose distributions are shown on an axial plane through the tumor (**c**) and on a lateral view (**d**). The patient had no evidence of disease and no symptoms 3 years after treatment.

Patient Setup

For external beam radiotherapy to nasal vestibule tumors, the patient is positioned supine, with the neck slightly flexed so as to align the anterior surface of the maxilla perpendicular to the couch of the treatment table. The patient is immobilized with a customized mask, and an anterior appositional field is generally appropriate. For treatment of the primary tumor, skin collimation is used to minimize scattering of radiation to the eye and to reduce the beam penumbra. To avoid heterogeneity due to the oblique incidence and surface irregularity, customized beeswax material is commonly used to generate a flat surface contour for electrons. To reduce heterogeneities and avoid dose perturbations from air cavities when electron beams are used, tissue-equivalent material or "bolus" is used to fill the nares. An intraoral Cerrobend (Wood's metal)-containing stent is commonly used to displace the tongue posteriorly and to partially shield the upper alveolar ridge from the radiation.

The right and left facial lymphatics are irradiated with anterior appositional fields using ~15-degree gantry rotation to the respective side. Each field abuts both the appositional primary lesion portal and the upper neck fields. To reduce the risk of excessive heterogeneity at the abutment sites, the dose is feathered by incorporated junction shifts twice during the course of treatment. The submandibular and subdigastric nodes are treated with lateral parallel-opposed photon fields, and when nodes are involved, the middle and low neck nodes are treated with an anterior field matched to the lateral upper neck field.

Brachytherapy

Well-differentiated nasal vestibule tumors that are smaller than 1.5 cm in diameter and circumscribed can be treated with brachytherapy using iridium 192 (^{192}Ir) wire implants (**Fig. 20.1**) or, in selected cases, an intra-cavitary ^{192}Ir mold. The prescribed dose is 60 to 66 Gy over 5 to 7 days.

For larger tumors (i.e., >1.5 cm in diameter), a brachy-therapy boost to a dose of 20 to 25 Gy delivered over 2 days after 50 Gy of external beam radiotherapy would be appropriate. High–dose rate brachytherapy can also be used as a boost as follows. First, a customized mold of the nasal vestibule is fabricated and the tumor is marked in the mold; then two to four plastic tubes are placed, 1.0 cm apart, in the mold alongside the tumor. After delivery of 50 Gy of external beam radiotherapy, the high–dose rate brachytherapy is delivered twice daily during week 6 to a dose of 18 Gy at 3 Gy per fraction.

Nasal Fossa Tumors

External Beam Radiotherapy

The depth of the neoplasm in the nasal cavity, as deter-mined by both imaging and physical examination, dic-tates the appropriate radiotherapy technique. For tumors located within 4 cm from the apex of the nose, electrons are commonly used, and linear accelerators can generate electrons at energies up to 20 MeV that can provide cov-erage for tumors to a depth of 5 cm. To spare the skin, the lower half of the nose and the upper lip are treated with an anterior appositional field using 20-MeV electrons and 6-MV photons weighted 4:1. For tumors located within 4 cm of the apex of the nose, this practice allows a target volume that should include an additional 1 cm posterior to the tumor. The right and left facial lymphatics are irra-diated with anterior appositional fields using ~15-degree gantry rotation to the respective side with 6-MeV elec-tron fields. The upper neck nodes are treated with paral-lel-opposed lateral photon fields. The techniques applied for these lesions are consistent with those applied for nasal vestibule tumors as described above. The primary tumor is treated to 60 Gy (at 90%) in 30 fractions, and the electively treated facial and upper neck nodes are treated to 50 Gy in 25 fractions.

A conformal external beam radiation technique that is best suited for tumors that extend within the nasal cavity more than 4 cm from the apex of the nose is intensity-modulated radiotherapy (IMRT) (**Fig. 20.2**). Using 7 to 10 coplanar or noncoplanar beams, this technique can opti-mize tight conformality around the target volumes, mini-mize dose heterogeneity within the target volumes and organs at risk, and minimize the overall dose to critical organ structures. For primary radiotherapy, with or with-out chemotherapy, IMRT allows treatment to be acceler-ated with a simultaneous boost, with definitive doses of 70 Gy in 33 fractions (2.12 Gy/fraction) to the primary clinical target volume or CTV1, which equals the gross tumor volume plus a 1.0- to 1.5-cm margin; 63 Gy to the intermediate-risk microscopic tumor volume (CTV2); and 57 Gy to the low-risk microscopic volume (CTV3). For patients who had received induction chemotherapy, the CTV1 was contoured to include the gross disease present before the chemotherapy.

Postoperative radiotherapy for patients with nega-tive margins and no gross residual disease is delivered with doses of 60 Gy in 30 fractions to the primary tumor bed with a 1.0- to 1.5-cm margin (CTV1); 57 Gy to the intermediate-risk microscopic volumes; and 54 Gy to the low-risk microscopic volumes. For postoperative radiotherapy for patients with positive margins or gross residual disease, doses of 66 to 70 Gy to the target vol-ume with a 1.0- to 1.5-cm margin would be appropriate. If perineural invasion is identified, the microscopic CTV should encompass the tract of the maxillary cranial nerve V2 to the foramen rotundum.

If IMRT is not available, three-dimensional (3D) con-formal radiotherapy with CT-based treatment planning should be used, with anterior oblique wedge-pair photon fields for lesions located in the anterior lower half of the nasal cavity or opposed-lateral fields for tumors located at the posterior part of the nasal fossa. Dose–volume histograms should be generated to evaluate the doses to critical organ structures such as the optic apparatus, brain, brainstem, and spinal cord. The dose schedule for primary radiation using 3D conformal radiotherapy is 66 to 70 Gy in 33 to 35 fractions (2 Gy/fraction) to CTV1, 60 Gy to CTV2, and 50 Gy to CTV3. Postoperative radio-therapy for patients without gross disease and negative surgical margins consists of 60 Gy in 30 fractions (2 Gy/fraction) prescribed to CTV1, 56 Gy to CTV2, and 50 Gy to CTV3. Postoperative radiotherapy for patients with posi-tive margins should include an additional boost of 6 Gy for a total dose of 66 Gy in 33 fractions.

Techniques for the delivery of proton radiotherapy are rapidly evolving. Theoretically, the advantage of proton therapy derives from the unique physical properties of protons that allow deposition of most of the particles' energy at the end of its range. Descriptions of the vari-ous techniques by which proton therapy can be delivered

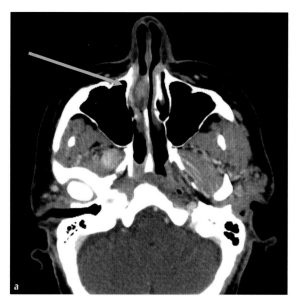

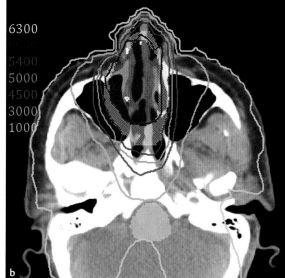

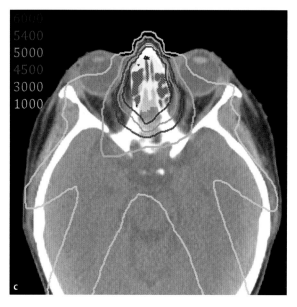

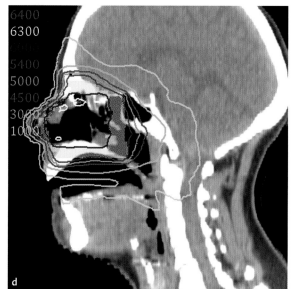

Fig. 20.2a–e A 60-year-old woman presented with nasal obstruction and epistaxis. She was found to have a lesion in the posterior right nasal septum. Biopsy was positive for squamous cell carcinoma; (**a**) shows the tumor (green arrow) in an axial slice of diagnostic CT scan. She underwent an endoscopic resection of the tumor. Margins were negative but contained high-grade dysplasia. She was then treated with postoperative IMRT. A mouth-opening, tongue-depressing stent was used to minimize dose to the oral structures. As the vCTV was relatively small, it was elected to omit CTV_{ID} but define CTV_{HD} fairly generously to include the septum and right nasal cavity. The remaining left nasal cavity, medial aspect of the right maxillary sinus, hard palate (floor of the nasal cavity), anterior sphenoid sinus, and ethmoid sinuses were defined as CTV_{ED}. CTV_{HD} and CTV_{ED} were prescribed 60 and 54 Gy, respectively, and treatment was delivered in 30 fractions. An axial view of the isodose distribution is shown through the midnose (**b**) along with CTV_{HD} (*red*) and CTV_{ED} (*yellow*). A second axial view (**c**) through the ethmoids and orbits shows only CTV_{ED} at this level. The doses to the optic nerves and lenses were <45 and <10 Gy, respectively. Isodose distributions in sagittal (**d**) and coronal (**e**) views through midplane of the head are also shown. The contour colorwash inside the 60-Gy line is removed so the underlying resected tissues can be appreciated. The mouth-opening stent can also be seen on these views. The patient has done well and is without disease 3 years later.

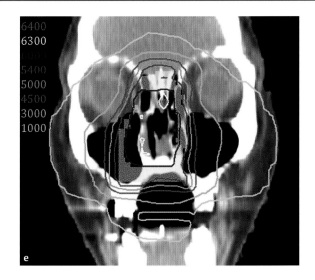

(e.g., passive scattering, single-field uniform dose optimization, and intensity-modulated proton therapy) are beyond the scope of this chapter. Nevertheless, with optimization of dosimetry, the conformality and heterogeneity within the target volumes provided by proton therapy should be equivalent to that which can be achieved with IMRT, with the added advantage of minimizing the unnecessary dose or "dose bath" to the surrounding normal tissue structures.

Patient Setup For External Beam Radiotherapy

The setup for patients with tumors up to 4 cm from the apex of the nose is similar to that described for nasal vestibule carcinomas when electrons are to be used. Several treatment devices can be used to optimize conformality, minimize dose heterogeneity, and protect critical organ structures. For example, lead skin collimators can be used to sharpen the penumbra; bolus material can be used to provide greater dose homogeneity within the air cavities; intraoral stents can be used to depress the tongue out of the treatment field; and tungsten eye shields can be used if the target volume puts the cornea at risk.

For IMRT or 3D conformal radiotherapy, the patient is positioned supine, with the head resting comfortably on a head-and-neck holder and the neck slightly flexed such that the nasal floor is perpendicular to the couch of the treatment table. Scars are marked with radiopaque wires with a 3- to 5-mm bolus encompassing each scar with a 1.0-cm margin. An intraoral stent is commonly used to depress the tongue out of the treatment field. A thermoplastic mask is necessary for rigid immobilization of the head and shoulders, and the shoulders can be depressed and fixed by using wrist straps tethered to a footboard. CT-based treatment simulation is used to generate images for treatment planning purposes.

Brachytherapy

For small anteroinferior septal lesions, a single-plane brachytherapy implant encompassing the gross disease with a 2-cm margin can be considered. As a general rule, the required activity for single-plane implants is 0.5 to 0.7 mCi per cm radium equivalent for sources spaced 1 cm apart. For low–dose rate brachytherapy implants, the dose schedule is 60 to 66 Gy over 5 to 7 days. The isodose contour that will cover the target volume should ensure that the volume of dose heterogeneity around the sources is minimized.

Tumors of the Paranasal Sinuses (Maxillary, Ethmoid, Sphenoid, and Frontal)

Treatment Principles

Paranasal Sinus Tumors

Surgery as single-modality therapy can produce excellent control rates for T1 maxillary sinus tumors. Surgery followed by postoperative radiotherapy is generally indicated for T2 and small T3 lesions. However, maxillary sinus tumors often present as locally advanced disease (large T3 or T4), and surgery followed by adjuvant radiotherapy has been the mainstay of treatment. Ethmoid sinus carcinomas are commonly managed with surgery and postoperative radiotherapy. For older patients, patients with significant comorbid conditions, and patients with poor performance status, primary radiotherapy, with or without chemotherapy, can be considered.

Use of neoadjuvant chemotherapy (i.e., before surgery) can in some cases reduce the tumor volume so as to facilitate less severe surgical resection and orbital exenteration. Chemotherapy before primary radiotherapy can also reduce the tumor volume and increase the distance between tumor borders and critical organ structures such as the brain, chiasm, optic nerve, and spinal cord, which can improve both treatment planning and the therapeutic ratio of the radiotherapy. Investigative studies are currently ongoing to determine whether the response to neoadjuvant chemotherapy can help in the choice of definitive treatment strategies. For example, if induction chemotherapy produces a complete response, then primary radiotherapy, with or without chemotherapy, can be considered; a less-than-complete response would prompt surgical excision of the lesion followed by adjuvant radiation therapy.

Concurrent chemoradiotherapy can also be used for patients with medical conditions that preclude surgery if those patients have good performance status. Depending on the patient's performance status and renal function, single-agent cisplatin or carboplatin can be used concurrently with external beam radiotherapy for locally advanced, unresectable squamous cell carcinoma. Neoadjuvant chemotherapy or concurrent chemoradiotherapy with etoposide and cisplatin or carboplatin can be used to treat sinonasal undifferentiated carcinoma, neuroendocrine carcinoma, or small cell carcinoma.

A 1991 review of outcomes after treatment of maxillary sinus carcinomas at MD Anderson Cancer Center[18] reported 5-year local and regional control rates according to pathological T category as follows: 91% local and 71% regional for T1–T2 tumors; 77% local and 80% regional for T3 tumors; and 65% local and 93% regional for T4 tumors. Five-year regional control rates according to N category were 84% for N0 disease and 82% for N1–N2 disease. The most common histological subtypes were squamous cell carcinoma (36 of 73 patients) and adenoid cystic carcinoma (20 patients); 5-year local and regional control rates were 62% (local) and 86% (regional) for squamous cell tumors and 82% (local) and 94% (regional) for adenoid tumors. Perineural invasion and nodal disease at presentation were poor prognostic factors.[18] An update of this report in 2007 showed that increasing the radiation portals to cover the skull base for patients with perineural invasion reduced the risk of local recurrence, and the addition of elective nodal irradiation for patients with squamous or undifferentiated tumors improved the rates of nodal control, distant metastasis, and recurrence-free survival.[19] Five-year outcomes from studies reported since 1998 after treatment of paranasal sinus malignancies continue to illustrate that local control remains problematic (**Table 20.3**).[19,20–24] The role of neoadjuvant or concurrent systemic therapy for such tumors is the subject of ongoing investigation.

The extent of neuroendocrine differentiation of sinonasal carcinomas influences the patterns of failure. In one study,[16] the 5-year actuarial rates of local, regional, and distant failure according to tumor histology were as follows: esthesioneuroblastoma—4% local failure, 9% regional failure, and 0% distant failure; neuroendocrine carcinoma—27% local, 13% regional, and 12% distant; sinonasal undifferentiated carcinoma—21% local, 16% regional, and 25% distant; and small cell carcinoma—33% local failure, 44% regional failure, and 75% distant failure.

Radiotherapy Techniques[17]

Sinus Tumors

IMRT is the preferred external beam radiotherapy technique because of the proximity of the tumor and postoperative resected cavities to the orbit, cranial nerve foramina, optic chiasm, brain, and brainstem. Delineation of the target volumes should be based on pretreatment imaging, physical examination, and both intraoperative and pathological findings. Definitive doses for primary radiotherapy are 66 to 70 Gy in 33 fractions (2.12 Gy/fraction) to the primary clinical target volume (CTV1, equal to the gross tumor volume plus a 1.0- to 1.5-cm margin); 63 Gy to the intermediate-risk microscopic tumor volume (CTV2); and 57 Gy to the low-risk microscopic volume (CTV3). During treatment planning, heterogeneity corrections should be incorporated into the dosimetric calculations to account for the significant amounts of air and bone within the sinuses.

Conventional treatment borders are determined primarily by the location and size of the tumor. For tumors of the infrastructure with no extension into the orbit or ethmoids, anterior and ipsilateral wedge-pair photon fields are commonly used. Placing the isocenter at the level of the orbital floor and shielding the upper half of the field avoids exposure of the contralateral eye from beam divergence. Lateral-opposed photon fields are preferred for tumors located in the infrastructure that spread across the midline through the hard palate. A three-field technique is preferred for tumors of the ethmoids or superstructure. Prescribed doses for conventional postoperative radiotherapy are 60 Gy to CTV1, 56 Gy to CTV2, and 50 Gy to CTV3, all delivered at 2 Gy/fraction.

Table 20.3 Recent studies of paranasal sinus cancer: control and survival rates at 5 years

Study authors and reference	No. of patients	Local control (%)	Regional control (%)	Distant control (%)	Overall survival (%)
Paulino et al 1998[23]	48	59	71	83	47
Le et al 1999[24]	97	43	90	66	34
Myers et al 2002[21]	170	46	96	67	52
Blanco et al 2004[20]	106	58	39[a]	71	27
Hoppe et al 2007[22]	85	62	87	82	67
Bristol et al 2007[19]	146	70	83	83	62

[a] Reported as locoregional control rate.

Patients presenting with squamous cell or poorly differentiated carcinoma and no adenopathy should receive elective nodal irradiation to the ipsilateral submandibular and subdigastric nodes to a dose of 50 to 54 Gy in 25 to 30 fractions.[19] Patients presenting with lymph node–positive disease require treatment of the whole ipsilateral neck or bilateral neck. The upper neck can be treated with IMRT to spare the parotid glands or with conventional electron beam therapy. To minimize unnecessary irradiation of the larynx, a monoisocentric technique with IMRT for the upper neck and an oblique low neck field using an asymmetric jaw for optimal matching is commonly used. For patients with negative surgical margins and nodal disease found at neck dissection, IMRT to a dose of 60 Gy in 30 fractions (at 2 Gy/fraction) is prescribed to the postoperative bed (CTV1), 57 Gy to CTV2 (at 1.9 Gy/fraction), and 54 Gy to CTV3 (at 1.8 Gy/fraction).

Patient Setup

For IMRT or 3D conformal radiotherapy, the patient is positioned supine, with the head resting comfortably on a head-and-neck holder and the neck slightly flexed such that the floor of the orbit is perpendicular to the couch of the treatment table. Scars are marked with radiopaque wires with a 3- to 5-mm bolus encompassing each scar with a 1.0-cm margin. An intraoral stent is commonly used to depress the tongue out of the treatment field. A thermoplastic mask is necessary for rigid immobilization of the head and shoulders, and the shoulders can be depressed and fixed by using wrist straps tethered to a footboard. CT-based treatment simulation is used to generate images for treatment planning purposes.

Future Directions in Radiotherapy

IMRT is rapidly becoming the standard-of-care external beam treatment technique for sinonasal malignancies.[22,25,26] The role of proton beam therapy for nasal and paranasal sinus tumors is currently being investigated; this form of therapy may confer additional advantages over IMRT by limiting the radiation dose bath to normal critical tissue structures. Well-designed clinical trials in a cooperative group setting will be necessary to provide the evidence required for widespread adoption of proton therapy over IMRT for these rare malignancies. Finally, further improvements in the local control of sinonasal malignancies will require incorporating systemic agents in neoadjuvant or concurrent therapy. The rarity of sinonasal cancer will most likely require international cooperative group trials to facilitate timely analyses of outcomes and design of future trials.

References

1. Greenlee RT, Hill-Harmon MB, Murray T, Thun M. Cancer statistics, 2001. CA Cancer J Clin 2001;51(1):15–36
2. Million RR. The myth regarding bone or cartilage involvement by cancer and the likelihood of cure by radiotherapy. Head Neck 1989;11(1):30–40
3. Wong CS, Cummings BJ, Elhakim T, Briant TD. External irradiation for squamous cell carcinoma of the nasal vestibule. Int J Radiat Oncol Biol Phys 1986;12(11):1943–1946
4. Chobe R, McNeese M, Weber R, Fletcher GH. Radiation therapy for carcinoma of the nasal vestibule. Otolaryngol Head Neck Surg 1988;98(1):67–71
5. McCollough WM, Mendenhall NP, Parsons JT, et al. Radiotherapy alone for squamous cell carcinoma of the nasal vestibule: management of the primary site and regional lymphatics. Int J Radiat Oncol Biol Phys 1993;26(1):73–79
6. Mak AC, van Andel JG, van Woerkom-Eijkenboom WM. Radiation therapy of carcinoma of the nasal vestibule. Eur J Cancer 1980;16(1):81–85
7. Langendijk JA, Poorter R, Leemans CR, de Bree R, Doornaert P, Slotman BJ. Radiotherapy of squamous cell carcinoma of the nasal vestibule. Int J Radiat Oncol Biol Phys 2004;59(5):1319–1325
8. Wallace A, Morris CG, Kirwan J, Amdur RJ, Werning JW, Mendenhall WM. Radiotherapy for squamous cell carcinoma of the nasal vestibule. Am J Clin Oncol 2007; 30(6):612–616
9. Dowley A, Hoskison E, Allibone R, Jones NS. Squamous cell carcinoma of the nasal vestibule: a 20-year case series and literature review. J Laryngol Otol 2008;122(10):1019–1023
10. Agger A, von Buchwald C, Madsen AR, et al. Squamous cell carcinoma of the nasal vestibule 1993–2002: a nationwide retrospective study from DAHANCA. Head Neck 2009;31(12):1593–1599
11. Poulsen M, Turner S. Radiation therapy for squamous cell carcinoma of the nasal vestibule. Int J Radiat Oncol Biol Phys 1993;27(2):267–272
12. Ang KK, Jiang GL, Frankenthaler RA, et al. Carcinomas of the nasal cavity. Radiother Oncol 1992;24(3):163–168
13. Badib AO, Kurohara SS, Webster JH, Shedd DP. Treatment of cancer of the nasal cavity. Am J Roentgenol Radium Ther Nucl Med 1969;106(4):824–830
14. Bosch A, Vallecillo L, Frias Z. Cancer of the nasal cavity. Cancer 1976;37(3):1458–1463
15. Hawkins RB, Wynstra JH, Pilepich MV, Fields JN. Carcinoma of the nasal cavity—results of primary and adjuvant radiotherapy. Int J Radiat Oncol Biol Phys 1988; 15(5):1129–1133
16. Rosenthal DI, Barker JL Jr, El-Naggar AK, et al. Sinonasal malignancies with neuroendocrine differentiation: patterns of failure according to histologic phenotype. Cancer 2004;101(11):2567–2573
17. Ang KK, Garden AS. Radiotherapy for Head and Neck Cancers: Indications and Techniques. 3rd ed. Philadelphia: Lippincott Williams and Williams; 2006
18. Jiang GL, Ang KK, Peters LJ, Wendt CD, Oswald MJ, Goepfert H. Maxillary sinus carcinomas: natural history and results of postoperative radiotherapy. Radiother Oncol 1991;21(3):193–200
19. Bristol IJ, Ahamad A, Garden AS, et al. Postoperative radiotherapy for maxillary sinus cancer: long-term outcomes and toxicities of treatment. Int J Radiat Oncol Biol Phys 2007;68(3):719–730
20. Blanco AI, Chao KSC, Ozyigit G, et al. Carcinoma of paranasal sinuses: long-term outcomes with radiotherapy. Int J Radiat Oncol Biol Phys 2004;59(1):51–58

21. Myers LL, Nussenbaum B, Bradford CR, Teknos TN, Esclamado RM, Wolf GT. Paranasal sinus malignancies: an 18-year single institution experience. Laryngoscope 2002;112(11):1964–1969

22. Hoppe BS, Stegman LD, Zelefsky MJ, et al. Treatment of nasal cavity and paranasal sinus cancer with modern radiotherapy techniques in the postoperative setting—the MSKCC experience. Int J Radiat Oncol Biol Phys 2007;67(3):691–702

23. Paulino AC, Marks JE, Bricker P, Melian E, Reddy SP, Emami B. Results of treatment of patients with maxillary sinus carcinoma. Cancer 1998;83(3):457–465

24. Le QT, Fu KK, Kaplan M, Terris DJ, Fee WE, Goffinet DR. Treatment of maxillary sinus carcinoma: a comparison of the 1997 and 1977 American Joint Committee on cancer staging systems. Cancer 1999;86(9):1700–1711

25. Myers LL, Nussenbaum B, Bradford CR, Teknos TN, Esclamado RM, Wolf GT. Paranasal sinus malignancies: an 18-year single institution experience. Laryngoscope 2002;112(11):1964–1969

26. Dirix P, Vanstraelen B, Jorissen M, Vander Poorten V, Nuyts S. Intensity-modulated radiotherapy for sinonasal cancer: improved outcome compared to conventional radiotherapy. Int J Radiat Oncol Biol Phys 2010;78(4):998–1004

21 Rehabilitation

Physical

In addition to reconstruction of the skull base and orbit, which have been covered in Chapter 19, there are several other aspects that should be considered when the upper jaw is involved. These may be divided into temporary and permanent, and the choice is dependent on the extent of the defect and factors related to the patient and facilities available.

A classification system has been proposed for maxillary and midface defects (**Fig. 21.1**)[1,2] that assists in these decisions, but whatever the choice, the involvement of a team that includes both prosthodontists and maxillofacial technicians is necessary as well as dietetic and psychological support.

In Class I where only a portion of the alveolus has been resected, a local flap and/or modification of an existing denture may suffice. Similarly, small midline palatal defects may be closed with mucosal flaps or a small obturator can be used (**Fig. 21.2**).

Class II, which represents a partial maxillectomy without loss of the orbital floor, also does well with obturation. At the time of surgery, a temporary obturator can be fashioned with material such as gutta percha on a modified preexisting or new denture plate, taking account of the surgical cavity and any hemostatic packing (**Fig. 21.3 a, b**). This allows the patient to eat, drink, and speak immediately following the surgery. It can be removed and modified over the immediate postoperative period as packing is removed and a new lightweight obturator can be made in due course to more accurately conform to the cavity as it alters with healing (**Figs. 21.4, 21.5, 21.6**).

To improve retention and stability, an implant-retained prosthesis may be used, particularly when the defect is larger (**Fig 21.7 a–d**). In contrast, a variety of free vascularized flaps may also be used, including fibula, iliac crest, and scapula flaps. The scapula flap may be based on the angular branch of the thoracodorsal artery or circumflex scapula artery, of which the former offers a longer pedicle.

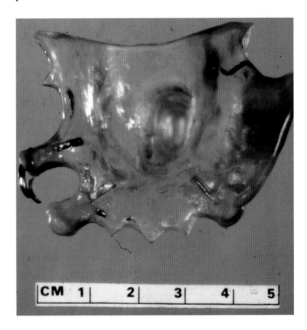

Fig. 21.2 Photograph of small lightweight definitive acrylic prosthesis to obturate a limited palatal defect and augment missing upper left dentition.

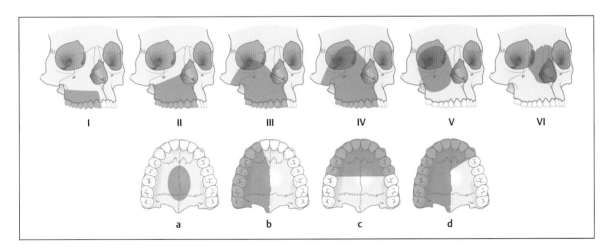

Fig. 21.1 Classification of maxillary and midface defects.[3] Classes I to VI show the vertical component of the defect and a to d the palatal and dentoalveolar component, which is associated with increasing difficulty in obtaining good results with a prosthesis.

(After Head and Neck Cancer: Multidisciplinary Guidelines. 4th ed. London: British Association of Otorhinolaryngology 2011:314 with permission.)

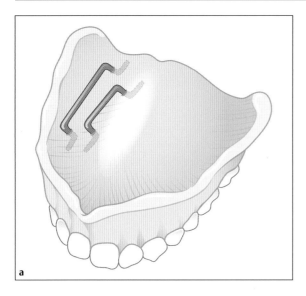

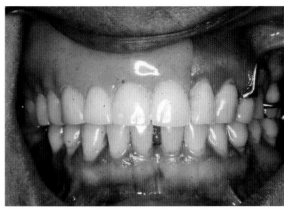

Fig. 21.4 Photograph showing a patient with a lightweight definitive maxillary obturator in place on the right side, constructed to take advantage of undercuts and further stabilized by stainless clasps fitted around the residual left upper dentition.

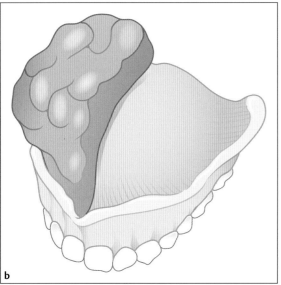

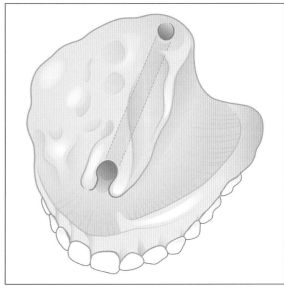

Fig. 21.3a, b

a Drawing of an existing removable prosthesis where the denture base has been modified to support and retain gutta percha applied at the end of the total maxillectomy operation.

b Drawing of the immediate replacement obturator, to make which the gutta percha (previously heated in near-boiling water for 3 to 4 minutes) is then heated with a flame to adhere to the denture surface and retention loops. This obturator is placed in the maxillectomy defect and molded to the tissues to neatly fill the defect.

Fig. 21.5 Different designs and materials have been used following maxillectomy. This drawing shows a lightweight hollow box acrylic obturator with a nasal airway.

Class III defects include the orbital floor and may extend into the nasal bridge. In the past if the orbital periosteum was intact, obturators alone were still the rehabilitation of choice, but in recent years pedicled or free vascularized flaps are most often used, often in combination with an implant-retained prosthesis (**Fig. 21.5**). Adequate support of the eye is essential if ectropion, conjunctival exposure, epiphora, and diplopia are to be avoided (Chapter 19). Many options of varying complexity have been described in the literature,[3] some representing the triumph of technique over common sense. The rectus abdominis, latissimus dorsi, scapula, rib, or fibula are commonly used, but it should be remembered that transplanted bone in the more complex osseomusculocutaneous flaps may not withstand postoperative radiotherapy.

Fig. 21.6 Photograph of a lightweight acrylic two-part maxillary obturator. This patient had significant trismus following postoperative radiotherapy and the design facilitates insertion in two parts.

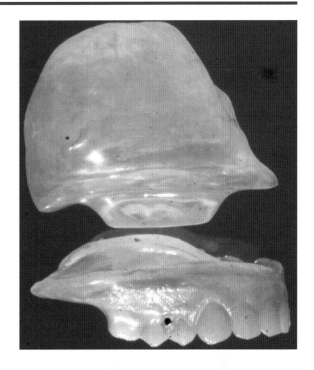

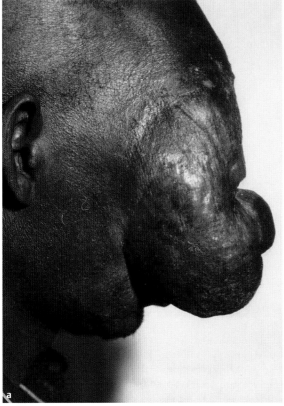

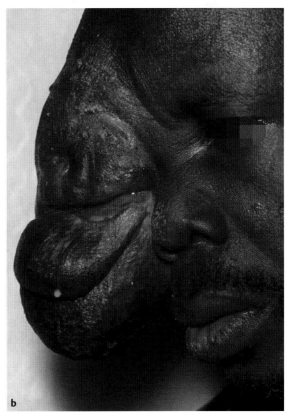

Fig. 21.7a–d

a, b A traffic policeman from Uganda with a 7-year history of gross proptosis, blindness, and then a steadily increasing mass. This proved to be a huge benign pleomorphic adenoma extending from the midpoint of the anterior cranial fossa inferiorly as

shown. After its removal by craniofacial resection, it appeared that it probably arose from the right lacrimal gland and had destroyed the orbit, skull base, upper maxilla, and anterior cranial bone.

Fig. 21.7c–d ▷

◁ continued

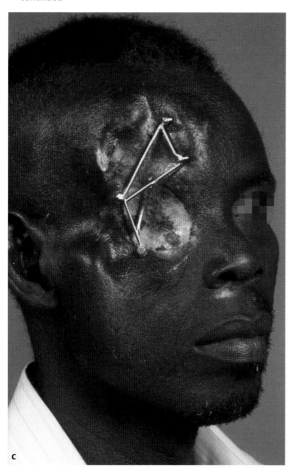

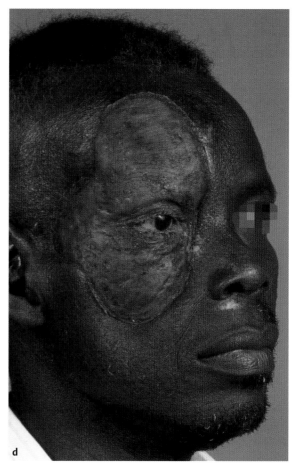

c   The patient tolerated the surgery extremely well and recovered to have the osseointegrated framework installed.

d   The initial prosthesis was a little too dark for skin color match, as the patient's facial skin lightened during his 6 weeks in a UK winter environment. A second, lighter prosthesis was provided. He remained alive and well at 5-year follow-up and was delighted with the result.

Class IV involves a more extensive orbital defect that may be treated with soft tissue alone in the form of a rectus abdominis flap, but inclusion of bone as in the iliac crest with the internal oblique can provide better implant options.

In Class V, where the orbit has been cleared and an orbital prosthesis is required, a less bulky repair is preferred such as temporalis muscle or a temporoparietal flap. Other options to consider are a radial forearm or anterolateral thigh flaps.

Class VI encompasses a large midfacial defect including skin, soft tissues, and nasal structure as in a rhinectomy. If there is sufficient bony support, an entire osseointegrated nasal prosthesis may be considered, although patients are often resistant to the concept of a "plastic nose." Reconstruction using a radial forearm flap with associated skin and fascia is an option. This may be augmented by glabellar or even forehead flaps in the older patient, though both require some form of internal support. Patients should understand that such complex reconstructive surgery may require several subsequent procedures to refine the result, especially if postoperative radiotherapy is given.

Psychological

Malignant disease in many parts of the body can become quite extensive, undergo substantial medical and surgical oncological treatment, and ultimately kill the patient and yet remain relatively discreet to the bitter end. By contrast, tumors in the sinonasal region may be initially quite innocuous in their symptoms, thus presenting late, but are often far from inconspicuous when major surgery and chemoradiotherapy is required, and in their terminal stages with large local recurrence. In the United Kingdom, we are extremely fortunate to have a well-established and well-organized system of palliative care, but even these services may be unable to cope with a fungating facial mass or major epistaxis.

There is an enormous literature on the psychological effects of facial disfigurement, which is beyond the scope of this book, but we should be aware of the significant effects that sinonasal tumors and their treatment have on our patients, impacting as they do on most of the senses (smell, vision, and taste) as well as the cosmetic impact and problems of crusting in the surgical cavity and/or dealing with a prosthesis.[4] The dramatic effects on quality of life are documented elsewhere (Chapter 19, pp. 510–512) and this is an area of considerable importance when assessing the success of treatment.

Previous studies have shown that even when the patients are cured by procedures with a relatively low morbidity such as craniofacial resection, they are still markedly affected by the associated loss of smell from resection of the olfactory epithelium, bulbs, and tract.[5] It may be that endoscopic techniques can go some way to ameliorating this by preservation of the contralateral side, but subsequent chemotherapy and radiotherapy are likely to undo any benefit that this may provide.[6–9] It may even be possible in the future to improve olfaction, given the ability of olfactory epithelium to regenerate and the progress in stem cell research.[10]

Access to a cancer nurse is very valuable as they have the time and training to discuss the patients' and their families' concerns and problems. Many departments now provide written information on the treatments that patients are about to undergo, which may go some way to allaying their fears. However, ready access to the clinicians is extremely important and regular follow-up during and after treatment is essential, not only for reassurance but also to detect residual disease or recurrence as early as possible. This is particularly important if cure is not possible when continued symptomatic care and psychological support are vital.

Palliative Care

The term "palliative" derives from *palliare*, which is Latin for "cloak." Thus, as patients approach the end of life, we should take care that we improve its quality rather than adversely affecting it with treatments that are unlikely to work, that have significant side effects, or that offer false hopes. There is still much that can be done and ideally this care should be delivered by a group that includes social workers, psychologists, and dietitians as well as the surgical and medical oncologists.

Treatments will include control of pain, adequate fluid and nutrition, management of airway, epistaxis, and visual loss, as well as control of anxiety and depression. In addition, judicious debulking of large tumors and long-term packing (e.g., with Whitehead's varnish–soaked gauze) may help in selected cases, particularly where bleeding is a problem. Short courses and/or hypofractionation regimes of radiotherapy may be used, particularly for pain from local disease or bony metastases. The potential side effects of this alone or in combination with chemotherapy must be balanced against any benefit and will not be appropriate in many cases.

Pain is not usually a major issue in sinonasal disease until the cranial nerves become involved. In addition to the WHO Pain Ladder proposals (**Table 21.1**), neuropathic pain may be helped by drugs such as amitriptyline, gabapentin, and carbamazepine. The latter is often helpful with the pain associated with nerve involvement in adenoid cystic carcinoma. A short course of corticosteroids—for example, dexamethasone 8 to 16 mg/day—may be considered for acute neuropathic pain and optic neuritis but is rarely effective in the longer term.[11]

Table 21.1 WHO pain ladder

1. Paracetamol ± nonsteroidal anti-inflammatory drugs
2. Weak opioid (codeine or tramadol) + step 1 drugs
3. Strong opioid replacing the weak + step 1 drugs

References

1. Brown JS, Shaw RJ. Reconstruction of the maxilla and midface: introducing a new classification. Lancet Oncol 2010;11(10):1001–1008
2. Head and Neck Cancer: Multidisciplinary Management Guidelines. 4th ed. London: British Association of Otorhinolaryngology; 2011:313–315
3. Suárez C, Ferlito A, Lund VJ, et al. Management of the orbit in malignant sinonasal tumors. Head Neck 2008; 30(2):242–250
4. Moolenburgh SE, Mureau MA, Versnel SL, Duivenvoorden HJ, Hofer SO. The impact of nasal reconstruction following tumour resection on psychosocial functioning, a clinical-empirical exploration. Psychooncology 2009; 18(7):747–752
5. Jones E, Lund VJ, Howard DJ, Greenberg MP, McCarthy M. Quality of life of patients treated surgically for head and neck cancer. J Laryngol Otol 1992;106(3):238–242
6. Ho WK, Kwong DL, Wei WI, Sham JS. Change in olfaction after radiotherapy for nasopharyngeal cancer—a prospective study. Am J Otolaryngol 2002;23(4):209–214
7. Hölscher T, Seibt A, Appold S, et al. Effects of radiotherapy on olfactory function. Radiother Oncol 2005;77(2):157–163
8. Müller A, Landis BN, Platzbecker U, Holthoff V, Frasnelli J, Hummel T. Severe chemotherapy-induced parosmia. Am J Rhinol 2006;20(4):485–486
9. Lund VJ, Stammberger H, Nicolai P, et al. European position paper on endoscopic management of tumours of the nose, paranasal sinuses and skull base. Rhinol Suppl 2010; (22):1–143
10. Vats A, Birchall M. Stem cells and regenerative medicine: potentials and realities for rhinology. Rhinology 2010;48(3):259–264
11. Hardy JR, Rees E, Ling J, et al. A prospective survey of the use of dexamethasone on a palliative care unit. Palliat Med 2001;15(1):3–8

Section II Nasopharynx

22 Anatomy and Pathologies

Anatomy

The pharynx, an incomplete muscular tubular structure, is divided into nasopharynx, oropharynx, and hypopharynx depending on its relationship with the oral cavity. Anatomically, the nasopharynx is above the oral cavity, the oropharynx is at the same level as the oral cavity, and the hypopharynx is below the oral cavity.

The nasopharynx is located behind the nasal cavity and it continues inferiorly into the oropharynx. It is a potential space enclosed by roof, floor, and posterior and lateral walls. The superior constrictor forms the muscular wall of the nasopharynx on the posterior and lateral walls only. The average anteroposterior distance ranges from 2 to 3 cm while both the transverse and vertical diameters range from 3 to 4 cm. There are considerable variations between individuals and, even in one person, its volume and shape change with the position of the patient and during various movements of the organs of the oral cavity.[1]

Anteriorly, the two choanae of the nasal cavity continue into the nasopharynx, where the posterior edge of the nasal septum that separates the choanae constitutes part of the anterior wall. The roof is formed by the continuation of the rostrum posterior to the undersurface of the body of the sphenoid, which slopes backward and downward to merge with the posterior wall. The posterior wall is formed by the anterior surface of the arch of the atlas and the upper portion of the body of the axis. The floor opens into the oropharynx and, when the soft palate moves upward to close this potential space, the pharyngeal isthmus, the upper surface of the soft palate becomes the floor of the nasopharynx (**Fig. 22.1**).

High on the lateral wall of the nasopharynx is the orifice of the eustachian tube, followed inferiorly by the superior constrictor muscle. The pharyngeal openings of the eustachian tube are enclosed by an incomplete cartilaginous ring, which is deficient inferolaterally. This cartilaginous ring on the medial side of the opening forms an elevation of mucosa; this is the torus tubarius. Medial to this elevation is the pharyngeal recess or fossa of Rosenmüller, which is a slitlike space of variable depth, shape, and size (**Fig. 22.2**). The opening of the recess may be narrow or wide and the recess may extend laterally, occasionally to above the superior constrictor muscle. The fossa of Rosenmüller is the most common site where NPC is found. Tumor in the fossa may infiltrate nearby structures before growing into the lumen of the nasopharynx. Due to the close proximity of the fossa to structures at the skull base, these structures may be affected early in the course of the disease and contribute to the presenting clinical features.

The epithelial lining of the nasopharynx mainly consists of pseudostratified ciliated columnar cells; this starts at the choana area and extends to the roof and lateral wall. In the posterior wall most of the lining epithelium is composed of stratified squamous cells. These epithelial cells lie on a distinct basement membrane and the lamina propria contains abundant lymphoid tissue (**Fig. 22.3**).

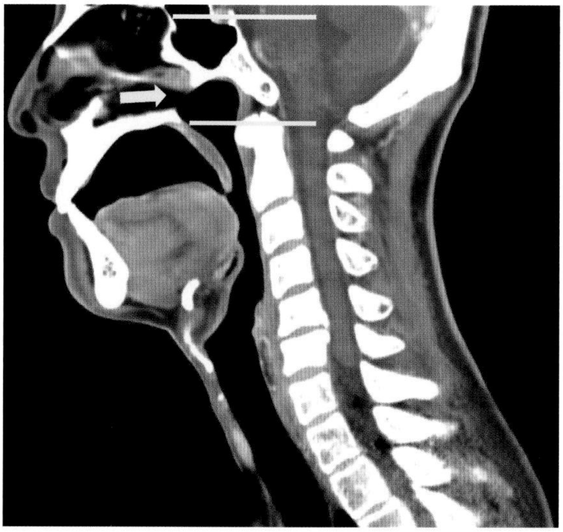

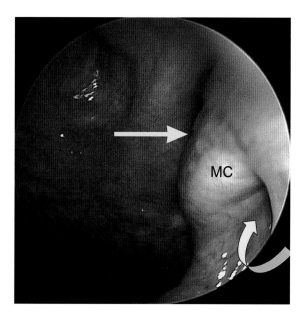

Fig. 22.1 CT image showing the boundaries of the nasopharynx. Upper line, level of the floor of the sphenoid sinus; lower line, level of the palate; arrow, the posterior choana.

Fig. 22.2 Endoscopic view of the nasopharynx showing the medial crura (MC), the eustachian tube orifice (curved arrow), and the fossa of Rosenmüller (arrow).

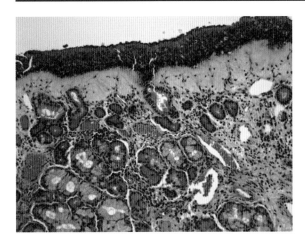

Fig. 22.3 Pseudostratified ciliated columnar cells lining of normal nasopharynx. Below the epithelium there is abundant glandular tissue with lymphocytes (hematoxylin and eosin, ×200).

The enclosing muscular layer comprises the superior constrictor muscle that is deficient in the upper part of the lateral wall where the eustachian tube passes medially, separating it from the upper edge of the muscle and the skull base. External to and enclosing the muscle is the pharyngobasilar fascia, which covers the posterior and lateral aspects of the superior constrictor. This fascia is attached to the basiocciput superiorly and forms a median raphe in the posterior midline. This pharyngobasilar fascia is a solid sheet of fibrous tissue that extends laterally to the medial pterygoid plate while inferiorly it merges with the buccopharyngeal fascia. Posteriorly, behind the superior constrictor are the prevertebral muscles with the prevertebral fascia and then the vertebrae.

The fascia around the nasopharynx form a few potential spaces and each of them contains important structures. These spaces to some extent influence the pathway of tumor spread.

1. The retropharyngeal space lies between the pharyngobasilar fascia and the prevertebral fascia, and is a part of the retrostyloid portion of the paranasopharyngeal space. It is found on both sides, paramedian in location, situated lateral to the median raphe of the pharyngobasilar fascia. The retropharyngeal space contains the lymph node of Rouvière, the first lymph node station that may be affected when a tumor extends through the lymphatic channel (**Fig. 22.4**).
2. The parapharyngeal space is lateral to the pharynx and is divided by the styloid process and its attachments into the prestyloid and retrostyloid compartments. The former is located lateral to the fossa of Rosenmüller and contains the maxillary artery and nerves. The more posteromedially retrostyloid located compartment contains the contents of the carotid sheath, the last four cranial nerves, the sympathetic trunk, and the

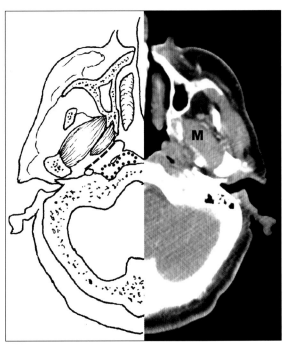

Fig. 22.4 CT (right) and line drawing (left) showing the medial pterygoid muscle (M); the dotted line joining the pterygoid plate and the styloid process is an imaginary line that divides the paranasopharyngeal space, the prestyloid space (lateral to the line), and the poststyloid space (medial to the line). The space enclosed by the dotted line is the retropharyngeal space.

upper deep cervical lymph nodes (**Fig. 22.5**). The tumor in the nasopharynx involves the prestyloid compartment by direct extension, and once there it may infiltrate the maxillary nerve and, extending upward, the trigeminal nerve. The retrostyloid compartment can be affected either by direct tumor extension and invasion or by lymphatic spread. The associated symptoms reflect the involvement of the respective cranial nerves.

The arterial supplies of the nasopharynx are abundant; these are the ascending pharyngeal, ascending palatine, and pharyngeal branches of the sphenopalatine artery, all of which originate from the external carotid artery. The venous plexus beneath the mucosal membrane communicates with the nearby pterygoid plexus. There is a well-developed submucosal plexus of lymph vessels in the nasopharynx that drains primarily into the retropharyngeal lymph nodes and sometimes directly to the cervical nodes. Efferents from the retropharyngeal group of nodes drain to the deep cervical lymph nodes. As the nasopharynx is a midline structure, the efferents of lymphatics draining the central area frequently reach lymph nodes on both sides of the neck.

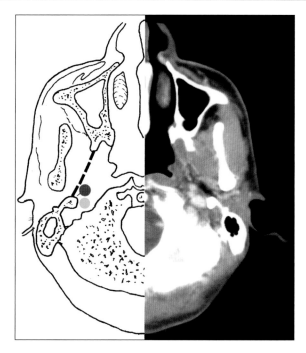

Fig. 22.5 CT (right) and line drawing (left) at a lower level. The space medial to the imaginary line joining the styloid process to the pterygoid plates (dashed line) contains the internal carotid artery (red disk), the last four cranial nerves, and the sympathetic trunk (blue disk).

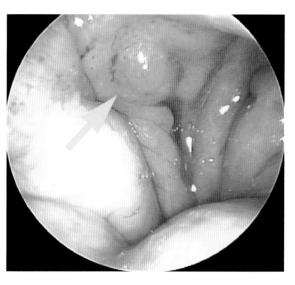

Fig. 22.6 Endoscopic view showing a retention cyst in the roof of the right nasopharynx (arrow).

Pathologies

Retention Cyst

When a duct of the seromucinous gland in the nasopharynx dilates following some obstruction, it forms a cyst (**Fig. 22.6**).[2] These cysts are usually small and incidentally noticed in a nasopharyngectomy specimen. When a cyst is infected or increases in size, it may become painful. Conservative treatment with antibiotics is usually effective, and if the condition frequently recurs, transnasal surgical removal is indicated.

Adenoids

The lymphoid tissue and nodules are present submucosally extending from the nasopharynx laterally to the eustachian tube orifices and then inferiorly to the soft palate and along the lateral wall to the tonsils. Medially the lymphoid tissue extends to the tongue base. This forms the Waldeyer's ring of lymphoid tissue and is regarded as the first line of defense.

Adenoids are aggregates of lymphoid follicles and nodules in the nasopharynx that have increased in size physiologically or have formed a mass in response to repeated inflammation, and that may produce symptoms.

This usually happens in children between 3 and 7 years of age. The symptoms related to the increase in size are nasal obstruction or decreased hearing due to serous otitis media when the eustachian tube openings are blocked. This might also account for obstructive sleep apnea in children.[3] When there is associated infection, additional symptoms may include nasal discharge, postnasal drip, otitis media, and generalized malaise. The diagnosis is usually made by the clinical features and endoscopic examination of the nasopharynx. The adenoids usually regress after adolescence, although in some patients the lymphoid tissue may persist as a mass in the nasopharynx even when they are adults. Biopsy under endoscopic view is indicated to differentiate it from other pathologies in the nasopharynx (**Fig. 22.7**).

The treatment should start with medication such as topical corticosteroids if there is an allergic element or mild decongestant nasal drops; if symptoms escalate despite medication, then adenoidectomy is indicated.

Thornwaldt's Cyst

Thornwaldt's cyst is a dilatation of the pharyngeal bursa that is the embryological remnant of connection between the notochord and the nasopharynx. It is located in the posterosuperior wall of the nasopharynx in the midline (**Fig. 22.8**). The cyst might be asymptomatic or, if it becomes infected, it may form an abscess and may have symptoms such as nasopharyngeal discharge, occipital headache, otalgia, or neck pain as the pharyngeal bursa is situated between the upper end of the longus capitis muscle.[4]

The diagnosis is through endoscopic examination and imaging such as MRI. Asymptomatic cysts may be left

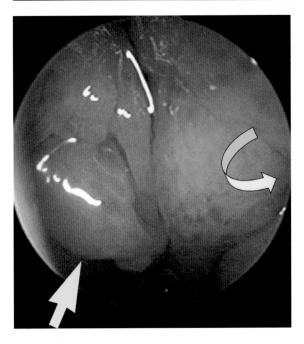

Fig. 22.7 Endoscopic view showing adenoid tissue in the nasopharynx (arrow). Curved arrow: left eustachian tube opening.

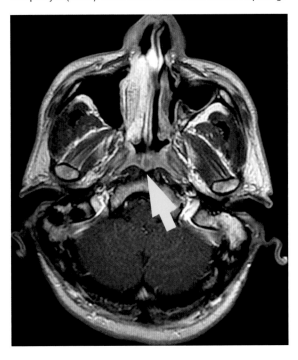

Fig. 22.8 MRI axial view showing a Thornwaldt's cyst in the midline (arrow).

alone and their size monitored regularly. When the cyst is large and gives rise to symptoms, surgical resection or marsupialization can be performed. A large cyst can be removed with powered instruments.[5]

Lesions from the Brain or Spinal Cord

Craniopharyngioma

As the nasopharynx lies below the skull base, developmental anomalies from the hypophysis cerebri (pituitary body) may present as a mass in the nasopharynx. The hypophysis is formed from two distinct sources, the hypophyseal diverticulum or Rathke's pouch, which is the cranial extension of the ectoderm of the primitive embryonic oral cavity of the stomodeum, and the infundibular diverticulum. The former develops into the anterior lobe, while the latter forms the posterior lobe of the pituitary gland. At the roof of the nasopharynx, there is a collection of adenohypophyseal tissue, the pharyngeal hypophysis, which also develops from the Rathke's pouch and comprises a collection of hormone-secreting endocrine tissue similar to the anterior pituitary. This is present in all individuals.[6] The Rathke's pouch gives rise to the craniopharyngeal duct, which normally degenerates.

The remnants of the Rathke's pouch may form a cyst in the roof of the nasopharynx, or the growth of the endocrine cells of the pharyngeal hypophysis may hypertrophy to form a pituitary adenoma in the roof of the nasophayrnx.[7]

Craniopharyngiomas are benign cystic neoplasms arising from the remnants of the lining of the craniopharyngeal duct, or from the pharyngeal hypophysis[8]; they contain brownish fluid and characteristically are situated in the suprasellar or sellar region.[9] Although most craniopharyngiomas are found close to the pituitary gland, they might present as a nasopharyngeal mass. The main symptoms are nasal obstruction and the extent of the mass can be assessed endoscopically and with various imaging studies. Transpalatal removal was the practice in the past,[10] but in recent years transsphenoidal removal[11] or craniofacial resection have been the primary choice of treatment with less morbidity.[12]

Chordoma

Chordomas are malignant neoplasms arising from the remnants of notochordal tissue. The common sites are the sacral, sphenoid, and clival regions. Thus the cranial chordomas are close to the nasopharynx and present with a mass in the nasopharynx (**Figs. 22.9 and 22.10**).[13] The age of presentation ranges from the twenties to the sixties and the symptoms range from headache to deterioration in vision due to cranial nerve involvement.[14] Imaging studies will show the extension of the lesion and the diagnosis is made through biopsy. Surgical resection can be performed followed by radiotherapy, but the prognosis has remained poor.[15] Proton beam therapy has been used in recent years with some success.[16]

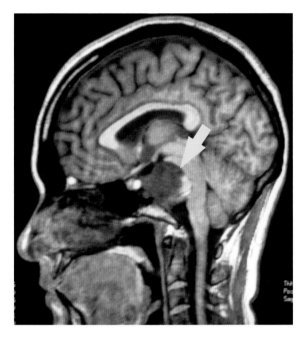

Fig. 22.9 MRI sagittal view showing a chordoma (arrow).

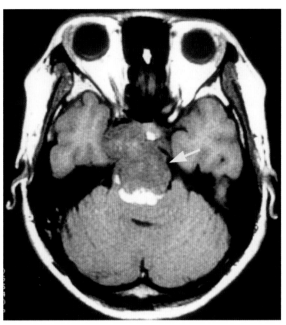

Fig. 22.10 MRI axial view showing the same chordoma as in Fig. 22.9 (arrow).

Benign Tumors

Benign neoplasms from the epithelial linings of the nasopharynx are uncommon. Occasionally, a hemangioma may involve the nasopharynx and the common presenting symptom is nasal obstruction, especially in an infant,[17] or mild epistaxis. Sometimes the lesion might be asymptomatic and the diagnosis is made while an endoscopic examination is being performed for other reasons (Fig. 22.11). The extent of the lesion can be determined by contrast imaging studies (Fig. 22.12). The management is usually conservative if the hemangioma is asymptomatic. Injection of sclerosant agent or surgical intervention is indicated only when there are symptoms such as frequent bleeding.

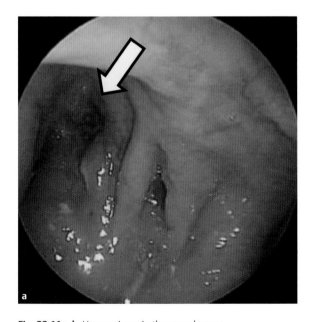

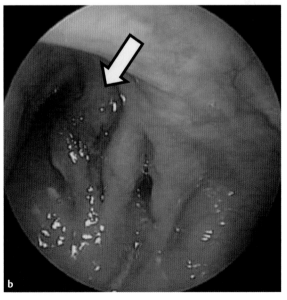

Fig. 22.11a, b Hemangioma in the nasopharynx.

a Collapsed (arrow).

b Distended with Valsalva maneuver (arrow).

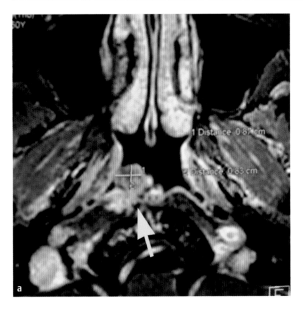

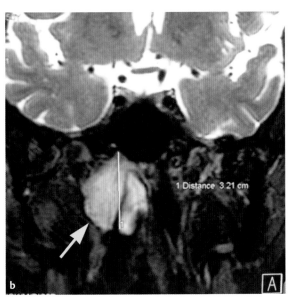

Fig. 22.12a, b MRI showing the hemangioma of **Fig. 22.11** (arrow).
a Axial view.

b Coronal view.

Benign salivary gland tumors such as pleomorphic adenoma arising from the minor salivary gland in the nasopharynx have been reported. They frequently present with nasal obstruction and the extent can be determined by imaging study (**Fig. 22.13**). The diagnosis is usually confirmed by biopsy of the mass. For small lesions, endoscopic removal is the treatment of choice; for large lesions, a transpalatal resection will ensure removal of all tissue to avoid recurrence (**Fig. 22.14**).

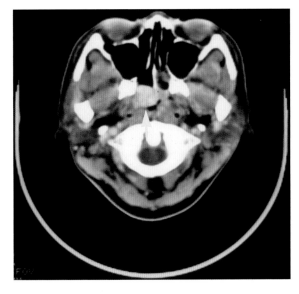

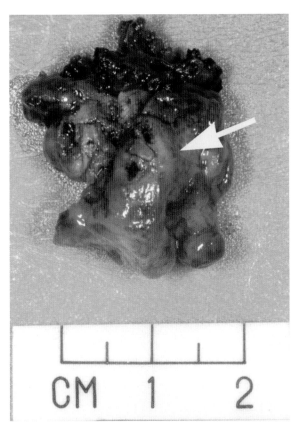

Fig. 22.13 CT showing a pedunculated minor salivary gland tumor arising from the lateral wall (arrow).

Fig. 22.14 Photograph of a specimen of benign salivary gland tumor with margin, showing the stalk (arrow).

Malignant Tumors

Nasopharyngeal Carcinoma

Nasopharyngeal carcinoma (NPC) is the commonest malignant lesion in the nasopharynx. This refers to the carcinoma arising from the crypt epithelium of the nasopharynx. This carcinoma was previously named lymphoepithelioma as the malignant cells of NPC are frequently intermingled with lymphoid cells in the nasopharynx (**Fig. 22.15**).[18] The degree of infiltration of lymphocytes has no correlation with prognosis.[19] Electron microscopy studies have determined that in these tumors, the carcinoma cells are of squamous origin, and this includes the nonkeratinizing squamous cell carcinoma and the undifferentiated carcinoma.[20]

The histological appearance of NPC has a wide range of forms and has caused some confusion; this prompted the World Health Organization (WHO) to propose a histological classification of nasopharyngeal carcinoma in 1978 that was revised in 1991.[21] This classification categorized NPCs into three types. Type I were the typical keratinizing squamous cell carcinomas, similar to those found in other parts of the head and neck region. The malignant cells showed squamous cell differentiation with the presence of extracellular keratin or intercellular cytoplasmic bridges (**Fig. 22.16**). Type II included nonkeratinizing squamous carcinomas, the stratified malignant cells presented in a plexiform or ribbon architecture (**Fig. 22.17**). Type III were the undifferentiated carcinomas; here the cells were in a syncytial form with indistinct cell borders (**Fig. 22.18**). Over the years, an alternative classification was proposed that grouped all NPCs into two histological types, the squamous cell carcinomas (SCCs) and undifferentiated carcinomas of the nasopharyngeal type (UCNTs).[22] This classification was found to correlate

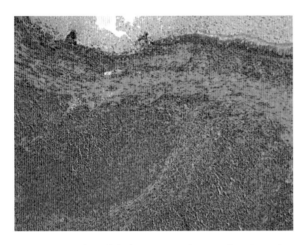

Fig. 22.15 Histology slide showing nasopharyngeal carcinoma in the submucosal region. (Hematoxylin and eosin, ×100.)

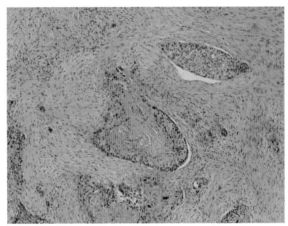

Fig. 22.16 Histology slide showing type I squamous cell nasopharyngeal carcinoma. (Hematoxylin and eosin, ×200.)

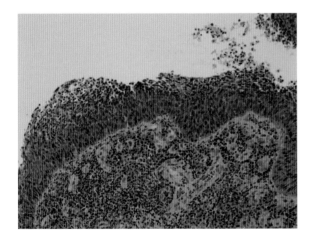

Fig. 22.17 Histology slide showing type II nonkeratinizing squamous cell nasopharyngeal carcinoma. (Hematoxylin and eosin, ×200.)

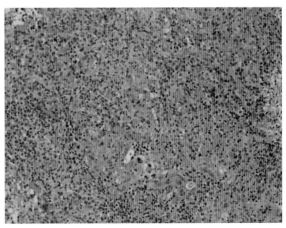

Fig. 22.18 Histology slide showing type III undifferentiated nasopharyngeal carcinoma. (Hematoxylin and eosin, ×200.)

with Epstein-Barr virus (EBV) serology tests among these patients. Those patients with SCCs have a lower EBV titer, while those with UCNTs have elevated titers. This second classification was applicable for epidemiological research and has also been shown to have prognostic bearing. The UCNTs have a higher local tumor control rate and a higher incidence of distant metastasis.[23,24] In North America, in 25% of patients the histology was type I, in 12% it was type II, and in the remaining 63% it was type III. The corresponding histological distribution in southern Chinese patients was 2%, 3%, and 95% respectively.[25]

As EBV is regularly detected in NPC patients from regions of high and low incidence, EBV-encoded RNA (EBER) in situ hybridization has been used frequently in the diagnosis of NPC (**Fig. 22.19**).

Other malignant tumors are the lymphomas, sarcoma, and malignant tumors arising from the salivary gland.

Lymphomas

Lymphomas arising from the lymphoid tissue of the Waldeyer's ring are usually the non-Hodgkin's large B-cell lymphoma.[26] Although the nasopharynx lies close to the Waldeyer's ring of lymphoid tissue, the lymphomas in the region are commonly T-cell (NK) lymphomas.[27] Patients usually present with a nasal mass or otological symptoms related to the mass. The diagnosis is generally reached following biopsy of the lesion. Radiotherapy is the treatment employed for small and low-stage tumor, while combined chemoradiotherapy is used for high-stage lesions. A 5-year disease-free survival rate of 57% has been reported.[28] Extramedullary plasmacytomas are neoplasms from plasma cells arising from extraosseous tissue. The nasopharynx is a common site for this tumor in the head and neck region. This tumor is radiosensitive and over 95% local control has been reported.[29]

Sarcoma

Rhabdomyosarcoma is the most common sarcoma in the nasopharynx and it usually affects young children. The common presenting symptom is nasal obstruction with or without otitis media. On endoscopic examination, a smooth, firm mass is seen occupying the entire nasopharynx. In common with other sarcomas, the tumor grows rapidly and invades surrounding structure.[30] The optimal treatment results are achieved with multimodality therapy, radiation, chemotherapy, and sometimes surgery.[31] The 5-year survival for patients treated in a specialized center is greater than 70%.[32]

Salivary Gland Tumors

Salivary gland tumors usually present with nasal obstruction, and investigation shows a mass in the nasopharynx. Adenoid cystic carcinoma presents in adults with epistaxis, diplopia, and insidious facial pain along the fifth cranial nerve distribution.[33] They are rare tumors and have a poor prognosis; the best chance of eradicating them is surgery followed by radiotherapy.[34] The other rare malignant tumor,[35] polymorphous adenocarcinoma arising from the minor salivary gland in the nasopharynx, has a better prognosis (**Fig. 22.20**). The tumor causes nasal obstruction and, when the surface ulcerates, there can be epistaxis. The treatment is surgical resection, and adequate removal of the disease gives long-term survival.[36]

References

1. Adams WS. The transverse dimensions of the nasopharynx in child and adult with observations on its contractile function. J Laryngol Otol 1958;72(6):465–471
2. Miller RH, Sneed WF. Tornwaldt's bursa. Clin Otolaryngol Allied Sci 1985;10(1):21–25

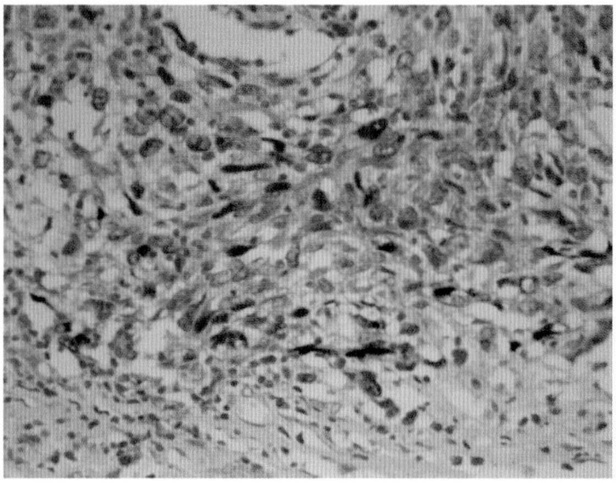

Fig. 22.19 Histology slide showing the use of Epstein-Barr virus–encoded RNA (EBER) in situ hybridization in the diagnosis of nasopharyngeal carcinoma (×400).

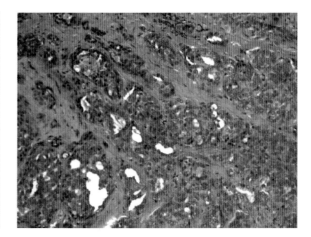

Fig. 22.20 Polymorphous adenocarcinoma of the salivary gland arising from the nasopharynx. (Hematoxylin and eosin, ×200.)

3. Vlastos IM, Houlakis M, Kandiloros D, Manolopoulos L, Ferekidis E, Yiotakis I. Adenoidectomy plus tympanostomy tube insertion versus adenoidectomy plus myringotomy in children with obstructive sleep apnoea syndrome. J Laryngol Otol 2011;125(3):274–278

4. Miyahara H, Matsunaga T. Tornwaldt's disease. Acta Otolaryngol Suppl 1994;517:36–39

5. Eloy P, Watelet JB, Hatert AS, Bertrand B. Thornwaldt's cyst and surgery with powered instrumentation. B-ENT 2006;2(3):135–139

6. Fuller GN, Batsakis JG. Pharyngeal hypophysis. Ann Otol Rhinol Laryngol 1996;105(8):671–672

7. Ali R, Noma U, Jansen M, Smyth D. Ectopic pituitary adenoma presenting as midline nasopharyngeal mass. Ir J Med Sci 2010;179(4):593–595

8. Lewin R, Ruffolo E, Saraceno C. Craniopharyngioma arising in the pharyngeal hypophysis. South Med J 1984; 77(12):1519–1523

9. Trippi AC, Garner JT, Kassabian JT, Shelden CH. A new approach to inoperable craniopharyngiomas. Am J Surg 1969;118(2):307–310

10. Johnson NE. Craniopharyngioma—review with a discussion of transpalatal approach. Laryngoscope 1962; 72:1731–1749

11. Mortini P, Losa M, Pozzobon G, et al. Neurosurgical treatment of craniopharyngioma in adults and children: early and long-term results in a large case series. J Neurosurg 2011;114(5):1350–1359

12. Magill JC, Ferguson MS, Sandison A, Clarke PM. Nasal craniopharyngioma: case report and literature review. J Laryngol Otol 2011;125(5):517–519

13. Campbell WM, McDonald TJ, Unni KK, Laws ER Jr. Nasal and paranasal presentations of chordomas. Laryngoscope 1980;90(4):612–618

14. Richter HJ Jr, Batsakis JG, Boles R. Chordomas: nasopharyngeal presentation and atypical long survival. Ann Otol Rhinol Laryngol 1975;84(3 Pt 1):327–332

15. Wu Z, Zhang J, Zhang L, et al. Prognostic factors for long-term outcome of patients with surgical resection of skull base chordomas—106 cases review in one institution. Neurosurg Rev 2010;33(4):451–456

16. Hug EB, Slater JD. Proton radiation therapy for chordomas and chondrosarcomas of the skull base. Neurosurg Clin N Am 2000;11(4):627–638

17. Strauss M, Widome MD, Roland PS. Nasopharyngeal hemangioma causing airway obstruction in infancy. Laryngoscope 1981;91(8):1365–1368

18. Godtfredsen E. On the histopathology of malignant nasopharyngeal tumors. Acta Pathol Microbiol Scand 1944;55(Suppl):38–319

19. Roth SL, Krueger GF, Bertram G, Sack H. Carcinoma of the nasopharynx. The significance of lymphocytic infiltration. Acta Oncol 1990;29(7):897–901

20. Prasad U. Cells of origin of nasopharyngeal carcinoma: an electron microscopic study. J Laryngol Otol 1974;88(11):1087–1094

21. Shanmugaratnam K, Sobin LH. Histological typing of tumours of the upper respiratory tract and ear. In: Shanmugaratnam, Sobin LH, eds. International Histological Classification of Tumours: No 19. Geneva: World Health Organization; 1991:32–33

22. Micheau C, Rilke F, Pilotti S. Proposal for a new histopathological classification of the carcinomas of the nasopharynx. Tumori 1978;64(5):513–518

23. Reddy SP, Raslan WF, Gooneratne S, Kathuria S, Marks JE. Prognostic significance of keratinization in nasopharyngeal carcinoma. Am J Otolaryngol 1995;16(2):103–108

24. Marks JE, Phillips JL, Menck HR. The National Cancer Data Base report on the relationship of race and national origin to the histology of nasopharyngeal carcinoma. Cancer 1998;83(3):582–588

25. Nicholls JM. Nasopharyngeal carcinoma: classification and histological appearances. Adv Anat Pathol 1997;4(2):71–84 doi: 10.1097/00125480-199703000-00001

26. Menárguez J, Mollejo M, Carrión R, et al. Waldeyer ring lymphomas. A clinicopathological study of 79 cases. Histopathology 1994;24(1):13–22

27. Chan JK, Ng CS, Lau WH, Lo ST. Most nasal/nasopharyngeal lymphomas are peripheral T-cell neoplasms. Am J Surg Pathol 1987;11(6):418–429

28. Laskar S, Muckaden MA, Bahl G, et al. Primary non-Hodgkin's lymphoma of the nasopharynx: prognostic factors and outcome of 113 Indian patients. Leuk Lymphoma 2006;47(10):2132–2139

29. Liebross RH, Ha CS, Cox JD, Weber D, Delasalle K, Alexanian R. Clinical course of solitary extramedullary plasmacytoma. Radiother Oncol 1999;52(3):245–249

30. Canalis RF, Jenkens HA, Hemenway WG, Lincoln C. Nasopharyngeal rhabdomyosarcoma. A clinical perspective. Arch Otolaryngol 1978;104(3):122–126

31. Healy JN, Borg MF. Paediatric nasopharyngeal rhabdomyosarcoma: A case series and literature review. J Med Imaging Radiat Oncol 2010;54(4):388–394

32. Walterhouse D, Watson A. Optimal management strategies for rhabdomyosarcoma in children. Paediatr Drugs 2007;9(6):391–400

33. Lee DJ, Smith RR, Spaziani JT, Rostock R, Holliday M, Moses H. Adenoid cystic carcinoma of the nasopharynx. Case reports and literature review. Ann Otol Rhinol Laryngol 1985;94(3):269–272

34. Liu TR, Yang AK, Guo X, et al. Adenoid cystic carcinoma of the nasopharynx: 27-year experience. Laryngoscope 2008;118(11):1981–1988

35. Wei YC, Huang CC, Chien CY, Hwang JC, Chen WJ. Polymorphous low-grade adenocarcinoma of the nasopharynx: a case report and brief review. J Clin Pathol 2008;61(10):1124–1126

36. Wenig BM, Harpaz N, DelBridge C. Polymorphous low-grade adenocarcinoma of seromucous glands of the nasopharynx. A report of a case and a discussion of the morphologic and immunohistochemical features. Am J Clin Pathol 1989;92(1):104–109

23 Nasopharyngeal Carcinoma: Epidemiology, Etiology, Screening, and Staging

Epidemiology

Nasopharyngeal carcinoma (NPC), unlike many other head and neck cancers, is an uncommon neoplasm in most parts of the world. The age-adjusted incidence for both sexes is less than 1 per 100,000 population per year in many countries.[1] On a global scale there are only 80,000 new patients per year, constituting 0.7% of all cancers, making it the 23rd-commonest new cancer in the world.[2] It has a very distinctive geographic distribution: a high incidence is seen in the southern part of China, especially among the inhabitants of Guangdong province, including Hong Kong. The reported incidence for males is 17.8 per 100,000 and for females is 6.7 per 100,000. A range of intermediate rates is observed in populations in Southeast Asia, and in natives of the Arctic region such as northern Canada,[3] North Africa, and the Middle East.[4] One report on the incidence of this tumor in the Eskimo population in Greenland from 1955 to 1976 gave 12.3 and 8.5 per 100,000 per year for males and females, respectively.[5] The incidence in northern African countries was 5.4 and 1.9 per 100,000 population, respectively, and these are roughly 10 times higher than the incidence in Europe.[6]

This geographic variation in the incidence of NPC is also seen within China: low rates of 1.1 per 100,000 population are seen in northern China, such as Harbin city. The distribution of the disease among different ethnic groups is also not uniform. In the southern province of Guangdong, the incidence of NPC is three times higher among Cantonese speakers than in Hakka, Hokkien, or Chiu Chau dialect groups.[7] In Malaysia, the incidence of NPC is again higher among the Cantonese Chinese than among the Hokkien and the Teochiu.[8] This may be associated with social and racial intermingling. In the Vietnamese city of Hanoi, the incidence of NPC is twice that in Ho Chi Minh City as there are more Chinese descendants in Hanoi.[9] In the United States, a study of 1,645 NPC patients also showed the highest incidence in Chinese, followed by Filipinos then the whites and blacks.[10] The survival was also the highest among the Chinese.[11]

The incidence of NPC remains high among Chinese who have migrated to North America, but is lower among Chinese born in North America than in those born in southern China.[12,13] A similar higher incidence was seen among Chinese who have immigrated to Australia[14] and the southern part of England.[15] Migrant studies also showed that the incidence of NPC is higher in the offspring of north Africans who have migrated to Israel than among native Israelis.[16]

These findings suggest that geographic, ethnic, and environmental influences together with other factors contribute to the etiology of nasopharyngeal carcinoma.[17]

In nearly all reports the incidence of nasopharyngeal carcinoma is 2 to 3 times higher in males than in females.[1] As for the distribution of the disease within age groups, in low-risk regions, NPC incidence increases with increasing age.[18] In high-risk regions, the peak incidence is around ages 50 to 59 years and declines thereafter[19,20]; there is also a minor peak among young adults,[21–23] consistent with exposure to carcinogenic agents in early life.

Etiology

Salt-Preserved Fish

Preservation of fish and other food material with salt makes them partially putrefied, resulting in the accumulation of significant levels of nitrosamines, which are known carcinogens.[24,25] Salted fish is a traditional weaning food for infants, especially among the Cantonese population. A case–control study has shown that weekly consumption of salted fish before 10 years of age is associated with a 3-fold increased risk of developing NPC.[26] The consumption of salted fish in childhood rather than adulthood,[27] and the duration and frequency of intake, were independently associated with increased risk of NPC.[28] However, even in low-risk regions such as the northern provinces of China[29] and the United States of America,[30] preserved food is a common dietary component. Thus consumption of salted fish per se is unlikely to be the cause of nasopharyngeal carcinoma. The consumption of fresh fruit and vegetables is associated with a low risk of nasopharyngeal carcinoma,[31] especially in childhood.[32] This might be related to the antioxidant effects of fresh fruit and vegetables rather than to the specific food items.[33]

Epstein-Barr Virus

The Epstein-Barr virus (EBV) is a double-stranded DNA virus that belongs to the herpesvirus family. The virus is ubiquitous in the human population; it may cause infections such as infectious mononucleosis and has also been found to be associated with certain lymphomas and NPC. It infects and persists latently in the global population; most of the infection is subclinical and transmission is common in crowded conditions. In Hong Kong, most children have been infected by the age of 10 years.[34] The B lymphocytes are the target of EBV infection and it is known to be associated with Burkitt's lymphoma.[35] The association of EBV with NPC was postulated as patients suffering from NPC also have higher EBV antibody titers than controls.[36] In particular, the IgA class of antibodies to viral capsid antigen and early antigen are elevated in NPC patients.[37,38]

There were reports showing that these antibodies titers were elevated for some time before the presentation of NPC[39,40] and that they are correlated with tumor staging[41] and prognosis.[42]

Recently, through PCR, cell-free EBV DNA was detected in the plasma of patients suffering from nasopharyngeal carcinoma.[43] The number of copies of this EBV DNA can be quantified[44] and this has been shown to be related to stage of the disease[45] and survival.[46]

However, EBV is unlikely to be the sole causative factor of NPC as it is ubiquitous in human populations. It is more likely that under specific circumstances the virus plays an oncogenic role together with other cofactors in leading to the development of NPC.

Genetic Factors

The high incidence of NPC among southeastern Chinese and their descendants suggests the presence of a genetic factor.[47] This familial aggregation is also seen in intermediate-incidence[48] and low-incidence populations.[49] The genetic evidence is further supported by the fact that NPC is 4 to 10 times more common in first-degree relatives of patients suffering from nasopharyngeal carcinoma than in controls.[50,51] This familial clustering might be the result of shared genetic susceptibility and related environmental factors; probably multiple genetic and environmental factors in combination are responsible, rather than a single gene.[52]

The human leukocyte antigen (HLA) genes were identified to be the genes responsible for the development of NPC. These genes encode proteins that present foreign antigens such as viral particles to the immune system for lysis. Individuals with HLA alleles that have reduced ability to present the viral particle, in this case the Epstein-Barr virus, for lysis have an increased risk of developing NPC.[53] In a meta-analysis of the studies on southern Chinese, the finding of patients with HLA alleles HLA-A2, B14, and B46 is associated with an increased risk of developing NPC.[54]

Meta-analysis of comparative genomic hybridization studies revealed several genomic spots where chromosomal losses and gains were identified in NPC.[55] These losses on chromosomes 3p, 9p, 11q, 13q, and 14q suggested that tumor suppressor genes at these loci might be involved in NPC development.[56,57]

Screening

In regions where NPC is endemic, EBV serology has been used for population screening aimed at detection of the disease in its early stage. In a prospective study performed in the early 1980s, 1,136 individuals were detected to have elevated IgA antibodies against the viral capsid antigen of EBV. They were examined regularly for 4 years. During this period, 35 NPC patients were detected, most of them (91.5%) were diagnosed in the early stages.[58] Comparable results were reported from a similar study conducted in Guangdong province, China.[59] The predictive value of EBV serology was also reported in a study from Taiwan that included 9,699 patients. Their EBV serological status was cross-checked with the cancer and death registry for a 15-year period. The results showed that the longer the follow-up period, the greater was the difference in cumulative incidence of nasopharyngeal carcinoma between those with elevated serology and those with negative serology.[40] In a prospective study of 42,048 patients, this raised level of antibody titer could be detected for up to 10 years before diagnosis of the tumor. The mean duration of this preclinical serological elevation window was 37 ± 28 months.[60]

Although this elevation of antibody titer of EBV has also been reported in low-risk regions,[61] its value in general population screening aiming to detect early stage disease for more effective treatment is not likely to be cost-effective, even in high-incidence regions. It might be applicable in the screening of family members such as first-degree relatives in a high-risk region. In a prospective study of 1,199 asymptomatic family members of NPC patients, screening identified 16 patients.[62] The sensitivity and specificity of EBV serology were 88.9% and 87.0%, respectively, and these patients have a 10 to 12% higher survival rate than those patients diagnosed without screening.[63]

When the NPC cell dies, the associated EBV is released and its quantity in the plasma can be detected by real-time polymerase chain reaction (PCR). This plasma cell-free EBV DNA is detectable in 96% of patients,[44] especially in the undifferentiated carcinoma cells. It correlates with the stage of the disease and has prognostic significance.[45] It is also of value in the diagnosis of recurrences and can be detected before the appearance of the recurrent tumor.[64] Studies on EBV DNA detection were mainly performed on patients suffering from NPC; its role as a screening tool in the general population has not been determined.[65]

Staging

As with other malignancies, a clinical staging system for nasopharyngeal carcinoma is essential for planning treatment and evaluating the results of therapy. A simple staging system for NPC was first described in 1952.[66] With

Table 23.1 The American Joint Committee on Cancer Staging[77]

Primary tumor in nasopharynx (T)	
T1	Tumor confined to the nasopharynx, or tumor extends to oropharynx and/or nasal cavity without parapharyngeal extension
T2	Tumor with parapharyngeal extension
T3	Tumor involves bony structures of skull base and/or paranasal sinuses
T4	Tumor with intracranial extension and/or involvement of cranial nerves, hypopharynx, orbit, or with extension to the infratemporal fossa/masticator space

Regional lymph nodes (N)	
The distribution and the prognostic impact of regional lymph node spread from nasopharynx cancer, particularly of the undifferentiated type, are different from those of other head and neck mucosal cancers and justify the use of a different N classification scheme.	
NX	Regional lymph nodes cannot be assessed
N0	No regional lymph node metastasis
N1	Unilateral metastasis in lymph node(s), 6 cm or less in greatest dimension, above the supraclavicular fossa, and/or unilateral or bilateral, retropharyngeal lymph nodes, 6 cm or less, in greatest dimension
N2	Bilateral metastasis in lymph node(s), 6 cm or less in greatest dimension, above the supraclavicular fossa
N3	Metastasis in a lymph node(s) >6 cm and/or to supraclavicular fossa
N3a	Greater than 6 cm in dimension
N3b	Extension to the supraclavicular fossa

Distant metastasis (M)	
M0	No distant metastasis
M1	Distant metastasis

Stage/prognostic group	
Stage 0	Tis N0 M0
Stage I	T1 N0 M0
Stage II	T1 N1 M0
	T2 N0 M0
	T2 N1 M0
Stage III	T1 N2 M0
	T2 N2 M0
	T3 N0 M0
	T3 N1 M0
	T3 N2 M0
Stage IVA	T4 N0 M0
	T4 N1 M0
	T4 N2 M0
Stage IVB	Any T N3 M0
Stage IVC	Any T Any N M1

this system, each stage covered too wide a range of tumor involvement and did not accurately reflect the clinical condition. Over the years a number of staging systems have been used for NPC; the Union for International Cancer Control/Union International Contre le Cancer (UICC) and the American Joint Committee on Cancer Staging (AJCC) systems are preferred in Europe and America, respectively, while Ho's system is frequently used in Asia.[67,68] The nodal classification in Ho's system has demonstrated its prognostic significance, but its stratification of the T stages into five stages differs from other staging systems for malignant disease. The lack of a universally accepted staging system reflects, to some extent, the inadequacies of the various existing staging classifications.[69]

The development of a revised staging system since the 2000s has taken into consideration the experiences gained from various centers around the world. It also takes into account several prognostic factors, such as the extension of primary tumor to the paranasopharyngeal space,[70] skull base erosion, the involvement of cranial nerves,[71] and also the position and size of the cervical nodes.[72]

Both the UICC and the AJCC systems assess tumor extent in the nasopharynx by considering the number of tumor-affected sites within the nasopharynx, while the Ho system classifies all tumors confined to the nasopharynx as T1 disease. The UICC and AJCC systems have been unified since 1992 and the clinical staging is the same in their recent published manuals.[73,74] In the staging system of 2009, T1 stage included all tumors that were confined to the nasopharynx or extended locally such as anteriorly to the nasal cavity, or inferiorly to the oropharynx. This is because the nasopharynx is an irregular structure and the margins of the walls are not precise, and the exact limit of the tumor is also difficult to define. There is also the additional problem of submucosal extension, which is difficult to determine even with endoscopy.[75] The whole nasopharynx and its vicinity are included in the radiation field; so as long as the tumor is superficial and confined to the mucosa, it is classified as T1 disease. On the other hand, lateral tumor extension to involve the paranasopharyngeal space is important and this can be accurately determined by cross-sectional imaging. Thus, T2 stage included tumor that had extended to the paranasopharyngeal space. The T3 stage covered tumors that had extended to the skull base or other paranasal sinuses. T4 stage covered tumors that had extended into the infratemporal fossa, orbit, hypopharynx, and cranium, or had affected the cranial nerves.

The disparity between the UICC/AJCC and Ho staging systems is greater in the N stage. The UICC/AJCC currently recognizes the size of the lymph node as an important factor. In N staging for other head and neck cancers, staging between N1 and N2 depends on whether the node is smaller or larger than 3 cm, and the difference between N2 and N3 is the nodal size of 6 cm. Another criticism

common to the various N-staging systems is that the retropharyngeal nodes, which are the first-echelon nodes, are not taken into account by any staging systems. These nodes, although difficult to examine clinically, can now be assessed by CT or MRI.[76]

These factors were addressed in the nodal staging section of the UICC/AJCC nasopharyngeal cancer staging system (**Table 23.1**). Here only a measurement of 6 cm is considered as a factor in size. Laterality and level of involvement such as the retropharyngeal region and the supraclavicular fossa are other important factors employed in the determination of N-staging. Under the current system, N1 refers to unilateral nodal involvement less than 6 cm in diameter and not reaching the supraclavicular fossa. The presence of bilateral retropharyngeal nodes, as long as they are less than 6 cm in diameter, remains N1. Bilateral nodal disease in the neck that has not reached N3 designation is classified as N2, irrespective of the size, number, and anatomical location of the nodes. Stage N3 disease refers to lymph nodes larger than 6 cm (N3a), or nodes that have extended to the supraclavicular fossa (N3b). There is agreement on M-staging, where M1 represents distant metastases, including any lymph node involvement below the level of the clavicle. The current unified staging system has enabled patients to be staged more precisely and simply; it also gives a better predictor of prognosis.[77–79]

References

1. Curado MP, Edwards B, Shin HR, et al, eds. Cancer Incidence in Five Continents, Vol. IX. Lyon: IARC; 2007: 141–143 (IARC Scientific Publications No.160)
2. Parkin DM, Bray F, Ferlay J, Pisani P. Global cancer statistics, 2002. CA Cancer J Clin 2005;55(2):74–108
3. Mallen RW, Shandro WG. Nasopharyngeal carcinoma in Eskimos. Can J Otolaryngol 1974;3(2):175–179
4. Al-Rajhi N, El-Sebaie M, Khafaga Y, AlZahrani A, Mohamed G, Al-Amro A. Nasopharyngeal carcinoma in Saudi Arabia: clinical presentation and diagnostic delay. East Mediterr Health J 2009;15(5):1301–1307
5. Nielsen NH, Mikkelsen F, Hansen JP. Nasopharyngeal cancer in Greenland. The incidence in an Arctic Eskimo population. Acta Pathol Microbiol Scand [A] 1977;85(6):850–858
6. Zanetti R, Tazi MA, Rosso S. New data tells us more about cancer incidence in North Africa. Eur J Cancer 2010;46(3):462–466
7. Li CC, Yu MC, Henderson BE. Some epidemiologic observations of nasopharyngeal carcinoma in Guangdong, People's Republic of China. Natl Cancer Inst Monogr 1985;69:49–52
8. Armstrong RW, Kannan Kutty M, Dharmalingam SK, Ponnudurai JR. Incidence of nasopharyngeal carcinoma in Malaysia, 1968–1977. Br J Cancer 1979;40(4):557–567
9. Nguyen QM, Nguyen HC, Parkin DM. Cancer incidence in Ho Chi Minh City, Viet Nam, 1995–1996. Int J Cancer 1998;76(4):472–479
10. Burt RD, Vaughan TL, McKnight B. Descriptive epidemiology and survival analysis of nasopharyngeal carcinoma in the United States. Int J Cancer 1992;52(4):549–556
11. Ou SH, Zell JA, Ziogas A, Anton-Culver H. Epidemiology of nasopharyngeal carcinoma in the United States: improved survival of Chinese patients within the

keratinizing squamous cell carcinoma histology. Ann Oncol 2007;18(1):29–35

12. Dickson RI, Flores AD. Nasopharyngeal carcinoma: an evaluation of 134 patients treated between 1971–1980. Laryngoscope 1985;95(3):276–283

13. Buell P. The effect of migration on the risk of nasopharyngeal cancer among Chinese. Cancer Res 1974;34(5):1189–1191

14. McCredie M, Williams S, Coates M. Cancer mortality in East and Southeast Asian migrants to New South Wales, Australia, 1975–1995. Br J Cancer 1999;79(7-8):1277–1282

15. Warnakulasuriya KA, Johnson NW, Linklater KM, Bell J. Cancer of mouth, pharynx and nasopharynx in Asian and Chinese immigrants resident in Thames regions. Oral Oncol 1999;35(5):471–475

16. Parkin DM, Iscovich J. Risk of cancer in migrants and their descendants in Israel: II. Carcinomas and germ-cell tumours. Int J Cancer 1997;70(6):654–660

17. Chang ET, Adami HO. The enigmatic epidemiology of nasopharyngeal carcinoma. Cancer Epidemiol Biomarkers Prev 2006;15(10):1765–1777

18. Levine PH, Connelly RR, Easton JM. Demographic patterns for nasopharyngeal carcinoma in the United States. Int J Cancer 1980;26(6):741–748

19. Lee AW, Foo W, Mang O, et al. Changing epidemiology of nasopharyngeal carcinoma in Hong Kong over a 20-year period (1980–99): an encouraging reduction in both incidence and mortality. Int J Cancer 2003;103(5):680–685

20. Zong YS, Zhang RF, He SY, Qiu H. Histopathologic types and incidence of malignant nasopharyngeal tumors in Zhongshan County. Chin Med J (Engl) 1983;96(7):511–516

21. Balakrishnan U. An additional younger-age peak for cancer of the nasopharynx. Int J Cancer 1975;15(4):651–657

22. Andejani AA, Kundapur V, Malaker K. Age distribution of nasopharyngeal cancer in Saudi Arabia. Saudi Med J 2004;25(11):1579–1582

23. Rothwell RI. Juvenile nasopharyngeal carcinoma in Sabah (Malaysia). Clin Oncol 1979;5(4):353–358

24. Preston-Martin S. N-nitroso compounds as a cause of human cancer. IARC Sci Publ 1987; (84):477–484

25. Zou XN, Lu SH, Liu B. Volatile N-nitrosamines and their precursors in Chinese salted fish—a possible etiological factor for NPC in china. Int J Cancer 1994;59(2):155–158

26. Yu MC, Ho JH, Lai SH, Henderson BE. Cantonese-style salted fish as a cause of nasopharyngeal carcinoma: report of a case-control study in Hong Kong. Cancer Res 1986;46(2):956–961

27. Gallicchio L, Matanoski G, Tao XG, et al. Adulthood consumption of preserved and nonpreserved vegetables and the risk of nasopharyngeal carcinoma: a systematic review. Int J Cancer 2006;119(5):1125–1135

28. Yu MC, Mo C-C, Chong W-X, Yeh F-S, Henderson BE. Preserved foods and nasopharyngeal carcinoma: a case-control study in Guangxi, China. Cancer Res 1988;48(7):1954–1959

29. Ning JP, Yu MC, Wang QS, Henderson BE. Consumption of salted fish and other risk factors for nasopharyngeal carcinoma (NPC) in Tianjin, a low-risk region for NPC in the People's Republic of China. J Natl Cancer Inst 1990;82(4):291–296

30. Farrow DC, Vaughan TL, Berwick M, Lynch CF, Swanson GM, Lyon JL. Diet and nasopharyngeal cancer in a low-risk population. Int J Cancer 1998;78(6):675–679

31. Ward MH, Pan WH, Cheng YJ, et al. Dietary exposure to nitrite and nitrosamines and risk of nasopharyngeal carcinoma in Taiwan. Int J Cancer 2000;86(5):603–609

32. Yu MC, Huang TB, Henderson BE. Diet and nasopharyngeal carcinoma: a case-control study in Guangzhou, China. Int J Cancer 1989;43(6):1077–1082

33. Weisburger JH. Mechanisms of action of antioxidants as exemplified in vegetables, tomatoes and tea. Food Chem Toxicol 1999;37(9-10):943–948

34. Kangro HO, Osman HK, Lau YL, Heath RB, Yeung CY, Ng MH. Seroprevalence of antibodies to human herpesviruses in England and Hong Kong. J Med Virol 1994;43(1):91–96

35. zur Hausen H, Schulte-Holthausen H, Klein G, et al. EBV DNA in biopsies of Burkitt tumours and anaplastic carcinomas of the nasopharynx. Nature 1970;228(5276):1056–1058

36. Henle W, Henle G, Ho HC, et al. Antibodies to Epstein-Barr virus in nasopharyngeal carcinoma, other head and neck neoplasms, and control groups. J Natl Cancer Inst 1970;44(1):225–231

37. Lin TM, Yang CS, Chiou JF, et al. Antibodies to Epstein-Barr virus capsid antigen and early antigen in nasopharyngeal carcinoma and comparison groups. Am J Epidemiol 1977;106(4):336–339

38. Henle G, Henle W. Epstein-Barr virus-specific IgA serum antibodies as an outstanding feature of nasopharyngeal carcinoma. Int J Cancer 1976;17(1):1–7

39. Ho HC, Kwan HC, Ng MH, de The G. Serum IgA antibodies to Epstein-Barr virus capsid antigen preceding symptoms of nasopharyngeal carcinoma. Lancet 1978;1(8061):436

40. Chien YC, Chen JY, Liu MY, et al. Serologic markers of Epstein-Barr virus infection and nasopharyngeal carcinoma in Taiwanese men. N Engl J Med 2001;345(26):1877–1882

41. Neel HB III, Pearson GR, Weiland LH, et al. Application of Epstein-Barr virus serology to the diagnosis and staging of North American patients with nasopharyngeal carcinoma. Otolaryngol Head Neck Surg 1983;91(3):255–262

42. de-Vathaire F, Sancho-Garnier H, de-Thé H, et al. Prognostic value of EBV markers in the clinical management of nasopharyngeal carcinoma (NPC): a multicenter follow-up study. Int J Cancer 1988;42(2):176–181

43. Mutirangura A, Pornthanakasem W, Theamboonlers A, et al. Epstein-Barr viral DNA in serum of patients with nasopharyngeal carcinoma. Clin Cancer Res 1998;4(3):665–669

44. Lo YM, Chan LY, Lo KW, et al. Quantitative analysis of cell-free Epstein-Barr virus DNA in plasma of patients with nasopharyngeal carcinoma. Cancer Res 1999;59(6):1188–1191

45. Lin JC, Wang WY, Chen KY, et al. Quantification of plasma Epstein-Barr virus DNA in patients with advanced nasopharyngeal carcinoma. N Engl J Med 2004;350(24):2461–2470

46. Lin JC, Chen KY, Wang WY, et al. Detection of Epstein-Barr virus DNA in the peripheral-blood cells of patients with nasopharyngeal carcinoma: relationship to distant metastasis and survival. J Clin Oncol 2001;19(10):2607–2615

47. Loh KS, Goh BC, Lu J, Hsieh WS, Tan L. Familial nasopharyngeal carcinoma in a cohort of 200 patients. Arch Otolaryngol Head Neck Surg 2006;132(1):82–85

48. Albeck H, Bentzen J, Ockelmann HH, Nielsen NH, Bretlau P, Hansen HS. Familial clusters of nasopharyngeal carcinoma and salivary gland carcinomas in Greenland natives. Cancer 1993;72(1):196–200

49. Levine PH, Pocinki AG, Madigan P, Bale S. Familial nasopharyngeal carcinoma in patients who are not Chinese. Cancer 1992;70(5):1024–1029

50. Yu MC, Garabrant DH, Huang TB, Henderson BE. Occupational and other non-dietary risk factors for nasopharyngeal carcinoma in Guangzhou, China. Int J Cancer 1990;45(6):1033–1039

51. Jia WH, Feng BJ, Xu ZL, et al. Familial risk and clustering of nasopharyngeal carcinoma in Guangdong, China. Cancer 2004;101(2):363–369

52. Jia WH, Collins A, Zeng YX, et al. Complex segregation analysis of nasopharyngeal carcinoma in Guangdong, China: evidence for a multifactorial mode of inheritance

(complex segregation analysis of NPC in China). Eur J Hum Genet 2005;13(2):248–252

53. Hildesheim A, Apple RJ, Chen CJ, et al. Association of HLA class I and II alleles and extended haplotypes with nasopharyngeal carcinoma in Taiwan. J Natl Cancer Inst 2002;94(23):1780–1789

54. Goldsmith DB, West TM, Morton R. HLA associations with nasopharyngeal carcinoma in Southern Chinese: a meta-analysis. Clin Otolaryngol Allied Sci 2002;27(1):61–67

55. Li X, Wang E, Zhao YD, et al. Chromosomal imbalances in nasopharyngeal carcinoma: a meta-analysis of comparative genomic hybridization results. J Transl Med 2006;4:4

56. Hu LF, Eiriksdottir G, Lebedeva T, et al. Loss of heterozygosity on chromosome arm 3p in nasopharyngeal carcinoma. Genes Chromosomes Cancer 1996;17(2):118–126

57. Chien G, Yuen PW, Kwong D, Kwong YL. Comparative genomic hybridization analysis of nasopharygeal carcinoma: consistent patterns of genetic aberrations and clinicopathological correlations. Cancer Genet Cytogenet 2001;126(1):63–67

58. Zeng Y, Zhang LG, Wu YC, et al. Prospective studies on nasopharyngeal carcinoma in Epstein-Barr virus IgA/VCA antibody-positive persons in Wuzhou City, China. Int J Cancer 1985;36(5):545–547

59. Zong YS, Sham JS, Ng MH, et al. Immunoglobulin A against viral capsid antigen of Epstein-Barr virus and indirect mirror examination of the nasopharynx in the detection of asymptomatic nasopharyngeal carcinoma. Cancer 1992;69(1):3–7

60. Ji MF, Wang DK, Yu YL, et al. Sustained elevation of Epstein-Barr virus antibody levels preceding clinical onset of nasopharyngeal carcinoma. Br J Cancer 2007;96(4):623–630

61. Breda E, Catarino RJ, Azevedo I, Lobão M, Monteiro E, Medeiros R. Epstein-Barr virus detection in nasopharyngeal carcinoma: implications in a low-risk area. Braz J Otorhinolaryngol 2010;76(3):310–315

62. Ng WT, Choi CW, Lee MC, Law LY, Yau TK, Lee AW. Outcomes of nasopharyngeal carcinoma screening for high risk family members in Hong Kong. Fam Cancer 2010;9(2):221–228

63. Choi CW, Lee MC, Ng WT, Law LY, Yau TK, Lee AW. An analysis of the efficacy of serial screening for familial nasopharyngeal carcinoma based on Markov chain models. Fam Cancer 2011;10(1):133–139

64. Lo YM, Chan LY, Chan AT, et al. Quantitative and temporal correlation between circulating cell-free Epstein-Barr virus DNA and tumor recurrence in nasopharyngeal carcinoma. Cancer Res 1999;59(21):5452–5455

65. Wong LP, Lai KT, Tsui E, Kwong KH, Tsang RH, Ma ES. Plasma Epstein-Barr virus (EBV) DNA: role as a screening test for nasopharyngeal carcinoma (NPC)? Int J Cancer 2005;117(3):515–516

66. Geist RM Jr, Portmann UV. Primary malignant tumors of the nasopharynx. Am J Roentgenol Radium Ther Nucl Med 1952;68(2):262–271

67. Ho JH. An epidemiologic and clinical study of nasopharyngeal carcinoma. Int J Radiat Oncol Biol Phys 1978;4(3-4):182–198

68. Ho JH. Stage classification of nasopharyngeal carcinoma: a review. IARC Sci Publ 1978; (20):99–113

69. Wei WI. A comparison of clinical staging systems in nasopharyngeal carcinoma. Clin Oncol 1984;10(3):225–231

70. Chua DT, Sham JS, Kwong DL, Choy DT, Au GK, Wu PM. Prognostic value of paranasopharyngeal extension of nasopharyngeal carcinoma. A significant factor in local control and distant metastasis. Cancer 1996;78(2):202–210

71. Sham JS, Cheung YK, Choy D, Chan FL, Leong L. Cranial nerve involvement and base of the skull erosion in nasopharyngeal carcinoma. Cancer 1991;68(2):422–426

72. Teo P, Yu P, Lee WY, et al. Significant prognosticators after primary radiotherapy in 903 nondisseminated nasopharyngeal carcinoma evaluated by computer tomography. Int J Radiat Oncol Biol Phys 1996;36(2):291–304

73. Sobin LH, Gospodarowicz MK, Wittekind CH, eds. TNM Classification of Malignant Tumours, 7th ed. New York: Wiley-Blackwell; 2009:30–38

74. Edge SB, Byrd DR, Compton CC, Fritz AG, Greene FL, Trotti A. AJCC Cancer Staging hand book, 7th ed. New York :Springer; 2010:63–79

75. Sham JS, Wei WI, Nicholls J, Chan CW, Choy D. Extent of nasopharyngeal carcinoma involvement inside the nasopharynx. Lack of prognostic value on local control. Cancer 1992;69(4):854–859

76. Chua DT, Sham JS, Kwong DL, Au GK, Choy DT. Retropharyngeal lymphadenopathy in patients with nasopharyngeal carcinoma: a computed tomography-based study. Cancer 1997;79(5):869–877

77. Lee AW, Foo W, Law SC, et al. Staging of nasopharyngeal carcinoma: from Ho's to the new UICC system. Int J Cancer 1999;84(2):179–187

78. Özyar E, Yildiz F, Akyol FH, Atahan IL; American Joint Committee on Cancer. Comparison of AJCC 1988 and 1997 classifications for nasopharyngeal carcinoma. Int J Radiat Oncol Biol Phys 1999;44(5):1079–1087

79. Chua DT, Sham JS, Wei WI, Ho WK, Au GK. The predictive value of the 1997 American Joint Committee on Cancer stage classification in determining failure patterns in nasopharyngeal carcinoma. Cancer 2001;92(11):2845–2855

24 Nasopharyngeal Carcinoma: Diagnostic Strategies

Clinical Features

Compared with other malignancies in the head and neck region, nasopharyngeal carcinoma (NPC) affects a relatively younger age group of patients[1] and this has remained much the same over the years.[2,3] In most countries it is 2 to 3 times more common in males than females.[4] The symptoms of NPC are related to the location of the tumor in the nasopharynx, the degree of its infiltration and effect on surrounding structures, and its metastases both regionally and distantly.

Commonly, NPC patients present with one or more of the four groups of symptoms.

1. **Nasal symptoms related to the presence of tumor mass in the nasopharynx.** This could be unilateral nasal obstruction when the tumor reaches a significant size or, when the tumor ulcerates, blood-stained nasal discharge frequently seen in the early-morning postnasal discharge. Severe epistaxis is rarely seen and only presents in advanced-stage disease when the tumor erodes a vessel.

2. **Aural symptoms include hearing loss, tinnitus and, less frequently, otalgia and otorrhea.** This is related to the location of the tumor at the fossa of Rosenmüller or its posterolateral extension to the paranasopharyngeal space, leading to eustachian tube dysfunction.[5] This might cause the collection of fluid in the middle ear, which is responsible for the conductive hearing loss. Serous otitis media was reported to be present in ~30% of patients at diagnosis.[6] In an ethnic Chinese patient, the presentation of serous otitis media after childhood should alert the attending clinician to the possible diagnosis of NPC.[7,8]

3. **Cranial nerve palsies, which are associated with the superior extension of the tumor.** The incidence of cranial nerve involvement on presentation is ~20% and is related to skull base erosion and direct tumor infiltration.[9] The patient might experience headache, diplopia, facial pain, and numbness. Cranial nerves III, IV, and VI are involved when a tumor extends upward and affects the cavernous sinus (**Fig. 24.1**). The trigeminal nerve will be affected when the tumor involves the foramen ovale region.[10] Cranial nerves IX to XII are frequently affected when the tumor extends to the paranasopharyngeal space below the base of the skull.

4. **Metastatic cervical lymph node presenting as neck masses.** This is the commonest mode of presentation of NPC, a painless unilateral mass in the upper neck.[11] Bilateral cervical nodal involvement is not uncommon as the nasopharynx is a central structure with a rich lymphatic supply and the tumor frequently crosses the midline (**Fig. 24.2**). The lymph nodes around the posterior belly of the digastric muscle and upper jugular groups are frequently affected before those in the middle and lower neck.[12] This orderly involvement of lymph nodes, from upper neck to lower neck has been shown to be of prognostic significance.[13]

A larger retrospective analysis of 4,768 patients suffering from nasopharyngeal carcinoma showed that the median duration between the onset of symptoms and establishing diagnosis was 8 months. The symptoms at presentation were neck mass (75.8%), nasal-related symptoms (73.4%), aural-related symptoms (62.4%), headache (34.8%), diplopia (10.7%), facial numbness (7.6%), weight loss (6.9%), and trismus (3.0%).[14] The physical signs elicited at diagnosis were enlarged neck node (74.5%), and cranial nerve palsy (20.0%). The cranial nerves most commonly involved were the fifth, sixth, third, and twelfth.[15] The presenting symptoms in young patients, those below 20 years of age, were in general similar to those in adults.

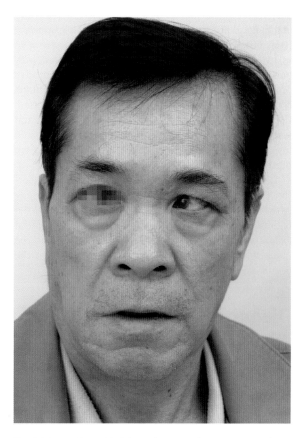

Fig. 24.1 A patient with right sixth nerve palsy presenting with diplopia.

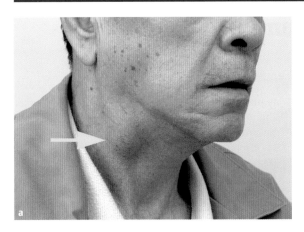
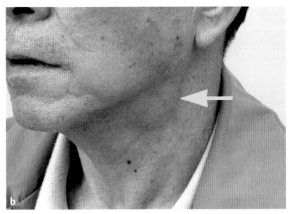

Fig. 24.2a, b Patient with bilateral lymph node metastases (same patient as in **Fig. 24.1**).

a Right upper neck lymph node.

b Left upper neck node.

Nasal and aural symptoms were more frequently seen than neck masses.[16]

Trismus and headache are less frequently seen as the presenting symptom, as they are related to extensive tumor involvement and usually accompany other symptoms. Trismus is caused by tumor extension laterally to involve the pterygoid muscles, while headache is due to involvement of the skull base. The incidence of distant metastasis on presentation in general is less than 5%. The frequent sites of metastasis are the vertebrae and femoral heads. Radiologically, 66% of the lesions are lytic, although mixed lytic and sclerotic lesions are seen in 13% of patients.[17] The main symptom associated with bone metastasis is localized bone pain. Less frequent sites of metastasis are the lungs and liver and these patients could have chest symptoms and deranged liver function. General symptoms of malignancy such as anorexia and weight loss are uncommon in NPCs, and disseminated disease should be suspected when these symptoms are present.

Unfortunately, symptoms of early-stage disease—those related to nasal and aural symptoms—are usually trivial and nonspecific, and thus are often ignored by the patient or misinterpreted by the physician. A full clinical examination of the nasopharynx is also not easy; thus the majority of NPC patients are only diagnosed when the tumor has reached advanced stages.

Diagnosis

Clinical

Symptoms of nasopharyngeal carcinoma vary greatly between different patients, even when they have in the same stage of disease. Some of the symptoms may be trivial and patients may not be aware of them, thus it is difficult to arrive at the diagnosis by taking history alone.

A full clinical examination of the head and neck region is essential, and particular effort should be exercised to detect the presence of serous otitis media, cervical lymphadenopathy, and any cranial nerve involvement.

When a patient is suspected to be suffering from nasopharyngeal carcinoma, a thorough examination of the nasopharynx is mandatory. The posterior nasal space in some patients can be adequately examined indirectly with a mirror, while in other patients the examination is limited by anatomical variation of the nasopharynx such as the approximation of the soft palate toward the posterior wall of the nasopharynx. Other patients may have an exaggerated gag reflex, making the examination difficult.

The nasopharynx can be examined directly under local anesthesia with either a rigid or a flexible endoscope. When a suspicious lesion is seen, a biopsy can be taken at the same time. The rigid 0° and 30° Hopkin rod endoscopes provide an excellent view of the nasopharynx on the side of the insertion (**Fig. 24.3**) and the superficial extent of the tumor can be determined (**Fig. 24.4**). The 30° endoscope can be used to view the opposite side of the nasopharynx when an anatomical variation, such as a deviated nasal septum, does not allow the introduction of the endoscope through the nasal passage (**Fig. 24.5**). Alternatively, the 70° endoscope introduced through the mouth beyond the soft palate can provide a centered view of the whole nasopharynx, including the extent of the tumor (**Fig. 24.6**). These rigid endoscopes with an outer diameter of 3 or 4 mm do not have a suction or biopsy channel. Therefore, a separate suction catheter has to be inserted alongside the endoscope to remove blood or mucus before an unobstructed view of the nasopharynx can be obtained. A pair of forceps also has to be inserted separately along the endoscope in the same nasal passage, or through the other nasal cavity to obtain a biopsy.

A flexible fiberoptic endoscope, with or without a suction and biopsy channel, allows a more thorough examination of the nasopharynx compared with a rigid

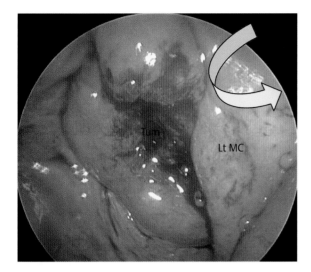

Fig. 24.3 0° Endoscopic view showing tumor (Tum) filling the left fossa of Rosenmüller. The left medial crura (Lt MC) and the opening of the eustachian tube (curved arrow) are shown.

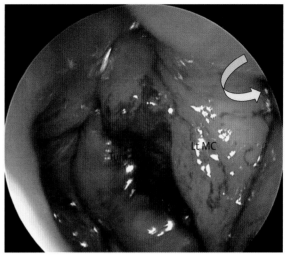

Fig. 24.4 30° Endoscopic view showing the same tumor (Tum) filling the fossa of Rosenmüller. The medial crura (Lt MC) and the opening of the eustachian tube (curved arrow) are shown.

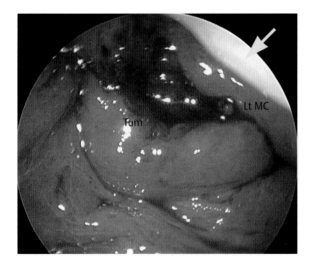

Fig. 24.5 30° Endoscope inserted through the right nasal cavity, viewing the same tumor (Tum) filling the fossa of Rosenmüller on the left side. The nasal septum is marked by an arrow and the left medial crura (Lt MC) is seen.

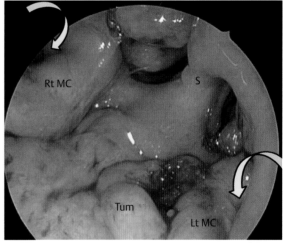

Fig. 24.6 70° Endoscope inserted behind the uvula showing the tumor (Tum) filling the left fossa of Rosenmüller. The posterior edge of the nasal septum (S) is seen. The left (Lt MC) and right (Rt MC) medial crura and the openings of the eustachian tubes (curved arrows) are shown.

endoscope. This is because the tip of the endoscope can be manipulated to turn round angles to reach the tumor. The image obtained from the flexible fiberoptic endoscope is inferior to that from the rigid endoscope, although with the flexible videoendoscopes the quality of images are much better (**Fig. 24.7**). The flexible endoscope can be inserted through one nasal cavity and then turned behind the nasal septum to examine the opposite nasopharynx. Thus, the entire nasopharynx can be adequately examined with the endoscope inserted once. When there is difficulty in passing the endoscope through the nasal cavity owing to the presence of a large tumor or other anatomical variation, the flexible endoscope can be inserted through the mouth and manipulated to above the soft palate to examine the entire nasopharynx (**Fig. 24.8**).

After adequate examination of the tumor following removal of mucus by suction, a biopsy is taken of any suspicious lesion in the nasopharynx as seen through the endoscope (**Fig. 24.9**). When a separate forceps (**Fig. 24.10**) is used for taking the biopsy, a large piece of tissue can be obtained for histological examination (**Fig. 24.11**). When a flexible endoscope is used, only a small biopsy forceps can be inserted through the narrow flexible

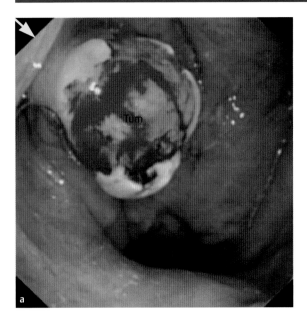

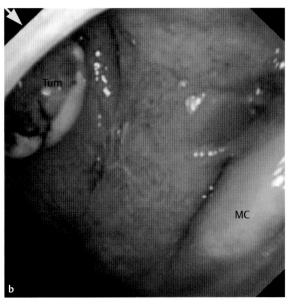

Fig. 24.7a, b Flexible video endoscopic view.

a Polypoid tumor (Tum) arising from the right lower fossa of Rosenmüller; the medial crura is just seen (arrow).

b Endoscope in the left nasal fossa; the tumor (Tum) is seen behind the nasal septum (arrow). The medial crura of the left eustachian tube (MC) is also seen.

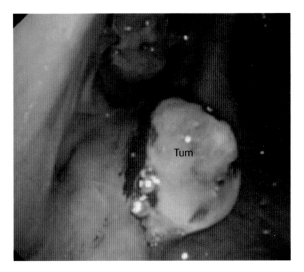

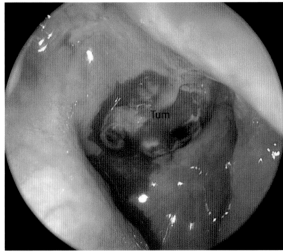

Fig. 24.8 Flexible video endoscope introduced behind the soft palate, curving upward to see the tumor (Tum) arising from the right lateral wall. The posterior edge of the nasal septum (S) is seen.

Fig. 24.9 0° Endoscopic view showing tumor (Tum) on the roof of the right nasopharynx.

Serology

endoscopic channel and the amount of tissue obtained may not be sufficient for diagnosis. However, the small biopsy forceps are useful for taking biopsies from the narrow confines of the pharyngeal recess. The mucosa overlying the lesion should be broken with the forceps and then one jaw of the forceps is inserted through the mucosal wound into the submucosa to obtain more tissue for histological examination.[18]

The ubiquitous Epstein-Barr Virus (EBV) has a strong association with NPC. EBV-specific antigens can be grouped into latent-phase antigens, early replicative antigens, and late antigens. Latent-phase antigens include the EBV-associated nuclear antigen (EBNA) and the latent membrane proteins (LMPs).[19] The early antigens are the early membrane antigen (EMA) and early intracellular antigen (EA).[20] The late antigens are the viral capsid antigen (VCA) and late membrane antigen (LMA).[21]

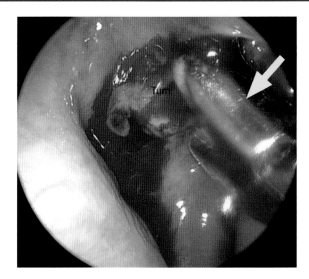

Fig. 24.10 0° Endoscopic view showing tumor (Tum) on the roof of the right nasopharynx; a biopsy forceps (arrow) is taking a biopsy.

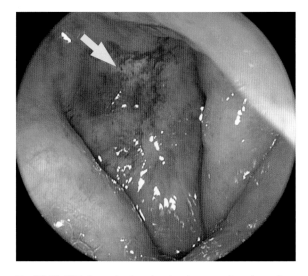

Fig. 24.11 0° Endoscopic view showing the tumor base (arrow) after the main tumor bulk had been removed.

The immunological response of a patient infected with EBV varies between individuals and depends on the manifestation of the associated disease. Patients suffering from NPC have a high level of immunoglobulin (IgA) response to VCA and EA. This has been used for decades as a diagnostic indicator for nasopharyngeal carcinoma.[22,23] The antibodies for viral capsid antigen (IgA anti-VCA) and early antigen (IgA anti-EA) have been used widely to screen for early nasopharyngeal carcinoma.[24,25] Determination of levels of these antibodies has been used in the screening of NPC in endemic areas.[26] The IgA anti-VCA is a more sensitive but less specific test than IgA anti-EA. Endoscopic examination and biopsy of the nasopharynx, aiming at early detection of NPC, were performed in patients with high IgA levels.[27]

A prospective study was performed in Guangdong, southeast China, to evaluate the efficacy of serology in detecting early nasopharyngeal carcinoma.[28] IgA levels against the VCA and EA of the Epstein-Barr virus were tested in 67,891 healthy persons. A total of 6,102 subjects (9%) were found to have an elevated serum antibody titer. On endoscopic examination and biopsy 48 (0.8%) of the seropositive subjects had NPC although they were asymptomatic. Of the remaining 6,054 seropositive patients, 130 were randomly recruited for endoscopic examination and biopsy of the nasopharynx. There were 71 men and 59 women, ages ranging from 30 to 61 years (median, 44 years). Positive biopsy was obtained from seven patients, confirming NPC.

From this prospective study, subclinical NPC was diagnosed in 5.4% of patients (7/130) with elevated IgA titer against EBV. Thus in high-risk regions, patients with elevated antibody levels should undergo an endoscopic examination of the nasopharynx.

The level of the IgA anti-EBV has also been shown to be related to the stage of the tumor, which is proportional to the tumor burden.[29] Most of the studies on the EBV serology for early diagnosis of NPC were performed in the 1980s. When IgA anti-VCA was compared with antibodies against other EBV antigens such as EBNA in the diagnosis of nasopharyngeal carcinoma, IgA anti-VCA has the lowest false-negative value.[30] A recent meta-analysis of 20 of these types of studies showed that IgA anti-VCA when elevated has a sensitivity of 91% and specificity of 92% in the diagnosis of nasopharyngeal carcinoma.[31] Although the level of IgA anti-VCA has been shown to decrease in NPC patients whose tumors have been eradicated,[32] its value in the monitoring of recurrence is not established.[33]

As EBV is frequently detected in nasopharyngeal undifferentiated carcinoma cells and on the lysis of these malignant cells, EBV DNA is released into the blood. This DNA has a short half-life but, with a high turnover rate of malignant cells, increasingly numerous copies of EBV DNA are released and this circulating free EBV DNA can now be detected by PCR in patients with NPC.[34] In 96% of patients suffering from NPC, EBV DNA can be detected in plasma.[35] This is further supported by the fact that increased copies of EBV DNA were found in the blood during the initial phase of radiotherapy, suggesting that the viral DNA was released into the circulation after cell death.[36] The quantity of free plasma EBV DNA as measured by real-time quantitative PCR has been shown to be related to the stage of the disease.[37] The detection of EBV DNA has increasingly been used for the diagnosis of NPC and this has been shown to be more accurate than measuring the antibody titers against the various EBV antigens.[38]

The use of serum EBV DNA has been shown to be sensitive and reliable for the detection of distant metastases.[39] The numbers of EBV DNA copies before and after treatment are significantly related to the rates of overall and disease-free survival.[40,41] There were reports stating that the levels of posttreatment EBV DNA, when compared with pretreatment EBV DNA, had a better prediction for progression-free survival,[42] and they have also been used to monitor any recurrent disease after treatment.[43] Elevated levels of EBV DNA were, however, detected in only 67% of patients with locoregional recurrence when the recurrence volume was small.[44] When EBV DNA was employed together with IgA against viral capsid antigen of EBV, the sensitivity of early diagnosis of nasopharyngeal carcinoma increased.[45]

Cytology

The applications of cytology in the diagnosis of NPC are twofold. First, exfoliative cytology has been employed to detect tumor cells from the primary carcinoma in the nasopharynx. Second, cytological examination of fine needle aspirates from a cervical lymph node contributes to the confirmation of metastasis to the neck gland.

The sensitivity of exfoliative cytology in the detection of NPC has been reported to be in the range 75 to 88%.[46,47] This involves scraping the mucosal surface of the nasopharynx with a swab either transnasally or transorally to obtain the cells for examination. As a biopsy of the nasopharynx can easily be obtained with the endoscope, exfoliative cytology is seldom used nowadays for diagnostic purposes. The procedure is simple and inexpensive, thus this exfoliative cytological technique might be considered as a screening procedure in NPC endemic regions.

Fine needle aspiration of enlarged cervical lymph nodes to obtain cells for cytological examination has a high success rate in confirming the diagnosis of metastatic NPC.[48,49] However, the same procedure employed for the diagnosis of recurrent cervical lymphadenopathy, after radiotherapy, is not impressive.[50] This is not surprising as it is difficult to obtain enough cells for a proper cytological examination after irradiation, and this is also true for other head and neck malignancies. The use of in situ hybridization for the determination of EBV EBER1 RNA (Epstein–Barr virus-encoded RNA1) may improve the sensitivity and specificity of cytological diagnosis of metastasis to the cervical lymph nodes.[51]

Imaging

Endoscopic examination of the nasopharynx and clinical examination provide information on local tumor extension on the mucosa and metastasis to neck lymph nodes. However, it cannot assess the deep extension of tumor such as involvement of musculature of the nasopharynx, erosion of bone at the skull base, and possible intracranial spread.

Cross-sectional imaging has revolutionized the management of NPCs. Computed tomography (CT) can identify the paranasopharyngeal extension of the tumor, which is a common mode of local extension of NPC.[52] CT is able to show soft tissue infiltration, which is not possible even with multidirectional tomography (**Fig. 24.12**).[53] The main application of CT is due to its sensitivity in detecting skull base erosion (**Fig. 24.13**).[54] Perineural spread through the foramen ovale is an important route of intracranial extension and this might lead to cavernous sinus involvement (**Fig. 24.14**).[55] CT should be performed when the status of the base of the skull needs to be evaluated.[56] The information provided through CT is important for staging and thus for choice of therapeutic measures.[57] Sometimes the primary tumor is submucosal in location and cannot be visualized with the endoscope, while at the same time the retropharyngeal lymph node is shown on CT. With the use of a CT navigation system, precise tissue biopsy is possible with the forceps inserted through the wall of the nasopharynx into the retropharyngeal node (**Fig. 24.15**).

CT has limitations in the assessment of nasopharyngeal carcinoma as it has poor tumor enhancement. In contrast, MRI has better tissue specificity and distinguishes tumor from inflammatory tissue, especially in the paranasal sinuses. In addition to its multiplanar capabilities (**Figs. 24.16, 24.17, 24.18**) MRI delineates fascial planes with clarity.[58] It is generally agreed that MRI may miss subtle bone erosion shown on CT but it is more sensitive

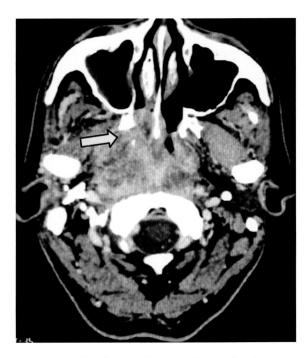

Fig. 24.12 Axial CT showing a large nasopharyngeal carcinoma eroding the right pterygoid plates (arrow).

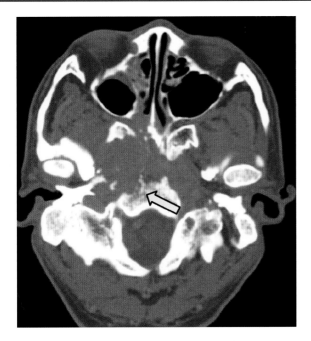

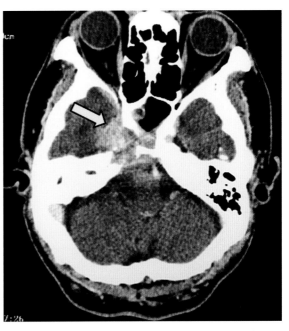

Fig. 24.13 Axial CT showing a large nasopharyngeal carcinoma eroding the skull base bone, including the clivus (arrow).

Fig. 24.14 Axial CT showing the large nasopharyngeal carcinoma (arrow) eroding the skull base bone to affect the cavernous sinus.

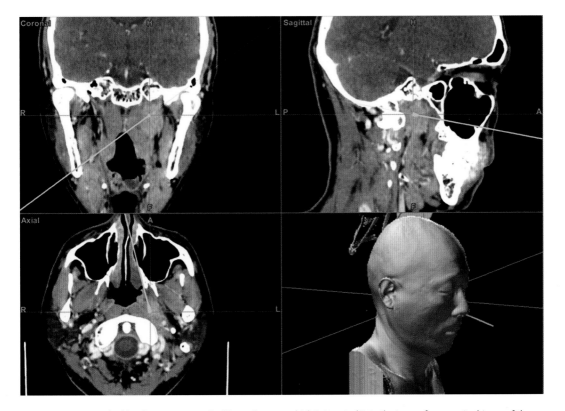

Fig. 24.15 CT navigation: the blue line represents the biopsy forceps, which is inserted into the tumor for a precise biopsy of the paranasopharyngeal tissue.

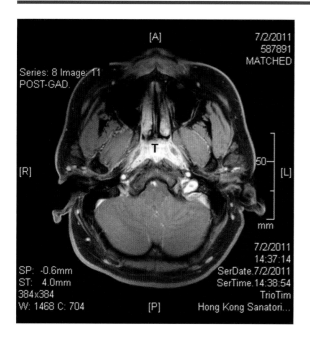

Fig. 24.16 MRI axial view, showing the tumor (T).

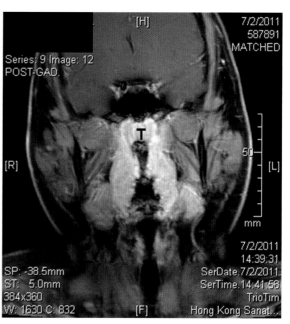

Fig. 24.17 MRI coronal view, showing the tumor (T).

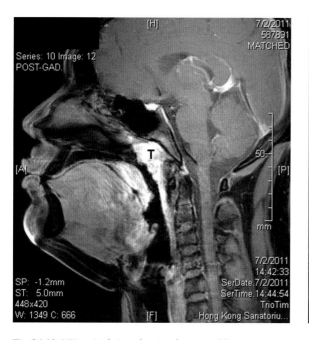

Fig. 24.18 MRI sagittal view, showing the tumor (T).

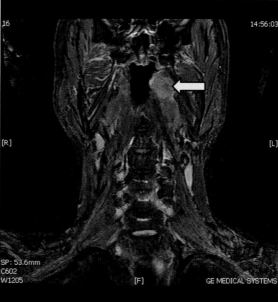

Fig. 24.19 MRI coronal view, showing the paranasopharyngeal lymph node (arrow).

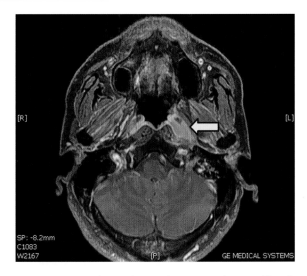

Fig. 24.20 MRI axial view, showing the paranasopharyngeal lymph node (arrow).

in detecting bone marrow infiltration[59] and in evaluation of retropharyngeal nodal metastases (**Figs. 24.19 and 24.20**).[60] Therefore, CT and MRI are more likely to be complementary rather than competing imaging techniques and this is especially true in the evaluation of the deep tissue planes of the nasopharynx. Cross-sectional imaging displays precisely the extent of the primary tumor. This enables radiotherapy treatment to be administered more accurately and effectively, which improves outcome.[61] It is particularly the case with the application of intensity-modulated radiotherapy (IMRT), which makes use of composite CT-MRI targets.[62] The radiation energy is focused on the tumor and spares adjacent normal tissues (**Fig. 24.21**).

Another contribution of cross-sectional imaging is in the determination of the extent of cervical nodal involvement (**Fig. 24.22**) and more importantly the extension of tumor into the paranasopharyngeal space or the involvement of the retropharyngeal nodes of Rouvière, which are the most cranially situated cervical nodes (**Figs. 24.23, 24.24, 24.25**). Accurate identification of nodal involvement by tumor has prognostic significance and is essential in the planning of radiation treatment.

Positron emission tomography (PET) reveals the primary nasopharyngeal carcinoma tumor and the metastatic lymph nodes (**Figs. 24.26 and 24.27**). However, it did not improve the accuracy of diagnosis or affect the staging of patients before treatment.[63] For locally advanced nasopharyngeal carcinoma, the fluorine-18 fluorodeoxyglucose (^{18}F-FDG) uptake as measured by standard uptake value (SUV_{max}) has been shown to have prognostic significance.[64] Those with SUV_{max} greater than 5 have a poor outcome.[65]

The conventional investigations for metastatic disease such as bone scans, ultrasound examination of the abdomen, and liver scans are of little value.[66,67]

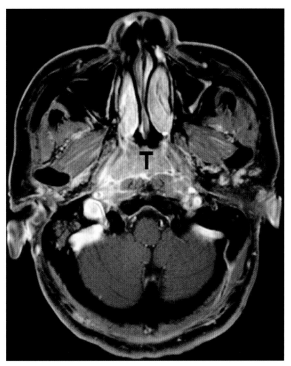

Fig. 24.21 MRI axial view, showing the local extent of the tumor (T).

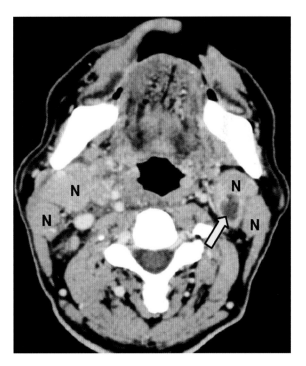

Fig. 24.22 CT showing bilateral cervical lymph nodes (N). One of the large nodes shows central necrosis (arrow).

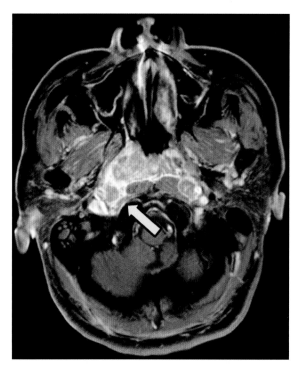

Fig. 24.23 MRI axial view, showing the primary tumor and the paranasopharyngeal lymph node (arrow).

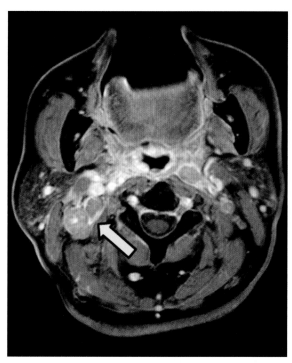

Fig. 24.24 MRI axial view, showing the paranasopharyngeal lymph node extending to the neck node behind the mandible (arrow).

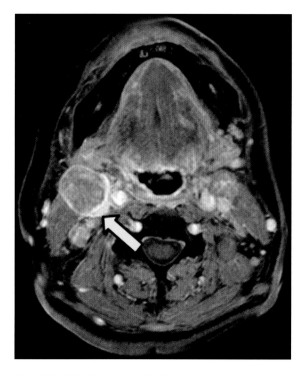

Fig. 24.25 MRI axial view, showing the lymph node extending all the way to involve the upper neck nodes (arrow).

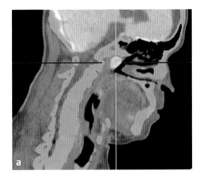
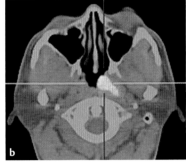
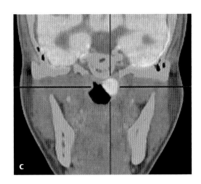

Fig. 24.26a–c PET showing hypermetabolic activity in the left nasopharyngeal tumor.

a Sagittal.   **b** Axial.   **c** Coronal.

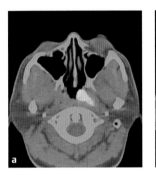
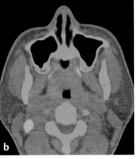
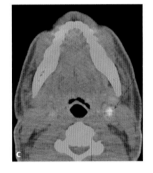
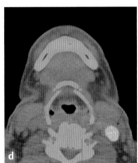

Fig. 24.27a–d PET of nasopharynx.

a Hypermetabolic activity in the left nasopharyngeal tumor.
b Hypermetabolic activity in the right upper neck node.

c Hypermetabolic activity in the left upper neck node.
d Hypermetabolic activity in the left lower neck node.

The role of PET in the detection of distant metastases in NPC and other malignancies was first noted in 2003.[68] A subsequent prospective study, however, showed that PET is not more sensitive than whole-body MRI in the detection of distant metastasis in the newly diagnosed nasopharyngeal carcinoma.[69] It has been suggested that PET was more sensitive than MRI at detecting residual and recurrent tumors in the nasopharynx[70]; a recent systematic review confirmed this and also that both sensitivity and specificity were better with dual-section and multi-section helical CT.[71]

References

1. Buell P. Nasopharynx cancer in Chinese of California. Br J Cancer 1965;19(3):459–470
2. Sham JS, Wei WI, Tai PT, Choy D. Multiple malignant neoplasms in patients with nasopharyngeal carcinoma. Oncology 1990;47(6):471–474
3. Lee AW, Foo W, Mang O, et al. Changing epidemiology of nasopharyngeal carcinoma in Hong Kong over a 20-year period (1980–99): an encouraging reduction in both incidence and mortality. Int J Cancer 2003;103(5):680–685
4. Curado MP, Edwards B, Shin HR, et al, eds. Cancer Incidence in Five Continents, Vol. IX. Lyon: IARC; 2007:141–143 (IARC Scientific Publication No.160)
5. Su CY, Hsu SP, Lui CC. Computed tomography, magnetic resonance imaging, and electromyographic studies of tensor veli palatini muscles in patients with nasopharyngeal carcinoma. Laryngoscope 1993;103(6):673–678
6. Dempster JH, Simpson DC. Nasopharyngeal neoplasms and their association with adult onset otitis media with effusion. Clin Otolaryngol Allied Sci 1988;13(5):363–365
7. Sham JST, Wei WI, Lau SK, Yau CC, Choy D. Serous otitis media. An opportunity for early recognition of nasopharyngeal carcinoma. Arch Otolaryngol Head Neck Surg 1992;118(8):794–797
8. Ho KY, Lee KW, Chai CY, Kuo WR, Wang HM, Chien CY. Early recognition of nasopharyngeal cancer in adults with only otitis media with effusion. J Otolaryngol Head Neck Surg 2008;37(3):362–365
9. Sham JST, Cheung YK, Choy D, Chan FL, Leong L. Cranial nerve involvement and base of the skull erosion in nasopharyngeal carcinoma. Cancer 1991;68(2):422–426
10. Cui C, Liu L, Ma J, et al. Trigeminal nerve palsy in nasopharyngeal carcinoma: correlation between clinical findings and magnetic resonance imaging. Head Neck 2009; 31(6):822–828
11. Huang SC. Nasopharyngeal cancer: a review of 1605 patients treated radically with cobalt 60. Int J Radiat Oncol Biol Phys 1980;6(4):401–407
12. Sham JST, Choy D, Wei WI. Nasopharyngeal carcinoma: orderly neck node spread. Int J Radiat Oncol Biol Phys 1990;19(4):929–933
13. Sham JS, Choy D, Choi PH. Nasopharyngeal carcinoma: the significance of neck node involvement in relation to the pattern of distant failure. Br J Radiol 1990;63(746):108–113
14. Lee AW, Foo W, Law SC, et al. Nasopharyngeal carcinoma: presenting symptoms and duration before diagnosis. Hong Kong Med J 1997;3(4):355–361

15. Ozyar E, Atahan IL, Akyol FH, Gürkaynak M, Zorlu AF. Cranial nerve involvement in nasopharyngeal carcinoma: its prognostic role and response to radiotherapy. Radiat Med 1994;12(2):65–68
16. Sham JS, Poon YF, Wei WI, Choy D. Nasopharyngeal carcinoma in young patients. Cancer 1990;65(11):2606–2610
17. Sham JST, Cheung YK, Chan FL, Choy D. Nasopharyngeal carcinoma: pattern of skeletal metastases. Br J Radiol 1990;63(747):202–205
18. Wei WI, Sham JS, Zong YS, Choy D, Ng MH. The efficacy of fiberoptic endoscopic examination and biopsy in the detection of early nasopharyngeal carcinoma. Cancer 1991;67(12):3127–3130
19. Reedman BM, Klein G. Cellular localization of an Epstein-Barr virus (EBV)-associated complement-fixing antigen in producer and non-producer lymphoblastoid cell lines. Int J Cancer 1973;11(3):499–520
20. Henle G, Henle W, Klein G. Demonstration of two distinct components in the early antigen complex of Epstein-Barr virus-infected cells. Int J Cancer 1971;8(2):272–282
21. Rowe M, Finke J, Szigeti R, Klein G. Characterization of the serological response in man to the latent membrane protein and the six nuclear antigens encoded by Epstein-Barr virus. J Gen Virol 1988;69(Pt 6):1217–1228
22. Ho HC, Ng MH, Kwan HC, Chau JC. Epstein-Barr-virus-specific IgA and IgG serum antibodies in nasopharyngeal carcinoma. Br J Cancer 1976;34(6):655–660
23. Liu MT, Yeh CY. Prognostic value of anti-Epstein-Barr virus antibodies in nasopharyngeal carcinoma (NPC). Radiat Med 1998;16(2):113–117
24. Ng MH, Chen HL, Luo RX, et al. Serological diagnosis of nasopharyngeal carcinoma by enzyme linked immunosorbent assay: optimization, standardization and diagnostic criteria. Chin Med J (Engl) 1998;111(6):531–536
25. Zeng Y, Zhong JM, Li LY, et al. Follow-up studies on Epstein-Barr virus IgA/VCA antibody-positive persons in Zangwu County, China. Intervirology 1983;20(4):190–194
26. Levine PH, Pearson GR, Armstrong M, et al. The reliability of IgA antibody to Epstein-Barr virus (EBV) capsid antigen as a test for the diagnosis of nasopharyngeal carcinoma (NPC). Cancer Detect Prev 1981;4(1–4):307–312
27. Zeng Y. Seroepidemiological studies on nasopharyngeal carcinoma in China. Adv Cancer Res 1985;44:121–138
28. Sham JS, Wei WI, Zong YS, et al. Detection of subclinical nasopharyngeal carcinoma by fibreoptic endoscopy and multiple biopsy. Lancet 1990;335(8686):371–374
29. Henle W, Ho HC, Henle G, Kwan HC. Antibodies to Epstein-Barr virus-related antigens in nasopharyngeal carcinoma. Comparison of active cases with long-term survivors. J Natl Cancer Inst 1973;51(2):361–369
30. Chan KH, Gu YL, Ng F, et al. EBV specific antibody-based and DNA-based assays in serologic diagnosis of nasopharyngeal carcinoma. Int J Cancer 2003;105(5):706–709
31. Li S, Deng Y, Li X, Chen QP, Liao XC, Qin X. Diagnostic value of Epstein-Barr virus capsid antigen-IgA in nasopharyngeal carcinoma: a meta-analysis. Chin Med J (Engl) 2010;123(9):1201–1205
32. Henle W, Ho JH, Henle G, Chau JC, Kwan HC. Nasopharyngeal carcinoma: significance of changes in Epstein-Barr virus-related antibody patterns following therapy. Int J Cancer 1977;20(5):663–672
33. Lynn TC, Tu SM, Kawamura A Jr. Long-term follow-up of IgG and IgA antibodies against viral capsid antigens of Epstein-Barr virus in nasopharyngeal carcinoma. J Laryngol Otol 1985;99(6):567–572
34. Mutirangura A, Pornthanakasem W, Theamboonlers A, et al. Epstein-Barr viral DNA in serum of patients with nasopharyngeal carcinoma. Clin Cancer Res 1998;4(3):665–669
35. Lo YM, Chan LY, Lo KW, et al. Quantitative analysis of cell-free Epstein-Barr virus DNA in plasma of patients with nasopharyngeal carcinoma. Cancer Res 1999;59(6):1188–1191
36. Lo YM, Leung SF, Chan LY, et al. Kinetics of plasma Epstein-Barr virus DNA during radiation therapy for nasopharyngeal carcinoma. Cancer Res 2000;60(9):2351–2355
37. Lo YM, Leung SF, Chan LY, et al. Plasma cell-free Epstein-Barr virus DNA quantitation in patients with nasopharyngeal carcinoma. Correlation with clinical staging. Ann N Y Acad Sci 2000;906:99–101
38. Shao JY, Li YH, Gao HY, et al. Comparison of plasma Epstein-Barr virus (EBV) DNA levels and serum EBV immunoglobulin A/virus capsid antigen antibody titers in patients with nasopharyngeal carcinoma. Cancer 2004;100(6):1162–1170
39. Hong RL, Lin CY, Ting LL, Ko JY, Hsu MM. Comparison of clinical and molecular surveillance in patients with advanced nasopharyngeal carcinoma after primary therapy: the potential role of quantitative analysis of circulating Epstein-Barr virus DNA. Cancer 2004;100(7):1429–1437
40. Lin JC, Wang WY, Chen KY, et al. Quantification of plasma Epstein-Barr virus DNA in patients with advanced nasopharyngeal carcinoma. N Engl J Med 2004; 350(24):2461–2470
41. Leung SF, Chan AT, Zee B, et al. Pretherapy quantitative measurement of circulating Epstein-Barr virus DNA is predictive of posttherapy distant failure in patients with early-stage nasopharyngeal carcinoma of undifferentiated type. Cancer 2003;98(2):288–291
42. Chan AT, Lo YM, Zee B, et al. Plasma Epstein-Barr virus DNA and residual disease after radiotherapy for undifferentiated nasopharyngeal carcinoma. J Natl Cancer Inst 2002;94(21):1614–1619
43. Lo YM, Chan LY, Chan AT, et al. Quantitative and temporal correlation between circulating cell-free Epstein-Barr virus DNA and tumor recurrence in nasopharyngeal carcinoma. Cancer Res 1999;59(21):5452–5455
44. Wei WI, Yuen AP, Ng RW, Ho WK, Kwong DL, Sham JS. Quantitative analysis of plasma cell-free Epstein-Barr virus DNA in nasopharyngeal carcinoma after salvage nasopharyngectomy: a prospective study. Head Neck 2004;26(10):878–883
45. Leung SF, Tam JS, Chan AT, et al. Improved accuracy of detection of nasopharyngeal carcinoma by combined application of circulating Epstein-Barr virus DNA and anti-Epstein-Barr viral capsid antigen IgA antibody. Clin Chem 2004;50(2):339–345
46. Lau SK, Hsu CS, Sham JS, Wei WI. The cytological diagnosis of nasopharyngeal carcinoma using a silk swab stick. Cytopathology 1991;2(5):239–246
47. Hanji D, Shujing S, Shuwei H, Gohao L. The cytological diagnosis of nasopharyngeal carcinoma from exfoliated cells collected by suction method. An eight-year experience. J Laryngol Otol 1983;97(8):727–734
48. Chan MKM, McGuire LJ, Lee JCK. Fine needle aspiration cytodiagnosis of nasopharyngeal carcinoma in cervical lymph nodes. A study of 40 cases. Acta Cytol 1989;33(3):344–350
49. Viguer JM, Jiménez-Heffernan JA, López-Ferrer P, Banaclocha M, Vicandi B. Fine-needle aspiration cytology of metastatic nasopharyngeal carcinoma. Diagn Cytopathol 2005;32(4):233–237
50. Toh ST, Yuen HW, Goh YH, Goh CH. Evaluation of recurrent nodal disease after definitive radiation therapy for nasopharyngeal carcinoma: diagnostic value of fine-needle aspiration cytology and CT scan. Head Neck 2007;29(4):370–377
51. Dictor M, Sivén M, Tennvall J, Rambech E. Determination of nonendemic nasopharyngeal carcinoma by in situ hybridization for Epstein-Barr virus EBER1 RNA: sensitivity and

specificity in cervical node metastases. Laryngoscope 1995;105(4 Pt 1):407–412

52. Sham JS, Cheung YK, Choy D, Chan FL, Leong L. Nasopharyngeal carcinoma: CT evaluation of patterns of tumor spread. AJNR Am J Neuroradiol 1991;12(2):265–270

53. Gonsalves CG, Briant TD, Harmand WM. Computed tomography of the paranasal sinuses, nasopharynx, and soft tissues of the neck. Comput Tomogr 1978;2(4):271–278

54. Cheung YK, Sham J, Cheung YL, Chan FL. Evaluation of skull base erosion in nasopharyngeal carcinoma: comparison of plain radiography and computed tomography. Oncology 1994;51(1):42–46

55. Chong VF, Fan YF, Khoo JB. Nasopharyngeal carcinoma with intracranial spread: CT and MR characteristics. J Comput Assist Tomogr 1996;20(4):563–569

56. Olmi P, Fallai C, Colagrande S, Giannardi G. Staging and follow-up of nasopharyngeal carcinoma: magnetic resonance imaging versus computerized tomography. Int J Radiat Oncol Biol Phys 1995;32(3):795–800

57. Hu YC, Chang CH, Chen CH, et al. Impact of intracranial extension on survival in stage IV nasopharyngeal carcinoma: identification of a subset of patients with better prognosis. Jpn J Clin Oncol 2011;41(1):95–102

58. Chong VF, Fan YF, Khoo JB. Computed tomographic and magnetic resonance imaging findings in paranasal sinus involvement in nasopharyngeal carcinoma. Ann Acad Med Singapore 1998;27(6):800–804

59. Cheng SH, Jian JJ, Tsai SY, et al. Prognostic features and treatment outcome in locoregionally advanced nasopharyngeal carcinoma following concurrent chemotherapy and radiotherapy. Int J Radiat Oncol Biol Phys 1998;41(4):755–762

60. Dillon WP, Mills CM, Kjos B, DeGroot J, Brant-Zawadzki M. Magnetic resonance imaging of the nasopharynx. Radiology 1984;152(3):731–738

61. Cellai E, Olmi P, Chiavacci A, et al. Computed tomography in nasopharyngeal carcinoma: Part II: impact on survival. Int J Radiat Oncol Biol Phys 1990;19(5):1177–1182

62. Emami B, Sethi A, Petruzzelli GJ. Influence of MRI on target volume delineation and IMRT planning in nasopharyngeal carcinoma. Int J Radiat Oncol Biol Phys 2003;57(2):481–488

63. King AD, Ma BB, Yau YY, et al. The impact of ^{18}F-FDG PET/CT on assessment of nasopharyngeal carcinoma at diagnosis. Br J Radiol 2008;81(964):291–298

64. Xie P, Yue JB, Fu Z, Feng R, Yu JM. Prognostic value of ^{18}F-FDG PET/CT before and after radiotherapy for locally advanced nasopharyngeal carcinoma. Ann Oncol 2010;21(5):1078–1082

65. Liu WS, Wu MF, Tseng HC, et al. The role of pretreatment FDG-PET in nasopharyngeal carcinoma treated with intensity-modulated radiotherapy. Int J Radiat Oncol Biol Phys 2012;82(2):561–566

66. Sham JS, Tong CM, Choy D, Yeung DW. Role of bone scanning in detection of subclinical bone metastasis in nasopharyngeal carcinoma. Clin Nucl Med 1991;16(1):27–29

67. Kraiphibul P, Atichartakarn V, Clongsusuek P, Kulapaditharom B, Ratanatharathorn V, Chokewattanaskul P. Nasopharyngeal carcinoma: value of bone and liver scintigraphy in the pre-treatment and follow-up period. J Med Assoc Thai 1991;74(7):276–279

68. Nakamoto Y, Osman M, Wahl RL. Prevalence and patterns of bone metastases detected with positron emission tomography using F-18 FDG. Clin Nucl Med 2003;28(4):302–307

69. Ng SH, Chan SC, Yen TC, et al. Pretreatment evaluation of distant-site status in patients with nasopharyngeal carcinoma: accuracy of whole-body MRI at 3-Tesla and FDG-PET-CT. Eur Radiol 2009;19(12):2965–2976

70. Yen RF, Hung RL, Pan MH, et al. 18-Fluoro-2-deoxyglucose positron emission tomography in detecting residual/recurrent nasopharyngeal carcinomas and comparison with magnetic resonance imaging. Cancer 2003;98(2):283–287

71. Liu T, Xu W, Yan WL, Ye M, Bai YR, Huang G. FDG-PET, CT, MRI for diagnosis of local residual or recurrent nasopharyngeal carcinoma, which one is the best? A systematic review. Radiother Oncol 2007;85(3):327–335

25 Treatment of Nasopharyngeal Carcinoma

D. T. T. Chua and W. I. Wei

Introduction

Nasopharyngeal carcinoma is a highly aggressive tumor with a tendency to invade the adjacent nasal cavity and paranasal sinus, skull base, and foramina, and spread early to the cervical lymphatics. The undifferentiated type of nasopharyngeal carcinoma, which is the predominant histological type in endemic regions, also has a high risk of distant metastases compared with other head and neck cancers. As a result, surgery has a limited role in the treatment of newly diagnosed nasopharyngeal carcinoma, and radiotherapy with or without chemotherapy is the usual treatment for this disease. In patients with locoregional recurrence, salvage surgery may be feasible, especially in those with disease confined to the nasopharynx and/or neck. Reirradiation using different techniques should be considered in patients that are not candidates for surgery. In advanced recurrence and distant metastases, palliative chemotherapy can often achieve durable control of symptoms and disease control. Occasional long-term survivors have been reported after aggressive systemic chemotherapy.

Radiotherapy

Radiotherapy is the mainstay of treatment for locoregionally confined nasopharyngeal carcinoma. The outcome of patients who received radiotherapy for nasopharyngeal carcinoma has improved significantly in the past four decades, from a gloomy 5-year survival rate of 25% in the 1950s,[1] to 50% in the 1970s to 1980s,[2] and to 75% in the 1990s.[3] The improvement of outcome can be attributed to earlier disease at presentation, introduction of new and advanced imaging techniques, improved radiotherapy techniques, and the use of combined chemoradiotherapy.

Techniques

In treating nasopharyngeal carcinoma, a large target volume is needed to cover the primary tumor and potential sites of spread. This volume includes not only the nasopharynx but also the paranasopharyngeal space, oropharynx, base of the skull, sphenoid sinus, posterior ethmoid sinus, and posterior half of the maxillary antrum. Extension of the treatment field to cover the cavernous sinus and cranial fossa may be needed in advanced disease. Cervical nodal irradiation is mandatory even in node-negative patients due to the high incidence of neck relapse in the absence of prophylactic nodal irradiation.[4]

A dose of 65 to 70 Gy is normally given to the primary tumor, 65 to 70 Gy to the involved neck nodes, and 50 to 60 Gy to the node-negative neck. In the past, radiotherapy for nasopharyngeal carcinoma was performed using two-dimensional treatment planning with two or three large fields to cover the primary ± upper neck and one or two fields to cover the lower neck (**Fig. 25.1**). Normal structures are protected by custom-made lead shields or a multileaf collimator. Treatment is usually delivered using a single fraction daily and five fractions per week.

Intracavitary brachytherapy was sometimes used to deliver a boost dose for T1 and T2 tumors after external beam radiotherapy and this has been reported to improve the tumor control rate by 16%.[5] Altered fractionation using accelerated hyperfractionation in which twice daily fractions were used failed to improve the tumor control despite a higher risk of developing neurologic toxicity.[6]

Intensity-Modulated Radiotherapy

One major advance in radiotherapy of nasopharyngeal carcinoma during the 2000s was the advent of intensity-modulated radiotherapy (IMRT). IMRT is a complicated technique that allows the delivery of a dose distribution closely conformed to the target and critical structures

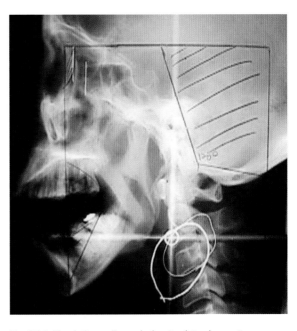

Fig. 25.1 Simulation radiograph showing lateral opposing treatment field for nasopharyngeal carcinoma using simple 2D planning.

through optimization of the intensity of multiple beams. The treatment design is based on the computer algorithm to calculate the best result that matches the user-defined parameters in a process called inverse planning. An advantage of IMRT is the ability to deliver highly conformal radiotherapy to an irregular target, such as the generation of a concave or U-shaped dose distribution, which is very useful if the target volume wraps around critical structures such as the brainstem and spinal cord, as in the case of nasopharyngeal carcinoma (**Fig. 25.2**); other advantages include the ability to treat primary and regional lymphatic in one volume, and the ability to deliver simultaneous integrated boost in the same setting. IMRT is ideal for treatment of nasopharyngeal carcinoma with the potential of improving dose distribution and therapeutic ratio. IMRT has already achieved excellent local control rates for newly diagnosed nasopharyngeal carcinoma, with a reported local control rate of 92 to 97% at 3 to 4 years.[7,8] Apart from improvement of tumor control, IMRT also reduces the risk of late complications such as xerostomia in early-stage disease.[9]

Combined Chemoradiotherapy

Combining chemotherapy and radiotherapy has many theoretical advantages in the treatment of nasopharyngeal carcinoma; this malignancy has a high incidence of distant metastases, which constitute the major cause of treatment failure and death, and chemotherapy is needed to address this issue. Local failure still constitutes another important cause of failure in advanced T stage despite improvement in outcome with modern radiotherapy, and

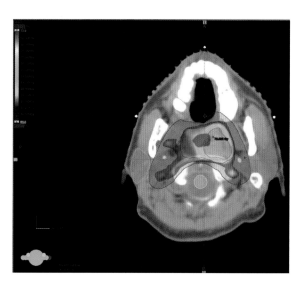

Fig. 25.2 Planning CT showing the U-shaped target typical of nasopharyngeal carcinoma and adequate coverage of the target by intensity-modulated radiotherapy.

the use of chemotherapy may allow rapid shrinkage of the tumor to facilitate radiotherapy. Some recurrent and metastatic disease has shown good response to chemotherapy, with occasional observation of long-term survivors, suggestive that the disease is highly chemosensitive. Unlike patients with other head and neck cancers, most patients with nasopharyngeal carcinoma are younger with good performance status and absence of comorbidities, and hence they should tolerate chemoradiotherapy better.

Randomized Trials

Many randomized trials have been conducted to explore the benefits of combined chemoradiotherapy in nasopharyngeal carcinoma. Most studies employed cisplatin-based regimens and the main difference has been the timing of chemotherapy in relation to radiotherapy: before (induction), during (concurrent), or after (adjuvant) radiotherapy.

Four randomized phase III studies have been reported comparing induction chemotherapy followed by radiotherapy versus radiotherapy alone in nasopharyngeal carcinoma.[10-13] None of these studies has demonstrated survival benefits after adding chemotherapy to radiotherapy. Two of these studies were recently updated and the data pooled for analysis; although significant improvement in disease-free survival in the chemotherapy arm was observed, overall survival was not improved.[14] Only two adjuvant chemotherapy phase III studies have been reported, and both showed no survival benefits.[15,16] The adjuvant chemotherapy trials had limitations since non-platinum chemotherapy was used in one study and chemotherapy compliance was rather poor in the other study. These studies showed that induction chemotherapy alone has a limited role in nasopharyngeal carcinoma, whereas the role of adjuvant chemotherapy remains undefined.

In recent years, concurrent chemoradiotherapy has emerged as the treatment of choice for locoregionally advanced nasopharyngeal carcinoma, largely due to the positive findings of the Intergroup 0099 trial, which was the first randomized trial to demonstrate survival benefit with the use of chemotherapy in nasopharyngeal carcinoma.[17] The Intergroup trial employed both concurrent and adjuvant chemotherapy in the study arm and reported an absolute improvement of survival of 31% (i.e. from 47% to 78%) at 3 years. The Intergroup study, however, has a high proportion of patients with WHO type I histology and a relatively poor outcome in the radiotherapy-alone arm. Thus there were initially some concerns in extrapolating the findings of the Intergroup study to patient groups in the Asian context where the disease is endemic and the majority of patients have undifferentiated carcinoma, WHO type III histology.

Subsequent randomized trials conducted in endemic regions have largely confirmed the benefits of concurrent

Table 25.1 Treatment outcomes for subgroups of NPC patients treated with intensity-modulated radiation therapy ± chemotherapy

Subgroup	5-year local relapse-free survival	5-year distant metastasis-free survival	5-year overall survival
Early disease group (T1–2N0–1M0)	97.1%	96.3%	95.6%
Advanced local disease group (T3–4N0–1M0)	87.2%	84.4%	80.1%
Advanced nodal disease group (T1–2N2–3M0)	94.7%	83.3%	84.8%
Advanced locoregional disease group (T3–4N2–3M0)	83%	62.3%	62.2%

chemoradiotherapy in locoregionally advanced nasopharyngeal carcinoma, although different regimens and schedules were being employed in these studies.[18–21] Interestingly, only one study employed the same chemotherapy regimens used in the Intergroup study, but the final report from that study showed no survival benefits, although there was improvement in failure-free survival and progression-free survival.[22] Nevertheless, current evidence indicates that concurrent chemoradiotherapy may have a role in advanced-stage nasopharyngeal carcinoma, but the optimal regimen and schedule remain to be defined. The design of most chemotherapy trials that employed both concurrent and adjuvant chemotherapy does not allow the role of adjuvant treatment to be separately defined, but one common observation in these trials was the low compliance rate of adjuvant chemotherapy, especially when given after concurrent chemoradiotherapy. On the other hand, it may be easier to combine induction with concurrent chemotherapy with the added benefit of rapid tumor shrinkage prior to radiotherapy, and preliminary reports showed that excellent control can be achieved using this approach in advanced T stage tumors.[23] Based on current evidence, chemoradiotherapy should be given to all patients with nodal disease and/or T3–4 disease, whereas radiotherapy alone should be reserved for those with T1–2 N0 disease. Following this treatment concept, the overall survival of patients with early and advanced-stage disease has been reported to be 96% and 62%, respectively (**Table 25.1**).[24]

Sequelae of Therapy

Although radical treatment of nasopharyngeal carcinoma often yields good response and cure, there are many complications that can adversely affect the quality of life of patients after treatment. Xerostomia is almost universal after conventional radiotherapy, and this leads to dry mouth, poor oral hygiene, and dental caries.[25] Hearing impairment is common and is the combined result of direct radiation damage to the hearing apparatus, persistent disturbance of eustachian tube function, and chemotherapy-induced ototoxicity.[26] Soft tissue fibrosis may lead to restriction of neck movement or mouth opening, often accompanied by discomfort.[27] Cranial nerve palsy is usually due to incomplete healing of damage caused by tumor; although cranial nerves, especially the lower four nerves, can also be damaged directly by radiation.[28] Dysphagia can occur as a result of cranial nerve palsy or pharyngeal stricture.[29] Hormonal insufficiency can develop due to damage to the hypothalamic-pituitary axis or end organs such as thyroid gland.[30] Carotid artery stenosis can develop following neck irradiation and may result in cerebral ischemia.[31] The most serious sequelae arise from the damage to higher functions that leads to memory loss, cognitive dysfunction, and neuropsychological dysfunction,[32–34] which can occur with or without radiological evidence of temporal lobe necrosis (**Fig. 25.3**).

Risk factors for development of these late sequelae include the use of large dose per fraction (hypofractionation); short interfraction time when multiple fractions per day are used; high cumulative dose; reirradiation, especially after a short time interval; and use of chemoradiotherapy. The advent of conformal radiotherapy such as IMRT has the potential for reducing late radiation

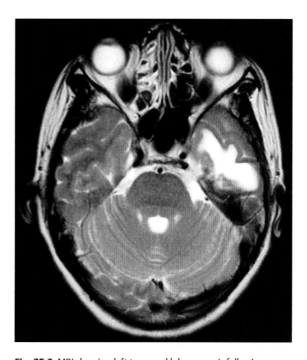

Fig. 25.3 MRI showing left temporal lobe necrosis following radiotherapy of nasopharyngeal carcinoma.

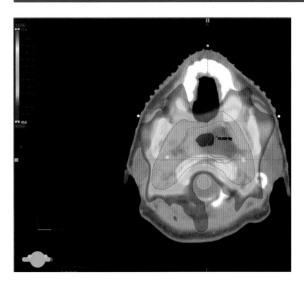

Fig. 25.4 Planning CT showing sparing of bilateral parotid glands with the use of intensity-modulated radiotherapy for nasopharyngeal carcinoma.

sequelae by reducing the dose delivered to critical structures. For example, it is possible to prevent xerostomia by selectively sparing the parotid glands using three-dimensional conformal radiotherapy or IMRT (**Fig. 25.4**).[35]

Circulating EBV DNA: A Prognostic Indicator

Circulating cell-free Epstein-Barr virus (EBV) DNA can be detected in most patients with nasopharyngeal carcinoma and the number of copies of EBV DNA can be measured by real-time quantitative polymerase chain reaction. The quantity of EBV DNA is related to the stage of disease, with high numbers of copies more commonly detected in advanced stage.[36] The quantity of EBV DNA measured before and after treatment is also an important predictive factor of outcome. One study reported that patients with posttreatment EBV DNA above 500 copies/mL had a higher chance of developing relapse and death.[37] Another study reported that pretreatment EBV DBA above 4,000 copies/mL in stage I–II patients was associated with a higher risk of distant failure.[38] These results suggested that pre- and post-therapy EBV DNA might provide important prognostic information that can allow clinicians to define a high-risk patient group that warrants more aggressive treatment. EBV DNA may also serve as a tumor marker for monitoring of treatment response and follow-up, but it is less useful in detecting local recurrence than distant metastases because up to one-third of patients with locoregional recurrence did not have elevated EBV DNA copies.[37]

Novel Approaches

Novel approaches are currently being developed for nasopharyngeal carcinoma and these focus on the unique association of the disease with EBV. Strategies targeted at EBV include immune therapy and more recently gene therapy. Approaches for immune therapy included therapeutic augmentation of cytotoxic T-lymphocyte responses[39] and adoptive transfer of autologous ex vivo expanded EBV-specific cytotoxic T lymphocytes.[40] Gene therapy with a novel replication-deficient adenovirus vector in which transgenic expression is under the transcriptional regulation of oriP of EBV has also been reported.[41]

In addition, therapy targeted on the epidermal growth factor receptor (EGFR) axis using monoclonal antibody[42] may also prove to be useful in nasopharyngeal carcinoma due to the high percentage of EGFR expression in this carcinoma.[43,44] Preliminary studies using small-molecule inhibitors of EGFR tyrosine kinase were disappointing, however.[45,46] Future studies on approaches targeting EBV or molecular targets in nasopharyngeal carcinoma may further improve the treatment outcome.

References

1. Moss WT. Therapeutic Radiology, 2nd ed. St Louis: Mosby; 1965
2. Lee AWM, Poon YF, Foo W, et al. Retrospective analysis of 5037 patients with nasopharyngeal carcinoma treated during 1976–1985: overall survival and patterns of failure. Int J Radiat Oncol Biol Phys 1992;23(2):261–270
3. Lee AW, Sze WM, Au JS, et al. Treatment results for nasopharyngeal carcinoma in the modern era: the Hong Kong experience. Int J Radiat Oncol Biol Phys 2005;61(4):1107–1116
4. Lee AW, Sham JS, Poon YF, Ho JH. Treatment of stage I nasopharyngeal carcinoma: analysis of the patterns of relapse and the results of withholding elective neck irradiation. Int J Radiat Oncol Biol Phys 1989;17(6):1183–1190
5. Leung TW, Tung SY, Wong VY, et al. High dose rate intracavitary brachytherapy in the treatment of nasopharyngeal carcinoma. Acta Oncol 1996;35(1):43–47
6. Teo PM, Leung SF, Chan AT, et al. Final report of a randomized trial on altered-fractionated radiotherapy in nasopharyngeal carcinoma prematurely terminated by significant increase in neurologic complications. Int J Radiat Oncol Biol Phys 2000;48(5):1311–1322
7. Lee N, Xia P, Quivey JM, et al. Intensity-modulated radiotherapy in the treatment of nasopharyngeal carcinoma: an update of the UCSF experience. Int J Radiat Oncol Biol Phys 2002;53(1):12–22
8. Kam MK, Teo PM, Chau RM, et al. Treatment of nasopharyngeal carcinoma with intensity-modulated radiotherapy: the Hong Kong experience. Int J Radiat Oncol Biol Phys 2004;60(5):1440–1450
9. Kwong DL, Pow EH, Sham JS, et al. Intensity-modulated radiotherapy for early-stage nasopharyngeal carcinoma: a prospective study on disease control and preservation of salivary function. Cancer 2004;101(7):1584–1593
10. Preliminary results of a randomized trial comparing neoadjuvant chemotherapy (cisplatin, epirubicin, bleomycin) plus radiotherapy vs. radiotherapy alone in stage IV(> or = N2, M0) undifferentiated nasopharyngeal carcinoma: a positive effect on progression-free survival. International

Nasopharynx Cancer Study Group. VUMCA I trial. Int J Radiat Oncol Biol Phys 1996;35(3):463–469

11. Chua DTT, Sham JST, Choy D, et al; Asian-Oceanian Clinical Oncology Association Nasopharynx Cancer Study Group. Preliminary report of the Asian-Oceanian Clinical Oncology Association randomized trial comparing cisplatin and epirubicin followed by radiotherapy versus radiotherapy alone in the treatment of patients with locoregionally advanced nasopharyngeal carcinoma. Cancer 1998;83(11):2270–2283

12. Ma J, Mai HQ, Hong MH, et al. Results of a prospective randomized trial comparing neoadjuvant chemotherapy plus radiotherapy with radiotherapy alone in patients with locoregionally advanced nasopharyngeal carcinoma. J Clin Oncol 2001;19(5):1350–1357

13. Hareyama M, Sakata K, Shirato H, et al. A prospective, randomized trial comparing neoadjuvant chemotherapy with radiotherapy alone in patients with advanced nasopharyngeal carcinoma. Cancer 2002;94(8):2217–2223

14. Chua DT, Ma J, Sham JS, et al. Long-term survival after cisplatin-based induction chemotherapy and radiotherapy for nasopharyngeal carcinoma: a pooled data analysis of two phase III trials. J Clin Oncol 2005;23(6):1118–1124

15. Rossi A, Molinari R, Boracchi P, et al. Adjuvant chemotherapy with vincristine, cyclophosphamide, and doxorubicin after radiotherapy in local-regional nasopharyngeal cancer: results of a 4-year multicenter randomized study. J Clin Oncol 1988;6(9):1401–1410

16. Chi KH, Chang YC, Guo WY, et al. A phase III study of adjuvant chemotherapy in advanced nasopharyngeal carcinoma patients. Int J Radiat Oncol Biol Phys 2002;52(5):1238–1244

17. Al-Sarraf M, LeBlanc M, Giri PG, et al. Chemoradiotherapy versus radiotherapy in patients with advanced nasopharyngeal cancer: phase III randomized Intergroup study 0099. J Clin Oncol 1998;16(4):1310–1317

18. Lin JC, Jan JS, Hsu CY, Liang WM, Jiang RS, Wang WY. Phase III study of concurrent chemoradiotherapy versus radiotherapy alone for advanced nasopharyngeal carcinoma: positive effect on overall and progression-free survival. J Clin Oncol 2003;21(4):631–637

19. Chan AT, Leung SF, Ngan RK, et al. Overall survival after concurrent cisplatin-radiotherapy compared with radiotherapy alone in locoregionally advanced nasopharyngeal carcinoma. J Natl Cancer Inst 2005;97(7):536–539

20. Wee J, Tan EH, Tai BC, et al. Randomized trial of radiotherapy versus concurrent chemoradiotherapy followed by adjuvant chemotherapy in patients with American Joint Committee on Cancer/International Union against cancer stage III and IV nasopharyngeal cancer of the endemic variety. J Clin Oncol 2005;23(27):6730–6738

21. Kwong DL, Sham JS, Au GK, et al. Concurrent and adjuvant chemotherapy for nasopharyngeal carcinoma: a factorial study. J Clin Oncol 2004;22(13):2643–2653

22. Lee AW, Tung SY, Chua DT, et al. Randomized trial of radiotherapy plus concurrent-adjuvant chemotherapy vs radiotherapy alone for regionally advanced nasopharyngeal carcinoma. J Natl Cancer Inst 2010;102(15):1188–1198

23. Rischin D, Corry J, Smith J, Stewart J, Hughes P, Peters L. Excellent disease control and survival in patients with advanced nasopharyngeal cancer treated with chemoradiation. J Clin Oncol 2002;20(7):1845–1852

24. Su SF, Han F, Zhao C, et al. Treatment outcomes for different subgroups of nasopharyngeal carcinoma patients treated with intensity-modulated radiation therapy. Chin J Cancer 2011;30(8):565–573

25. Pow EH, McMillan AS, Leung WK, Wong MC, Kwong DL. Salivary gland function and xerostomia in southern Chinese following radiotherapy for nasopharyngeal carcinoma. Clin Oral Investig 2003;7(4):230–234

26. Ho WK, Wei WI, Kwong DL, et al. Long-term sensorineural hearing deficit following radiotherapy in patients suffering from nasopharyngeal carcinoma: a prospective study. Head Neck 1999;21(6):547–553

27. Leung SF, Zheng Y, Choi CY, et al. Quantitative measurement of post-irradiation neck fibrosis based on the young modulus: description of a new method and clinical results. Cancer 2002;95(3):656–662

28. Lin YS, Jen YM, Lin JC. Radiation-related cranial nerve palsy in patients with nasopharyngeal carcinoma. Cancer 2002;95(2):404–409

29. Chang YC, Chen SY, Lui LT, et al. Dysphagia in patients with nasopharyngeal cancer after radiation therapy: a videofluoroscopic swallowing study. Dysphagia 2003; 18(2):135–143

30. Fang FM, Chiu HC, Kuo WR, et al. Health-related quality of life for nasopharyngeal carcinoma patients with cancer-free survival after treatment. Int J Radiat Oncol Biol Phys 2002;53(4):959–968

31. Cheng SW, Ting AC, Lam LK, Wei WI. Carotid stenosis after radiotherapy for nasopharyngeal carcinoma. Arch Otolaryngol Head Neck Surg 2000;126(4):517–521

32. Lam LC, Leung SF, Chan YL. Progress of memory function after radiation therapy in patients with nasopharyngeal carcinoma. J Neuropsychiatry Clin Neurosci 2003; 15(1):90–97

33. Cheung M, Chan AS, Law SC, Chan JH, Tse VK. Cognitive function of patients with nasopharyngeal carcinoma with and without temporal lobe radionecrosis. Arch Neurol 2000;57(9):1347–1352

34. Lee PW, Hung BK, Woo EK, Tai PT, Choi DT. Effects of radiation therapy on neuropsychological functioning in patients with nasopharyngeal carcinoma. J Neurol Neurosurg Psychiatry 1989;52(4):488–492

35. Jen YM, Shih R, Lin YS, et al. Parotid gland-sparing 3-dimensional conformal radiotherapy results in less severe dry mouth in nasopharyngeal cancer patients: a dosimetric and clinical comparison with conventional radiotherapy. Radiother Oncol 2005;75(2):204–209

36. Lin JC, Wang WY, Chen KY, et al. Quantification of plasma Epstein-Barr virus DNA in patients with advanced nasopharyngeal carcinoma. N Engl J Med 2004;350(24):2461–2470

37. Chan AT, Ma BB, Lo YM, et al. Phase II study of neoadjuvant carboplatin and paclitaxel followed by radiotherapy and concurrent cisplatin in patients with locoregionally advanced nasopharyngeal carcinoma: therapeutic monitoring with plasma Epstein-Barr virus DNA. J Clin Oncol 2004;22(15):3053–3060

38. Leung SF, Chan AT, Zee B, et al. Pretherapy quantitative measurement of circulating Epstein-Barr virus DNA is predictive of posttherapy distant failure in patients with early-stage nasopharyngeal carcinoma of undifferentiated type. Cancer 2003;98(2):288–291

39. Duraiswamy J, Sherritt M, Thomson S, et al. Therapeutic LMP1 polyepitope vaccine for EBV-associated Hodgkin disease and nasopharyngeal carcinoma. Blood 2003;101(8):3150–3156

40. Chua D, Huang J, Zheng B, et al. Adoptive transfer of autologous Epstein-Barr virus-specific cytotoxic T cells for nasopharyngeal carcinoma. Int J Cancer 2001;94(1):73–80

41. Li JH, Chia M, Shi W, et al. Tumor-targeted gene therapy for nasopharyngeal carcinoma. Cancer Res 2002; 62(1):171–178

42. Chan AT, Hsu MM, Goh BC, et al. Multicenter, phase II study of cetuximab in combination with carboplatin in patients with recurrent or metastatic nasopharyngeal carcinoma. J Clin Oncol 2005;23(15):3568–3576

43. Chua DT, Nicholls JM, Sham JS, Au GK. Prognostic value of epidermal growth factor receptor expression in patients

with advanced stage nasopharyngeal carcinoma treated with induction chemotherapy and radiotherapy. Int J Radiat Oncol Biol Phys 2004;59(1):11–20

44. Ma BB, Poon TC, To KF, et al. Prognostic significance of tumor angiogenesis, Ki 67, p53 oncoprotein, epidermal growth factor receptor and HER2 receptor protein expression in undifferentiated nasopharyngeal carcinoma—a prospective study. Head Neck 2003;25(10):864–872

45. Chua DT, Wei WI, Wong MP, Sham JS, Nicholls J, Au GK. Phase II study of gefitinib for the treatment of recurrent and metastatic nasopharyngeal carcinoma. Head Neck 2008;30(7):863–867

46. Ma B, Hui EP, King A, et al. A phase II study of patients with metastatic or locoregionally recurrent nasopharyngeal carcinoma and evaluation of plasma Epstein-Barr virus DNA as a biomarker of efficacy. Cancer Chemother Pharmacol 2008;62(1):59–64

26 Nasopharyngeal Carcinoma: Salvage of Residual or Recurrent Tumor

Incidence and Diagnosis

As nasopharyngeal carcinoma is radiosensitive and it has a high incidence of metastases to the cervical lymph nodes, the field of external radiation covers both the nasopharynx and the neck. Despite the improved efficacy of concomitant chemoradiotherapy in the management of nasopharyngeal carcinoma, there were still some patients who developed local or regional failure. The incidence of local failure was around 8.3%[1] and patients may present with residual or recurrent tumor. Regional recurrence in the cervical nodes was around 4.7%[1] and this might be associated with tumor recurrence in the nasopharynx or distant metastasis. Most reported series on treatment failures are from single-center experiences with small numbers of patients. The Hong Kong NPC Group reported a comprehensive review on outcome of NPC after primary treatment in the contemporary era of chemoradiotherapy.[2] There were 319 local failures as the first failure for 2,915 patients treated between 1996 and 2000. Among these 319 patients, 275 (86%) had isolated local failure. The incidence of isolated failure in the neck nodes reduced from 10% in 1978 to 5% in 1985,[3] and in more recent years it has been around 1.6%.[4]

Early detection of residual or recurrent disease is essential in achieving a successful salvage. Regular clinical examination is important; and whenever there is suspicion of disease, investigation should be performed. Copies of Epstein-Barr virus DNA in blood have been reported to increase in number before the manifestation of macroscopic disease. Imaging studies such as CT and MRI cannot give unequivocal evidence of disease but a progressive enlarging mass would be worrisome. These imaging studies also provide information on the extent of the recurrent disease. PET scan has also been shown to be superior to the conventional imaging studies in the diagnosis of disease,[5] especially for tumor lying below the mucosa. However, endoscopic examination of the nasopharynx with biopsy of the tumor remains the "gold standard" in confirming the presence of disease. Sequential biopsy of the nasopharynx after treatment has shown that it takes ~10 weeks for the primary tumor to regress completely after radiotherapy. Thus only tumor that has persisted for 12 weeks after treatment is considered to be residual disease.

It is notoriously difficult to confirm residual or recurrent tumor in the cervical lymph nodes after radiotherapy. Fine needle aspiration is not helpful as the fibrosis developed after radiation reduces the yield of the aspiration and also in some of the recurrent lymph nodes

only clusters of tumor cells are present.[6] Sometimes even Tru-cut biopsies may not be able to obtain enough tissue for definitive diagnosis. Imaging techniques such as CT or MRI may have features that are suggestive of disease, such as the hypodense center of the node or evidence of central necrosis. They also evaluate the local extent of the neck disease (**Fig. 26.1**). The probability of disease escalates when the node increases in size on sequential imaging. The definitive diagnosis, however, still depends on histological confirmation and sometimes this is only available after salvage surgery.

Management of Residual or Recurrent Disease

Salvage treatment, even by aggressive procedures for locally recurrent NPC, is indicated especially when the disease is confined to the nasopharynx. The survival after salvage treatment for extensive disease remains poor, but it is still higher than in patients receiving supportive treatment only. Even for those patients who develop synchronous locoregional failures, aggressive treatment should be considered for selected patients.[7]

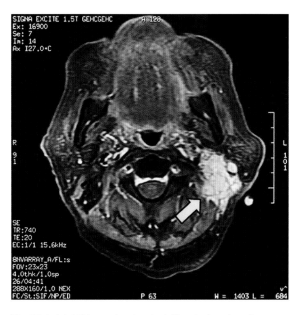

Fig. 26.1 Axial CT scan showing the infiltrative lymph node (arrow); the edge is irregular, infiltrating deep neck tissue and the overlying skin.

Disease in the Neck

When further doses of external radiotherapy were employed to treat these cervical lymph node metastases, the 5-year actuarial control rate of local disease for lymph nodes smaller than 4 cm in diameter was 51% and the overall 5-year survival rate was 19.7%.[8] Excision of the lymph node followed by second course of radiotherapy as the salvage treatment was employed by others but the results were not conclusive because of the small patient numbers.[9] The associated morbidities of radiotherapy were also significant.

Radical neck dissection has been employed for salvage of recurrent metastatic neck lymph node in nasopharyngeal carcinoma. The 5-year actuarial control rate of disease in the neck was 66%, and the 5-year actuarial survival for this group of patients was 38%.[10] Whether such an extensive operation such as radical neck dissection is necessary to achieve control of the neck disease is debatable, as frequently the cervical metastasis presents clinically as a solitary node and, sometimes, subsequent examination of the radical neck dissection specimen reveals no tumor in any of the lymph nodes removed.[6]

The optimal management of localized metastasis in the neck lymph nodes depends on the pathological behavior of the tumor and a prospective study was performed to clarify this point. Classical radical neck dissection specimens were obtained from 43 nasopharyngeal carcinoma patients who developed localized disease in the neck after radiotherapy. The whole radical neck dissection specimen was fixed and sequentially sliced at 3-mm intervals. A histological slide was made from each tissue slice. From these 43 radical neck dissection specimens, a total of 1,075 histological sections were obtained and a total of 2,137 lymph nodes were examined, of which 294 contained tumor. In three patients, no malignant cells were identified in any of the neck nodes examined; there was only reactive hyperplasia with fibrosis.

For the remaining 40 patients, significantly more tumor-bearing lymph nodes were identified histologically than detected clinically. The tumor-bearing lymph nodes were found mostly in the upper part of the neck and in the posterior triangle. The distribution of the neck nodes was level I 5% (15/294), level II 34% (99/294), level III 16% (48/294), level IV 7% (19/294), and level V 38% (113/294). Surgical clearance of lymph nodes at all levels in the neck is important, especially in the upper neck. These tumor-bearing lymph nodes also showed extracapsular spread in 46% (135/294). In view of the extensive nature of these lymph node metastases (Fig. 26.2), a radical neck dissection is recommended as the salvage treatment for cervical nodal metastasis after radiotherapy in patients with NPC. However, a recent review suggested that as the neck nodes in level I were frequently not affected in these patients, a less extensive neck dissection, sparing level I might be applicable in patients with localized involvement of the neck lymph nodes.[11]

When the residual or recurrent disease in the neck is extensive, such as when the nodes have infiltrated the floor of the neck or the overlying skin, then brachytherapy should be applied in addition to the radical neck dissection as a salvage procedure. During the radical neck dissection the skin over the tumor in the neck is removed with the specimen (Fig. 26.3) and hollow nylon tubes are placed over the operative site for after-loading brachytherapy with iridium wire (Fig. 26.4). The cutaneous defect in the neck is covered with either a deltopectoral flap or a pectoralis major myocutaneous flap (Fig. 26.5). With this additional brachytherapy, the 3-year actuarial control rate of neck disease was around 60%[12] and this was similar to the disease control rate when a radical neck dissection was performed for less extensive neck disease.

Disease in the Nasopharynx

When residual or recurrent tumor is detected in the nasopharynx after radiation or concurrent chemoradiotherapy, it can be managed with a second course of external radiotherapy. The recommended radiation dosage has to be greater than the initial dose to eradicate those tumor cells that survived the initial irradiation. In an early report, survival of up to 50% has been reported.[13] The response of the surrounding tissues to further radiation limits the radiation dose. The neuroendocrine injury,[14] temporal lobe necrosis,[15] cranial nerve palsies, and other problems such as trismus and deafness, can be incapacitating. However, with the development of precision radiotherapy, such as intensity-modulated radiotherapy (IMRT) and stereotactic radiotherapy, a second course of external radiotherapy could be given with sufficient efficacy and acceptable side effects. In a report, following a second course of radiation, a salvage rate of 32% was achieved, the cumulative incidence of late post-reirradiation sequelae was 24%, with

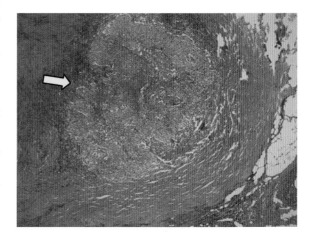

Fig. 26.2 A metastatic lymph node showing that the malignant cells are infiltrating the capsule and surrounding neck tissue (arrow). (Hematoxylin and eosin ×50.)

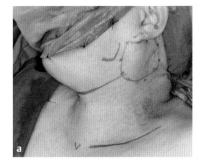

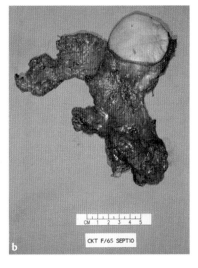

Fig. 26.3a, b

a Radical neck dissection incisions for an extensive metastatic cervical lymph node; the skin overlying the lymph node will be removed.

b Radical neck dissection specimen; the skin over the lymph node was removed en bloc.

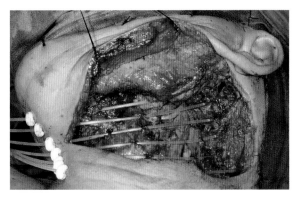

Fig. 26.4 Hollow nylon tubes are placed onto the tumor bed, at 1 cm spacing, planning for additional after-loading brachytherapy.

treatment mortality of 1.8%.[16] Stereotactic radiotherapy for the treatment of recurrent disease has been reported to achieve a 2-year local tumor control rate of 72%.[17] The number of patients treated with this method was small and long-term follow-up information is not available.[18]

External Beam Reirradiation

Retreatment of nasopharyngeal carcinoma by external beam radiation is difficult and poses special challenges to the clinician and the patient. Reirradiation of nasopharyngeal carcinoma is difficult due to the large numbers of critical structures in the vicinity of the recurrent disease that were already irradiated to a high dose during the primary course of radiotherapy. Whenever possible, brachytherapy or stereotactic radiosurgery should be considered first for retreatment of the nasopharynx. The reported 5-year survival rates after external beam reirradiation using conventional technique ranged from 8% to 36%.[19,20] A high incidence of late complications, mostly neurologic damage and soft tissue fibrosis, has commonly been observed after external beam reirradiation.

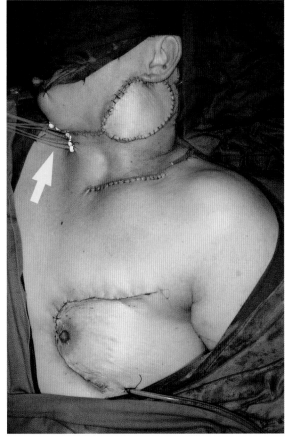

Fig. 26.5 The skin defect is covered with a pectoralis major myocutaneous flap. The ends of the nylon tubes can be seen (arrow).

The use of three-dimensional conformal radiotherapy and more recently IMRT has improved the outlook of patients receiving external reirradiation. In one study using three-dimensional conformal radiotherapy for retreatment of nasopharyngeal carcinoma, the 5-year local control rate was 71% but the actuarial incidence of major late toxicities was still high with all patients developing at least grade 3 toxicities and nearly half had grade 4 toxicities at 5 years.[21] Several preliminary reports using IMRT for reirradiation of nasopharyngeal carcinoma reported good short-term control with a relatively low incidence of severe late toxicities, but long-term outcome is not yet available.[22,23]

Prognostic Factors with Reirradiation

Important prognostic factors in patients receiving external reirradiation for recurrent NPC include T stage, time to recurrence, and the reirradiation dose for local control and/or survival. The most consistent prognostic factor reported has been the T stage of the recurrence, and patients treated for advanced T stage have had poor local control and survival after reirradiation. There appears to be an important relationship between reirradiation dose and treatment outcome, with most series reporting poor tumor control with a dose below 60 Gy,[23,24] although the optimal dose has yet to be defined.

Chemoradiotherapy may also improve treatment outcome in locally recurrent nasopharyngeal carcinoma in settings similar to those of newly diagnosed cases. One study employed induction chemotherapy to shrink the tumor volume followed by reirradiation using IMRT, and reported 75% local control rate at 1 year.[25] Another study employed concurrent chemoradiotherapy and reported a 1-year progression-free rate of 42%.[26] In patients with advanced local recurrence in which treatment planning for reirradiation is difficult, induction rather than concurrent chemotherapy is preferred as induction may allow tumor shrinkage to take place and facilitate subsequent radiotherapy planning and whole-target coverage but there is no evidence of improved survival.

Stereotactic Radiosurgery

Stereotactic radiosurgery is the technique in which a small target is stereotactically localized and irradiated by multiple convergent beams using a large single dose of radiation. The technique was originally developed for treatment of functional neurologic disorders, but was later found to be useful for vascular malformations, benign intracranial/skull base neoplasms, and cerebral metastases. Stereotactic radiosurgery has also been employed in nasopharyngeal carcinoma to deliver a boost dose after a second course of radiotherapy or as a salvage treatment of local recurrence. Stereotactic radiosurgery alone has been reported to achieve a crude local control rate of 53 to 86% for locally recurrent nasopharyngeal carcinoma.[27,28] For recurrent disease confined to the nasopharynx or adjacent soft tissues, the reported local control rate at 2 years was 72%.[17] When stereotactic radiosurgery

was administered as a boost dose after reirradiation, the 3-year control rate ranged from 52% to 58%.[29,30]

The same technique may also be used to deliver multiple fractions of radiation and is termed "stereotactic radiotherapy" (**Fig. 26.6**), but the control rates appeared to be similar to those with radiosurgery. These results indicate that radiosurgery is an effective salvage treatment for local failures of nasopharyngeal carcinoma, although there are no data comparing the relative efficacy and complications of radiosurgery with other salvage treatments. In practice, selection of treatment modalities depends mainly on extent of disease and expertise available. For recurrent disease confined to the nasopharynx or adjacent soft tissues, the results of radiosurgery appear to be comparable to those of brachytherapy or surgery, and can be considered as a treatment option. The advent of IMRT appeared to improve the outcome of recurrent nasopharyngeal carcinoma, and reirradiation using modern techniques is recommended for patients with extensive local recurrence while reserving radiosurgery as a boost treatment or for further recurrence.

Complications

Although most studies report a relatively low risk of late complications following radiosurgery, massive hemorrhage remains the most severe form of complication with a potential fatal outcome.[18] Massive hemorrhage that developed after radiosurgery is usually due to radiation damage to the carotid artery as a result of using large fraction dose and a high cumulative dose. To minimize

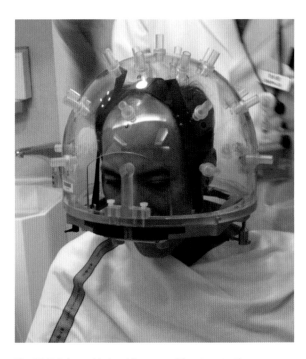

Fig. 26.6 Relocatable head frame used for stereotactic radiotherapy.

the risk of hemorrhage, radiosurgery should only be used in the absence of direct tumor encasement of the carotid artery, otherwise the patient should be treated by fractionated radiotherapy using a small fraction dose.

Brachytherapy

Brachytherapy delivers a high dose of radiation to the residual or recurrent tumor but the radiation dose decreases rapidly with distance from the radiation source; thus the radiation delivered to surrounding tissue is much smaller. Brachytherapy also delivers continuous low-dose radiation, giving a radiobiological advantage over fractionated external radiation. Intracavitary brachytherapy has been used for nasopharyngeal carcinomas.[31] The radiation source was placed either in a tube or a mold[32] and this was then inserted into the nasopharynx to place it close to the tumor. As the nasopharynx has an irregular contour and residual or recurrent tumor has an uneven surface, it is difficult to apply the radiation source accurately to provide a tumoricidal dose. For this form of application of brachytherapy to be effective, accurate insertion of the implant into the tumor is essential. Thus interstitial radioactive implants have been used to treat small, localized residual or recurrent tumor in the nasopharynx.[33]

The radiation source frequently employed for interstitial brachytherapy is radioactive gold 198 grains ([198]Au). These gold grains can be implanted into the nasopharyngeal tumor either transnasally or through the split-palate approach.[34] The latter gives the surgeon a direct view of the tumor and enables the implantation of the radioactive gold grains into the tumor precisely according to a geometric distribution so that a 1 cm thick layer of tissue is irradiated. The number of gold grains permanently implanted depends on the size and location of the tumor. During the surgical procedure, lead shielding is used to protect all medical personnel in the operating room.

Gold grain implantation is an effective salvage method for small tumors localized in the nasopharynx, without bone invasion, and not encroaching onto the eustachian tube cartilage.[35] Five-year local tumor control rates of 87% for residual and 63% for recurrent NPC after radiotherapy have been reported, while the 5-year disease-free survival rates were 68% and 60%, respectively.[36] There were no other significant sequelae associated with this form of treatment and it is recommended for management of small recurrent NPC localized in the nasopharynx.

Nasopharyngectomy

Another salvage option for residual or recurrent tumor in the nasopharynx is surgical resection. This is indicated when the localized disease cannot be managed adequately by brachytherapy, either because the tumor is too extensive and extends into paranasopharyngeal space or because of its location—for example, close to the cartilage of the eustachian tube crus where gold grains cannot be implanted.

Nasopharyngectomy in those patients who have localized disease in the nasopharynx is a good option for salvage. There are reports of removal of small recurrent tumor with the use of the endoscope.[37-40] The tumor has to be located at an appropriate site in the nasopharynx before an oncological resection can be performed with rigid instruments. Small tumor located in the posterior wall of the nasopharynx (**Fig. 26.7**) was removed adequately with an endoscope and instruments inserted through the nasal (**Fig. 26.8**) and oral cavities, curving upward behind the soft palate (**Fig. 26.9**). The wound usually healed well (**Fig. 26.10**). Microwave coagulation therapy has also been reported to have success and the procedure can be performed transnasally.[41] In general the use of rigid endoscopic instruments limits the lateral resection margin of the tumor or the deep margin of laterally situated tumors. This limitation can be circumvented

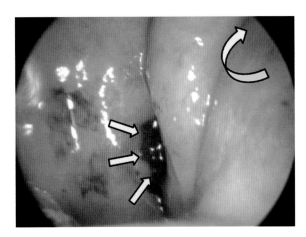

Fig. 26.7 A small tumor (arrows) situated at the lower part of the fossa of Rosenmüller, medial to the medial crura (MC) and the eustachian tube opening (curved arrow).

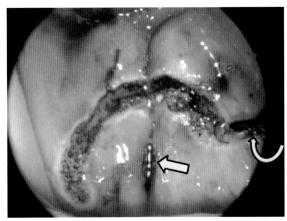

Fig. 26.8 The diathermy needle (curved arrow) employed to cut at a distance from the tumor (arrow).

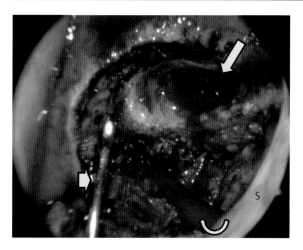

Fig. 26.9 The tumor (arrow) was removed using two instruments: the diathermy (curved arrow) inserted through the left nasal cavity behind the nasal septum (S), and the sucker/dissector (arrow head) inserted behind the uvula.

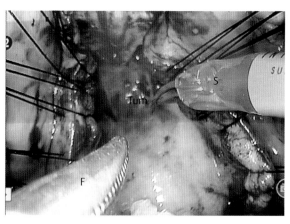

Fig. 26.11 With splitting of the soft palate, the tumor (Tum) in the nasopharynx can be seen; this is resected using scissors/diathermy (S) on the right and forceps (F) on the left, incorporated into the EndoWrist of the robot.

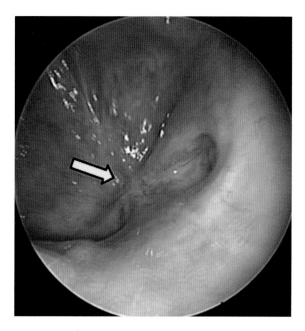

Fig. 26.10 Three years post resection, there was a scar (arrow) medial to the lower part of the medial crura.

to some extent when the da Vinci Robot is employed for resection (**Fig. 26.11**). Adequate tumor resection has been reported with the versatile EndoWrist of the da Vinci Robot inserted through a split-palate approach.[42]

A successful surgical salvage depends on adequate tumor removal with a negative resection margin.[43] Thus, for more extensive tumor in the nasopharynx, the region has to be exposed widely so that an oncological resection can be performed. This challenge is related to the anatomy of the nasopharynx, as it lies in the center of the head. It is difficult to gain adequate exposure of the pathology in

the nasopharynx and its vicinity so that adequate tumor extirpation is possible.

The residual or recurrent tumor in the nasopharynx is situated anterior to the brainstem and the upper cervical spine, thus a posterior approach to the pathology is impractical. To approach the lesion from the superior aspect, the trans–skull base approach is needed. Removal of tumors in the nasopharynx has been reported, but the associated morbidities, such as meningitis and encephalocele, could be serious consequences because the subarachnoid space is exposed to the pathogens of the nasal cavity[44]; as a consequence this approach is no longer used.

Several other approaches to the nasopharynx have been reported. The various anterior approaches to the nasopharynx described in the past, via either the transantral or the transnasal route, do not provide adequate exposure of the nasopharynx for adequate tumor removal.[45] From the anterior aspect, even with down fracture of the hard palate as in a Le Fort I[46] or the midfacial degloving route with removal of the medial wall of the maxilla, the exposure of the lateral aspect of the nasopharynx is not satisfactory.[47]

The infratemporal fossa or lateral approach to the nasopharynx has also been described.[48] To reach the nasopharynx, a mastoidectomy has to be performed and then exposure of the infratemporal fossa is achieved. Some important structures, such as the internal carotid artery, the fifth cranial nerve, and the floor of middle cranial fossa have to be mobilized or removed. A recent study on 11 patients salvaged with this approach reported a 2-year disease-free survival rate of 72%.[49] Although tumors in the nasopharynx on the side of the approach and those that have extended laterally to the paranasopharyngeal space can be removed, it is difficult to remove a tumor that has crossed the midline, and the associated morbidity of this lateral approach is not negligible.

From the inferior aspect, the transpalatal, transmaxillary, and transcervical routes have been reported to be applicable for the removal of recurrent nasopharyngeal carcinoma.[50,51] With the inferior approach, it is difficult to carry out dissection of paranasopharyngeal pathologies under direct vision, especially when the tumor is close to the internal carotid artery. This approach is useful for tumors situated in the central part of the nasopharynx. As long as the internal carotid artery is safeguarded, the associated morbidity of the operation is low.

The anterolateral or maxillary swing approach to the nasopharynx (**Fig. 26.12**) provides adequate exposure of the nasopharynx and the paranasopharyngeal space.[52]

Following a Weber–Fergusson incision (**Fig. 26.13**) and three osteotomies, the maxilla attached to the anterior cheek flap is swung laterally as an osteocutaneous flap. The osteotomies are on the anterior wall of the maxilla below the inferior orbital rim (**Fig. 26.14**) and on the hard palate (**Fig. 26.15**) in the midline and separating the pterygoid plates from the maxillary tuberosity. The soft palate is left intact while the swung maxilla receives its blood supply from the soft tissue of the anterior cheek flap. When the whole osteocutaneous complex is swung laterally, the nasopharynx, the cartilaginous crura of the eustachian tube (**Fig. 26.16**), the recurrent or residual tumor (**Fig. 26.17**), and the paranasopharyngeal space tissue are all widely exposed. Pathological tissues in this region can then be removed en bloc as required as an oncological resection (**Fig. 26.18**). The posterior part of the nasal septum, the rostrum, and the anterior wall of the sphenoidal sinus can also be removed to achieve an additional tumor clearance margin and to increase the

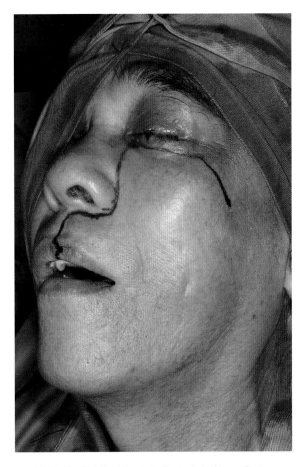

Fig. 26.13 The facial incision is similar to that of a maxillectomy and is marked.

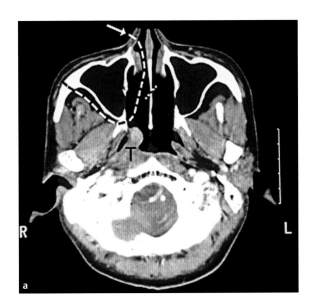

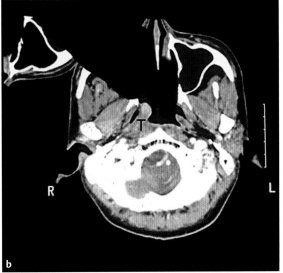

Fig. 26.12a, b Schematic computed tomography.

a Osteotomies on the right maxilla are marked with dotted line. The posterior half of the nasal septum is also removed to expose the tumor (T).

b The right maxilla is swung laterally as an osteocutaneous flap; the blood supply comes from the anterior cheek flap. The tumor (T) is completely exposed with the maxilla swung laterally.

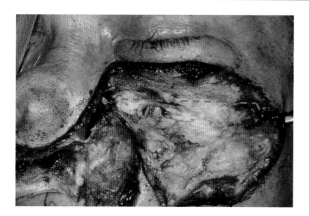

Fig. 26.14 The osteotomy on the anterior wall of the maxilla and the lower half of the zygomatic arch is marked with a blue dotted line.

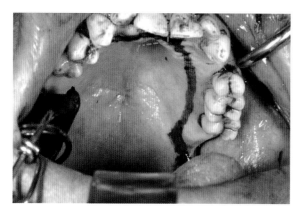

Fig. 26.15 The curved incision on the palate allows the lifting of the palatal flap and the osteotomy on the hard palate goes between the two medial incisors (blue line). The soft tissue incision and the osteotomy are in different planes, thus avoiding palatal fistula.

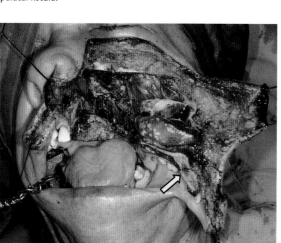

Fig. 26.16 The left maxilla is swung laterally to expose the nasopharynx and its vicinity. The hard palate with the left medial incisor is indicated by the arrow.

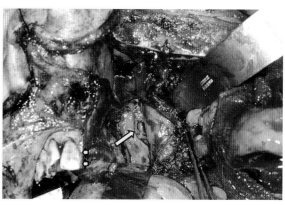

Fig. 26.17 After the left maxilla is swung laterally, the tumor can be seen (arrow). The right medial incisor is indicated by arrow heads.

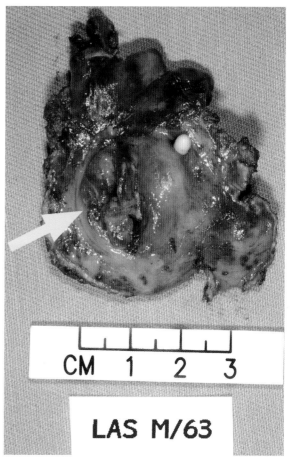

Fig. 26.18 Specimen showing tumor (arrow) removed with margin. The yellow tube marks the left eustachian tube orifice.

exposure of the lateral wall on the contralateral side. The internal carotid artery below the base of the skull can be dissected free from the residual or recurrent nasopharyngeal carcinoma (**Fig. 26.19**). After tumor extirpation, the maxilla is returned and fixed onto the facial skeleton with miniplates (**Fig. 26.20**). The complications in these patients are in general minor; some patients develop trismus and others a palatal fistula. With modification of surgical techniques, the palatal fistula rate associated with the maxillary swing approach has been markedly reduced.[53] These morbidities are still acceptable and the quality of life of these patients has been satisfactory (**Fig. 26.21**).[54,55]

Between 1989 and 2009, this maxillary swing nasopharyngectomy was employed as the surgical salvage procedure for 246 patients with residual or recurrent primary NPC after radiotherapy. With a follow-up period ranging from 6 to 18 years (median 38 months), the 5-year actuarial local tumor control rate was 74%, and the 5-year actuarial survival was 56%.[56]

For more extensive tumors, those lying close to the internal carotid artery, the vessel would be exposed after

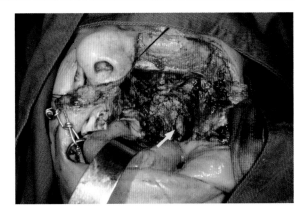

Fig. 26.20 After resection of the tumor and the paranasopharyngeal tissue, the internal carotid artery is exposed (arrow).

tumor extirpation. Vascularized tissue should be used to cover the vessel and the adjacent region. This will promote healing and, if indicated, further radiation can be delivered to the region. The free microvascular muscle transfer employing either the rectus abdominis or the vastus lateralis muscle (**Fig. 26.22**) can performed following tumor resection. The free muscle with its vascular pedicle, at the level of the soft palate, is passed behind the lateral pharyngeal wall to the neck, where it is anastomosed to the recipient artery and veins.

The mortalities associated with most of these salvage surgical procedures have been low considering that all the patients concerned had had previous radiotherapy. For surgical salvage, as long as the residual or recurrent tumor can be removed adequately, the long-term results have been satisfactory.[57–60]

The success of salvage of residual or recurrent nasopharyngeal carcinoma depends very much on the early diagnosis of the disease. When the disease is localized to the mucosa, interstitial brachytherapy offers a good chance of eradicating the tumor. For thicker, localized tumor in an appropriate position, resection with the help of the endoscope or the da Vinci Robot, or these in combination, is applicable.[61] For larger tumors that are still localized to the nasopharynx and the paranasopharyngeal space, surgical resection with an open approach still provides a chance of cure.

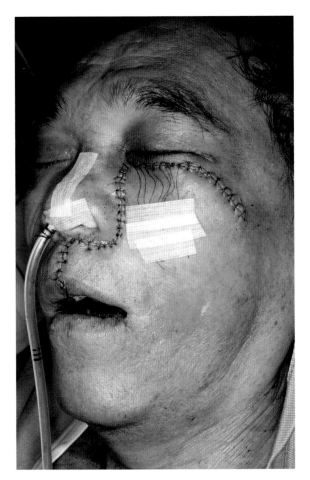

Fig. 26.19 The maxilla is returned and fixed to the rest of facial skeleton with miniplates and sutures.

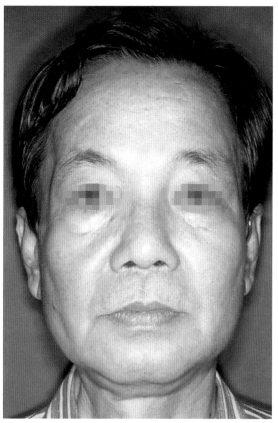

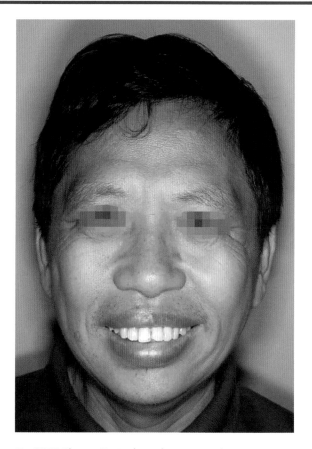

Fig. 26.21 Three patients who underwent nasopharyngectomy with the maxillary swing approach; the facial scar is not obvious.

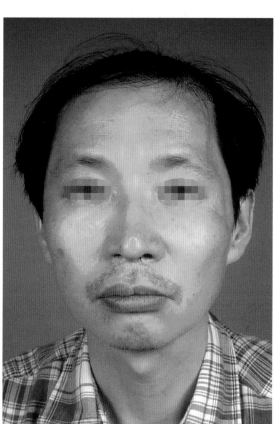

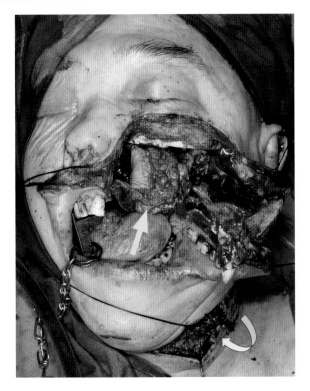

Fig. 26.22 Vastus lateralis muscle from the thigh is moved to fill the defect in the nasopharynx and to cover the carotid artery. The skin and subcutaneous tissue is shown (arrow); the pedicle is tunneled to the neck (curved arrow) to be anastomosed to the neck vessels.

References

1. Ng WT, Lee MC, Hung WM et al. Clinical outcomes and patterns of failure after intensity-modulated radiotherapy for nasopharyngeal carcinoma. Int J Radiat Oncol Biol Phys 2011;79(2):420–428
2. Yu KH, Leung SF, Tung SY, et al; Hong Kong Nasopharyngeal Carcinoma Study Group. Survival outcome of patients with nasopharyngeal carcinoma with first local failure: a study by the Hong Kong Nasopharyngeal Carcinoma Study Group. Head Neck 2005;27(5):397–405
3. Huang SC, Lui LT, Lynn TC. Nasopharyngeal cancer: study III. A review of 1206 patients treated with combined modalities. Int J Radiat Oncol Biol Phys 1985;11(10):1789–1793
4. Lee AW, Sze WM, Au JS, et al. Treatment results for nasopharyngeal carcinoma in the modern era: the Hong Kong experience. Int J Radiat Oncol Biol Phys 2005;61(4):1107–1116
5. Kao CH, Tsai SC, Wang JJ, Ho YJ, Yen RF, Ho ST. Comparing 18-fluoro-2-deoxyglucose positron emission tomography with a combination of technetium 99m tetrofosmin single photon emission computed tomography and computed tomography to detect recurrent or persistent nasopharyngeal carcinomas after radiotherapy. Cancer 2001;92(2):434–439
6. Wei WI, Ho CM, Wong MP, Ng WF, Lau SK, Lam KH. Pathological basis of surgery in the management of postradiotherapy cervical metastasis in nasopharyngeal carcinoma. Arch Otolaryngol Head Neck Surg 1992;118(9):923–929, discussion 930
7. Chua DT, Wei WI, Sham JS, Cheng AC, Au G. Treatment outcome for synchronous locoregional failures of nasopharyngeal carcinoma. Head Neck 2003;25(7):585–594
8. Sham JS, Choy D. Nasopharyngeal carcinoma: treatment of neck node recurrence by radiotherapy. Australas Radiol 1991;35(4):370–373
9. Tu GY, Hu YH, Xu GZ, Ye M. Salvage surgery for nasopharyngeal carcinoma. Arch Otolaryngol Head Neck Surg 1988;114(3):328–329
10. Wei WI, Lam KH, Ho CM, Sham JS, Lau SK. Efficacy of radical neck dissection for the control of cervical metastasis after radiotherapy for nasopharyngeal carcinoma. Am J Surg 1990;160(4):439–442
11. Khafif A, Ferlito A, Takes RP, Thomas Robbins K. Is it necessary to perform radical neck dissection as a salvage procedure for persistent or recurrent neck disease after chemoradiotherapy in patients with nasopharyngeal cancer? Eur Arch Otorhinolaryngol 2010;267(7):997–999
12. Wei WI, Ho WK, Cheng AC, et al. Management of extensive cervical nodal metastasis in nasopharyngeal carcinoma after radiotherapy: a clinicopathological study. Arch Otolaryngol Head Neck Surg 2001;127(12):1457–1462
13. Wang CC. Re-irradiation of recurrent nasopharyngeal carcinoma—treatment techniques and results. Int J Radiat Oncol Biol Phys 1987;13(7):953–956
14. Lam KSL, Ho JH, Lee AW, et al. Symptomatic hypothalamic-pituitary dysfunction in nasopharyngeal carcinoma patients following radiation therapy: a retrospective study. Int J Radiat Oncol Biol Phys 1987;13(9):1343–1350
15. Lee AW, Ng SH, Ho JH, et al. Clinical diagnosis of late temporal lobe necrosis following radiation therapy for nasopharyngeal carcinoma. Cancer 1988;61(8):1535–1542
16. Lee AW, Law SC, Foo W, et al. Retrospective analysis of patients with nasopharyngeal carcinoma treated during 1976-1985: survival after local recurrence. Int J Radiat Oncol Biol Phys 1993;26(5):773–782
17. Chua DT, Sham JS, Kwong PW, Hung KN, Leung LH. Linear accelerator-based stereotactic radiosurgery for limited, locally persistent, and recurrent nasopharyngeal carcinoma: efficacy and complications. Int J Radiat Oncol Biol Phys 2003;56(1):177–183
18. Xiao J, Xu G, Miao Y. Fractionated stereotactic radiosurgery for 50 patients with recurrent or residual nasopharyngeal carcinoma. Int J Radiat Oncol Biol Phys 2001;51(1):164–170
19. Oksüz DÇ, Meral G, Uzel Ö, Cağatay P, Turkan S. Reirradiation for locally recurrent nasopharyngeal carcinoma: treatment results and prognostic factors. Int J Radiat Oncol Biol Phys 2004;60(2):388–394
20. Chang JT, See LC, Liao CT, et al. Locally recurrent nasopharyngeal carcinoma. Radiother Oncol 2000;54(2):135–142
21. Zheng XK, Ma J, Chen LH, Xia YF, Shi YS. Dosimetric and clinical results of three-dimensional conformal radiotherapy for locally recurrent nasopharyngeal carcinoma. Radiother Oncol 2005;75(2):197–203
22. Lu TX, Mai WY, Teh BS, et al. Initial experience using intensity-modulated radiotherapy for recurrent nasopharyngeal carcinoma. Int J Radiat Oncol Biol Phys 2004;58(3):682–687
23. Chua DT, Sham JS, Leung LH, Au GK. Re-irradiation of nasopharyngeal carcinoma with intensity-modulated radiotherapy. Radiother Oncol 2005;77(3):290–294
24. Lee AW, Foo W, Law SC, et al. Reirradiation for recurrent nasopharyngeal carcinoma: factors affecting the therapeutic ratio and ways for improvement. Int J Radiat Oncol Biol Phys 1997;38(1):43–52
25. Chua DT, Sham JS, Au GK. Induction chemotherapy with cisplatin and gemcitabine followed by reirradiation for locally recurrent nasopharyngeal carcinoma. Am J Clin Oncol 2005;28(5):464–471

26. Poon D, Yap SP, Wong ZW, et al. Concurrent chemoradiotherapy in locoregionally recurrent nasopharyngeal carcinoma. Int J Radiat Oncol Biol Phys 2004;59(5):1312–1318

27. Cmelak AJ, Cox RS, Adler JR, Fee WE Jr, Goffinet DR. Radiosurgery for skull base malignancies and nasopharyngeal carcinoma. Int J Radiat Oncol Biol Phys 1997;37(5):997–1003

28. Chua DT, Sham JS, Hung KN, Kwong DL, Kwong PW, Leung LH. Stereotactic radiosurgery as a salvage treatment for locally persistent and recurrent nasopharyngeal carcinoma. Head Neck 1999;21(7):620–626

29. Chen HJ, Leung SW, Su CY. Linear accelerator based radiosurgery as a salvage treatment for skull base and intracranial invasion of recurrent nasopharyngeal carcinomas. Am J Clin Oncol 2001;24(3):255–258

30. Pai PC, Chuang CC, Wei KC, Tsang NM, Tseng CK, Chang CN. Stereotactic radiosurgery for locally recurrent nasopharyngeal carcinoma. Head Neck 2002;24(8):748–753

31. Wang CC, Busse J, Gitterman M. A simple afterloading applicator for intracavitary irradiation of carcinoma of the nasopharynx. Radiology 1975;115(3):737–738

32. Law SC, Lam WK, Ng MF, Au SK, Mak WT, Lau WH. Reirradiation of nasopharyngeal carcinoma with intracavitary mold brachytherapy: an effective means of local salvage. Int J Radiat Oncol Biol Phys 2002;54(4):1095–1113

33. Harrison LB, Weissberg JB. A technique for interstitial nasopharyngeal brachytherapy. Int J Radiat Oncol Biol Phys 1987;13(3):451–453

34. Wei WI, Sham JS, Choy D, Ho CM, Lam KH. Split-palate approach for gold grain implantation in nasopharyngeal carcinoma. Arch Otolaryngol Head Neck Surg 1990;116(5):578–582

35. Choy D, Sham JS, Wei WI, Ho CM, Wu PM. Transpalatal insertion of radioactive gold grain for the treatment of persistent and recurrent nasopharyngeal carcinoma. Int J Radiat Oncol Biol Phys 1993;25(3):505–512

36. Kwong DL, Wei WI, Cheng AC, et al. Long term results of radioactive gold grain implantation for the treatment of persistent and recurrent nasopharyngeal carcinoma. Cancer 2001;91(6):1105–1113

37. Roh JL. Transpalatal endoscopic resection of residual nasopharyngeal carcinoma after sequential chemoradiotherapy. J Laryngol Otol 2004;118(12):951–954

38. Wen YH, Wen WP, Chen HX, Li J, Zeng YH, Xu G. Endoscopic nasopharyngectomy for salvage in nasopharyngeal carcinoma: a novel anatomic orientation. Laryngoscope 2010;120(7):1298–1302

39. Chen MK, Lai JC, Chang CC, Liu MT. Minimally invasive endoscopic nasopharyngectomy in the treatment of recurrent T1-2a nasopharyngeal carcinoma. Laryngoscope 2007;117(5):894–896

40. Chen MY, Wen WP, Guo X, et al. Endoscopic nasopharyngectomy for locally recurrent nasopharyngeal carcinoma. Laryngoscope 2009;119(3):516–522

41. Mai HQ, Mo HY, Deng JF, et al. Endoscopic microwave coagulation therapy for early recurrent T1 nasopharyngeal carcinoma. Eur J Cancer 2009;45(7):1107–1110

42. Wei WI, Ho WK. Transoral robotic resection of recurrent nasopharyngeal carcinoma. Laryngoscope 2010; 120(10):2011–2014

43. Vlantis AC, Tsang RK, Yu BK, et al. Nasopharyngectomy and surgical margin status: a survival analysis. Arch Otolaryngol Head Neck Surg 2007;133(12):1296–1301

44. Van Buren JM, Ommaya AK, Ketcham AS. Ten years' experience with radical combined craniofacial resection of malignant tumors of the paranasal sinuses. J Neurosurg 1968;28(4):341–350

45. Wilson CP. Observations on the surgery of the nasopharynx. Ann Otol Rhinol Laryngol 1957;66(1):5–40

46. Belmont JR. The Le Fort I osteotomy approach for nasopharyngeal and nasal fossa tumors. Arch Otolaryngol Head Neck Surg 1988;114(7):751–754

47. To EW, Teo PM, Ku PK, Pang PC. Nasopharyngectomy for recurrent nasopharyngeal carcinoma: an innovative transnasal approach through a mid-face deglove incision with stereotactic navigation guidance. Br J Oral Maxillofac Surg 2001;39(1):55–62

48. Fisch U. The infratemporal fossa approach for nasopharyngeal tumors. Laryngoscope 1983;93(1):36–44

49. Danesi G, Zanoletti E, Mazzoni A. Salvage surgery for recurrent nasopharyngeal carcinoma. Skull Base 2007;17(3):173–180

50. Fee WE Jr, Roberson JB Jr, Goffinet DR. Long-term survival after surgical resection for recurrent nasopharyngeal cancer after radiotherapy failure. Arch Otolaryngol Head Neck Surg 1991;117(11):1233–1236

51. Morton RP, Liavaag PG, McLean M, Freeman JL. Transcervico-mandibulo-palatal approach for surgical salvage of recurrent nasopharyngeal cancer. Head Neck 1996;18(4):352–358

52. Wei WI, Lam KH, Sham JS. New approach to the nasopharynx: the maxillary swing approach. Head Neck 1991;13(3):200–207

53. Ng RW, Wei WI. Elimination of palatal fistula after the maxillary swing procedure. Head Neck 2005;27(7):608–612

54. Wei WI. Cancer of the nasopharynx: functional surgical salvage. World J Surg 2003;27(7):844–848

55. Ng RW, Wei WI. Quality of life of patients with recurrent nasopharyngeal carcinoma treated with nasopharyngectomy using the maxillary swing approach. Arch Otolaryngol Head Neck Surg 2006;132(3):309–316

56. Wei WI, Chan JY, Ng RW, Ho WK. Surgical salvage of persistent or recurrent nasopharyngeal carcinoma with maxillary swing approach—Critical appraisal after 2 decades. Head Neck 2011;33(7):969–975

57. Shu CH, Cheng H, Lirng JF, et al. Salvage surgery for recurrent nasopharyngeal carcinoma. Laryngoscope 2000;110(9):1483–1488

58. Wei WI. Nasopharyngeal cancer: current status of management: a New York Head and Neck Society lecture. Arch Otolaryngol Head Neck Surg 2001;127(7):766–769

59. Fee WE Jr, Moir MS, Choi EC, Goffinet D. Nasopharyngectomy for recurrent nasopharyngeal cancer: a 2- to 17-year follow-up. Arch Otolaryngol Head Neck Surg 2002;128(3):280–284

60. Hao SP, Tsang NM, Chang KP, Hsu YS, Chen CK, Fang KH. Nasopharyngectomy for recurrent nasopharyngeal carcinoma: a review of 53 patients and prognostic factors. Acta Otolaryngol 2008;128(4):473–481

61. Yin Tsang RK, Ho WK, Wei WI. Combined transnasal endoscopic and transoral robotic resection of recurrent nasopharyngeal carcinoma. Head Neck 2012;34(8):1190–1193

Index

Note: Illustrations are comprehensively referred to in the text. Therefore significant material in illustrations has usually been given a page reference only in the absence of its concomitant mention in the text referring to that figure. Page references to tables are in bold and those to figures are in italics. 'vs.' indicates differential diagnosis.